2024–2027 Report of the Committee on Infectious Diseases
33rd Edition

Author:

Committee on Infectious Diseases,
American Academy of Pediatrics

David W. Kimberlin, MD, FAAP, Editor

Ritu Banerjee, MD, PhD, FAAP, Associate Editor
Elizabeth D. Barnett, MD, FAAP, Associate Editor
Ruth Lynfield, MD, FAAP, Associate Editor
Mark H. Sawyer, MD, FAAP, Associate Editor

American Academy of Pediatrics
345 Park Blvd
Itasca, IL 60143

Suggested citation: American Academy of Pediatrics. [Chapter title.] In: Kimberlin DW, Banerjee R, Barnett ED, Lynfield R, Sawyer MH, eds. *Red Book: 2024 Report of the Committee on Infectious Diseases*. American Academy of Pediatrics; 2024:[page numbers]

33rd Edition
1st Edition – 1938
2nd Edition – 1939
3rd Edition – 1940
4th Edition – 1942
5th Edition – 1943
6th Edition – 1944
7th Edition – 1945
8th Edition – 1947
9th Edition – 1951
10th Edition – 1952
11th Edition – 1955
12th Edition – 1957
13th Edition – 1961
14th Edition – 1964
15th Edition – 1966
16th Edition – 1970
16th Edition Revised – 1971
17th Edition – 1974
18th Edition – 1977
19th Edition – 1982
20th Edition – 1986
21st Edition – 1988
22nd Edition – 1991
23rd Edition – 1994
24th Edition – 1997
25th Edition – 2000
26th Edition – 2003
27th Edition – 2006
28th Edition – 2009
29th Edition – 2012
30th Edition – 2015
31st Edition – 2018
32nd Edition – 2021

ISSN No. 1080-0131
ISBN No. 978-1-61002-734-2
eBook: 978-61002-735-9
MA1140

Quantity prices on request. Address all inquiries to:
American Academy of Pediatrics
345 Park Blvd
Itasca, IL 60143

or Phone:
1-888-227-1770 Publications

The recommendations in this publication do not indicate an exclusive course of treatment or serve as a standard of medical care. Variations, taking into account individual circumstances, may be appropriate.

Publications from the American Academy of Pediatrics benefit from expertise and resources of liaisons and internal (AAP) and external reviewers. However, publications from the American Academy of Pediatrics may not reflect the views of the liaisons of the organizations or government agencies that they represent.

Dr David Kimberlin has disclosed a financial relationship with Elsevier as an editor. Associate Editor disclosures were not relevant to their work related to the *Red Book*. Disclosures are reviewed and mitigated through a Conflict of Interest process approved by the AAP Board of Directors.

The American Academy of Pediatrics has neither solicited nor accepted any commercial involvement in the development of the content of this publication.

3-366/0424 1 2 3 4 5 6 7 8 9 10

Committee on Infectious Diseases 2021–2024

Collaborators

Andrew Abbott, MD, MPH, Centers for Disease Control and Prevention, Atlanta, GA

Mark J. Abzug, MD, University of Colorado School of Medicine and Children's Hospital Colorado, Aurora, CO

Anna M. Acosta, MD, Centers for Disease Control and Prevention, Atlanta, GA

Laura Adams, DVM, MPH, Centers for Disease Control and Prevention, Atlanta, GA

AdeSubomi O. Adeyemo, PharmD, MPH, Centers for Disease Control and Prevention, Atlanta, GA

Paula Ehrlich Agger, MD, MPH, Food and Drug Administration, Silver Spring, MD

N. Peart Akindele, MD, Food and Drug Administration, Laurel, MD

Upton D. Allen, MBBS, MSc, University of Toronto, Toronto, Ontario, Canada

Maria C. Allende, MD, MPH, Food and Drug Administration, Silver Spring, MD,

Krow Ampofo, MB, ChB, University of Utah School of Medicine, Salt Lake City, UT

Evan J. Anderson, MD, Emory University School of Medicine, Atlanta, GA

Jon K. Andrus, MD, University of Colorado and George Washington University, Washington, DC

Kristina M. Angelo, DO, MPH&TM, Centers for Disease Control and Prevention, Atlanta, GA

E. Gloria Anyalechi, MD, MPH, Centers for Disease Control and Prevention, Lilburn, GA

Grace D. Appiah, MD, Centers for Disease Control and Prevention, Atlanta, GA

Brian S. Appleby, MD, Case Western Reserve University, Cleveland, OH

Stephen S. Arnon, MD, MPH, California Department of Public Health, Richmond, CA

Naomi E. Aronson, MD, Uniformed Services University of the Health Sciences, Bethesda, MD

Negar Ashouri, MD, CHOC Children's Hospital, Orange, CA

T. Prescott Atkinson, MD, PhD, University of Alabama at Birmingham, Birmingham, AL

Kevin A. Ault, MD, University of Kansas Medical Center, Kansas City, KS

Lorraine C. Backer, PhD, MPH, Centers for Disease Control and Prevention, Chamblee, GA

John W. Baddley, MD, MSPH, University of Maryland School of Medicine, Baltimore, MD

Bethany M. Baer, MD, Food and Drug Administration, Silver Spring, MD

Gerri R. Baer, MD, Food and Drug Administration, Rockville, MD

Carol J. Baker, MD, University of Texas Health Science Center, McGovern Medical School, Houston, TX

Valerie D. Bampoe, DrPH, Centers for Disease Control and Prevention, Lawrenceville, GA.

Lindley Barbee, MD, MPH, Centers for Disease Control and Prevention, Seattle, WA

Roxanne Y. Barrow, MD, MPH, Centers for Disease Control and Prevention, Douglasville, GA

Albert E. Barskey, MPH, Centers for Disease Control and Prevention, Atlanta, GA

William J. Barson, MD, MS, Nationwide Children's Hospital and The Ohio State University, Columbus, OH

Margaret C. Bash, MD, MPH, Food and Drug Administration, Bethesda, MD

Melisse Baylor, MD, Food and Drug Administration, Silver Spring, MD

Judy A. Beeler, MD, Food and Drug Administration, Silver Spring, MD

Amy M. Beeson, MD, Centers for Disease Control and Prevention, Denver, CO

Ermias Belay, MD, Centers for Disease Control and Prevention, Atlanta, GA

Roy Benaroch, MD, Emory University, Dunwoody, GA

William E. Benitz, MD, Stanford University School of Medicine, Palo Alto, CA

Henry H. Bernstein, DO, MHCM, Cohen Children's Medical Center/Northwell Health, Princeton, NJ

Nicolette C. Bestul, MPH, Centers for Disease Control and Prevention, Brookhaven, GA

Holly Biggs, MD, MPH, Centers for Disease Control and Prevention, Atlanta, GA

Jessica M. Biggs, PharmD, BCPPS, University of Maryland Medical Center, Baltimore, MD

Danae Bixler, MD, MPH, Centers for Disease Control and Prevention, Brookhaven, GA

Amy E. Blain, MPH, Centers for Disease Control and Prevention, Atlanta, GA

Daniel B. Blatt, MD, University of Louisville School of Medicine, Louisville, KY

Joseph A. Bocchini, Jr, MD, Tulane University, Shreveport, LA

Daniel J. Bonthius, MD, PhD, Levine Children's Hospital, Charlotte, NC

Suresh B. Boppana, MD, University of Alabama at Birmingham, Birmingham, AL

LaTasha R. Boswell, BSN, MPH, Centers for Disease Control and Prevention, Duluth, GA

William A. Bower, MD, Centers for Disease Control and Prevention, Atlanta, GA

Dave Boxrud, MS, Centers for Disease Control and Prevention, Roseville, MN

John S. Bradley, MD, University of California San Diego/Rady Children's Hospital San Diego, San Diego, CA

Denise Bratcher, DO, Children's Mercy Kansas City, Kansas City, MO

Timothy Patrick Brennan, PhD, MD, MS, Food and Drug Administration, Silver Spring, MD

Deborah Jane Briggs, PhD, Kansas State University, Manhattan, KS

Benjamin J. Briggs, MD, PhD, University of Rochester Medical Center, Rochester, NY

Amadea K. Britton, MD, SM, Centers for Disease Control and Prevention, Brookline, MA

Karen R. Broder, MD, Centers for Disease Control and Prevention, Decatur, GA

Beau Benjamin Bruce, MD, PhD, Centers for Disease Control and Prevention, Atlanta, GA

Michael G. Bruce, MD, MPH, Centers for Disease Control and Prevention, Anchorage, AK

Fernando J. Bula-Rudas, MD, Johns Hopkins All Children's Hospital, St. Petersburg, FL

Rachel M. Burke, PhD, MPH, Centers for Disease Control and Prevention, Atlanta, GA

Jane C. Burns, MD, University of California San Diego, La Jolla, CA

Gale R. Burstein, MD, MPH, Erie County Department of Health, Buffalo, NY

Mario Alejandro Bustos-Paz, MD, Universidad del Valle. Cali, Colombia, Jamundí, Valle del Cauca, Colombia

Carrie L. Byington, MD, University of California Health, Oakland, CA

Angela P. Campbell, MD, MPH, Centers for Disease Control and Prevention, Atlanta, GA

Doug Campos-Outcalt, MD, MPA, College of Public Health, College of Medicine-Phoenix, University of Arizona, Phoenix, AZ

Paul T. Cantey, MD, MPH, Centers for Disease Control and Prevention, Atlanta, GA

Joseph B. Cantey, MD, MPH, University of Texas Health San Antonio, San Antonio, TX

Michael Cappello, MD, Yale School of Medicine, New Haven, CT

Delicia Carey, PhD, Centers for Disease Control and Prevention, Marietta, GA

Emily Cartwright, MD, Centers for Disease Control and Prevention, Atlanta, GA

Pam Cassiday, MS, Centers for Disease Control and Prevention, Atlanta, GA

Ellen Gould Chadwick, MD, Northwestern University Feinberg School of Medicine, Ann & Robert H. Lurie Children's Hospital of Chicago, Chicago, IL

Rana Chakraborty, MD, MSc, FRCPCH, DPhil (Oxon), Mayo Clinic, Rochester, MN

Philip Chan, MD, Centers for Disease Control and Prevention, Atlanta, GA

Rebecca Chancey, MD, DTMH, Centers for Disease Control and Prevention, Atlanta, GA

Kirk M. Chan-Tack, MD, Food and Drug Administration, Silver Spring, MD

Min-hsin Chen, PhD, Centers for Disease Control and Prevention, Atlanta, GA

Preeti Chhabra, PhD, Centers for Disease Control and Prevention, Atlanta, GA

Kathleen Chiotos, MD, MSCE, Children's Hospital of Philadelphia, Philadelphia, PA

Mary J. Choi, MD, MPH, Centers for Disease Control and Prevention, Atlanta, GA

Nancy Chow, PhD, MS, Centers for Disease Control and Prevention, Atlanta, GA

John C. Christenson, MD, Indiana University School of Medicine, Indianapolis, IN

Paul R. Cieslak, MD, Oregon Health Authority Public Health Division, Portland, OR

Susan E. Coffin, MD, MPH, Children's Hospital of Philadelphia & UPenn School of Medicine, Philadelphia, PA

Adam L. Cohen, MD, MPH, Centers for Disease Control and Prevention, Atlanta, GA

Jeffrey I. Cohen, MD, National Institute of Allergy and Infectious Diseases, National Institutes of Health, Bethesda, MD

Jennifer P. Collins, MD, MSc, Centers for Disease Control and Prevention, Atlanta, GA

Joseph Wayne Conlan, BSc, PhD, National Research Council Canada, Ottawa, Ontario, Canada

Roxanne Connelly, BS, MS, PhD, Centers for Disease Control and Prevention, Fort Collins, CO

Mark Connelly, MD, Food and Drug Administration, Silver Spring, MD

Erin E. Conners, PhD, MPH, Centers for Disease Control and Prevention, Atlanta, GA

Laura A. Cooley, MD, MPHTM, Centers for Disease Control and Prevention, Atlanta, GA

Caitlin Cossaboom, DVM, PhD, MPH, Centers for Disease Control and Prevention, Atlanta, GA

Tamera Coyne-Beasley, MD, MPH, University of Alabama at Birmingham, Birmingham, AL

Lisa M. Cranmer, MD, MPH, Emory University School of Medicine, Atlanta, GA

Sue E. Crawford, PhD, Baylor College of Medicine, Houston, TX

C. Buddy Creech, MD, MPH, Vanderbilt University Medical Center, Nashville, TN

Matthew Crist, MD, MPH, Centers for Disease Control and Prevention, Atlanta, GA

Stephen N. Crooke, PhD, Centers for Disease Control and Prevention, Atlanta, GA

Sam Crowe, PhD, MPH, Centers for Disease Control and Prevention, Decatur, GA

Charles L. Daley, MD, National Jewish Health, Denver, CO

Jency M. Daniel, MD, FAAP, Children's National Hospital, Dix Hills, NY

Richard N. Danila, PhD, MPH, Minnesota Department of Health, St. Paul, MN

Toni Darville, MD, University of North Carolina at Chapel Hill, Chapel Hill, NC

Irini Daskalaki, MD, Princeton University, Princeton, NJ

Alma C. Davidson, MD, Food and Drug Administration, Silver Spring, MD

Bionca M. Davis, MN, MPH, Centers for Disease Control and Prevention, Anchorage, AK

Fatimah Sultana Dawood, MD, Centers for Disease Control and Prevention, Atlanta, GA

Roberta Lynn DeBiasi, MD, MS, Children's National Health System/The George Washington University School of Medicine and Health Sciences, Washington, DC

Walter Dehority, MD, MSc, The University of New Mexico School of Medicine, Albuquerque, NM

Maureen H. Diaz, PhD, MPH, Centers for Disease Control and Prevention, Atlanta, GA

Kathleen L. Dooling, MD, MPH, Centers for Disease Control and Prevention, Atlanta, GA

Dorothy E. Dow, MD, MSc, Duke University Medical Center, Durham, NC

Naomi A. Drexler, MPH, DrPH, Centers for Disease Control and Prevention, Atlanta, GA

Amanda J. Driscoll, PhD, MHS, University of Maryland School of Medicine, Baltimore, MD

Jan Drobeniuc, MD, PhD, Centers for Disease Control and Prevention, Atlanta, GA

Jonathan Duffy, MD, MPH, Centers for Disease Control and Prevention, Atlanta, GA

Allison Ross Eckard, MD, Medical University of South Carolina, Mount Pleasant, SC

Judith K. Eckerle, MD, University of Minnesota, Minneapolis, MN

Chris Edens, PhD, Centers for Disease Control and Prevention, Atlanta, GA

Brian R. Edlin, MD, Centers for Disease Control and Prevention, New York, NY

Leslie D. Edwards, MHS, BSN, Centers for Disease Control and Prevention, Martinsville, VA

Morven S. Edwards, MD, Baylor College of Medicine, Houston, TX

Lawrence F. Eichenfield, MD, University of California San Diego and Rady Children's Hospital San Diego, San Diego, CA

Samer El-Kamary, MD, MPH, Food and Drug Administration, Silver Spring, MD

Sean P. Elliott, MD, Tucson Hospitals Medical Education Program, Tucson, AZ

Roselyn E. Epps, MD, Food and Drug Administration, Silver Spring, MD

Mathew D. Esona, PhD, Centers for Disease Control and Prevention, Atlanta, GA

Darcie L. Everett, MD, MPH, Food and Drug Administration, Silver Spring, MD

Tarayn A. Fairlie, MD, MPH, Centers for Disease Control and Prevention, Atlanta, GA

Dino Ariel Feigelstock, PhD, Food and Drug Administration, Silver Spring, MD

Anat R. Feingold, MD, MPH, Cooper University Hospital, Camden, NJ

Meghan Ferris, MD, MPH, Food and Drug Administration, Silver Spring, MD

Dorian L. Fink, MD, PhD, Food and Drug Administration, Silver Spring, MD

Marc Fischer, MD, MPH, Centers for Disease Control and Prevention, Anchorage, AK

Brian T. Fisher, DO, MSCE, Children's Hospital of Philadelphia, Philadelphia, PA

Patricia Flanagan, MD, FAAP, Brown University/Hasbro Children's Hospital, Providence, RI

Katherine E. Fleming-Dutra, MD, Centers for Disease Control and Prevention, Atlanta, GA

Patricia Michelle Flynn, MD, MS, St. Jude Children's Research Hospital, Memphis, TN

Kaitlin Forsberg, MPH, Centers for Disease Control and Prevention, Atlanta, GA

Rebecca J. Free, MD, MPH, Centers for Disease Control and Prevention, Atlanta, GA

Robert W. Frenck, Jr, MD, Cincinnati Children's Hospital Medical Center, Cincinnati, OH

Cindy Friedman, MD, Centers for Disease Control and Prevention, Atlanta, GA

Yasuko Fukuda, MD, FAAP, Pacific Pediatrics, San Francisco, CA

Sara Gagneten, PhD, Food and Drug Administration, Silver Spring, MD

Ruth Gallego, RN, MPH, CHES, Centers for Disease Control and Prevention, Atlanta, GA

Renee L. Galloway, MPH, Centers for Disease Control and Prevention, Atlanta, GA

Anthony J. Garcia-Prats, MD, MSCE, PhD, University of Wisconsin-Madison, School of Medicine and Public Health, Madison, WI

Shikha Garg, MD, MPH, Centers for Disease Control and Prevention, Atlanta, GA

Paul A. Gastañaduy, MD, MPH, Centers for Disease Control and Prevention, Atlanta, GA

Nicholas Geagan, DO, Food and Drug Administration, Washington, DC

Jay E. Gee, PhD, Centers for Disease Control and Prevention, Atlanta, GA

Anne A. Gershon, MD, Columbia University Vagelos College of Physicians and Surgeons, New York, NY

Michael Gewitz, MD, FAAP, FACC, FAHA, Maria Fareri Children's Hospital at WMC Health/NY Medical College, Mt Kisco, NY

Mayurika Ghosh, MD, Food and Drug Administration, White Oak, MD

Francis Gigliotti, MD, University of Rochester School of Medicine and Dentistry, Rochester, NY

Janet R. Gilsdorf, MD, University of Michigan, Ann Arbor, MI

Carol A. Glaser, DVM, MD, California Department of Public Health, Richmond, CA

Dominique Geneine Godfrey, BS, MPH, Centers for Disease Control and Prevention, Atlanta, GA

Jeremy Gold, MD, MS, Centers for Disease Control and Prevention, Atlanta, GA

Carolyn V. Gould, MD, MSCR, Centers for Disease Control and Prevention, Fort Collins, CO

Luisa Gregori, PhD, Food and Drug Administration, Silver Spring, MD

Patricia M. Griffin, MD, Centers for Disease Control and Prevention, Atlanta, GA

Daniel Griffin, MD, PhD, CTropMed, CTH, Columbia University, New York, NY

Lisa A. Grohskopf, MD, MPH, Centers for Disease Control and Prevention, Atlanta, GA

Alice Y. Guh, MD, MPH, Centers for Disease Control and Prevention, Atlanta, GA

Bruce Gutelius, MD, MPH, Centers for Disease Control and Prevention, Atlanta, GA

Julie R. Gutman, MD, MSc, Centers for Disease Control and Prevention, Decatur, GA

Judith A. Guzman-Cottrill, DO, Oregon Health and Science University, Portland, OR

Jesse Hackell, MD, Boston Children's Heath Physicians and New York Medical College, Pomona, NY

Jill K. Hacker, PhD, MPH, California Department of Public Health, Richmond, CA

Melissa B. Hagen, MD, MPH, Centers for Disease Control and Prevention, Atlanta, GA

Aron J. Hall, DVM, MSPH, Centers for Disease Control and Prevention, Atlanta, GA

Elisha Hall, PhD, RD, Centers for Disease Control and Prevention, Duluth, GA

Scott A. Halperin, MD, Dalhousie University, IWK Health Centre, Halifax, Nova Scotia, Canada

Davidson H. Hamer, MD, Boston University School of Public Health, Boston, MA

Shannon S. Hamilton, DO, Riley Hospital for Children, Indiana University, Indianapolis, IN

Laura Hammitt, MD, Johns Hopkins Bloomberg School of Public Health, Durango, CO

Jin-Young Han, MD, PhD, Weill Cornell Medicine, New York, NY

Elizabeth Hannapel, MPH, Centers for Disease Control and Prevention, Atlanta, GA

Kathleen H. Harriman, PhD, MPH, RN, California Department of Public Health, Richmond, CA

Jason B. Harris, MD, MPH, Massachusetts General Hospital, Wellesley, MA

Joshua D. Hartzell, MD, MS-HPEd, Walter Reed National Military Medical Center, Bethesda, MD

Julia C. Haston, MD, MSc, Centers for Disease Control and Prevention, Atlanta, GA

Kristen Heitzinger, PhD, MPH, Centers for Disease Control and Prevention, Atlanta, GA
Katherine Hendricks Walters, MD, Centers for Disease Control and Prevention, Atlanta, GA
Maureen Hess, MPH, RD, Food and Drug Administration, Rockville, MD
Lauri Hicks, DO, Centers for Disease Control and Prevention, Decatur, GA
Susan L. Hills, MBBS, MTH, Centers for Disease Control and Prevention, Fort Collins, CO
Alison F. Hinckley, PhD, Centers for Disease Control and Prevention, Fort Collins, CO
Hiwot Hiruy, Food and Drug Administration, Silver Spring, MD
Michelle C. Hlavsa, RN, MPH, Centers for Disease Control and Prevention, Atlanta, GA
Aimee C. Hodowanec, MD, Food and Drug Administration, Silver Spring, MD
Megan G. Hofmeister, MD, MS, MPH, Centers for Disease Control and Prevention, Atlanta, GA
Jae Ho Hong, MD, AAHIVS, Food and Drug Administration, Silver Spring, MD
Karen W. Hoover, MD, MPH, Centers for Disease Control and Prevention, Atlanta, GA
Christopher H. Hsu, MD, PhD, MPH, Centers for Disease Control and Prevention, Atlanta, GA
Katherine K. Hsu, MD, MPH, Massachusetts Department of Public Health, Boston University Medical Center, Jamaica Plain, MA
Christine Hughes, MPH, Centers for Disease Control and Prevention, Atlanta, GA
Michael J. Hughes, MPH, Centers for Disease Control and Prevention, Atlanta, GA
David A. Hunstad, MD, Washington University School of Medicine, St. Louis, MO
Jennifer C. Hunter, DrPH, MPH, Centers for Disease Control and Prevention, Atlanta, GA
Christelle Ilboudo, MD, Children's Mercy Kansas City, Kansas City, MO
Stuart N. Isaacs, MD, Perelman School of Medicine at the University of Pennsylvania, Philadelphia, PA
Mary Anne Jackson, MD, University of Missouri Kansas City School of Medicine, Kansas City, MO
Ruth Ann Jajosky, DMD, MPH, Centers for Disease Control and Prevention, Lilburn, GA
Tara C. Jatlaoui, MD, MPH, Centers for Disease Control and Prevention, Atlanta, GA
John A. Jereb, MD, Centers for Disease Control and Prevention, Atlanta, GA
Ravi Jhaveri, MD, Ann & Robert H. Lurie Children's Hospital of Chicago/Northwestern University Feinberg School of Medicine, Chicago, IL
Jefferson M. Jones, MD, MPH, Centers for Disease Control and Prevention, Atlanta, GA
Nicola L. Jones, MD, FRCPC, PhD, University of Toronto, Toronto, Ontario, Canada
S. Patrick Kachur, MD, MPH, Columbia University Irving Medical Center, New York, NY
Alexander Kallen, MD, MPH, Centers for Disease Control and Prevention, Decatur, GA
Mary L. Kamb, MD, MPH, Centers for Disease Control and Prevention, Atlanta, GA
Satoshi Kamidani, MD, Centers for Disease Control and Prevention, Atlanta, GA
Saleem Kamili, PhD, Centers for Disease Control and Prevention, Atlanta, GA
Bill G. Kapogiannis, MD, National Institute of Child Health and Human Development, Bethesda, MD
Rama Kapoor, MD, Food and Drug Administration, Silver Spring, MD
Kevin R. Kazacos, DVM, PhD, DACVM, Purdue University, Punta Gorda, FL
Amelia Keaton, MD, MS, Centers for Disease Control and Prevention, Atlanta, GA
John M. Kelso, MD, Scripps Clinic, San Diego, CA
Gilbert J. Kersh, PhD, Centers for Disease Control and Prevention, Atlanta, GA

Maryam Keshtkar-Jahromi, MD, MPH, FIDSA, National Institutes of Health, Rockville, MD

David L. Kettl, MD, Food and Drug Administration, Silver Spring, MD

Yury Khudyakox, Centers for Disease Control and Prevention, Atlanta, GA

Sarah Kidd, MD, MPH, Centers for Disease Control and Prevention, Atlanta, GA

Marie Killerby, VetMB, MPH, Centers for Disease Control and Prevention, Nashville, TN

Mary Kim, MD, Food and Drug Administration, Silver Spring, MD

Anne Kimball, MD, MPH, Centers for Disease Control and Prevention, Atlanta, GA

Charles H. King, MD, MS, Case Western Reserve University, Cleveland, OH

Miwako Kobayashi, Centers for Disease Control and Prevention, Atlanta, GA

Natalia A. Kozak-Muiznieks, PhD, Centers for Disease Control and Prevention, Atlanta, GA

Peter J. Krause, MD, Yale School of Public Health and Yale School of Medicine, New Haven, CT

Andrew Thaddeus Kroger, MD, MPH, Centers for Disease Control and Prevention, Atlanta, GA

Elisabeth Krow-Lucal, PhD, MPH, Centers for Disease Control and Prevention, Atlanta, GA

Zuzana Kucerova, MD, PhD, Centers for Disease Control and Prevention, Atlanta, GA

Kiersten J. Kugeler, PhD, MPH, Centers for Disease Control and Prevention, Fort Collins, CO

Allison Lale, MD, MPH, Centers for Disease Control and Prevention, Atlanta, GA

Adam J. Langer, DVM, MPH, Centers for Disease Control and Prevention, Atlanta, GA

Tatiana M. Lanzieri, MD, MPH, Centers for Disease Control and Prevention, Atlanta, GA

Ralph Eli LeBlanc, MD, PhD, Food and Drug Administration, Baltimore, MD

Christine C. Lee, PhD, Centers for Disease Control and Prevention, Atlanta, GA

Sooji Lee, MSPH, MS, Centers for Disease Control and Prevention, Peachtree Corners, GA

Joohee Lee, MD, Food and Drug Administration, Silver Spring, MD

Lucia H. Lee, MD, Food and Drug Administration, Silver Spring, MD

Myron M. Levine, MD, DTPH, Centers for Disease Control and Prevention, Baltimore, MD

Nicole Politi Lindsey, MS, Centers for Disease Control and Prevention, Fort Collins, CO

John J. LiPuma, MD, University of Michigan, Ann Arbor, MI

Shawn R. Lockhart, PhD, Centers for Disease Control and Prevention, Atlanta, GA

Naeemah Logan, MD, Centers for Disease Control and Prevention, Atlanta, GA

Benjamin Lorenz, MD, Food and Drug Administration, Silver Spring, MD

Matthew Lozier, PhD, MPH, Centers for Disease Control and Prevention, Atlanta, GA

Xiaoyan Lu, Centers for Disease Control and Prevention, Atlanta, GA

Carolina Lúquez, PhD, Centers for Disease Control and Prevention, Atlanta, GA

Joseph Daniel Lutgring, MD, Centers for Disease Control and Prevention, Atlanta, GA

Meghan Lyman, MD, Centers for Disease Control and Prevention, Atlanta, GA

Maria Fernanda Machicao, BS, Cohen Children's Medical Center, New Hyde Park, NY

Yvonne A. Maldonado, MD, Stanford University, Stanford, CA

Jason H. Malenfant, MD, MPH, Centers for Disease Control and Prevention, Oakville, Ontario, Canada

Mona Marin, MD, Centers for Disease Control and Prevention, Atlanta, GA

Laurie E. Markowitz, MD, Centers for Disease Control and Prevention, Atlanta, GA

Gabriela M. Maron, MD, MS, St. Jude Children's Research Hospital, Memphis, TN

Gary S. Marshall, MD, Norton Children's and the University of Louisville School of Medicine, Louisville, KY

Chung K. Marston, Centers for Disease Control and Prevention, Atlanta, GA

Diana L. Martin, PhD, Centers for Disease Control and Prevention, Atlanta, GA

Haley Martin, Centers for Disease Control and Prevention, Atlanta, GA

Stacey W. Martin, MSc, Centers for Disease Control and Prevention, Fort Collins, CO

Kimberly C. Martin, DO, MPH, Food and Drug Administration, Silver Spring, MD

Emily T. Martin, PhD, MPH, University of Michigan School of Public Health, Ann Arbor, MI

Grace E. Marx, MD, MPH, Centers for Disease Control and Prevention, Fort Collins, CO

Jonathan Alexander Mayhew, MD, Indiana University, Indianapolis, IN

Alastair Kenneth McAlpine, MBChB, FRCPC, BC Children's Hospital, Vancouver, British Columbia, Canada

James B. McAuley, MD, MPH, Whiteriver Indian Hospital - Indian Health Service, Whiteriver, AZ

Andrea M. McCollum, PhD, MS, Centers for Disease Control and Prevention, Atlanta, GA

David W. McCormick, MD, MPH, Centers for Disease Control and Prevention, Fort Collins, CO

Anita K. McElroy, MD, PhD, University of Pittsburgh, Pittsburgh, PA

Haley McKeel, BS, Centers for Disease Control and Prevention, Atlanta, GA

Susan L. F. McLellan, MD, MPH, University of Texas Medical Branch, Galveston, TX

Brian J. McMahon, MD, Alaska Native Tribal Health Consortium, Anchorage, AK

Meredith L. McMorrow, MD, MPH, Centers for Disease Control and Prevention, Atlanta, GA

Lucy A. McNamara, PhD, MS, Centers for Disease Control and Prevention, Decatur, GA

Michael M. McNeil, MD, MPH, Centers for Disease Control and Prevention, Atlanta, GA

Paul S. Mead, MD, MPH, Centers for Disease Control and Prevention, Atlanta, GA

Elissa Meites, MD, MPH, Centers for Disease Control and Prevention, Atlanta, GA

Asuncion Mejias, MD, PhD, MsCS, Nationwide Children's Hospital and The Ohio State University, Columbus, OH

Ann J. Melvin, MD, MPH, Seattle Children's Hospital, Seattle, WA

Kevin Messacar, MD, University of Colorado, Children's Hospital Colorado, Aurora, CO

Marisa H. Miceli, MD, University of Michigan, Ann Arbor, MI

Ian C. Michelow, MD, DTM&H, Warren Alpert Medical School of Brown University, Providence, RI

Claire M. Midgley, PhD, Centers for Disease Control and Prevention, Atlanta, GA

Elaine R. Miller, MPH, BSN, Centers for Disease Control and Prevention, Atlanta, GA

Sara A. Mirza, PhD, MPH, Centers for Disease Control and Prevention, Atlanta, GA

John F. Modlin, MD, Geisel School of Medicine at Dartmouth, Norwich, VT

Heidi Moline, MD, MPH, Centers for Disease Control and Prevention, Atlanta, GA

Tina Hhoie Mongeau, MD, MPH, Food and Drug Administration, Potomac, MD

Martha P. Montgomery, MD, MHS, Centers for Disease Control and Prevention, Taiwan

Susan P. Montgomery, DVM, MPH, Centers for Disease Control and Prevention, Atlanta, GA

Anne Chadwick Moorman, MPH, Centers for Disease Control and Prevention, Atlanta, GA

Estelle Mei-Shan Morin, MDCM, FRCPC, BC Children's Hospital, Vancouver, British Columbia, Canada

Pedro Moro, MD, MPH, Centers for Disease Control and Prevention, Atlanta, GA

Anna-Barbara Moscicki, MD, University of California, Los Angeles, Los Angeles, CA

Barbara E. Murray, MD, University of Texas Health Science Center at Houston, Houston, TX

Neil Murthy, MD, MPH, MSJ, Centers for Disease Control and Prevention, Decatur, GA

Oidda Ikumboka Museru, MSN, MPH, Centers for Disease Control and Prevention, Grayson, GA

Christina A. Muzny, MD, MSPH, University of Alabama at Birmingham, Birmingham, AL

Angela Leigh Myers, MD, MPH, Children's Mercy Kansas City, Kansas City, MO

James Nataro MD, PhD, MBA, University of Virginia, Charlottesville, VA

Mark Needles, MD, Food and Drug Administration, Silver Spring, MD

Maria, E. Negron, DVM, PhD, MS, Centers for Disease Control and Prevention, Atlanta, GA

Christina A. Nelson, MD, MPH, Centers for Disease Control and Prevention, Fort Collins, CO

Noele P. Nelson, MD, PhD, MPH, Centers for Disease Control and Prevention, Atlanta, GA

Steven R. Nesheim, MD, Centers for Disease Control and Prevention (Retired), Atlanta, GA

Jason G. Newland, MD, MEd, Washington University School of Medicine, St. Louis, MO

Han Jin Ng, Centers for Disease Control and Prevention, Atlanta, GA

Fei Fan Ng, Centers for Disease Control and Prevention, Atlanta, GA

Megin Nichols, DVM, MPH, Centers for Disease Control and Prevention, Atlanta, GA

William L. Nicholson, BS, MS, PhD, Centers for Disease Control and Prevention, Atlanta, GA

Lise E. Nigrovic, MD, MPH, Boston Children's Hospital, Boston, MA

Dawn Nolt, MD, MPH, Oregon Health and Science University, Portland, OR

Laura E. Norton, MD, MS, University of Minnesota Medical School, Minneapolis, MN

Thomas B. Nutman, MD, National Institutes of Health, Bethesda, MD

Elizabeth O'Shaughnessy, MB, BCh, BAO, Food and Drug Administration, Silver Spring, MD

Andrew J. O'Carroll, DVM, MPH, Food and Drug Administration, Silver Spring, MD

Theresa Jean Ochoa, MD, PhD, Universidad Peruana Cayetano Heredia, Lima, Perú

Christine Olson, MD, MPH, Centers for Disease Control and Prevention, Decatur, GA

Jesse Garrett O'Shea, MD, MSc, Centers for Disease Control and Prevention, Atlanta, GA

Belinda Ostrowsky, MD, MPH, Centers for Disease Control and Prevention, New York, NY

Melissa Otis, BSN, RN, Centers for Disease Control and Prevention, Buford, GA

Gary D. Overturf, MD, University of New Mexico, Albuquerque, NM

Christopher D. Paddock, MD, MPHTM, Centers for Disease Control and Prevention, Atlanta, GA

Diane E. Pappas, MD, JD, University of Virginia Department of Pediatrics, Orange, VA

Umesh D. Parashar, MBBS, MPH, Centers for Disease Control and Prevention, Atlanta, GA

Ina U. Park, MD, MS, UC San Francisco School of Medicine, Berkeley, CA

Colin R. Parrish, PhD, Cornell University, Ithaca, NY

Sheral S. Patel, MD, Food and Drug Administration, Silver Spring, MD

Nehali Patel, MD, St. Jude Children's Research Hospital, Memphis, TN

Lucia Pawloski, PhD, Centers for Disease Control and Prevention, Atlanta, GA

Gabriela Paz-Bailey, MD, PhD, MSc, DTM&H, Centers for Disease Control and
Prevention, Atlanta, GA
Stephen I. Pelton, MD, Boston University School of Medicine, Boston Medical Center,
Boston, MA
Ludmila Perelygina, PhD, Centers for Disease Control and Prevention, Atlanta, GA
John R. Perfect, MD, Duke University Medical Center, Durham, NC
Kiran M. Perkins, MD, MPH, Centers for Disease Control and Prevention, Atlanta, GA
Brett W. Petersen, MD, MPH, Centers for Disease Control and Prevention, Atlanta, GA
Jeannine M. Petersen, PhD, Centers for Disease Control and Prevention, Fort Collins, CO
Andreas Pikis, MD, Food and Drug Administration, Bethesda, MD
Swetha Geetha Pinninti, MD, University of Alabama at Birmingham, Birmingham, AL
Ana Yecê Neves Pinto, PhD, MD, Evandro Chagas Institute, Ananindeua, Pará, Brasil
Paul J. Planet, MD, PhD, University of Pennsylvania, Children's Hospital of Philadelphia,
Philadelphia, PA
Ian D. Plumb, MBBS, MSc, Centers for Disease Control and Prevention, Atlanta, GA
Claudette Lapage Poole, MD, MSPH, University of Alabama at Birmingham,
Birmingham, AL
Roberto Posada, MD, Mount Sinai Hospital/Icahn School of Medicine at Mount Sinai,
New York, NY
Caroline Q. Pratt, MNS, MPH, Centers for Disease Control and Prevention, Hayesville, NC
Nathan Price, MD, University of Arizona, Tucson, AZ
Gerardo Priotto, MD, MPH, World Health Organization, Genève, Switzerland
Bobbi S. Pritt, MD, MSc, DTMH, Mayo Clinic, Rochester, MN
Gary W. Procop, MD, MS, American Board of Pathology & Cleveland Clinic, Tampa, FL
Michae, A. Purdy, PhD, Centers for Disease Control and Prevention, Atlanta, GA
Laura Ann Sideli Quilter, MD, MPH, Centers for Disease Control and Prevention,
Atlanta, GA
Elizabeth M. Quincer, MD, Emory University School of Medicine, Atlanta, GA
Octavio Ramilo, MD, Nationwide Children's Hospital, Columbus, OH
Agam K. Rao, MD, Centers for Disease Control and Prevention, Atlanta, GA
Anuja Rastogi, MD, MHS, Food and Drug Administration, Clarksburg, MD
Mobeen Hasan Rathore, MD, University of Florida Center for AIDS/HIV, Research,
Education and Service, Jacksonville, FL
Logan Christopher Ray, MPH, Centers for Disease Control and Prevention, Atlanta, GA
Suja, C. Reddy, MD, Centers for Disease Control and Prevention, Atlanta, GA
Susan Reef, Centers for Disease Control and Prevention, Atlanta, GA
Rebecca Reindel, MD, Food and Drug Administration, Silver Spring, MD
Hilary Reno, MD, PhD, Centers for Disease Control and Prevention, St. Louis, MO
Melissa Reyes, MD, MPH, Food and Drug Administration, Silver Spring, MD
Frank O. Richards Jr, MD, FASTM, The Carter Center, Atlanta, GA
Virginia A. Roberts, MSPH, Centers for Disease Control and Prevention, Atlanta, GA
Joan L. Robinson, MD, University of Alberta, Edmonton, Alberta, Canada
Carina A. Rodriguez, MD, University of South Florida, Tampa, FL
Jorge Martin Rodriguez, MD, University of Alabama at Birmingham, Birmingham, AL
Dawn M. Roellig, PhD, MS, Centers for Disease Control and Prevention, Atlanta, GA
Alix Taylor Rosenberg, BS, Cohen Children's Medical Center, New Hyde Park, NY

Hannah G. Rosenblum, MD, Centers for Disease Control and Prevention, Atlanta, GA
Shannon Ross, MD, MSPH, The University of Alabama at Birmingham, Birmingham, AL
Paul A. Rota, PhD, Centers for Disease Control and Prevention, Atlanta, GA
Sandra Roush, MT, MPH, Centers for Disease Control and Prevention, Lilburn, GA
Regina K. Rowe, MD, PhD, University of Rochester, Rochester, NY
Sharon L. Roy, MD, MPH, Centers for Disease Control and Prevention, Atlanta, GA
Lorry G. Rubin, MD, Cohen Children's Medical Center of New York of Northwell
    Health, New Hyde Park, NY
Candace D. Rutt, PhD, Centers for Disease Control and Prevention, Atlanta, GA
Nicole Salazar-Austin, MD, ScM, Johns Hopkins University School of Medicine,
    Baltimore, MD
Johanna Salzer, DVM, PhD, Centers for Disease Control and Prevention, Atlanta, GA
Jason B. Sauberan, PharmD, Neonatal Research Institute, Sharp Mary Birch Hospital for
    Women and Newborns, San Diego, CA
Christian Sauder, PhD, Food and Drug Administration, Silver Spring, MD
Muskaan Sawhney, BS, University of Illinois Urbana-Champaign, New Hyde Park, NY
John Scribner Schieffelin, MD, MSPH, Tulane University School of Medicine, New
    Orleans, LA
Sarah Schillie, MD, MPH, MBA, Centers for Disease Control and Prevention, Decatur, GA
Stephanie Schrag, DPhil, Centers for Disease Control and Prevention, Atlanta, GA
Shera Carlson Schreiber, MD, Food and Drug Administration, Bethesda, MD
Stacey Schultz-Cherry, PhD, St. Jude Children's Research Hospital, Memphis, TN
Dorothy E. Scott, MD, Food and Drug Administration, Silver Spring, MD
Justin Benjamin Searns, MD, University of Colorado, Children's Hospital Colorado,
    Aurora, CO
W. Evan Secor, PhD, Centers for Disease Control and Prevention, Atlanta, GA
Talal B. Seddik, MD, Stanford University, School of Medicine, Walnut Creek, CA
Isaac See, MD, Centers for Disease Control and Prevention, Atlanta, GA
Warren M. Seigel, MD, MBA, FAAP, FSAHM, NYC Health and Hospital/South
    Brooklyn Health, Kew Gardens, NY
Andi L. Shane, MD, MPH, MSc, Emory University School of Medicine and Children's
    Healthcare of Atlanta, Atlanta, GA
Shashi Sharma, PhD, MSN, RN, Centers for Disease Control and Prevention,
    Woodbridge, VA
Virginia Sheikh, MD, MHS, Food and Drug Administration, Silver Spring, MD
Avinash K. Shetty, MBBS, MD, DCH, Wake Forest University School of Medicine,
    Winston-Salem, NC
Tom T. Shimabukuro, MD, MPH, MBA, Centers for Disease Control and Prevention,
    Atlanta, GA
Masako Shimamura, MD, Nationwide Children's Hospital, Columbus, OH
Azadeh Shoaibi, PhD, MHS, Food and Drug Administration, Silver Spring, MD
Trevor Shoemaker, PhD, MPH, Centers for Disease Control and Prevention, Atlanta, GA
Timothy R. Shope, MD, MPH, Children's Hospital of Pittsburgh of UPMC, Gibsonia, PA
Stanford T. Shulman, MD, Lurie Childrens Hospital/Northwestern, Evanston, IL
Upinder Singh, MD, Stanford University School of Medicine, Stanford, CA
Rosalyn J. Singleton, MD, MPH, Alaska Native Tribal Health Consortium, Anchorage, AK

Tami H. Skoff, MS, Centers for Disease Control and Prevention, Atlanta, GA
John W. Sleasman, MD, Duke University School of Medicine, Durham, NC
Dallas J. Smith, PharmD, Centers for Disease Control and Prevention, Atlanta, GA
Jessica Coquese Smith, MPH, Centers for Disease Control and Prevention, Glen Rose, TX
Thomas D. Smith, MD, Food and Drug Administration, Silver Spring, MD
Kirk Smith, DVM, MS, PhD, Minnesota Department of Health, St. Paul, MN
Lizzy Smith-Jeffcoat, MPH, Centers for Disease Control and Prevention, Atlanta, GA
Paul W. Spearman, MD, Cincinnati Children's Hospital, Cincinnati, OH
Kevin B. Spicer, MD, PhD, MPH, Centers for Disease Control and Prevention,
    Shelbyville, KY
Philip R. Spradling, MD, Centers for Disease Control and Prevention, Colorado Springs,
    CO
Mary Allen Staat, MD, MPH, Cincinnati Children's Hospital Medical Center, Cincinnati,
    OH
J. Erin Staples, MD, PhD, Centers for Disease Control and Prevention, Fort Collins, CO
Victoria A. Statler, MD, MSc, Norton Children's and University of Louisville School of
    Medicine, Louisville, KY
William M. Stauffer, MD, MSPH, FASTMH, University of Minnesota, Lake Elmo, MN
William J. Steinbach, MD, University of Arkansas for Medical Sciences, Little Rock, AR
Jonathan Steinberg, RN, MPH, Centers for Disease Control and Prevention, Anchorage,
    AK
David S. Stephens, MD, Emory University, Atlanta, GA
Patricia A. Stinchfield, RN, MS, CPNP, Children's Minnesota, St. Paul, MN
Shannon Stokley, DrPH, Centers for Disease Control and Prevention, Atlanta, GA
Anne Straily, DVM, MPH, Centers for Disease Control and Prevention, Atlanta, GA
Nancy A. Strockbine, PhD, Centers for Disease Control and Prevention, Atlanta, GA
John R. Su, MD, PhD, MPH, Centers for Disease Control and Prevention, Atlanta, GA
David E. Sugerman, MD, MPH, Centers for Disease Control and Prevention, Atlanta, GA
Diya Surie, MD, Centers for Disease Control and Prevention, Atlanta, GA
Peter G. Szilagyi, MD, MPH, University of California, Los Angeles, Agoura Hills, CA
Pranita D. Tamma, MD, MHS, Johns Hopkins University School of Medicine, Baltimore,
    MD
Kathrine R. Tan, MD, MPH, Centers for Disease Control and Prevention, Atlanta, GA
Mary R. Tanner, MD, Centers for Disease Control and Prevention, Suwanee, GA
Jacqueline E. Tate, PhD, Centers for Disease Control and Prevention, Atlanta, GA
Eyasu H. Teshale, Centers for Disease Control and Prevention, Lilburn, GA
Natalie J. Thornburg, PhD, Centers for Disease Control and Prevention, Atlanta, GA
Melissa Tobin-D'Angelo, MD, MPH, Georgia Department of Public Health, Atlanta, GA
Suxiang Tong, PhD, Centers for Disease Control and Prevention, Atlanta, GA
Sanet Torres-Torres, MD, San Jorge Children Hospital, San Juan, Puerto Rico
Sean R. Trimble, MPH, Centers for Disease Control and Prevention, Canton, GA
Erin Tromble, MD, Centers for Disease Control and Prevention, Tucson, AZ
Stephanie Barrett, Troy, MD, Food and Drug Administration, Silver Spring, MD
Richard W. Truman, PhD, Truman Properties, LLC, Baton Rouge, LA
Sharon V. Tsay, MD, Centers for Disease Control and Prevention, Atlanta, GA
Ellen K. Turner, MD, Food and Drug Administration, Cherry Hill, NJ

Anna Uehara, PhD, MScGH, Centers for Disease Control and Prevention, Atlanta, GA
Elizabeth R. Unger, PhD, MD, Centers for Disease Control and Prevention, Atlanta, GA
John A. Vanchiere, MD, PhD, Louisiana State University Health Sciences Center,
    Shreveport, Shreveport, LA
Kayla L. Vanden Esschert, MPH, Centers for Disease Control and Prevention, Decatur,
    GA
Antonio Vieira, DVM, MPH, PhD, Centers for Disease Control and Prevention, Atlanta,
    GA
Joseph M. Vinetz, MD, Yale University School of Medicine, New Haven, CT
Jan Vinje, PhD, Centers for Disease Control and Prevention, Atlanta, GA
Prabha Viswanathan, MD, Food and Drug Administration, Silver Spring, MD
Duc J. Vugia, MD, MPH, California Department of Public Health, Richmond, CA
Timothy J. Wade, MPH, PhD, United States Environmental Protection Agency, Research
    Triangle Park, NC
Ryan Wallace, DVM, MPH, Centers for Disease Control and Prevention, Atlanta, GA
Emmanuel B. Walter, MD, MPH, Duke University School of Medicine, Durham, NC
Louise Francois Watkins, MD, MPH, Centers for Disease Control and Prevention,
    Atlanta, GA
Kathryn Weakley, MD, University of Louisville, Louisville, KY
Michelle Weinberg, MD, MPH, Centers for Disease Control and Prevention, Atlanta, GA
Geoffrey A. Weinberg, MD, University of Rochester School of Medicine and Dentistry,
    Rochester, NY
Eric Weintraub, MPH, Centers for Disease Control and Prevention, Atlanta, GA
Thomas Weiser, MD, MPH, Indian Health Service, Portland, OR
Scott J. Weissman, MD, Seattle Children's Hospital, Seattle, WA
Daniel Lowell Weller, PhD, Centers for Disease Control and Prevention, Atlanta, GA
Mark K. Weng, MD, MSc, Centers for Disease Control and Prevention, Atlanta, GA
A. Clinton White, Jr, MD, University of Texas Medical Branch, Galveston, TX
Amy Whitesell, MPH, Centers for Disease Control and Prevention, Atlanta, GA
Richard James Whitley, MD, University of Alabama at Birmingham, Birmingham, AL
Melisa A. Willby, PhD, Centers for Disease Control and Prevention, Atlanta, GA
Charnetta Williams, MD, Centers for Disease Control and Prevention, Atlanta, GA
Samanth L. Williams, MPH, Centers for Disease Control and Prevention, Atlanta, GA
Margaret Williams, Centers for Disease Control and Prevention, Atlanta, GA
Susana Williams Keeshin, MD, University of Utah, Salt Lake City, UT
Carla Winston, PhD, MA, Centers for Disease Control and Prevention, Atlanta, GA
Robin Wisch, MD, Food and Drug Administration, Silver Spring, MD
A. Patricia Wodi, MD, Centers for Disease Control and Prevention, Marietta, GA
Joshua Wolf, MBBS, PhD, FRACP, St. Jude Childrens Research Hospital, Memphis, TN
JoEllen S. Wolicki, BSN, University of Detroit/Mercy, Atlanta, GA
Susan K. Wollersheim, MD, Food and Drug Administration, Silver Spring, MD
Jane Woo, MD, MPH, Food and Drug Administration, Silver Spring, MD
Kate Russell Woodworth, MD, MPH, Centers for Disease Control and Prevention,
    Atlanta, GA
Kimberly Workowski, MD, Emory University, Atlanta, GA
Alexandra S. Worobec, MD, Food and Drug Administration, Silver Spring, MD
Caitlin M. Worrell, MPH, Centers for Disease Control and Prevention, Atlanta, GA

Mary A. Worthington, PharmD, BCPS, BCPPS, Samford University McWhorter School of Pharmacy, Birmingham, AL
Karen Wu, DVM, MSPH, Centers for Disease Control and Prevention, Decatur, GA
Pablo Yagupsky, MD, Soroka University Medical Center, Ben-Gurion University of the Negev, Beer-Sheva, Israel
Albert C. Yan, MD, Children's Hospital of Philadelphia & Perelman School of Medicine at the University of Pennsylvania, Philadelphia, PA
Sixun Yang, MD, PhD, Food and Drug Administration, Silver Spring, MD
April M. Yarbrough, PharmD, BCPS, Children's of Alabama, Birmingham, AL
Sarah Yashar-Gershman, AB, Cohen Children's Medical Center, New Hyde Park, NY
Jonathan S. Yoder, MPH, Centers for Disease Control and Prevention, Atlanta, GA
Danielle M. Zerr, MD, MPH, Seattle Children's Hospital, Seattle, WA
Rachel Zhang, MD, Food and Drug Administration, North Bethesda, MD

AAP Committee on Adolescence
AAP Committee on Bioethics
AAP Committee on Coding and Nomenclature
AAP Committee on Drugs
AAP Committee on Fetus and Newborn
AAP Committee on Hospital Care
AAP Committee on Medical Liability and Risk Management
AAP Committee on Native American Child Health
AAP Committee on Nutrition
AAP Committee on Pediatric and Adolescent HIV
AAP Committee on Pediatric Emergency Medicine
AAP Committee on Practice and Ambulatory Medicine
AAP Committee on Substance Use and Prevention
AAP Council on Child Abuse and Neglect
AAP Council on Children and Disasters
AAP Council on Children With Disabilities
AAP Council on Clinical Information Technology
AAP Council on Environmental Health and Climate Change
AAP Council on Foster Care, Adoption, and Kinship Care
AAP Council on Genetics
AAP Council on Immigrant Child and Family Health
AAP Council on Quality Improvement and Patient Safety
AAP Council on School Health
AAP Council on Sports Medicine and Fitness
AAP FamilY Partnerships Network
AAP Pediatric Practice Management Alliance
AAP Section on Administration and Practice Management
AAP Section on Adolescent Health
AAP Section on Allergy and Immunology
AAP Section on Breastfeeding
AAP Section on Cardiology and Cardiac Surgery
AAP Section on Critical Care
AAP Section on Dermatology

AAP Section on Emergency Medicine
AAP Section on Epidemiology, Public Health, and Evidence
AAP Section on Gastroenterology, Hepatology, and Nutrition
AAP Section on Global Health
AAP Section on Hematology/Oncology
AAP Section on Home Care
AAP Section on Hospital Medicine
AAP Section on Infectious Diseases
AAP Section on Lesbian, Gay, Bisexual, and Transgender Health and Wellness
AAP Section on Minority Health, Equity, and Inclusion
AAP Section on Neonatal-Perinatal Medicine
AAP Section on Nephrology
AAP Section on Neurology
AAP Section on Ophthalmology
AAP Section on Orthopaedics
AAP Section on Otolaryngology–Head and Neck Surgery
AAP Section on Pediatric Pulmonology and Sleep Medicine
AAP Section on Radiology
AAP Section on Rheumatology
AAP Section on Surgery

Committee on Infectious Diseases, 2021–2024

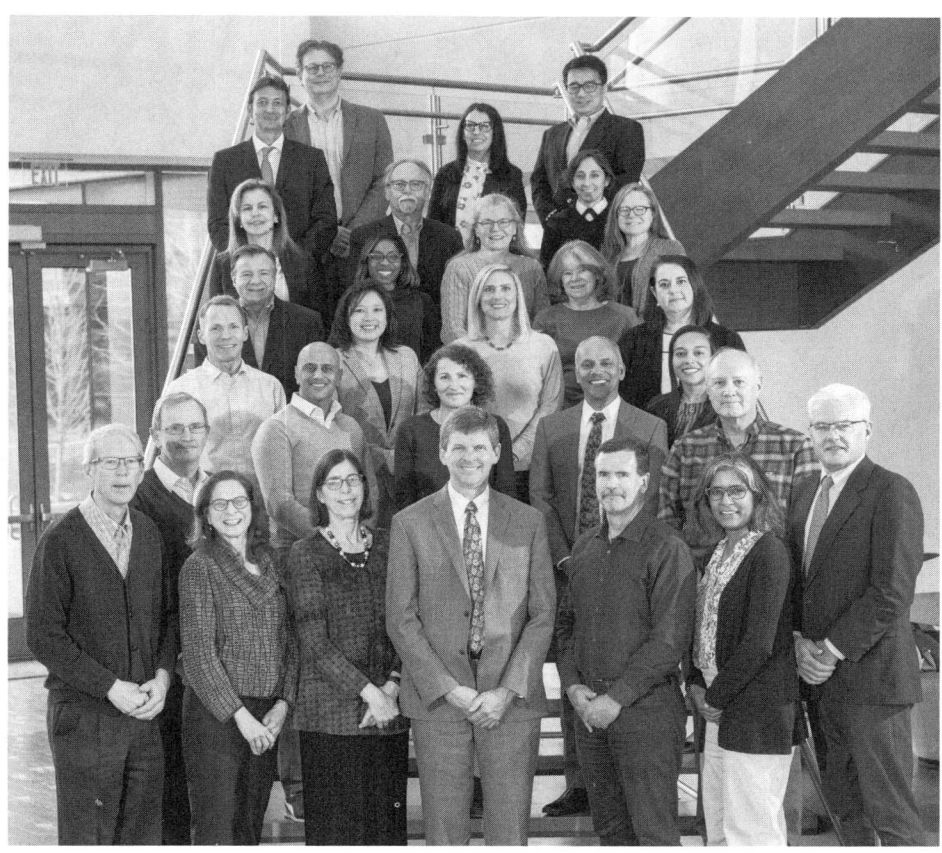

FIRST ROW, LEFT TO RIGHT: Mark H. Sawyer, Ruth Lynfield, Elizabeth D. Barnett, David W. Kimberlin, Sean T. O'Leary, Ritu Banerjee, James D. Campbell

SECOND ROW, LEFT TO RIGHT: Robert W. Frenck, Jr, Samir S. Shah, Mary T. Caserta, Chandy C. John, Denee J. Moore, Jeffrey R. Starke

THIRD ROW, LEFT TO RIGHT: Jeffrey S. Gerber, Pia S. Pannaraj, Angela L. Myers, Melinda Wharton, Monica I. Ardura

FOURTH ROW, LEFT TO RIGHT: Charles R. Woods, Jr, Lakshmi Panagiotakopoulos, Lisa M. Kafer, Laura Sauvé

FIFTH ROW, LEFT TO RIGHT: Athena P. Kourtis, José R. Romero, Cristina Cardemil

SIXTH ROW, LEFT TO RIGHT: Eduardo López Medina, Adam Ratner, Jennifer M. Frantz, David Kim

NOT PICTURED: Henry H. Bernstein, Kristina A. Bryant, Karen M. Farizo, Jennifer Thompson, Claudia Espinosa, Aaron Milstone, C. Mary Healy

2024 *Red Book* Dedication for Sarah S. Long, MD, FAAP

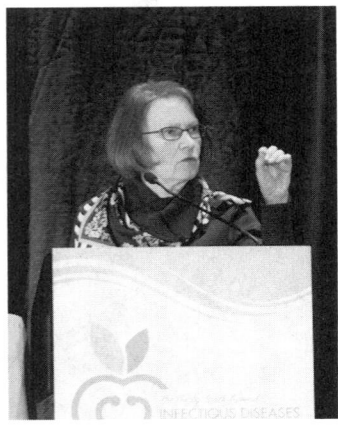

In 1750 and living in Philadelphia, Benjamin Franklin is reported to have said: "Tell me and I forget. Teach me and I remember. Involve me and I learn." These words likely resonate with each of us. As we think back across our careers, we marvel at our good fortune to have touched lives with gifted educators who inspired us by doing exactly this – teaching, involving, motivating us to realize our full potentials. For so many of us in pediatrics and pediatric infectious diseases, the name that is synonymous with gifted teacher is another Philadelphian—a woman who has blazed a path across decades and lit fires in our minds and our hearts. In recognition of her lifetime of commitment to children and those of us who take care of them, the 2024 *Red Book* is dedicated to Dr. Sarah Long.

Dr. Long's infectious energy and high expectations are best understood through the lens of her origin. Born in Alaska 15 years before statehood, she has had a frontier spirit throughout all the journeys of her life. When Alaska became a state in 1959, she moved with her family to Washington, DC, where her father was Chief of Staff to Alaska's first US Senator. From there, she moved to Pennsylvania and attended St. Francis College in the 1960s before entering Jefferson Medical College (now Sidney Kimmel Medical College) as one of only 10 women in a class of almost 200, graduating in 1970. She stayed in Philadelphia for her pediatric residency training at St. Christopher's Hospital for Children. Always inquisitive, she spent her summers in medical school working at the National Institutes of Health, with a subsequent research fellowship as an NIH trainee at Temple University. She began her first faculty position in 1975 as Chief of Infectious Diseases at St. Christopher's Hospital for Children, Temple University School of Medicine, and Drexel University College of Medicine in Philadelphia, a position that she held for the next 44 years.

Dr. Long's recognition for her gifts as an educator are innumerable. She received outstanding teaching awards across every decade beginning in 1977, including the Infectious Diseases Society of America National Clinical Teacher Award in 2012. She was selected by the National Institutes of Health Medical Research Scholars Program to give the

2021 Great Teacher's Lecture. And across the decades, she has delivered over 90 named, memorial, and honorary society lectureships and visiting professorships across the globe, in addition to an average of more than 30 annual lectures nationally and internationally for more than 3 decades. She continues to serve in the IDWeek Clinical Educator Mentor Coaching Program.

In service to the American Academy of Pediatrics (AAP), Dr. Long served on the Committee on Infectious Diseases (COID, or the *Red Book* Committee) from 2002 through 2008. She was Associate Editor of the 2006, 2009, 2012, 2015, and 2018 editions of the *Red Book*. Across those 20 years, she established the doctrine (known by COID members and liaisons as the "Long Doctrine") by which all current and future iterations of the *Red Book* are anchored, namely that the *Red Book* represents settled science upon which sound clinical decision making can be based. She received the AAP Section on Infectious Diseases Lifetime Contribution to Infectious Diseases Award in 2009, a full decade before she closed out her chapter of service to the Academy.

Dr. Long also served the American Board of Pediatrics (ABP) across the 1990s and into the 2000s, as a member of the ABP Board of Directors, as Secretary-Treasurer, and ultimately as Board Chair. She was the inaugural Chair of the ABP Subspecialty Board of Infectious Diseases when pediatric infectious diseases was designated a subspecialty of pediatrics, where she literally wrote the first pediatric infectious diseases subspecialty examination (her Board Certificate is, appropriately, #01). For all of these activities and more, she received the ABP Board of Directors Proclamation of Distinguished Service in 2015.

Dr. Long also provided key leadership to the Pediatric Infectious Diseases Society (PIDS) and the Infectious Diseases Society of America (IDSA), serving on PIDS Council (now called the PIDS Board of Directors) from 1989 through 1993 and as PIDS President from 1999 through 2001. She Co-Chaired the 48th ICAAC/46th IDSA joint meeting with incredible dexterity and has served as Director of the IDSA Foundation Board of Directors since 2019. She received the PIDS Distinguished Service Award in 2003 and the PIDS Distinguished Physician Award in 2016.

In the mid-1990s, Dr. Long developed the seminal textbook in the field, *Principles and Practice of Pediatric Infectious Diseases*, literally creating it from scratch. Before stepping down in 2023, she served as the Chief Editor for each of its 6 editions published to date (1997, 2003, 2008, 2012, 2018, and 2023), and very appropriately, the 7th edition will now officially be known as *Long's Principles and Practice of Pediatric Infectious Diseases* (which is what we've all been calling it from the beginning!). She has served as Associate Editor of *The Journal of Pediatrics* since 1996 and has published over 320 peer-reviewed publications and close to 200 book chapters. Since 2020, Dr. Long has been a member of the Centers for Disease Control and Prevention (CDC) Advisory Committee on Immunization Practices (ACIP), on which she adroitly helped guide COVID-19 vaccine recommendations across the course of the worst pandemic the world has seen in over a century, in addition to chairing the Maternal/Child RSV Work Group as it developed recommendations for use of the first licensed RSV vaccines.

Even with all of these accomplishments and more not listed, Dr. Long's most meaningful contributions are really at the one-on-one level. Since 2013, she has served on the Program Committee for the Infectious Diseases in Children Symposium held in New York City each November. Even among the tremendously talented speakers featured at that meeting each year, Dr. Long's lectures are head and shoulders above the rest. It is common to see her surrounded by literally scores of meeting attendees who are general pediatricians and nurse practitioners from around the country, hanging on each clinical insight or teaching point that she provides. Watching these interactions and others at large meetings across the country, I cannot help but think back to Mr. Franklin's words. Sarah teaches them, and they remember. Sarah involves them, and they learn.

Sarah's first fellow was Margaret (Meg) C. Fisher, MD, FAAP, who herself went on to be a tremendous pediatric infectious diseases physician, educator, and AAP Board of Directors member. In 2019, Sarah received the Margaret C. Fisher Eternal Spirit of St. Christopher's Award, from the house staff of St. Christopher's Hospital for Children, taking her contributions full circle. She started at St. Christopher's, she reached out and changed the world, and her hometown family said thank you. Dr. Long, we join in that chorus. Thank you for teaching and involving us all.

PREVIOUS *RED BOOK* DEDICATION RECIPIENTS:
2021 Louis Z. Cooper, MD, FAAP
2018 Larry K. Pickering, MD, FAAP, and Carol J. Baker, MD, FAAP
2015 Stanley Plotkin, MD, FAAP
2012 Samuel L. Katz, MD, FAAP
2009 Ralph Feigin, MD, FAAP
2006 Caroline Breese Hall, MD, FAAP
2003 Georges Peter, MD, FAAP
2000 Edgar O. Ledbetter, MD, FAAP
1997 Georges Peter, MD, FAAP
1988 Jean D. Lockhart, MD, FAAP

Preface

The *Red Book*, now in its 33rd edition, has been a unique and valuable source of information on infectious diseases and immunizations for pediatric practitioners since 1938. With the practice of pediatrics and pediatric infectious diseases changing rapidly and the limited time available to the practitioner, the *Red Book* remains an essential resource to quickly obtain current, accurate, and easily accessible information about vaccines and vaccine recommendations, emerging infectious diseases, diagnostic modalities, and treatment recommendations. The Committee on Infectious Diseases of the American Academy of Pediatrics (AAP), the editors of the *Red Book*, and the 500 *Red Book* contributors are dedicated to providing the most current and accurate information available in the concise, practical format for which the *Red Book* is known.

As with the 2021 edition, the print version of the *Red Book* will be provided to every AAP member as part of their member benefit. This commitment reflects the Academy's strong interest in its members' needs. In addition, AAP members also will continue to have access to *Red Book* content on *Red Book Online* (**www.aapredbook.org**). AAP policy statements, clinical reports, and technical reports as well as recommendations endorsed by the AAP are posted on *Red Book Online* as they become available during the 3 years between *Red Book* editions, and online chapters are modified as needed to reflect these changes. The Outbreaks section of *Red Book Online* is a valuable resource that concisely summarizes current infectious disease outbreaks that affect the pediatric population and that have been identified in multiple US states; other outbreak types may be covered occasionally as situations warrant. *Red Book* users also are encouraged to sign up for e-mail alerts on **www.aapredbook.org** to receive new information and policy updates between editions. In the 2021 *Red Book*, we introduced the Systems-Based Treatment Table, available in both the print edition and *Red Book Online*. The Systems-Based Treatment Table has quickly become a valuable and highly used resource among pediatric practitioners. With this edition, we have expanded and updated the table to include more conditions and the latest information on optimal treatments and durations for specific conditions, and the table has been placed at the beginning of the book before Section 1 for ease of reference. Another important resource is the visual library of *Red Book Online*, which is continually updated and expanded to include more images of infectious diseases, examples of classic radiologic and other findings, and recent information on epidemiology of infectious diseases.

The Committee on Infectious Diseases relies on information and advice from many experts, as evidenced by the lengthy list of contributors to *Red Book*. We especially are indebted to the many contributors from other AAP Committees, Sections, and Councils; the American Academy of Family Physicians; the American College of Obstetricians and Gynecologists; the American Thoracic Society; the Canadian Paediatric Society; the Centers for Disease Control and Prevention; the US Food and Drug Administration; the National Institutes of Health; the National Vaccine Program Office; the Pediatric Infectious Diseases Society; la Sociedad Latinoamericana de Infectología Pediátrica; the World Health Organization; and many other organizations and individuals who have made this edition possible. In addition, suggestions made by individual AAP members to improve the presentation of information on specific issues and on topic selection have been incorporated whenever possible.

Most important to the success of this edition is the dedication and work of the editors, whose commitment to excellence is unparalleled. This new edition was made possible under the able leadership of David W. Kimberlin, MD, Editor, along with Associate Editors Ritu Banerjee, MD, PhD, Elizabeth D. Barnett, MD, Ruth Lynfield, MD, and Mark H. Sawyer, MD. We also are indebted to Tina Tan, MD, for her work on the *Red Book Atlas of Pediatric Infectious Diseases* and *Red Book: A Quick Diagnosis Deck*, and to Kristina Bryant, MD, for her extensive efforts on *Red Book Online*. We also extend heartfelt thanks to Henry H. Bernstein, DO, MHCM, for his many years of service as Editor of *Red Book Online*. Finally, we would like to extend our thanks to many staff at the AAP who contribute to the production of the *Red Book*. Specifically, we would like to thank Jennifer Frantz, MPH, for her many years of service as Senior Manager of Infectious Diseases Policy and Programs; Gillian Gibbs, MPH, who now serves in that role; Linda Rutt, for keeping all of the draft chapters flowing through a very complex production sequence; and Jennifer Shaw, for her extraordinary copyediting skills.

As noted in previous editions of the *Red Book*, some omissions and errors are inevitable in a book of this type. We ask that AAP members continue to assist the committee actively by suggesting specific ways to improve the quality of future editions. The committee membership and editorial staff hope that the 2024 *Red Book* will enhance your practice and benefit the children you serve.

Sean T. O'Leary, MD, MPH, FAAP
Chairperson, Committee on Infectious Diseases

Introduction

The Committee on Infectious Diseases (COID) of the American Academy of Pediatrics (AAP) is responsible for developing and revising guidance from the AAP for management and control of infectious diseases in infants, children, and adolescents. Every 3 years, the COID issues the *Red Book: Report of the Committee on Infectious Diseases,* which contains a composite summary of current recommendations representing the policy of the AAP on various aspects of infectious diseases, including updated vaccine recommendations for the most recent US Food and Drug Administration (FDA)-licensed vaccines for infants, children, and adolescents. These recommendations represent a consensus of opinions based on consideration of the best available evidence by members of the COID, in conjunction with liaison representatives from the Centers for Disease Control and Prevention (CDC), the FDA, the National Institutes of Health (NIH), the National Vaccine Program Office, the Canadian Paediatric Society, the American Thoracic Society, the Pediatric Infectious Diseases Society, the American Academy of Family Physicians, the American College of Obstetricians and Gynecologists, *Red Book* consultants, and scores of collaborators. This edition of the *Red Book* is based on information available as of February 2024.

To aid physicians and other health care professionals in assimilating current changes in recommendations in the *Red Book,* a listing of major changes between the 2021 and 2024 editions has been compiled (see Summary of Major Changes, p xxxvii). However, this list only begins to cover the many in-depth changes that have occurred in each chapter and section. Throughout the *Red Book,* internet addresses enable rapid access to new information available following the publication date. In addition, specific chapters within the *Red Book* may be updated prior to the publication of the next edition to incorporate new information from AAP policy statements and clinical reports, publications in the CDC *Morbidity and Mortality Weekly Report (MMWR),* society guidelines (eg, from the Infectious Diseases Society of America or the American Thoracic Society), management recommendations from the World Health Organization, and similar authoritative guidance documents from organizations of similar stature. When updates to existing *Red Book* chapters are made, the new material is posted on *Red Book Online* with clear delineation of how the chapter has been updated with the new information. This and other *Red Book Online* content can be accessed at **www.publications. aap.org/redbook.**

The *Red Book* is your personal access to literally hundreds of pediatric infectious disease consultant, on your bookshelf and ready for you 24 hours a day, 7 days a week. Arguably, it is most valuable in those circumstances in which definitive data from randomized controlled trials are lacking. It is in those situations that guidance from experts in the field is most critical, and the COID has literally thousands of years of cumulative expertise to bring to bear on such recommendations. This is all the more important as we move into the post-pandemic era, in which the rapid retrieval of accurate and reliable information is critical to the care of patients and the workflow of physician practices. A major emphasis of the 2024 *Red Book* is to provide more guidance in the format of tables, figures, and algorithms to allow for busy clinicians in offices, hospitals, and via telehealth to quickly find management recommendations from the hundreds of contributors to *Red Book* content.

One significant change since the publication of the 2021 *Red Book* is our appreciation that "Words Matter," to use the phrase embraced by the AAP.[1] Throughout the 2024 edition of the *Red Book*, we have sought to use inclusive, anti-biased language contextualized to the unique moment in history in which we practice medicine. For some chapters, however, the terms "male" and "female" are used for clarity of recommendations; when so utilized, a footnote has been added at the beginning of the chapter to indicate that these terms refer to the sex assigned at birth. Likewise, the word chestfeeding may be used by nonbinary, transgender, and other parents to identify how they feed their infants. It may refer to human milk or human milk substitute feeding, from a person who lactates or not. Because of this broad and variable definition, chestfeeding and breastfeeding are not always synonymous, and the words are not interchangeable. Published literature findings on breastfeeding may not hold the same outcomes for chestfeeding, so throughout the 2024 edition, the words breastfeeding and human milk are used.

Preparation of the *Red Book* is a team effort in the truest sense of the term. Within weeks following the publication of each *Red Book* edition, all *Red Book* chapters are sent for updates to primary reviewers who are leading national and international experts in their specific areas. For the 2024 *Red Book*, one third of primary reviewers were new to this process, ensuring that the most up-to-date information has been included in this new edition. Following review by the primary reviewer, each chapter is returned to the assigned Associate Editor for incorporation of the reviewer's edits. The chapter then is disseminated to content experts at the CDC, NIH, and FDA and to members of all AAP Sections, Committees, and Councils who agree to review specific chapters for their additional edits as needed, after which it again is returned to the assigned Associate Editor for harmonization and incorporation of edits as appropriate. Two designated COID reviewers then complete a final review of the chapter, and it is returned to the assigned Associate Editor for inclusion of any needed additional modifications. Chapters requiring consideration by the full committee then are debated at the COID "Marathon Meeting," where the chapters are finalized. Copyediting by the Editor and Senior Medical Copy Editor, Jennifer Shaw, follows, and the book then is reviewed by the *Red Book* reviewers appointed by the AAP Board of Directors. In all, over 1000 hands have touched the 2024 *Red Book* prior to its publication! That so many contributors dedicate so much time and expertise to this product is a testament to the role the *Red Book* plays in the care of children.

Through the deliberative and inclusive process that defines the production of the *Red Book*, the COID endeavors to provide current, relevant, evidence-based recommendations for the prevention and management of infectious diseases in infants, children, and adolescents. Seemingly unanswerable scientific questions, the complexity of medical practice, ongoing innovative technology, continuous new information, and inevitable

---

[1] American Academy of Pediatrics. Words Matter: AAP Guidance on Inclusive, Anti-biased Language. May 14, 2021. Available at: **www.aap.org/en/about-the-aap/american-academy-of-pediatrics-equity-and-inclusion-efforts/words-matter-aap-guidance-on-inclusive-anti-biased-language/**

differences of opinion among experts all are addressed during production of the *Red Book*. In some cases, other committees and experts may differ in their interpretation of data and resulting recommendations, and occasionally no single recommendation can be made because several options for management are equally acceptable. In such circumstances, the language incorporated in the chapter acknowledges these differing acceptable management options by use of the phrases "most experts recommend..." and "some experts recommend..." Both phrases indicate valid recommendations, but the first phrase signifies more agreement and support among the experts. Inevitably in clinical practice, questions arise that cannot be answered easily on the basis of currently available data. When this happens, the COID still provides guidance and information that, coupled with clinical judgment, will facilitate well-reasoned, clinically relevant decisions. Through this process of lifelong learning, the committee seeks to provide a practical guide for physicians and other health care professionals in their care of infants, children, and adolescents.

Information on use of antimicrobial agents is included in the package inserts (product labels) prepared by manufacturers, including contraindications and adverse events. The *Red Book* does not attempt to provide this information comprehensively, because it is available readily in package inserts. As in previous editions of the *Red Book*, recommended dosage schedules for antimicrobial agents are provided (see Section 4, Antimicrobial Agents and Related Therapy) and may differ from those of the manufacturer as provided in the package insert. Antimicrobial agents recommended for specific infections in the *Red Book* may or may not have an FDA indication for treatment of that infection. Physicians also can reference additional information in the package inserts of vaccines licensed by the FDA (which also may differ from COID and CDC recommendations for use) and of immune globulins, as well as recommendations of other committees (see Sources of Information About Vaccines and Immunization, p 21), many of which are included in the *Red Book*.

This book could not have been prepared without the dedicated professional competence of numerous people. The AAP staff has been outstanding in its committed work and contributions, particularly Jennifer Shaw, Senior Medical Copy Editor; Linda Rutt, Division Coordinator; Jennifer Frantz and Gillian Gibbs, Senior Managers, who served as the administrative directors for the COID and coordinated preparation of the *Red Book;* Theresa Wiener, Manager of Publishing and Production Services; and all of the directors and staff of the AAP publishing and marketing groups who make the full *Red Book* product line possible.

Lakshmi Panagiotakopoulos, MD, of the CDC, and Karen M. Farizo, MD, of the FDA, devoted time and effort in providing significant input from their organizations. Patricia Flanagan, MD, Yasuko Fukuda, MD, and Warren Seigel, MD, served as *Red Book* reviewers appointed by the AAP Board of Directors, spending scores of hours reviewing the final chapters for consistency and accuracy. I am especially indebted to the Associate Editors, Ritu Banerjee, MD, PhD, Elizabeth D. Barnett, MD, Ruth Lynfield, MD, and Mark H. Sawyer, MD, for their expertise, tireless work, good humor, and immense contributions in their editorial and committee work. Members of the COID contributed countless hours and deserve appropriate recognition for their patience, dedication, revisions, and reviews. The COID appreciates the guidance and dedication of Sean O'Leary, MD,

COID Chairperson, whose knowledge, dedication, insight, and leadership are reflected in the quality and productivity of the committee's work. There are many additional contributors whose professional work and commitment have been essential in the committee's preparation of the *Red Book*. Please forgive any omissions I have made in expressing my gratitude.

And last but certainly not least, I thank my wife, Kim, for always being there and for her patience, understanding, and never-ending support as this edition of the *Red Book* came to fruition.

David W. Kimberlin, MD, FAAP, Editor

Table of Contents

SECTION 2
RECOMMENDATIONS FOR CARE OF CHILDREN
IN SPECIAL CIRCUMSTANCES

SECTION 3
SUMMARIES OF INFECTIOUS DISEASES

SECTION 4
ANTIMICROBIAL AGENTS AND RELATED THERAPY

SECTION 5
ANTIMICROBIAL PROPHYLAXIS

APPENDICES

Summary of Major Changes in the 2024 *Red Book*

MAJOR CHANGES: GENERAL

1. All chapters in the last edition of the *Red Book* were assessed for relevance in the dynamic environment that is the practice of pediatric medicine today. The revisions to the **Discussing Vaccines With Patients and Parents** chapter included discussions of safety monitoring mechanisms, allowing for elimination of 6 chapters included in the last *Red Book* that reviewed each of these safety systems separately. Chapters on **COVID-19** and **Mpox** have been broken out from the chapters in which they were discussed in the 2021 edition, creating 2 new chapters. This means we have a net decrease of 4 chapters in the 2024 *Red Book* compared with the prior edition.

2. Every chapter in the 2024 *Red Book* has been modified since the last edition. The listing below outlines the more major changes throughout the 2014 edition.

3. A major focus of the 2024 *Red Book* is to streamline the retrieval of information needed to care for the patient sitting in front of the clinician, either in the office or hospital room or remotely via telehealth. To accomplish this, we have greatly expanded the use of tables, figures, and algorithms that can rapidly be accessed to gather the information needed at that moment.

4. Appropriate chapters throughout the *Red Book* have been updated to be consistent with 2024 American Academy of Pediatrics (AAP) and Centers for Disease Control and Prevention (CDC) vaccine recommendations, CDC recommendations for immunization of health care personnel, and drug recommendations from *2024 Nelson's Pediatric Antimicrobial Therapy*.[1]

5. To ensure that the information presented in the *Red Book* is based on the most accurate and up-to-date scientific data, the primary reviewers of each *Red Book* chapter were selected for their specific academic expertise in each particular area. In this edition of the *Red Book*, 35% of the primary reviewers were new for their assigned chapters. This ensures that the *Red Book* content is viewed with fresh eyes with each publication cycle.

6. Throughout the *Red Book*, the number of websites where additional current and future information can be obtained has been updated. All websites are in bold type for ease of reference, and all have been verified for accuracy and accessibility.

7. Reference to evidence-based policy recommendations from the AAP, the Advisory Committee on Immunization Practices (ACIP) of the CDC, the National Institutes of Health (NIH), and other select professional organizations have been updated throughout the *Red Book*.

---

[1] Bradley JS, Nelson JD, Barnett ED, et al, eds. *2024 Nelson's Pediatric Antimicrobial Therapy.* 30th ed. Itasca, IL: American Academy of Pediatrics; 2024

8. Standardized approaches to disease prevention through immunizations, antimicrobial prophylaxis, and infection-control practices have been updated throughout the *Red Book*.
9. Policy updates released after publication of this edition of the *Red Book* will be posted on *Red Book Online*.

SYSTEMS-BASED TREATMENT TABLE

1. The **Systems-Based Treatment Table** that was introduced in Section 4 of the 2021 edition of the *Red Book* has been moved to the front of the book for easier access. It also has been reordered so that the grouped recommendations by body system are more easily and quickly accessed. Empiric antibiotic options for several of the infections in this table have been expanded.

SECTION 1. ACTIVE AND PASSIVE IMMUNIZATION

1. Internet resources for vaccine information have been updated in **Sources of Information About Immunization.**
2. The **Discussing Vaccines With Patients and Parents** chapter has been completely rewritten to align with the forthcoming AAP clinical report "Strategies for Improving Vaccine Communication and Uptake." This chapter includes discussion of safety surveillance systems, allowing for elimination of separate chapters covering these in the prior edition of the *Red Book*.
3. In the **Active Immunization** chapter and across the *Red Book*, terminology has changed from "live and inactivated vaccines" to "live and non-live vaccines." In addition, detailed information on mRNA vaccines has been added.
4. New-generation vaccines containing mRNA encoding for antigens or viral vectors that express antigens have been added to the **Vaccine Ingredients** chapter.
5. Guidance on storage of a frozen vaccine that has been thawed and on beyond-use date/time (BUD) has been added to the **Vaccine Handling and Storage** chapter.
6. In the **Vaccine Administration** chapter, a Vaccine Administration Errors section has been added, and the Patient Care Before, During, and After Vaccine Administration section has been expanded.
7. A listing of vaccines that are more likely to be painful has been added to the **Managing Injection Pain** chapter.
8. A strong statement discouraging creation of unique vaccination schedules outside of the reviewed and recommended schedules has been added to the **Immunization Schedule and Timing of Vaccines** chapter.
9. Recommendation has been added to **Minimum Ages and Minimum Intervals Between Vaccine Doses** for what to do if intervals between doses are longer than recommended.
10. *Haemophilus influenzae* type b, rotavirus, and quadrivalent meningococcal vaccines have been added to the list of approved vaccines in the **Interchangeability of Vaccine Products** chapter that may be used interchangeably during a vaccine series from different manufacturers.

11. Recommendations have been added to the chapter on **Simultaneous Administration of Multiple Vaccines** for spacing between mpox vaccine and COVID-19 vaccines.

12. In the **Combination Vaccines** chapter, use of DTaP-IPV (Quadracel) as a 4th or 5th dose in the IPV series has been expanded to include patients who previously had received Vaxelis.

13. In the **Unknown or Uncertain Immunization Status** chapter, specific acceptable approaches are provided for when the immunogenicity of vaccines or the completeness of the vaccine series are unknown, especially for vaccines administered outside of the United States.

14. Guidance is provided in the **Vaccine Dose** chapter on appropriate dosing for a child receiving a COVID-19 vaccine when the child's age changes between doses.

15. The chapter on **Active Immunization After Receipt of Antibody-Containing Products** has been modified to better reflect the chapter contents. An interval between receipt of an antibody product and administration of dengue vaccine has been added. "Different anatomic site" language for hepatitis B vaccine (HepB) and hepatitis B immune globulin (HBIG) has been clarified.

16. Recommendations have been updated to the **Hypersensitivity Reactions After Immunization** chapter for skin testing for reactions to excipients in vaccines.

17. Bioavailability adjustments for immune globulin subcutaneous (IGSC) compared with immune globulin intravenous (IGIV) are provided in the **Passive Immunization** chapter.

18. A link to a listing of all immune globulin intramuscular (IGIM) products available in the United States has been added to the **Immune Globulin Intramuscular** chapter.

19. Use of IGIV in multisystem inflammatory syndrome in children (MIS-C) has been added to the **Immune Globulin Intravenous** chapter.

20. Dose-adjustment instructions on transitioning from IGIV to IGSC are provided in the **Immune Globulin Subcutaneous** chapter.

21. Language has been added to **Immunization in Special Clinical Circumstances** chapter stressing the need for caregivers of preterm and very low birth weight infants to receive COVID-19 vaccine.

22. In the **Immunization in Pregnancy** chapter, COVID-19 vaccine has been added to the list of vaccines specifically recommended for routine administration during pregnancy. Tdap vaccines have been approved by the US Food and Drug Administration (FDA) for use in pregnancy since the last edition, and these have been added. Guidance on use of mpox vaccine during pregnancy has been added.

23. The definition of severe immunosuppression from human immunodeficiency virus (HIV) has been standardized across the *Red Book*, including the chapter on **Immunization and Other Considerations in Immunocompromised Children**. Recommendations have been added for vaccine administration to persons who have received CD19-targeted chimeric antigen receptor (CAR) T-cell therapy.

24. Guidance is provided in the **Immunization in Children With a Personal or Family History of Seizures** chapter on what information should be provided to parents of children with a personal history of febrile seizures.

25. Asplenia and persistent compliment component deficiency have been added to the **Immunization in Children With Chronic Diseases** chapter.

26. Discussion of pertussis and COVID-19 vaccination has been added to the chapter on **Immunization in American Indian/Alaska Native Children and Adolescents.**

27. Recent detections of circulating vaccine-derived poliovirus in the United States have been added to the **Immunization in Health Care Personnel** chapter. COVID-19 vaccination of health care personnel is addressed.

28. A new table has been added to the chapter on **Children Who Received Immunizations Outside the United States or Whose Immunization Status is Unknown or Uncertain** showing when antibody testing for vaccine-preventable diseases should be performed in unimmunized or underimmunized children.

29. Tick-borne encephalitis (TBE) and COVID-19 vaccines have been added to the **International Travel** chapter. Rabies preexposure prophylaxis recommendations have been updated. Availability of the yellow fever vaccine in the United States has been updated.

SECTION 2. RECOMMENDATIONS FOR CARE OF CHILDREN IN SPECIAL CLINICAL CIRCUMSTANCES

1. The **Breastfeeding and Human Milk** chapter was updated to align with information in the 2022 AAP policy statement on breastfeeding. This chapter includes recommendations on COVID-19, group B *Streptococcus*, cytomegalovirus (CMV), hepatitis C virus (HCV), HIV, mpox, and tick-borne encephalitis infections in breastfeeding individuals or transmission in human milk.

2. COVID-19 has been added to the **Children in Group Child Care and Schools** chapter.

3. On the basis of experience from the COVID-19 pandemic, recommendations on prevention of airborne and droplet transmission are presented in the **Infection Prevention and Control for Hospitalized Children** chapter more in terms of points along a continuum rather than discrete modes of transmission. Discussion of source control of sick visitors is expanded.

4. Identification of patients known to be infected or colonized with highly resistant organisms is emphasized in the **Infection Prevention and Control in Ambulatory Settings** chapter. Guidance on drawing up of medications is provided.

5. The preexposure HIV prophylaxis description has been expanded in the **Sexually Transmitted Infections in Adolescents and Children** chapter. *Trichomonas* treatment and expedited partner therapy information have been updated.

6. The **Medical Evaluation for Infectious Diseases for Internationally Adopted, Refugee, and Other Immigrant Children** chapter has had a number of modifications. When to test for hepatitis A has been clarified. Testing recommendations for syphilis have been updated. Acceptable assays for tuberculosis (TB) testing have been expanded. Circumstances in which repeat testing for HIV

following resettlement have been added. Presumptive treatment recommendations for malaria are provided.

7. Testing recommendations following possible exposure to HCV are updated and expanded in the **Injuries From Needles Discarded in the Community** chapter.

8. Risk of B virus infection following macaque bites, of *Salmonella* and *Aeromonas* infection following reptile bites, and of *Vibrio* species infection following shark bites has been added to the **Bite Wounds** chapter.

9. A table has been added to the **Prevention of Mosquito-borne and Tick-borne Infections** chapter summarizing mosquito- and tick-borne infections in the United States.

SECTION 3. SUMMARIES OF INFECTIOUS DISEASES

1. *Actinomyces* as a cause of adverse pregnancy outcomes and neonatal bacteremia has been added to the **Actinomycosis** chapter.

2. **Adenovirus** has been added as a cause of severe hepatitis and liver failure. Discussion of the antiviral treatment of adenovirus infections has been expanded. Management of adenovirus in immunocompromised patients has been added.

3. Secnidazole has been added as a treatment option for mild to moderate intestinal **Amebiasis.**

4. *Acanthamoeba* as a cause of rhinosinusitis has been added to the **Amebic Meningoencephalitis and Keratitis** chapter. Treatment options for *Acanthamoeba* infections have been expanded.

5. Treatment and postexposure prophylaxis of **Anthrax** has been aligned with new CDC recommendations. New vaccine information is also provided.

6. Dengue and yellow fever vaccine information has been updated in the **Arboviruses** chapter. Tick-borne encephalitis vaccine has been added. Cache Valley virus has been added.

7. Description of invasive disease, which occurs rarely, has been added to the ***Arcanobacterium haemolyticum* Infections** chapter.

8. Mention of the cost of albendazole and mebendazole for ***Ascaris lumbricoides* Infections** has been added.

9. Use of polymerase chain reaction (PCR) assay in patients with **Aspergillosis** who have underlying hematologic malignancies and hematopoietic cell transplantation recipients has been added.

10. Typing by amplification and sequencing of small regions of the **Astrovirus** capsid gene for assessment of outbreaks has been added.

11. The expanding geographic area with **Babesiosis** is detailed. New information is provided in the Diagnosis section.

12. The pathogenesis of disease caused by diarrheal toxins of ***Bacillus cereus*** has been clarified.

13. Discussion of nucleic acid amplification tests (NAATs) is expanded in the **Bacterial Vaginosis** chapter.

14. Antibacterial treatment options for ***Bacteroides, Prevotella,* and Other Anaerobic Gram-Negative Bacilli Infections** have been updated.

15. Descriptions of diagnostic modalities for ***Balantidium coli* Infections** have been expanded. Foodborne sources of infection have been updated.

16. Information on PCR diagnosis of ***Bartonella henselae* (Cat-Scratch Disease)** has been added. Antibiotics and prolonged treatment durations have been expanded.

17. The Clinical Manifestations and Epidemiology sections of the ***Baylisascaris* Infections** chapter have been greatly expanded.

18. Diagnostic approaches to detection and interpretation of ***Blastocystis* species** in stool have been updated.

19. Newer formulations of itraconazole with enhanced bioavailablity are discussed in the **Blastomycosis** chapter.

20. Greater detail is provided on duration of shedding of **Bocavirus** and its impact on interpreting positive diagnostic tests.

21. The Clinical Manifestations, Epidemiology, and Treatment sections of ***Borrelia* Infections Other Than Lyme Disease** have been greatly expanded.

22. Clinical Manifestations of **Brucellosis** have been expanded. Secondary treatment options have been added.

23. *Burkholderia pseudomallei* epidemiology and chronicity are addressed more fully in the ***Burkholderia* Infections** chapter. Postexposure prophylaxis following laboratory exposure to *Burkholderia* species has been added.

24. Treatment recommendations for ***Campylobacter* Infections** are provided with greater specificity. Epidemiologic data have been updated.

25. Treatment recommendations for invasive **Candidiasis**, including congenital and neonatal *Candida* disease, have been updated. Diagnosis and Treatment of *Candida auris* have been expanded. Fluconazole prophylaxis recommendations for extremely low birthweight neonates have been updated.

26. Avoidance of corticosteroids during the acute phase of **Chikungunya** disease, and use of disease-modifying anti-rheumatic drugs (DMARDs) during the chronic phase, have been added. Clinical Manifestations in children have been enhanced.

27. Epidemiology and diagnosis of ***Chlamydia pneumoniae*** have been updated.

28. Mention and definition of Horder spots have been added to the ***Chlamydia psittaci*** chapter. Rare human-to-human spread has now been documented.

29. Routine screening recommendations for ***Chlamydia trachomatis*** have been updated.

30. Ancillary testing in patients with suspected **Botulism** has been outlined. A PCR assay to detect botulinum neurotoxin genes (BoNT) in clostridial species in cultures is discussed.

31. New data on the clinical effectiveness of fidaxomicin on lowering recurrence rates of ***Clostridioides difficile*** disease has been added. Success rates following fecal transplant have been updated.

32. Seasonal occurrence of ***Clostridium perfringens*** outbreaks has been added.

33. Serologic, molecular, and antigen detection testing availability and performance for **Coccidioidomycosis** have been updated.

34. Information on **COVID-19** has been moved to its own chapter. Discussion of the severity of disease caused by the other human **Coronaviruses,** especially in immunocompromised people, has been expanded.

35. Prevalence of ***Cryptococcus*** disease in children compared with adults has been added. Treatment of HIV-positive adults with a single dose of liposomal amphotericin following by flucytosine and fluconazole is mentioned.

36. Molecular diagnostic testing for **Cryptosporidiosis** has been updated. Antimicrobial options for immunocompromised hosts have been expanded.

37. Description of the skin rash of **Cutaneous Larva Migrans** has been expanded.

38. Additional treatment options in persons with HIV who are infected with **Cyclosporiasis** have been added.

39. Discussion of targeted screening for congenital **Cytomegalovirus** infection is expanded. Maribavir has been added to the list of approved CMV antiviral drugs. Treatment recommendations for congenital CMV have been liberalized with regard to timing of initiation of therapy and use in patients with isolated sensorineural hearing loss.

40. Recent CDC recommendations for use of Dengvaxia have been incorporated in the **Dengue** chapter. Diagnostic testing has been updated.

41. Antimicrobial treatment of **Diphtheria** is provided in greater detail. Treatment options for eradication of carriage have been expanded. Updates to national notification requirements have been added.

42. In the ***Ehrlichia, Anaplasma,* and Related Infections** chapter, the increasing number of cases of *Anaplasma* infections in the United States and the rarity of rash in these patients is emphasized. Hemophagocytic lymphohistiocytosis occurring with ehrlichiosis is described.

43. In the **Serious Neonatal Bacterial Infections Caused By *Enterobacterales*** chapter, the order name has been changed from *Enterobacteriaceae* to *Enterobacterales*. Treatment recommendations for extended-spectrum beta-lactamases and carbapenem-resistant *Enterobacterales* using new antibiotics and beta-lactamase inhibitor combinations are provided.

44. Clinical manifestations associated with specific **Enterovirus** types are added. Recommendations for return to school or child care are provided.

45. Etiology and treatment of **Epstein-Barr Virus**-associated post-transplant lymphoproliferative disease (PTLD) has been expanded.

46. In the ***Escherichia coli* Diarrhea** chapter, description of disease caused by enteropathogenic *E coli* (EPEC) is expanded. Long-term sequelae following hemolytic-uremic syndrome are added.

47. Treatment recommendations for **Other Fungal Diseases** have been modified for 8 of the 10 pathogens listed in the table that comprise this chapter.

48. Discussion of rapid diagnostic tests for ***Fusobacterium*** species has been added.

49. Sources of recent ***Giardia duodenalis*** outbreaks are updated.

50. Discussion of antibiotic resistance in **Gonococcal Infections** has been expanded. Routine screening recommendations have been updated.

51. Discussion of otitis media treatment has been streamlined in the ***Haemophilus influenzae* Infections** chapter.

52. The listing of characteristic laboratory findings in **Hantavirus Pulmonary Syndrome** is expanded.

53. Indications for testing for ***Helicobacter pylori*** have been added to the chapter.

54. In the **Hemorrhagic Fevers Caused by Arenaviruses** chapter, wording supporting the use of intravenous ribavirin for treatment of Lassa fever has been softened.

55. In the **Hemorrhagic Fevers Caused by Bunyaviruses** chapter, duration of observation following exposure to Crimean-Congo hemorrhagic fever (CCHF) has been modified. An inactivated vaccine for CCHF is available in Eastern Europe.

56. In the **Hemorrhagic Fevers Caused by Filoviruses: Ebola and Marburg** chapter, vaccine information against differing Ebola species has been updated.

57. Increasing cases of **Hepatitis A** infection among people using injection drugs and people lacking housing are described.

58. New **Hepatitis B** vaccines (for adults) have been added to the chapter. A statement has been added that routine nursery procedures, such as skin-to-skin care, delayed bathing, and breastfeeding within the first hour, may continue as recommended by the facility.

59. Antiviral treatments for **Hepatitis C** have been updated, including options for children as young as 3 years and for pregnant people. Testing recommendations for infants whose birthing parent is HCV positive have been updated.

60. Antiviral therapies for **Hepatitis D** have been added to the chapter.

61. In the **Herpes Simplex** chapter, exclusion of athletes with active herpes gladiatorum or rugbiorum infections is provided. Antiviral suppression in these athletes is endorsed. Management of neonates whose birthing parent has a first episode genital herpes in the final trimester of pregnancy but no lesions at delivery has been modified.

62. Details of central nervous system manifestations of **Histoplasmosis** have been added.

63. Diagnostic modalities for **Hookworm Infections** have been updated and expanded.

64. Description of diagnostic studies suggesting inherited chromosomally integrated HHV-6 (iciHHV6) has been expanded in the **Human Herpesvirus 6 (Including Roseola) and 7** chapter.

65. Diagnostic approaches for management in infants whose birthing parent has **Human Immunodeficiency Virus Infection** and in adolescents have been updated. Postexposure management of people with HIV following measles and varicella exposure has been clarified. Postexposure management following hepatitis A exposure has been added.

66. Epidemiologic information and cervical cancer screening recommendations in **Human Papillomaviruses** have been updated.

67. The **Influenza** chapter has been brought into alignment with the annual influenza policy statements published by the AAP since 2021.

68. Contrasts between **Kawasaki Disease** and MIS-C are provided. Descriptions of adjunctive therapies for primary treatment and management of IGIV resistance have both been expanded.

69. Management options for ***Kingella kingae* Infections** in outbreak settings have been added.

70. Diagnostic modalities for ***Legionella pneumophila* Infections** have been updated. Control measures for prevention of *Legionella* infections have been expanded.

71. Mention of cases of **Leishmaniasis** in Indigenous populations in the southwestern United States has been added.

72. The **Leprosy** chapter includes mention of the open-access *International Textbook of Leprosy* as a resource.
73. Use of matrix-assisted laser desorption/ionization–time-of-flight (MALDI-TOF) mass spectrometry for rapid identification of ***Listeria monocytogenes* Infections** is discussed.
74. The diagnostic testing required for **Lyme Disease** has been modified for greater clarity.
75. A listing of extracerebral involvement has been added to the **Lymphocytic Choriomeningitis Virus** chapter.
76. Clinical and laboratory parameters defining severe **Malaria** have been added. The need to confirm the diagnosis of malaria prior to initiating therapy has been emphasized.
77. Distinguishing between someone with fever and rash from measles, mumps, and rubella (MMR) vaccine versus someone with **Measles** infection has been added. The postexposure prophylaxis tables have been modified.
78. Text and a new table have been added to the **Meningococcal Infections** chapter providing guidance for when ciprofloxacin-resistant isolates are detected.
79. A diagnostic pearl to improve visualization of the umbilicated lesions of **Molluscum Contagiosum** is provided.
80. Wording has been added to distinguish between ***Moraxella catarrhalis*** respiratory colonization versus disease.
81. **Mpox** is an entirely new chapter to the 2024 *Red Book*.
82. In the ***Mycoplasma pneumoniae* and Other *Mycoplasma* Species Infections** chapter, disease caused by *Mycoplasma genitalium* has been expanded, as have treatment recommendations for this pathogen. The increasing antibiotic resistance of all *Mycoplasma* species is discussed.
83. Discussion of risk factors for **Nocardiosis** is expanded. Treatment options have been updated.
84. Mention of nitazoxanide as a possible treatment in immunocompromised transplant recipients has been added to the **Norovirus and Sapovirus Infections** chapter, albeit in "some experts recommend" language.
85. Treatment of **Onchocerciasis (River Blindness, Filariasis)** has been updated.
86. Sensitivity and specificity of diagnostic tests for **Paracoccidioidomycosis** have been added.
87. Cerebral **Paragonimiasis** is discussed in greater detail.
88. Use of corticosteroids and nebulized epinephrine in the management of **Parainfluenza Viral Infections** has been added.
89. Modes of human infection and clinical manifestations in humans have been updated for many of the **Parasitic Diseases** in the table of this chapter.
90. Molecular diagnostic testing for **Parechovirus Infections** has been updated.
91. Persistence of low concentrations of noninfectious **Parvovirus B19** DNA for months or years is emphasized.
92. Manifestations of ***Pasteurella* Infections** in neonates has been added. Treatment duration for endocarditis has been added.
93. The treatment section of the **Pediculosis Capitis** chapter has been updated with the recommendations from the 2022 clinical report published by the AAP. A new treatment algorithm figure has been added.

94. The cause of pruritis from body lice has been added to the **Pediculosis Corporis** chapter.
95. A time period has been added to the **Pediculosis Pubis** chapter for persistence of pubic lice on bedding, towels, and clothing.
96. Treatment recommendations for **Pelvic Inflammatory Disease** during pregnancy are provided.
97. Tdap vaccines have been approved by the FDA for use in pregnancy since the last edition of the *Red Book*, and the **Pertussis (Whooping Cough)** chapter has been updated accordingly.
98. Modes of transmission for **Pinworm Infections** have been updated.
99. Treatment of **Pityriasis Versicolor** with topical retinoids has been added.
100. The diagnosis and treatment sections of the **Plague** chapter have been aligned with the 2021 CDC recommendations.
101. Extrapulmonary manifestations of ***Pneumocystis jirovecii* Infections** have been added. Intravenous steroid dosing for people unable to take oral steroids has been added.
102. The **Poliovirus Infections** chapter has been updated to include risk of circulating vaccine-derived polioviruses to undervaccinated communities in the United States. Proof of vaccination that is accepted by the United States is listed.
103. Options for treatment of **Polyomaviruses** has been expanded.
104. The utility of brain magnetic resonance imaging (MRI) in Creutzfeldt-Jakob disease has been added to the **Prion Diseases** chapter.
105. Duration of therapy recommendations for ***Pseudomonas aeruginosa* Infections** have been updated.
106. Outcomes of **Q Fever** among pregnant people have been added. A treatment option for chronic Q fever in children is provided.
107. The pre- and postexposure prophylaxis sections of the **Rabies** chapter have been harmonized with recent CDC guidance. A new table on preexposure prophylaxis has been developed.
108. Information has been added to the **Rat-Bite Fever** chapter on anticoagulants in blood culture media that can inhibit growth of *Streptobacillus moniliformis*.
109. The unusual **Respiratory Syncytial Virus** circulation patterns in 2021 and 2022 are discussed. Precaution measures are updated. New active and passive immunization products that likely are nearing FDA approval are mentioned.
110. The average number of **Rhinovirus Infections** a child experiences each year is provided.
111. Guidance on duration of antibiotic therapy for **Rickettsialpox** has been updated.
112. Identification of groups at higher risk of death from **Rocky Mountain Spotted Fever**, including children younger than 10 years and patients with glucose-6-phosphate dehydrogenase (G6PD) deficiency, has been added.
113. Reduction in risk of seizures with use of **Rotavirus** vaccine has been added to the chapter.
114. Manifestations of persistence of **Rubella** virus in patients with primary immunodeficiencies have been added.

115. Treatment options for *Salmonella* Typhi have been updated in the **Salmonella Infections** chapter. Details on the extensively drug-resistant (XDR) *S* Typhi outbreak in Pakistan, and its impact on international travelers, are updated as well.

116. The treatment section of the **Scabies** chapter has been updated to include additional alternative therapeutic options.

117. Information on hybridization and local transmission of *Schistosoma haematobium* and *Schistosoma bovis* has been added to the **Schistosomiasis** chapter.

118. The increasing number of antibiotic-resistant **Shigella** isolates detected in the United States is detailed, and treatment options updated accordingly.

119. Antiviral therapy options and new information on vaccines that protect against **Smallpox** have been added.

120. Hyperthermia has been added as a treatment option for pregnant people with **Sporotrichosis,** in whom antimicrobial therapy should be avoided.

121. Discussion of the enterotoxins that produce **Staphylococcal Food Poisoning** has been expanded.

122. Treatment durations for **Staphylococcus aureus** osteomyelitis have been decreased, in alignment with the Pediatric Infectious Diseases Society/Infectious Diseases Society of America guidance document that was recently published. Decolonization approaches are discussed in greater detail. New drugs with anti-staphylococcal activity are summarized.

123. New antibiotics with utility in **Coagulase-Negative Staphylococcal Infections** are listed. Situations in which combination therapy can be considered are provided. Durations of treatment are updated.

124. Diagnosis of poststreptococcal acute glomerulonephritis is specifically stated in the **Group A Streptococcal Infections** chapter. Eradication of nephritogenic strains has been added. The increasing degree of clindamycin resistance is addressed, and use of linezolid for blocking protein (toxin) production in cases of clindamycin resistance has been added.

125. New long-term outcome data for survivors of **Group B Streptococcal Infections** during infancy have been added. Treatment of sequential parenteral-oral therapy of bacteremia without a focus and isolated urinary tract infections has been liberalized somewhat. Testing of human milk for an infant with late-onset GBS is discouraged.

126. The treatment section of the **Non-Group A or B Streptococcal and Enterococcal Infections** chapter has been modified to include updated duration recommendations.

127. PCV15 and PCV20 have been added to the **Streptococcus pneumoniae (Pneumococcal) Infections** chapter. A table with susceptibility breakpoints by drug and site of infection has been added.

128. Treatment for suspected or confirmed hyperinfection/dissemination syndrome has been added to the **Strongyloidiasis** chapter. Management of eligible refugees who arrive in the United States through the US Refugee Resettlement Program versus other immigrants, including internationally adopted children, has been added.

129. The increasing incidence of **Syphilis** and congenital syphilis is documented. Performance characteristics of treponemal tests are discussed. Neonates known to be exposed to syphilis at delivery should not have delayed bathing.

130. Transmission and obligate versus intermediate host descriptions have been expanded in the **Tapeworm Diseases** chapter.

131. Treatment of *Echinococcus* has been updated in the **Other Tapeworm Infections** chapter.

132. Management of patients who experience anaphylactic reaction to **Tetanus** vaccine has been added. Progress toward global elimination of maternal and neonatal tetanus has been updated.

133. Treatment recommendations, including drugs available in the United States, have been updated in the **Tinea Capitis** and **Tinea Corporis** chapters.

134. Description of the clinical manifestations of **Tinea Cruris** have been expanded.

135. Use of efinaconazole and tavaborole in children as young as 6 years for **Tinea Pedis and Tinea Unguium** has been added.

136. The specific classes of immunoglobulin that constitute hypergammaglobulinemia for the diagnosis of **Toxocariasis** have been clarified.

137. Benefits of each type of imaging modality (ultrasonography, magnetic resonance imaging [MRI], computed tomography [CT]) for congenital ***Toxoplasma gondii* Infections** are provided.

138. Discussion of the role of steroids in severe systemic **Trichinellosis** has been added. Mention of the cost of albendazole and mebendazole has been included.

139. Use of NAAT for diagnosis of ***Trichomonas vaginalis* Infections** has been updated. Treatment options have been expanded, and discussion of management of recurrent infection is provided.

140. Combination therapy for **Trichuriasis** is added as a management option.

141. Fexinidazole has been added as a treatment option for some patients with **African Trypanosomiasis**.

142. Newer diagnostic modalities for **American Trypanosomiasis (Chagas Disease)**, including next-generation techniques using cell-free pathogen DNA and newer immunoassays, have been added.

143. New **Tuberculosis** treatment durations aligning with WHO recommendations have been added. IGRA testing at any pediatric age has been expanded (previously was 2 years and older). Terminology of TB infection versus TB disease is emphasized.

144. Identification of macrolide resistance in the treatment of **Nontuberculous Mycobacteria** through detection of the erm gene with sequencing or line-probe assay has been added. Initiation recommendations for *Mycobacterium avium* complex (MAC) prophylaxis in patients starting antiretroviral therapy (ART) are provided.

145. **Tularemia** treatment options have been reorganized for clarity.

146. Serologic responses in patients with Brill-Zinsser disease have been added to the **Louse-borne Typhus** chapter.

147. Sensitivity of PCR assay in whole blood, serum, and skin biopsies has been added to the **Murine Typhus** chapter.

148. The anti-inflammatory characteristics of azithromycin have been added to the ***Ureaplasma urealyticum* and *Ureaplasma parvum* Infections** chapter.

149. Birth in the United States before 1980 is added to those things that provide evidence of immunity to **Varicella-Zoster Virus Infections.** The types of highly immunocompromised patients who should not receive varicella vaccine are specifically listed.

150. Vaxchora now is available in children down to 2 years of age for the prevention of **Cholera**.
151. The anticipated impact of climate change on incidence of *Vibrio* infections has been added to the **Other *Vibrio* Infections** chapter.
152. Discussion of community-level mosquito control measures for prevention of **West Nile Virus** is expanded.
153. Description of disease caused by *Yersinia pseudotuberculosis* has been expanded in the ***Yersinia enterocolitica* and *Yersinia pseudotuberculosis* Infections** chapter.
154. Testing recommendations for **Zika** virus have been updated. A new table to aid with interpreting test results has been added. Restrictions on blood donations have been loosened.

SECTION 4. ANTIMICROBIAL AGENTS AND RELATED THERAPY

1. Adverse events from use of fluoroquinolones have been updated in **Antimicrobial Agents and Related Therapy.**
2. Recommendations are provided in the **Antimicrobial Resistance and Antimicrobial Stewardship: Appropriate and Judicious Use of Antimicrobial Agents** chapter to enhance clear and effective communication across clinical settings in order to improve antimicrobial stewardship efforts.
3. Several new antibiotics have been added to the **Tables of Antimicrobial Drug Dosages.** For the neonatal dosing table, gestational ages are provided with more precise breakpoints.
4. Treatment options for **Sexually Transmitted Infections** are now listed as those that are preferred and those that are alternatives to the preferred option.
5. Differences in formulations of posaconazole and itraconazole are provided in the **Antifungal Drugs for Systemic Fungal Infections** chapter. Ibrexafungerp has been added. The durations of time on drug before checking trough concentrations for the azoles and flucytosine are clarified.
6. New dosing recommendations are provided for many of the antifungal medications in the table that contains the **Recommended Doses of Parenteral and Oral Antifungal Drugs.**
7. The listing of drugs in the **Topical Drugs for Superficial Fungal Infections** table have been aligned with what is currently available in the United States.
8. Antivirals for COVID-19 and mpox have been added to the **Non-HIV Antiviral Drugs** table. Age indications for many antiviral drugs, including HCV and influenza drugs, have been lowered to reflect current indications for use by the FDA.
9. Updated dosing recommendations based on new guidance have been incorporated throughout the **Drugs for Parasitic Infections** table.

SECTION 5. ANTIMICROBIAL PROPHYLAXIS

1. Results of the NIH RIVUR study have been added to the discussion of UTI prophylaxis in the **Antimicrobial Prophylaxis** chapter.

2. The decline of MRSA infections in children and, therefore, a decreased need to cover for these resistant bacteria prophylactically is detailed in the **Antimicrobial Prophylaxis in Pediatric Surgical Patients** chapter.
3. The **Prevention of Bacterial Endocarditis** chapter has been harmonized with the 2021 updated statement on infectious endocarditis from the American Heart Association.
4. Options for periods of shortage of erythromycin ointment have been updated in the **Neonatal Ophthalmia Prevention** chapter.

APPENDICES

1. Web links have been updated in the **Directory of Resources**. A link to the CDC's website on vaccine shortages and delays has been added. The European Society for Pediatric Infectious Diseases has been added.
2. The listing of **Codes for Commonly Administered Pediatric Vaccines, Toxoids, and Immune Globulins** has been expanded to include specific codes for wound prophylaxis for tetanus, respiratory syncytial virus (RSV) prophylaxis with palivizumab, and hepatitis B immune globulin (HBIG) use in perinatal hepatitis B exposure.
3. The diseases listed in the **Nationally Notifiable Infectious Diseases in the United States** table have been updated to those required in 2023.
4. In the **Guide to Contraindications and Precautions to Immunizations** appendix, moderate or severe acute illness, with or without fever, has been identified as the only precaution applicable to all vaccines.
5. Sources of foodborne infections have been updated in the **Prevention of Disease From Contaminated Food Products** appendix.
6. The incubation periods for hemolytic-uremic syndrome and botulism have been tightened in the **Clinical Syndromes Associated With Foodborne Diseases** table.
7. Sources and modes of transmission have been updated throughout the **Diseases Transmitted by Animals (Zoonoses)** table. Leishmaniasis, *Streptococcus suis*, Cache Valley virus, Heartland virus, and Lujo hemorrhagic fever have been added.

Systems-Based Treatment Table[a]

System	Condition	Common Pathogens	Empiric Antibiotic Therapy	Antibiotic Duration	Notes	Key Resources
Bloodstream Infection in Nonneonates (***uncomplicated**) *Defined by ≤3 days bacteremia in nonneutropenic host without complex source (eg, endocarditis, septic thrombophlebitis, osteomyelitis) or ongoing undrained purulent focus	Common sources include vascular catheter-associated infection, urinary tract infection, intra-abdominal infection, pneumonia, skin/soft tissue infection	*Staphylococcus aureus*	<u>MSSA</u> Cefazolin OR Oxacillin OR Nafcillin <u>MRSA</u> Vancomycin OR Linezolid OR Daptomycin OR Ceftaroline	14 days from first negative blood culture	Vascular catheter removal generally recommended for persistent hemodynamic instability or ongoing (≥3 days) bacteremia	RCTs for duration of gram-negative BSI: Yahav et al[1] von Dach et al[2] Molina et al[3] Observational studies: Sutton et al[4] Punjabi et al[5] Tamma et al[6] Heil et al[7] Mponponsuo et al[8] Tamma et al[9]
		Enterococcus faecalis	Ampicillin	7 days from first negative blood culture		
		Enterococcus faecium	Vancomycin OR Linezolid OR Daptomycin	7 days from first negative blood culture		

Systems-Based Treatment Table,[a] continued

System	Condition	Common Pathogens	Empiric Antibiotic Therapy	Antibiotic Duration	Notes	Key Resources
Bloodstream Infection in Nonneonates (***uncomplicated**) *Defined by ≤3 days bacteremia in nonneutropenic host without complex source (eg, endocarditis, septic thrombophlebitis, osteomyelitis) or ongoing undrained purulent focus		**Enterobacterales (eg, *Escherichia coli*, *Klebsiella* species, *Enterobacter* species)**	Choice depends on results of antibiotic susceptibility testing	7 days from first negative blood culture	Duration of therapy is regardless of whether vascular catheter is removed, and should not be extended solely based on presence of antibiotic resistance or retained vascular catheter Duration of therapy is based on duration of active therapy (ie, adequate dose and antibiotic susceptibility) Transition to oral antibiotics may be considered for uncomplicated gram-negative bacteremia if all of the following criteria are met: (1) susceptibility to an appropriate, highly available oral agent is demonstrated; (2) the patient is hemodynamically stable; (3) reasonable source control measures have occurred; (4) intestinal absorption is intact; and (5) there is confidence in patient adherence	
		Pseudomonas aeruginosa	Choice depends on results of antibiotic susceptibility testing	7 days from first negative blood culture		

Systems-Based Treatment Table,[a] continued

System	Condition	Common Pathogens	Empiric Antibiotic Therapy	Antibiotic Duration	Notes	Key Resources
		Coagulase-negative **Staphylococcus** (not including *Staphylococcus Lugdunensis*, which should be managed like *S aureus*)	Vancomycin OR Oxacillin (if susceptible)	5–7 days from first negative blood culture, OR observation following removal of foreign body source (eg, catheter)	A single positive culture absent hardware generally reflects skin contamination	
Bone/Joint	Osteomyelitis (acute, hematogenous)	**S aureus** *Streptococcus pyogenes* *Kingella kingae*	<u>Mild-Moderate</u> Cefazolin OR Oxacillin OR Nafcillin <u>Severe and low suspicion of MRSA</u> Cefazolin OR Oxacillin OR Nafcillin <u>Severe and high suspicion of MRSA</u> Vancomycin	3–4 wk Chronic osteomyelitis typically requires more prolonged antibiotic treatment and may require consideration of alternate antibiotic choice	*Kingella* infection not effectively treated by clindamycin and not reliably susceptible to oxacillin/nafcillin Early switch to oral route recommended with clinical improvement, even for patients with transient bacteremia For empiric management of children with osteomyelitis and severe sepsis, combination therapy of vancomycin PLUS oxacillin/nafcillin can be considered	Woods et al[10]

Systems-Based Treatment Table,[a] continued

System	Condition	Common Pathogens	Empiric Antibiotic Therapy	Antibiotic Duration	Notes	Key Resources
Bone/Joint						
	Septic arthritis	**S aureus** S pyogenes K kingae	Mild-Moderate Cefazolin OR Oxacillin OR Nafcillin Severe and low suspicion of MRSA Cefazolin OR Oxacillin OR Nafcillin Severe and high suspicion of MRSA Vancomycin OR Clindamycin OR Linezolid OR Daptomycin	2–3 wk	_Kingella_ not effectively treated by clindamycin and not reliably susceptible to oxacillin/nafcillin Early switch to oral route recommended with clinical improvement, even for patients with transient bacteremia	Woods et al[11]
			OR Clindamycin OR Linezolid OR Daptomycin			

Systems-Based Treatment Table,[a] continued

System	Condition	Common Pathogens	Empiric Antibiotic Therapy	Antibiotic Duration	Notes	Key Resources
Central Nervous System	Meningitis (non-neonates)	Streptococcus pneumoniae Neisseria meningtidis Haemophilus influenzae	Ceftriaxone PLUS Vancomycin	These are empiric recommendations; specific choice and duration of antibiotic therapy should be guided by culture and susceptibility results S pneumoniae: 10–14 days H influenzae: 7–10 days N meningitidis: 5–7 days	Longer courses are necessary for patients with parenchymal brain infection (cerebritis, rhombencephalitis, brain abscess) Dexamethasone is beneficial for treatment of infants and children with Hib meningitis to diminish the risk of hearing loss, if administered before or concurrently with the first dose of antimicrobial agent(s) For all children with bacterial meningitis presumed to be caused by S pneumoniae, vancomycin should be administered in addition to ceftriaxone because of the possibility of resistant S pneumoniae Consider adding acyclovir for patients with concurrent encephalitis	Streptococcus pneumoniae (Pneumococcal) Infections, p 810 Meningococcal Infections, p 585 Haemophilus influenzae Infections, p 400

Systems-Based Treatment Table,[a] continued

System	Condition	Common Pathogens	Empiric Antibiotic Therapy	Antibiotic Duration	Notes	Key Resources
Ear, Nose, and Throat	Mastoiditis	**S pneumoniae** **S pyogenes** **S aureus** H influenzae <u>Also consider for chronic:</u> Microaerophilic streptococci Fusobacterium P aeruginosa	Consider surgical drainage/excision Ampicillin-sulbactam OR Ceftriaxone (Allergy[b]: Clindamycin) <u>If follows chronic AOM:</u> Cefepime OR Levofloxacin Consider MRSA based on local prevalence	2–4 wk depending on adequate débridement, intracranial extension, extent of osteomyelitis, associated thrombosis	Transition to oral with clinical improvement Ampicillin-sulbactam may not be optimal for intracranial infections	*Haemophilus influenzae* Infections, p 400 *Fusobacterium* Infections, p 388 *Pseudomonas aeruginosa* Infections, p 697 *Staphylococcus aureus*, p 767 Group A Streptococcal Infections, p 785 Non-Group A or B Streptococcal and Enterococcal Infections, p 806 *Streptococcus pneumoniae* (Pneumococcal) Infections, p 810

Systems-Based Treatment Table,[a] continued

System	Condition	Common Pathogens	Empiric Antibiotic Therapy	Antibiotic Duration	Notes	Key Resources
Ear, Nose, and Throat	Acute sinusitis	**S pneumoniae** H influenzae Moraxella catarrhalis	Amoxicillin OR Amoxicillin-clavulanate (Allergy[b]: Clindamycin OR Levofloxacin)	5–7 days	Diagnosis of acute bacterial sinusitis requires the presence of one of the following criteria: (1) persistent nasal discharge or daytime cough without evidence of clinical improvement for ≥10 days; consider watchful waiting in this scenario (2) worsening or new onset of nasal discharge, daytime cough, or fever after initial improvement (3) temperature ≥39°C with purulent nasal discharge and/or facial pain for at least 3 consecutive days	*Haemophilus influenzae* Infections, p 400 *Moraxella catarrhalis* Infections, p 604 *Streptococcus pneumoniae* (Pneumococcal) Infections, p 810 Chow et al[12] Wald et al[13]
	Acute otitis media	**S pneumoniae** H influenzae M catarrhalis	Amoxicillin OR Amoxicillin-clavulanate[c] (Allergy: Cefdinir OR Cefpodoxime OR Cefuroxime OR Ceftriaxone for 1 (first occurrence) to 3 (treatment failure) days	>6 y: 5 days 2–5 y: 7 days <2 y or severe symptoms: 10 days	Consider observation without antibiotics for 48–72 hours for children 24 months or older without severe symptoms; if symptoms persist or worsen, use same antibiotic recommendations as for those receiving immediate therapy Consider *S aureus* and *Pseudomonas* infection for chronic otitis media	*Haemophilus influenzae* Infections, p 400 *Moraxella catarrhalis* Infections, p 604 *Streptococcus pneumoniae* (Pneumococcal) Infections, p 810 Lieberthal et al[14] Rosenfeld et al[15]

Systems-Based Treatment Table,[a] continued

System	Condition	Common Pathogens	Empiric Antibiotic Therapy	Antibiotic Duration	Notes	Key Resources
Ear, Nose, and Throat	Streptococcal pharyngitis	*S pyogenes*	First line: Penicillin OR Amoxicillin (Allergy,[b]: Cephalexin OR Clindamycin OR Azithromycin)	10 days	Children with rhinorrhea, cough, hoarseness, or oral ulcers should not be tested or treated for GAS infection; testing also generally is not recommended for children <3 y Management of recurrent GAS pharyngitis and pharyngeal carriers is detailed in Group A Streptococcal Infections (p 785) Tetracyclines, TMP-SMX, and fluoroquinolones should not be used for treating GAS pharyngitis Return to school after afebrile and ≥12 h of antibiotic therapy	Group A Streptococcal Infections, p 785 Shulman et al[16]
	Retropharyngeal abscess	*S aureus* *S pyogenes* Anaerobes *Streptococcus anginosus* *H influenzae* (often polymicrobial)	Mild-moderate: Ampicillin/sulbactam OR Clindamycin Severe: Ampicillin/sulbactam PLUS EITHER Vancomycin OR Linezolid	14 days	Longer duration of therapy may be required for complex infections with insufficient source control	

Systems-Based Treatment Table,[a] continued

System	Condition	Common Pathogens	Empiric Antibiotic Therapy	Antibiotic Duration	Notes	Key Resources
Genitourinary	UTI - pyelonephritis	*E coli* *Klebsiella* species *Proteus* species *Enterobacter* species *Citrobacter* species *Enterococcus* species *Staphylococcus saprophyticus*	Cephalexin OR TMP-SMX OR Ampicillin PLUS Gentamicin OR Ceftriaxone OR Ciprofloxacin	7–10 days (hospitalized) 5–10 days (outpatient) 3–5 days (simple cystitis in adolescents) Longer durations may be required for complicated cases such as renal abscess without drainage	Drug selection should be based on local antibiogram or patient's prior urine isolates Initial short course of IV therapy (2–4 days) is as effective as longer courses of IV therapy Avoid nitrofurantoin for upper urinary tract infection or bacteremia	Mattoo et al[17] Gupta et al[18]
Intra-abdominal	Intra-abdominal infection	*E coli* **Anaerobes** *Klebsiella* species (often polymicrobial)	Drainage Mild-moderate: Ceftriaxone PLUS Metronidazole Severe or hospital onset: Piperacillin-tazobactam OR Ciprofloxacin PLUS Metronidazole	4–7 days (from source control)	May need longer duration if insufficient source control Mild-moderate infection includes complicated appendicitis with rupture, absent sepsis	Mazuski et al[19]

Systems-Based Treatment Table,[a] continued

System	Condition	Common Pathogens	Empiric Antibiotic Therapy	Antibiotic Duration	Notes	Key Resources
Neonatal Fever (Term Neonates)	Suspected UTI	**E coli** *Enterococcus* species GBS	Ampicillin PLUS Gentamicin	These are empiric recommendations; specific choice and duration of antibiotic therapy should be guided by culture results		
	Unclear source	**GBS** **E coli** HSV	Neonates 0–7 days of age: Ampicillin PLUS Gentamicin Neonates 8–28 days of age: Ampicillin PLUS Gentamicin OR Ampicillin PLUS Cefotaxime (Ceftazidime or Cefepime if Cefotaxime not available)	These are empiric recommendations; specific choice and duration of antibiotic therapy should be guided by culture results	Consider adding empiric acyclovir with surface, blood, and CSF HSV sampling for infants at increased risk of HSV, including the presence of skin vesicles, seizures, CSF pleocytosis with a negative Gram stain, leukopenia, hepatitis, thrombocytopenia, hypothermia, mucous membrane ulcers, or maternal history of genital HSV lesions or fever from 48 hours before to 48 hours after delivery. For further discussion of HSV, see Herpes Simplex (p 467).	

Systems-Based Treatment Table,[a] continued

System	Condition	Common Pathogens	Empiric Antibiotic Therapy	Antibiotic Duration	Notes	Key Resources
Neonatal Fever (Term Neonates)	Suspected meningitis	**GBS** **E coli** HSV	Neonates 0–7 days of age: Ampicillin PLUS Gentamicin (some experts will add a third or fourth generation cephalosporin if the cerebrospinal fluid gram stain shows gram-negative organisms) Neonates 8–28 days of age: Ampicillin PLUS Cefotaxime (Ceftazidime or Cefepime if Cefotaxime not available) (some experts will add an aminoglycoside if the cerebrospinal fluid Gram stain shows gram-negative organisms)	These are empiric recommendations; specific choice and duration of antibiotic therapy should be guided by culture results GBS: 14 days penicillin G E coli: 21 days of non-aminoglycoside antibiotic to which isolate is susceptible	Some experts suggest repeat lumbar puncture to document CSF sterility Consider adding empiric acyclovir with surface, blood, and CSF HSV sampling for infants at increased risk of HSV, including the presence of skin vesicles, seizures, CSF pleocytosis with a negative Gram stain, leukopenia, hepatitis, thrombocytopenia, hypothermia, mucous membrane ulcers, or maternal history of genital HSV lesions or fever from 48 hours before to 48 hours after delivery. For further discussion of HSV, see Herpes Simplex (p 467).	Puopolo et al[20] Puopolo et al[21]

Systems-Based Treatment Table,[a] continued

System	Condition	Common Pathogens	Empiric Antibiotic Therapy	Antibiotic Duration	Notes	Key Resources
Ophthalmologic	Preseptal cellulitis (ie, nonsinus origin)	**S pyogenes** S aureus	Mild-moderate: Cefazolin OR Cephalexin (Allergy[b]: Clindamycin) Severe: Vancomycin OR Linezolid OR Ceftaroline OR Daptomycin	5–7 days	Switch to oral with 24 hours improvement in fever, swelling, and erythema Consider empiric MRSA coverage if high local MRSA rates	
	Orbital cellulitis	**S aureus S pneumoniae Anaerobes** S anginosus H influenzae M catarrhalis S pyogenes	Surgical drainage (if abscess): Ampicillin/ sulbactam (Allergy[b]: Clindamycin) Severe: Add Vancomycin OR Linezolid OR Ceftaroline OR Daptomycin	10–14 days May extend to 3–4 wk with extensive bone involvement and/or insufficient source control	Consider empiric MRSA coverage if high local MRSA rates	

Systems-Based Treatment Table,[a] continued

System	Condition	Common Pathogens	Empiric Antibiotic Therapy	Antibiotic Duration	Notes	Key Resources
Respiratory	Community-acquired pneumonia (CAP)	**S pneumoniae** *Mycoplasma pneumoniae* *S pyogenes* *S aureus* *H influenzae* *M catarrhalis* Respiratory viruses, including influenza virus, adenovirus, parainfluenza virus, respiratory syncytial virus, coronaviruses, human metapneumovirus	Amoxicillin OR Ampicillin OR Penicillin for fully immunized patients in regions without high prevalence of PCN-resistant pneumococcus (Allergy[b]): Clindamycin OR Levofloxacin) Ceftriaxone for hospitalized patients in regions with high levels PCN-resistant pneumococcus Add macrolide if atypical pathogen (eg, *Mycoplasma* or *Chlamydia* species) suspected Add Vancomycin OR Clindamycin OR Linezolid if MRSA suspected	5 days for uncomplicated CAP with resolution of fever, tachypnea, and supplemental oxygen requirement May extend duration when complicated by empyema, necrotizing pneumonia, or pulmonary abscess	Respiratory viruses cause the majority of CAP, especially in young children; thus, antibiotic therapy may not be indicated for all patients Early switch to oral route encouraged when tolerated Transient *S pneumoniae* bacteremia in otherwise uncomplicated pneumonia does not warrant prolonged or IV antibiotic therapy Consider *S aureus* superinfection in patients with influenza	Bradley et al[22]

Systems-Based Treatment Table,[a] continued

System	Condition	Common Pathogens	Empiric Antibiotic Therapy	Antibiotic Duration	Notes	Key Resources
Skin and Soft Tissue Infections	Cellulitis (nonpurulent)	*S pyogenes* *S aureus*	Mild-moderate: Cefazolin OR Oxacillin/nafcillin OR Cephalexin (Allergy[b]: Clindamycin OR TMP/SMX OR Doxycycline) Severe: Vancomycin OR Linezolid OR Ceftaroline OR Daptomycin Necrotizing fasciitis: Surgical débridement B-lactam PLUS Clindamycin (+/- Vancomycin)	5–7 days Tailor duration based on resolution of signs and symptoms	For bite wounds, see p 202 Necrotizing fasciitis may require gram-negative or anaerobic coverage in the correct clinical scenario For severe infections, consider coverage of MRSA based on local prevalence	*Staphylococcus aureus*, p 767 Group A Streptococcal Infections, p 785 *Bacteroides, Prevotella*, and Other Anaerobic Gram-Negative Bacilli Infections, p 261 Stevens et al[23]

Systems-Based Treatment Table,[a] continued

System	Condition	Common Pathogens	Empiric Antibiotic Therapy	Antibiotic Duration	Notes	Key Resources
Skin and Soft Tissue Infections	Purulent cellulitis/ Abscess	*S aureus*	Drainage Mild-moderate: Cefazolin/cephalexin OR TMP/SMX OR Clindamycin OR Doxycycline Consider MRSA based on local prevalence Severe: Vancomycin OR Linezolid OR Ceftaroline OR Daptomycin	5–7 days Tailor duration based on resolution of signs and symptoms Surgical drainage alone may be adequate for small, completely drained abscesses	Conversion to oral antibiotic therapy after transient[d] *S aureus* bacteremia with source control is appropriate but might warrant more prolonged therapy	*Staphylococcus aureus*, p 767 Stevens et al[23]

Systems-Based Treatment Table,[a] continued

System	Condition	Common Pathogens	Empiric Antibiotic Therapy	Antibiotic Duration	Notes	Key Resources
	Lymphadenitis	Acute/unilateral: **S pyogenes** **S aureus** Subacute/chronic: *Bartonella* species Nontuberculous mycobacteria (NTM)	For acute/unilateral lymphadenitis: Consider surgical drainage Cefazolin/ Cephalexin (Allergy[b]: Clindamycin) Consider MRSA based on local prevalence	5–7 days Tailor duration based on resolution of signs and symptoms	For management of NTM or *Bartonella* infection, please see those chapters (p 920 and p 263) Bacterial adenitis is typically unilateral; bilateral disease is typically viral in etiology	*Bartonella henselae* (Cat-Scratch Disease), p 263 *Staphylococcus aureus,* p 767 Group A Streptococcal Infections, p 785 Nontuberculous Mycobacteria, p 920

AAP indicates American Academy of Pediatrics; AOM, acute otitis media; CAP, community-acquired pneumonia; CSF, cerebrospinal fluid; GAS, group A *Streptococcus*; GBS, group B *Streptococcus*; HSV, herpes simplex virus; IV, intravenous; MRSA, methicillin-resistant *Staphylococcus aureus*; MSSA, methicillin-susceptible *Staphylococcus aureus*; NTM, nontuberculous mycobacteria; PCN, penicillin; TMP-SMX, trimethoprim-sulfamethoxazole; UTI, urinary tract infection.

Boldface indicates primary pathogen(s) targeted by empiric antibiotic therapy.

[a] Empiric antibiotic selection should be based on local antibiotic resistance prevalence.

[b] Antibiotic allergy incudes anaphylaxis or cutaneous response (eg, hives) within 6 hours of drug exposure, or severe cutaneous reaction at any time (eg, Steven Johnson syndrome [SJS], toxic epidermal necrolysis [TEN], drug reaction w/eosinophilia and systemic symptoms [DRESS], erythema multiforme, or serum sickness like reaction). Isolated gastrointestinal tract symptoms, family history of drug allergy, or later-onset nonspecific maculopapular rash do not indicate IgE-mediated drug allergy (see **www.allergyparameters.org/published-practice-parameters-guidelines/alphabetical-listing/drug-allergy-download/**).

[c] Amoxicillin-clavulanate should be used if the patient has received amoxicillin treatment in last 30 days, has concurrent purulent conjunctivitis, or has a history of recurrent AOM unresponsive to amoxicillin.

[d] Oral antibiotics may be considered for bacteremia if bacteremia clears within 72 hours of source control and initiation of effective antibiotic therapy.

1. Yahav D, Franceschini E, Koppel F, et al. Seven versus 14 days of antibiotic therapy for uncomplicated gram-negative bacteremia: a noninferiority randomized controlled trial. *Clin Infect Dis.* 2019;69(7):1091-1098

2. von Dach E, Albrich WC, Brunel AS, et al. Effect of C-reactive protein-guided antibiotic treatment duration, 7-day treatment, or 14-day treatment on 30-day clinical failure rate in patients with uncomplicated gram-negative bacteremia: a randomized clinical trial. *JAMA.* 2020;323(21):2160-2169

3. Molina J, Montero-Mateos E, Praena-Segovia J, et al. Seven-versus 14-day course of antibiotics for the treatment of bloodstream infections by Enterobacterales: a randomized, controlled trial. *Clin Microbiol Infect.* 2022;28(4):550-557

4. Sutton JD, Stevens JW, Chang NN, et al. Oral β-lactam antibiotics vs fluoroquinolones or trimethoprim-sulfamethoxazole for definitive treatment of Enterobacterales bacteremia from a urine source. *JAMA Netw Open.* 2020;3(10):e2020166

5. Punjabi C, Tien V, Meng L, Deresinski S, Holubar M. Oral fluoroquinolone or trimethoprim-sulfamethoxazole vs. β-lactams as step-down therapy for Enterobacteriaceae bacteremia: systematic review and meta-analysis. *Open Forum Infect Dis.* 2019;6(10):ofz364

6. Tamma PD, Conley AT, Cosgrove SE, et al. Association of 30-day mortality with oral step-down vs continued intravenous therapy in patients hospitalized with Enterobacteriaceae bacteremia. *JAMA Intern Med.* 2019;179(3):316-323

7. Heil EL, Bork JT, Abbo LM, et al. Optimizing the management of uncomplicated gram-negative bloodstream infections: consensus guidance using a modified Delphi process. *Open Forum Infect Dis.* 2021;8(10):ofab434

8. Mponponsuo K, Brown KA, Fridman DJ, et al. Highly versus less bioavailable oral antibiotics in the treatment of gram-negative bloodstream infections: a propensity-matched cohort analysis. *Clin Microbiol Infect.* 2023;29(4):490-497

9. Tamma PD, Aitken SL, Bonomo RA, Mathers AJ, van Duin D, Clancy CJ. IDSA guidance on the treatment of antimicrobial-resistant gram-negative infections: version 1.0. Infectious Diseases Society of America; 2022. Available at: www.idsociety.org/practice-guideline/amr-guidance/

10. Woods CR, Bradley JS, Chatterjee A, et al. Clinical practice guideline by the Pediatric Infectious Diseases Society (PIDS) and the Infectious Diseases Society of America (IDSA): 2021 Guideline on diagnosis and management of acute hematogenous osteomyelitis in pediatrics. DOI: **https://doi.org/10.1093/jpids/piab027**

11. Woods CR, Bradley JS, Chatterjee A, et al. Clinical practice guideline by the Pediatric Infectious Diseases Society (PIDS) and the Infectious Diseases Society of America (IDSA): 2023 guideline on diagnosis and management of acute bacterial arthritis in pediatrics. *J Pediatr Infect Dis Soc.* Published online November 6, 2023. DOI: **https://doi.org/10.1093/jpids/piad089**

12. Chow AW, Benninger MS, Brook I, et al. IDSA clinical practice guideline for acute bacterial rhinosinusitis in children and adults. *Clin Infect Dis.* 2012;54(8):e72-e112. DOI: **https://doi.org/10.1093/cid/cis370**

13. Wald ER, Applegate KE, Bordley C, et al. Clinical practice guideline for the diagnosis and management of acute bacterial sinusitis in children aged 1 to 18 years. *Pediatrics.* 2013;132(1):e262-e280. DOI: **https://doi.org/10.1542/peds.2013-1071**

14. Lieberthal AS, Carroll AE, Chonmaitree T, et al. Clinical practice guideline: diagnosis and management of acute otitis media. *Pediatrics.* 2013;131(3):e964-e999. DOI: **https://doi.org/10.1542/peds.2013-3791**

15. Rosenfeld RM, Shin JJ, Schwartz SR, et al. Clinical practice guideline: otitis media with effusion (update). *Otolaryngol Head Neck Surg.* 2016;154(1 Suppl):S1-S41. DOI: 10.1177/0194599815623467

16. Shulman ST, Bisno AL, Clegg HW, et al. Clinical practice guideline for the diagnosis and management of group a streptococcal pharyngitis: 2012 update by the Infectious Diseases Society of America. *Clin Infect Dis.* 2012;55(10):e86-e102. DOI: **https://doi.org/10.1093/cid/cis629**

17. Mattoo TK, Shaikh N, Nelson CP. Contemporary management of urinary tract infection in children. *Pediatrics.* 2021;147(2):e2020012138. DOI: **https://doi.org/10.1542/peds.2020-012138**

18. Gupta K, Hooton TM, Naber KG, et al. International Clinical Practice Guidelines for the Treatment of Acute Uncomplicated Cystitis and Pyelonephritis in Women: A 2010 Update by the Infectious Diseases Society of America and the European Society for Microbiology and Infectious Diseases. *Clin Infect Dis.* 2011;52(5):e103-e120. DOI: **https://doi.org/10.1093/cid/ciq257**

19. Mazuski JE, Tessier JM, May AK, et al. The Surgical Infection Society revised guidelines on the management of intra-abdominal infection. *Surg Infect (Larchmt).* 2017;18(1):1-76

20. Puopolo KM, Lynfield R, Cummings JJ; American Academy of Pediatrics, Committee on Fetus and Newborn and Committee on Infectious Diseases. Management of infants at risk for group B streptococcal disease. *Pediatrics.* 2019;144(2):e2019 1881. DOI: **https://doi.org/10.1542/peds.2019-2350**

21. Puopolo KM, Benitz WE, Zaoutis TE; American Academy of Pediatrics, Committee on Fetus and Newborn and Committee on Infectious Diseases. Management of neonates born at ≥35 0/7 weeks' gestation with suspected or proven early onset bacterial sepsis. *Pediatrics.* 2018;142(6):e20182894. DOI: **https://doi.org/10.1542/peds.2018-2894**

22. Bradley JS, Byington CL, Shah SS, et al. The management of community-acquired pneumonia in infants and children older than 3 months of age: clinical practice guidelines by the Pediatric Infectious Diseases Society and the Infectious Diseases Society of America. *Clin Infect Dis.* 2011;53(7):e25-e76. DOI: **https://doi.org/10.1093/cid/cir531**

23. Stevens DL, Bisno AL, Chambers HF, et al. Practice guidelines for the diagnosis and management of skin and soft tissue infections: 2014 update by the Infectious Diseases Society of America. *Clin Infect Dis.* 2014;59(2):e10-e52. DOI: **https://doi.org/10.1093/cid/ciu296**

Active and Passive Immunization

PROLOGUE

Vaccination is the act of introducing a vaccine into the body to stimulate the immune system to produce protection from a specific disease. Immunization is the process by which a person becomes protected against a disease through vaccination. The ultimate goal of immunization is elimination of disease, decrease of infection transmission, and ideally, eradication of the pathogen that causes the infection and disease; the immediate goal is prevention of disease in people or groups. To accomplish these goals, physicians must make timely immunization a high priority in the care of infants, children, adolescents, and adults. The global eradication of smallpox in 1977, elimination of poliomyelitis disease from the Americas in 1991, elimination of endemic measles transmission in the United States in 2000 and in the Americas in 2002, elimination of rubella and congenital rubella syndrome from the United States in 2004 and from the Americas in 2015, and global eradication of type 2 wild poliovirus in 2015 and type 3 wild poliovirus in 2019 serve as models for fulfilling the promise of disease control through immunization. These accomplishments were achieved by combining a comprehensive immunization program providing consistent, high levels of vaccine coverage with intensive surveillance and effective public health disease-control measures. The resurgence of measles and mumps over recent years and the 2022 case of paralytic poliomyelitis in the United States, however, illustrate how precarious the substantial gains to date can be without vigilant commitment by physicians, public health officials, and members of the public. Worldwide eradication of polio, measles, and rubella remains possible through implementation of proven prevention strategies, and in the case of polio even now is tantalizingly close, but diligence must prevail until eradication is achieved, or success itself is imperiled.

High immunization rates, in general, have reduced dramatically the incidence of all vaccine-preventable diseases (see Table 1.1) in the United States. Yet, because pathogens that cause vaccine-preventable diseases persist in the United States and elsewhere around the world, ongoing immunization efforts must be not only maintained but also strengthened. All vaccine-preventable diseases are, at most, 18 hours away by air travel from any part of the world.

Discoveries in immunology, molecular biology, and medical genetics have resulted in groundbreaking advances in vaccine research. Licensing of new, improved, and even more safe vaccines; establishment of an adolescent immunization platform; development of vaccines against cancer (eg, human papillomavirus and hepatitis B vaccines); and application of novel vaccine-delivery systems promise to continue the advances in preventive medicine achieved during the latter half of the 20th century. The extremely rapid pace of development of COVID-19 vaccines beginning in early 2020 is a testament to the scientific investments in vaccinology over 70 years. From the launch of the COVID-19 vaccination program in December 2020 through November 2022, an estimated 3.2 million American lives and $1.15 trillion were saved. The advent of population-based postlicensure studies of vaccines facilitates detection of rare adverse

Table 1.1. Comparison of Prevaccine Era Estimated Average Annual Morbidity With Current Estimates

Disease	Prevaccine Era Annual Case Estimate[a]	2020 Reported Cases[b]	Percent Decrease
Diphtheria	21 053	1	>99
Haemophilus influenzae type b (Hib) <5 y of age	20 000	15	>99
Hepatitis A	117 333	9946	92
Hepatitis B (acute)	66 232	2155	97
Measles	530 217	12	>99
Mumps	162 344	694	>99
Pertussis	200 752	6124	97
Polio (paralytic)	16 316	0	100
Pneumococcus (invasive)			
All ages	63 067	11 946	81
<5 y	16 069	561	97
Rubella	47 745	6	>99
Congenital rubella syndrome	152	0	100
Smallpox	29 005	0	100
Tetanus	580	17	97
Varicella	4 085 120	2928	>99

[a]Roush SW, Murphy TV; Vaccine-Preventable Disease Table Working Group. Historical comparisons of morbidity and mortality for vaccine-preventable diseases in the United States. *JAMA.* 2007;298(18):2155-2163.
[b]Centers for Disease Control and Prevention. Nationally Notifiable Diseases and Conditions, United States: Annual Tables. Available at: **https://wonder.cdc.gov/nndss/static/2020/annual/2020-table1.html.**

events temporally associated with immunization that were undetected during large prelicensure clinical trials as well as detection of changes over time in vaccine effectiveness that directly inform recommendations on use of specific vaccines.

Each edition of the *Red Book* provides recommendations for immunization of infants, children, adolescents, and young adults. These recommendations, which are harmonized among the American Academy of Pediatrics (AAP), the Advisory Committee on Immunization Practices (ACIP) of the Centers for Disease Control and Prevention (CDC), and the American Academy of Family Physicians (AAFP), are based on careful analysis of disease epidemiology, benefits, and risks of immunization; feasibility of implementation; and cost-benefit analysis. ACIP recommendations utilize Grading of Recommendations Assessment, Development and Evaluation (GRADE), when feasible, in evaluating the evidence of benefits and risks for a given vaccine, further ensuring that the recommendations are evidence based and objectively assessed.

Use of trade names and commercial sources in the *Red Book* is for identification purposes only and does not imply endorsement by the AAP. Internet sites referenced in the *Red Book* are provided as a service to readers and may change without notice; citation of websites does not constitute AAP endorsement.

SOURCES OF INFORMATION ABOUT VACCINES AND IMMUNIZATION

In addition to the latest print edition of the *Red Book*, the following sources can assist providers in remaining up-to-date with information pertaining to vaccines and immunization recommendations and finding answers to questions that arise in practice. For many of these resources, providers can sign up for e-mail alerts to receive new information as soon as it is available.

- **American Academy of Pediatrics (AAP)**—*Red Book Online* includes the print edition content plus updates and is available on the Internet (**http://redbook.solutions.aap.org/Redbook.aspx**) to AAP members and subscribers. The website has links to the latest implementation guidance, immunization schedules, and the Vaccine Status Table, which provides information on recently submitted, approved, and recommended vaccines and biologics. New recommendations are summarized in *AAP News* (**www.aappublications.org/news**), the official newsmagazine of the AAP, and are published in *Pediatrics* (**http://pediatrics.aappublications.org**), the official journal of the Academy. The AAP also maintains a website (**www.aap.org/en/patient-care/immunizations/**) that contains useful links to immunization resources for providers as well as a website with information geared toward parents (**https://healthychildren.org/english/safety-prevention/immunizations/pages/default.aspx**).

- **Centers for Disease Control and Prevention (CDC)**—The CDC Vaccines & Immunizations website (**www.cdc.gov/vaccines/**) contains a wealth of information, including annually updated immunization schedules; vaccine safety information; recommendations from the Advisory Committee on Immunization Practices (ACIP); vaccine supply updates; vaccine coverage and disease surveillance data; recommendations for specific patient populations; information about storage, handling, and administration of vaccines; legal requirements; and education and training. ACIP recommendations become "official" when they are published in the *Morbidity and Mortality Weekly Report (MMWR)*, but the CDC may post provisional recommendations that can assist providers in making decisions on use of new vaccines prior to the publication of final recommendations. Noteworthy CDC Internet resources are listed in Table 1.2. CDC experts also are available to answer immunization-related questions by email at **nipinfo@cdc.gov**.

- **Food and Drug Administration (FDA)**—The FDA website includes information on the scientific and regulatory vaccine development process, vaccine safety and effectiveness, vaccine shortages, advisory committee meetings, and a repository of current FDA-approved prescribing information (**www.fda.gov/vaccines-blood-biologics/vaccines/**). The FDA-approved prescribing information (also referred to as the "label" or "package insert") contains detailed information for health care providers to ensure safe and effective use. The approved indications in the package insert are supported by the safety and effectiveness data evaluated by the FDA. The FDA does not issue guidelines or recommendations for vaccine use, and in some instances recommendations of the AAP or ACIP may differ from FDA-approved prescribing information.

Table 1.2. CDC Immunization Web Page Quick Reference

Content	URL
Glossary, acronyms, abbreviations, foreign language terms	www.cdc.gov/vaccines/terms/
Information for parents	www.cdc.gov/vaccines/parents/index.html
Provider resources for conversations with parents	www.cdc.gov/vaccines/hcp/conversations/conv-materials.html
ACIP recommendations	www.cdc.gov/vaccines/hcp/acip-recs/index.html
General best practice guidelines	www.cdc.gov/vaccines/hcp/acip-recs/general-recs/index.html
Schedules	www.cdc.gov/vaccines/schedules/hcp/index.html
Child and Adolescent Vaccine Assessment Tool	www2a.cdc.gov/vaccines/childquiz/
Vaccine Information Statements	www.cdc.gov/vaccines/hcp/vis/index.html
Vaccines for Children Program	www.cdc.gov/vaccines/programs/vfc/index.html
Travel	wwwnc.cdc.gov/travel/destinations/list
CDC Health Information for International Travel (also known as the Yellow Book)	wwwnc.cdc.gov/travel/page/yellowbook-home
Epidemiology and Prevention of Vaccine-Preventable Diseases (also known as the Pink Book)	www.cdc.gov/vaccines/pubs/pinkbook/index.html
Pink Book Series	www.cdc.gov/vaccines/ed/webinar-epv/index.html
Manual for the Surveillance of Vaccine-Preventable Diseases	www.cdc.gov/vaccines/pubs/surv-manual/index.html
Morbidity and Mortality Weekly Report (MMWR)	www.cdc.gov/mmwr/index.html

- **Immunize.org** (formerly the **Immunization Action Coalition [IAC]**)— Working in partnership with the CDC, the organization maintains a website (**www. immunize.org**) replete with copyright-free information about virtually every aspect of vaccine practice. Unique content includes Vaccine Information Statement (VIS) translations in multiple languages; *Ask the Experts*, a repository of answers to challenging immunization questions; handouts for patients and staff; *Unprotected People Stories*, containing personal accounts of encounters with vaccine-preventable diseases; updated information about state mandates and exemptions; expansive image and video libraries; and screening tools for contraindications and precautions. The organization also maintains websites for the public (**www.vaccineinformation. org**) and for immunization coalitions (**www.immunizationcoalitions.org**). Their weekly e-mail newsletter, *IZ Express*, is available free of charge.

- **Vaccine Manufacturers**—Vaccine manufacturers maintain websites with current information about their FDA-approved vaccines, contact information for medical questions, and updated package inserts.
- **Other Resources**—Table 1.3 lists major national and international organizations that are involved in vaccine development, regulation of vaccines, immunization policy, education, implementation, and advocacy, along with their respective websites. The Directory of Resources in Appendix I (p 1134) also is a source of contact information for these and other organizations.

Table 1.3. Internet Resources for Vaccine Information for Health Care Professionals and Parents

Resource	URL
Government	
Centers for Disease Control and Prevention: Vaccines & Immunization	**www.cdc.gov/vaccines/**
Centers for Disease Control and Prevention Vaccine Safety	**www.cdc.gov/vaccinesafety/**
National Institute of Allergy and Infectious Diseases	**www.niaid.nih.gov**
US Food and Drug Administration	**www.fda.gov/vaccines-blood-biologics/vaccines**
National Vaccine Injury Compensation Program	**www.hrsa.gov/vaccine-compensation/index.html**
Vaccine Adverse Event Reporting System	**www.vaers.hhs.gov/index**
US Department of Health and Human Services	**www.hhs.gov/vaccines**
International	
Pan American Health Organization	**www.paho.org/hq**
World Health Organization	**www.who.int/en**
Professional Associations	
American Academy of Pediatrics	**www.aap.org**
American Academy of Family Physicians	**www.aafp.org**
American Medical Association	**www.ama-assn.org**
American College Health Association	**www.acha.org**
American College of Nurse Midwives	**www.midwife.org**
American College of Physicians	**www.acponline.org**
American College of Obstetricians and Gynecologists	**www.acog.org**
American Association of Nurse Practitioners	**www.aanp.org**
American Immunization Registry Association	**www.immregistries.org**
American Nurses Association	**www.nursingworld.org**
American Osteopathic Association	**www.osteopathic.org**
American Pharmacists Association	**www.pharmacist.com**
American Public Health Association	**www.apha.org**

Table 1.3. Internet Resources for Vaccine Information for Health Care Professionals and Parents, continued

Resource	URL
American Society for Health System Pharmacists	www.ashp.org
Association for Prevention Teaching and Research	www.aptrweb.org
Association of State and Territorial Health Officials	www.astho.org
Association of Immunization Managers	www.immunizationmanagers.org
Council of State and Territorial Epidemiologists	www.cste.org
Infectious Diseases Society of America	www.idsociety.org
National Association of County and City Health Officials	www.naccho.org
National Association of Pediatric Nurse Practitioners	www.napnap.org
National Foundation of Infectious Diseases	www.nfid.org
National Medical Association	www.nmanet.org
Pediatric Infectious Diseases Society	www.pids.org
Society for Adolescent Health and Medicine	www.adolescenthealth.org
Society for Healthcare Epidemiology of America	www.shea-online.org
Society of Teachers of Family Medicine	www.stfm.org
Advocacy, Communication, Education, and Implementation	
American Academy of Pediatrics	www.healthychildren.org/English/safety-prevention/Pages/default.aspx
	https://pedialink.aap.org/visitor/home
	www.aap.org/en/patient-care/immunizations/communicating-with-families-and-promoting-vaccine-confidence/
Children's Hospital of Philadelphia Vaccine Education Center	www.chop.edu/centers-programs/vaccine-education-center
Comprehensive Vaccine Education Program (Pediatric Infectious Diseases Society)	https://pids.org/education-training/vaccine-education-program/
Families Fighting Flu	www.familiesfightingflu.org
Global Alliance for Vaccines and Immunization	www.gavi.org
Immunization for Women (American College of Obstetricians and Gynecologists)	www.immunizationforwomen.org
Immunize.org	www.immunize.org
National HPV Vaccination Roundtable	www.hpvroundtable.org
National Meningitis Association	www.nmaus.org
Unity Consortium	www.unity4teenvax.org/
Vaccinate Your Family (formerly Every Child by Two)	www.vaccinateyourfamily.org
Voices for Vaccines	www.voicesforvaccines.org

DISCUSSING VACCINES WITH PATIENTS AND PARENTS[1]

Vaccine Uptake: Definitions and Understanding Common Influences of Vaccine Behavior

It is critical to be clear about the terms used when discussing vaccine uptake. A helpful approach is to categorize terms within the attitudes, intentions, and behaviors framework. Vaccine attitudes signify how one thinks and feels about vaccination. Vaccine attitudes shape vaccine intentions, which reflect one's willingness to act on these attitudes. Vaccine intentions, in turn, shape vaccine behavior, which comprises the actions one takes with respect to vaccination. Vaccine confidence, which describes the belief that vaccines are safe, effective, and part of a trustworthy medical system, is a vaccine attitude. Vaccine hesitancy, a motivational state of being conflicted about or opposed to getting vaccinated, is a vaccine intention. And vaccine uptake, defined as receipt of a vaccine, is a vaccine behavior. Barriers to accessing vaccines as well as intentional vaccine refusal and delay are two important predictors of vaccine behavior.

Vaccine hesitancy may result in a range of behaviors, from refusal of all vaccinations, to receipt of all recommended vaccinations while still having concerns about vaccinations. In 2019, the Centers for Disease Control and Prevention (CDC) National Immunization Survey found that 20% of US parents reported that they were "hesitant about childhood shots." Several frameworks for categorization of parents and caregivers with respect to their vaccine attitudes, intentions, and behaviors have emerged, with an example shown in Table 1.4. A small proportion of parents (1%–3%) refuse all vaccines and may have more fixed beliefs and attitudes about vaccines. On-time routine vaccination decreased in the years immediately following the COVID-19 pandemic; however, it is uncertain whether this decrease is more related to missed well-visit appointments rather than changes in vaccine hesitancy during the pandemic. Some US and Canadian surveys have shown that vaccine hesitancy has not changed significantly since the onset of the pandemic. In contrast to the small number who adamantly refuse any vaccine, the majority of hesitant parents likely have some ambivalence toward vaccination decisions and many may be receptive to information and guidance about routine childhood vaccines that improve their confidence and uptake for their children.

A World Health Organization framework organizes determinants of vaccine hesitancy into contextual, individual and group, and vaccine factors.[2] At the contextual level, both access to trusted sources of vaccine information and the spread of misinformation may influence beliefs about vaccines and the diseases they prevent. Individual and group preferences for "natural" or "organic" approaches to health are

---

[1] American Academy of Pediatrics, Committee on Infectious Diseases, Committee on Practice and Ambulatory Medicine, Committee on Bioethics. Clinical report. Strategies for improving vaccine communication and uptake. *Pediatrics*. 2024; in press

[2] World Health Organization, SAGE Working Group. Report of the SAGE Working Group on Vaccine Hesitancy. Geneva, Switzerland: World Health Organization; 2014. Available at: **www.asset-scienceinsociety.eu/sites/default/files/sage_working_group_revised_report_vaccine_hesitancy.pdf**

Table 1.4. Determinants of Vaccine Hesitancy Matrix (World Health Organization)

Contextual influences Influences from historic, sociocultural, environmental, health system/institutional, economic, or political factors	• Communication and media environment • Influential leaders, immunization program gatekeepers, and anti- or provaccination groups • Historical influences • Religion/culture/gender/socioeconomic • Politics/policies • Geographic barriers • Perception of the pharmaceutical industry
Individual and group influences Influences from personal perception of the vaccine or influences of the social/peer environment	• Personal, family, and/or community members' experience with vaccination, including pain • Beliefs, attitudes about health and prevention • Knowledge/awareness • Health system and providers—trust and personal experience • Risk/benefit (perceived, heuristic) • Immunization as a social norm vs not needed/harmful
Vaccine/vaccination-specific issues Directly related to vaccine or vaccination	• Benefit/risk (epidemiologic and scientific evidence) • Introduction of a new vaccine or new formulation or a new recommendation for an existing vaccine • Mode of administration • Design of vaccination program/mode of delivery (eg, routine program or mass vaccination campaign) • Reliability and/or source of supply of vaccine and/or vaccination equipment • Vaccination schedule • Costs • The strength of the recommendation and/or knowledge base and/or attitude of health care professionals

Adapted from: World Health Organizatoin, SAGE Working Group. *Report of the SAGE Working Group on Vaccine Hesitancy.* Geneva, Switzerland: World Health Organization; 2014.

also associated with vaccine hesitancy, and these preferences often overlap with distrust for health care professionals and medical systems. Psychological factors underlying vaccine attitudes include valuing autonomy, conspiratorial thinking, and cognitive biases in how people weigh probabilities of present and future risks. In contrast, social norms can help promote vaccine uptake.

Receiving a vaccine is strongly associated with perceived disease risk or susceptibility. Refusing a vaccine, conversely, may be associated with a lower perceived disease risk and has been linked to increased risk of diseases like measles, pertussis, and invasive pneumococcal infection at the individual and community level. Geographic clustering of vaccine refusal further increases the risk of communicable disease outbreaks in certain communities even when vaccination rates at a state or national level remain high overall. For example, large outbreaks of measles in the United States in the 2010s frequently occurred in undervaccinated communities with shared religious and cultural beliefs.

Disruption to routine pediatric vaccination during the COVID-19 pandemic has left many children vulnerable to vaccine-preventable diseases and more locations susceptible to outbreaks in the United States and around the world. Although evidence remains inconclusive, disease resurgence may help bolster vaccine uptake; media coverage of recent measles outbreaks has been associated with more provaccine communication and positive parental vaccine attitudes. In contrast, pediatric COVID-19 vaccine uptake has been slow as parents consider a new vaccine for a new disease amidst ongoing spread of both disease and misinformation. COVID-19 is a reminder that disease prevalence is only one of many factors that contribute to vaccine acceptance.

Distrust of health systems based on historic and ongoing discrimination and inequitable access to care are intertwined challenges that contribute to racial and ethnic disparities in vaccine uptake. Although there has been progress in reducing racial, ethnic, and socioeconomic disparities in childhood vaccination coverage, the COVID-19 pandemic made clear how much work is yet to be done. Solutions to reduce disparities and promote vaccine uptake must build trust, improve access to care and access to information for all communities, increase diversity and representation among the ranks of scientists and health care professionals, and acknowledge the contribution of structural and interpersonal racism to health disparities. Promising approaches include partnering with trusted messengers to promote vaccination as well as community engagement to understand barriers to vaccine uptake and to build on existing sources of information and connection. Vaccine conversations with parents from historically minoritized groups may also require more explicit acknowledgement of the medical mistreatment and exclusion experienced by these groups and the damaging effect this has had on trust in medical and public health authorities.

Understanding Vaccine Evaluation and Safety as an Approach to Addressing Parental Concerns

Among parents or caregivers who refuse or question vaccines, safety has consistently been shown to be a top concern. Therefore, it is important for pediatricians and other clinicians who care for children to have knowledge of the processes for vaccine licensure and vaccine safety monitoring in order to address parents' questions and concerns. Because vaccines are generally given to healthy individuals to prevent disease, they are held to a higher safety standard than other medications. Prior to a vaccine being added to the routine immunization schedule, there is a multistep process including preclinical animal studies, clinical trials in humans, submission of an application to the US Food and Drug Administration (FDA) for licensure (or, as in the case of COVID-19 vaccines, for emergency use authorization [EUA]), approval or authorization by the FDA, and recommendations for use by the Advisory Committee on Immunization Practices (ACIP). In each of these steps, safety is a top consideration.

Prelicensure clinical trials and progression through the phases of clinical development are under the oversight of FDA. Prelicensure, phase 1 trials are conducted for the purpose of understanding the safety profile and side effects of a vaccine generally among 20 to 100 healthy volunteers. If there are no safety concerns in this phase, a vaccine may move into phase 2 trials, generally among several hundred volunteers, when, in addition to further expanding an understanding of the vaccine's safety profile, immunogenicity is assessed. For vaccines with acceptable phase 2 safety data and promising immunogenicity data, phase 3 trials may proceed, often with thousands of volunteers, to assess both effectiveness and detection of less common adverse events in a larger population. After completion of phase 3 trials, the manufacturer of the vaccine may submit an application to the FDA for licensure. The FDA then reviews the application; if it determines that the vaccine is safe and effective and confirms that the manufacturing and facility information assure product quality and consistency, it may grant a license for use. The reviews conducted by the FDA are publicly posted on the FDA website. The ACIP then examines the available data submitted to the FDA as well as other contributory data to decide whether the benefits of vaccination outweigh any possible risks for the target population. Although some of the deliberations are internal to the FDA and CDC, this process is highly transparent, with public ACIP meetings and the opportunity for written or oral public comment. The process for authorization of COVID-19 vaccines under EUA and subsequent ACIP recommendation was very similar to fully licensed vaccine products, albeit on an accelerated timeline because of the urgent nature of the emergency (eg, pandemic) under which they were being considered.

Although prelicensure trials can identify common adverse events within a limited timeframe after vaccination, it is not feasible to conduct clinical trials large enough to detect all rare vaccine-related events (ie, <1 event per 10 000 vaccinees). Therefore, the United States has developed a robust postlicensure vaccine safety surveillance system. Two of the most widely known components of this surveillance network are the **Vaccine Adverse Event Reporting System (VAERS)** and the **Vaccine Safety Datalink (VSD)**, both of which were established in 1990. A surveillance system managed by the CDC and FDA, VAERS is the US government's early warning system for vaccine adverse events. Although VAERS is crucial to vaccine safety surveillance, it cannot generally assess causality. It therefore serves as a hypothesis-*generating* system. On the other hand, the VSD, a collaboration between CDC and 13 integrated health care organizations, is a hypothesis-*testing* system and can assess causality. Using electronic health records (EHRs) with highly accurate data, if a signal for a possible vaccine adverse event is identified through VAERS or other monitoring sources, further studies can then be conducted in the VSD to determine whether an association with the vaccine in question exists using several different types of methods, such as case-control (comparing the incidence of the possible adverse event in vaccinated and unvaccinated individuals) and self-controlled case series (in which only individuals who experienced the outcome of interest are examined using risk intervals around the time of vaccination). The VSD has been able to identify rare adverse events after vaccination, such as the association between measles, mumps, and rubella vaccine (MMR) and immune thrombocytopenic purpura and the increased risk of febrile seizures after measles, mumps, rubella, and varicella vaccine (MMRV). Equally importantly, the VSD has been able to demonstrate the lack of association of numerous vaccines with purported vaccine adverse events.

In addition to VAERS and the VSD, the FDA has its own active surveillance effort involving the **Biologics Effectiveness and Safety (BEST)** system, which covers more than 100 million people and comprises large-scale claims data, EHRs, and linked claims-EHR databases. The system makes use of multiple data sources and enables rapid queries to detect or evaluate adverse events as well as studies to answer specific safety questions for vaccines.

In addition to the VSD, VAERS, and BEST, the United States has several other important systems monitoring vaccine safety, including the **Clinical Immunization Safety Assessment Project (CISA)**, various surveillance systems through the US Department of Defense, and, with onset of the COVID-19 pandemic, **v-safe**, the after-vaccination checker. The United States also collaborates internationally to study vaccine safety through partnerships with the World Health Organization, the European Medicines Agency, and the Pan-American Health Organization, among others. Details of several of the major US vaccine safety surveillance systems are shown in Table 1.5.

The safety of the recommended childhood vaccines and the recommended schedule has been affirmed by multiple independent reviews, including from the National Academy of Medicine (NAM) and the Agency for Healthcare Research and Quality (AHRQ). The 2013 report from the NAM includes a review of the evidence for known vaccine adverse events and was used to inform the vaccine injury compensation program. The 2021 update to the AHRQ report identified no new safety risks associated with the recommended vaccination schedule, and pediatricians can use this information to explain the reasons for the timing of the recommended schedule. Many vaccine-preventable diseases like measles, pertussis, rotavirus, and pneumococcal and *Haemophilus influenzae* infection are associated with higher morbidity and mortality in infancy and early childhood. Delaying vaccination leaves children unprotected at the age when they are most at risk. Vaccines are studied to ensure safety and adequate immune response at the age when they are recommended. For example, immune response to human papillomavirus (HPV) vaccine is stronger when given at an earlier age, and delaying vaccination may result in the need for more doses to achieve adequate protection.

Pursuing a nonrecommended vaccination schedule is associated with lower likelihood of being up-to-date on early childhood vaccinations and involves using an approach that is less well studied than the recommended schedule. It is also important to have children fully vaccinated before they attend group settings with other children (eg, any type of group child care setting, preschool, or elementary school where the risk of exposure to a vaccine-preventable disease increases). When using a nonrecommended vaccine schedule, this goal can be compromised. Deviation from the recommended schedule, therefore, is generally discouraged. After making a reasonable effort to discuss the recommended vaccination schedule with a family, deviation from the recommended schedule may be considered if it is the only way to move forward to vaccinate a child.

Some parents and caregivers have concerns about the number of vaccinations children receive or the specific components in vaccines. Clinicians can respond to the concern among some parents that "too many" vaccines are given at once with evidence-based, valid, culturally sensitive statements to promote vaccine uptake. It may be helpful to explain that there are fewer antigens in the current schedule than historical schedules that included the whole-cell pertussis vaccine. The immune system has the capacity to respond to a large number of stimuli at once and responds to the many immunogenic substances it encounters outside vaccinations through routine childhood food, environmental, and circulating disease exposures.

Parents and caregivers sometimes raise concerns about vaccines causing the infection they are actually working to prevent. Pediatricians can explain that non-live vaccines contain only a portion of the bacteria or virus they are working to prevent and

Table 1.5. Examples of Major Vaccine Safety Surveillance Systems in the United States

Surveillance System	Data Source	Population Under Surveillance	Management	Characteristics	Strengths	Limitations
Vaccine Adverse Event Reporting System (VAERS)	Online reporting system; Health care providers and vaccine manufacturers are required by law to report certain events after vaccination	Entire United States	FDA, CDC	• "Nation's early warning system" • Passive, spontaneous reporting • Hypothesis-generating • 85%–90% of reports are nonserious • Serious reports are followed up	• Accepts reports from anyone • All data are publicly available	• Generally cannot assess causality • Prone to both overreporting and underreporting
Vaccine Safety Datalink (VSD)	Electronic health record data from 13 large health care organizations across the United States	12.5 million	CDC, in collaboration with integrated health care organizations	• Active surveillance system • Hypothesis-testing • Can conduct medical record review to verify outcomes • Multiple methods developed to conduct valid, accurate vaccine safety studies	• Can estimate potential causal associations • Capable of real-time monitoring • High-quality data	• Limited ability to assess adverse events with delayed or insidious onset • May not be able to control for all confounders • Represents an insured population

Table 1.5. Examples of Major Vaccine Safety Surveillance Systems in the United States, continued

Surveillance System	Data Source	Population Under Surveillance	Management	Characteristics	Strengths	Limitations
Biologics Effectiveness and Safety System (BEST)	Large-scale claims data, electronic health records (EHRs), and linked claims-EHR databases	100 million	FDA	• Enables rapid queries to detect or evaluate adverse events as well as studies to answer specific safety questions for vaccines	• Very large population • Possible to study the safety of vaccines in subpopulations with preexisting conditions or in pregnant persons	• Limited evaluation of pediatric vaccines to date • Statistical signals must be further evaluated through rigorous epidemiologic study
Clinical Immunization Safety Assessment (CISA)	Generally medical records from clinicians	Not applicable	CDC, in collaboration with medical research centers	• In depth clinical, pathophysiological, and vaccinology expertise to assess causal relationships between vaccines and adverse events	• US health care providers with a complex vaccine safety question about a specific patient may contact CISA to request a consult	• Limited in scope

BEST indicates Biologics Effectiveness and Safety System; CDC, Centers for Disease Control and Prevention; CISA, Clinical Immunization Safety Assessment; EHR, electronic health records; FDA, US Food and Drug Administration; VAERS, Vaccine Adverse Event Reporting System; VSD, Vaccine Safety Datalink.

that most common vaccine side effects are from the immune system response and are not a sign of infection. Some vaccines contain only the genetic material for a specific protein and direct the body to produce a small amount of that protein. Live vaccines are contraindicated for some immunocompromised people because of the risk of vaccine-strain viral replication causing vaccine associated disease; however, these vaccines do not cause infection or disease in immunocompetent people.

Other common concerns focus on specific vaccine ingredients. In the United States, mercury was removed from most vaccine products in the early 2000s. Thimerosal (which contains ethylmercury) is still used as a preservative to prevent contamination in some influenza vaccines supplied in multidose vials, but other routine childhood vaccines in the United States, including single-dose vial influenza vaccines, do not contain ethylmercury. Concerns about neurologic effects of mercury exposure are based on risks associated with methylmercury, whereas ethylmercury is metabolized more quickly and not associated with the same risks. Alleged correlations between methylmercury and autism have been debunked.

Aluminum is used in some vaccines as an adjuvant that facilitates a strong immune response. The amount of aluminum in vaccines is safe, regulated, and comparable to the amount of aluminum infants are exposed to through human milk and formula feeding.

Fetal cell lines have been used in the development, testing, and production of some vaccines and other medications, but vaccines do not contain cells or DNA from aborted fetuses. Most major religions have issued statements that the use of fetal cells in vaccine development does not prohibit use of these vaccines, and some have pointed out the moral good of vaccination to protect the health of children and the people around them.

The CDC's *Epidemiology of Vaccine Preventable Disease: The Pink Book* and collection of *Morbidity and Mortality Weekly Reports (MMWRs)* containing ACIP vaccination recommendations are useful resources for more detailed information about vaccine contraindications and precautions, ingredients, schedules, and side effects. A summary of common misconceptions with accompanying facts is provided in Table 1.6.

Evidence-Based Communication Strategies to Increase Uptake of Childhood Vaccines[1]

Pediatricians are the most common source of vaccine information for parents and caregivers, are the most trusted source for vaccine-safety information, and can positively influence a parent's vaccine behavior, even among parents with concerns about vaccines. Vaccine-related facts that pediatricians may use when discussing vaccines with parents are important. How those facts are communicated is also important. It is important to establish an honest dialogue, take time to listen, and solicit and welcome questions. Recent evidence has further improved the understanding of specific clinician communication strategies that can improve uptake of childhood vaccines. Although many techniques for working with vaccine-hesitant parents have been suggested, relatively few have been studied to determine efficacy in improving vaccination uptake, although recent years have seen an uptick in large, funded randomized trials.

---

[1] American Academy of Pediatrics, Committee on Infectious Diseases, Committee on Practice and Ambulatory Medicine, Committee on Bioethics. Clinical report. Strategies for improving vaccine communication and uptake. Pediatrics. 2024; in press

Table 1.6. Common Misconceptions/Myths About Vaccines and Immunizations

Claims	Facts
"Natural" methods of enhancing immunity, such as contracting the disease, are better than vaccinations.	Vaccinations are the safest way to achieve immunity; having immunity the "natural way" means being sick with a potentially very serious, even lethal, infectious disease. Immunity from a preventive vaccine provides protection against disease when a person is exposed to it in the future. That immunity is usually similar to what is acquired from natural infection, although several doses of a vaccine may have to be administered for a child to develop an adequate immune response.
Giving multiple vaccines at the same time causes an "overload" of the immune system.	Vaccination does not overburden a child's immune system; the recommended vaccines use only a small portion of the immune system's "memory." Although the number of unique vaccines administered has risen over recent decades, the number of antigens administered has decreased because of advances in science and manufacturing. The National Academy of Medicine (NAM) has concluded that there is no evidence that the immunization schedule is unsafe.
Vaccines are ineffective.	Vaccines have spared millions of people the effects of devastating diseases.
Prior to the use of vaccinations, these diseases had begun to decline because of improved nutrition and hygiene.	In the 19th and 20th centuries, some infectious diseases began to be better controlled because of improvements in sanitation, clean water, pasteurized milk, and pest control. However, vaccine-preventable diseases decreased dramatically after the vaccines for those diseases were approved and were administered to large numbers of children.
Vaccines cause poorly understood illnesses or disorders, such as autism, sudden infant death syndrome (SIDS), immune dysfunction, diabetes, neurologic disorders, allergic rhinitis, and eczema.	These claims are false. Multiple, high-quality scientific studies have failed to substantiate any link between vaccines and these health conditions. See NAM and Agency for Healthcare Research and Quality (AHRQ) reports.[a,b]
Vaccines weaken the immune system.	Vaccines strengthen the immune system. Vaccinated children have decreased risk of infections. Importantly, natural infections like influenza, measles, and chickenpox can weaken the immune system, increasing the risk of other infections.

Table 1.6. Common Misconceptions/Myths About Vaccines and Immunizations, continued

Claims	Facts
Giving many vaccines at the same time is untested.	With some exceptions, administering multiple vaccines at the same time is as effective and safe as administering vaccines separately. Routine administration of all age-appropriate doses of vaccines at the same time is important to keep children up-to-date with all recommended vaccines.
Vaccines can be delayed, separated, and spaced out without consequences.	Many vaccine-preventable diseases occur in early infancy. Optimal vaccine-induced immunity may require a series of vaccines over time. Any delay in receiving age-appropriate immunization increases the risk of diseases that vaccines are administered to prevent. Spacing out vaccine may also have psychological consequences, because many more office visits will be associated with injections.

Adapted from Myers MG, Pineda D. *Do Vaccines Cause That? A Guide for Evaluating Vaccine Safety Concerns*. Galveston, TX: Immunizations for Public Health; 2008:79.
[a] **www.nap.edu/catalog/13164/adverse-effects-of-vaccines-evidence-and-causality; www.nap.edu/catalog/13563/the-childhood-immunization-schedule-and-safety-stakeholder-concerns-scientific-evidence**
[b] Agency for Healthcare Research and Quality, Safety of Vaccines Used for Routine Immunization in the United States: An Update. Available at: **https://effectivehealthcare.ahrq.gov/products/safety-vaccines/research**

USE A STRONG VACCINE RECOMMENDATION AND THE PRESUMPTIVE FORMAT FOR INITIATING THE VACCINE DISCUSSION

One of the clinician vaccine communication strategies with strong evidence for increased uptake of childhood and adolescent vaccines is providing a vaccine recommendation. The strength and quality of this recommendation is also important. There is higher vaccine receipt among children whose parents or caregivers receive a very strong clinician vaccine recommendation than those who do not. The ability to confidently provide such strong recommendations is based on decades of broad national and international pediatric health care experience, data collection, and rigorous, well-designed studies of vaccine safety, efficacy, and effectiveness.

A related communication strategy with similarly strong evidence for increased vaccine uptake is a clinician's use of a presumptive format to initiate the vaccine discussion. A presumptive format is one in which the clinician asserts a position regarding vaccines using a closed-ended statement, such as "Sara is due for several vaccines today" or "Well, we have to do some shots." This is in contrast to a participatory format, in which an open-ended question is used to more explicitly invite the parent to voice an opinion, such as "How do you feel about vaccines today?" Clinician use of a presumptive format is associated with increased vaccine uptake, even among vaccine-hesitant parents. In addition, clinicians' repeated use of a presumptive (as compared with participatory) format with vaccine-hesitant parents or caregivers over several visits, given the longitudinal nature of vaccine administration and discussions, yields significantly less underimmunization among children. Overall, implementation of the presumptive format in practice has been perceived by clinicians as time-saving, easy to use, and a way to promote vaccination as part of routine care. Engaging all team members in the office setting or inpatient unit who communicate with parents about vaccines on the rationale and technique for initiating the vaccine discussion using the presumptive format could maximize its effect.

FOR PARENTS WHO EXPRESS HESITANCY, USE ADDITIONAL EVIDENCE-BASED COMMUNICATION STRATEGIES

Although a strong recommendation and use of a presumptive format for initiating the vaccine discussion with parents and caregivers are effective, they are not a panacea; despite use of these strategies, a proportion of vaccine-hesitant parents will still voice initial resistance to vaccinating their child. There are additional vaccine communication strategies needed with parents who continue to express hesitancy. One such strategy is motivational interviewing. Motivational interviewing is a patient-centered framework for behavior change that helps leverage one's inherent motivation for behaviors. Evidence from observational studies to support the use of motivational interviewing in the vaccination context is growing. The strongest evidence for motivational interviewing has come from a large cluster randomized controlled trial.[1] Clinicians in intervention practices were trained to use the presumptive format for initiating the discussion for all parents regarding HPV vaccine, followed by use of motivational interviewing in discussions with parents who voiced initial reluctance in having their child receive the HPV vaccine. Clinicians in control practices provided usual care. Investigators found a significant increase in HPV vaccine initiation and completion among children of parents who received care in intervention (versus control) practices.

Other adjunctive clinician vaccine communication strategies with some evidence supporting their effectiveness include: (a) pursuing adherence to the recommended vaccines due for the child at a visit despite initial parental reluctance; and (b) bundling the discussion of all vaccines a child is eligible for at the visit at once. Pursuing adherence refers to responding immediately to a parent's initial reluctance to the vaccines for which their child is due with a reiteration of the importance of the recommended vaccines for the child, such as "Your child really needs these shots." In several observational studies, parental verbal acceptance of vaccines for their child was significantly higher when clinicians pursued their vaccine recommendations (versus acquiesced) after initial parent reluctance. Bundling the discussion of all vaccines for which a child is due at a visit at once is supported by observational work in which investigators found concurrent discussion of the influenza vaccine with other vaccines for which a child was also due was associated with higher influenza vaccine uptake. Clinicians may also mention that they use strategies to minimize the pain associated with vaccination, as this is a common concern among parents and caregivers.

Finally, clinicians can emphasize their own experiences when discussing the need for vaccination, including personal experience with vaccine-preventable diseases and the fact that they and their families are vaccinated because of their confidence in the safety and efficacy of the vaccines.

---

[1] Dempsey AF, Pyrznawoski J, Lockhart S, et al. Effect of a health care professional communication training intervention on adolescent human papillomavirus vaccination: a cluster randomized clinical trial. *JAMA Pediatr.* 2018;172(5):e180016

LEVERAGE SYSTEMS, ORGANIZATIONAL APPROACHES, AND COMMUNITY INITIATIVES TO IMPROVE PARENTAL ACCESS TO VACCINES

Pediatrician-parent communication is only one of the many efforts required to achieve and maintain high vaccination coverage. There are many established and long-standing evidence-based practices for increasing vaccination coverage, such as standing orders for vaccination, reminder/recall, use of immunization information systems, school and child care entry requirements, and audit and feedback, among others. There are also emerging community-based approaches designed to build trust and address the concerns of specific populations, including religious and vulnerable populations. These may include community- and school-based vaccination programs, which may help to demonstrate vaccination as a social norm and encourage greater uptake. Effectively implementing these strategies has the potential to save time in the clinical encounter by reducing the time needed to discuss vaccines.

Policies for Families Who Refuse or Delay Vaccination

Dismissal of child patients of vaccine-refusing parents or caregivers can be a difficult decision arrived at after considering multiple factors and documented attempts to counsel vaccine-refusing families. However, if repeated attempts to help understand and address parental values and vaccine concerns fails to engender trust, move parents toward vaccine acceptance, or strengthen the therapeutic alliance, dismissal can be an acceptable option. When considering the dismissal of a vaccine-refusing parent, it is important to verify that less drastic alternatives are not feasible. The consideration, design, and implementation of office policies for dismissal will ideally take into account practice setting, patient population, availability of other nearby reputable sources of medical care for children, and the framing of the policy (stressing the importance of vaccination). Transparency and equitable application of such policies is also important. Dismissal must be conducted in a manner consistent with applicable state laws prohibiting abandonment of patients. Although these laws vary from state to state, official notification of the parents or legal guardian is required, along with the provision of information for finding a new physician. The parental refusal of recommended vaccines and attempts to counsel the family should be documented in the patient's medical record. Furthermore, the dismissing physician is obligated to continue current treatment and provide emergency care for a reasonable period of time, usually 30 days.

Vaccine Injury Compensation

Although vaccines are extremely safe products, serious adverse events, such as allergic reactions, are rare but can result from vaccine administration. The Vaccine Injury Compensation Program (VICP) was established in 1988 as an alternative to civil litigation and to simplify the process of settling vaccine injury claims. The VICP is a no-fault system in which compensation may be sought if people believe they have experienced an injury as a result of administration of a vaccine listed in the current Vaccine Injury Table, the link to which can be found at **www.hrsa.gov/vaccine-compensation.** People seeking compensation for alleged injuries from covered vaccines must first file claims with the VICP before pursuing civil litigation against manufacturers or vaccine providers. If the claimant accepts the judgment of the VICP, neither vaccine providers nor manufacturers can be sued in civil litigation. If the claimant rejects the VICP judgment, he or she has the option of filing a claim against the vaccine company and the health care professional who administered the vaccine, although this seldom happens.

The VICP compensates for injuries that have occurred as a result of the administration of a vaccine routinely recommended for children and adolescents, although the vaccine recipient and beneficiary can be of any age. Vaccines not routinely recommended for children, including zoster vaccines, pneumococcal polysaccharide vaccine (PPSV23), and travel vaccines, are not covered by the VICP. The 21st Century Cures Act, signed into law in December 2016, amended the VICP to include coverage for vaccines recommended for routine use in pregnant people, ensuring that both a person who received a covered vaccine while pregnant and the child (in utero at the time) are covered by the program.

Claims must be filed within 36 months after the first symptom appeared following immunization, and death claims must be filed within 2 years of a death and within 4 years after the first symptom of the vaccine injury that resulted in the death. To ensure that legal expenses are not a barrier to entry into the program, the VICP may pay attorney's fees and other legal costs related to a claim, regardless of the judgment, if certain minimal requirements are met and the claim is determined to have been filed on a reasonable basis and in good faith.

The VICP compensates for vaccine-related injuries that are included on the Vaccine Injury Table, the link to which can be found at **www.hrsa.gov/vaccine-compensation.** The table lists the vaccines covered by the VICP as well as injuries, disabilities, illnesses, and conditions for which compensation may be awarded. The Vaccine Injury Table defines the time during which the first symptoms or significant aggravation of an injury must appear after immunization. If the claim pertains to conditions not listed in the Vaccine Injury Table, claimants still may file a claim. The average time from filing a claim to a judgement is under 3 years.

In 2009, a separate program, the Countermeasure Injury Compensation Program (CICP), was created to cover medical countermeasures developed and/or used in response to public health emergencies, such as in a pandemic (eg, COVID-19), epidemic, or security threat (eg, smallpox, anthrax, botulism) **(www.hrsa.gov/cicp).** CICP awards are paid by the Covered Countermeasure Process Fund, which is funded by Congress via emergency appropriations to the US Department of Health and Human Services. The CICP requires a higher burden of proof regarding injury causation, has a shorter time limit to file a claim (within 1 year following the date of vaccination), and does not compensate for pain, suffering, emotional distress, or attorney's fees. Denied claims cannot be appealed.

A vaccine covered by the CICP can be transferred to the VICP once the vaccine is approved by the US Food and Drug Administration (FDA) using the biologics license application (ie, the normal process), is recommended by the Centers for Disease Control and Prevention (CDC) Advisory Committee on Immunization Practices (ACIP) to be included in the CDC vaccine schedule, and is authorized by the Secretary of Health and Human Services. In addition, Congress has to authorize an excise tax on it.

Information about the VICP and the Vaccine Injury Table can be obtained from: Parklawn Building, 5600 Fishers Lane, 8N146B Rockville, MD 20857; telephone: 800-338-2382; email: **vaccinecompensation@hrsa.gov**; website: **www.hrsa. gov/vaccine-compensation/index.html.** People wishing to file a claim for a vaccine injury should telephone or write to: United States Court of Federal Claims, 717 Madison Place, NW, Washington, DC 20439; telephone: 202-357-6400. Information on the VICP is also available to caregivers through Vaccine Information Statements (**www.cdc.gov/vaccines/hcp/vis/index.html),** which are required to be provided before administering each dose of each vaccine covered by the program.

···

ACTIVE IMMUNIZATION

Active immunization involves administration of all or part of a microorganism or a modified product of a microorganism (eg, a toxoid, a purified antigen, an antigen produced by genetic engineering, or nucleic acid encoding an antigen) to evoke an immunologic response and clinical protection that mimics that of infection with the microorganism but usually presents little or no risk to the recipient. Immunization can result in antitoxin, anti-adherence, anti-invasive, or neutralizing activity or other types of protective humoral or cellular responses in the recipient. Some vaccines provide nearly complete and lifelong protection against disease, some provide protection against the more severe manifestations and/or consequences of the infection if exposed, and some must be readministered periodically to maintain protection. The immunologic response to vaccination is dependent on the type and dose of antigen, the effect of adjuvants, and host factors related to age, preexisting antibody, nutrition, concurrent disease, and genetics of the host. The effectiveness of a vaccine is assessed by evidence of protection against the disease it is designed to prevent. For some infectious diseases, induction of antibodies following vaccination is an indirect measure that predicts protection (eg, antitoxin against *Clostridium tetani* or neutralizing antibody against measles virus), but for others, serum antibody concentration does not always predict protection.

Vaccines are categorized as live (viral or bacterial microbes, which almost always are attenuated), or non-live (also viral or bacterial) vaccines. Non-live vaccines can include those produced by inactivating the entire microbe, or fractional vaccines such as recombinant vaccines produced through genetic technologies that contain a portion of the microbe. Also included under the category of non-live vaccines are toxoids, which generate an antibody response to toxins produced by a microbe rather than to the microbe itself. Several recently developed non-live vaccines do not contain antigen but employ DNA or RNA to instruct the recipient's own cellular mechanism to generate antigenic material, which then stimulates the immune response that confers protection against the pathogen.

Recommendations for vaccines routinely advised for immunocompetent and immunocompromised children and adolescents are updated annually in the harmonized schedule developed by the American Academy of Pediatrics (AAP), Centers for Disease Control and Prevention (CDC), American Academy of Family Physicians (AAFP), American College of Obstetricians and Gynecologists (ACOG), American College of Nurse Midwives (ACNM), American Academy of Physician Associates (AAPA), and National Association of Pediatric Nurse Practitioners (NAPNAP) (**http://redbook.solutions.aap.org/SS/Immunization_Schedules.aspx**), and for simplicity are referred to as being "on the annual immunization schedule." Vaccines approved for use in the United States are listed in Table 1.7. The US Food and Drug Administration (FDA) maintains and updates a website that lists vaccines approved for immunization and distribution in the United States with supporting documents (**www.fda.gov/vaccines-blood-biologics/vaccines/vaccines-licensed-use-united-states**). Appendix II (Codes for Commonly Administered Pediatric Vaccines, Toxoids, and Immune Globulins, p 1139) provides information on the billing codes for commonly administered pediatric vaccines and toxoids used for vaccine administration. A regularly updated listing of *Current Procedural Terminology* (CPT) product codes for commonly administered pediatric vaccines can be found at **https://downloads.aap.org/AAP/PDF/coding_vaccine_coding_table.pdf.**

Among currently approved vaccines in the United States, there are 3 live attenuated bacterial vaccines (oral typhoid, oral cholera, and bacille Calmette-Guérin vaccines) and several live attenuated viral vaccines. Although active bacterial or viral replication ensues after administration of these vaccines, few or no symptoms of illness occur because the pathogen has been attenuated. Sufficient antigenic characteristics of the virus or bacteria are retained during attenuation so that a protective immune response develops in the vaccine recipient.

A replication-incompetent virus that expresses an antigen of interest is another type of vaccine. An example is the adenovirus type 26-vectored COVID-19 vaccine, which expresses the SARS-CoV-2 spike protein, or the replication-deficient modified vaccinia Ankara smallpox and mpox vaccine (JYNNEOS).

Vaccines for some viruses (eg, hepatitis A, hepatitis B, human papillomavirus) and most bacteria are inactivated, component, subunit (purified components) preparations or inactivated toxins. Some vaccines contain purified bacterial polysaccharides conjugated chemically to immunobiologically active proteins (eg, tetanus toxoid, diphtheria toxoid, nontoxic variant of mutant diphtheria toxin, meningococcal outer membrane protein complex).

Viruses and bacteria in inactivated, subunit, and conjugate vaccine preparations are not capable of replicating in the host; therefore, these vaccines must contain sufficient antigen content and possibly include an adjuvant to stimulate a desired response. In the case of conjugate polysaccharide vaccines, the linkage between the polysaccharide and the carrier protein enhances vaccine immunogenicity by converting the vaccine from a T-lymphocyte–independent antigen to a T-lymphocyte–dependent antigen. Maintenance of long-lasting immunity with non-live viral or non-live bacterial vaccines (including toxoid vaccines) may require periodic administration of booster doses. Although non-live vaccines may not elicit the range of immunologic response provided by live attenuated agents, efficacy of approved non-live vaccines in children is high. For example, an injected non-live viral vaccine may evoke sufficient serum antibody or cell-mediated immunity but evoke only minimal mucosal antibody in the form of secretory immunoglobulin (Ig) A. Mucosal protection after administration of non-live vaccines generally is inferior to mucosal immunity induced by live attenuated vaccines. Nonetheless, the demonstrated efficacy for such vaccines against invasive infection is high. Bacterial polysaccharide conjugate vaccines (eg, *Haemophilus influenzae* type b, pneumococcal, and meningococcal ACWY conjugate vaccines) reduce nasopharyngeal colonization through exudated IgG.

Table 1.7. Vaccines Approved or Authorized by Emergency Use Authorization for Immunization and Distributed in the United States and Their Routes of Administration[a]

Vaccine	Type	Route of Administration
Anthrax	Inactivated[b]	IM or SC
BCG	Live bacteria	Percutaneous using multiple puncture device
Cholera	Live attenuated bacteria	Oral
COVID-19	mRNA	IM
Dengue[c]	Live attenuated chimeric viruses	SC
DTaP	Toxoids and inactivated bacterial components	IM
DTaP, hepatitis B, and IPV	Toxoids and inactivated bacterial components, recombinant viral antigen, inactivated virus	IM
DTaP-IPV	Toxoids and inactivated bacterial components, inactivated virus	IM
DTaP, hepatitis B, Hib, and IPV	Toxoids and inactivated bacterial components, recombinant viral antigen, polysaccharide-protein conjugate, inactivated virus	IM
DTaP-IPV-Hib	Toxoids and inactivated bacterial components, inactivated virus, polysaccharide-protein conjugate	IM
Hepatitis A (HepA)	Inactivated virus	IM
Hepatitis B (HepB)	Recombinant viral antigen	IM
Hepatitis A-hepatitis B	Inactivated virus and recombinant viral antigens	IM
Hib conjugate (tetanus toxoid)[d]	Bacterial polysaccharide-protein conjugate	IM
Hib conjugate (meningococcal protein conjugate)	Bacterial polysaccharide-protein conjugate	IM
Human papillomavirus (9vHPV)	Recombinant viral antigens	IM
Influenza (IIV)	Inactivated viral components	IM
Influenza (IIV)	Inactivated viral components	ID[e]
Influenza (LAIV)	Live attenuated viruses	Intranasal
Japanese encephalitis	Inactivated virus	IM
Meningococcal ACWY conjugate (MCV4 or MenACWY)	Bacterial polysaccharide-protein conjugate	IM

Table 1.7. Vaccines Approved or Authorized by Emergency Use Authorization for Immunization and Distributed in the United States and Their Routes of Administration,[a] continued

Vaccine	Type	Route of Administration
Meningococcal serogroup B (MenB)	Bacterial recombinant protein	IM
MMR	Live attenuated viruses	SC or IM[f]
MMRV	Live attenuated viruses	SC or IM
Pneumococcal polysaccharide (PPSV)	Bacterial polysaccharide	IM or SC
Pneumococcal conjugate (PCV)	Bacterial polysaccharide-protein conjugate	IM
Poliovirus (IPV)	Inactivated viruses	SC or IM
Rabies	Inactivated virus	IM
Rotavirus (RV1 and RV5)	Live attenuated virus	Oral
Tetanus-diphtheria (Td)	Toxoids	IM
Tdap	Toxoids and inactivated bacterial components	IM
Typhoid	Bacterial capsular polysaccharide	IM
Typhoid	Live attenuated bacteria	Oral
Varicella (VAR)	Live attenuated virus	SC or IM
Yellow fever	Live attenuated virus	SC
Zoster (RZV)	Recombinant viral antigens	IM

BCG indicates bacille Calmette-Guérin; ID, intradermal; SC, subcutaneous; IM, intramuscular; DTaP, diphtheria and tetanus toxoids and acellular pertussis, adsorbed; IPV, inactivated poliovirus; Hib, *Haemophilus influenzae* type b; PRP-T, polyribosylribitol phosphate-tetanus toxoid; HPV, human papillomavirus; MMR, live measles, mumps, rubella; MMRV, live measles, mumps, rubella, varicella (monovalent measles, mumps, and rubella components are not being produced in the United States); Td, tetanus and diphtheria toxoids (for children 7 years of age or older and adults); Tdap, tetanus toxoid, reduced diphtheria toxoid, and acellular pertussis; RZV, recombinant zoster vaccine.

[a] Other vaccines approved in the United States but not distributed include adenovirus (types 4, 7), anthrax, Ebola, plague, smallpox (ACAM2000), H5N1 influenza vaccines, influenza A (H1N1) monovalent 2009 vaccine, JE-virus vaccine (JE-VAX), pneumococcal conjugate vaccine (PCV7 and PCV13), HepB-Hib (Comvax), quadrivalent HPV vaccine (Gardasil), and bivalent HPV vaccine (Cervarix). The FDA maintains a website listing currently approved vaccines in the United States (**www.fda.gov/vaccines-blood-biologics/vaccines/vaccines-licensed-use-united-states**). The AAP maintains a website (**http://publications.aap.org/redbook/resources/15449**) showing status of licensure and recommendations for newer vaccines.

[b] Anthrax vaccine is not approved for use in children (**https://pediatrics.aappublications.org/content/133/5/e1411**). Federal/state authorities would oversee emergency use under an investigational new drug application for children, should the need arise.

[c] Dengue vaccine is approved only for individuals 6 through 16 years of age with laboratory-confirmed prior dengue infection and living in areas with endemic infection.

[d] See Table 3.12, p 406.

[e] Intradermal influenza vaccine is recommended only for people 18 through 64 years of age.

[f] PRIORIX is administered only SC, while M-M-R-II can be administered SC or IM.

Viruses and bacteria in non-live vaccines cannot replicate in or be excreted by the vaccine recipient as infectious agents and, thus, do not present the same safety concerns for immunosuppressed vaccine recipients or contacts of vaccine recipients as might live attenuated vaccines. For example, live rotavirus vaccines pose risk and are contraindicated in children with severe combined immunodeficiency disease. Furthermore, the AAP, the Advisory Committee on Immunization Practices (ACIP) of the CDC, and the Healthcare Infection Control Practices Advisory Committee (HICPAC) recommend against administering live attenuated influenza vaccine to close contacts and caregivers of severely immunosuppressed people who require a protected environment.

Messenger RNA (mRNA) vaccines contain mRNA that encodes for an antigen based on a pathogen-specific protein (or portion of a protein), and expression of the antigen by host cells induces an immune response to the antigen. For example, mRNA COVID-19 vaccines encode for all or a portion of the spike protein of SARS-CoV-2.

Recommendations for dose, vaccine storage and handling (see Vaccine Handling and Storage, p 45), route and technique of administration (see Vaccine Administration, p 52), and immunization schedules should be followed for predictable, effective protection (also see disease-specific chapters in Section 3). Adherence to recommended guidance in terms of sequence, timing, route of administration, and dosage is critical to the success of immunization practices at both the individual and the societal levels.

Vaccine Ingredients

As part of the licensure process, the US Food and Drug Administration (FDA) reviews laboratory and clinical data on vaccines to ensure their safety and effectiveness. For each licensed vaccine, the FDA-approved prescribing information, commonly known as the package insert, contains information on the vaccine and lists antigens and other ingredients, each of which serves a specific purpose. A catalog of package inserts for vaccines currently licensed for use in the United States is available at **www.fda.gov/vaccines-blood-biologics/vaccines/vaccines-licensed-use-united-states.** A summary table of ingredients other than antigens (excipients) that are used in vaccines can be accessed at **www.cdc.gov/vaccines/pubs/pinkbook/downloads/appendices/B/excipient-table-2.pdf.** Additional information is available at **www.fda.gov/vaccines-blood-biologics/safety-availability-biologics/common-ingredients-us-licensed-vaccines.**

Allergic reactions may occur if the vaccine recipient is allergic to any ingredient in the vaccine. Therefore, careful screening for allergy to a vaccine or a vaccine component is indicated. Standardized screening checklists are available to assist clinicians in screening for allergies and other potential contraindications to vaccines. An example can be found at **www.immunize.org/catg.d/p4060.pdf.** The safety of vaccines licensed for use in the United States is continuously monitored by the FDA and the Centers for Disease Control and Prevention (CDC). In addition to antigens, vaccines may also contain conjugates, adjuvants, stabilizers, preservatives, antibiotics, and diluents. These and other vaccine ingredients (eg, cell culture media) are listed in vaccine package inserts. Vaccine package inserts can be found at **www.fda.gov/vaccines-blood-biologics/vaccines/vaccines-licensed-use-united-states** and **www.immunize.org/fda/.**

ANTIGENS

Antigens in vaccines, sometimes referred to as immunogens, are viruses, bacteria, viral or bacterial components, or toxoids that result in active immunization, which is the process by which a person becomes protected from a disease. New generation vaccines contain messenger RNA (mRNA) encoding for antigens or for viral vectors that express antigens. Some vaccines consist of one or more antigens that are highly defined constituents (eg, tetanus and diphtheria toxoids). Some vaccines consist of multiple antigens, which vary in chemical composition, structure, and number (eg, acellular components in pertussis vaccines; polysaccharide protein conjugates in multivalent pneumococcal conjugate vaccine and serogroups A, C, W, and Y meningococcal conjugate vaccines; and recombinant proteins in 9-valent human papillomavirus vaccine). Other vaccines contain live attenuated viruses (eg, measles, mumps, and rubella vaccine [MMR]), live reassorted viruses (eg, rotavirus vaccine [RV]), or killed whole cell viruses (eg, non-live poliovirus vaccine and hepatitis A vaccine [HepA]). FDA-approved or authorized vaccines to prevent COVID-19 contain nucleoside-modified mRNA encoding the viral spike glycoprotein of SARS-CoV-2, a recombinant spike protein, or a replication-incompetent adenovirus vector expressing spike protein.

CONJUGATES

Conjugates are proteins that chemically combine with polysaccharide antigens to increase immunogenicity and induce immunological memory. Conjugates improve immune response for children younger than 18 months who do not consistently respond to polysaccharide antigens. Conjugates also boost antibody response to multiple doses of a vaccine. Some vaccines (eg, *Haemophilus influenzae* type b [Hib] and certain pneumococcal and meningococcal vaccines) include polysaccharide antigens chemically conjugated to protein carriers with proven immunologic potential (eg, non-toxic mutant of diphtheria toxin [CRM_{197}], tetanus toxoid protein, and meningococcal outer membrane protein complex).

ADJUVANTS

Adjuvants are vaccine ingredients that improve the immune response to antigens but do not themselves provide immunity. Adjuvants stimulate an immune response via cytokine release. Not all vaccines use adjuvants. For example, live vaccines such as MMR, varicella (VAR), and RV vaccines do not include adjuvants. Because the purpose of adjuvants is to generate stronger immune response, adjuvanted vaccines may cause local and systemic reactions more frequently compared with nonadjuvanted vaccines. Adjuvants have been used in vaccines in the United States for decades. Aluminum salts, a class of adjuvants that has been used safely in the United States since the 1930s and remains widely in use, are often in vaccines that contain subunit antigens of a cell (eg, hepatitis B vaccine [HepB]) or toxoids (eg, diphtheria and tetanus toxoids). Newer adjuvants currently in use in the United States are generally limited to certain vaccines approved for use only in adults. They include oil-in-water emulsions (used in adjuvanted non-live influenza vaccine [IIV]), deacylated monophosphoryl lipid A and saponin in a liposomal formulation (used in recombinant zoster vaccine), and cytosine-phosphate-guanine enriched oligodeoxynucleotide motifs (used in Heplisav-B, which is a HepB formulation). Adjuvants can also allow for "antigen sparing," in which a reduced amount of antigen can stimulate an equivalent immune response because of the presence of an adjuvant. Adjuvants also permit the production of multifold numbers of vaccine doses from a limited antigen supply when large numbers of people need them, such as during an influenza pandemic.

STABILIZERS

Stabilizers are ingredients used in vaccines to help ensure that vaccine potency is not affected by adverse conditions such as heat and abnormal pH during the vaccine manufacturing process or during transport and storage. Stabilizers used in vaccines include sugars (eg, lactose or sucrose in Hib), amino acids (eg, arginine or monosodium salt of glutamic acid in live attenuated influenza vaccine), or proteins (eg, gelatin in VAR and MMR).

PRESERVATIVES

Preservatives are included in multidose vials of vaccines as a safety measure to prevent the growth of microorganisms that may be introduced into the vaccine when the vial is penetrated repeatedly to withdraw doses of the vaccine. Examples of preservatives include thimerosal, formaldehyde, and phenol derivatives. Thimerosal is an ethyl mercury-containing organic compound that has been widely used as a preservative in many vaccines since the 1930s to help prevent contamination. Although there are minor side effects associated with vaccines containing thimerosal, such as redness and swelling at the injection site, thimerosal in vaccines has a long and strong safety record. Regardless, all routinely recommended vaccines for infants and children in the United States are available thimerosal free. IIV for pediatric use is available in thimerosal-free or thimerosal-containing (for multidose vials) formulations. Additional information on thimerosal in vaccines is available from the FDA at **www.fda.gov/vaccines-blood-biologics/safety-availability-biologics/thimerosal-and-vaccines.** Formaldehyde is used in vaccines to detoxify bacterial toxins (eg, diphtheria and tetanus toxoids) and inactivate viruses (eg, several IIV formulations). Although almost all formaldehyde is removed during the production of vaccines that use formaldehyde, very low amounts may remain. Formaldehyde exposure at such a residual level is far less than what occurs naturally in the environment. Phenols are used as a preservative in the 23-valent pneumococcal polysaccharide vaccine.

ANTIBIOTICS

As a class of preservatives, antibiotics are sometimes used during the vaccine manufacturing process to inhibit bacterial growth, and trace amounts can remain in the final product. Antibiotics such as neomycin, gentamicin, and polymyxin B are used during production of several IIV formulations. Other vaccines that have trace amounts of antibiotics include MMR and HepA.

DILUENTS

Some vaccines are supplied as a lyophilized powder that must be reconstituted with their supplied liquid diluent prior to use. For some vaccines, the diluent is sterile water (eg, measles, mumps, rubella, and varicella [MMRV]) and for others it is sodium chloride (eg, Hib). Certain multicomponent vaccines include a lyophilized component with some vaccine antigens and a diluent with the other vaccine antigens in solution (eg, diphtheria and tetanus toxoids and acellular pertussis, adsorbed; non-live poliovirus; Hib [Pentacel]; and serogroups A, C, W, and Y meningococcal conjugate vaccine [Menveo]). Certain adjuvanted vaccines include a lyophilized component with the vaccine antigen and a diluent with the adjuvant component (eg, recombinant zoster vaccine). Diluents are specifically formulated for each vaccine. Therefore, only the specific diluent supplied for each vaccine should be used.

Vaccine Handling and Storage

For vaccines to be optimally effective, they must be stored properly from the time of manufacturing until they are administered. Immunization providers are responsible for proper storage and handling from the time the vaccine arrives at their facility until the vaccine is administered. All staff should be knowledgeable about the importance of proper storage and handling of vaccines and the implications of improper storage and handling. The administration of improperly stored and handled vaccines is a frequent error reported to the Vaccine Adverse Event Reporting System (VAERS) (see Understanding Vaccine Evaluation and Safety as an Approach to Addressing Parental Concerns, p 27).

Recommendations for handling and storage of vaccines are summarized in the package insert for each product (**www.fda.gov/vaccines-blood-biologics/vaccines/vaccines-licensed-use-united-states**) and should be reviewed. Additional information can be obtained directly from manufacturers. Contact information for manufacturers is available online (**www.cdc.gov/vaccines/hcp/admin/storage/downloads/manufact-dist-contact.pdf**). The Centers for Disease Control and Prevention (CDC) has online training and other resources including:

- You Call the Shots: Vaccine Storage and Handling is a free, online training module focused on storage and handling requirements (**www.cdc.gov/vaccines/ed/youcalltheshots.html**).
- Vaccine Storage and Handling toolkit is a useful resource for quality-control systems for safe handling and storage of vaccines in an office or clinic setting (**www.cdc.gov/vaccines/hcp/admin/storage/toolkit/storage-handling-toolkit.pdf**).

A written detailed vaccine-specific storage and handling plan should be available for reference by all staff members and kept on or near the unit used for storing vaccines. The plan should be updated annually and when new vaccines are added to the inventory. It should outline standard operating procedures for both routine management of vaccines and emergency measures for vaccine retrieval and storage, and should include documentation of these activities.

Most, but not all vaccines are designated for optimal storage between +2°C and +8°C (+36°F and +46°F). For the most current information, check the manufacturer's package insert. It is imperative that great care be taken to avoid exposing refrigerated vaccines to freezing temperatures, even for brief periods. Such exposure can compromise the integrity of refrigerated vaccines even without generating ice crystals or other changes in physical appearance of the vaccine. Visual inspection cannot reliably detect a vaccine that has been compromised by freeze exposure; thus, only the careful monitoring of the temperatures used to store these vaccines will allow identification of potentially altered vaccines. Refrigerator or freezer thermostats should be set at the factory-set or midpoint temperature, which will decrease the likelihood of temperature excursions.

Vaccines exposed to temperatures outside their approved storage ranges are generally considered ineffective, especially when no records exist about the temperature excursion or light exposure. They should be segregated in a bag or container, marked **"Do Not Use,"** and kept under the appropriate storage conditions (vaccine refrigerator or freezer). If it is a frozen vaccine that has been thawed, store in the refrigerator between 2°C and 8°C (36°F and 46°F) until manufacturer guidance is received, as refreezing the vaccine may damage it. The affected vaccines should not be used until the specifics of the temperature excursion are reviewed and it has been determined the vaccines can be administered. Protocols after the event vary depending on individual state or agency policies. Providers should contact their state immunization program, vaccine manufacturer, or both for guidance. Advice regarding disposition of improperly handled or stored vaccines should be documented. In general, manufacturers analyze information about the magnitude of the temperature excursion and the total amount of time that temperatures were out of range, as well as information about the vaccine in question, to determine whether a vaccine is likely to still be viable. Ideally, a temperature excursion should be immediately identified and immunization using affected vaccine halted until a vaccine viability determination can be made. If vaccine exposed to a temperature excursion is administered and subsequently determined not to be viable, the doses administered using the nonviable vaccine should be considered invalid. Providers should refer to state or agency policy on management of patients in receipt of invalid doses because of temperature excursion and vaccine administration errors. Manufacturers can be asked about possible replacement of nonviable vaccine.

Many vaccines should be protected from light prior to preparation and administration. Protection from light exposure can be accomplished by keeping each vial or syringe in its original carton while in recommended storage and until immediate use.

The diluent component of vaccines that need reconstitution may require storage at a different temperature than the antigen component and generally cannot be frozen. For appropriate storage of the diluent component, the recommendations in the package insert should be followed.

PERSONNEL

A primary staff vaccine coordinator and an alternate vaccine coordinator should be trained and responsible for vaccine storage and handling. In addition, a physician or manager with understanding of the importance of appropriate vaccine storage should be engaged with the responsible vaccine coordinating staff. The CDC offers online training on vaccine storage and handling, and information can be found at **www2a.cdc.gov/nip/isd/ycts/mod1/courses/sh/ce.asp.** Vaccine coordinators and all staff handling vaccines should have training and education on vaccine storage and handling as part of new employee orientation, annually (refresher training), when new vaccines are added to the inventory, and when recommendations for storage and handling of vaccines are updated (**www.cdc.gov/vaccines/ed/courses.html**). Document staff training with dates and participant names. The vaccine coordinator should be responsible for:
- Ordering vaccines.
- Overseeing proper receipt and storage of vaccine deliveries.
- Documenting vaccine inventory information.

- Organizing vaccines in storage units.
- Setting up temperature-monitoring devices.
- Checking and recording storage unit temperatures on a log (at the start of each workday if using a device that displays minimum/maximum temperatures or the current temperature at the start and end of the workday if using a device that does not display minimum/maximum temperatures).
- Reviewing and analyzing temperature data at least weekly for any shifts in temperature trends.
- Daily physical inspection of the storage unit.
- Rotating stock at least weekly so that vaccines closest to expiration date are used first.
- Contacting the state Vaccines for Children (VFC) program vaccine coordinator if it appears that VFC vaccines will expire before they will be used in the practice.
- Monitoring expiration dates and ensuring expired vaccines are removed from the refrigerator/freezer.
- Responding to potential storage temperature excursions and calling the manufacturer, VFC program, or both to obtain guidance for temperature excursion events.
- Overseeing proper vaccine transport, either routine or in an emergency.
- Maintaining all appropriate vaccine storage and handling documentation, such as inventory and temperature logs, including temperature excursion responses.
- Maintaining storage equipment and records, including VFC program documentation.
- Informing all people who will be handling vaccines about specific storage requirements and stability limitations of the products they will encounter. The details of proper storage conditions should be posted on or near each refrigerator or freezer used for vaccine storage or should be readily available to staff. Receptionists, mail clerks, and other staff members who also may receive shipments should be educated in these matters as well.
- Overseeing emergency preparations, such as tracking inclement weather conditions and ensuring appropriate handling of vaccines during a disaster or power outage.

EQUIPMENT

STORAGE UNITS

- Store vaccines in refrigerator and freezer units that can maintain the appropriate temperature range and are large enough to maintain the largest anticipated inventory without crowding. Use purpose-built or pharmaceutical-grade units designed to either refrigerate or freeze. These units can be compact, under-the-counter style, or large.
- Household-grade units can be an acceptable alternative to pharmaceutical-grade or purpose-built vaccine storage units in some situations. However, these units should be replaced with stand-alone units as soon as is practical. Household-grade units are primarily designed for home use. The freezer compartment is not recommended to store vaccines, and certain areas of the refrigerator should be avoided as well, including directly under cooling vents, in deli, fruit, or vegetable drawers, or in door shelves, because of instability of temperatures and air flow in these areas. A separate freezer unit is necessary if the facility provides frozen vaccines.
- Dormitory-style or bar-style combined refrigerator/freezer units are not acceptable for vaccine storage under any circumstances and are not allowed for vaccine storage of VFC program products. These units have a single exterior door and an evaporator

plate/cooling coil, usually located in an icemaker/freezer compartment. These units pose a significant risk of freezing vaccine, even when used for temporary storage.

- Inspection of door seals, vacuuming coils, and other maintenance of refrigeration units should be performed at least annually.
- Use refrigerators with wire—not glass—shelving to improve air circulation in the unit, and do not place bins or boxes against rear or side walls of the refrigerator.

TEMPERATURE MONITORING DEVICE

- The CDC recommends that each vaccine storage unit and each transport unit (emergency or nonemergency) should be monitored by a digital data logger (DDL). At least one back-up DDL is recommended in case of breakage.
- Recommended DDL features include:
  - Accuracy of $+/- 0.5°C$ (1°F)
  - The temperature-monitoring device should be capable of continuous frequent measurements (no less frequently than every 30 minutes)
  - Detachable probe that best reflects vaccine temperatures, such as those in a temperature buffer (eg, biosafe glycol, glass beads, sand, Teflon)
  - Display current minimum and maximum temperatures, and these should be readable without opening the unit door
  - An alarm for out-of-range temperatures and a low-battery indicator
- The buffered probe(s) should be located in the center of the vaccines, away from the walls, vents, and floor of the vaccine storage unit. Temperature data should be displayed graphically and should be able to be stored for 3 years.
- The temperature-monitoring device with buffered probe should have a Certificate of Calibration Testing (also known as Report of Calibration). Such temperature-monitoring devices have been individually tested for accuracy against a recognized reference standard by a laboratory with accreditation from an International Laboratory Accreditation Cooperation (ILAC) Mutual Recognition Arrangement (MRA) signatory body, or by a laboratory or manufacturer with documentation that calibration testing performed meets ISO/IEC 17025 international standards for calibration testing and traceability. These devices are sold with an individually numbered certificate documenting this testing. Providers who receive VFC vaccines or other vaccines purchased with public funds should consult their state's immunization program regarding the required methods and timeframe for temperature-monitoring device calibration testing. The National Institute of Standards and Technology maintains a website devoted to vaccine storage education (**www.nist.gov/programs-projects/reliable-vaccine-storage**). Calibration testing and traceability must be performed every 1 to 2 years from the last calibration testing date (date certificate issued) or suggested calibration timelines from the manufacturer of the device must be used. Temperature accuracy of temperature-monitoring devices can be checked using an ice melting point test (**www.nist.gov/pml/div685/grp01/upload/Ice-Melting-Point-Validation-Method-for-Data-Loggers.pdf**). Providers should check with their state VFC program for specific requirements related to calibration testing of temperature-monitoring devices. Do not drill through the refrigerator or freezer to route a temperature probe.
- Providers should use a remote alarm notification system that sends an alert if the temperature is out of range. These alarms usually have the capability to send

notifications via email, telephone, or text. Redundant, multiple alerts are recommended to ensure receipt. Provision should be made to ensure alerts are still sent if there is loss of power and/or internet.

PROCEDURES

- Maintain a vaccine inventory log, which should include vaccine name, number of doses, arrival condition of the vaccine, manufacturer and lot numbers, and expiration date. If the shipment includes lyophilized (freeze-dried) vaccines, ensure they came with the correct type and quantity of diluents.
- Formally accept vaccine on receipt of shipment: .
  - Ensure that the expiration date of the delivered product has not passed and identify any soon-to-expire products.
  - Examine the merchandise and its shipping container for any evidence of damage during transport.
  - Determine whether the interval between shipment from the supplier and arrival of the product at its destination is within the allowable limit noted on the shipping insert or container and whether the product has been exposed to excessive heat or cold that might alter its integrity. Review vaccine time and temperature indicators, both chemical and electronic, if included in the vaccine shipment.
  - Find and inspect any temperature excursion devices (electronic or temperature-tape) in the shipment for evidence of temperature excursions. Do not accept the shipment if reasonable suspicion exists that the delivered product may have been damaged by environmental insult or improper handling during transport.
    - However, if you are a VFC provider, do not refuse vaccine shipments. In the case of vaccine shipment compromise or a problem with the temperature monitors, the VFC provider must contact the McKesson Specialty Contact Center and/or the VFC program immediately using the telephone number dedicated to receiving provider calls about vaccine usability: 1-877-TEMP123.
  - Contact the vaccine supplier or manufacturer when unusual circumstances raise questions about the stability of a delivered vaccine. Store suspect vaccine under proper conditions and label it **"Do Not Use"** until the usability has been determined.
- Inspect the refrigerator and freezer:
  - A **"Do Not Unplug"** sign should be affixed directly next to the refrigerator electrical outlet and to the circuit breaker controlling that circuit.
- Train and designate staff to respond immediately to temperature recordings outside the recommended range and to document response and outcome.
- Establish routine procedures:
  - Store vaccine where temperature remains constant.
  - Store vaccines according to temperatures specified in the package insert.
  - Check and record the minimum/maximum temperature at the beginning of each workday.
  - Rotate vaccine supplies so that the shortest-dated vaccines are in front to reduce wastage because of expiration.
  - Inspect the unit weekly for outdated vaccine and either dispose of or return expired products appropriately.

- Promptly remove expired (outdated) vaccines and diluents from inventory and dispose of them appropriately or return to manufacturer to avoid accidental use.
- Store both opened and unopened vials in the original packaging, which facilitates temperature stability, inventory management, and rotation of vaccine by expiration date and avoids light exposure. Mark the outside of boxes of opened vaccines with a large "X" to indicate that they have been opened.
- Keep opened vials of vaccine in a tray so that they are readily identifiable.
- Indicate on the label of each vaccine vial the date and time the vaccine was reconstituted or first opened.
- Prepare vaccine just prior to administration. Avoid reconstituting multiple doses of vaccine or drawing up multiple doses of vaccine in multiple syringes. Predrawing vaccine increases the possibility of medication errors and causes uncertainty of vaccine stability.
- Because different vaccines can share similar components/names (eg, diphtheria and tetanus and acellular pertussis vaccines [DTaP and Tdap], or pneumococcal, meningococcal, and influenza products), care should be taken during storage to ensure that the different products are stored separately in a manner to avoid confusion and possible medication errors. CDC vaccine storage labels (**www.cdc. gov/vaccines/hcp/admin/storage/guide/vaccine-storage-labels.pdf**) help to easily identify and organize vaccines within the storage unit.
- Each vaccine and diluent vial should be inspected carefully for damage or contamination prior to use.
- The expiration date should be checked prior to preparation and administration. For all licensed vaccines, the expiration date is printed on the carton. Additionally, the expiration date may be printed on the container (eg, vial or syringe) label or may be accessed by scanning a barcode. For vaccines authorized for use under emergency use authorization, the expiration date may not be printed on the carton or container labels; instead, the date of manufacture is printed on the carton. In such cases, the expiration date must be accessed elsewhere (eg, barcode scan, website). The Fact Sheet for Health Care Providers may also provide the calculated expiration date based on the date of manufacture. Ensure staff are knowledgeable regarding how to determine the expiration date of the vaccines and diluents in the facility's inventory. Expired vaccine or diluent should never be used. When the expiration date has only a month and year, the product may be used up to and including the last day of that month. If a day is included with the month and year, the product may only be used through the end of that day. Regardless of expiration date, vaccine and diluent should only be used as long as their appearance is as described in the product package insert and they have been stored and handled properly.
- Beyond-use date/time (BUD): Some vaccines have a BUD, which is calculated based on the date the vial is first entered and the storage information in the package insert. If the vaccine has no BUD, use the expiration date provided by the manufacturer. The BUD replaces but never exceeds the product's expiration date. Once calculated, the BUD should be noted on the label along with the initials of the person making the calculation. Examples of BUDs include some vaccines in multidose vials, a reconstituted vaccine, and manufacturer-shortened expiration dates. BUD information is available in the product package insert.

- All reconstituted vaccines should be administered as soon as possible after reconstitution and within the time interval specified in the package insert.
- Always store vaccines in the refrigerator or freezer as indicated until immediately prior to administration.
- Do not keep food or drink in refrigerators in which vaccine is stored. This will reduce frequent opening of the unit that leads to thermal instability.
- Do not store radioactive materials in the same refrigerator in which vaccines are stored.
- Discuss with all clinic or office personnel any violation of protocol for handling vaccines or any accidental temperature excursion. Determine the root cause and put strategies in place to prevent it from happening again. Follow temperature excursion procedures until the vaccine manufacturers can be contacted to determine the disposition of the affected vaccine.

SUMMARY

Best equipment and practices for storage of refrigerated vaccines are as follows:
1. Purpose-built or pharmaceutical-grade refrigerator is recommended for vaccine storage.
   a. Wire shelving—not glass—and an interior circulating fan.
2. A digital data logger with a buffered probe should be placed in the center of the vaccines within each storage unit.
   a. Displays with current temperature and resettable maximum and minimum temperatures visible on the outside of the unit.
   b. Audible temperature alarm with capability for rapid user notification via phone/text message/email should temperature excursion be detected.
3. Household-grade units can be used to store vaccines. However, the freezer compartment of this type of unit is not recommended to store vaccines. If the facility provides vaccines that must be stored frozen, a separate freezer unit is necessary.
   a. Extra space in a household-grade unit should be filled with water bottles to serve as a cold mass and to prolong safe storage in the event of refrigerator failure. Follow manufacturer's guidance for purpose-built and pharmaceutical-grade vaccine storage units because this practice may not be necessary or recommended in those units.

VACCINE TRANSPORT

Transport of vaccines is not routinely recommended but may be necessary in emergency situations (eg, entire stock is being relocated for its protection) and may be appropriate for off-site clinics or when relocation of stock is required (eg, another site needs your excess supply). Vaccines should only be transported, even for short distances, using appropriate packing materials that provide the maximum protections. Portable vaccine refrigerator or freezer units are preferred, but qualified containers and packouts may also be used for either emergency or other necessary vaccine transport. The conditioned water bottle transport system may only be used for emergency transport. The manufacturer's original shipping container may only be used in an emergency as a last resort. Soft-sided food and beverage coolers should never be used; however, soft-sided containers engineered specifically for vaccine transport may be used. Phase change materials at +4°C to +5°C (+39°F to +41°F) can be purchased to maintain proper temperatures. Follow the manufacturer's instructions for use to reduce the risk of freezing vaccines during transport.

- Do not use frozen gel packs or coolant packs from original vaccine shipments to pack refrigerated vaccines. They can still freeze vaccines even if they are conditioned or appear to be "sweating."
- Use a continuous temperature-monitoring device, preferably a digital data logger with a probe that best reflects vaccine temperatures such as a buffered probe, for monitoring and recording temperatures while transporting vaccines. Place the buffered probe directly with the vaccines.
  - Keep the temperature-monitoring device display outside of the transport unit so the temperature can be seen easily without opening the container.
  - Use a temperature log to record transport unit temperatures.
- Ensure staff are trained on emergency procedures, and roles and responsibilities are clearly detailed in a written plan that is easily accessible to all staff.

EMERGENCY VACCINE STORAGE AND HANDLING

In addition to emergency transport instructions, practices should develop a written plan for emergency management of vaccine in the event of a catastrophic event or malfunction of the storage unit, train personnel, and make the plan easily accessible. Refrigerators vary and may maintain their +2°C to +8°C temperature for only 2 to 3 hours without power. This plan should include establishing an agreement with at least one alternate storage facility even if you have a generator or battery-powered back-up equipment. Ensure 24-hour access to alternate facilities as well as after-hours access to your own facility. Refer to emergency transport plans in the event you need to move vaccine to an alternate facility.

After a power outage or mechanical failure, it should not be assumed that vaccine exposed to temperature above the recommended range is unusable without first contacting the vaccine manufacturer (or, for VFC vaccines, the McKesson Specialty Contact Center at 1-877-TEMP123 and/or VFC program) for guidance before discarding vaccine. Guidance on vaccine transport is available from CDC (**www.cdc.gov/vaccines/hcp/admin/storage/toolkit/index.html**).

Vaccine Administration

GENERAL CONSIDERATIONS

Proper vaccine administration is critical to ensure safe and effective delivery of the vaccine antigen to the recipient. Practices are advised to identify an individual(s) to serve as vaccine champion whose job description includes keeping vaccine operations and staff education current. Health care personnel who administer vaccines should be trained in proper vaccine preparation, administration, infection control practices, and care of patients before and after vaccine administration, including considerations for needle anxiety, needlestick pain, and potential injection site pain after vaccination. The complete Advisory Committee on Immunization Practices (ACIP) guidance for vaccine administration is available as a resource at **www.cdc.gov/vaccines/hcp/acip-recs/general-recs/administration.html**.

TRAINING AND EDUCATION. Competency-based training on vaccination, including a post-vaccine administration observation component, should be integrated into existing staff education programs such as new staff orientation and annual continuing education requirements. Numerous in-person and online vaccination training opportunities are available, including the web-based education and training modules available at **www.aap.org/en-us/advocacy-and-policy/aap-health-initiatives/immunizations/Practice-Management/Pages/Vaccine-Administration.aspx** and **www.cdc.gov/vaccines/ed/index.html.** Additionally, demonstration videos and other resources can be found at **www.aap.org/en/patient-care/immunizations/implementing-immunization-administration-in-your-practice/vaccine-administration, www.cdc.gov/vaccines/hcp/admin/resource-library.html,** and **immunize.org/clinic/administering-vaccines.asp.**

INFECTION CONTROL. Health care personnel who administer vaccines should take appropriate precautions to protect themselves and minimize the risk of disease spread. Proper hand hygiene is required before preparing and administering vaccines and with each new patient contact. The use of gloves is not required when administering vaccines unless the health care provider has an open lesion on the hand, if contact with body fluids is anticipated, or when gloves are required because of isolation precautions for the patient. Proper hand hygiene should be practiced whether or not gloves are used, and gloves should be changed between patients. Syringes and needles must be sterile and not reused. Discard used syringes and needles promptly in a proper puncture-proof, labeled container located in the room where the vaccine is administered. To prevent inadvertent needlesticks or reuse, needles should not be recapped after use; the use of safety needles is preferred.

VACCINE PREPARATION. Vaccines and diluents should be used only if they have been stored and handled properly. Vaccines should be prepared following the manufacturer's guidance and immediately before administration using aseptic technique. If the vaccine requires reconstitution or dilution, only the diluent supplied for that vaccine should be used. Each vaccine and diluent should be carefully inspected for damages on the container or vial and evidence of contamination (eg, unusual coloration or sediments). The expiration date for both the vaccine and diluent should be checked to ensure that the vaccine and diluent have not expired. Some vaccines in a multidose vial should be used within a certain timeframe after the initial puncture to the vial septum ("beyond use date/time," or BUD); the BUD on the package insert should be identified and noted on the vial. Vaccine should not be administered after the BUD. Changing needles between drawing vaccine into a syringe and its administration is not necessary unless the needle has been damaged.

PATIENT CARE BEFORE, DURING, AND AFTER VACCINE ADMINISTRATION. Before administering any vaccine, patients should be screened for contraindications and precautions, even if the patient has previously received that vaccine. The patient's health condition or recommendations regarding contraindications or precautions for vaccination may change from one visit to the next. To assess patients correctly and consistently, a standardized, comprehensive screening tool is recommended. An example of screening checklist for contraindications for vaccines can be found at

www.immunize.org/catg.d/p4060.pdf. Health care personnel are required to provide the vaccine information sheet (VIS) for the patient, and the VIS can also be used as a tool to inform and counsel the patient on the vaccine. Because of the rare possibility of a severe allergic reaction to a vaccine or its components, health care personnel who administer vaccines should be able to recognize, treat, and report allergic reactions, including anaphylaxis (see Hypersensitivity Reactions After Immunization, p 71).

A patient should be comfortably seated or lying down before an injection and, if necessary, safely restrained (see Managing Injection Pain, p 57). Syncope can occur following vaccine administration, particularly in adolescents and young adults. Health care personnel should take appropriate measures to prevent injuries if weakness, dizziness, or loss of consciousness occurs. However, syncope can occur without presyncopal symptoms, so patients should be seated or lying down during vaccination. A 15-minute observation period (with the patient sitting or lying down) is advised after all vaccine administration to avoid the risk of injury if syncope occurs. Syncope following vaccination is not a contraindication to that or any other vaccine in the future. Any clinically significant adverse event that occurs during or following vaccine administration should be reported to the Vaccine Adverse Event Reporting System (VAERS) (see Understanding Vaccine Evaluation and Safety as an Approach to Addressing Parental Concerns, p 27).

Patient education should include a discussion of comfort and care after vaccination. These instructions should include information for dealing with common side effects such as injection site pain, fever, and fussiness (especially in infants) and should provide guidance about when to seek medical attention and when to notify the health care provider about concerns that arise following vaccination.

SITES AND ROUTES OF VACCINE ADMINISTRATION

Each vaccine has a specific administration route: parenteral, oral, or intranasal. Parenteral routes include intramuscular (IM) and subcutaneous (SC) injections; intradermal (ID) vaccines are not routinely used in children in the United States. Additional information is available at **www.aap.org/en/patient-care/immunizations/implementing-immunization-administration-in-your-practice/vaccine-administration** and **www.cdc.gov/vaccines/hcp/admin/admin-protocols.html.**

PARENTERAL VACCINATION. Approved sites and routes of administration can be found in package inserts of vaccines and in Table 1.7 (p 40). When multiple parenteral vaccines are indicated, separate injection sites should be used. If the same limb must be used as the injection site for 2 or more vaccinations, separate injections by at least 1 inch so that local reactions can be differentiated if they develop. Multiple vaccines should not be mixed in a single syringe. In sequencing the vaccinations, vaccines that are more reactive/likely to cause an injection site reaction (eg, diphtheria and tetanus toxoids and acellular pertussis, pneumococcal conjugate vaccine) should be administered in different limbs if possible, and vaccines that are more painful (eg, human papillomavirus; measles, mumps, and rubella [MMR]) should be administered last (see Simultaneous Administration of Multiple Vaccines, p 63).

IM Administration. Most vaccines are administered intramuscularly. Vaccines administered intramuscularly should be injected in a 90° angle at a site that minimizes risks
for neural, vascular, or tissue injury. Vaccinators should be familiar with the anatomy
of the area of the identified site (vastus lateralis or deltoid muscles) to correctly identify where to inject vaccine. For IM injections, the site of choice between thigh and
arm depends on the age of the vaccine recipient, degree of muscle development, and
thickness of adipose tissue at the injection site. In children younger than 2 years, the
anterolateral aspect of the upper thigh provides the largest muscle and is the preferred
site. In older children, the deltoid muscle is usually large enough for IM injection.
Decisions on needle length should be based on the size of the muscle and the thickness of adipose tissue at the injection site. Needles should be long enough to reach the
muscle mass and prevent vaccine from seeping into subcutaneous tissue and causing
local reactions but not so long as to reach underlying nerves, blood vessels, or bone.
Aspiration after injection is not needed and can increase pain at the injection site. The
use of a 22- to 25-gauge needle generally is recommended for IM injections. Suggested
needle lengths are described in Table 1.8. Note that the upper, outer aspect of buttocks
generally should not be used for vaccination, because the gluteal region is covered by a
significant layer of subcutaneous fat. Because of diminished immunogenicity, hepatitis
B and rabies vaccines should not be administered in the buttocks at any age. Localized
swelling, redness, and pain can occur at the IM injection site, but serious complications are rare. Reported adverse events include infections, bleeding, nerve injury, and
shoulder injury related to vaccine administration (SIRVA) from inadvertent injection
into the joint space. In general, vaccines containing adjuvants (eg, aluminum) are recommended to be injected deep into the muscle mass. If administered subcutaneously
or intradermally, these vaccines can cause local irritation, inflammation, granuloma
formation, and tissue necrosis. For patients with a known bleeding disorder or receiving anticoagulant therapy, bleeding complications following IM injection can occur.
Additional information on vaccinating patients with bleeding disorders and other special populations such as preterm infants and pregnant women are available at **www.
cdc.gov/vaccines/hcp/acip-recs/general-recs/special-situations.html.**

SC Administration. Several routinely recommended vaccines are administered subcutaneously, including the PRIORIX MMR vaccine. In contrast, M-M-R-II; measles, mumps,
rubella, and varicella (MMRV); and varicella (VAR) vaccines may be administered subcutaneously or intramuscularly. Non-live poliovirus and pneumococcal polysaccharide vaccines can be administered subcutaneously or intramuscularly (pneumococcal conjugate
vaccines are administered intramuscularly). SC injections place the vaccine in the tissue
between the dermal and muscle layers. SC administration is made at the anterolateral
aspect of the thigh or the upper outer triceps area by inserting the needle in a pinched-up
fold of skin at a 45° angle. A 23- to 25-gauge needle of ⅝ inch length is generally recommended. Like other vaccines that are administered parenterally, localized swelling, redness, and pain can occur at the injection site, but serious complications are rare.

ORAL VACCINATION. Only rotavirus vaccines and oral typhoid vaccine are approved
for oral administration in children. For infants, oral vaccines should be administered
slowly down one side of the inside of the cheek between the cheek and gum toward
the back of the mouth, allowing the infant to swallow, but not so far as to trigger the
gag reflex. Do not squirt the vaccine directly into the throat. Detailed information on
oral delivery of vaccines is included in package inserts. Breastfeeding does not appear

Table 1.8. Site and Needle Length by Age for Intramuscular Immunization[a]

Age Group	Needle Length, inches (mm)	Suggested Injection Site
Newborns (preterm and term) and infants <1 mo of age	⅝ (16)[b]	Anterolateral thigh muscle
Infants, 1–12 mo of age	1 (25)	Anterolateral thigh muscle
Toddlers, 1–2 years	1–1¼ (25–32)	Anterolateral thigh muscle (preferred)
	⅝[b]–1 (16–25)	Deltoid muscle of the arm
Children, 3–10 years	⅝[b]–1 (16–25)	Deltoid muscle of arm (preferred)
	1–1¼ (25–32)	Anterolateral thigh muscle
Children, 11–18 years	⅝[b]–1 (16–25)	Deltoid muscle of arm (preferred)
	1–1½ (25–38)	Anterolateral thigh muscle
Adults		
Weight <130 lb	1 (25)[c]	Deltoid muscle of the arm
Weight 130–152 lb	1 (25)	Deltoid muscle of the arm
Weight 153–200 lb	1–1½ (25–38)	Deltoid muscle of the arm
Weight 201–260 lb	1–1½ (25–38)[d]	Deltoid muscle of the arm
Weight >260 lb	1½ (38)	Deltoid muscle of the arm

[a] Adapted from General Best Practice Guidelines for Immunization: Best Practices Guidance of the Advisory Committee on Immunization Practices (ACIP), Vaccine Administration, Table 6-2 (**www.cdc.gov/vaccines/hcp/acip-recs/general-recs/administration.html#t6_2**).
[b] If the skin is stretched tightly and subcutaneous tissues are not bunched.
[c] Some experts recommend a ⅝-inch needle for adults who weigh less than 130 lb. If used, skin must be stretched tightly (do not bunch subcutaneous tissue).
[d] Consider individual body composition (eg, adiposity, muscle mass) in determining needle length.

to diminish response to rotavirus vaccines, and the infant can eat or drink immediately following oral vaccination. If a dose of rotavirus vaccine is regurgitated, spat out, or vomited out, do not readminister the vaccine. Currently, there are no data available on the benefits or risks of repeating the dose. The infant should receive the remaining recommended doses of rotavirus vaccine following the routine schedule.

INTRANASAL VACCINATION. Live attenuated influenza vaccine (LAIV) is the only vaccine currently approved for intranasal administration. LAIV is approved for use for healthy, nonpregnant people 2 years through 49 years of age. The vaccine is prepared inside a special sprayer device that divides the dose into equal parts for delivery into each nostril and should be delivered in single brisk movement on each side rather than slowly. Patients should be sitting upright, the vaccinator should put a hand behind the patient's head, and the patient should be asked to breathe normally. The dose does not need to be repeated if the patient sneezes after vaccination. LAIV can be administered during minor illnesses, but if nasal congestion might impede delivery of LAIV then administer injectable influenza vaccine or defer LAIV until after the resolution of nasal congestion.

VACCINE ADMINISTRATION ERRORS

Vaccines, like other medications, can inadvertently be administered in error. Vaccine administration errors can have many consequences, including inadequate immunologic protection, possible injury to the patient, cost, inconvenience, and reduced confidence in the health care delivery system. Common vaccine administration errors include use of expired vaccine or diluent, doses administered too early, and the use of improperly stored vaccines. Guidance for handling common vaccine administration errors is included in ACIP's General Best Practice Guidelines for Immunization (**www.cdc.gov/vaccines/hcp/acip-recs/general-recs/administration. html**). When a vaccine administration error occurs, health care personnel should determine how it happened and put strategies in place to prevent it occurring again in the future. In addition, they are encouraged to report vaccine administration errors to VAERS (see Understanding Vaccine Evaluation and Safety as an Approach to Addressing Parental Concerns, p 27).

Managing Injection Pain

Children of all ages benefit from a planned approach to decrease pain and anxiety related to immunization. The Advisory Committee on Immunization Practices (ACIP),[1] the Canadian Medical Association,[2] and the World Health Organization[3] provide guidance on a variety of pain mitigation interventions during vaccination. Parents, children 3 years and older, and health care providers administering vaccine injections should be educated about age-appropriate, evidence-based techniques for reducing injection pain or distress. Combination vaccines should be used when feasible to reduce the number of injections and their attendant pain.

PHYSICAL AND PSYCHOLOGICAL TECHNIQUES FOR MINIMIZING INJECTION PAIN AND ANXIETY

Strategies to reduce pain include tactile stimulation (rubbing the site near the injection before and after the vaccination) and holding the child, which is routinely recommended in children younger than 3 years (along with patting or rocking the child after the injection). Allowing children 3 years and older to sit up rather than lie down can also assist in decreasing child anxiety. If multiple vaccines are to be given, they should be administered in order from least to most painful (painful vaccines include measles, mumps, rubella; pneumococcal conjugate vaccine; human papillomavirus; and diphtheria, tetanus, and acellular pertussis). The appropriately sized needle should be plunged rapidly through the skin and removed rapidly without aspiration. Aspiration

[1] Kroger A, Hahta L, Hunter P. General Best Practice Guidelines for Immunization. Vaccine Recommendations and Guidelines of the Advisory Committee on Immunization Practices (ACIP). Available at: **www.cdc.gov/vaccines/hcp/acip-recs/general-recs/index.html**

[2] Taddio A, McMurtry M, Shah V, et al. Reducing pain during vaccine injections: clinical practice guideline. *CMAJ*. 2015;187(13):975-982

[3] World Health Organization. Reducing pain at the time of vaccination: WHO position paper – September 2015. *Wkly Epidemiol Rec*. 2015;90(39):505-510

before injection is not necessary, because large blood vessels are not present at the recommended injection sites and pain may be increased with longer needle dwell time in the tissue. For children younger than 3 years, breastfeeding, feeding sweet-tasting solutions (eg, sucrose or glucose solution 1-2 minutes before the vaccine), and applying topical anesthetics (all ages) at the site of injection are other strategies that have been used before vaccine administration to decrease pain (**www.cdc.gov/vaccines/ hcp/acip-recs/general-recs/administration.html**).

Distraction strategies, including pinwheels, deep breathing exercises, music, and videos or video games, have been used in older children to decrease anxiety and pain. Adolescents should be seated or lying down during vaccination to reduce the risk of injury should syncope develop. Warming a vaccine by rubbing it between the hands is not recommended because of concern for altering vaccine effectiveness.

PHARMACOLOGIC TECHNIQUES FOR MINIMIZING INJECTION PAIN

If topical anesthesia is used, planning ahead is necessary to ensure the anesthetic is applied sufficiently in advance to develop effective anesthesia. Strategies can include applying the anesthetic en route to the office visit or immediately on arrival. Lidocaine 4% (LMX4) is approved by the US Food and Drug Administration (FDA) for children older than 2 years, is available over the counter, and takes effect 30 minutes after application. Lidocaine 2.5%/prilocaine 2.5% (EMLA), available by prescription, is approved by the FDA for neonates >37 weeks' estimated gestational age, infants, and children and takes effect 60 minutes after application. These products should be applied under occlusion. Topical application of ethyl chloride, a coolant sprayed onto a cotton ball and placed over the injection site for 15 seconds prior to administering the injection, has been shown to decrease injection pain in school-aged children. Note that for some children, topical anesthesia may not penetrate deeply enough to alleviate pain from intramuscular injections. Administration of oral analgesics, such as acetaminophen, prior to vaccinations has not been shown to reduce pain and may have a detrimental effect on the immune response to the vaccine(s) being administered. Age-appropriate doses of acetaminophen can be used after immunization to treat pain and to reduce the discomfort of fever.

Immunization Schedule and Timing of Vaccines

The purpose of a vaccine is to prompt the development of immunity against a disease in a person without the person developing the disease. The balance between timely protection and optimal immunologic response is the basis of the immunization schedule. The immunization schedule—including dose, frequency, and timing, along with the age and health status of the person—considers available clinical and epidemiologic data on vaccine safety and efficacy as well as programmatic considerations (such as incorporating vaccinations into scheduled health maintenance visits; **www.cdc.gov/ vaccines/schedules/hcp/imz/child-adolescent.html**). The schedule must be read with its accompanying notes and special considerations. For those who fall behind or start late, catch-up vaccination should occur at the earliest opportunity following the recommended catch-up immunization schedule for children and adolescents who start late or who are more than 1 month behind (**www.cdc.gov/vaccines/schedules/ hcp/imz/catchup.html**).

RECOMMENDED IMMUNIZATION SCHEDULE

The "Recommended Child and Adolescent Immunization Schedule for Ages 18 Years or Younger, United States" represents the recommendation of the Advisory Committee on Immunization Practices (ACIP), a federal advisory committee administered by the Centers for Disease Control and Prevention (CDC), with approval by the CDC. The immunization schedule is also approved by the American Academy of Pediatrics (AAP), the American Academy of Family Physicians (AAFP), the American College of Obstetricians and Gynecologists (ACOG), the American College of Nurse-Midwives (ACNM), the American Academy of Physician Associates (AAPA), and the National Association of Pediatric Nurse Practitioners (NAPNAP). The immunization schedule is reviewed annually and published in February each year. Creating unique vaccination schedules outside of the aforementioned reviewed and recommended schedules is not advised and may not provide effective protection against vaccine-preventable diseases.

AGE INDICATIONS FOR VACCINES

The age at which a vaccine is indicated depends on the immunologic maturity and health status of the patient, risk of exposure to the pathogen for which the vaccine is effective, vaccine safety, and optimal booster effect if the vaccine is a part of a series. In general, a vaccine is recommended for the youngest age of patients who are at risk for disease for which the vaccine is safe and provides protection. With a parenterally administered live vaccine for infants, the inhibitory effect of residual maternal antibody determines the optimal age at which the infant should receive the vaccine. For example, a measles-containing vaccine provides suboptimal seroconversion during the first year of life of an infant because of an interference by maternal antibody acquired through transplacental passage as well as the infant's own immature immune system.

MULTIPLE DOSES OF THE SAME VACCINE

Some vaccines are administered as a series of doses to provide optimal protection. For example, one dose of the measles, mumps, and rubella vaccine (MMR) is 93% effective against measles, 78% effective against mumps, and 97% effective against rubella. Two doses of MMR increases vaccine effectiveness to 97% for measles, 88% for mumps and >97% for rubella. The protection provided by some vaccines wanes over time, and booster doses are periodically indicated. For example, tetanus and diphtheria toxoids require booster doses to maintain protective antibody concentrations. For multidose primary vaccination series, administration of doses at recommended intervals optimizes the immunologic response and minimizes possible adverse reactions (eg, local and systemic reactions to diphtheria and tetanus toxoids administration).

MULTIPLE VACCINES ADMINISTERED AT THE SAME TIME

In general, it is safe to administer different vaccines at the same time. Administration of multiple vaccines at the same time, as recommended in the immunization schedule, promotes adherence to completion of vaccination series (ie, reduced medical visits) and ensures optimal protection. Simultaneous administration of vaccines is also important for scheduling immunizations for children with lapsed or missed immunizations, for children requiring early or rapid protection, and for people preparing for international travel (see Simultaneous Administration of Multiple Vaccines, p 63).

Table 1.9. Guidelines for Spacing of Live and Non-Live Vaccines

Antigen Combination	Recommended Minimum Interval Between Doses
2 or more non-live[a]	May be administered simultaneously or at any interval
Non-live plus live	May be administered simultaneously or at any interval
2 or more live[b]	28-day minimum interval if not administered simultaneously

[a]See text below for the 3 exceptions to this.
[b]An exception is made for live oral vaccines, which can be administered simultaneously or at any interval before or after non-live or live parenteral vaccines.

More than 1 live-virus vaccine (eg, MMR, varicella, and live attenuated influenza vaccines) may be administered at the same time. However, immune responses may be impaired when 2 or more parenterally or nasally administered live-virus vaccines are not administered simultaneously but within 28 days (4 weeks) of each other; therefore, live-virus vaccines not administered on the same day should be given at least 28 days apart whenever possible (Table 1.9). Live oral vaccines—Ty21a typhoid vaccine and rotavirus vaccine—may be administered simultaneously with or at any interval before or after non-live or live injectable vaccine or nasally administered vaccine (Table 1.9).

No minimum interval is required between administration of different non-live vaccines, with 3 exceptions:

1. When both pneumococcal conjugate vaccine (PCV) and 23-valent pneumococcal polysaccharide vaccine (PPSV23) are indicated, PCV should be administered first, followed by PPSV23 at least 8 weeks later, to optimize immune response (see *Streptococcus pneumoniae* (Pneumococcal) Infections, p 810).
2. When MenACWY-D (Menactra) is administered 30 days after diphtheria and tetanus toxoids and acellular pertussis vaccine (DTaP), it interferes with the immune response for all four meningococcal serogroups. Therefore, MenACWY-D (Menactra) should be administered either before or at the same time as DTaP; alternatively, Menveo or MenQuadfi (if ≥2 years of age) may be administered because they do not have any interference with DTaP (see Meningococcal Infections, p 585).
3. Because of their high risk for invasive pneumococcal disease, children with functional or anatomic asplenia or HIV infection should not be vaccinated with MenACWY-D (Menactra) before age 2 years to avoid interference with the immune response to PCV (see Meningococcal Infections, p 585). Only MenACWY-CRM (Menveo) should be used in this group; MenACWY-TT (MenQuadfi) should not be used in this situation because it is only approved in children ≥2 years of age.

COMBINATION VACCINES

Combination vaccine products may be administered when they are age appropriate and any of the component vaccine is indicated and other components are not contraindicated. The use of a combination vaccine generally is preferred over separate injections of its equivalent component vaccines (see Combination Vaccines, p 65).

Web-based childhood immunization schedulers using the current vaccine recommendations are available for parents, caregivers, and health care professionals to facilitate making schedules for children and adolescents are at **www.cdc.gov/vaccines,** and associated vaccination recommendations by the AAP can be found at **www.aap. org/en/patient-care/immunizations/vaccination-recommendations-by-the-aap/.** State and certain city immunization information systems (also known as vaccine registries) will generally forecast immunizations that are due according to the immunization schedule.

Minimum Ages and Minimum Intervals Between Vaccine Doses

Immunizations generally are recommended for members of the youngest age group at risk of experiencing the disease for whom efficacy, effectiveness, immunogenicity, and safety of the vaccine have been demonstrated. Most vaccines in the childhood and adolescent immunization schedule require 2 or more doses for stimulation of an adequate and persisting immune response. The schedule is determined based on studies demonstrating safety and effectiveness of individual vaccines evaluated in the context of the existing childhood immunization schedule (**www.cdc.gov/vaccines/schedules/index.html**).

Vaccines generally should not be administered at intervals less than the recommended minimum or at an age earlier than the recommended minimum (ie, accelerated schedules). If intervals between doses are longer than recommended, the vaccine series can continue and does not need to be started over. Administering doses of a multidose vaccine at intervals shorter or at an age earlier than those recommended for routine vaccination might be necessary in circumstances in which an infant or child is behind schedule and needs to be brought up to date quickly or when international travel is anticipated. In these situations, the minimum intervals and ages for catch-up vaccinations can be used (**www.cdc.gov/vaccines/schedules/hcp/imz/catchup.html#table-catchup**). For example, during a measles outbreak or for international travel, measles vaccine may be administered as early as 6 months of age. However, if a measles-containing vaccine is administered before 12 months of age, the dose is not counted toward the 2-dose measles vaccine series, and the child should be reimmunized at 12 through 15 months of age with a measles-containing vaccine; a third dose of a measles-containing vaccine then is indicated at 4 through 6 years of age but can be administered as early as 4 weeks after the second dose (see Measles, p 570).

Certain circumstances, such as the need for an additional office visit or a patient or parent poorly adherent to scheduled visits, could lead to consideration of administering a vaccine up to 4 days before the minimum interval or age. In general, vaccine doses administered (intentionally or inadvertently) 4 days or fewer before the minimum interval or age can be counted as valid. Health care professionals should be aware that state and school guidelines may consider such doses invalid and require additional vaccinations. Doses administered 5 days or more before the minimum interval or age should not be counted as valid doses and should be repeated as age appropriate. The repeat dose should be spaced by the recommended minimum interval after the invalid dose. Because of the unique schedule for rabies vaccine, consideration of days of a shortened interval between doses must be individualized.

The latest recommendations can be found in the annual immunization schedule (**http://redbook.solutions.aap.org/SS/Immunization_Schedules.aspx**).

Additional information from the Centers for Disease Control and Prevention (CDC) can be found on the CDC website (**www.cdc.gov/vaccines/hcp/acip-recs/general-recs/index.html**).

Interchangeability of Vaccine Products

Similar vaccines made by different manufacturers can vary in several ways: the type, number, and amount of antigenic components; the formulation of adjuvants and conjugating agents; and the choice of stabilizers and preservatives. These differences may lead to variation in the immune response elicited. When possible, effort should be made to complete a series with vaccine made by the same manufacturer. If different brands of a particular vaccine require a different number of doses for series completion (eg, *Haemophilus influenzae* type b [Hib] and rotavirus [RV] vaccines) and a provider mixes brands in the primary series, the higher number of doses is recommended for series completion. Although data documenting the effects of interchanging vaccines are limited, available results are reassuring for adequate immune responses, and most experts have considered vaccines interchangeable when administered according to their recommended schedule and dosing regimen. Approved vaccines that may be used interchangeably during a vaccine series from different manufacturers, according to recommendations from the AAP or ACIP, include Hib conjugate, hepatitis B (HepB), hepatitis A (HepA), RV, and quadrivalent meningococcal conjugate vaccines.

Adolescents 18 years or older who start their HepB series with Heplisav-B should complete it with the same product. Of note, data are limited on safety and immunogenicity when PreHevbrio is interchanged with HepB vaccines from other manufacturers.

Regarding the 2 serogroup meningococcal B vaccines (ie, Bexsero and Trumenba), because each use very different protein antigens and because there are no data on their interchangeability, the same vaccine must be used for all doses to complete the full meningococcal serogroup B series.

Approved rotavirus vaccines (RV5 [RotaTeq3-dose series] and RV1 [Rotarix 2-dose series]) are considered interchangeable as long as recommendations concerning conversion from a 2-dose regimen (RV1) to a 3-dose regimen (RV5) are followed (see Rotavirus, p 730). If any dose in the series is either RotaTeq or unknown, default to a 3-dose series.

Similarly, approved Hib conjugate vaccines are considered interchangeable, as long as recommendations for a total of 3 doses in the first year of life are followed (ie, if 2 doses of Hib-OMP PedvaxHIB are not administered, 3 doses of a Hib-containing vaccine are required). The combination diphtheria and tetanus and acellular pertussis (DTaP)-non-live poliovirus (IPV)-Hib-HepB vaccine (Vaxelis) is not recommended for use as a booster dose; a different Hib-containing vaccine should be used for the booster dose at age 12 to 15 months.

When a vaccine with increased serotype content is recommended as an option (eg, 15-valent or 20-valent pneumococcal conjugate vaccine [PCV15 or PCV20] as an alternative for 13-valent pneumococcal conjugate vaccine [PCV13]) or replaces a previously recommended product (eg, 9-valent human papillomavirus vaccine [9vHPV] for quadrivalent human papillomavirus vaccine [4vHPV]), the vaccines are considered interchangeable, so the series can be completed with the broader serotype product.

Minimal data on safety and immunogenicity and no data on efficacy are available for interchangeability of DTaP vaccines from different manufacturers. When feasible, DTaP from the same manufacturer should be used for the primary series (see Pertussis, p 656). However, in circumstances in which the DTaP product received previously is not known or the previously administered product is not readily available, any of the DTaP vaccines may be used according to licensure for dose and age. Matching of booster doses of DTaP and adolescent tetanus and diphtheria toxoids and acellular pertussis vaccine (Tdap) by manufacturer is not necessary. Single-component vaccines from the same manufacturer of combination vaccines, including DTaP-IPV-Hib-HepB (Vaxelis), DTaP-HepB-IPV (Pediarix), and DTaP-IPV/Hib (Pentacel) are interchangeable (see Combination Vaccines, p 65).[1]

In general, written documentation of immunizations received outside of the United States can be accepted as valid evidence of previous immunization if the vaccines, dates of administration, number of doses, intervals between doses, and age of the child at the time of immunization are comparable to current US or World Health Organization schedules (**www.who.int/immunization/policy/immunization_tables/en/**; see Immunizations Received Outside the United States, p 119).

Simultaneous Administration of Multiple Vaccines

Simultaneous administration of most vaccines according to the recommended immunization schedule is safe and effective. Infants and children have sufficient immunologic capacity to respond to multiple vaccine antigens administered at the same time. The immune response to one vaccine generally does not interfere with responses to other vaccines. For example, simultaneous administration of non-live poliovirus vaccine; measles, mumps, and rubella vaccine (MMR); varicella vaccine; or diphtheria and tetanus and acellular pertussis vaccine (DTaP) results in rates of seroconversion and of adverse events similar to those observed when these vaccines are administered at separate visits.

There is no contraindication to simultaneous administration of multiple vaccines routinely recommended for infants and children, with 2 exceptions:
1. When both pneumococcal conjugate vaccine (PCV) and 23-valent pneumococcal polysaccharide vaccine (PPSV23) are indicated, PCV should be administered first, followed by PPSV23 at least 8 weeks later, to optimize immune response (see *Streptococcus pneumoniae* (Pneumococcal) Infections, p 810).
2. In children for whom quadrivalent meningococcal conjugate vaccine is indicated,

---

[1] Kroger A, Bahta L, Long S, Sanchez P. General best practice guidelines for immunization. Best practices guidance of the Advisory Committee on Immunization Practices (ACIP). Available at: **www.cdc.gov/vaccines/hcp/acip-recs/general-recs/downloads/general-recs.pdf.**

MenACWY-D (Menactra) should not be administered concomitantly OR within 4 weeks of administration of PCV vaccine, to avoid potential interference with the immune response to PCV. Therefore, because of their high risk for invasive pneumococcal disease, children with functional or anatomic asplenia or HIV infection should not be vaccinated with MenACWY-D (Menactra) before age 2 years to avoid interference with the immune response to PCV (see Meningococcal Infections, p 585). Only MenACWY-CRM (Menveo) should be used in this group; MenACWY-TT (MenQuadfi) should not be used in this situation because it is only approved in children ≥2 years of age.

A slightly increased risk of febrile seizures is associated with the first dose of measles, mumps, rubella, and varicella vaccine (MMRV) compared with MMR and monovalent varicella vaccine administered simultaneously at separate sites among children 12 through 23 months of age; after dose 1 of MMRV, 1 additional febrile seizure is expected to occur per approximately 2300 to 2600 young children immunized, compared with MMR and monovalent varicella administered simultaneously at separate sites. Evidence from epidemiologic studies indicated that during the 2 influenza seasons spanning 2010–2012, there was an increased risk of febrile seizures in young children, mostly concentrated in children 6 through 23 months of age, when non-live influenza vaccine (IIV) was administered simultaneously with PCV13 or DTaP-containing vaccines. This risk occurred on the day of vaccination to the day after; there did not appear to be an increased risk when IIV was administered without PCV13 or DTaP-containing vaccines. The risk was small with, at most, 1 additional febrile seizure per 3333 children vaccinated with any combination of simultaneous administration of these vaccines. A Sentinel Program Center for Biologics Evaluation and Research (CBER)/Post-licensure Rapid Immunization Safety Monitoring (PRISM) surveillance report evaluating influenza vaccines and febrile seizures found no evidence of an elevated risk of febrile seizures in children 6 through 23 months of age following IIV administration during the 2013–2014 and 2014–2015 influenza seasons, noting that the risk of seizures after PCV13 or concomitant PCV13 and IIV was low compared with a child's lifetime risk of febrile seizures from other causes. Overall, simultaneous administration of IIV and PCV continues to be recommended when both vaccines are indicated because of the preponderance of benefit relative to the risk.

In adolescents or young adults whose sex assigned at birth is male, it is reasonable to consider waiting 4 weeks after orthopoxvirus (mpox) vaccination (either JYNNEOS or ACAM2000) before receiving a Moderna, Novavax, or Pfizer-BioNtech COVID-19 vaccine because of the known risk for myocarditis and/or pericarditis after both these COVID-19 vaccines and the unknown risk after orthopoxvirus vaccine.

Individual vaccines should never be mixed in the same syringe unless they are specifically approved and labeled for administration in 1 syringe. Separate sites should be used, and injections into the same extremity should be separated by at least 1 inch so that any local reactions can be differentiated. If a non-live vaccine and an immune globulin product are indicated concurrently (eg, hepatitis B vaccine and hepatitis B immune globulin, rabies vaccine and rabies immune globulin, tetanus-containing vaccine and tetanus immune globulin), they should be administered at separate anatomic sites (eg, different extremities).

Combination Vaccines

Combination vaccine products may be administered when they are age appropriate and any of the component vaccine is indicated and other components are not contraindicated. The use of a combination vaccine generally is preferred over separate injections of its equivalent component vaccines because they can decrease the number of injections during a single clinic visit. Table 1.10 lists combination vaccines approved for use and the age groups for which they are approved in the United States. Factors that could be clinically considered, in consultation with the parent, for their use include the routinely recommended schedule for vaccines based on age, health status, and other indications; vaccine safety and availability; cost; the number of injections needed; and whether the patient is likely to return for follow-up and complete the vaccine series. Not all providers stock all vaccines that are routinely recommended. In addition, the use of combination vaccines can involve complex economic and logistic considerations.

When patients have received the recommended series of immunizations for a particular antigen, administering an extra dose of this antigen as part of a combination vaccine is permissible and doing so will reduce the number of injections required, as long as the vaccines are age appropriate and there are no contraindications.

Table 1.10. Combination Vaccines Approved by the US Food and Drug Administration (FDA)[a]

Vaccine[b]	Trade Name (Year Approved)	FDA Licensure	
		Age Group	Use in Immunization Schedule
HepA-HepB	Twinrix (2001)	≥18 y	Three doses on a 0-, 1-, and 6-mo schedule
DTaP-HepB-IPV	Pediarix (2002)	6 wk through 6 y	Three-dose series at 2, 4, and 6 mo of age
MMRV[c]	ProQuad (2005)	12 mo through 12 y	Two doses usually at 12–15 mo and 4–6 y of age (see Varicella-Zoster Infections, p 938); separate by at least 1 mo between measles-containing vaccine and ProQuad and at least 3 mo between varicella-containing vaccine and ProQuad
DTaP-IPV	Kinrix (2008)	4 y through 6 y	Booster for fifth dose of DTaP and fourth dose of IPV in children who have received 3 doses of Pediarix or Infanrix and a fourth dose of Infanrix
DTaP-IPV/Hib	Pentacel (2008)	6 wk through 4 y	Four-dose series administered at 2, 4, 6, and 15 mo through 18 mo of age

Table 1.10. Combination Vaccines Approved by the US Food and Drug Administration (FDA),[a] continued

| Vaccine[b] | Trade Name (Year Approved) | FDA Licensure | |
		Age Group	Use in Immunization Schedule
DTaP-IPV	Quadracel (2015)	4 y through 6 y	Single dose approved for use in children 4 through 6 years of age as a fifth dose in DTaP series and as a fourth or fifth dose in IPV series, in children who have received Pentacel, Daptacel, or Vaxelis vaccine
DTaP-IPV-Hib-HepB	Vaxelis (2018)	6 wk through 4 y	Three dose series administered at 2, 4, and 6 months of age[d]

DTaP indicates diphtheria and tetanus toxoids and acellular pertussis vaccine; HepA, hepatitis A vaccine; HepB, hepatitis B vaccine; HepA-HepB, hepatitis A and hepatitis B combination vaccine; Hib, *Haemophilus influenzae* type b vaccine; IPV, non-live poliovirus vaccine; MMRV, measles, mumps, rubella, and varicella vaccine.

[a] Excludes measles, mumps, rubella vaccine (MMR); DTaP; tetanus and diphtheria toxoids and acellular pertussis vaccine (Tdap), and tetanus and diphtheria toxoids (Td), for which individual component vaccines are not available. IPV is not available as a single-antigen vaccine.

[b] Dash (-) indicates products in which the active components are supplied in their final (combined) form by the manufacturer; slash (/) indicates products in which active components must be mixed by the user.

[c] The American Academy of Pediatrics expresses no preference between MMR plus monovalent varicella vaccine or MMRV for toddlers receiving their first immunization of this kind. Parents should be counseled about the rare possibility of their child developing a febrile seizure 1 to 2 weeks after immunization with MMRV for the first immunizing dose.

[d] A fourth dose of acellular pertussis vaccine is needed to complete the pertussis primary series in infants who receive 3 doses of Vaxelis.

Confusing ambiguities in the names of vaccines and vaccine combinations benefit from development of electronic systems that automate bar code scanning, which reduce potential recording errors enhancing the convenience and accuracy of transferring vaccine-identifying information into health records and immunization information systems.

Lapsed Immunizations

A lapse in an immunization series does not require restarting the series or adding doses to the series. If a dose in a vaccine series is missed or delayed, it should be administered at the next opportunity, and the series should resume for completion as recommended from the time of the catch-up vaccination. The catch-up schedule for children who have fallen behind on immunizations can be found at **www.cdc.gov/vaccines/schedules/hcp/imz/catchup.html.** Not all childhood vaccine series are required to be completed if there is an extended gap between doses or a delay in series initiation. A summary of recommended intervals between doses in vaccine series can be found at **www.cdc.gov/vaccines/hcp/acip-recs/general-recs/timing.html#t-02.** Although this summary discusses typically straightforward recommendations for several catch-up vaccinations, 2 distinct recommendations are described below.

1. For rotavirus vaccination, the doses in the series are age limited, and catch-up vaccination may not be indicated (see Rotavirus Infections, p 730). The rotavirus vaccination series should not start at or after age 15 weeks, 0 days, and the final dose in the series should not be administered after age 8 months, 0 days.

2. Children 6 months through 8 years of age who are receiving influenza vaccine for the first time or have received only 1 dose before the current influenza season should receive 2 doses of influenza vaccine separated by at least 4 weeks. Detailed influenza vaccination recommendations can be found in the Influenza chapter (p 511) and in the annual influenza policy statement of the American Academy of Pediatrics, which can be accessed through **https://redbook.solutions.aap.org/ss/influenza-resources.aspx.**

Health records of children for whom immunizations have been missed or delayed should be flagged as a reminder to resume their immunization series at the next opportunity and to implement reminder/recall communications to the family. An interactive app developed by the Centers for Disease Control and Prevention is available for downloading and has up-to-date information on the childhood immunization schedule, including catch-up timing of missed vaccines (**www.cdc.gov/vaccines/schedules/hcp/schedule-app.html**).

Unknown or Uncertain Immunization Status

Many children, adolescents, and young adults do not have adequate documentation of their vaccinations, which reinforces the need to record all vaccinations in state-based immunization information systems (IISs). Parent, guardian, or child recollection of immunization history may not be accurate. Additionally, many immigrant children have missing or unavailable vaccination records at the time of arrival in the United States. Health care providers should only accept written/electronic, dated, and authentic records as evidence of immunization, as long as the vaccines, dates of administration, number of doses, intervals between doses, and age of the child at the time of immunization are comparable to current US or World Health Organization schedules (**www.who.int/immunization/policy/immunization_tables/en/**). The 2 exceptions to this are influenza vaccine and pneumococcal polysaccharide vaccine (PPSV23); self-reported doses of these vaccines are acceptable.

When vaccine history is uncertain, there should be an immediate attempt to locate missing records by contacting previous health care providers, reviewing state or local IISs, and asking parents and guardians to search personally held records. In general, when in doubt, a person with unknown or uncertain immunization status should be considered disease susceptible, and recommended immunizations should be initiated without delay on a schedule appropriate for the person's current age. If the primary series has been started but not completed, the series should be completed if it is age appropriate, but there is no need to repeat doses or restart the full course.

Health care providers may use one of multiple approaches if the immunogenicity of vaccines or the completeness of series, especially those administered outside of the United States, is in question. Repeating the vaccinations is a safe, acceptable option that prevents the need to obtain and interpret serologic tests. If avoiding unnecessary injections is desired, judicious use of serologic testing may help determine which vaccinations are needed for certain antigens (eg, measles, rubella, hepatitis A, and tetanus) (see Serologic Testing to Document Immunization Status, p 121, and Table 1.19, p 122). Curtailing the number of excess doses administered to patients controls costs incurred by patients, providers, insurers, vaccination programs, and other stakeholders and could potentially decrease adverse reactions to vaccines. However, commercial serologic testing takes time, can lead to a failed immunization opportunity, and may not always be sufficiently sensitive to indicate protection. Importantly, no evidence suggests that administration of vaccines to already immune recipients is harmful. In addition, serologic testing may not satisfy some school immunization requirements.

Vaccine Dose

Recommended vaccine doses are those that have been determined to be both safe and effective for their specified indication in prelicensure clinical trials; variations from the recommended route or site of administration or volume or number of doses of any vaccine are ill-advised, because they may not be safe or effective. Reducing or exceeding a recommended dose volume or collecting residual volumes to make up a dose is never recommended. Reducing or dividing doses of any vaccine, including vaccines administered to preterm or low birth weight infants, can result in inadequate immune responses. A previous immunization with a dose that was less than the standard dose or one administered by a nonstandard route should not be counted as valid, and the person should be reimmunized as recommended for age.

A special situation is a child who transitions between doses recommended for age groups for primary series doses of COVID-19 vaccine (**www.cdc.gov/ vaccines/covid-19/clinical-considerations/interim-considerations-us. html#transitioning-younger-older**). For example, if a child turns 12 years of age between their first and second dose of Pfizer-BioNTech COVID-19 vaccine and they received the second vaccine in a dose appropriate for 5- to 11-year old children, the vaccine dose does not need to be repeated. Another special situation is with influenza vaccine, where recommendations for 2 versus 1 dose depend on age of the child and whether they had received influenza vaccine at any time in the past. Children who receive the first dose before their ninth birthday should receive 2 doses, even if they turn 9 years of age during the same influenza season.

Active Immunization After Receipt of Antibody-Containing Products

Donor-derived antibodies contained in polyclonal immune globulin (IG) preparations, including hyperimmune globulins like hepatitis B immune globulin (HBIG), can inactivate certain live-virus vaccines and reduce their immunogenicity. As such, these vaccines should be deferred for varying periods of time when IG preparations have been administered. Other blood products, such as plasma or packed red blood cells, also may contain antibodies capable of inactivating live vaccines. However, because the concentration of antibodies in these blood products is generally low, the length of vaccine deferral is less.

In the United States, the issue of interference by passively administered antibodies is most relevant for measles, mumps, and rubella vaccine (MMR); varicella vaccine (VAR); and measles, mumps, rubella, and varicella vaccine (MMRV). Table 1.11 shows the suggested intervals between receipt of blood products, including IG, and vaccine administration. This varies depending on the product type, the calculated amount of immunoglobulin G (IgG) in the product, and the dose of the product. Although there is some evidence that passive antibodies can interfere with the response to certain non-live vaccines, these vaccines may be administered at any time in relation to receipt of antibody-containing blood products. When both IG and vaccine are indicated to provide short- and long-term protection, respectively (eg, HBIG and hepatitis B vaccine [HepB] for an infant whose birthing parent is a carrier of hepatitis B virus), the products should always be administered in different anatomic sites (eg, different extremities used for HBIG and HepB). For additional information, see chapters on specific diseases in Section 3. The respiratory syncytial virus monoclonal antibodies palivizumab and nirsevimab do not interfere with the immunogenicity of any vaccine.

Live intranasal (live attenuated influenza vaccine [LAIV]) and oral (rotavirus vaccine [RV], and Ty21A typhoid vaccine) vaccines do not need to be deferred, because parenterally administered antibodies are unlikely to achieve significant concentrations at mucosal surfaces. Also, donor blood in the United States is unlikely to have neutralizing antibodies to *Salmonella* Typhi, yellow fever, and currently circulating strains of influenza. Immunogenicity and safety of recombinant live attenuated dengue vaccine after administration of immune globulin intravenous (IGIV) and other immunoglobulin-containing products has not been studied. Clinicians considering dengue vaccine for persons who recently received blood products (including IGIV) or other immunoglobulin containing products should delay prevaccination testing and administration of vaccine doses by 12 months.

Table 1.11. Recommended Intervals Between Receipt of Blood Products and Administration of MMR, Varicella, or MMRV Vaccines[a]

Indications or Blood Product	Route	Usual Dose	Interval, mo[b,c]
Blood transfusion			
Washed RBCs	IV	10 mL/kg (negligible IgG/kg)[d]	0
RBCs, adenine-saline added	IV	10 mL/kg (10 mg IgG/kg)[d]	3
Packed RBCs	IV	10 mL/kg (60 mg IgG/kg)[d]	6
Whole blood	IV	10 mL/kg (80–100 mg IgG/kg)[d]	6
Plasma or platelet products	IV	10 mL/kg (160 mg IgG/kg)	7
Hyperimmune globulin			
Botulinum immune globulin	IV	1 mL/kg (50 mg IgG/kg)	6
Cytomegalovirus immune globulin	IV	150 mg/kg (maximum)	6
Hepatitis B immune globulin	IM	0.06 mL/kg (10 mg IgG/kg)	3
Rabies immune globulin	IM	20 IU/kg (22 mg IgG/kg)	4
Tetanus immune globulin	IM	250 U (10 mg IgG/kg)	3
Varicella immune globulin	IM	125 U/10 kg (60–200 mg IgG/kg) (max 625 U)	5

Table 1.11. Recommended Intervals Between Receipt of Blood Products and Administration of MMR, Varicella, or MMRV Vaccines,[a] continued

Indications or Blood Product	Route	Usual Dose	Interval, mo[b,c]
Immune globulin			
Hepatitis A prophylaxis			
Contact prophylaxis	IM	0.1 mL/kg (16.5 mg IgG/kg)	6
International travel (short-term <1 month stay)	IM	0.1 mL/kg (16.5 mg IgG/kg)	6
International travel (long-term ≥1 month stay)	IM	0.2 mL/kg (33 mg IgG/kg)	6
Measles prophylaxis			
Not pregnant or immunocompromised[e]	IM	0.5 mL/kg (80 mg IgG/kg; maximum 15 mL)	6
Pregnant or immunocompromised[f]	IV	400 mg/kg	8
Varicella prophylaxis	IV	400 mg/kg	8
Replacement for immunodeficiency[g]	IV	300–400 mg/kg	8
Treatment of immune thrombocytopenic purpura	IV	400 mg/kg OR 1000 mg/kg	8 / 10
Treatment of Kawasaki disease	IV	2000 mg/kg	11

Adapted from General Best Practice Guidelines for Immunization: Best Practices Guidance of the Advisory Committee on Immunization Practices (ACIP), Vaccine Administration, Table 3–6 (**www.cdc.gov/vaccines/hcp/acip-recs/general-recs/timing.html#t-06**).

IM indicates intramuscular; IV, intravenous; MMR, measles, mumps, and rubella; MMRV, measles, mumps, rubella, and varicella; RBCs, red blood cells.

[a] Live vaccines may be contraindicated in patients receiving certain blood products because of immunosuppression caused by their underlying disease.

[b] These intervals should provide sufficient time for decreases in passive antibodies that would allow for an adequate immune response to measles vaccine. Physicians should not assume that children are protected fully against measles during these intervals, and if measles virus is circulating in the community or if the child is traveling to an area where measles may be circulating, a measles-containing vaccine should be administered but not counted as a valid dose (measles vaccine should be readministered after the appropriate interval has passed from the receipt of blood product in accordance with the routine immunization schedule). If a blood product must be given within 14 days after administration of a measles- or varicella-containing vaccine, these vaccine doses are considered invalid and the vaccines should be readministered after the appropriate interval.

[c] The interval between dengue vaccine and blood/passive antibody products should be 12 months.

[d] The given intervals are applicable for neonates, even though transfusion volume may be 15 mL/kg of washed, adenine-saline added, or packed RBCs. Whole blood transfusions of >10 mL/kg may be used for cardiopulmonary surgery, exchange transfusions, or responding to trauma.

[e] This table is not intended for determining the correct indications and dosages for using antibody-containing products. Unvaccinated people might not be protected fully against measles during the entire recommended interval, and additional doses of IG or measles vaccine might be indicated after measles exposure. Concentrations of measles antibody in an IG preparation can vary by manufacturer's lot. Rates of antibody clearance after receipt of an IG preparation also might vary. Recommended intervals are extrapolated from an estimated half-life of 30 days for passively acquired antibody and an observed interference with the immune response to measles vaccine for 5 months after a dose of 80 mg IgG/kg.

[f] Immune globulin intravenous is recommended for pregnant people without evidence of measles immunity and for severely immunocompromised hosts regardless of immunologic or vaccination status, including patients with severe primary immunodeficiency; patients who have received a bone marrow transplant until at least 12 months after finishing all immunosuppressive treatment, or longer in patients who have developed graft-versus-host disease; patients on treatment for acute lymphocytic leukemia within and until at least 6 months after completion of immunosuppressive chemotherapy; individuals who have received a solid organ transplant; and people with HIV infection who have severe immunosuppression, defined as CD4+ T-lymphocyte percentage <15% for children ≤5 years of age and a CD4+ T-lymphocyte percentage <15% or a CD4+ T-lymphocyte count <200/mm³ for children >5 years, and those who have not received MMR vaccine since receiving effective antiretroviral therapy.

[g] Patients who receive immune globulin subcutaneous (IGSC) at regular (eg, 1–4 week) intervals should not be vaccinated with MMR, varicella, MMRV, or dengue vaccines (see footnote **c**) while on therapy. If IGSC therapy is discontinued and vaccination is not otherwise contraindicated, vaccination with MMR, varicella, or MMRV may occur ≥8 months later.

Hypersensitivity Reactions After Immunization

Anaphylactic reactions to vaccines are rare. However, medications, equipment, and competent staff necessary to respond to these medical emergencies, to maintain patency of the airway, and to manage cardiovascular collapse should be available to treat anaphylaxis in all settings in which vaccines are administered (see Treatment of Anaphylactic Reactions, p 84). This recommendation includes administration of vaccines in schools, pharmacies, or other nontraditional vaccination settings.

In general, children who have experienced an immediate-type hypersensitivity reaction to a vaccine should be evaluated by an allergist before receiving subsequent doses of the suspect vaccine or other vaccines containing an ingredient in common. This evaluation may help determine whether an adverse event following immunization (AEFI) was allergic, or perhaps attributable to other mimics such as a vasovagal reaction or immunization stress-related response. Even when the child truly is allergic and no alternative vaccines are available, in almost all cases the risk of remaining unimmunized or inadequately immunized exceeds the risk of careful, graded increase in vaccine dose that is administration under observation where personnel, medications, and equipment are available and prepared to treat anaphylaxis, should it occur.

IMMEDIATE-TYPE ALLERGIC REACTIONS

Immediate allergic reactions may be caused by the immunizing agent (vaccine antigen) itself or, more often, by other vaccine components, particularly protein excipients. Almost all anaphylactic reactions to vaccines occur within minutes to 1 to 2 hours after vaccination.

ALLERGIC REACTIONS TO EGG PROTEIN (OVALBUMIN). Current measles and mumps vaccines (and some rabies vaccines) are derived from chicken embryo fibroblast tissue cultures and do not contain significant amounts of egg proteins. Studies indicate that children with egg allergy, even those with a history of severe reactions to egg ingestion, have no increased risk of anaphylaxis to these vaccines (eg, measles, mumps, and rubella [MMR] or measles, mumps, rubella, and varicella [MMRV]) compared with children without egg allergy. Most immediate hypersensitivity reactions after MMR or MMRV vaccination are attributable to other vaccine components, such as gelatin. Therefore, children with egg allergy may receive MMR or MMRV vaccines without special precautions.

Most non-live influenza vaccines (IIVs) and the live attenuated influenza vaccine (LAIV) also are produced in eggs and contain residual amounts of egg protein (ovalbumin). However, data have shown that these vaccines are well tolerated by recipients who have egg allergy, including patients with severe egg allergy, likely because the concentration of ovalbumin in the vaccines is below the threshold required to induce an allergic reaction. All children with egg allergy of any severity can receive any influenza vaccine without any additional precautions beyond those recommended for all vaccines.[1]

The yellow fever vaccine may contain a larger amount of egg protein than influenza vaccines, but there are fewer reports on administering the vaccine to patients with egg allergy. A history of egg allergy should be sought prior to administration, and

[1] American Academy of Pediatrics, Committee on Infectious Diseases. Recommendations for prevention and control of influenza in children, 2022-2023. *Pediatrics*. 2022;150(4):e2022059274

consultation with an allergist is recommended if there is such a history. The vaccine package insert describes a protocol involving skin testing the patient with the vaccine and, if positive, administering the vaccine in graded doses.

ALLERGIC REACTIONS TO GELATIN. Some vaccines, such as MMR, MMRV, varicella, yellow fever, LAIV, and some rabies vaccines, contain gelatin of porcine or bovine origin as a stabilizer. Children who are allergic to gelatin (which is very rare) should receive IIV (or recombinant influenza vaccine if age-appropriate) instead of LAIV. The Vero cell culture-derived Japanese encephalitis (JE-VC) vaccine and the recombinant zoster vaccine do not contain gelatin stabilizers. People with a history of food allergy to gelatin may develop anaphylaxis after receipt of gelatin-containing vaccines. In addition, people without any apparent clinical allergy to oral ingestion of gelatin may experience an immediate hypersensitivity reaction following injection of a vaccine containing gelatin. In those very rare situations in which a patient is believed to be allergic to gelatin, evaluation by an allergist should occur, with immediate-type allergy skin testing before receiving gelatin-containing vaccines. If gelatin allergy is confirmed, gelatin-containing vaccines should be administered in graded doses under observation, with competent personnel, medications, and equipment available to manage anaphylaxis.

ALLERGIC REACTIONS TO YEAST. Hepatitis B and human papillomavirus vaccines are manufactured using recombinant technology in *Saccharomyces cerevisiae* (baker's or brewer's yeast). Allergy to yeast is rare; however, patients claiming such an allergy should be evaluated by an allergist before receiving yeast-containing vaccines to confirm the yeast allergy. If the history and testing suggest immediate hypersensitivity, the vaccine should be administered, in graded doses, under observation, with competent personnel, medications, and equipment available to manage anaphylaxis.

ALLERGIC REACTIONS TO LATEX. Dry natural rubber latex contains naturally occurring proteins that may be responsible for allergic reactions, although such reactions to dry natural rubber latex are much less common than reactions to natural rubber latex. Some vaccine vial stoppers and syringe plungers contain dry natural rubber latex. However, allergic reactions to such vaccines in recipients with latex allergy are exceedingly rare, likely because little, if any, latex allergen from the vial or syringe is present in the liquid vaccine being administered. Other vaccine vials and syringes contain synthetic rubber, which does not pose risk to the child with latex allergy. Information about latex used in vaccine packaging is available in the manufacturer's package inserts or on the Centers for Disease Control and Prevention website (**www.cdc.gov/ vaccines/pubs/pinkbook/downloads/appendices/B/latex-table.pdf**). Patients with latex allergy should receive vaccines with natural rubber latex in the packaging in the normal manner, but under observation, with competent personnel, medications, and equipment available to manage the rare allergic reaction, should it occur.

DELAYED-TYPE ALLERGIC REACTIONS

With most cell-mediated, delayed-type hypersensitivity (DTH) allergic reactions, the allergens are small molecules. The molecules present in vaccines capable of producing such reactions include preservatives like thimerosal, adjuvants like aluminum, and antimicrobial agents.

ALLERGIC REACTIONS TO THIMEROSAL. Most patients with DTH reactions to thimerosal tolerate injection of vaccines containing thimerosal uneventfully or with only a temporary nodule or swelling at the injection site. This is not a contraindication to receive a vaccine that contains thimerosal. Thimerosal was removed from childhood vaccines in 2001. Only multidose vials of influenza vaccines currently contain thimerosal, and many thimerosal-free influenza vaccines in prefilled syringes are available.

ALLERGIC REACTIONS TO ALUMINUM SALTS. Sterile abscesses or persistent nodules have occurred at the site of injection of certain adjuvanted vaccines. These abscesses may result from a DTH response to the aluminum salts used as vaccine adjuvants such as aluminum hydroxide, aluminum phosphate, alum (potassium aluminum sulfate), or mixed aluminum salts. In some instances, these reactions may be caused by inadvertent subcutaneous inoculation of a vaccine intended for intramuscular use (Table 1.7, p 40). Aluminum-related abscesses recur frequently with subsequent dose(s) of vaccines containing aluminum. Only if such reactions were severe would they constitute a contraindication to further vaccination with aluminum-containing vaccines.

ALLERGIC REACTIONS TO ANTIMICROBIAL AGENTS. Many vaccines contain trace amounts of streptomycin, neomycin, or polymyxin B. Some people have DTH reactions to these agents and may develop an injection site papule 2- to 4 days after vaccine administration. This minor reaction is not a contraindication to future doses of vaccines containing these agents. The rare patients with a history of an anaphylactic reaction to one of these antimicrobial agents should be evaluated by an allergist before receiving vaccines containing them. No vaccine currently approved for use in the United States contains penicillin or its derivatives, cephalosporins, or fluoroquinolones.

OTHER VACCINE REACTIONS

Large local injection site swelling after administration of tetanus-containing vaccines had been believed to be common if such vaccines were given at short intervals between doses. However, recent studies indicate that the reactions are uncommon, even with short intervals between immunizations. These reactions are self-limited and do not contraindicate future doses of vaccines at appropriate intervals. Therefore, when indicated, a tetanus-containing vaccine should be administered regardless of interval since the last tetanus-containing vaccine.

PASSIVE IMMUNIZATION

Passive immunization entails administration of preformed antibody to a recipient and, unlike active immunization, confers immediate protection but for only a limited period of time. Passive immunization is indicated in the following general circumstances for prevention or amelioration of infectious diseases:

- For prophylaxis, when a person susceptible to a disease is exposed to or has a high likelihood of exposure to a specific infectious agent. This is especially important when that person has a high risk of complications from the disease or when time does not permit adequate protection by active immunization alone (eg, rabies immune globulin, varicella zoster immune globulin, hepatitis B immune globulin, tetanus immune globulin).

- As replacement, when people are deficient in synthesis of antibody as a result of primary immune deficiency (eg, severe combined immunodeficiency) or secondary immune deficiency in which antibody production is defective, alone or in combination with other immunodeficiencies (eg, immunosuppressive therapy or human immunodeficiency virus [HIV] infection).
- Therapeutically, when a disease is already present, whereby administration of preformed antibodies (ie, passive immunization) may ameliorate or aid in suppressing the effects of a toxin (eg, foodborne, wound, or infant botulism; diphtheria; or tetanus), ameliorate or suppress clinical disease (eg, anthrax, vaccinia, post-transplantation hepatitis B, post-transplantation cytomegalovirus [CMV]), or suppress certain inflammatory responses (eg, Kawasaki disease or multisystem inflammatory syndrome in children [MIS-C]).

Passive immunization can be accomplished with several types of products. The choice is dictated by the types of products available, the type of antibody desired, the route of administration, timing, and other considerations. These products include standard immune globulin intramuscular (IGIM); standard immune globulin intravenous (IGIV); hyperimmune globulins, some of which are for intramuscular use (eg, hepatitis B, rabies, tetanus, varicella) and some of which are for intravenous use (eg, botulism, CMV, vaccinia); antibodies of animal origin (eg, foodborne botulism, black widow spider, coral snake, rattlesnake, and scorpion antitoxins); and monoclonal antibodies (eg, respiratory syncytial virus [RSV], and SARS-CoV-2). Although the use of immune globulin subcutaneous (IGSC) for replacement has become increasingly common, IGSC usually is not preferred for initial prophylactic or therapeutic use because of the slower absorption and diminished bioavailability compared with IGIV. For patients requiring replacement therapy, bioavailability differences can be compensated for by giving a 1.3 to 1.37 times higher dose of IGSC (product-specific calculation) and monitoring trough levels to ensure equivalence with the prior IGIV dose.

Indications for administration of IG preparations other than those relevant to infections, Kawasaki disease, or MIS-C are not reviewed in the *Red Book*.

Immune Globulin Intramuscular (IGIM)

Immune globulin intramuscular (IGIM) is derived from pooled plasma of adults by a cold ethanol fractionation procedure (Cohn fraction II). IGIM consists of at least 90% immunoglobulin (Ig) G with trace amounts of IgA and IgM. It is treated with solvent/detergent to inactivate lipid-enveloped viruses, is sterile, and is not known to transmit any virus or other infectious agent. IGIM is a concentrated protein solution (approximately 16.5%, or 165 mg/mL) containing specific antibodies that reflect the infection prevalence and immunization status of the population from whose plasma the IGIM was prepared. Many donors (1000 to 60 000 donors per lot of final product) are used to include a broad spectrum of antibodies. Products sold in the United States are derived from plasma collected exclusively in US-licensed facilities. See **www.fda.gov/vaccines-blood-biologics/approved-blood-products/immune-globulins** for more information on products licensed in the United States.

IGIM is licensed and recommended for intramuscular administration. Therefore, IGIM should be administered deep into a large muscle mass (see Sites and Routes of Vaccine Administration, p 54). Ordinarily, no more than 5 mL should be administered at one site in an adult, adolescent, or large child; a lesser volume per site (1–3 mL) should be given to small children and infants. Health care professionals should refer to the package insert for total maximal dose at one time. Peak serum concentrations usually are achieved 2 to 3 days after administration.

Standard human IGIM should never be administered intravenously. Intradermal use of IGIM is not recommended. For information on hyperimmune globulins for intramuscular use (eg, hepatitis B, rabies, tetanus, varicella), see chapters on specific diseases in Section 3.

INDICATIONS FOR THE USE OF IGIM

HEPATITIS A PROPHYLAXIS. IGIM is indicated for **postexposure prophylaxis (PEP)** to provide short-term protection against hepatitis A infection in previously unvaccinated patients. PEP with IGIM alone should be used for infants younger than 12 months and for people who have serious allergy to the hepatitis A (HepA) vaccine or its components. For patients older than 40 years, depending on the clinician's risk assessment **(stacks.cdc.gov/view/cdc/59777)**, IGIM may be administered in addition to HepA vaccine. For patients 12 months through 40 years of age, HepA vaccine alone is preferred for PEP against hepatitis A infection (see Table 3.17, p 432).

For unvaccinated patients traveling to areas with high or intermediate hepatitis A endemicity, IGIM alone can be used for **preexposure prophylaxis (PrEP)** in infants younger than 6 months and people who have serious allergy to HepA vaccine or its components. For protection of infant travelers 6 through 11 months of age, preexposure HepA vaccine is preferred to IGIM because IGIM would interfere with the measles vaccine that also is required for international travel; this HepA dose does not count toward completing the immunization requirement. For healthy travelers 12 months through 40 years of age, HepA vaccine alone is recommended. For people older than 40 years, immunocompromised people of all ages, and people with chronic liver disease or other chronic medical condition, HepA vaccine should be administered, and in addition, IGIM can be considered (see Table 3.19, p 435).

IGIM is not indicated for people with clinical manifestations of hepatitis A infection or for people exposed to hepatitis A virus more than 14 days earlier.

MEASLES PROPHYLAXIS. IGIM administered to exposed, measles-susceptible (immunocompromised or not previously vaccinated) people can prevent or attenuate infection if administered within 6 days of exposure (see Measles, p 570). The effectiveness of IGIM is titer dependent. Vaccine-eligible people 12 months or older exposed to measles should preferably receive measles, mumps, and rubella vaccine (MMR), if it can be administered within 72 hours of initial exposure (see Table 3.32, p 575). Measles vaccine and IGIM should not be administered at the same time. Subsequent vaccination with MMR is recommended in nonimmune people exposed to measles who received IGIM for PEP. The appropriate interval between IGIM administration and measles immunization varies with the dose of IGIM and the specific product (see Table 1.11, p 69).

RUBELLA PROPHYLAXIS. Administration of IGIM to susceptible people experimentally exposed to rubella virus can prevent clinical rubella. However, there have also been many reports of the failure of IGIM to prevent the anomalies of congenital rubella. For this reason, the routine use of IGIM for the prevention of rubella in an exposed pregnant patient is not recommended.

REPLACEMENT THERAPY IN ANTIBODY DEFICIENCY DISORDERS. Most experts no longer consider IGIM appropriate for replacement therapy in immunodeficiency because of the pain of administration and the inability to achieve therapeutic blood concentrations of IgG. If IGIM is used for this indication, the usual dose (limited by muscle mass and the volume that should be administered) is 100 mg/kg (equivalent to 0.66 mL/kg) every 3 weeks. Customary practice is to administer twice this dose initially and to adjust the interval between administration of the doses (2–4 weeks) on the basis of trough IgG concentrations and clinical response (absence of or decrease in infections).

ADVERSE REACTIONS TO IGIM

- Almost all recipients experience local discomfort and many experience pain at the site of IGIM administration that is related to the volume administered per injection site. Discomfort is lessened if the preparation is at room temperature at the time of injection. Less common reactions include nausea, flushing, chills, headache, and aseptic meningitis.
- Serious reactions are uncommon; these reactions can be anaphylactic or anaphylactoid in nature and manifest as chest pain or constriction, dyspnea, or hypotension and shock.
- Both IGIM and immune globulin subcutaneous have been associated with thrombosis, particularly for individuals at increased risk. To minimize risk of thrombosis, recipients should be adequately hydrated before IGIM administration.
- An increased risk of systemic reactions, including renal dysfunction, hemolysis, and transfusion-related acute lung injury (TRALI), may result from inadvertent intravenous administration. Standard IGIM should not be administered intravenously.
- People requiring repeated doses of IGIM have been reported to experience systemic reactions, such as fever, chills, sweating, and shock.
- IGIM should not be administered to people with known selective IgA deficiency (serum IgA concentration <7 mg/dL; IgG and IgM concentrations normal). Because IGIM contains trace amounts of IgA, people who have selective IgA deficiency may develop anti-IgA antibodies on rare occasions and on a subsequent dose of IGIM may experience an anaphylactic reaction with systemic symptoms such as fever, chills, and shock. In rare cases in which reactions related to anti-IgA antibodies have occurred, subsequent use of a licensed immune globulin intravenous (IGIV) preparation with the lowest IgA concentration may decrease the likelihood of further reactions. Because these reactions are rare, routine screening for anti-IgA antibodies is not recommended.

PRECAUTIONS FOR THE USE OF IGIM

- Caution should be used when administering IGIM to a patient with a history of adverse reactions to IGIM. In this circumstance, some experts recommend administering a test dose (1%–10% of the intended dose) before the full dose.
- Although systemic reactions to IGIM are rare (see Adverse Reactions to IGIM), epinephrine and other means of treating serious, acute reactions should be immediately available. Health care professionals administering IGIM should have training in the management of anaphylaxis and shock.

- Unless the benefit will outweigh the risk, IGIM should not be used in patients with severe thrombocytopenia or any coagulation disorder that would preclude IM injection. In such cases, use of IGIV is recommended.

Immune Globulin Intravenous (IGIV)

Immune globulin intravenous (IGIV) is a highly purified preparation of immunoglobulin (Ig) G antibodies extracted from the pooled plasma of 1000 to 60 000 qualified adult donors using methods that vary by manufacturer. IGIV contains more than 95% IgG, with trace amounts of IgA and IgM. IGIV is available as a lyophilized powder or as a formulated liquid solution, with final concentrations of IgG of 5% or 10% depending on the product. IGIV does not contain thimerosal or any other preservative. IGIV products vary in their sodium content, type of stabilizing excipients (eg, sugars, amino acids), osmolarity/osmolality, pH, IgA content, isoagglutinins, trace amounts of other plasma proteins, and recommended infusion rate. Each of these factors may contribute to tolerability and the risk of serious adverse events. All IGIV preparations must have a minimum concentration of antibodies to measles virus, *Corynebacterium diphtheriae* toxoid, poliovirus, and hepatitis B virus. Antibody concentrations against other pathogens, such as *Streptococcus pneumoniae*, cytomegalovirus, and respiratory syncytial virus (RSV), vary widely among products and even between lots from the same manufacturer. One product, Asceniv, is produced from donors with high anti-RSV titers and has a specification for amount of anti-RSV antibody; it is approved for treatment of primary immunodeficiency in patients 12 years and older, but the clinical impact of the high anti-RSV titers on this or other patient populations is unknown.

INDICATIONS FOR THE USE OF IGIV

IGIV preparations available in the United States currently are licensed by the US Food and Drug Administration (FDA) for use in 8 conditions for either immune prophylaxis for primary and secondary immune deficiency or for immune modulation, as in Kawasaki disease and immune-mediated thrombocytopenia (Table 1.12). IGIV

Table 1.12. Uses of Immune Globulin Intravenous (IGIV) Approved by the US Food and Drug Administration[a]

Primary immunodeficiency disorders such as common variable immunodeficiency, X-linked agammaglobulinemia, Wiskott-Aldrich syndrome

Kawasaki disease, for prevention of coronary aneurysms

Immune-mediated thrombocytopenia, to increase platelet count

Secondary immunodeficiency attributable to therapy for B-cell chronic lymphocytic leukemia or autoimmunity

Chronic inflammatory demyelinating polyneuropathy, to improve neuromuscular disability

Multifocal motor neuron neuropathy, to improve muscle strength

Reduction of serious bacterial infection in children with HIV infection

Dermatomyositis in adults

[a] Not all IGIV products are approved by the FDA for all indications and not all products are approved for children or for all ages of the pediatric population.

products may be useful for other conditions, including multisystem inflammatory syndrome in children (MIS-C), although demonstrated efficacy from controlled trials is often not available. Blood sample(s) needed for diagnostic serologic tests for infectious diseases or to evaluate for immunologic disorders must be obtained before IGIV administration, because IgG antibodies present in IGIV may confound test interpretation over many months. Administration of IGIV can increase the erythrocyte sedimentation rate (ESR).

All IGIV products are licensed to prevent serious bacterial infections in primary humoral immunodeficiency, but not all licensed products are approved for the other indications listed in Table 1.12. Not all products are licensed for the entire pediatric age spectrum, and in some cases only a single product has certain indications. Therapeutic differences among IGIV products from different manufacturers may exist, but there are no comparative clinical trials of currently available products. Most experts believe that licensed IGIV and immune globulin subcutaneous (IGSC) products are equally efficacious except for Kawasaki disease, which should be treated with IGIV. IGIV (but not IGSC) is among the recommended therapies for MIS-C (see Coronavirus Disease-2019 [COVID-19], p 324). However, IGSC has slower absorption and diminished bioavailability compared with IGIV. Hyperimmune globulins (eg, BabyBIG, varicella-zoster immune globulin) as well as animal-derived immune globulin products are not discussed in this chapter. Among the licensed IGIV products, but not necessarily for each product individually, indications for prevention or treatment of infectious diseases in children and adolescents include the following:

- **Replacement therapy in antibody-deficiency disorders.** The typical dose of IGIV in primary immune deficiency is 400 to 600 mg/kg but may be as high as 800 mg/kg or higher, administered by IV infusion approximately every 21 to 28 days. Because of the half-life of administered IgG, dosing intervals greater than 28 days are not recommended. Dose and frequency of infusions should be based on clinical effectiveness in an individual patient and in conjunction with an expert on primary immune deficiency disorders. When possible, the same brand of IGIV should be administered longitudinally, because changing products is associated with an increased risk of adverse reactions.

- **Kawasaki disease.** Administration of IGIV at a dose of 2 g/kg as a single dose within the first 10 days of onset of fever, when combined with salicylate therapy, decreases the frequency of coronary artery abnormalities and shortens the duration of symptoms. IGIV treatment for children with symptoms of Kawasaki disease for more than 10 days is recommended, although data on efficacy are not available (see Kawasaki Disease, p 522). Repeat doses of IGIV may be indicated for refractory Kawasaki disease.

- **Pediatric human immunodeficiency virus (HIV) infection.** In children with HIV infection and hypogammaglobulinemia, IGIV may be used to prevent serious bacterial infection.[1]

---

[1] Guidelines for the Prevention and Treatment of Opportunistic Infections in Children With and Exposed to HIV. Department of Health and Human Services. Available at: **https://clinicalinfo.hiv.gov/en/guidelines/hiv-clinical-guidelines-pediatric-opportunistic-infections/bacterial-infections**. Accessed May 20, 2023

- **Immune thrombocytopenia (ITP).**[1] Several IGIV products are licensed for the treatment of ITP and are considered first line therapy by some experts. Studies have demonstrated a more rapid rise in platelet count with IGIV therapy compared with other treatments.
- **MIS-C.** Although optimal treatment for MIS-C is unknown, most experts recommend administration of IGIV at a dose of 2 g/kg, with infusion length/frequency based on cardiac function, weight, and fluid status of the patient. Steroids and immunomodulatory biologic therapies (ie, anakinra) can be administered concurrently. A recent study found that initial treatment with both IGIV and steroids led to earlier resolution of fever compared with IGIV alone. See Coronavirus Disease 2019 (COVID-19), p 324, for additional information.
- **Guillain-Barré syndrome (GBS), chronic inflammatory demyelinating polyneuropathy (CIDP), and multifocal motor neuropathy (MMN).** In GBS, IGIV treatment has been demonstrated to have efficacy equivalent to that of plasmapheresis and is easier to administer. IGIV has been licensed by the US Food and Drug Administration for treatment of CIDP and MMN in adults. IGIV is equivalent to steroids and plasmapheresis in treatment of CIDP, although individual patients may respond better to one treatment than another. MMN, unlike GBS and CIDP, responds only to IGIV, not steroids or plasmapheresis.
- **Toxic shock syndrome.** IGIV has been administered to patients with severe staphylococcal or streptococcal toxic shock syndrome and necrotizing fasciitis, although its use is controversial. Therapy appears most likely to be beneficial when used early in the course of illness.
- **Low birth weight infants.** Results of most clinical trials have indicated that IGIV does not decrease the incidence or mortality rate of late-onset infections in infants who weigh less than 1500 g at birth. IGIV is not recommended for routine use in preterm infants to prevent early-onset or late-onset infection.
- **Other potential uses.** IGIV may be useful for sustained hypogammaglobulinemia secondary to anti-B cell therapy for autoimmunity or malignancy, severe anemia caused by parvovirus B19 infection, neonatal alloimmune thrombocytopenia that is unresponsive to other treatments, neonatal enteroviral sepsis syndrome, immune-mediated neutropenia, decompensation in myasthenia gravis, dermatomyositis, polymyositis, stiff person syndrome, transplant rejection, and severe thrombocytopenia that is unresponsive to other treatments.

TRANSMISSION OF INFECTION BY IGIV

Following an outbreak of hepatitis C virus infection associated with IGIV in the United States in 1993, changes in the preparation of IGIV, including additional viral clearance steps (such as solvent/detergent exposure, pH 4 incubation, trace enzyme exposure, nanofiltration, and heat treatment), have been instituted to prevent transmission of hepatitis C virus and other enveloped viruses, nonenveloped viruses, and prions via immune globulin (IG) preparations. Most manufacturers use 3 or 4 different pathogen removal/inactivation procedures. All products currently available in the United States are believed to be free of known pathogens,

---

[1] Neunert C, Terrell DR, Arnold DM, et al. American Society of Hematology 2019 guidelines for immune thrombocytopenia. *Blood Adv.* 2019;3(23):3829-3866

and the risk of transmission of infection with IGIV administration is extremely low. Transmission of HIV by any IGIV product licensed in the United States has never been reported.

ADVERSE REACTIONS TO IGIV

INFUSION REACTIONS. Reactions such as fever, headache, myalgia, chills, nausea, and vomiting often are related to the rate of IGIV infusion and may occur in as many as 25% of patients. These systemic adverse events usually are mild to moderate and self-limited (Table 1.13). There have been numerous documented cutaneous reactions to IGIV, including urticaria, eczematous or lichenoid eruptions, petechiae, erythroderma, nonspecific macular or maculopapular rashes, and pruritus. Serum sickness reactions with arthritis have also been reported. The cause of most acute reactions is uncertain. Product-to-product variations in adverse effects occur among individual patients, but it is not possible at this time to predict the reactogenicity of one product relative to others.

SERIOUS ADVERSE REACTIONS. Acute, severe reactions including hypersensitivity and anaphylactoid reactions occur infrequently and are marked by flushing, changes in blood pressure, tachycardia, and shock. Anaphylactic reactions induced by anti-IgA are very rare and only occur in some patients with selective IgA deficiency (ie, total absence of circulating IgA, IgA <7 mg/dL, with normal anti-protein antibody forming ability) who have been previously sensitized to IgA, rarely in patients with common variable immunodeficiency who develop IgE antibodies to IgA, and in a small number of patients with primary humoral immunodeficiency. Infusion of licensed IGIV

Table 1.13. Managing IGIV Reactions[a]

Timing	Symptoms	Management
During infusion	Anaphylactic/ anaphylactoid	Stop the infusion. Administer epinephrine and fluid support, diphenhydramine, and glucocorticoid.
	Headache, fever, chills, myalgias, cough, mild hypotension	Slow the infusion until symptoms resolve. Administer diphenhydramine, NSAID; consider glucocorticoid. When symptoms resolve, the infusion rate may be increased. Pretreatment with an NSAID, antihistamine, or glucocorticoid or a combination may lessen or prevent a reaction.
After infusion	Headache	Administer NSAID, triptan, glucocorticoid. Consider additional hydration with normal saline before/after infusion, using an alternative product or changing to IGSC if there are repeated reactions.
	Myalgia/malaise	Administer NSAID, glucocorticoid. Consider an alternative product or change to IGSC if there are repeated reactions.

NSAID indicates nonsteroidal anti-inflammatory drug.
[a] There are no studies of the management of IGIV adverse effects, only expert opinion.

products with a low concentration of IgA may reduce the likelihood of further reactions but rarely is needed. Because of the extreme rarity of these reactions, screening for anti-IgA antibodies is not recommended.

Other potentially life-threatening adverse reactions include thrombosis, isoimmune hemolysis, renal insufficiency and failure, aseptic meningitis, noncardiogenic pulmonary edema, and transfusion-related acute lung injury (TRALI). Products are screened for antibody to A and B blood group antigens (hemolysis risk) and coagulation factor 11 (FXIa) contamination (thrombosis risk). Although products now are tested for presence of thrombogenic substances, occasional events still may occur, particularly in patients with underlying thrombosis risk factors. Renal failure is rare and occurs mainly in patients with preexisting renal dysfunction and diabetes mellitus. It has been mostly, but not exclusively, associated with products containing sucrose excipient. Acute renal failure also may occur secondary to acute hemolysis mediated by isoagglutinins.

Hemolytic events are observed mainly in patients with A, B, or AB blood types receiving high doses of IGIV (approximately 80% of patients received $\geq$1.5 g/kg). Patients receiving high doses of IGIV should be monitored for hemolysis, which can be acute or can evolve over 5 to 10 days. Complications of severe hemolysis include need for transfusion, renal failure, and rarely, disseminated intravascular coagulation. If transfusion is needed, type O blood cells are recommended.

Aseptic meningitis syndrome beginning several hours to days following IGIV treatment is rare and may be associated with severe headache, nuchal rigidity, fever, nausea, and vomiting. Pleocytosis frequently is present in the cerebrospinal fluid. Aseptic meningitis is more common with high-dose IGIV (ie, 2 g/kg) and in those with a history of migraines.

Reactions are more likely to occur during the first infusion, when infusion rates are fast, if there was a long interval since previous infusion, when patients are switched to a new product, and in the setting of active infection. Risk factors for these adverse reactions include hypertension, coronary artery disease, diabetes mellitus, history of thrombosis, other thrombotic risk factors, oral contraception use, prior renal compromise, and underlying hyperviscosity. The risk of some reactions can be mitigated by limiting the dose and infusion rate or by subcutaneous administration using IGSC (see Immune Globulin Subcutaneous, p 82). The infusion rate and type of adverse events are factors that should be considered when deciding on a route of IG administration.

PRECAUTIONS FOR THE USE OF IGIV

- Patients receiving IGIV should be adequately hydrated before and during the infusion to reduce the risk of renal dysfunction, which can occur in volume depleted patients.
- Caution should be used when administering IGIV to a patient with a history of adverse reactions to IG.
- Because acute anaphylactic or anaphylactoid reactions to IGIV can occur (see Adverse Reactions to IGIV, p 80), experienced personnel, medications, and equipment to manage anaphylaxis should be immediately available. If an anaphylactic or anaphylactoid reaction occurs, the risk versus benefit of further infusions should be evaluated. If IG therapy is continued, IGSC or enzyme-facilitated subcutaneous infusion (see Immune Globulin Subcutaneous, p 82) is recommended because of

the decreased incidence of systemic adverse events compared with IGIV. Whichever modality of administration is used, the product that elicited the reaction should not be used again.

- As practitioners have gained experience with IGSC (see Immune Globulin Subcutaneous, p 82), many experts recommend a change to subcutaneous administration instead of manipulating methods of IV infusion or administering premedications to patients who have had reactions to IGIV.
- Most of the infusion-related adverse events associated with IGIV are associated with the rate of infusion. The initial infusion rate for most products is 4 mg/kg/min with a maximum infusion rate of 8 mg/kg/min, although some patients can tolerate up to 12 mg/kg/min. Reducing either the rate of infusion or the IGIV dose often can alleviate mild to moderate infusion-related nonallergic adverse reactions (excluding life-threatening subacute adverse events). Patients sensitive to one product often tolerate alternative products. Patients who experience aseptic meningitis with IGIV often tolerate IGSC. Although there are no studies to support the practice, most experts pretreat patients who have experienced significant reactions with a nonsteroidal anti-inflammatory agent such as ibuprofen or aspirin, acetaminophen, antihistamines, or a glucocorticoid to modify or relieve symptoms. Clinicians should balance the benefits of routine, long-term glucocorticoid premedication with the known accumulating risks of ongoing exposure. Significant adverse effects of IGIV administration should prompt consultation with an immunologist or other specialist experienced in managing this problem.
- Seriously ill patients with compromised cardiac function who are receiving large volumes of IGIV may be at increased risk of vasomotor or cardiac complications manifested as elevated blood pressure, cardiac failure, or both. In this setting, a low-sodium, high-IgG concentration product should be used if available. In hospitalized patients, these and other IGIV adverse event risks can be mitigated by using very slow infusion rates (approximately 30 mL/hour of a 10% IGIV product).

Immune Globulin Subcutaneous (IGSC)

Subcutaneous (SC) administration of immune globulin (IG) using manual syringe push or mechanical or battery-driven pumps has been shown to be safe and effective immune globulin prophylaxis in the treatment of adults and children with primary immunodeficiencies. Because the SC delivery method does not require intravenous or implanted venous access devices, most parents or patients can be taught to infuse immune globulin subcutaneous (IGSC) at home. Compared with immune globulin intravenous (IGIV), IGSC uses smaller doses administered more frequently (ie, daily to biweekly), providing a slow release of IG into systemic circulation. This leads to a more consistent steady state IgG concentration. When transitioning patients from IGIV to IGSC, the majority of clinicians use 1:1 dosing and monitor serum immunoglobulin (Ig) G concentrations and frequency of clinical infections to adjust the IGSC dose. Immunoglobulin replacement therapy doses are generally started around 400 to 600 mg/kg/month. Patients with chronic lung disease or bronchiectasis may benefit from higher doses (750–800 mg/kg/month).

Both mild and severe systemic reactions are substantially less frequent with IGSC than with IGIV therapy, and premedication is rarely required for IGSC. The most common adverse effects of IGSC are infusion-site reactions, including local swelling,

Table 1.14. Comparison of Routes for Immune Globulin Administration

Attribute	IGIV	Conventional IGSC	IGHY
Infusion frequency	Typically every 3–4 weeks	Most often daily to every 2 weeks	Every 2–4 weeks
Administration requirements	IV access, usually by a health care provider	No IV access, self-administered	No IV access, self-administered or by a health care provider
Sites/month	1	4–30	1–2
Systemic adverse events	Higher than with IGSC	Lower than with either IGIV or IGHY	Lower than with IGIV
Local adverse events	Infrequent	Common	Similar to conventional IGSC

IGIV indicates immune globulin intravenous; IGHY recombinant human hyaluronidase plus IGSC; IGSC, immune globulin subcutaneous; IV, intravenous.

redness, itching, soreness, induration, and local heat. These most often occur during or soon after completion of infusion and generally resolve over 1 to 2 days. Such reactions occur more frequently during the first months of treatment. Many local site reactions are associated with infusion needle length. Selection of 6-mm, 9-mm, or 12-mm needles is based on an individual's subcutaneous tissue composition. The most common systemic reaction is headache. Systemic reactions should be treated as discussed for IGIV (p 80). Infusing daily to several times a week decreases or eliminates systemic adverse effects in most patients.

Factors involved in selection of IGSC versus IGIV are listed in Table 1.14. Several products, with concentrations of 10%, 16.5%, and up to 20%, are licensed in the United States for conventional SC use (**www.fda.gov/vaccines-blood-biologics/approved-blood-products/immune-globulins**). IGSC is well tolerated in patients with thrombocytopenia and those receiving anticoagulant therapy. High-dose IGSC has been shown to be effective for immunomodulation in autoimmune neurologic conditions, and a 20% IGSC product has been licensed for the treatment of chronic inflammatory demyelinated polyneuropathy. Because there are limited data on the efficacy of IGSC for conditions requiring high-dose IG, only IGIV should be used for the treatment of Kawasaki disease or multisystem inflammatory syndrome in children (MIS-C).

Because the subcutaneous space limits infusion volume, multiple infusion sites and frequent infusions are needed to achieve an adequate steady state IgG level using conventional IGSC. Dosing volumes/site are product-dependent. The prescribing information for each product should be consulted to determine the starting volumes for new patients and the maximum volume/site that can be given. Pretreatment with recombinant human hyaluronidase (a spreading factor) permits the subcutaneous infusion of larger volumes (up to 600 mL) of IG at a single site, although many clinicians prefer to limit infusions to 300 mL/site. Products have been developed that include both the hyaluronidase for pre-infusion and the IGSC and are known as IGHY. The efficacy of IGHY products is comparable with that of standard IGSC and of IGIV. The infusion frequency and number of needlesticks required for IGHY are similar to those for IGIV, and IGHY has less than half the frequency of systemic adverse events compared with IGIV. The peak serum IgG concentration achieved following IGHY administration occurs several days following infusion and is far lower than that of IGIV. Unlike the consistent steady-state serum concentration achieved following conventional IGSC, trough concentrations associated with IGHY are comparable to those following administration of IGIV.

TRANSMISSION OF INFECTION BY IGSC

The transmission of infections by IGSC products is considered to be the same as with IGIV and is exceedingly low.

PRECAUTIONS FOR THE USE OF IGSC AND IGHY

- Caution should be used when administering IGSC to a patient with a history of adverse reactions to any form of immunoglobulin replacement. In this circumstance, most experts recommend use of an alternative product. Some suggest administering a fraction (1/30) of the monthly dose daily.
- Immediate, systemic reactions to IGSC are substantially less common and usually less severe than those with IGIV (see Adverse Reactions to IGIV, p 80). Epinephrine should be immediately available (ie, epinephrine autoinjector) where the IGSC is administered. Health care professionals administering IGSC should have training in the management of emergencies (particularly anaphylactic shock). Parents and patients should be trained in the use of epinephrine autoinjector in case of anaphylaxis outside of a medical setting.
- Life-threatening, subacute systemic adverse reactions (eg, thrombosis, hemolysis, renal injury) appear to be less common following IGSC than with IGIV but may occur (see Adverse Reactions to IGIV, p 80).

Treatment of Anaphylactic Reactions

Health care professionals administering vaccines or other biologic products must be able to recognize and treat systemic anaphylaxis. Medications, equipment, and competent staff necessary to maintain the patency of the airway and to manage cardiovascular collapse must be available.[1,2] In the event of a severe reaction requiring interventions beyond the capacity of the initial treatment team, emergency medical services should be requested to initiate additional emergency care prior to and during transport to a site for higher level of care.

The emergency treatment of anaphylactic reactions is epinephrine administered intramuscularly in the anterolateral thigh. Delayed administration of epinephrine is believed to be the major contributor to fatalities. Mild symptoms such as skin reactions alone (eg, pruritus, erythema, localized urticaria, or angioedema) may be the first signs of an anaphylactic reaction but in isolation are not dangerous and can be treated with antihistamines. However, using clinical judgment, an injection of epinephrine may be administered, depending on the clinical situation (Table 1.15). Epinephrine should be

---

[1] Shenoi RP, Timm N; American Academy of Pediatrics, Committee on Drugs. Drugs used to treat pediatric emergencies. *Pediatrics*. 2020;145(1): e20193450

[2] Sicherer SH; American Academy of Pediatrics, Section on Allergy and Immunology. Epinephrine for first-aid management of anaphylaxis. *Pediatrics*. 2017;139(3):e20164006

Table 1.15. Epinephrine in the Treatment of Anaphylaxis[a]

Epinephrine autoinjector (0.1 mg per dose for children weighing <10 kg; 0.15 mg per dose for children weighing 10 through 25 kg; or 0.3 mg per dose for children weighing 26 kg through 50 kg), IM (anterolateral thigh), repeated every as often as every 5 min if necessary

OR

Epinephrine 1 mg/mL (1:1000) (aqueous): IM (anterolateral thigh), 0.01 mg/kg (0.01 mL/kg) per dose, up to 0.5 mg (0.5 mL), repeated every as often as every 5 min if necessary

A continuous infusion should be started if inadequate response to repeated intramuscular doses. 1 mg (1 mL) of 1 mg/mL (1:1000) dilution of epinephrine added to 250 mL of 5% dextrose in water, resulting in a concentration of 4 µg/mL, is infused initially at a rate of 0.1 µg/kg per minute and increased gradually to 1 µg/kg per minute to maintain blood pressure.

[a]In addition to epinephrine, maintenance of the airway and administration of oxygen are critical.

injected promptly for anaphylaxis, which is likely (although not exclusively) occurring when 1 of the following 3 criteria are fulfilled:
1. Acute onset of an illness (minutes to hours) with involvement of the skin, mucosal tissue, or both with either respiratory involvement or reduced blood pressure and/or associated symptoms of end-organ dysfunction; or
2. Two or more of the following that occur rapidly after exposure to a likely allergen for the patient, including (i) involvement of skin-mucosal tissue, (ii) respiratory involvement, (iii) reduced blood pressure or associated symptoms, or (iv) gastrointestinal symptoms; or
3. Reduced blood pressure as a result of exposure to a known allergen trigger.[1]

If a patient is known to have had a previous severe allergic reaction to the biologic product/serum, onset of skin, cardiovascular, or respiratory symptoms alone may warrant treatment with epinephrine. Epinephrine should be administered via the intramuscular (IM) route, because higher in vivo concentrations are achieved more rapidly compared with subcutaneous administration. Use of readily available commercial epinephrine autoinjectors (available in 3 dosages based on patient weight: 0.1, 0.15, and 0.3 mg/dose; see Table 1.15) are preferred and have been shown to reduce time to drug administration and dosing errors.

Aqueous epinephrine (1 mg/mL [1:1000], 0.01 mg/kg; maximum dose, 0.5 mg) or autoinjector can be administered as often as every 5 minutes, as necessary, to control symptoms and maintain blood pressure. Repeat doses of epinephrine are required in up to 35% of cases of anaphylaxis cases. Most patients being treated for anaphylaxis should be placed in a supine position. Patients having difficulty breathing may be asked to sit up, and patients who are vomiting may be asked to lie on their side. When the patient's condition improves and remains stable, an oral antihistamine can be given for an additional 24 to 48 hours but is not always necessary. Corticosteroids have no proven role in the treatment of acute anaphylaxis.

[1] Shaker MS, Wallace DV, Golden DBK, et al. Anaphylaxis—a 2020 practice parameter update, systematic review, and Grading of Recommendations, Assessment, Development and Evaluation (GRADE) analysis. *J Allergy Clin Immunol.* 2020:145(4):1082-1123

Maintenance of the airway and administration of oxygen should be instituted promptly. Severe or potentially life-threatening systemic anaphylaxis involving severe bronchospasm, laryngeal edema, other airway compromise, shock, and cardiovascular collapse necessitates additional therapy. Rapid intravenous (IV) bolus infusion of isotonic fluids adequate to maintain blood pressure may be required to compensate for the loss of circulating intravascular volume.

Epinephrine is administered intramuscularly in the anterolateral thigh immediately while IV access is being established. IV epinephrine may be indicated for continuous infusion but should be used with extreme caution and only after failure of symptoms to respond to multiple intramuscular doses (see Table 1.15). Administration of epinephrine intravenously can lead to lethal arrhythmia, and cardiac monitoring is recommended. A slow, continuous, low-dose epinephrine infusion is preferable to repeated bolus administration, because the dose can be titrated to the desired effect, and accidental administration of large boluses of epinephrine can be avoided.

Nebulized albuterol is indicated for bronchospasm. In some cases, the use of other inotropic agents, such as dopamine, may be necessary for blood pressure support. H_1 antihistamines may be used as adjunctive therapy. These and other secondary drugs used for anaphylaxis are detailed in Table 1.16.

All patients showing signs and symptoms of systemic anaphylaxis, regardless of severity, should be observed in an appropriate facility, even after remission of immediate symptoms. Anaphylactic reactions are monophasic in 90% of cases, but can be biphasic or persistent over 24 to 36 hours despite early and aggressive management. Although a specific period of observation has not been established, a reasonable period of observation would be 1 hour for a mild episode in a person with no risk factors for biphasic anaphylaxis (eg, severe initial reaction, drug or unknown trigger) and as long as 24 hours for a severe episode.

Table 1.16. Dosages of Commonly Used Secondary Drugs in the Treatment of Anaphylaxis

Drug	Dose
H1 receptor-blocking agents (antihistamines)	
Diphenhydramine	Oral, IM, IV: 1 mg/kg, every 4–6 h (40 mg, maximum single dose <12 y; 50 mg, maximum single dose for 12 y and older)
Cetirizine	Oral: 2.5 mg, 6–23 mo; 5 mg, 2–5 y; 10 mg, ≥6 y (single dose daily)
B$_2$-agonist	
Albuterol	Nebulizer solution: 0.5% (5 mg/mL), 0.05–0.15 mg/kg per dose in 2–3 mL isotonic sodium chloride solution, maximum 5 mg/dose every 20 min over a 1-h to 2-h period, or 0.5 mg/kg/h by continuous nebulization (15 mg/h, maximum dose)
Vasopressor	
Dopamine	5–20 µg/kg/min, IV drip

IM indicates intramuscular; IV, intravenous.

Anaphylaxis occurring in people who are taking beta-adrenergic–blocking agents or angiotensin-converting enzyme inhibitors can be more profound and significantly less responsive to epinephrine and other beta-adrenergic agonist drugs. More aggressive therapy with epinephrine may override receptor blockade in some patients. In a patient who is taking a beta-blocker who has not responded to at least 2 doses of intramuscular epinephrine, glucagon can be administered via the IM or IV route at a dose of 0.5 mg for children weighing less than 25 kg and 1 mg for children weighing more than 25 kg.

At the time of discharge, all patients should be provided with an epinephrine auto-injector, a written emergency plan to treat future reactions, and follow-up appointment with an allergist. The patient and/or parent(s) should be trained on the use of the specific autoinjector provided.

IMMUNIZATION IN SPECIAL CLINICAL CIRCUMSTANCES

Immunization in Preterm and Low Birth Weight Infants

Infants born preterm (at less than 37 weeks of gestation) or low birth weight (less than 2500 g) who are clinically stable should, with few exceptions, receive all routinely recommended childhood vaccines at the same chronologic age as term and normal birth weight infants. Although studies have shown decreased immune responses to several vaccines administered to neonates with very low birth weight (less than 1500 g) and neonates of very early gestational age (less than 29 weeks of gestation), most preterm infants, including infants who receive corticosteroids for bronchopulmonary dysplasia, produce sufficient vaccine-induced immunity to prevent disease. Vaccine dosages administered to term infants should not be reduced or divided when administered to preterm or low birth weight infants.

Preterm and low birth weight infants tolerate most childhood vaccines as well as term infants do. Some studies show that cardiorespiratory events may increase in extremely (less than 1000 g) and very (less than 1500 g) low birth weight infants who receive selected vaccines. Apnea within 24 hours prior to immunization, younger age, or weight less than 2000 g at the time of immunization and 12-hour Score for Neonatal Acute Physiology II[1] greater than 10 have been associated with development of postimmunization apnea, and it may be prudent to monitor infants with these characteristics for 48 hours after immunization if they are still in the hospital.

Medically stable preterm infants who remain in the hospital at 2 months of chronologic age should receive all inactivated vaccines recommended at that age (see Recommended Child and Adolescent Immunization Schedule for Ages 18 Years or Younger [**http://redbook.solutions.aap.org/SS/Immunization_Schedules.aspx**]). A medically stable infant is defined as one who does not require ongoing management for serious infection; metabolic disease; or acute renal, cardiovascular, neurologic, or respiratory tract illness and who demonstrates a clinical course of sustained recovery and a pattern of steady growth. All immunizations required at 2 months of

---

[1] Zupancic JAF, Richardson DK, Horbar JD, Carpenter JH, Lee SK, Escobar GJ. Vermont Oxford Network SNAP Pilot Project Participants. Revalidation of the Score for Neonatal Acute Physiology in the Vermont Oxford Network. *Pediatrics*. 2007;119(1):e156-e163

age can be administered simultaneously to preterm or low birth weight infants, with the possible exception of live oral rotavirus vaccine in hospitalized infants (see below and Rotavirus, p 730). The number of vaccine injections at 2 months of age can be minimized by using combination vaccines. When limited injection sites preclude simultaneous administration, vaccines recommended at 2 months of age may be administered at different times with any interval between doses of different inactivated parenteral vaccines. The choice of needle lengths used for intramuscular (IM) vaccine administration is determined by available muscle mass of the preterm or low birth weight infant (see Table 1.8, p 56).

Hepatitis B vaccine administered to preterm or low birth weight infants weighing 2000 g or more at birth produces an immune response comparable to that in term infants. Medically stable infants weighing less than 2000 g demonstrate a lower hepatitis B antibody response. Hepatitis B vaccine schedules for infants weighing <2000 g and infants weighing ≥2000 g whose birthing parent's hepatitis B surface antigen (HBsAg) status is positive, negative, or unknown are provided in Hepatitis B, Special Considerations, including Table 3.22 (p 451). Only monovalent hepatitis B vaccine should be used for preterm or term infants younger than 6 weeks. Administration of a total of 4 doses of hepatitis B vaccine is permitted when a combination vaccine containing hepatitis B vaccine is administered after the birth dose.

Because all preterm infants are considered at increased risk of complications of influenza, 2 doses of inactivated influenza vaccine, administered 1 month apart, should be offered for all preterm infants beginning at 6 months of chronologic age (see Influenza, p 511). Influenza vaccine should be given to all pregnant people during pregnancy (may be administered at any time during pregnancy) to protect the pregnant person and to provide passive protection of young infants. Because preterm infants younger than 6 months and infants of any age with chronic complications of preterm birth are extremely vulnerable to influenza virus infection, it is very important that household contacts, child care providers, and hospital nursery personnel caring for preterm infants receive influenza vaccine annually (see Influenza, p 511).

Preterm infants younger than 6 months, who are too young to have completed the primary immunization series, are at increased risk of pertussis infection and pertussis-related complications. Tetanus toxoid, reduced diphtheria toxoid, and acellular pertussis (Tdap) vaccine should be administered to all pregnant people (ideally between weeks 27 and 36 of gestation, to maximize passive antibody transfer to the infant) during every pregnancy. Tdap should be administered immediately postpartum for birthing parents who were not immunized during pregnancy. Health care personnel caring for pregnant people and infants, as well as household contacts and child care providers of all infants who have not previously received Tdap, also should be vaccinated with Tdap (see Pertussis, p 656). Preterm infants, infants born with certain congenital heart defects, and certain infants with chronic lung disease of prematurity or hemodynamically significant heart disease may benefit from immunoprophylaxis with a monoclonal antibody product (respiratory syncytial virus monoclonal antibody) during respiratory syncytial virus season (see Respiratory Syncytial Virus, p 713). Routine childhood immunizations should be administered on schedule in infants receiving palivizumab or nirsevimab.

Rotavirus vaccine virus is shed by some infants in the weeks after vaccination. There are limited published studies on the transmission of vaccine virus in hospital settings, including neonatal intensive care units, that have not documented nosocomial transmission. Individual institutions may consider administering rotavirus vaccine at the recommended chronologic age to otherwise eligible infants during hospitalization, including in the neonatal intensive care unit. Otherwise, the first dose of rotavirus vaccine should be administered at the time of discharge to eligible infants.

Preterm or very low birth weight infants are at increased risk for respiratory illness from SARS-CoV-2 infection (see Coronavirus Disease-2019 [COVID-19], p 324). Extra efforts should be made to provide COVID-19 vaccines to all caregivers of preterm and very low birth weight infants to decrease the risk to infants and to the infants themselves beginning at 6 months of age.

Immunization in Pregnancy[1]

Immunization is an essential component of care in pregnancy. Several vaccine-preventable diseases, such as influenza and COVID-19, are associated with increased morbidity and mortality during pregnancy, and others, like pertussis, can affect newborn infants who are too young to begin active vaccination until months after birth. The benefits of vaccinating the pregnant individual and providing protection for the infant through transplacentally acquired antibodies have led to recommendations for select vaccinations during pregnancy.[2] Vaccines routinely recommended during pregnancy are safe for the pregnant person and the fetus. Obstetric care providers play a critical role in reviewing pregnant patients' vaccination history and ensuring that they receive recommended vaccines. Pediatric care providers are also frequently asked about vaccines during pregnancy by expectant parents and play an important role in reinforcing the importance of vaccines. This chapter covers active immunization during pregnancy. Immunity passively transferred to the infant via human milk is discussed in the chapter Breastfeeding and Human Milk (p 135).

Four vaccines are specifically recommended for routine administration during pregnancy—tetanus and diphtheria toxoids and acellular pertussis vaccine (Tdap), non-live influenza vaccine (IIV), COVID-19 vaccine, and respiratory syncytial virus (RSV) vaccine.

- **Tdap With Each Pregnancy.** Tdap administered during the third trimester of pregnancy reduces pertussis infection in infants. The Centers for Disease Control and Prevention (CDC), the American Academy of Pediatrics (AAP), the American College of Obstetricians and Gynecologists (ACOG), and the American Academy of Family Physicians (AAFP) recommend administration of Tdap during every pregnancy to ensure that infants have high concentrations of pertussis-specific antibodies at the time of birth. The recommended timing for administration of Tdap is as early as possible during the interval between 27 and 36 weeks' gestation, to maximize the pregnant individual's antibody response and passive antibody transfer to the infant. Tdap may be safely administered at any time during pregnancy if needed for wound management, pertussis outbreaks, or other extenuating circumstances. If Tdap was not administered during the current pregnancy, previously unimmunized individuals should be receive Tdap immediately postpartum (see Pertussis, p 656). Tdap, COVID-19, and IIV can be administered together safely, and Tdap can be safely administered after a recent dose of Td regardless of interval.

---

[1] See adult immunization schedule available at **www.cdc.gov/vaccines/schedules/hcp/adult.html.**

[2] **www.cdc.gov/vaccines/pregnancy/index.html**

- **Influenza Vaccine Each Influenza Season.** Pregnancy increases risks of severe influenza infection even among those who do not have underlying medical conditions. Influenza vaccination is recommended for everyone 6 months of age or older who does not have a contraindication, and pregnancy is a specific indication for vaccination with IIV or recombinant influenza vaccine (RIV). In addition to protecting the pregnant person, influenza vaccination in pregnancy also protects infants younger than 6 months of age who are too young to be vaccinated with IIV. IIV or RIV may be administered at any time during pregnancy (see Influenza, p 511). Pregnancy is a contraindication for live attenuated influenza vaccine (LAIV).
- **COVID-19 vaccine.** The CDC, ACOG, and Society for Maternal-Fetal Medicine recommend COVID-19 vaccines (primary series and boosters) for persons who are pregnant, breastfeeding, trying to get pregnant now, or might become pregnant in the future. There is an increased risk of severe COVID-19 infection and death during pregnancy as well as an increased risk for adverse pregnancy and neonatal outcomes. Accumulating data have supported the safety and effectiveness of COVID-19 vaccination in persons who are pregnant. COVID-19 vaccination can be administered in any trimester. The latest guidance on the use of COVID-19 vaccines currently approved or authorized in the United States is available at **www.cdc.gov/vaccines/ covid-19/clinical-considerations/interim-considerations-us.html.**
- **RSV vaccine.** On December 21, 2022, Pfizer Inc submitted a biologics license application (BLA) to the US Food and Drug Administration (FDA) to support licensure of its RSVpreF vaccine (Abrysvo) in pregnant people for prevention of RSV in their infants. Vaccine efficacy for prevention of severe RSV-associated lower respiratory tract disease within 90 days after birth was 81.8% (99.5% confidence interval [CI]: 40.6, 96.3), and within 180 days after birth was 69.4% (97.6% CI: 44.3, 84.1). Safety assessments for both the pregnant and infant populations were similar for vaccine and placebo recipients. A slightly higher percentage of preterm births occurred in the vaccine recipients compared with placebo recipients (5.6% [95% CI: 4.9%, 6.4%] versus 4.7% [95% CI: 4.1%, 5.5%]), but this did not reach statistical significance. On August 21, 2023, the FDA approved RSVpreF vaccine for use in pregnant people as a single dose to be given at 32 through 36 weeks' gestation, and in September 2023, the CDC recommended its use for pregnant people during 32 through 36 weeks' gestation, using seasonal administration, to prevent RSV lower respiratory tract infection in infants.

LIVE ATTENUATED VACCINES

Pregnancy is generally a contraindication for most live-virus vaccines, given the theoretical risks to the developing fetus. The background rate of major and minor structural fetal malformations in otherwise uncomplicated pregnancies, commonly accepted as 3% to 5%, needs to be considered when discussing concerns regarding a birth defect diagnosed before or after birth that could be inappropriately attributed to a vaccine. This consideration is particularly important when vaccination with a live or live-attenuated vaccine has occurred after completion of embryogenesis in the first trimester. Inadvertent administration of live-virus vaccines in early pregnancy has not been shown to result in specific embryopathy and is not an indication to consider pregnancy termination. However, pregnancy should be avoided for 4 weeks after receiving a live-virus vaccine because of the theoretical risk to the fetus.

- **Measles, Mumps, and Rubella Vaccine.** Measles, mumps, and rubella (MMR), varicella (VAR), and measles, mumps, rubella, and varicella (MMRV) vaccines are contraindicated for pregnant people. Efforts should be made to immunize individuals without evidence of immunity against these viruses before they become pregnant or in the immediate postpartum period. Following receipt of MMR, individuals should avoid pregnancy for at least 4 weeks. No case of embryopathy caused by live rubella vaccine has been reported; however, a rare theoretical risk of embryopathy from inadvertent administration cannot be excluded. Because pregnancy might result in a higher risk for severe measles disease and complications, immune globulin intravenous (IGIV) should be administered to pregnant people who do not have evidence of measles immunity and have been exposed to measles (see Measles, p 570, and Table 3.33, p 576). IGIV does not prevent rubella or mumps infection after exposure and is not recommended for that purpose.
- **Varicella Vaccine.** Like MMR, varicella-containing vaccines (VAR, MMRV) are live vaccines and are contraindicated in pregnancy. This contraindication is based on a theoretical risk for congenital varicella syndrome, although there is no association between inadvertent administration of VAR or MMRV and adverse pregnancy outcome based on available safety surveillance. A pregnant person living in a household is not a contraindication for another household member to be vaccinated against varicella. Pregnant individuals who do not have evidence of immunity to varicella are at risk for severe disease and related complications. Varicella-zoster immune globulin is recommended for pregnant people without evidence of immunity who have been exposed and should ideally be administered within 96 hours of exposure for greatest effectiveness but can be administered up to 10 days after exposure (see Varicella-Zoster Virus Infections, p 938, and Fig 3.22, p 945). The purpose of using varicella-zoster immune globulin during pregnancy is to prevent complications in the pregnant person rather than to protect the fetus/infant. If varicella-zoster immune globulin is not available, some experts suggest use of IGIV. Published data on the benefit of acyclovir as postexposure prophylaxis among immunocompromised individuals are limited, although the use of acyclovir during pregnancy is not contraindicated if clinically indicated.
- **Live Attenuated Influenza Vaccine (LAIV).** Although influenza vaccination is recommended during pregnancy, LAIV, as a live vaccine, is contraindicated even though there have been no demonstrated harms because of inadvertent LAIV administration during pregnancy. Any licensed non-live influenza vaccine (IIV, RIV) that is otherwise appropriate for age should be used instead.
- **Yellow Fever Vaccine.** Unlike most other live vaccines, the yellow fever vaccine is not contraindicated in pregnancy. It nevertheless poses a theoretical risk, and pregnancy is a precaution to yellow fever vaccine administration because of rare cases of transmission of the vaccine virus in utero, albeit without adverse effects in the infant. Whenever possible, pregnant people should defer travel to areas where yellow fever is endemic. If travel to an area with endemic disease is unavoidable and risks for yellow fever virus exposure are believed to outweigh the vaccination risks, a pregnant individual should be vaccinated. Breastfeeding also is a precaution for yellow fever vaccine administration (see Breastfeeding and Human Milk, p 135).
- **Typhoid Vaccine.** There are 2 types of typhoid vaccine currently available in the United States—a live attenuated vaccine for oral administration and a

polysaccharide vaccine for parenteral administration. No information is available on the safety of either typhoid vaccine in pregnancy. Generally, live vaccines should be avoided in pregnancy. If travel to an endemic area is unavoidable in pregnancy, inactivated typhoid vaccine may be considered.

- **Cholera Vaccine.** Pregnant people are at increased risk for poor outcomes from cholera infection. No information is available on the safety of live attenuated cholera vaccine in pregnancy. The vaccine is not absorbed from the recipient's gastrointestinal tract. Thus, administration of the vaccine to a pregnant person is not expected to result in fetal vaccine virus exposure. When considering cholera vaccination during pregnancy, for travel to areas of cholera transmission, the benefit of protection offered by the vaccine should be weighed against the risk of possible adverse events.
- **Smallpox-Mpox Vaccine.** The use of live replicating smallpox virus (vaccinia) vaccine (ACAM2000) is limited to laboratory workers who work with the virus or other orthopoxviruses that infect humans (eg, mpox) and is contraindicated in pregnant or breastfeeding people. Smallpox causes more severe disease in pregnant than nonpregnant individuals, but it is unknown whether mpox is more severe during pregnancy. The live, nonreplicating smallpox/mpox vaccine (JYNNEOS) can be offered to people who are pregnant or breastfeeding who are otherwise eligible, although data on safety are limited.

NON-LIVE VACCINES

- **Pneumococcal Vaccines.** Generally, pneumococcal vaccines should be deferred during pregnancy; however, pregnant people with underlying conditions that warrant pneumococcal immunization may be vaccinated when the benefit of the vaccination is considered to outweigh any potential risks.
- **Meningococcal Vaccines.** Serogroups A, C, W, and Y meningococcal conjugate vaccine (MenACWY) should be administered to pregnant people if indicated. Because limited data are available for MenB vaccination during pregnancy, vaccination with MenB should be deferred unless the pregnant individual is at increased risk and, after consultation with the pregnant person's health care provider, the benefits of vaccination are considered to outweigh the potential risks.
- **Hepatitis A and Hepatitis B Vaccines.** Infection with hepatitis A virus or hepatitis B virus can result in severe disease in the pregnant person and, in the case of hepatitis B, chronic infection in the infant. If not already vaccinated with hepatitis A vaccine (HepA), the vaccine should be administered in pregnancy if the patient is at risk for hepatitis A infection during pregnancy. No adverse effect on the developing fetus has been observed after immunization with hepatitis B vaccine (HepB) during pregnancy. Pregnancy and lactation are not contraindications to HepB immunization, and if not already vaccinated with HepB, the vaccine should be administered in pregnancy. Data about safety during pregnancy are not yet available for Heplisav B or PreHevbrio; until such data are available, other HepB vaccines are recommended for immunization during pregnancy.
- **Non-live Poliovirus Vaccine.** Although data on safety of inactivated poliovirus (IPV) vaccine for a pregnant person or developing fetus are limited, no adverse effect has been found. IPV vaccine can be administered to pregnant people who never have received poliovirus vaccine, are immunized partially, or are immunized completely but require a booster dose (see Poliovirus Infections, p 682).

- **Human Papillomavirus Vaccine.** The HPV vaccine is not recommended for use during pregnancy because of limited information about safety. The health care professional should inquire about pregnancy in patients who are known to be sexually active, but a pregnancy test is not required before starting the HPV vaccination series. If a vaccine recipient becomes pregnant, subsequent doses should be postponed until the person is no longer pregnant. If a dose has been administered inadvertently during pregnancy, no intervention is needed. Data to date show no evidence of adverse effect of any HPV vaccine on outcomes of pregnancy. Health care professionals can report inadvertent administrations of 9vHPV to pregnant people by calling the vaccine manufacturer at 1-800-986-8999.
- **Rabies Vaccine.** The serious consequences of rabies dictate prompt postexposure prophylaxis and the rabies vaccine should be administered regardless of pregnancy status. Studies have shown that there is no association between rabies vaccination and increases in spontaneous abortions, preterm births, or other adverse pregnancy outcomes. If the risk of exposure to rabies during pregnancy is substantial, preexposure vaccine may be indicated.
- **Japanese Encephalitis Vaccine.** No studies in humans have assessed the safety of Japanese encephalitis virus vaccine for pregnant people. Individuals at risk for Japanese encephalitis exposure should be immunized before pregnancy, if possible. Immunization during pregnancy may be considered if travel to an area with endemic infection is unavoidable and the risk of disease outweighs the risk of adverse events in pregnancy (see Arboviruses, p 237).
- **Tick-borne Encephalitis Vaccine.** No studies in humans have assessed the safety of tick-borne encephalitis virus vaccine for pregnant people. Individuals at risk of tick-borne encephalitis exposure should be immunized before pregnancy, if possible. Immunization during pregnancy may be considered if travel to an area with endemic infection is unavoidable and the risk of disease outweighs the risk of adverse events in pregnancy (see Arboviruses, p 237).
- **Anthrax Vaccine.** Anthrax vaccine is not licensed for use in pregnant people; however, in a postevent setting that poses a high risk of exposure to aerosolized *Bacillus anthracis* spores, pregnancy is neither a precaution nor a contraindication to its use in postexposure vaccine (see Anthrax, p 232).
- **Ebola Vaccine.** Limited human data from clinical trials with Ebola vaccines have not identified vaccine-associated risks during pregnancy. The decision regarding whether to vaccinate a pregnant person should consider the risk for exposure to Ebola virus (see Hemorrhagic Fevers Caused by Filoviruses: Ebola and Marburg, p 423).

Immunization and Other Considerations in Immunocompromised Children

The safety and effectiveness of vaccines in people with immunodeficiency depends on the nature and extent of their immunosuppression. Even though these individuals represent a heterogeneous population, their immunodeficiency can be classified into primary and secondary disorders. Primary disorders of the immune system generally are inherited and can involve any part of the immune defenses. Secondary disorders of the immune system are acquired, including conditions related to infection, malignancies, and chronic diseases and their treatments (see Table 1.17). The Infectious Diseases Society of

Table 1.17. Immunization of Children and Adolescents With Primary and Secondary Immune Deficiencies

Category	Example of Specific Immunodeficiency	Vaccine Contraindications[a]	Comments
Primary			
B lymphocyte (humoral)	Severe antibody deficiencies (eg, X-linked agammaglobulinemia and common variable immunodeficiency)	OPV,[b] BCG, smallpox vaccine, LAIV, YF vaccine, dengue vaccine, and live-bacteria vaccines[c]; no data for rotavirus vaccines	Effectiveness of any vaccine is uncertain if dependent only on humoral response (eg, PPSV23). Replacement IG therapy interferes with response to live vaccines MMR and VAR. Annual IIV is the only vaccine administered routinely to patients with profound hypogammaglobulinemia receiving IG replacement therapy. All non-live vaccines are safe to administer as part of immune response assessment prior to instituting IG therapy.
	Less severe antibody deficiencies (eg, selective IgA deficiency and IgG subclass deficiencies)	OPV,[b] BCG, dengue vaccine, YF vaccine	All non-live and, with the exception of dengue vaccine, all live vaccines[d] on the standard annual schedule are safe, likely are effective (although responses may be attenuated), and should be administered.[e] PPSV23 should be administered beginning at 2 years of age.[f]
T lymphocyte (cell-mediated and humoral)	Complete defects (eg, severe combined immunodeficiency, complete DiGeorge syndrome)	All live-bacteria and live-virus vaccines (including rotavirus vaccine)[c,d,g]	All non-live vaccines probably are ineffective. Annual IIV is the only vaccine administered routinely to patients receiving IG replacement therapy; if there is some residual antibody-producing capacity.

Table 1.17. Immunization of Children and Adolescents With Primary and Secondary Immune Deficiencies, continued

Category	Example of Specific Immunodeficiency	Vaccine Contraindications[a]	Comments
T lymphocyte (cell-mediated and humoral)	Partial defects (eg, most patients with DiGeorge syndrome, hyper-IgM syndrome, Wiskott-Aldrich syndrome, ataxia telangiectasia)	All live-bacteria and live-virus vaccines[c,d,g]	All non-live vaccines on the standard annual schedule are safe, may be effective depending on the degree of the immune defect, and should be administered.[e] Those with ≥500 CD3+ T lymphocytes/mm^3, ≥200 CD8+ T lymphocytes/mm^3, and normal mitogen response could be considered to receive MMR and VAR vaccine (but not MMRV). PPSV23 should be administered beginning at 2 years of age.[f] Consider MenACWY-CRM series beginning in infancy[h] and the MenB series beginning at 10 years of age depending on splenic dysfunction.
	Interferon-alpha; interferon-gamma; interleukin 12 axis deficiencies; STAT1 deficiencies	All live-bacteria vaccines[c] and YF vaccine; other live-virus vaccines[d] if severely lymphopenic	All non-live vaccines on the standard annual schedule are safe, likely are effective, and should be administered.[e] Based on experience in HIV-infected children with the measles vaccine, MMR and VAR (but not MMRV) probably are safe and may be preferable to the risk of disease. Non-live typhoid vaccine (Typhoid Vi) should be used for people living in areas with endemic typhoid.
Complement	Persistent complement component, properdin, mannan-binding lectin, or factor B deficiency; secondary deficiency because receiving eculizumab	None	All non-live and live vaccines on the standard annual schedule are safe, likely are effective, and should be administered.[e] PPSV23 should be given beginning at 2 years of age[f]; MenACWY-CRM series beginning in infancy[h]; and the MenB series beginning at 10 years of age. Meningococcal vaccination may be ineffective in patients receiving eculizumab; prophylactic antimicrobial therapy such as amoxicillin or penicillin can be considered for duration of treatment and until immune competence has returned.

Table 1.17. Immunization of Children and Adolescents With Primary and Secondary Immune Deficiencies, continued

Category	Example of Specific Immunodeficiency	Vaccine Contraindications[a]	Comments
Phagocytic function	Chronic granulomatous disease	Live-bacteria vaccines[c]	All non-live and live-virus vaccines[d] on the standard annual schedule are safe, likely are effective, and should be administered.[e,i]
	Phagocytic deficiencies that are ill-defined or accompanied by defects in T-lymphocyte and natural killer cell dysfunction (such as Chediak-Higashi syndrome, leukocyte adhesion defects, and myeloperoxidase deficiency)	All live-bacteria[c] and live-virus vaccines[d]	All non-live vaccines on the standard annual schedule are safe, likely are effective, and should be administered. PPSV23 should be administered beginning at 2 years of age.[f] Consider MenACWY-CRM series beginning in infancy[h] and the MenB series beginning at 10 years of age depending on splenic dysfunction.
Secondary			
	HIV/AIDS	OPV,[b] smallpox vaccine, BCG, LAIV, MMRV, MMR, VAR, dengue, YF vaccine in highly immunocompromised children	All non-live vaccines on the standard annual schedule are safe, may be effective, and should be administered.[e] Rotavirus vaccine should be administered on the standard schedule. MMR and VAR are recommended for children with HIV infection who are asymptomatic or have only low-level immunocompromise.[j] PPSV23 should be administered beginning at 2 years of age.[f] MenACWY-CRM series should be administered beginning in infancy.[h] Hib is indicated for under- or unimmunized children ≥5 years of age.[k]

Table 1.17. Immunization of Children and Adolescents With Primary and Secondary Immune Deficiencies, continued

Category	Example of Specific Immunodeficiency	Vaccine Contraindications[a]	Comments
	Malignancy, transplantation, autoimmune disease, immunosuppressive or radiation therapy	All live-virus and live-bacteria vaccines, depending on immune status[c,d]	Refer to text for guidance. All non-live vaccines on the standard annual schedule are safe and may be effective depending on degree of immunocompromise[e] Annual IIV is recommended unless receiving intensive chemotherapy or anti-B cell antibodies. PPSV23 should be administered beginning at 2 years of age.[f] Hib vaccine is indicated in under- or unimmunized children <5 years of age only.[e]
	Asplenia (functional, congenital anatomic, surgical)	LAIV	All non-live and live-virus vaccines on the standard annual schedule are safe, likely are effective, and should be administered.[e] PPSV23 should be administered beginning at 2 years of age[f]; MenACWY-CRM series beginning in infancy[h], and the MenB series beginning at 10 years of age.[k] Hib is indicated for under- or unimmunized children ≥5 years of age.[k]
	Chronic renal failure	None	All non-live and live-virus vaccines, except LAIV, on the standard annual immunization schedule are safe, likely are effective, and should be administered.[e] PPSV23 should be administered beginning at 2 years of age.[f] HepB is indicated if not previously immunized.
	CNS anatomic barrier defect (cochlear implant, congenital dysplasia of the inner ear; persistent CSF communication with naso-oropharynx)	LAIV	All non-live and live-virus vaccines on the standard annual immunization schedule are safe and effective and should be administered.[e] PPSV23 should be administered beginning at 2 years of age.[f]

Table 1.17. Immunization of Children and Adolescents With Primary and Secondary Immune Deficiencies, continued

Category	Example of Specific Immunodeficiency	Vaccine Contraindications[a]	Comments

AIDS indicates acquired immunodeficiency syndrome; BCG, bacille Calmette-Guérin; CNS, central nervous system; CSF, cerebrospinal fluid; HepB, hepatitis B vaccine; Hib, *Haemophilus influenzae* type b vaccine; HIV, human immunodeficiency virus; IG, immune globulin; IgA, immunoglobulin A; IgG, immunoglobulin G; IIV, non-live influenza vaccine; LAIV, live attenuated influenza vaccine; Men-ACWY, serogroups A, C, W, and Y meningococcal conjugate vaccine; MenACWY-CRM, MenACWY (Menveo); MenB, serogroup B meningococcal conjugate vaccine; MMR, measles, mumps, and rubella vaccine; MMRV, measles, mumps, rubella, and varicella vaccine; OPV, oral poliovirus vaccine; PPSV23, 23-valent pneumococcal polysaccharide vaccine; STAT1, signal transducer and activator of transcription 1; VAR, varicella vaccine; YF, yellow fever.

[a] This table refers to contraindications for nonemergency vaccination as recommended by the Advisory Committee on Immunization Practices, Centers for Disease Control and Prevention).

[b] OPV vaccine not available in the United States.

[c] Live-bacteria vaccines: BCG, Ty21a *Salmonella* Typhi vaccine, cholera vaccine.

[d] Live-virus vaccines: MMR, VAR, MMRV, OPV, YF vaccine, dengue vaccine, vaccinia (smallpox vaccine), and rotavirus vaccine. Except for severe T-lymphocyte deficiency, data to contraindicate rotavirus vaccine are lacking; the immunocompromised state generally is considered a precaution for rotavirus vaccine. LAIV is not indicated for any person with a potentially immunocompromising condition.

[e] Children who are under- or unimmunized for age should receive routinely recommended vaccines, according to age and the catch-up schedule, with urgency to administer needed Hib and pneumococcal conjugate vaccine (PCV).

[f] PPSV23 is begun at ≥2 years of age for patients with complement deficiency other than those with a deficiency limited to terminal complement components. If PCV is required (ie, for children <6 years who have not received all required doses, and for those ≥6 years of age who never received PCV), PCV dose(s) should be administered first, followed by PPSV23 at least 8 weeks later; a second dose of PPSV23 is given 5 years after the first. If one or more of the PCV doses is with PCV20, however, PPSV23 is not needed and should not be administered (see *Streptococcus pneumoniae* [Pneumococcal] Infections, p 810).

[g] Regarding T-lymphocyte immunodeficiency as a contraindication to rotavirus vaccine, data only exist for severe combined immunodeficiency syndrome.

[h] Age and schedule of doses depend on the product; repeated doses are required (see Meningococcal Infections, p 585).

[i] Additional pneumococcal vaccine is not indicated for children with chronic granulomatous disease beyond age-based standard recommendations for PCV, because these children are not at increased risk of pneumococcal disease.

[j] HIV-infected children should be considered for varicella vaccine if CD4+ T-lymphocyte count is ≥15% and should receive MMR vaccine if they are aged ≥12 months and do not have: 1) evidence of current severe immunosuppression (ie, to not have severe immunosuppression, individuals aged ≤5 years must have CD4+ T-lymphocyte percentages ≥15% for ≥6 months; and individuals aged >5 years must have both CD4+ T-lymphocyte percentages ≥15% and CD4+ T-lymphocyte counts ≥200 lymphocytes/mm³ for ≥6 months); and 2) other current evidence of measles, rubella, and mumps immunity. In cases when only CD4+ T-lymphocyte counts or only CD4+ T-lymphocyte percentages are available for those older than age 5 years, the assessment of severe immunosuppression can be based on the CD4+ T-lymphocyte values (count or percentage) that are available. In cases when CD4+ T-lymphocyte counts at the time CD4+ T-lymphocyte counts were measured; i.e., absence of severe immunosuppression is defined as ≥6 months above age-specific CD4+ T-lymphocyte count criteria: CD4+ T-lymphocyte count >750 lymphocytes/mm³ while aged ≤12 months, and CD4+ T-lymphocyte count ≥500 lymphocytes/mm³ while aged 1 through 5 years. MMRV should not be administered to children with HIV infection, regardless of degree of immunosuppression, because of lack of safety data in this population.

[k] A single dose of Hib is indicated for unimmunized children and adolescents ≥5 years of age (children and adolescents who have not received a primary series and booster dose or at least 1 dose of Hib after 14 months of age are considered unimmunized) who have anatomic or functional asplenia (including sickle cell disease), who will undergo splenectomy, or who have HIV infection.

America (IDSA), in collaboration with the Centers for Disease Control and Prevention (CDC), the American Academy of Pediatrics (AAP), and other professional societies and organizations, has developed immunization guidelines for children and adults with primary and secondary immune deficiencies.[1] Health care providers should consult these guidelines for vaccinating children and adults with specific health conditions (eg, hematopoietic cell or solid organ transplant recipients) and life circumstances (eg, international travel or providing care for people with immune deficiencies). This chapter includes general principles and specific recommendations when the primary care physician is more likely to deliver care without the patient's continuous management by a subspecialist. Subspecialists who care for immunocompromised patients share responsibility with the primary care physician for ensuring appropriate vaccinations for immunocompromised patients and members of their households and other close contacts.

GENERAL PRINCIPLES

Certain generalizations regarding degree of immune suppression in patients with a primary or secondary immunodeficiency are useful for the health care provider and were adopted in the IDSA guideline.

High-level immunosuppression includes patients who:
- Have combined B- and T-lymphocyte primary immunodeficiency (eg, severe combined immunodeficiency [SCID])
- Receive cancer chemotherapy
- Receive chemotherapeutic agents (eg, cyclophosphamide, methotrexate, mycophenolate) or combination immunosuppressive drugs for rheumatologic conditions
- Have human immunodeficiency virus (HIV) infection and a CD4+ T-lymphocyte percentage <15% for children ≤5 years of age; for children >5 years of age, have either a CD4+ T-lymphocyte count <200 lymphocytes/mm^3 or a CD4+ lymphocyte percentage <15%
- Receive daily corticosteroid therapy at a dose ≥20 mg/day (or ≥2 mg/kg/day for patients weighing <10 kg) of prednisone or equivalent for ≥14 days
- Receive certain biologic immune modulators (eg, tumor necrosis factor-alpha [TNF-α] antagonists, anti–B-lymphocyte monoclonal antibodies, anti-T-lymphocyte monoclonal antibodies, or checkpoint inhibitors)
- Are within 2 months of solid organ transplantation (SOT)
- Are within 2 to 3 months of receiving hematopoietic cell transplant (HCT) at a minimum and frequently for a much longer period (HCT recipients can have prolonged high degrees of immunosuppression depending on type of transplant [allogeneic > autologous], type of donor and cell source, and post-transplant complications [eg, graft versus host disease {GVHD}] and their treatments)

Low-level immunosuppression includes patients who:
- Have HIV infection and a CD4+ T-lymphocyte percentage ≥15% for children ≤5 years of age; for children >5 years of age, have both a CD4+ T-lymphocyte count ≥200 lymphocytes/mm^3 and a CD4+ lymphocyte percentage ≥15%
- Receive a lower daily dose of systemic corticosteroids than for high-level immunosuppression for ≥14 days or receive alternate-day corticosteroid therapy

[1] Rubin LG, Levin MJ, Ljungman P, et al. 2013 IDSA clinical practice guideline for vaccination of the immunocompromised host. *Clin Infect Dis.* 2014;58(3):309-318. Available at: **https://academic.oup.com/cid/article/58/3/e44/336537**

- Receive methotrexate at a dosage of ≤0.4 mg/kg/week, azathioprine at a dosage of ≤3 mg/kg/day, or 6-mercaptopurine at a dosage of ≤1.5 mg/kg/day

TIMING OF VACCINES. For patients in whom initiation of immunosuppressive medication is planned, vaccinations should be administered before immunosuppression, when feasible. Live vaccines should be administered as indicated no closer than 4 weeks before initiation of immunosuppression or transplantation. If administration is not possible within this time restriction, immunization should be deferred until after recovery and/or reduction of profound immunosuppression. Non-live vaccines should be administered at least 2 weeks before immunosuppression or transplantation, if feasible.

Certain vaccines may be administered to children while they are modestly immunosuppressed, especially when the immunosuppressed state is likely to be lengthy or lifelong. Examples include some children with HIV infection and those having received solid organ transplants. Currently, there is no universally approved revaccination guidelines for nontransplanted childhood cancer survivors, and therefore the exact timing of when to revaccinate and/or catch-up children with cancer remains unclear. The IDSA recommends catch-up vaccination at 3 months following cessation of chemotherapy, but other societies recommend waiting 6 months. Patients who have received chemotherapies associated with longer-term immunocompromise, such as blinatumomab, rituximab, obinutuzumab, or alemtuzumab, may require longer delays. Some non-live vaccines have been administered during maintenance chemotherapy for children with acute leukemia, including non-live influenza vaccine (IIV) and COVID-19 vaccine. However, as described later in this chapter, live vaccines are generally contraindicated in immunocompromised people. Expert consultation is warranted if a live vaccine is being considered for immunocompromised people, including certain children after SOT, with HIV infection, and after HCT.

The interval between cessation of immunosuppressive therapy and immune reconstitution varies. Therefore, it is often not possible to make a definitive recommendation for an interval after cessation of immunosuppressive therapy when non-live vaccines can be administered effectively or when or whether live vaccines can be administered safely and effectively. Immunodeficiency that follows use of certain recombinant human proteins with anti-inflammatory properties, such as the anti-B-lymphocyte monoclonal antibody rituximab and the anti-leukemic monoclonal antibody blinatumomab, is prolonged and patients who receive such treatment are unlikely to respond to vaccines for at least 6 months and often much longer (see Biologic Response-Modifying Drugs Used to Decrease Inflammation, p 104).

Vaccinations after reduction or cessation of immunosuppression following transplantation vary depending on the vaccine, underlying disorder, specific immunosuppressive therapy, and presence or absence of GVHD.[1] Timing for non-live and live vaccines could vary from as early as 3 months after cessation of chemotherapy for acute leukemia to 24 months or longer for measles, mumps, and rubella vaccine (MMR) or varicella vaccine (VAR) after HCT in a patient without ongoing immunosuppression or GVHD. Timing also may be delayed for SOT recipients with graft rejection.

---

[1] Rubin LG, Levin MJ, Ljungman P, et al. 2013 IDSA clinical practice guideline for vaccination of the immunocompromised host. *Clin Infect Dis.* 2014;58(3):309-318. Available at: **https://academic.oup.com/cid/article/58/3/e44/336537**

LIVE VACCINES. In general, people who are severely immunocompromised or in whom immune function is uncertain should not receive live vaccines because of the risk of disease caused by the vaccine strains. However, there are particular immune deficiency disorders in which some live vaccines are safe and, for certain immunocompromised children and adolescents, the benefits may outweigh risks for use of particular live vaccines (see Table 1.17, p 94).

NON-LIVE VACCINES. Non-live vaccines do not convey substantial increased risk to an immunocompromised child compared with an immunocompetent child and, therefore, the decision to administer a non-live vaccine to children with immunodeficiency is based on an assessment of the likelihood of benefit. Non-live vaccines administered during certain immunosuppressive therapies (eg, receipt of anti-CD20 biologics, induction or consolidation chemotherapies) generally are not counted as valid in the recommended immunization schedule. Annual vaccination with non-live influenza vaccine (IIV) is recommended for immunocompromised patients 6 months of age and older. Other than IIV, non-live vaccines are generally not routinely administered to patients receiving immunoglobulin therapy for major antibody deficiency disorders or severe combined immunodeficiencies because of lack of added benefit.

Non-live vaccines not administered universally or at specific ages sometimes may be specifically indicated for children with inherited and acquired immunodeficient conditions because of their high risk for infection. These might include pneumococcal conjugate vaccine (PCV), followed by 23-valent pneumococcal polysaccharide vaccine (PPSV23) after the age of 6 years if not previously vaccinated with PCV; serogroups A, C, W, and Y meningococcal conjugate vaccine (MenACWY) beginning in infancy; serogroup B meningococcal conjugate vaccine (MenB) beginning at 10 years of age; and *Haemophilus influenzae* type b vaccine (Hib) after the age of 5 years. Some immunocompromised children and adolescents are at high risk of serious infection with SARS-CoV-2 and should receive booster doses of COVID-19 vaccine. Depending on the age of the person, the type of vaccine, and severity of immunocompromise, recommendations for primary series, additional doses, and use of boosters may vary. Clinicians should review the latest information available from the CDC and the Advisory Committee on Immunization Practices (ACIP).

Table 1.17 (p 94) provides guidance for some immunocompromising conditions. Additional information can be found in the IDSA clinical practice guideline for vaccination of the immunocompromised person (**https://academic.oup.com/cid/article/58/3/e44/336537**) and in the annually updated child and adolescent immunization schedule (**https://redbook.solutions.aap.org/SS/Immunization_Schedules.aspx**).

Because patients with congenital or acquired immunodeficiencies may not have an adequate response to vaccines, they may remain susceptible to infections despite having been immunized. Positive serologic test results are not always reliable markers of protection. Health care providers should generally assume susceptibility to infections when considering postexposure intervention strategies for these patients.

PRIMARY IMMUNODEFICIENCIES

Vaccine recommendations for primary immunodeficiency disorders depend on the specific immunologic abnormality and degree of impairment (Table 1.17, p 94). For B-lymphocyte primary immunodeficiency, vaccines to be avoided include oral poliovirus, yellow fever, live attenuated influenza, and live bacterial vaccines; safety and efficacy of rotavirus vaccine is unknown in this population. All live-virus and non-live vaccines can be administered to children with isolated immunoglobulin (Ig) A and IgG subclass deficiencies. Non-live vaccines other than IIV are not routinely administered to patients with major antibody deficiencies or SCID during immune globulin therapy. For these patients, non-live vaccines can be administered as part of immunologic assessment prior to immune globulin intravenous (IGIV) therapy without safety concerns. For patients with common variable immunodeficiency, MenACWY should be administered beginning at 2 months of age because of their splenic dysfunction and lack of substantial meningococcal antibodies in IGIV.

Live-virus vaccines such as MMR and VAR should not be administered to patients with major antibody deficiencies, SCID, and T-lymphocyte immunodeficiencies, including any of the following conditions: DiGeorge syndrome with CD3+ T-lymphocyte count <500 cells/mm^3,[1] other combined immunodeficiencies with similar CD3+ T-lymphocyte counts,[1] Wiskott-Aldrich syndrome, or X-linked lymphoproliferative disease or familial disorders that predispose to hemophagocytic lymphohistiocytosis.

Patients with primary complement deficiencies of early classic pathway, alternate pathway, or severe mannose-binding lectin deficiency should receive all routine non-live and live vaccines on the immunization schedule. For patients with complement deficiencies other than isolated terminal complement component deficiencies, PPSV23 should be administered at 2 years of age (and ≥8 weeks after last dose of PCV) and again 5 years after the initial dose. The MenACWY series should be initiated at age 2 months or older and the MenB series should be administered starting at age 10 years. MenACWY and MenB booster doses are indicated for those at chronic, increased risk for meningococcal disease (eg, functional [eg, sickle cell disease] and anatomical [eg, splenectomy] asplenia, HIV infection, persistent complement component deficiency) (see Meningococcal Infections, p 585). Both meningococcal vaccines are recommended for patients receiving eculizumab, which inhibits the complement cascade by binding to complement component 5 (C5).

Patients with phagocytic cell deficiencies (eg, chronic granulomatous disease [CGD], leukocyte adhesion deficiency [LAD], Chediak-Higashi syndrome, cyclic neutropenia) and patients with innate immune defects that result in defects of cytokine generation or response or cellular activation (eg, defects of interferon-gamma/interleukin [IL]-12 axis) should receive all non-live vaccines on the annual immunization schedule. Live-virus vaccines (eg, MMR) should be administered to patients with CGD and cyclic neutropenia, but live-bacterial vaccines (eg, oral typhoid vaccine [Ty21a]) should not be administered to these patients. Live-bacterial vaccines should not be administered to patients with interferon-gamma/IL-12 axis deficiencies. Live-bacterial and live-virus vaccines should not be administered to patients with LAD, Chediak-Higashi syndrome, or defects within the interferon-gamma or IL-12 pathway.

---

[1] Rubin LG, Levin MJ, Ljungman P, et al. 2013 IDSA clinical practice guideline for vaccination of the immunocompromised host. *Clin Infect Dis*. 2014;58(3):309-318. Available at: **https://academic.oup.com/cid/article/58/3/e44/336537**

SECONDARY (ACQUIRED) IMMUNODEFICIENCIES

Several factors should be considered in immunization of children with secondary immunodeficiencies (Table 1.17, p 94), including the underlying disease, the specific immunosuppressive regimen (dose and schedule), and the patient's infectious disease and immunization history. Live vaccines generally are contraindicated because of a proven or theoretical increased risk of vaccine virus disease. For example, in children with an immunocompromising condition or HIV infection and CD4+ T-lymphocyte percentage <15% or count <200/mm^3, MMR and VAR are contraindicated. LAIV should not be administered to children with HIV infection. Rotavirus vaccine should be administered to HIV-exposed and HIV-infected infants, irrespective of CD4+ T-lymphocyte percentage or count, according to the schedule for uninfected infants (see Human Immunodeficiency Virus Infection, p 489). Rotavirus vaccine may be indicated for infants with acquired immunocompromising conditions if the potential benefit of protection outweighs the risk of adverse reaction.

HOUSEHOLD MEMBERS OF IMMUNOCOMPROMISED PATIENTS

Household contacts of immunocompromised patients should receive all age- and exposure-appropriate vaccines, with the exception of smallpox vaccine, to minimize the exposure of the immunocompromised patient to vaccine-preventable infections. LAIV may be administered to healthy household and other close contacts of people with altered immunocompetence. However, if the person with altered immunocompetence is in a protected environment, then LAIV recipients should avoid close contact with the immunocompromised person for 7 days.

Live vaccines, when indicated for travel (eg, yellow fever and oral typhoid vaccines), should also be administered to household contacts, with the exception of oral poliovirus vaccine (OPV), which still is available in many countries outside of the United States. Although the risk of transmission is low, immunocompromised patients should avoid contact with people who develop skin lesions after receipt of VAR until the lesions clear. When transmission of vaccine-strain varicella virus has occurred, the virus is expected to maintain its attenuated characteristics and susceptibility to acyclovir. Therefore, administration of varicella-zoster immune globulin or IGIV to an immunocompromised person after exposure to a person with skin lesions that developed after varicella vaccination is not indicated. All members of the household should wash their hands after changing the diaper of an infant who received rotavirus vaccine to minimize rotavirus transmission, as shedding of the virus may occur up to 1 month after the last dose; immunocompromised patients ideally should not change diapers of infants at all for several weeks after rotavirus vaccine.

SPECIAL SITUATIONS/HOSTS

CORTICOSTEROIDS. Before starting corticosteroid therapy for inflammatory or autoimmune diseases, patients should be current in their vaccinations based on their age and other indications. Non-live vaccines should ideally be administered at least 2 weeks before and live vaccines should be administered at least 4 weeks before initiating corticosteroid therapy.

Guidance for Administration of Non-live Vaccines During Corticosteroid Therapy. Non-live vaccines can still be administered to patients while they are receiving steroid therapy long-term. Non-live vaccine administration can be deferred temporarily until corticosteroids are discontinued if the hiatus is expected to be brief and adherence to return appointment is likely. Non-live vaccines need not be avoided because of concern for exacerbation of an inflammatory or immune-mediated condition.

Guidance for Administration of Live Vaccines During Corticosteroid Therapy. Recommendations depend on potency, route of administration, and duration of corticosteroid therapy:

- **High doses of systemic corticosteroids given daily for 14 days or more.** Children receiving ≥2 mg/kg per day of prednisone or its equivalent, or ≥20 mg/day if they weigh 10 kg or more, for 14 days or more should not receive live vaccines until 4 weeks after discontinuation of treatment.
- **High doses of systemic corticosteroids given daily or on alternate days for fewer than 14 days.** Children receiving ≥2 mg/kg per day of prednisone or its equivalent, or ≥20 mg/day if they weigh 10 kg or more, can receive live-virus vaccines immediately after discontinuation of treatment.
- **Low or moderate doses of systemic corticosteroids or locally administered corticosteroids in children who have a disease (eg, systemic lupus erythematosus) that itself is immunosuppressive, or who are receiving immunosuppressive medication other than corticosteroids,** should not receive live vaccines during therapy, except in special circumstances during which the potential benefit of protection and the risk of adverse reaction are weighed.
- **Low or moderate doses of systemic corticosteroids given daily or on alternate days.** Children receiving <2 mg/kg per day of prednisone or its equivalent, or <20 mg/day if they weigh 10 kg or more, can receive live vaccines during corticosteroid treatment.
- **Physiologic maintenance doses of corticosteroids.** Children who are receiving only maintenance physiologic doses of corticosteroids can receive live vaccines.
- **Topical therapy, local injections, or aerosol use of corticosteroids.** Application of low-potency topical corticosteroids to localized areas on the skin; administration by aerosolization; application on conjunctiva; or intra-articular, bursal, or tendon injections of corticosteroids usually do not result in immunosuppression that limits the use of live vaccines.

BIOLOGIC RESPONSE-MODIFYING DRUGS USED TO DECREASE INFLAMMATION.
Biologic response modifiers (BRMs) are drugs used to treat immune-mediated conditions, including juvenile idiopathic arthritis, rheumatoid arthritis, and inflammatory bowel disease. Their immune-modulating effects can last for weeks to months after discontinuation. These BRMs are often used in combination with other immunosuppressive drugs, such as methotrexate or corticosteroids.

Vaccination status of patients who need BRMs should be assessed and recommended vaccines should be administered in advance where feasible (Table 1.18). Recommended vaccines include PPSV23 for patients 2 years or older unless they have received one or more doses of PCV20 already; if PCV is required (ie, for children <6 years of age who have not received all required doses, and for those ≥6 years of age who never received PCV), PCV dose(s) should be administered first, followed by PPSV23 at least 8 weeks later if indicated (eg, if the child has not received any doses of PCV20).

Most BRMs are considered highly immunosuppressive, and live vaccines are contraindicated during therapy; non-live vaccines, including IIV, should be administered as per the immunization schedule and should not be withheld because of concern for an exaggerated inflammatory response. The interval following therapy

Table 1.18. Recommendations for Evaluation Prior to Initiation of Biologic Response-Modifying Drugs

- Perform tuberculin skin test (TST) or interferon-gamma release assay (IGRA) (see Tuberculosis, p 888)
- Consider chest radiograph on the basis of clinical and epidemiologic findings
- Document vaccination status and, if required, administer:
  - Non-live vaccines (including annual IIV) a minimum of 2 weeks before initiation of biologic response-modifying drug
  - Live-virus vaccines a minimum 4 weeks before initiation of biologic response modifier therapy, unless contraindicated by condition or other therapies
- Counsel household members regarding risk of infection and ensure vaccination (see Household Members of Immunocompromised Patients, p 103)
- Consider serologic testing for *Histoplasma* species, *Toxoplasma* species, and other intracellular pathogens depending on risk of past exposure
- Perform serologic testing for hepatitis B virus and vaccinate/revaccinate if HBsAb is <10 mIU/mL
- Consider serologic testing for varicella-zoster virus and Epstein-Barr virus
- Counsel regarding:
  - Food safety (**www.cdc.gov/foodsafety**)
  - Maintenance of dental hygiene
  - Risks of exposure to garden soil, pets, and other animals
  - Avoiding high-risk activities (eg, excavation sites or spelunking because of risk of *Histoplasma capsulatum*)
  - Avoiding travel to areas with endemic pathogenic fungi (eg, certain areas of southwestern United States for risk of *Coccidioides* species) or to areas where tuberculosis is endemic

IIV indicates non-live influenza vaccine; HBsAb, hepatitis B surface antibody.
Modified from Le Saux N; Canadian Paediatric Society, Infectious Diseases and Immunization Committee. *Paediatr Child Health.* 2012;17(3):147-150 and Davies HD; American Academy of Pediatrics, Committee on Infectious Diseases. Infectious complications with the use of biologic response modifiers in infants and children. *Pediatrics.* 2016;138(2):e20161209 (Reaffirmed March 2021).

until live vaccines can be administered safely has not been established and is likely to vary by agent.

Infants exposed in utero to maternally administered BRMs can have detectable drug concentrations for many months following delivery, resulting in concern for immunosuppression among infants in the 12 months after the last maternal dose during pregnancy. Data are sparse on the safety of rotavirus vaccines in infants who were exposed in utero to BRMs administered to the expectant parent during pregnancy. Considering that rotavirus disease is rarely life-threatening in the United States, rotavirus vaccines should be avoided in infants for the first 12 months after the last in utero exposure to most BRMs. Exceptions include certolizumab, which is not transferred across the placenta because of its structure as a pegylated Fab fragment, and likely infliximab, although the data are sparser; rotavirus vaccination of infants can be considered when either of these BRMs were administered during pregnancy. As more data become available for the other BRMs, recommendations are likely to change,[1]

[1] Fitzpatrick T, Alsager K, Sadarangani M, et al; Special Immunization Clinic Network investigators. Immunological effects and safety of live rotavirus vaccination after antenatal exposure to immunomodulatory biologic agents: a prospective cohort study from the Canadian Immunization Research Network. *Lancet Child Adolesc Health.* 2023;7(9):648-656

so consultation with an immunologist or a pediatric infectious diseases physician is recommended. Because MMR, VAR, and measles, mumps, rubella, and varicella vaccine (MMRV) are recommended routinely at 12 months of age, previous receipt of BRMs during pregnancy does not preclude the infant from receiving these live vaccines at the recommended time. For measles prevention in infants younger than 12 months following exposure during outbreak settings or for travel, MMR or immune globulin intramuscular should be used. The choice depends on several factors (eg, age, time elapsed since exposure, which BRM was administered during pregnancy). International travel for infants who were exposed to BRMs in utero (other than certolizumab) should be discouraged for the 12 months following the last dose administered during pregnancy. These recommendations may not apply to management of infants born in other countries, where risks of wild-type infection may differ from the United States and where additional live vaccines may be administered in early infancy (eg, bacille Calmette-Guérin [BCG], OPV).

HEMATOPOIETIC CELL TRANSPLANTATION. Patients for whom HCT is planned should receive all routinely recommended non-live vaccines (including IIV) at least 2 weeks before the start of the conditioning period, when possible. Routinely recommended live vaccines should be administered if the patient is not already immunosuppressed and the interval to the start of the conditioning period is at least 4 weeks. By vaccinating the nonimmune patient before HCT, some protection likely will persist in the months after transplant. The HCT donor, if known and feasible, should be current with routinely recommended vaccines, but vaccination of the donor solely for benefit of the recipient is not recommended. Administration of MMR, MMRV, and VAR should be avoided within 4 weeks of hematopoietic stem cell harvest but may be contraindicated even prior to that because of pre-existing immunocompromise.

Household members of HCT recipients should be fully immunized (see Household Members of Immunocompromised Patients, p 103). Timing of immune reconstitution of HCT recipients varies greatly depending on type of transplantation, interval since transplantation, receipt of immunosuppressive medications, and presence or absence of GVHD and other complications. Routine and additional vaccinations are an important part of patient management in collaboration with the patient's specialty care providers. Revaccination for certain non-live vaccines, such as pneumococcal vaccines and IIV, can be given starting 3 to 6 months after transplantation. Live vaccines can be given as early as 2 years following transplantation but may be delayed if HCT recipients still have active GVHD and/or high degree of immunosuppression.

Following CD19-targeted chimeric antigen receptor T-cell (CAR-T) therapy, patients may have prolonged B-lymphocyte aplasia. The safety and immunogenicity of vaccinations after CAR-T therapy is not known, and currently no guidelines exist. On the basis of expert opinion, for patients in remission and who do not require additional chemotherapy or HCT, non-live vaccines may be administered if 6 months or longer has transpired following CAR-T therapy and it has been 2 months or more since last IG treatment; live vaccines may be administered if 1 year or longer has transpired following CAR-T therapy. Current mRNA COVID-19 vaccines should be offered beginning at 3 months after CAR-T therapy; refer to the most updated recommendations of primary and booster doses of COVID-19 vaccines from the CDC and ACIP (**www.cdc.gov/coronavirus/2019-ncov/vaccines/recommendations/ immuno.html**).

SOLID ORGAN TRANSPLANTATION. Children and adolescents with chronic heart, lung, liver, or kidney disease should receive all vaccinations as appropriate for age and health condition. Similarly, SOT candidates should be current with their vaccination status and, if feasible, should receive non-live vaccines at least 2 weeks prior and live vaccines 4 week prior to SOT. SOT candidates younger than 2 years should receive pneumococcal vaccination with PCV as described in the annual immunization schedule. If PCV is required (ie, for children <6 years of age who have not received all required doses, and for those ≥6 years of age who never received PCV), PCV dose(s) should be administered first, followed by PPSV23 at least 8 weeks later; a second dose of PPSV23 is given 5 years after the first. SOT candidates who have negative hepatitis B surface antigen (HBsAg) and hepatitis B surface antibody (anti-HBsAb) test results should complete the hepatitis B vaccine (HepB) series, followed by serologic testing to confirm immunity. Additional doses of HepB may be indicated if serologic test results are negative. Patients 12 months or older who have not completed the hepatitis A vaccine (HepA) series or have negative hepatitis A serologic test results should complete the HepA series. MMR can be administered to infants 6 through 11 months of age who are SOT candidates and who are not immunocompromised, with a second dose provided 4 weeks later. MMR doses given before 12 months of age cannot be counted toward the standard 2-dose series. As such, if an infant ≥12 months of age has received MMR and is still awaiting a transplant that will not occur within 4 weeks, 2 doses of MMR should be administered at least 4 weeks apart. Living SOT donors should be current on their vaccination status, with considerations for required vaccines the same as for HCT donors (see Hematopoietic Cell Transplantation, p 106). Donors should avoid receiving live vaccines within 4 weeks before donation. Household members of SOT recipients should be current on their vaccination status.[1]

HIV INFECTION (ALSO SEE HUMAN IMMUNODEFICIENCY VIRUS INFECTION, P 489). HIV-infected children and adolescents should receive all non-live vaccines as indicated on the annual immunization schedule. PPSV23 should be administered to people with HIV 2 years or older, at least 8 weeks after the last required PCV dose. Meningococcal conjugate vaccine (MenACWY) should be administered beginning at 8 weeks of age. Depending on age of the patient and the vaccine manufacturer, the number of doses and the intervals between doses can vary. A booster dose of MenACWY is recommended 3 to 5 years after the primary series, depending on age at vaccination. Children with HIV should not receive Menactra before the age of 2 years to avoid interference with the immunologic response to the infant series of pneumococcal conjugate vaccine; only MenACWY-CRM (Menveo) should be used in this group (see Meningococcal Infections, p 585, Table 3.39, p 592, and Table 3.40, p 594). Currently, MenB is not specifically recommended for people with HIV infection. Rotavirus vaccine should be administered to HIV-exposed and HIV-infected infants, irrespective of CD4+ T-lymphocyte percentage or count, according to the schedule for uninfected infants (see Human Immunodeficiency Virus Infection, p 489). MMR and VAR should be administered to children 12 months or older who are clinically stable and who have a CD4+ T-lymphocyte percentage ≥15% for children ≤5 years of age, or have both a CD4+ T-lymphocyte count ≥200 lymphocytes/mm^3 and a CD4+ lymphocyte percentage ≥15% for children >5 years of age (see General Principles, p 99).

[1] Suresh S, Upton J, Green M, et al. Live vaccines after pediatric solid organ transplant: proceedings of a consensus meeting, 2018. *Pediatr Transplant.* 2019;23(7):e13571

Children with HIV infection should not receive MMRV or LAIV. Mpox vaccination may be indicated for at-risk individuals with HIV and other immunocompromising conditions (**www.cdc.gov/poxvirus/mpox/clinicians/people-with-HIV. html**). JYNNEOS is the only mpox vaccine authorized for pre- and postexposure prophylaxis in eligible immunocompromised individuals.

In the United States, BCG is usually contraindicated for people with HIV. In areas of the world with a high incidence of tuberculosis, the World Health Organization (WHO) recommends administering BCG vaccine to children with HIV infection who are asymptomatic.

ASPLENIA AND FUNCTIONAL ASPLENIA. An asplenic state can result from the following: (1) surgical removal of the spleen (eg, after trauma, for treatment of hemolytic conditions); (2) functional asplenia (eg, from sickle cell disease or thalassemia); or (3) congenital asplenia or polysplenia. Special recommendations for patients with asplenia apply to all 3 categories. All infants, children, adolescents, and adults with asplenia have an increased risk of fulminant septicemia, especially associated with encapsulated bacteria, which is associated with a high mortality rate. In comparison with immuno-competent children who have not undergone splenectomy, the incidence of and mortality rate from septicemia are increased in children who have had splenectomy after trauma and in children with sickle cell disease by as much as 350-fold, and the rate may be even higher in children who have had splenectomy for thalassemia. The risk of invasive bacterial infection is higher in younger children than in older children, and the risk may be greater during the years immediately after surgical splenectomy. Fulminant septicemia, however, has been reported in adults as long as 25 years after splenectomy.

Streptococcus pneumoniae is the most common pathogen causing septicemia in children with asplenia. Less common vaccine-preventable causes include *Haemophilus influenzae* type b and *Neisseria meningitidis.*

Pneumococcal vaccination is vital for children with asplenia (see *Streptococcus pneumoniae* [Pneumococcal] Infections, p 810). Following administration of an appropriate number of primary series or catch-up doses of PCV, PPSV23 should be administered to children 24 months or older at least 8 weeks after the last PCV dose unless one or more of the PCV doses was with PCV20. If PPSV23 is used, a second dose of PPSV23 should be administered 5 years later (see *Streptococcus pneumoniae* [Pneumococcal] Infections, p 810).

Previously unimmunized children with asplenia younger than 5 years should receive appropriate number of doses of and intervals for Hib according to the catch-up schedule as described in the annual immunization schedule. Unimmunized children 5 years or older should receive a single dose of Hib.

MenACWY and Men B should be administered to children with asplenia, as recommended for those with primary complement component deficiencies (see Primary Immunodeficiencies, p 101), with one important caveat. MenACWY-D (Menactra) may interfere with antibody response to some serotypes contained in PCV when the vaccines are administered concurrently or closely together. Therefore, because of their high risk for invasive pneumococcal disease, children with functional or anatomic asplenia should not be vaccinated with MenACWY-D (Menactra) before age 2 years to avoid interference with the immune response to PCV (see Meningococcal Infections, p 585). Only MenACWY-CRM (Menveo) should be used in this group; MenACWY-TT (MenQuadfi) should not be used in this situation because it is only approved in children ≥2 years of age. For children 2 years of age and older, any of the

MenACWY vaccines (Menveo, MenQuadfi, or Menactra) can be used. For patients with asplenia who are younger than 7 years, an additional dose of meningococcal conjugate vaccine is recommended 3 years after the primary series and then every 5 years; for patients with asplenia who received the last dose of the primary series at 7 years and older, the initial booster dose following the primary series should be at 5 years instead of 3 years, and then every 5 years thereafter. Use of MenACWY vaccine (beginning in infancy) and MenB vaccine (beginning at 10 years of age) can be considered on a case-by-case basis for children with other primary or secondary splenic dysfunction.

When surgical splenectomy is planned, Hib, pneumococcal, and meningococcal vaccine history should be reviewed, and needed vaccines should be administered at least 2 weeks before surgery. If the patient is 2 years or older and is PPSV23 naïve, PPSV23 should be administered at least 8 weeks after indicated dose(s) of PCV and at least 2 weeks before surgery. If splenectomy is performed on an emergency basis or if needed vaccines were not administered before splenectomy, they should be administered as soon as possible when the patient's condition is stable.

In addition to immunization, antibiotic prophylaxis against pneumococcal infections is recommended for many children with asplenia (see *Streptococcus pneumoniae* [Pneumococcal] Infections, p 810).

CENTRAL NERVOUS SYSTEM ANATOMIC BARRIER DEFECTS. Patients of all ages scheduled to receive a cochlear implant as well as patients with congenital dysplasias of the inner ear or persistent cerebrospinal fluid (CSF) communication with the naso-oropharynx should receive vaccines recommended routinely on the annual immunization schedule. In addition, they should receive PCV as recommended for children with asplenia and at 24 months or older should receive PPSV23 (≥8 weeks after receipt of PCV). Indicated doses of PCV and PPSV23 should ideally be administered at least 2 weeks before cochlear implant surgery, when feasible.

There is no well-established evidence for use of antimicrobial prophylaxis for patients with CSF communication with the naso-oropharynx or middle ear. Risk of bacterial meningitis is highest in the first 7 to 10 days following acute traumatic breach. Some physicians recommend empiric parenteral antimicrobial therapy in the immediate post-traumatic period. Parenteral antimicrobial therapy also is given in the perioperative period for cochlear implantation and reparative neurosurgical procedures. Routine chronic antimicrobial prophylaxis is not indicated for persistent CSF communications or following cochlear implantation.

Immunization in Children With a Personal or Family History of Seizures

Studies have demonstrated a short-term increased risk of a febrile seizure (ie, generalized, brief, self-limited) following receipt of several vaccines (eg, diphtheria, tetanus, and whole-cell pertussis vaccine [DTwP]; measles, mumps, and rubella vaccine [MMR]; measles, mumps, rubella, and varicella vaccine [MMRV]; 13-valent pneumococcal conjugate vaccine [PCV13], and non-live influenza vaccine [IIV]). An increased incidence of febrile seizures has not been found with the currently recommended diphtheria, tetanus, and acellular pertussis (DTaP) vaccines. Children 6 months to 2 years of age may experience a small increased risk for febrile seizure when IIV is given simultaneously with PCV13 or DTaP. However, children this age should still continue to receive IIV, PCV13, and DTaP when these vaccines are due. Infants and children with a personal or family history of seizures of any etiology might be at greater risk of having a febrile seizure after receipt of these vaccines compared with children without such histories. Children who develop epilepsy soon after they receive immunization should be considered for genetic testing, because many genetic causes of early-life epilepsies present around the age at which vaccines are routinely given. No evidence indicates that febrile seizures cause permanent brain damage or epilepsy, aggravate neurologic disorders, or affect the prognosis for children with underlying disorders.

Parents of children with a personal history of febrile seizures should be informed that some vaccines could be associated with an increased risk of febrile seizures. However, vaccination generally should not be deferred in these children. Postimmunization seizures in these children are uncommon, and if they occur, they usually are febrile in origin, have a benign outcome, and are not likely to be confused with manifestations of a previously unrecognized neurologic disorder. In the case of pertussis immunization during infancy, vaccine administration could coincide with or hasten the recognition of a disorder associated with seizures, such as infantile spasms or Dravet syndrome, which could cause confusion about the role of pertussis immunization. Hence, pertussis immunization in infants with an *evolving* neurologic condition generally is deferred until the condition is stabilized. DTaP should be administered to infants and children with a *stable* neurologic condition, including well-controlled seizures, and to most children with a history of seizures (febrile or afebrile) occurring <3 days after a previous dose of DTwP or DTaP. However, a history of encephalopathy (eg, coma, decreased level of consciousness, prolonged seizures) not attributable to another cause occurring <7 days after a previous dose of DTwP or DTaP remains a contraindication to receiving DTaP.

Immunization in Children With Chronic Diseases

Chronic disease is defined as a medical condition that currently is not curable and that has been present for at least 3 months, will likely last longer than 3 months, or has occurred at least 3 times in the past year and likely will recur. Chronic diseases may increase children's susceptibility to infections or increase the severity of infection-related manifestations. Unless specifically contraindicated, immunizations recommended for healthy children should generally be administered to children with chronic diseases.

The importance of COVID-19 and annual influenza vaccinations, when indicated, should be particularly emphasized in children with chronic diseases and their household contacts. Children with hemophilia or other bleeding disorders should be immunized following the Centers for Disease Control and Prevention (CDC) guidelines for vaccinating persons with increased bleeding risk.[1] For children with chronic and immunocompromising conditions or therapies, see Immunization and Other Considerations in Immunocompromised Children (p 93) and the "Recommended Child and Adolescent Immunization Schedule for Ages 18 Years or Younger, United States," which is updated annually (**www.cdc.gov/vaccines/schedules/hcp/imz/child-adolescent.html** and **https://redbook.solutions.aap.org/SS/Immunization_Schedules.aspx**).

---

[1] **www.cdc.gov/vaccines/hcp/acip-recs/general-recs/special-situations.html**

Children with certain chronic diseases such as allergic, respiratory, cardiovascular, hematologic, metabolic, and renal disorders are at increased risk of complications from pneumococcal infection and may need to receive pneumococcal conjugate vaccine and 23-valent pneumococcal polysaccharide vaccine (PPSV23), or both, as recommended for age and condition (see *Streptococcus pneumoniae* [Pneumococcal] Infections, p 810). Children with certain immunocompromising conditions, such as asplenia or persistent complement component deficiencies, are particularly susceptible to severe infections by encapsulated bacteria and are routinely recommended to receive *Haemophilus influenzae* type b vaccine (Hib), serogroups A, C, W, and Y meningococcal vaccine (MenACWY), serogroup B meningococcal vaccine (MenB), and pneumococcal conjugate vaccine and PPSV23. See Table 3 in the Recommended Child and Adolescent Immunization Schedule by Medical Condition, United States, at **https://redbook.solutions.aap.org/SS/Immunization_Schedules. aspx,** and Immunization and Other Considerations in Immunocompromised Children, p 93.

All children with chronic liver disease are at risk of severe clinical manifestations of acute hepatitis virus infections and should receive hepatitis A (HepA) and hepatitis B (HepB) vaccines if not previously vaccinated (see Hepatitis A, p 430, and Hepatitis B, p 437). Household members of children with chronic diseases also should be up-to-date on recommended vaccines based on their age and health conditions (**https://redbook.solutions.aap.org/SS/Immunization_Schedules. aspx**).

In 2012, the National Academy of Medicine (NAM) assessed whether vaccines (measles, mumps, and rubella; acellular pertussis-containing diphtheria and tetanus; tetanus toxoid; influenza; hepatitis A; hepatitis B; and human papillomavirus vaccines) were a potential trigger for a flare or the onset of chronic inflammatory diseases. The NAM review concluded that the evidence was inadequate to establish or refute a causal relationship between these vaccines and onset or exacerbation of multiple sclerosis, systemic lupus erythematosus, vasculitis, rheumatoid arthritis, or juvenile idiopathic arthritis.[1] Additionally, NAM concluded that clinical evidence overall indicated that vaccines should not be withheld because concerns about their potential trigger for chronic inflammatory diseases.

Immunization in American Indian/Alaska Native Children and Adolescents

Indigenous populations worldwide have high morbidity and mortality from infectious diseases, including vaccine-preventable infections (**wwwnc.cdc.gov/eid/ article/7/7/pdfs/01-7732.pdf**). This chapter focuses on the US population of American Indian and Alaska Native (AI/AN) people and considerations for use of vaccines and biologic products that are special to these populations. For AI/AN people, persistent elevated rates of infectious diseases are driven by barriers to care seeking related to geographic isolation and historical trauma, socioeconomic factors such as poverty, household crowding, substandard housing, and poor indoor air quality.

---

[1] Stratton K, Andrew F, Rusch E, Clayton E. *Adverse Effects of Vaccines: Evidence and Causality*. Washington, DC: National Academies Press; 2012

Historically, compared with children from other US racial or ethnic groups, AI/AN children living on reservation lands or in Alaska Native villages have higher rates of certain vaccine-preventable diseases, such as *Haemophilus influenzae* type b, *Streptococcus pneumoniae*, hepatitis A, and hepatitis B. Although the rate of mortality from pneumonia and influenza among AI/AN infants has steadily declined over recent decades, disparities persist.

During the past 2 decades, childhood immunizations for hepatitis A and hepatitis B in the US have eliminated disease disparities for these pathogens in most populations of AI/AN children. Significant decreases have been documented in varicella hospitalizations and invasive disease caused by *H influenzae* type b and *S pneumoniae*. However, the historically high rates of infection and ongoing disparities highlight the importance of ensuring that recommendations for universal childhood immunization be implemented for all AI/AN children. Specific vulnerabilities are as follows.

- **_H influenzae_ type b.** There are important differences among the currently available *Haemophilus influenzae* type b (Hib) vaccines that should be considered by clinicians caring for AI/AN children. Before routine use of Hib, the incidence of invasive *H influenzae* type b disease was up to 10 times higher among young AI/AN children compared with non-AI/AN children. Because of the historically high risk of invasive *H influenzae* type b disease within the first 6 months of life in many AI/AN infant populations, the CDC Advisory Committee on Immunization Practices (ACIP) and the American Academy of Pediatrics (AAP) recommend the preferential use of PedvaxHIB, which contains polyribosylribitol phosphate-meningococcal outer membrane protein (PRP-OMP), as the first dose in the Hib series. The administration of the PRP-OMP-containing vaccine leads to more rapid development of protective concentrations of antibody compared with Hib containing polyribosylribitol phosphate-tetanus toxoid (PRP-T), and failure to use Hib containing PRP-OMP has been associated with excess cases of *H influenzae* type b disease in Alaska Native infants. Until information is available on the kinetics of antibody development following the first dose of the PRP-OMP-containing combination vaccine (DTaP-IPV-Hib-HepB [Vaxelis]), there is no preferential recommendation for its use in AI/AN infants. If the first dose of PRP-OMP-containing PedvaxHIB or Vaxelis is delayed by >1 month, the recommended catch-up schedule should be followed (available at **https://redbook.solutions.aap.org/SS/Immunization_Schedules.aspx**). A booster dose (dose 3) in the PRP-OMP Hib schedule or dose 4 in other Hib schedules is recommended at age 12 through 15 months; regardless of vaccine used in the primary Hib series, there is no preferred Hib formulation for the booster dose **(www.cdc.gov/mmwr/preview/mmwrhtml/rr6301a1.htm)**. Availability of more than one Hib product in a clinic, however, has been shown to lead to errors in vaccine administration. To avoid confusion for health care professionals who serve AI/AN children predominantly, it may be prudent to stock only PRP-OMP-containing Hib.

- **_S pneumoniae_.** Recommendations for pneumococcal conjugate vaccine (PCV) for AI/AN children are the same as for other children in the United States. Before introduction of heptavalent pneumococcal conjugate vaccine (PCV7), the incidence of invasive pneumococcal disease (IPD) in certain AI/AN children (Alaska Native, Navajo, and White Mountain Apache) was 5 to 24 times higher than the incidence among other children in the United States. Use of PCV7 in AI/AN infants resulted in near-elimination of IPD caused by vaccine serotypes and decreased incidence of overall IPD caused by all serotypes of *S pneumoniae*. Although the use of 13-valent pneumococcal conjugate vaccine (PCV13) has further reduced the incidence of IPD in AI/AN children, rates of overall IPD among some AI/AN children (Alaska Native, Navajo, and White Mountain Apache) remain more than fourfold higher than those among children in the general US population.

- **Hepatitis A and hepatitis B viruses.** Before the introduction of hepatitis vaccines, rates of hepatitis A and hepatitis B in the AI/AN population exceeded those of the general US population. In 1970, Alaska Native people had an overall prevalence of hepatitis B surface antigen (HBsAg) positivity of >6%, leading to high rates of hepatocellular carcinoma. Universal infant immunization with the hepatis B vaccine and population-wide screening and vaccination eliminated symptomatic hepatitis B virus infection and hepatocellular carcinoma in Alaska Native people younger than age 20 years. Similarly, after initiation of universal childhood hepatitis A vaccination, hepatitis A virus infection rates among AI/AN people declined 20-fold during 1997-2001 to a rate lower than that of the general US population.

- **Influenza virus.** The disparity in influenza-related mortality rates in the AI/AN population compared with the general US population was confirmed during the 2009 H1N1 epidemic; the H1N1 death rate among AI/AN people in 12 states (representing 50% of the AI/AN population in the United States) was 4 times higher than the H1N1 death rate for all other racial and ethnic populations combined. For this reason, the AI/AN population is listed among the groups at risk of severe complications from influenza. When vaccine or antiviral medication supplies are limited or delayed, AI/AN people are considered a high-risk priority group. Studies have also documented the value of influenza immunization during pregnancy to protect both the pregnant person and infant too young to be vaccinated.

- **Respiratory syncytial virus (RSV).** The rates of hospitalization for RSV have been much higher for AI/AN infants in rural Alaska and southwest Indian Health Service (IHS) regions than for other infants in the United States. Hospitalization rates for AI/AN infants attributable to RSV infection in these areas are similar to rates among medically high-risk and preterm infants in the overall US population. Use of RSV-specific monoclonal antibody prophylaxis (palivizumab or nirsevimab), as recommended by the AAP, should be optimized among high-risk AI/AN infants (see Respiratory Syncytial Virus, p 713). The RSV season may be different in northern latitudes, including Alaska, and RSV prophylaxis should reflect local seasonality and risk factors in these areas. The new RSVpreF vaccine (Abrysvo) is approved and recommended for use in pregnant people as a single intramuscular injection administered between 32 through 36 weeks' gestation. Among the general US population, vaccination during pregnancy reduces RSV-associated lower respiratory tract disease, including severe disease, throughout the first 6 months following the infant's birth. This efficacy of this vaccine has not been specifically studied in AI/AN populations.

- **Rotavirus.** In the 1990s, the percentage of AI/AN infants hospitalized with diarrheal illnesses was nearly twice that of the general infant population in the United States. Following introduction of rotavirus vaccination, diarrhea-associated hospitalizations of AI/AN children younger than 5 years have declined substantially, reinforcing the importance of this vaccine for AI/AN infants.

- **Pertussis.** A study of pertussis-related mortality from 1991-2008 showed that AI/AN infants aged ≥42 days had the highest risk for fatal outcome (odds ratio [OR], 3.7; 95% confidence interval [CI]: 1.8–7.8) compared with white infants, higher than infants of any other racial or ethnic group. This risk nearly doubled when other factors were controlled, including age, receipt of antibiotics, or receipt of at least 1 dose of diphtheria, tetanus, and acellular pertussis vaccine (DTaP). These disparities emphasize the importance of AI/AN infant immunization and immunization of AI/AN pregnant people with pertussis-containing vaccine.
- **COVID-19.** AI/AN people have had substantially higher rates of COVID-19 cases and COVID-19–related deaths compared with people from most other racial and ethnic groups, underscoring the importance of vaccination for this population. Further data are needed to understand the severity of COVID-19 for AI/AN children regarding hospitalization, death, prolonged illness, and multisystem inflammatory syndrome in children (MIS-C) and other COVID-19 sequelae. See Coronavirus Disease 2019 (COVID-19), p 324.

Immunization in Adolescent and College Populations

Immunization recommendations for adolescents and college students have become routine and are reflected on the adolescent immunization schedule that is published annually (**www.cdc.gov/vaccines/schedules/index.html**). The adolescent and young adult population presents many immunization challenges, including less frequent visits for preventive care, missed opportunities to immunize when they present for sports physicals and sick visits, and scheduling conflicts because of age-appropriate activities. In addition, the ability of minors to consent to immunization varies by state. Providers should know and abide by the laws in their state governing minor consent for immunizations. The Society for Adolescent Health and Medicine has a position paper on adolescents consenting for vaccination and the potential impact on immunization rates (**www.adolescenthealth.org/SAHM_Main/media/Advocacy/Positions/Oct-13-Consent-Vaccination.pdf**). Updates on state laws are available from the Centers for Disease Control and Prevention (CDC).[1]

All youth should have an annual comprehensive preventive health visit. Visits at 11 through 12 years of age and 16 through 18 years of age are especially important for administration of age-appropriate vaccines.[2] Additionally, all adolescent visits should be seen as opportunities to review each adolescent's immunization record in order to administer vaccines that may be due or overdue according to the recommended immunization schedule. The use of patient reminder-recall systems, provider reminders, and standing orders have been shown to increase immunization rates. Linking to statewide or regional immunization information systems will facilitate keeping adolescents appropriately immunized. Lapses in the immunization schedule do not necessitate reinitiation of a vaccine series or extra doses for any vaccine.

Tetanus toxoid, reduced diphtheria toxoid, and acellular pertussis vaccine (Tdap); serogroups A, C, W, and Y meningococcal vaccine (MenACWY); and human

---

[1] **www.cdc.gov/phlp/publications/topic/vaccinationlaws.html**

[2] American Academy of Pediatrics, Committee on Practice and Ambulatory Medicine, Bright Futures Periodicity Schedule Workgroup. 2023 recommendations for preventive pediatric health care. *Pediatrics.* 2023;151(4):e2023061451

papillomavirus (HPV) vaccine should be administered at the 11- through 12-year-old visit, although the HPV vaccine series can be started as early as 9 years of age (see below). Only 2 doses of human papillomavirus (HPV) vaccine are required for individuals whose first dose was given before their 15th birthday, while 3 doses are required for those starting HPV vaccination at 15 years or older and for immunocompromised persons (see Human Papillomaviruses, p 503). If possible, making appointments for subsequent doses of HPV vaccine at the conclusion of the first visit can enhance series completion. Providers can choose to begin the HPV vaccine series as early as 9 years of age if they deem this the optimal age to attain acceptance and completion prior to the risk of acquisition of HPV. When HPV vaccine is begun at 9 or 10 years, other adolescent vaccines (eg, MenACWY and Tdap) still are recommended to be initiated at 11 to 12 years. A MenACWY booster dose is recommended at 16 years of age. Serogroup B meningococcal vaccine (MenB) is not routinely recommended for adolescents in the absence of an outbreak or an underlying high-risk condition (eg, complement deficiency or asplenia) (see Meningococcal Infections, p 585), although vaccine providers may choose to administer a MenB vaccine to adolescents and young adults 16 through 23 years of age through shared clinical decision making with patients or their parents. When administered, the preferred age for MenB to be given is 16 through 18 years.

VACCINATION OF COLLEGE-AGED PEOPLE

A history should be obtained from all older adolescents to assess missing vaccines and risk factors that would require consideration for administration of additional vaccines, such as hepatitis A vaccine (HepA), MenB, *Haemophilus influenzae* type b vaccine (Hib), pneumococcal conjugate vaccine (PCV), and 23-valent pneumococcal polysaccharide vaccine (PPSV23). Specific indications for each of these vaccines are provided in the respective disease-specific chapters in Section 3.

Residential schools, colleges, and universities should establish a system to ensure all students are protected against vaccine-preventable diseases and also to identify unimmunized or underimmunized students in the event of an outbreak. Because outbreaks of vaccine-preventable diseases, including measles, mumps, meningococcal disease, and COVID-19, have occurred at colleges and universities, the American College Health Association encourages a comprehensive institutional prematriculation immunization policy consistent with recommendations from the CDC Advisory Committee on Immunization Practices **(www.acha.org/ACHA/Resources/Topics/Vaccine.aspx).** Many colleges and universities are mandated by state law to require vaccination for specific vaccines, either for all matriculating students or only those living in campus housing. Information regarding state laws requiring prematriculation immunization is available **(www.immunize.org/laws).**

The suspected occurrence of illness attributable to a vaccine-preventable disease in a school or college should be reported promptly to local health officials for aid in management, for assessment of public health implications, and to comply with state law (see Appendix III, Nationally Notifiable Infectious Diseases in the United States, p 1141).

Immunization in Health Care Personnel

People whose occupations place them in contact with patients with contagious diseases are at risk of contracting vaccine-preventable diseases and, if infected, transmitting them to their coworkers and patients. For the purposes of this section, health care personnel (HCP) are defined as those who have face-to-face contact with patients or anyone who works in a building where patient care is delivered or is employed or contracted by a health care facility (eg, laboratory personnel). The definition of HCP includes trainees and volunteers. All HCP should protect themselves and susceptible patients by receiving appropriate immunizations. Physicians, health care facilities, and schools for health care professionals should play an active role in promoting policies to maximize immunization of HCP. Vaccine-preventable diseases of special concern to people involved in the health care of children are as follows (see the disease-specific chapters in Section 3 for further recommendations).

- **Pertussis.** Pertussis outbreaks involving adults occur in the community and the workplace. HCP frequently are exposed to *Bordetella pertussis*, have substantial risk of illness, and can be sources for spread of infection to patients, colleagues, families, and the community. HCP of all ages who work in hospitals or ambulatory care settings should receive a dose of tetanus toxoid, reduced diphtheria toxoid, and acellular pertussis vaccine (Tdap) as soon as is feasible if they previously have not received Tdap. Hospitals and ambulatory care facilities should provide Tdap for HCP using approaches that maximize immunization rates.

  Either Td or Tdap can be used regardless of prior receipt of Tdap for the routine decennial tetanus-diphtheria booster and for wound prophylaxis when indicated. In addition, if there is an increased risk of pertussis in a health care setting, as evidenced by documented or suspected health care-associated transmission of pertussis, revaccination of HCP with Tdap vaccine may be considered (**www.cdc.gov/ vaccines/vpd/pertussis/tdap-revac-hcp.html**). In these cases, it is important to consider that vaccinating HCP with Tdap is not a substitute for infection prevention and control measures, including postexposure antimicrobial prophylaxis, and therefore, revaccinated HCP still should receive postexposure antimicrobial prophylaxis when applicable. If implemented, HCP who work with infants or pregnant people should be prioritized for revaccination.

- **Hepatitis B.** Hepatitis B vaccine (HepB) is recommended for all HCP whose work- and training-related activities involve reasonably anticipated risk of exposure to blood or other infectious body fluids. The Occupational Safety and Health Administration (OSHA) of the US Department of Labor issued a regulation requiring employers of personnel at risk of occupational exposure to hepatitis B to offer HepB immunization to personnel at the employer's expense. The employer shall ensure that employees who decline to accept HepB immunization offered by the employer sign a declination statement. To determine the need for revaccination and to guide postexposure prophylaxis, postvaccination serologic testing should be performed for all recently vaccinated HCP at risk of occupational percutaneous or mucosal exposure to blood or body fluids. Postvaccination serologic testing is performed 1 to 2 months after administration of the last dose of the vaccine series using a method that allows detection of the protective concentration of hepatitis B surface antibody (anti-HBs [$\geq$10 mIU/mL]). People determined to have anti-HBs concentrations of $\geq$10 mIU/mL at any time after receipt of the primary vaccine series are considered immune and the result should be documented. Future testing is not required.

  Although vaccine-induced anti-HBs wanes over time, protection persists for immunocompetent vaccine responders (eg, those with anti-HBs $\geq$10 mIU/mL at their postvaccination serologic testing). Therefore, testing HCP for anti-HBs years after vaccination (eg, when HepB vaccination was received as part of routine infant immunization) might not distinguish vaccine responders from nonresponders. Preexposure assessment of anti-HBs results at the time of hiring or matriculation, followed by one or more additional doses of HepB vaccine when needed helps to ensure that remotely vaccinated HCP will be protected. HCP who lack documentation of prior immunity to hepatitis B and who have anti-HBs <10 mIU/mL should be reimmunized with a single dose of vaccine and retested for anti-HBs within 1 to 2 months after that dose. HCP whose anti-HBs remains <10 mIU/mL should receive additional doses to complete the second vaccine series. For the 3-dose vaccine series using Engerix-B, PreHevbrio, or Recombivax HB, this would require 2 additional doses of vaccine, and for the 2-dose series using Heplisav-B, this would require 1 additional dose. For very recently vaccinated HCP with anti-HBs <10 mIU/mL, in whom the low antibody concentration is more likely to reflect a failure to respond rather than waning antibody concentration, it may be more practical to revaccinate with an entire second series (3 doses of Engerix-B, PreHevbrio, or Recombivax HB; 2 doses of Heplisav-B) followed by anti-HBs testing 1 to 2 months after the last dose. Heplisav-B or PreHevbrio may be used for revaccination following an initial HepB vaccine series that consisted of doses from a different manufacturer.[1,2]

People who do not respond to the second series and remain hepatitis B surface antigen (HBsAg) negative should be considered susceptible to hepatitis B virus infection and will need to receive hepatitis B immune globulin (HBIG) prophylaxis after any known or probable exposure to blood or body fluids infected with hepatitis B virus.

- **Influenza.** Because HCP can transmit influenza to patients and because health care-associated outbreaks of influenza do occur, annual influenza immunization should be considered a patient safety responsibility and a requirement for employment in a health care facility unless an individual has a recognized medical contraindication to immunization.[3] HCP should be educated about the benefits of influenza immunization and the potential health consequences of influenza illness for themselves and their patients. Influenza vaccine should be offered at no cost, and efforts should be made to ensure that vaccine is readily available to HCP on all shifts. A signed declination form should be obtained from personnel who decline for reasons other than medical contraindications in any facility that does not have a mandatory vaccine policy. Mandatory education about the benefits of vaccination should be required for all people who decline influenza immunization. Any approved influenza vaccine product is appropriate if otherwise indicated with the exception of live attenuated vaccine, which should not be used for personnel who will have close contact

[1] Schillie S, Vellozzi C, Reingold A, et al. Prevention of hepatitis B virus infection in the United States: recommendations of the Advisory Committee on Immunization Practices. *MMWR Recomm Rep.* 2018;67(RR-1):1–31

[2] Schillie S, Harris A, Link-Gelles R, et al. Recommendations of the Advisory Committee on Immunization Practices for Use of a Hepatitis B Vaccine with a Novel Adjuvant. *MMWR Morb Mortal Wkly Rep.* 2018;67(15):455-4580

[3] American Academy of Pediatrics, Committee on Infectious Diseases. Policy statement: Influenza immunization for all health care personnel: keep it mandatory. *Pediatrics.* 2015;136(4):809-818

with patients with altered immunocompetence who are in a protected environment; HCP receiving LAIV should avoid close contact with these immunocompromised people for 7 days following vaccination.

- **COVID-19.** Because HCP can transmit SARS-CoV-2 to patients and because health care-associated transmission of COVID-19 does occur, COVID-19 immunization should be considered a patient safety responsibility and a requirement for employment in a health care facility unless an individual has a recognized medical contraindication to immunization. HCP should be educated about the benefits of COVID-19 immunization and the potential health consequences of COVID-19 illness for themselves and their patients. COVID-19 vaccine should be offered at no cost, and efforts should be made to ensure that vaccine is readily available to HCP on all shifts. A signed declination form should be obtained from personnel who decline for reasons other than medical contraindications in any facility that does not have a mandatory vaccine policy. Mandatory education about the benefits of vaccination should be required for all people who decline COVID-19 immunization. HCP can receive any FDA-approved or -authorized vaccine. It is important that HCP be up to date with their COVID-19 vaccine series based on the latest CDC guidance.[1]

- **Measles.** Because measles in HCP has contributed to spread of this disease during outbreaks, evidence of immunity to measles should be required for HCP. Evidence of immunity is established by laboratory confirmation of infection, laboratory evidence of immunity (positive serologic test result for measles antibody), or documented receipt of 2 appropriately spaced doses of live virus-containing measles vaccine, the first of which was administered on or after the first birthday. People born before 1957 generally are considered immune to measles. However, because measles cases have occurred in HCP in this age group, health care facilities should consider offering 2 doses of measles-containing vaccine to HCP who lack proof of immunity to measles. In communities with documented measles outbreaks, 2 doses of MMR vaccine are recommended for unvaccinated HCP born before 1957 unless evidence of serologic immunity is demonstrated.

- **Mumps.** All people who work in health care facilities should be immune to mumps. Evidence of immunity is established by laboratory confirmation of infection, laboratory evidence of immunity (positive serologic test result for mumps antibody), documented receipt of 2 appropriately spaced doses of live virus-containing mumps vaccine, the first of which was administered on or after the first birthday, or birth before 1957. During an outbreak, a second dose of MMR vaccine should be offered to HCP born during or after 1957 who have only received 1 dose of MMR vaccine. HCP born before 1957 without a history of MMR immunization should obtain a mumps antibody titer to document their immune status and, if negative, should receive 2 appropriately spaced doses of MMR vaccine.

- **Rubella.** Transmission of rubella from HCP to pregnant individuals has been reported. Although the disease is mild in adults, the risk to a fetus necessitates documentation of rubella immunity in all HCP. People should be considered immune on the basis of a positive serologic test result for rubella antibody or documented proof of 1 dose of rubella-containing vaccine. A history of rubella disease is unreliable and should not be used in determining immune status. All susceptible HCP who may be exposed to patients with rubella or who take care of pregnant patients, as well as people who work in educational institutions or provide child care, should be immunized with 1 dose of MMR to prevent infection for themselves and to prevent transmission of rubella to pregnant patients.

- **Varicella.** Evidence of varicella immunity is recommended for all HCP. Evidence of immunity to varicella in HCP includes any of the following: 1) documentation of 2 doses of varicella vaccine at least 28 days apart, the first of which was administered on or after the first birthday; 2) history of varicella diagnosed or verified by a physician (for a patient reporting a history of or presenting with an atypical case, a mild case, or both, the physician should seek either an epidemiologic link with a typical varicella case or evidence of laboratory confirmation, if it was performed at the time of acute disease); 3) history of herpes zoster diagnosed by a physician; or 4) laboratory evidence of immunity or laboratory confirmation of disease. Birth in the United States before 1980 should not be considered as evidence of immunity for HCP, pregnant women, or immunocompromised people (**www.cdc.gov/ chickenpox/hcp/immunity.html**). The Centers for Disease Control and Prevention's Advisory Committee on Immunization Practices (ACIP) and Health Infection Control Practices Advisory Committee (HICPAC) do not recommend serologic testing of HCP for immunity to varicella after receiving varicella-zoster virus vaccine, because commercially available serologic assays may not be sufficiently sensitive to detect immunization-induced antibody.

- **Meningococcus.** Meningococcal vaccination is not recommended for HCP performing direct patient care. However, clinical microbiologists routinely exposed to isolates of *Neisseria meningitidis* are at increased risk of severe meningococcal disease if exposed to a clinical isolate and should be vaccinated with serogroups A, C, W, and Y meningococcal vaccine (MenACWY) and serogroup B meningococcal vaccine (MenB).

- **Poliovirus.** The recent detections of circulating vaccine-derived poliovirus in the United States, decades after poliovirus was eliminated from the country, raises the possibility of the infection of HCPs with either wild-type or vaccine-related polioviruses while caring for patients in areas of the United States where poliovirus has been detected and circulating. The majority of adults born after 1955 are protected against poliomyelitis because they were vaccinated during childhood. HCPs who have had 3 or more doses of poliovirus vaccine previously and are at increased risk of exposure to poliovirus may receive 1 lifetime booster dose of non-live poliovirus vaccine (IPV). Unvaccinated or incompletely vaccinated HCPs should complete the poliovirus vaccination series with IPV (**www.cdc.gov/vaccines/vpd/polio/ hcp/recommendations.html**).

Children Who Received Immunizations Outside the United States or Whose Immunization Status is Unknown or Uncertain

IMMUNIZATIONS RECEIVED OUTSIDE THE UNITED STATES

People immunized in other countries, including international students, internationally adopted children, refugees, and other immigrants, should be immunized according to recommended schedules (including minimal ages and intervals) in the United

States (**www.cdc.gov/vaccines/schedules/index.html**). The Immigration and Nationality Act (INA) of 1996 requires all people immigrating to the United States as legal permanent residents (ie, green card holders) to provide "proof of vaccination" with vaccines recommended by the Centers for Disease Control and Prevention (CDC) Advisory Committee on Immunization Practices (ACIP) before entry into the United States. Vaccines required for immigration must fulfill the following criteria: 1) must be an age-appropriate vaccine as recommended by the ACIP for the general US population; and 2) either must protect against a disease that has the potential to cause an outbreak or protect against a disease that has been eliminated or is in the process of being eliminated in the United States. For example, human papillomavirus (HPV) vaccine is not required. For vaccination instructions, including the list of required vaccines, see **www.cdc.gov/ immigrantrefugeehealth/panel-physicians/vaccinations.html.**

Internationally adopted children who are 10 years and younger may obtain a waiver of exemption from the INA regulations pertaining to immunization of immigrants before arrival in the United States (**www.cdc.gov/immigrantrefu-geehealth/adoption/overseas-exam.html**). Children adopted from countries that are not part of the Hague Convention can receive waivers to have their immunizations delayed until arrival in the United States (**https://travel.state.gov/content/ travel/en/Intercountry-Adoption/Adoption-Process/understanding-the-hague-convention.html**). When an exemption is granted, adoptive parents are required to sign an affidavit indicating their intention to comply with ACIP-recommended immunizations within 30 days after the child arrives in the United States.

Refugees are not required to meet immunization requirements of the INA at the time of initial entry into the United States but must show proof of immunization when they apply for permanent residency, typically 1 year after arrival. Some refugees bound for the United States are immunized in their country of departure before arrival in the United States. Clinicians may review the CDC Refugee Health Guidelines for the current overseas immunization schedule for US-bound refugees at **www.cdc. gov/immigrantrefugeehealth/guidelines/refugee-guidelines.html.** Guidance on evaluating and updating immunizations during the domestic medical examination for refugees after arrival in the United States is available at **www.cdc. gov/immigrantrefugeehealth/guidelines/domestic/immunizations-guidelines.html.**

An increasing number of vaccines are being incorporated into routine immunization schedules in countries outside the United States. In general, written documentation of immunizations can be accepted as evidence of previous immunization if the vaccines, dates of administration, number of doses, intervals between doses, and age of the child at the time of immunization are comparable to current US or World Health Organization schedules (**www.who.int/immunization/policy/ immunization_tables/en/**). Doses of vaccines that do not comply with US schedules may need to be repeated (such as MMR before age 1 year). Any vaccination documented on the official Department of State health immigration form (DS-3025) should be accepted. Inaccuracies, inconsistencies, and fraudulent data (such as doses given before the date of birth, or different names or dates of birth on vaccine records compared with other official documents) should be considered during review of records.

Record review also should include consideration of ACIP recommendations for poliovirus vaccination, which require protection against all 3 poliovirus types by age-appropriate vaccination with non-live poliovirus (IPV) or trivalent oral poliovirus (tOPV) vaccines. Some countries may have provided monovalent or bivalent oral poliovirus (OPV) vaccine during poliovirus vaccination campaigns after April 1, 2016. If OPV was administered before April 1, 2016, OPV can be counted as tOPV. If OPV was administered on or after April 1, 2016, it may not be counted as tOPV and is not valid toward US vaccination requirements; in the absence of adequate written vaccination records documenting the doses as tOPV, vaccination or revaccination in accordance with the age-appropriate US IPV schedule is recommended (see Poliovirus Infections, p 682, for further recommendations).

Studies performed in internationally adopted children are inconclusive with regard to the extent to which the child's immunization record reflects protection. Many children adopted internationally lived in institutional settings where there was extremely limited capacity to store, administer, and record vaccines safely and accurately. Vaccine records of internationally adopted children should be assessed considering these capacities in the child's prior location. Re-immunizing or using serologic verification may be indicated when these uncertainties exist, even if there is a written immunization record.

Limited country-specific data are available regarding serologic verification of immunization records for other categories of immigrant children. Evaluation of concentrations of antibody to vaccine-preventable diseases can be useful in some circumstances to ensure that vaccines were administered and were immunogenic and to document immunity from past infection (see Serologic Testing to Document Immunization Status).

UNKNOWN OR UNCERTAIN IMMUNIZATION STATUS IN US CHILDREN

There are circumstances in which the immunization status for a child born in the United States is uncertain or unknown because of lack of documentation, an incomplete or inaccurate record, or a recording inconsistent with a recommended product or schedule. Serologic testing can be considered to assist in determining whether antibody concentrations are present for some of the vaccine-preventable diseases (see Serologic Testing to Document Immunization Status). A combined strategy of serologic testing for antibodies to some vaccine antigens and immunization for others may be used, or the vaccines may be repeated, administering those appropriate for the child's current age.

SEROLOGIC TESTING TO DOCUMENT IMMUNIZATION STATUS

Usefulness, validity, and interpretation of serologic testing to guide management of vaccinations can be complex and varies by age (Table 1.19). Cost and effort of testing versus cost of administering a given immunization, complexity of interpretation of results, and likelihood of adherence for completing the immunization series should be considered in these decisions. If serologic testing is not available, is too costly, or if a positive result would not mitigate need for further immunization, the prudent course is to repeat or administer the immunizations in question. Some state laws stipulate that only certain serologic tests are accepted for school attendance; testing may not be worthwhile in this circumstance, as vaccine will still be needed. Considerations for specific vaccines are discussed below.

Table 1.19. Utility of Antibody Testing for Vaccine-Preventable Diseases in Unimmunized or Underimmunized Children[a]

Vaccine	Immunize Without Testing in Most Circumstances	Antibody Testing Available and Appropriate in Specific Circumstances	Antibody Testing Available but not Generally Performed	Considerations for Use of Testing	Notes
COVID-19	X		X		
Dengue		X		A positive test result or a history of laboratory-confirmed dengue infection is required prior to immunization with dengue vaccine	Recommended for individuals 9 through 16 years of age who reside in areas with endemic dengue and who have a history of a laboratory-confirmed dengue infection or a positive result of a highly accurate serodiagnostic screening test
Diphtheria	X		X	To confirm receipt of documented vaccine; to document response to vaccine	May not be affordable by all patients; may result in immunization delay
Hepatitis A	X	X		Not useful for children <1 y because of transplacentally acquired antibody; most appropriate for older children, history of jaundice, or birth in or migration through high-prevalence areas	Testing may be cost-effective in circumstances of high pretest probability of positive antibody

Table 1.19. Utility of Antibody Testing for Vaccine-Preventable Diseases in Unimmunized or Underimmunized Children,[a] continued

Vaccine	Immunize Without Testing in Most Circumstances	Antibody Testing Available and Appropriate in Specific Circumstances	Antibody Testing Available but not Generally Performed	Considerations for Use of Testing	Notes
Hepatitis B	X	X		May identify immunity from prior hepatitis B infection or from prior vaccination	An anti-HBs of ≥10 mIU/mL is considered protective only when measured after documented vaccine series completion
Hib	X		X	To confirm receipt of documented vaccine in children ≥6 mo; to document response to vaccine	May not be affordable by all patients; may result in immunization delay; not appropriate for children ≥5 y
HPV	X		X		
Influenza	X		X		
Measles	X		X	Not useful for children <1 y because of transplacentally acquired antibody	May not be affordable by all patients; may result in immunization delay; most informative if tests for mumps and rubella also performed
Meningococcus	X		X		
Mumps	X		X	Not useful for children <1 y because of transplacentally acquired antibody	May not be affordable by all patients; may result in immunization delay; most informative if tests for measles and rubella also performed

Table 1.19. Utility of Antibody Testing for Vaccine-Preventable Diseases in Unimmunized or Underimmunized Children,[a] continued

Vaccine	Immunize Without Testing in Most Circumstances	Antibody Testing Available and Appropriate in Specific Circumstances	Antibody Testing Available but not Generally Performed	Considerations for Use of Testing	Notes
PCV	X				
Pertussis	X		X		
Poliovirus	X		X		
Rotavirus	X		X		
Rubella	X		X	Not useful for children <1 year because of transplacentally acquired antibody	May not be affordable by all patients; may result in immunization delay; most informative if tests for measles and mumps also performed
Tetanus	X		X	To confirm receipt of documented vaccine; to document response to vaccine	May not be affordable by all patients; may result in immunization delay
Varicella	X	X		Not useful for children <1 y because of transplacentally acquired antibody; most appropriate for older children or history of varicella in patient or close family members	Testing may be cost-effective in circumstances of high pretest probability of positive antibody

anti-HBs indicates hepatitis B surface antibody; Hib, *Haemophilus influenzae* type b; HPV, human papillomavirus vaccine; PCV, pneumococcal conjugate vaccine.
[a] See the disease-specific chapters in Section 3 for additional information.

When validity of immunization records is in doubt, or when documentation of response to vaccine is desired for other reasons in children 6 months or older, serologic testing to document antibodies to diphtheria and tetanus toxoids (ie, ≥0.1 IU/mL) or *Haemophilus influenzae* type b for a child younger than 60 months (ie, ≥1.0 µg/mL) may be considered to determine whether the child likely has received and responded to dose(s) of the vaccine in question. Even if the child has a "protective" level of antibodies, the immunization series should be completed as appropriate for that child's age. If a child does not have a protective level of antibodies, the series should be restarted, with the understanding that for some vaccine-preventable diseases, fewer doses of vaccine are needed to complete the series as a child ages. The immunization record, plus presence of antibody to diphtheria and tetanus toxoids, can be used as proxy for receipt of pertussis-containing vaccine dose(s).

Hepatitis A, measles, mumps, rubella, and varicella antibody concentrations could be measured in children 12 months or older to determine whether the child is immune; these antibody tests should not be performed in children younger than 12 months because of the potential presence of maternal antibody. Prevaccination serologic testing is not recommended for hepatitis A, but children who were born or migrated through regions with high prevalence of hepatitis A may have had hepatitis A infection, and presence of immunoglobulin (Ig) G-specific antibody to hepatitis A virus in such patients would preclude need for hepatitis A vaccine. Usefulness of measuring measles antibody alone is limited, because many foreign-born children will need mumps and rubella vaccines as these vaccines are administered less frequently in resource-limited countries and they are available in the Unites States only as MMR vaccine. Two doses of MMR vaccine should be administered for mumps coverage, even if measles antibodies are present. Rubella coverage is achieved following 1 dose of a rubella-containing vaccine. Documented receipt of 2 doses of varicella vaccine or positive varicella antibody is the best indication of immunity to varicella. *H influenzae* type b vaccine (Hib) is not indicated for immunocompetent children 5 years or older, even if none was administered previously; serologic testing should not be performed, because children in this age group frequently have antibody concentrations <1.0 µg/mL yet are not susceptible to *H influenzae* type b infection. Age-appropriate pneumococcal vaccine dose(s) should be administered if a completed series is not documented; serologic testing should not be performed for validation or evidence of immunity. Serologic tests to assess immunity to poliovirus and rotavirus are not recommended.

Hepatitis B requires additional considerations when considering testing for antibody. Hepatitis B antibody testing is not indicated routinely before immunization of children or adolescents. High seroconversion rates and protective concentrations of hepatitis B surface antibody (anti-HBs [≥10 mIU/mL]) are achieved when HepB vaccine is administered in any of the recommended schedules, including schedules begun soon after birth in term infants. Serologic testing for identifying HBV infection (positive HBsAg) is indicated in specific circumstances, including an infant whose birthing parent is HBsAg positive, foreign-born individuals, and those in risk groups for hepatitis B infection. Before immunizing with hepatitis B vaccine without testing, children should be assessed for risk of hepatitis B infection and tested for infection if risk is present (see Serologic Testing section of Hepatitis B chapter, p 448).

International Travel

Children are at risk for illness when traveling internationally, and some may require medical care or hospitalization. US-born children of immigrants are especially likely to travel at young ages to visit relatives. A pretravel consultation with a health care professional who is knowledgeable or specializes in travel medicine can mitigate risk of travel-associated health problems but requires advance planning to allow time to complete necessary vaccinations and obtain necessary medications. Parents should be made aware that there is increased risk of exposure to vaccine-preventable diseases when traveling outside the United States, even in middle and high-income countries perceived to be without substantial risk of infectious diseases. Routine immunizations should be up-to-date before international travel; some may be administered early or on an accelerated schedule to optimize protection. Vaccines to prevent typhoid fever, yellow fever, meningococcal disease, rabies, Japanese encephalitis (JE), tick-borne encephalitis (TBE), and cholera may be indicated depending on the age of the child, destination, season of travel, duration of the trip, and activities during travel (see disease-specific chapters in Section 3). Families should arrange travel consultation to occur at least 4 to 6 weeks before planned departure, because travel vaccines may not be available at all sites and some vaccines, such as JE, TBE, and rabies vaccines, require multiple doses before departure.

Travelers also may be at risk for exposure to malaria, dengue, chikungunya, Zika, other mosquito-borne and tick-borne infections, diarrheal and respiratory illnesses, and skin conditions for which vaccines are not available. Although a dengue vaccine was licensed in 2019 by the US Food and Drug Administration (FDA) for use in individuals 9 through 16 years of age who reside in areas with endemic dengue and who have laboratory confirmation of a previous dengue infection, no dengue vaccine is licensed currently for travelers. Antimalarial chemoprophylaxis is recommended for travelers to areas with endemic malaria, and insect precautions should be addressed for all travelers at risk of vectorborne diseases. Attending to hand hygiene, choosing safer foods, and limiting exposure to animals, contaminated sand, soil, and water may reduce travelers' risk of acquiring other diseases.

Up-to-date information, including CDC Travel Health Notices about current disease outbreaks that may affect international travelers, is available on the CDC Travelers' Health website (**wwwnc.cdc.gov/travel/**). Country-level information can be quickly accessed at **wwwnc.cdc.gov/travel/destinations/list.** Disease Outbreak News can be found on the WHO website (**www.who.int/emergencies/disease-outbreak-news**). *Health Information for International Travel* (the "Yellow Book," **wwwnc.cdc.gov/travel/page/yellowbook-home**) is revised every 2 years by the CDC and is available to travelers and health professionals. Local and state health departments and travel clinics[1] also can provide updated information. Many colleges have clinics where pretravel counseling and immunizations can be obtained. Information about cruise ship sanitation inspection scores and reports can be found on the CDC website (**www.cdc.gov/nceh/vsp/default.htm**).

---

[1] Sources for travel clinics: Center for Disease Control and Prevention (**wwwnc.cdc.gov/travel/page/find-clinic**), American Society of Tropical Medicine and Hygiene (**www.astmh.org/for-astmh-members/clinical-consultants-directory**), and International Society for Travel Medicine (**www.istm.org/AF_CstmClinicDirectory.asp**).

RECOMMENDED IMMUNIZATIONS

Infants and children traveling internationally should be up-to-date with immunizations recommended for their age. Some vaccines may be administered before the age of routine immunization (hepatitis A vaccine [HepA]; meningococcal conjugate vaccine; measles, mumps, and rubella vaccine [MMR]) or be administered on an accelerated schedule (MMR) to optimize immunity before departure.

COVID-19. SARS-CoV-2 is the respiratory virus that causes COVID-19. Immunization is recommended for all children ≥6 months of age and should be completed before travel. Risk of acquiring COVID-19 during travel depends on personal safety measures, destination, and characteristics of the trip (see Coronavirus Disease-2019 [COVID-19], p 324). Some countries may have vaccination or testing requirements for entry (see **https://travel.state.gov/content/travel/en/international-travel/International-Travel-Country-Information-Pages.html**).

HEPATITIS A. HepA is recommended routinely in a 2-dose series ≥6 months apart for all children at 12 through 23 months of age in the United States, with catch-up vaccination recommended through 18 years of age. HepA also is recommended for all people ≥6 months of age who are unimmunized and traveling to areas with intermediate or high rates of hepatitis A infection (see Table 3.19, p 435), although some travel medicine experts provide vaccine even to those traveling to areas with low prevalence. For children 6 through 11 months of age, a dose of HepA does not count toward the routine 2-dose series, which should be started at age 12 months. Immune globulin intramuscular (IGIM) is recommended for hepatitis A preexposure prophylaxis prior to travel for infants <6 months of age. People with chronic liver disease as well as adults aged >40 years, immunocompromised people, and people with other chronic medical conditions planning to depart to an area with high or intermediate hepatitis A endemicity in <2 weeks should receive the initial dose of HepA vaccine and also simultaneously may receive IGIM at a separate anatomic injection site (**www.cdc.gov/mmwr/volumes/67/wr/mm6743a5.htm**). The dose of IGIM administered for hepatitis A prevention may interfere with the immune response to varicella and MMR vaccines for several months (see Table 1.11, p 69, for details). A combination HepA-HepB (hepatitis B) vaccine (Twinrix) is available for people 18 years and older.

HEPATITIS B. HepB is recommended for all children and adults through age 59 years in the United States and for people traveling to areas where the prevalence of chronic hepatitis B virus infection is 2% or greater (see Hepatitis B, p 437). Ideally, HepB vaccination should be administered ≥6 months before travel so that a 3-dose regimen can be completed. If fewer than 4 months are available before departure, the alternative 4-dose schedule of 0, 1, 2, and 12 months, licensed for the Engerix-B vaccine (see Table 3.21, p 445), can be considered. Individual health care providers also may choose to use an accelerated schedule (eg, 0, 1, and 2 months; or 0, 2, and 4 months) for travelers who will depart before an approved immunization schedule can be completed. An accelerated schedule of Twinrix (doses at days 0, 7, and 21–30, with a booster at 12 months) is available for those ≥18 years of age. People who receive immunization on an accelerated schedule that is not licensed by the FDA also should receive a dose at 12 months after initiation of the series to promote long-term immunity. For adults, the 2-dose regimen of Heplisav-B can be completed in 1 month.

MEASLES. Travelers are an important source of measles cases in the United States. People traveling anywhere outside the United States should be immune to measles to provide personal protection and minimize importation. Immunity to measles is defined by laboratory confirmation of prior infection; laboratory evidence of immunity (positive serologic test result for measles antibody); documented receipt of 2 appropriately spaced doses of live virus-containing measles vaccine, the first of which was administered on or after the first birthday; or birth in the United States before 1957 (see Measles, p 570). Children who travel anywhere outside the United States should be vaccinated beginning at 6 months of age. Children 6 through 11 months of age should receive 1 dose of MMR vaccine at least 2 weeks before departure if possible, and then should receive a second dose of measles-containing vaccine at 12 through 15 months of age (at least 28 days after the initial measles immunization) and a third dose at 4 through 6 years of age. Children 12 months or older as well as adults who have received 1 dose and are traveling outside the United States should receive their second dose before departure, provided the interval between doses is 28 days or more. MMR should not be administered to pregnant individuals, and pregnancy should be avoided for 28 days following the receipt of MMR. Live-virus vaccines (MMR, varicella, yellow fever) generally either should be administered on the same day or should be separated by at least 4 weeks, and attention should be paid to the timing of immune globulin product administration if these are indicated (see Simultaneous Administration of Multiple Vaccines, p 63, and Table 1.11, p 69).

POLIOVIRUS. Significant efforts have been made to achieve global eradication of poliovirus, but spread continues in some areas. Travelers should be up-to-date with poliovirus immunization for age before travel. Travelers to countries with wild-type or vaccine-derived poliovirus circulation (**http://polioeradication. org/polio-today/polio-now/public-health-emergency-status/**) within the past 12 months may require additional doses of vaccine according to current CDC guidance. Travelers 18 years or older visiting regions identified on the CDC Travelers' Health website (**wwwnc.cdc.gov/travel**) as being at risk for circulation of poliovirus should receive a single lifetime booster dose of non-live poliovirus vaccine (IPV). Current recommendations should be verified before departure (**wwwnc.cdc.gov/travel/yellowbook/2024/infections-diseases/ poliomyelitis**).

TRAVEL-RELATED IMMUNIZATIONS

Other immunizations may be required or recommended for international travelers depending on factors such as destination, planned activities, and length of stay (see **wwwnc.cdc.gov/travel/**, **wwwnc.cdc.gov/travel/destinations/list**, and disease-specific chapters in Section 3).

CHOLERA. An oral cholera vaccine (Vaxchora [CVD 103-HgR, PaxVax Bermuda Ltd, Redwood City, CA]) is approved in the United States for use in people 2 through 64 years of age. Vaccine is not recommended routinely for most travelers. Immunization is recommended for travelers going to areas with active cholera transmission (**wwwnc.cdc.gov/travel/news-announcements/ cholera-vaccine-for-travelers**).

INFLUENZA. Influenza immunization is recommended for travelers ≥6 months of age and may be needed outside the times when annual influenza immunization is recommended in the United States. Influenza season is different in the northern and southern hemispheres and epidemic strains may differ. Antigenic composition of influenza vaccines used in Northern and Southern hemispheres may be different, and timing of administration may vary (see Influenza, p 511).

JAPANESE ENCEPHALITIS.[1] Japanese encephalitis (JE) virus, a mosquito-borne Flavivirus, is the most common vaccine-preventable cause of encephalitis in Asia. Risk of JE is low for most travelers to Asia but varies based on destination, duration, season, accommodations, and activities (**wwwnc.cdc.gov/travel/ yellowbook/2024/infections-diseases/japanese-encephalitis**). Travelers to countries with endemic JE in Asia, Oceania, and Australia should be informed about the disease and should use personal protective measures to reduce the risk of mosquito bites, especially during the night. JE vaccine can reduce the risk for infection further, and is recommended for those taking up residence in a JE endemic country, longer-term travelers (eg, a month or longer), and frequent travelers to areas with endemic JE. JE vaccine also should be considered for shorter-term travelers if they plan to travel outside of an urban area and have an itinerary or activities that will increase their risk of mosquito exposure in an area with endemic infection. Information on the location of JE virus transmission and detailed information on vaccine recommendations and adverse events can be obtained from the Centers for Disease Control and Prevention (CDC **[www.cdc.gov/vaccines/hcp/ acip-recs/vacc-specific/je.html]**).

An inactivated Vero cell culture-derived JE virus vaccine (Ixiaro) is approved and available in the United States for use in adults and children 2 months and older. The primary vaccination series for children and adolescents aged <18 years is 2 doses administered 28 days apart. An interval of as short as 7 days may be used for travelers 18 to 65 years of age with imminent departures. A booster dose may be administered at 1 year or longer after the primary series if ongoing exposure or reexposure is expected.

MENINGOCOCCUS. Meningococcal conjugate vaccines against serogroups A, C, W, and Y (MenACWY) are recommended for use in people age ≥2 months traveling to areas where there is a high burden of meningococcal disease, such as the "meningitis belt" of sub-Saharan Africa where disease is more common during the dry season (December to June), or other areas of the world with ongoing meningococcal outbreaks. Meningococcal conjugate vaccines vary in conjugating protein, ages of approved use, and dosing schedules. The following MenACWY vaccines are available for travelers: MenACWY-CRM (Menveo; ages 2 months through 55 years of age), and MenACWY-TT (MenQuadfi; ages 2 years and older). Completion of the entire series before travel is preferred. Booster doses are recommended for people who are at continuous or repeated increased risk of meningococcal infection—after 3 years for those who received their last dose at <7 years of age and after 5 years for those who received their last dose at ≥7 years of age, and every 5 years thereafter for people at

[1] Hills SL, Walter EB, Atmar RL, Fischer M. Japanese encephalitis vaccine: recommendations of the Advisory Committee on Immunization Practices. *MMWR Recomm Rep.* 2019;68(RR-2):1–33

continued risk. The Kingdom of Saudi Arabia requires an International Certificate of Vaccination or Prophylaxis (ICVP) documenting immunization against meningococcal serogroups A, C, W, and Y for pilgrims attending the Hajj or Umrah pilgrimages (**www.saudiembassy.net/hajj-and-umrah-health-requirements**). Immunization against serogroup B meningococcal disease is not recommended routinely for travel unless there are other indications to provide this vaccine or there is an outbreak at the travel destination (see Meningococcal Infections, p 585).

RABIES. The mainstay of prevention of rabies is education of families about avoidance of animals and the need for immediate medical care if a bite or other exposure occurs. Rabies preexposure prophylaxis should be considered for children who will be traveling to areas with endemic rabies where they may encounter wild or domestic animals (particularly dogs). Preexposure prophylaxis consists of a 2-dose series of rabies vaccine administered on days 0 and 7, by intramuscular injection (see Rabies, p 702, and **www.cdc.gov/mmwr/volumes/71/wr/mm7118a2.htm**). Postexposure prophylaxis includes cleaning wounds thoroughly with soap and water and then receiving postexposure prophylaxis promptly (PEP; see Rabies, p 702). For individuals who have not received the 2 doses of vaccine for preexposure prophylaxis, PEP consists of rabies immune globulin (RIG), 20 IU/kg infiltrated into the wound (if this dose is too much to infiltrate the full amount into the wound, the remaining RIG is injected intramuscularly), plus 4 doses of rabies vaccine (days 0, 3, 7, and 14). For those who have received preexposure prophylaxis, 2 doses of rabies vaccine (days 0 and 3) is sufficient for PEP. The need for boosters after completion of the 2-dose preexposure series will depend on the ongoing or future risk for exposure and rabies antibody titers, if done. The WHO has recommended use of intradermal rabies immunization as an alternative to intramuscular administration to reduce costs, but the FDA and the Advisory Committee on Immunization Practices (ACIP) of the CDC have not endorsed this recommendation. Travelers can be informed that the treatment they may be offered for an exposure outside the United States may differ from what they would receive in the United States.

TICK-BORNE ENCEPHALITIS. Tick-borne encephalitis (TBE) occurs in parts of the region stretching from western and northern Europe through northern and eastern Asia. Risk for TBE for most travelers to areas with endemic infection is very low, but some individuals are at increased risk for infection based on the season and location of travel and their activities, including consumption of unpasteurized dairy products. All people who travel to areas with endemic TBE should be advised to take precautions to avoid tick bites (see Prevention of Mosquito-borne and Tick-borne Infections, p 207) and to avoid unpasteurized milk and cheese. An inactivated TBE vaccine is available in the United States for use in adults and children 1 year and older. The primary vaccination series for children and adolescents aged <16 years consists of doses on day 0 (dose 1), at 1–3 months after the first vaccination (dose 2), and 5–12 months after the second vaccination (dose 3). The schedule for people 16 years and older is similar, but dose 2 can be administered as early as 14 days after dose 1. A booster dose may be administered at least 3 years after completion of the primary series if ongoing exposure or reexposure is expected. TBE vaccine is recommended for people who are moving or traveling to an area with endemic TBE and will have extensive exposure to ticks based on their planned outdoor activities and itinerary. TBE vaccine also may be considered for others who might engage in outdoor activities in areas ticks are likely to be found, with the decision to vaccinate based on an assessment of their planned activities and itinerary, risk factors for a poorer medical outcome, and personal perception and tolerance of risk. Information on the location of TBE virus transmission and detailed information on risk factors for infection and vaccine considerations can be found on the CDC website (**www.cdc.gov/tick-borne-encephalitis/index.html**).

TUBERCULOSIS. Risk of being infected with *Mycobacterium tuberculosis* during international travel depends on the activities of the traveler, duration of travel, and the epidemiology of tuberculosis at the destination. Risk of acquiring infection during usual tourist activities appears to be low, and pre- or post-travel testing is not recommended routinely. Risk may be higher for travelers living or working among the general population of a country with a high prevalence of tuberculosis (**www.who. int/publications/digital/global-tuberculosis-report-2021/tb-disease- burden/incidence**). Children with a history of significant travel to countries with endemic tuberculosis infection who have substantial contact with the resident population should be tested with an interferon-gamma release assay (IGRA) or a tuberculin skin test (TST). Some experts define significant travel as birth, travel, or residence in a country with an elevated tuberculosis rate for at least 1 month. If the child is well and has no history of exposure, the IGRA or TST should be delayed for 10 weeks after return. Pretravel administration of bacille Calmette-Guérin vaccine generally is not recommended.

TYPHOID. Typhoid vaccine is recommended for travelers who may be exposed to contaminated food or water. Two typhoid vaccines are available in the United States: an oral vaccine containing live attenuated *Salmonella enterica* serovar Typhi (Ty21a strain), approved for people 6 years and older (the capsules must be swallowed whole), and a parenteral Vi capsular polysaccharide (ViCPS) vaccine, approved for people 2 years and older. The Ty21a vaccine consists of 1 enteric-coated capsule taken every other day for a total of 4 capsules; the series should be completed at least 1 week before anticipated exposure. The ViCPS vaccine is administered as a single intramuscular injection that should be given at least 2 weeks before anticipated exposure. Typhoid immunization is not 100% effective; both vaccines protect 50% to 80% of recipients and do not provide adequate protection against paratyphoid fever. Revaccination is recommended 5 years after Ty21a vaccine and 2 years after ViCPS vaccine if continued or subsequent exposure to *Salmonella enterica* serovar Typhi is expected. Reimmunization includes the 4-capsule Ty21a oral vaccine or receiving 1 intramuscular dose for the ViCPS parenteral vaccine. For specific recommendations, see *Salmonella* Infections (p 742). The oral live-attenuated Ty21a vaccine capsules should be refrigerated, should be taken on an empty stomach, and should not be administered together with Vaxchora (begin the oral typhoid vaccine 8 hours after the dose of cholera vaccine) or during use of any antimicrobial agent other than the antimalarial agents mefloquine, chloroquine, or atovaquone-proguanil (**www.cdc. gov/mmwr/preview/mmwrhtml/mm6411a4.htm**). Typhoid immunization is not a substitute for careful selection of food and beverages.

YELLOW FEVER. Yellow fever (YF) occurs in parts of sub-Saharan Africa and tropical South America. YF is reported rarely among unimmunized travelers but may be fatal. Prevention measures against YF include immunization and protection against mosquito bites (see Prevention of Mosquito-borne and Tick-borne Infections, p 207). Current country requirements and recommendations for YF immunization can change and are available at the CDC Travelers' Health website (**wwwnc.cdc.gov/travel/**). Travelers should verify entry requirements for their destination. YF vaccine should be administered at least 10 days before travel.

The yellow fever vaccine YF-VAX (Sanofi Pasteur) is available in the United States and is recommended for people 9 months and older who are traveling to or living in areas of South America and Africa in which risk exists for YF virus transmission. Booster doses of yellow fever vaccine are no longer recommended for most travelers, because a single dose of YF vaccine provides long-lasting protection.[1] An additional dose of YF vaccine is recommended for people who were pregnant when they received their initial dose of vaccine and people who received a hematopoietic stem cell transplant after receiving a dose of YF vaccine. People infected with HIV when they received their first dose of YF vaccine should receive a dose every 10 years if ongoing risk for infection is present (**wwwnc.cdc.gov/travel/yellowbook/2024/ infections-diseases/yellow-fever**).

YF immunization should be limited to people at risk of exposure to YF or who require proof of vaccination for country entry because of risk of rare but serious adverse events including vaccine-associated neurologic and viscerotropic (multiple-organ system failure) disease.

OTHER CONSIDERATIONS. Travelers outside the United States may be exposed to mosquito-borne diseases, such as malaria, which can be life threatening; dengue or chikungunya viruses; or Zika virus, which poses a risk to fetuses of individuals infected during pregnancy. Prevention strategies include mosquito-bite prevention (see Prevention of Mosquito-borne and Tick-borne Infections, p 207) and, for malaria, use of antimalarial chemoprophylaxis. For recommendations on appropriate use of chemoprophylaxis, including recommendations for pregnant people, infants, and breastfeeding individuals, see Malaria (p 561) and Table 3.31 (p 566).

Travelers' diarrhea affects up to 60% of travelers but may be mitigated by good hand hygiene and attention to foods and beverages ingested (such as avoiding ice). Chemoprophylaxis generally is not recommended. Educating families about self-treatment, particularly oral rehydration, is critical. Packets of oral rehydration salts can be obtained before travel and are available in most pharmacies throughout the world, including in resource-limited countries, where diarrheal diseases are common. Some families may choose to carry an antimicrobial agent (eg, azithromycin) for treatment of travelers' diarrhea when offered by their travel medicine professional. Taking antimicrobial agents increases risk of colonization with resistant bacteria, so treatment should be reserved for moderate to severe cases of travelers' diarrhea. Bacteria that cause travelers' diarrhea (eg, *Campylobacter* species) may be resistant to fluroquinolones, so this class should be used with caution. Antimotility agents may be considered for older children and adolescents (see *Escherichia coli* Diarrhea, p 376) for mild to moderate diarrhea (and may be used along with an antimicrobial agent) but generally should be avoided in cases of bloody diarrhea or diarrhea associated with fever. Bismuth subsalicylate

---

[1] Staples JE, Bocchini JA, Rubin L, Fischer M. Yellow fever vaccine booster doses: recommendations of the Advisory Committee on Immunization Practices, 2015. *MMWR Morb Mortal Wkly Rep.* 2015;64(23):647–650

has been shown to reduce risk and severity of travelers' diarrhea and is available over the counter. Dosing information is available for children ≥12 years of age; it should not be used in children younger than 12 years because of the risk of Reye syndrome (**wwwnc.cdc.gov/travel/yellowbook/2024/preparing/travelers-diarrhea**).

Travelers should be aware of potential acquisition of respiratory tract viruses, including COVID-19 and influenza. They should be counseled on the wearing of face masks while on airplanes and in enclosed, poorly ventilated spaces during respiratory virus season. Hand hygiene and avoidance of close contact with animals (dead or live) should also be emphasized. Swimming, water sports, and ecotourism involving exposure to fresh water carry risks of acquisition of infections from environmental contamination (notably schistosomiasis, giardiasis, and leptospirosis from lakes, streams, or rivers) and exposure to beaches contaminated with dog or cat feces can lead to risk of hookworm skin infection (cutaneous larva migrans, creeping eruption).

Recommendations for Care of Children in Special Circumstances

BREASTFEEDING AND HUMAN MILK

Breastfeeding provides numerous health benefits to infants, including protection against morbidity and mortality from infectious diseases of bacterial, viral, and parasitic origin. In addition to providing an optimal source of infant nutrition, human milk contains immune-modulating factors, including secretory antibodies, glycoconjugates, anti-inflammatory components, prebiotics, probiotics, and antimicrobial compounds such as lysozyme and lactoferrin, which contribute to the formation of a health-promoting microbiota and an optimally functioning immune system. Breastfed infants have high concentrations of protective bifidobacteria and lactobacilli in their gastrointestinal tracts, which diminish the risk of colonization and infection with pathogenic organisms. Protection by human milk is established most clearly for pathogens causing gastrointestinal tract infection. In addition, there is substantial evidence that human milk provides protection against otitis media and upper and lower respiratory tract infections. Breastfeeding decreases the severity of upper and lower respiratory tract respiratory infections, including bronchiolitis, resulting in more than 70% reduction in hospitalizations. Evidence indicates that human milk may modulate the development of the immune system of infants. Human milk (including pasteurized donor human milk) is superior to formula for preterm and very low birth weight infants, as it is associated with decreased rates of serious infections and necrotizing enterocolitis and better feeding tolerance and neurodevelopmental outcomes.[1-4]

AAP Recommendations on Breastfeeding

The American Academy of Pediatrics (AAP) recommends exclusive breastfeeding for the first 6 months of life, with introduction of complementary foods at about 6 months of age, while continuing breastfeeding up to 2 years of age or longer as mutually

---

[1] World Health Organization. *Guidelines on Optimal Feeding of Low Birth-Weight Infants in Low- and Middle-Income Countries.* Geneva, Switzerland: World Health Organization; 2011. Available at: **www.who.int/publications/i/item/9789241548366**

[2] Meek JY, Noble L; American Academy of Pediatrics, Section on Breastfeeding. Policy statement. Breastfeeding and the use of human milk. *Pediatrics.* 2022;150(1):e2022057988

[3] Abrams SA, Landers S, Noble LM, Poindexter BB; American Academy of Pediatrics, Committee on Nutrition, Section on Breastfeeding, Committee on Fetus and Newborn. Policy statement. Donor human milk for the high-risk infant: preparation, safety, and usage options in the United States. *Pediatrics.* 2017;139(1):e20163440

[4] Parker MG, Stellwagen MG, Noble L, Kim JH, Poindexter BB, Puopolo KM; American Academy of Pediatrics, Section on Breastfeeding, Committee on Nutrition, Committee on Fetus and Newborn. Clinical report. Promoting human milk and breastfeeding for the very low birth weight infant. *Pediatrics.* 2021;148(5):e2021054272

desired by breastfeeding parent and infant.[1] The AAP publishes policy statements[1-3] and a manual on infant feeding[4] that provide additional information about the benefits of breastfeeding, recommended feeding practices, and potential contaminants of human milk. In the *Pediatric Nutrition Handbook*[5] and in the AAP policy statements on human milk and pasteurized donor human milk, issues regarding immunization of lactating parents and breastfeeding infants, transmission of infectious agents via human milk, and potential effects on breastfed infants of antimicrobial agents administered to lactating parents are addressed.

Contraindications to Breastfeeding

Breastfeeding provides the most complete nutrition for infants, including preterm and ill newborn infants, and therefore, health care providers should carefully consider a parent's decision not to start, to interrupt, or to stop breastfeeding. Providers should engage in shared decision making with parents. In certain situations, parents should be counseled that avoidance of breastfeeding is the only option that completely eliminates the risk of pathogen transmission. These include the breastfeeding parent's infection with human immunodeficiency virus (HIV), human T-cell lymphotropic virus type I or type II, or Ebola virus. For additional considerations related to breastfeeding and HIV, see the Human Immunodeficiency Virus section (p 139). Temporary suspension of breastfeeding is recommended when the breastfeeding parent has active herpetic (herpes simplex virus) lesions on the breast (see p 138) or untreated brucellosis. Parents with infections that require airborne precautions (varicella, measles) should avoid contact with the infant, but the infant can be fed the parent's expressed human milk.

Transmission of Infectious Agents via Human Milk

BACTERIA

Postpartum mastitis occurs in one third of breastfeeding people in the United States and leads to breast abscesses in up to 10% of cases. Assessment of the parent's breasts for trauma or maternal oversupply of milk and of the infant's latch should be considered and addressed as underlying mitigating causes. Both mastitis and breast abscesses have been associated with the presence of bacterial pathogens in human milk. In cases

[1] Abrams SA, Landers S, Noble LM, Poindexter BB; American Academy of Pediatrics, Committee on Nutrition, Section on Breastfeeding, Committee on Fetus and Newborn. Policy statement. Donor human milk for the high-risk infant: preparation, safety, and usage options in the United States. *Pediatrics.* 2017;139(1):e20163440

[2] Meek JY, Noble L; American Academy of Pediatrics, Section on Breastfeeding. Policy statement: Breastfeeding and the use of human milk. *Pediatrics.* 2022;150(1):e2022057988

[3] Parker MG, Stellwagen MG, Noble L, Kim JH, Poindexter BB, Puopolo KM; American Academy of Pediatrics, Section on Breastfeeding, Committee on Nutrition, Committee on Fetus and Newborn. Clinical report. Promoting human milk and breastfeeding for the very low birth weight infant. *Pediatrics.* 2021;148(5):e2021054272

[4] American Academy of Pediatrics. *Breastfeeding Handbook for Physicians.* 2nd ed. Schanler RJ, Krebs NF, Mass SB, eds. Elk Grove Village, IL: American Academy of Pediatrics; 2013

[5] American Academy of Pediatrics, Committee on Nutrition. *Pediatric Nutrition Handbook.* Kleinman RE, Greer FR, eds. 8th ed. Itasca, IL: American Academy of Pediatrics; 2019

of breast abscess or cellulitis, breastfeeding on the affected breast should continue, even if a drain is present, as long as the infant's mouth is not in direct contact with purulent drainage or infected tissue. In general, infectious mastitis resolves with continued lactation during appropriate antimicrobial therapy and does not pose a significant risk for the infant. Breastfeeding on the affected side in cases of mastitis generally is recommended; however, even when breastfeeding is interrupted on the affected breast, breastfeeding may continue on the unaffected breast.

Breastfeeding individuals with tuberculosis who have been treated appropriately for 2 or more weeks or who are not considered contagious (negative sputum) may breastfeed. Breastfeeding individuals with tuberculosis disease suspected of being contagious should refrain from breastfeeding and from other close contact with the infant because of potential spread of *Mycobacterium tuberculosis* through respiratory tract droplets or airborne transmission (see Tuberculosis, p 888). However, expressed human milk can be fed to the infant, as long as there is no evidence of tuberculosis mastitis, which is extremely rare.

Expressed human milk can become contaminated with a variety of bacterial pathogens. Outbreaks of gram-negative bacterial infections in neonatal intensive care units occasionally have been attributed to contaminated milk processing equipment and, rarely, bacteria from the parent's pumping equipment. Breast pumps and components should be thoroughly cleaned between pumping sessions. Liquid human milk fortifiers are preferred, because receipt of powdered human milk fortifiers and powdered infant formula has been associated with invasive bacteremia and meningitis attributable to *Cronobacter* species (formerly *Enterobacter sakazakii*), resulting in death in approximately 40% of cases. Consequently, the AAP has advised against the use of powdered infant formulas/human milk fortifiers in preterm or immunocompromised infants. Routine culturing or heat treatment of a parent's milk fed to the infant has not been demonstrated to be necessary or cost-effective (see Human Milk Banks, p 143). Because of the immune-protective factors in human milk, there is a hierarchical preference for the parent's freshly expressed milk, followed by the parent's previously refrigerated or frozen milk, followed by pasteurized donor milk as the third best option for feeding of sick and/or preterm infants.[1]

VIRUSES

CYTOMEGALOVIRUS. Cytomegalovirus (CMV) may be shed intermittently in human milk. Nearly all term infants who acquire CMV through breastfeeding do not develop clinical illness. In contrast, among very preterm infants, postnatal acquisition of CMV can be associated with sepsis-like illness. The long-term impact of postnatally acquired CMV through human milk among preterm infants is unclear and studies have yielded mixed results. Decisions about breastfeeding of preterm infants by parents known to be CMV seropositive should include consideration of the potential benefits of human milk and the risk of CMV transmission. Parents who give birth to infants at <32 weeks' gestation can be screened for CMV. When available, Holder

---

[1] Abrams SA, Landers S, Noble LM, Poindexter BB; American Academy of Pediatrics, Committee on Nutrition, Section on Breastfeeding, Committee on Fetus and Newborn. Policy statement. Donor human milk for the high-risk infant: preparation, safety, and usage options in the United States. *Pediatrics*. 2017;139(1):e20163440

pasteurization (62.5°C [144.5°F] for 30 minutes) and short-term pasteurization (72°C [161.6°F] for 5 seconds) of human milk appear to inactivate CMV; however, this is impractical in many settings. Short-term pasteurization may be less harmful to the beneficial constituents of human milk. Freezing human milk at −20°C (−4°F) for the sole purpose of reducing CMV infectivity is not advised, because although it may reduce the viral load of CMV, it does not change the risk of CMV sepsis-like syndrome, and freezing reduces the bioactivity of human milk. There is insufficient evidence to support withholding the parent's own milk because of risk for CMV transmission.[1]

EBOLA VIRUS. Ebola virus has been detected in human milk during and in the first month after infection. The duration of Ebola virus shedding in human milk is unknown. Genomic analysis in a case of fatal Ebola in a 9-month-old strongly suggested Ebola virus transmission through human milk. When safe alternatives to breastfeeding and infant care exist, a parent with confirmed or suspected Ebola virus infection should not have close contact with the infant (including breastfeeding) to reduce the risk of transmitting Ebola virus to the child. There is not enough evidence to provide guidance on precisely when it is safe to resume breastfeeding after recovery. Where available, testing of human milk for the presence of Ebola virus RNA can help to guide decisions about when breastfeeding can be safely resumed. Additional recommendations may be found at **www.cdc.gov/vhf/ebola/clinicians/evd/neonatal-care.html** and **www.cdc.gov/vhf/ebola/clinicians/evd/pregnant-women.html.**

HEPATITIS B VIRUS. Hepatitis B surface antigen (HBsAg) has been detected in human milk from HBsAg-positive people. However, studies have indicated that breastfeeding by HBsAg-positive people does not significantly increase the risk of infection among their infants. In the United States, infants born to known HBsAg-positive people should receive the initial dose of hepatitis B vaccine within 12 hours of birth, and Hepatitis B Immune Globulin should be administered concurrently but at a different anatomic site. This combination effectively will eliminate any theoretical risk of transmission through breastfeeding (see Hepatitis B, p 437). There is no need to delay initiation of breastfeeding until after the infant is immunized.

HEPATITIS C VIRUS. Hepatitis C virus (HCV) RNA and antibody to HCV have been detected in human milk from people infected with HCV, but transmission of HCV via breastfeeding has not been documented in people with HCV infection in the absence of HIV infection. According to current guidelines from the Centers for Disease Control and Prevention (CDC), American Association for the Study of Liver Diseases, and Infectious Diseases Society of America, parental HCV infection is not a contraindication to breastfeeding. However, parents infected with HCV should abstain from breastfeeding from a breast with cracked or bleeding nipples.

HERPES SIMPLEX VIRUS TYPE 1. Breastfeeding parents with herpetic lesions can transmit herpes simplex virus (HSV) to their infants by direct contact with the lesions. Transmission may be reduced with meticulous hand hygiene and covering of lesions with which the infant might come into contact. Parents with herpetic lesions on a

---

[1] Parker MG, Stellwagen LM, Noble L, et al; American Academy of Pediatrics, Section on Breastfeeding, Committee on Nutrition, Committee on Fetus and Newborn. Promoting human milk and breastfeeding for the very low birth weight infant. *Pediatrics.* 2021;148(5):e2021054272

breast or nipple should refrain from breastfeeding an infant from the affected breast until lesions have resolved, but may breastfeed from the unaffected breast when lesions on the affected breast are covered completely to avoid transmission. In addition, a parent with active herpes lesions on the breast can feed expressed milk from that breast to the infant, as there is no concern of herpes transmission via the milk. However, no part of the breast pump or expressed milk should come in contact with the lesions during expression, if the milk will be fed to the infant. If the pump does come in contact with the herpetic lesions, the parent should still express milk to maintain milk supply and prevent mastitis, but the expressed milk should be discarded.

HUMAN IMMUNODEFICIENCY VIRUS.[1] All pregnant people in the United States should be screened for human immunodeficiency virus (HIV) infection as part of a prenatal testing panel (see Human Immunodeficiency Virus Infection, p 489). Transmission of HIV by breastfeeding accounted for one third to one half of perinatal transmission of HIV worldwide in the pre-antiretroviral therapy (ART) era. Transmission is more likely among pregnant people who acquire HIV infection late in pregnancy or during the postpartum period. In resource-limited settings, the World Health Organization recommends that people living with HIV breastfeed their infants exclusively for the first 6 months of life, because infant morbidity associated with formula feeding is unacceptably high and safe alternatives to human milk may not be readily available.

Replacement (formula) feeding is recommended for all infants born to people living with HIV infection in the United States, because this is the option that eliminates risk of transmission of HIV to the infant.[2] Replacement feeding should be recommended if the birth parent is not receiving ART or is not adherent and has a detectable viral load. Parents with HIV infection with fully suppressed viral load and who are adherent with ART who wish to breastfeed should be supported in their decision to do so. If a parent chooses to breastfeed, an appropriate plan of management can be developed, including encouraging adherence with ART during breastfeeding, use of antiretrovirals in the infant as prophylaxis while breastfeeding, exclusive breastfeeding for 6 months followed by weaning and introduction of complementary foods, lactation counseling, frequent viral load monitoring in the breastfeeding parent, and frequent infant testing for HIV infection (**https://clinicalinfo.hiv.gov/en/guidelines/ perinatal/counseling-and-managing-women-living-hiv-united-states-who-desire-breastfeed**).

HUMAN T-LYMPHOTROPIC VIRUS TYPE 1. Human T-lymphotropic virus type 1 (HTLV-1), which is endemic in Japan, the Caribbean, and parts of South America, is associated with development of malignant neoplasms and neurologic disorders among adults. Epidemiologic and laboratory studies suggest that vertical transmission of human HTLV-1 occurs primarily through breastfeeding, although freezing/thawing of expressed human milk may decrease infectivity of human milk. People in the United States who are HTLV-1 seropositive should be advised to not breastfeed or donate to human milk banks.

---

[1] American Academy of Pediatrics, Committee on Pediatrics AIDS, Section on Breastfeeding. Policy statement. Infant feeding for persons living with HIV in the United States. *Pediatrics*. 2023; in press

[2] Meek JY, Noble L; American Academy of Pediatrics, Section on Breastfeeding. Technical report. Breastfeeding and the use of human milk. *Pediatrics*. 2022;150(1):e2022057989

HUMAN T-LYMPHOTROPIC VIRUS TYPE 2. Human T-lymphotropic virus type 2 (HTLV-2) is a retrovirus that has been detected among American and European injection drug users and some American Indian/Alaska Native people. Although apparent vertical transmission has been reported, the rate and timing of transmission have not been established. Until additional data about possible transmission through breastfeeding become available, parents in the United States who are HTLV-2 seropositive should be counseled regarding the risk of transmission of HTLV-2 with breastfeeding and advised not to donate to human milk banks. Routine screening for both HTLV-1 or HTLV-2 during pregnancy is not recommended.

MPOX. The mpox virus is spread by close contact, and neonatal mpox infection may be severe; thus, breastfeeding should be delayed until all mpox lesions have resolved, the scabs have fallen off, and a fresh layer of intact skin has formed. It is unknown whether mpox virus is present in human milk. Expressed milk from infected parents should be discarded until their lesions have healed and they can resume direct breastfeeding.

RUBELLA. Wild and vaccine strains of rubella virus have been isolated from human milk. However, the presence of rubella virus in human milk has not been associated with significant disease in infants, and transmission is more likely to occur via other routes. Parents with rubella or those who have been immunized recently with a live attenuated rubella virus-containing vaccine may continue to breastfeed.

SARS-COV-2. SARS-CoV-2 has been detected rarely in human milk, but viable infectious virus has not been detected in human milk samples and there have been no documented cases of transmission to breastfeeding infants. Given these findings, direct breastfeeding is encouraged. Acutely infected breastfeeding parents should properly wash their hands with soap and water before handling the infant and be advised to wear a mask while nursing. When not nursing, the infant can be cared for by a healthy caregiver, if available, and/or maintained in the same room at least 6 feet away from the breastfeeding parent. Parents shedding SARS-CoV-2 may express milk after appropriate breast and hand hygiene, and this milk may be fed to the infant by designated caregivers. Breast pumps and components should be thoroughly cleaned between pumping sessions using disinfectant wipes on the pump and washing pump attachments with hot, soapy water.

TICK-BORNE ENCEPHALITIS. Tick-borne encephalitis (TBE) virus has not been identified in human milk, but likely transmission of tick-borne encephalitis virus via human milk has been reported in 2 cases, 1 probable and 1 possible. A non-live TBE vaccine is available for travelers to areas in Europe and Asia where TBE virus is endemic. Breastfeeding is not a contraindication or precaution to vaccination.

VARICELLA. Expressed/pumped milk from a parent with varicella or zoster can be fed to the infant, provided no lesions are on the breast. Breastfeeding is not a contraindication or precaution to vaccination (see Varicella-Zoster Infections, p 938).

WEST NILE VIRUS. West Nile virus RNA has been detected in human milk collected from a person with disease attributable to West Nile virus. The breastfed infant developed West Nile virus immunoglobulin M antibodies but remained asymptomatic. Such transmission appears to be rare, and no adverse effects on infants have been described.

Because the benefits of breastfeeding outweigh the risk of WNV disease in breastfeeding infants, parents should be encouraged to breastfeed even in areas with ongoing WNV transmission.

ZIKA VIRUS. Although Zika virus has been detected in human milk, only a few probable cases of transmission of Zika virus via breastfeeding have been reported. The infants did not develop clinical disease. To date there is no consistent evidence that infants acquire Zika virus through breastfeeding. Cases have occurred in areas where Zika virus infection is endemic and where mosquito-borne transmission could not be excluded. Current evidence suggests that the benefits of breastfeeding outweigh the theoretical risks of Zika virus transmission through human milk. The World Health Organization and CDC recommend infants born to people with suspected, probable, or confirmed Zika virus infection or to individuals who live in or have traveled to areas with Zika virus should continue to breastfeed.

Immunization of Breastfeeding Parents and Infants

EFFECT OF IMMUNIZATION OF BIRTH PARENT

Parents who have not received recommended immunizations before or during pregnancy may be immunized during the postpartum period, regardless of lactation status. With the exception of yellow fever vaccine (see below),[1] no evidence exists to validate any clinical concern about the presence of other live vaccine viruses in human milk if the parent is immunized while lactating. Lactating parents should be immunized as recommended for adults and adolescents (**www.cdc.gov/vaccines**). If previously unimmunized or if traveling to an area with endemic poliovirus circulation, a lactating parent may receive inactivated (non-live) poliovirus vaccine (IPV). Breastfeeding parents who are susceptible to any of the viruses contained in the measles, mumps, and rubella vaccine (MMR) should be immunized during the early postpartum period. Breastfeeding is not a contraindication to varicella immunization. In lactating parents who receive live attenuated varicella vaccine, neither varicella DNA in human milk (by polymerase chain reaction assay) nor varicella antibody in the infant can be detected. If not administered during pregnancy, tetanus toxoid, reduced diphtheria toxoid, and acellular pertussis vaccine (Tdap) should be administered immediately postpartum. Nonimmunized breastfeeding parents should receive COVID-19 and influenza vaccine.[2,3] Inactivated (non-live) influenza vaccine (IIV) or live attenuated influenza vaccine (LAIV) may be administered during the postpartum period, if not otherwise contraindicated. All

---

[1] Centers for Disease Control and Prevention. Yellow fever vaccine: recommendations of the Advisory Committee on Immunization Practices (ACIP). *MMWR Recomm Rep.* 2010;59(RR-7):1-27

[2] Grohskopf LA, Alyanak E, Broder KR, Walter EB, Fry AM, Jernigan DB. Prevention and control of seasonal influenza with vaccines: recommendations of the Advisory Committee on Immunization Practices—United States, 2019–20 influenza season. *MMWR Recomm Rep.* 2019;68(RR-3):1–21. For annual updates, see **www.cdc.gov/vaccines**

[3] American Academy of Pediatrics, Committee on Infectious Diseases. Recommendations for prevention and control of influenza, 2023-2024. *Pediatrics.* 2023;152(4):e2023063772. For updates, see **https://redbook. solutions.aap.org/ss/influenza-resources.aspx**

licensed and authorized vaccines against COVID-19 are safe while breastfeeding. JYNNEOS is a live, non-replicating viral vaccine licensed for prevention of both smallpox and mpox disease; JYYNNEOS can be offered to people who are pregnant or breastfeeding who are otherwise eligible.

Breastfeeding is a precaution for yellow fever vaccine administration. Three cases of yellow fever vaccine-associated neurologic disease have been reported in exclusively breastfed infants whose parents received yellow fever vaccine while lactating. All 3 infants were younger than 1 month at the time of exposure and had a diagnosis of encephalitis. The risk of potential yellow fever vaccine virus exposure through breastfeeding is unknown and is likely dependent on how old the infant is when the lactating parent is vaccinated and when the infant is breastfed after the parent's vaccination. Pregnant and breastfeeding people should avoid travel to areas with yellow fever. If travel is unavoidable and the risks of vaccination are believed to outweigh the likelihood of yellow fever virus exposure, a pregnant or breastfeeding person should be issued a medical waiver to fulfill health regulations. If the risk of yellow fever virus exposure outweighs the vaccination risks, a pregnant or breastfeeding person should be vaccinated. Although there are no data, some experts recommend that breastfeeding people who receive yellow fever vaccine should temporarily suspend breastfeeding and pump and discard expressed milk for at least 2 weeks. Others recommend that the benefits of breastfeeding in an area with endemic infection or during outbreaks are likely to far outweigh the risk of potential transmission of vaccine virus to infants.

The world's first Ebola vaccine, ERVEBO, is a vesicular stomatitis platform-based live-virus (sVSV-ZEBOV) vaccine. No information is yet available on the safety of this vaccine during lactation. Similarly, no data are available on the live attenuated cholera vaccine in breastfeeding people. However, the live attenuated cholera vaccine is not absorbed from the gastrointestinal tract, so maternal exposure to the vaccine is not expected to result in exposure of the fetus. Pregnant people and their clinicians should consider the risks associated with traveling to areas of active cholera transmission.

EFFICACY AND SAFETY OF IMMUNIZATION IN BREASTFED INFANTS

Infants should be immunized according to the recommended childhood and adolescent immunization schedule (**https://redbook.solutions.aap.org/SS/ Immunization_Schedules.aspx**), regardless of the mode of infant feeding. Theoretically, high concentrations of poliovirus antibody in human milk could interfere with the immunogenicity of oral, but not non-live, poliovirus vaccine. However, in areas using oral poliovirus, vaccinated lactating parents should be counseled to breastfeed. There is in vitro evidence that human milk from people who live in areas with endemic rotavirus contains antibodies that can neutralize live rotavirus vaccine virus. However, in licensing trials, the effectiveness of rotavirus vaccine in breastfed infants was comparable to that in nonbreastfed infants. Postmarketing immunogenicity studies conducted outside the United States did not demonstrate improved antibody response following rotavirus vaccine when breastfeeding was temporarily withheld before and after vaccine administration. Furthermore, breastfeeding reduces the likelihood of rotavirus disease in infancy.

Human Milk Banks

In some circumstances, ill or preterm hospitalized infants are not able to receive their own parents' milk. These infants may be fed pasteurized donor human milk from an accredited milk bank to accrue the health benefits it offers.[1,2] The potential for transmission of infectious agents through donor human milk requires appropriate selection and screening of donors and careful collection, processing, and storage of human milk.[3,4] Currently, US nonprofit donor milk banks that belong to the Human Milk Banking Association of North America (**www.hmbana.org/**) voluntarily follow pasteurization guidelines drafted in consultation with the US Food and Drug Administration and the CDC. Other pasteurization methods also are acceptable, but use of nonpasteurized donor milk is not recommended. These guidelines include screening all donors for hepatitis B virus, hepatitis C virus, HIV 1 and 2, HTLV 1 and 2, and syphilis. Donor milk is dispensed after it is heat treated at 62.5°C (144.5°F) for 30 minutes (Holder pasteurization) and no viable bacteria are present after pasteurization.

Although milk banks support infants and children in the hospital and at home, informal milk sharing has become more common. Parents should be informed of the safety risks of milk obtained from unscreened donors and milk that has not been safely collected, pasteurized, processed, handled, and stored. Parents who decide to use shared milk should be instructed on minimizing risk by screening donors for contraindicated illnesses and medications and ensuring that the milk was safely collected, stored, and delivered. Milk obtained through the internet should be discouraged, as the donors cannot be screened and there are risks of contamination with chemicals and prescription and/or illicit drugs and even adulteration with cow milk.

Inadvertent Human Milk Exposure

Policies have been developed to deal with occasions when an infant inadvertently is fed expressed human milk not obtained from the infant's parent. These policies require documentation, counseling, and observation of the affected infant for signs of infection and potential testing of the source of the human milk for infections that could be transmitted via the milk. Recommendations for management of a situation involving an accidental exposure may be found on the CDC website (**www.cdc.gov/ breastfeeding/recommendations/other_mothers_milk.htm**). Decisions about medical management and diagnostic testing of the infant who received another

---

[1] World Health Organization, United Nations Children's Fund. Guideline: Updates on HIV and Infant Feeding: The Duration of Breastfeeding, and Support from Health Services to Improve Feeding Practices Among Mothers Living with HIV. Geneva, Switzerland: World Health Organization; 2016

[2] American Academy of Pediatrics. COVID-19 Interim Guidance. Post-Hospital Discharge Guidance for Breastfeeding Parents or Newborn Infants With Suspected or Confirmed SARS-CoV-2 Infection. Last updated August 2, 2022. Available at: **www.aap.org/en/pages/2019-novel-coronavirus-covid-19-infections/ clinical-guidance/breastfeeding-guidance-post-hospital-discharge/**

[3] Abrams SA, Landers S, Noble LM, Poindexter BB; American Academy of Pediatrics, Committee on Nutrition, Section on Breastfeeding, Committee on Fetus and Newborn. Policy statement. Donor human milk for the high-risk infant: preparation, safety, and usage options in the United States. *Pediatrics*. 2017;139(1):e20163440

[4] Parker MG, Stellwagen MG, Noble L, Kim JH, Poindexter BB, Puopolo KM; American Academy of Pediatrics, Section on Breastfeeding, Committee on Nutrition, Committee on Fetus and Newborn. Clinical report. Promoting human milk and breastfeeding for the very low birth weight infant. *Pediatrics*. 2021;148(5):e2021054272

parent's milk should be based on the details of the individual situation and be determined collaboratively between the infant's physician and parent(s) or guardian(s). A summary of the recommendations includes the following:

1. Inform the donor about the inadvertent exposure, and ask:
   - When was the milk expressed and how it was handled?
   - Would the donor be willing to share information about current medication use, recent infectious disease history, and presence of cracked or bleeding nipples during milk expression with the other family or the infant's treating physician?
2. Discuss inadvertent administration of the donor milk with the parent(s) or legal guardian of the recipient infant.
   - Inform them that their child was given another person's expressed human milk.
   - Inform them that the risk of transmission of infectious diseases (eg, HIV, hepatitis B, or hepatitis C) is small.
   - If possible, provide the family with information on when the milk was expressed and how the milk was handled prior to being delivered to the caregiver.
   - Encourage the parent(s) or guardian(s) to notify the infant's treating physician of the situation and share any specific details known.

Antimicrobial Agents and Other Drugs in Human Milk

Antimicrobial agents often are prescribed for lactating people. Although these drugs may be detected in human milk, the potential risk to an infant must be weighed against the known benefits of continued breastfeeding. As a general guideline, an antimicrobial agent is safe to administer to a lactating person if the drug is safe to administer to an infant. Only in rare cases will interruption of breastfeeding be necessary because of antimicrobial use by the lactating parent. A breastfed infant who requires antimicrobial therapy should receive the recommended doses, independent of administration of the agent to the breastfeeding parent.

Current information about drugs and lactation can be found on the NIH's Drugs and Lactation Database (LactMed) (**www.ncbi.nlm.nih.gov/books/NBK501922/**). Data for drugs, including antimicrobial agents, administered to lactating people are provided in several categories, including drug concentrations in infants and lactating people, effects in breastfed infants, possible effects on lactation, alternative drugs to consider, and references. Information on potential risks for drugs and vaccines administered during lactation, including potential effects on the breastfed child, can also be found in US Food and Drug Administration-approved labeling for the medication.

Anti-TNF Biologic Response Modifiers in Human Milk

Available evidence supports a lack of any significant transfer of anti-tumor necrosis factor (anti-TNF) drugs to human milk. Anti-TNF drugs include adalimumab, certolizumab pegol, etanercept, golimumab, and infliximab. People receiving treatment with anti-TNF drugs should be advised to continue breastfeeding. Infants of breastfeeding parents who are receiving anti-TNF drugs should receive recommended vaccines, including live virus vaccines, as indicated and according to the recommended schedule, unless vaccination is being withheld because of in utero exposure to the biologic response modifier (see Biologic Response-Modifying Drugs Used to Decrease Inflammation, p 104).

CHILDREN IN GROUP CHILD CARE AND SCHOOLS

Infants and young children who are cared for in group child care settings (child care centers and home-based child care) and schools[1] have an increased rate of communicable infectious diseases. Children in group child care settings and schools transmit infections among themselves and spread these infections to their families and child care or school staff. Risk of communicable diseases decreases gradually as children advance through school. Respiratory infections are more common than gastrointestinal tract or skin infections. Health department interventions are often necessary when outbreaks of infectious diseases occur in these settings.

Children in child care are more likely to receive antimicrobial agents; hence, they may also be colonized or infected with antimicrobial-resistant organisms. Younger age, more time in group child care settings, and exposure to larger group size are all strongly associated with more frequent infections. As children get older and increase their time in group care, they develop lasting immunity to common infections earlier compared with peers with less exposure.

Compared with children in child care, school-aged children experience a lower incidence of infectious diseases because of increased immunity as well as improved infection control measures such as hand hygiene and respiratory etiquette. However, schools remain important sites of transmission of common infectious diseases including rhinovirus infections, influenza, pertussis, COVID-19, and others, including additional vaccine-preventable diseases.

Modes of Spread of Infectious Diseases

RESPIRATORY TRACT DISEASES

Children, especially young children in child care, spread respiratory pathogens efficiently because of suboptimal social distancing and respiratory etiquette (Table 2.1). Pathogens spread by the respiratory route include bacteria, sometimes associated with invasive infections, and viruses. Viral infections of the respiratory tract are common in children in group child care settings. Possible modes of transmission of respiratory tract pathogens include aerosols, respiratory droplets, direct contact with secretions, or indirect contact with contaminated fomites. The most common viral pathogens responsible for respiratory tract disease in child care settings include respiratory syncytial virus (RSV) and human metapneumovirus as well as viruses that also affect children in schools, including parainfluenza virus, influenza virus, adenovirus, rhinovirus, and SARS-CoV-2. Respiratory tract viruses are associated with exacerbations of asthma and an increase in the incidence of otitis media and can cause significant complications for children with chronic respiratory tract disease, such as cystic fibrosis and chronic lung disease of prematurity, and for children who are immunocompromised.

---

[1] American Academy of Pediatrics. *Managing Infectious Diseases in Child Care and Schools: A Quick Reference Guide.* Shope TR, Hashikawa AN, eds. 6th ed. Itasca, IL: American Academy of Pediatrics; 2023

Table 2.1. Modes of Transmission of Organisms

Usual Route of Transmission[a]	Bacteria	Viruses	Other[b]
Fecal-oral	*Campylobacter* species, *Salmonella* species; *Shigella* species; *Shiga* toxin-producing *Escherichia coli*, including *E coli* O157:H7	Astrovirus, enteric adenovirus, enteroviruses, hepatitis A virus, norovirus, rotaviruses, sapovirus	*Cryptosporidium* species, *Enterobius vermicularis*, *Giardia duodenalis*
Respiratory	*Bordetella pertussis*, group A *Streptococcus*, *Haemophilus influenzae* type b, *Kingella kingae*, *Mycobacterium tuberculosis* (children ≥10 years and adults), *Neisseria meningitidis*, *Streptococcus pneumoniae*	Adenovirus, coronavirus (including SARS-CoV-2), influenza virus, human metapneumovirus, measles virus, mumps virus, parainfluenza virus, parvovirus B19, respiratory syncytial virus, rhinovirus, rubella virus, varicella-zoster virus	...
Person-to-person contact	Group A *Streptococcus*, *Staphylococcus aureus*	Herpes simplex virus, varicella-zoster virus	Agents causing pediculosis, scabies, and ringworm[c]
Contact with blood, urine, and/or saliva	...	Cytomegalovirus, herpes simplex virus, hepatitis C virus	...
Bloodborne	...	Hepatitis B virus, hepatitis C virus, human immunodeficiency virus	...

[a] The potential for transmission of microorganisms in the child care setting by food and animals also exists (see Appendix VI, Clinical Syndromes Associated With Foodborne Diseases, p 1150, and Appendix VII, Diseases Transmitted by Animals [Zoonoses], p 1157).
[b] Parasites, fungi, mites, and lice.
[c] Transmission also may occur from contact with objects in the environment.

Seasonal outbreaks of common respiratory infections, such as hand-foot-and-mouth disease (enterovirus) and bronchiolitis, are common in group child care settings, and influenza outbreaks occur annually in child care settings and schools. Other respiratory pathogens that can cause sporadic outbreaks include group A streptococcal pharyngitis, *Neisseria meningitidis*, *Mycoplasma pneumoniae* (in schools), and some vaccine-preventable diseases such as pertussis, varicella, measles, mumps, rubella, COVID-19 and, rarely, *Haemophilus influenzae* type b. The incidence of vaccine-preventable diseases has markedly decreased since routine immunizations were implemented. Seasonal outbreaks of influenza continue to be common and, notably, most states do not require influenza vaccine for these settings. Communities with low vaccination rates continue to be at increased risk for vaccine-preventable disease outbreaks. More detailed recommendations for management and exclusion and return to care for these conditions are available in Table 2.2 and Table 2.3, as well as the relevant disease-specific chapters in Section 3 and other resources from the American Academy of Pediatrics (AAP).[1,2]

ENTERIC DISEASES

Diarrheal illness is much more common in child care settings than in schools, because young children and adult caregivers spread enteric diseases primarily by contact with pathogens during diapering and toileting procedures. Enteric diseases can also occur in schools if a person fails to maintain good hygiene after toilet use or if contaminated food is shared among classmates. Organisms spread by the fecal-oral route include common viruses, bacterial pathogens, and parasites. Seasonal enteric pathogens include noroviruses (which are a frequent cause of illness in children), enteric adenoviruses, and astroviruses (see Table 2.1). Rotavirus vaccination has dramatically decreased seasonal outbreaks attributable to this virus, but illness still occurs. Hepatitis A virus can cause outbreaks in child care settings and schools but similarly is much less common since widespread implementation of routine hepatitis A immunization. Bacterial enteropathogens such as *Shigella* species and *Escherichia coli* O157:H7 can cause significant outbreaks in group child care settings and require a very small infective dose of organisms, whereas *Salmonella* species and *Campylobacter* species are less frequent causes of outbreaks. Parasites like *Giardia duodenalis* and *Cryptosporidium* species can cause outbreaks in child care settings, particularly where shared pools are used in water play activities, because their spores are resistant to chlorination in water sources and to alcohol-based hand sanitizers (see Prevention of Illnesses Associated with Recreational Water Use, p 214). More detailed recommendations for management, exclusion, and return to care for these conditions are available in the relevant disease-specific chapters in Section 3 or other references,[1,2] and local public health authorities should be consulted.

---

[1] American Academy of Pediatrics. *Managing Infectious Diseases in Child Care and Schools: A Quick Reference Guide.* Shope TR, Hashikawa AN, eds. 6th ed. Itasca, IL: American Academy of Pediatrics; 2023

[2] American Academy of Pediatrics, American Public Health Association, National Resource Center for Health and Safety in Child Care and Early Education. *Caring for Our Children: National Health and Safety Performance Standards: Guidelines for Out-of-Home Child Care.* 4th ed. Itasca, IL: American Academy of Pediatrics; and Washington, DC: American Public Health Association; 2019

Table 2.2. General Recommendations for Exclusion of Children From Group Child Care and School

Symptom(s)	Management
Illness preventing participation in activities, as determined by child care staff	Exclusion until the child can participate in activities
Illness that requires a level of care that is greater than staff can provide without compromising health and safety of others	Exclusion until the child no longer requires extra care to the extent staff cannot adequately attend to the health and safety of others in their care
Severe illness suggested by fever with behavior changes, lethargy, irritability, persistent crying, difficulty breathing, progressive rash with above symptoms	Medical evaluation and exclusion until severe symptoms have resolved and child can participate in activities and does not require excessive care
Persistent abdominal pain (2 hours or more) or intermittent abdominal pain associated with fever, dehydration, or other systemic signs and symptoms	Medical evaluation and exclusion until severe symptoms have resolved and child can participate and does not require excessive care
Vomiting 2 or more times in preceding 24 hours	Exclusion until symptoms have resolved, unless vomiting is determined to be caused by a noncommunicable condition and child is able to remain hydrated and participate in activities
Diarrhea if stool not contained in diaper or if fecal accidents occur in a child who is normally continent, if stool frequency exceeds 2 stools above normal for that child, or stools contain blood or mucus	Medical evaluation for stools with blood or mucus; exclusion until stools are contained in the diaper or when toilet-trained children no longer have accidents using the toilet, and when stool frequency becomes no more than 2 stools above that child's normal frequency for the time the child is in the program, even if the stools remain loose
Oral lesions	Exclusion if unable to contain drool or if unable to participate because of other symptoms
Skin lesions	Exclusion if lesions are weeping and cannot be covered with a waterproof dressing

BLOODBORNE INFECTIONS

Bloodborne infections are a potential concern in group child care settings and schools. Hepatitis B virus (HBV) transmission from an infected child biting a susceptible child has occurred in child care, but this is rare, especially given high hepatitis B immunization rates. Human immunodeficiency virus (HIV) transmission in a child care setting has never been documented. School-aged children infected with HIV, HBV, or hepatitis C virus (HCV) do not need to be identified to school personnel. Rather, policies and procedures to manage all potential exposures to blood or blood-containing materials should be established and universally implemented. Care required for school-aged children with physical or intellectual disabilities may expose caregivers to urine,

Table 2.3. Disease- or Condition-Specific Recommendations for Exclusion of Children from Group Child Care[a]

Condition	Management of Case	Management of Contacts
COVID-19	See CDC (www.cdc.gov/coronavirus/2019-ncov/community/schools-childcare/child-care-guidance.html), state, and local health department recommendations	See CDC (www.cdc.gov/coronavirus/2019-ncov/community/schools-childcare/child-care-guidance.html), state, and local health department recommendations
Hand-foot-and-mouth disease (caused by enteroviruses)	Because hand-foot-and-mouth disease is normally mild, children can continue to attend child care and school as long as they have no fever, have no uncontrolled drooling, and are able to participate normally in classroom activities. In some cases, the health department may require children with hand-foot-and-mouth disease to stay home to control an outbreak.	In the event of an enterovirus A71 outbreak, consult the local or state health department for recommendations on exclusion and return to care.
Hepatitis A virus (HAV)	Serologic testing to confirm HAV infection in suspected cases. Exclusion until 1 week after onset of illness.	Hepatitis A outbreaks in child care are now rare because of the widespread adoption of universal childhood vaccination. In facilities with diapered children, if 1 or more cases confirmed in child or staff attendees or 2 or more cases in households of staff or attendees, hepatitis A vaccine (HepA) or immune globulin intramuscular (IGIM) should be administered within 14 days of exposure to all unimmunized staff and attendees. In centers without diapered children, HepA or IGIM should be administered only to unimmunized classroom contacts of index case. Asymptomatic contacts may return after receipt of IGIM or HepA (see Hepatitis A, p 430, for further discussion on indications for HepA or IGIM).

Table 2.3. Disease- or Condition-Specific Recommendations for Exclusion of Children from Group Child Care,[a] continued

Condition	Management of Case	Management of Contacts
Herpes simplex virus	Only children with HSV gingivostomatitis (ie, primary infection) who do not have control of oral secretions should be excluded from child care. Exclusion of children with cold sores (ie, recurrent infection) from child care or school is not indicated. HSV lesions on other parts of the body should be covered with clothing or a bandage, if practical, for children attending school or child care.	Avoid the sharing of respiratory secretions through contact with objects and washing and sanitizing mouthed toys, bottle nipples, and utensils that have come in contact with saliva.
Impetigo	No exclusion if treatment has been initiated and as long as lesions on exposed skin are covered.	No intervention unless additional lesions develop.
Measles	Exclusion until 4 days after beginning of rash and when the child is able to participate.	In outbreak setting, people without documentation of immunity should be immunized within 72 hours of exposure or excluded. Immediate readmission to group child care may occur following immunization. Unimmunized people and those who do not receive vaccine within 72 hours of exposure should be excluded for at least 21 days after onset of rash in the last case of measles. For use of immune globulin, see Measles (p 570).

Table 2.3. Disease- or Condition-Specific Recommendations for Exclusion of Children from Group Child Care,[a] continued

Condition	Management of Case	Management of Contacts
Mumps	Exclusion until 5 days after onset of parotid gland swelling.	In outbreak setting, people without documentation of immunity should be immunized or excluded. Immediate readmission may occur following immunization. Unimmunized people should be excluded until at least 26 days after onset of parotitis in the last person with mumps. A second dose of measles, mumps, and rubella vaccine (MMR) (or measles, mumps, rubella, and varicella vaccine [MMRV], if age appropriate) should be offered to all students (including those in postsecondary school) and to all health care personnel born in or after 1957 who have only received 1 dose of MMR vaccine. A second dose of MMR also may be considered during outbreaks for preschool-aged children who have received 1 MMR dose. People previously vaccinated with 2 doses of a mumps-containing vaccine who are identified by public health as at increased risk for mumps because of an outbreak should receive a third dose of a mumps-containing vaccine to improve protection against mumps disease and related complications (see Mumps, p 611).
Pediculosis capitis (head lice) infestation	Children should not be excluded or sent home early from school or child care because of head lice, because head lice have a low contagion in these settings. "No-nit" policies requiring that children be free of nits before they return to a child care facility or school should be discouraged.	Household and close contacts should be examined and treated if infested. No exclusion necessary.
Pertussis	Exclusion until completion of 5 days of the recommended course of antimicrobial therapy if pertussis is suspected; children and providers who refuse treatment should be excluded until 21 days have elapsed from cough onset (see Pertussis, p 656).	Immunization and chemoprophylaxis should be administered as recommended for household and child care contacts. Contacts should be observed for respiratory tract symptoms for 21 days and if they develop symptoms, then they should be treated (see Pertussis, p 656).

Table 2.3. Disease- or Condition-Specific Recommendations for Exclusion of Children from Group Child Care,[a] continued

Condition	Management of Case	Management of Contacts
Rubella	Exclusion for 7 days after onset of rash for postnatal infection.	In outbreak setting, children without evidence of immunity should be immunized or excluded for 21 days after onset of rash of the last case in the outbreak. Pregnant contacts should be evaluated (see Rubella, p 735).
Infection with *Salmonella* serotypes Typhi or Paratyphi	Exclusion until 3 consecutive stool cultures obtained at least 48 hours after cessation of antimicrobial therapy are negative, stools are contained in the diaper or child is continent, and stool frequency is no more than 2 stools above that child's normal frequency for the time the child is in the program.	When *Salmonella* serotype Typhi infection is identified in a child care staff member, local or state health departments should be consulted regarding regulations for length of exclusion and testing, which may vary by jurisdiction.
Infection with nontyphoidal *Salmonella* species, *Salmonella* of unknown serotype	Exclusion until stools are contained in the diaper or child is continent and stool frequency is no more than 2 stools above that child's normal frequency for the time the child is in the program. Stool consistency does not need to return to normal to be able to return to child care. Negative stool culture results generally are **not** required for nonserotype Typhi or Paratyphi *Salmonella* species.	Symptomatic contacts should be excluded until stools are contained in the diaper or child is continent and stool frequency is no more than 2 stools above that child's normal frequency for the time the child is in the program. Stool cultures are not required for asymptomatic contacts.
Scabies	Treatment at end of program day and readmission on completion of first treatment. Children should not be excluded or sent home early from school because of scabies, because scabies has a low contagion within classrooms.	Close contacts with prolonged skin-to-skin contact should receive prophylactic therapy. Bedding and clothing in contact with skin of infected people should be laundered (see Scabies, p 750).

Table 2.3. Disease- or Condition-Specific Recommendations for Exclusion of Children from Group Child Care,[a] continued

Condition	Management of Case	Management of Contacts
Infection with Shiga toxin-producing *Escherichia coli* (STEC), including *E coli* O157:H7	Exclusion until 2 stool cultures (obtained at least 48 hours after any antimicrobial therapy, if administered, has been discontinued) are negative, and stools are contained in the diaper or child is continent, and stool frequency is no more than 2 stools above the child's normal frequency. Report to and consult with local or state public health officials. Some state health departments have less stringent exclusion policies for children who have recovered from less virulent STEC infection.	Meticulous hand hygiene; stool cultures should be performed for any symptomatic contacts. In outbreak situations involving virulent STEC strains, stool cultures of asymptomatic contacts may aid controlling spread. Center(s) with cases should be closed to new admissions during STEC outbreak (see *Escherichia coli* Diarrhea, p 376).
Shigellosis	Exclusion until the state or local health department has deemed it safe to return to work per state or local child care exclusion regulations. Following this, children can return to child care facilities if stools are contained in the diaper or when toilet-trained children are continent and when stool frequency becomes no more than 2 stools above that child's normal baseline for the time the child is in the program, even if the stools remain loose.	Meticulous hand hygiene; stool cultures should be performed for any symptomatic contacts (see *Shigella* Infections, p 756).
Staphylococcus aureus skin infections	Exclusion only if skin lesions are draining and cannot be covered with a watertight dressing.	Meticulous hand hygiene; cultures of contacts are not recommended.

Table 2.3. Disease- or Condition-Specific Recommendations for Exclusion of Children from Group Child Care,[a] continued

Condition	Management of Case	Management of Contacts
Streptococcal pharyngitis	Exclusion until at least 12 hours after treatment has been initiated. In the setting of an outbreak, exclusion for at least 24 hours after treatment has been initiated should be considered, and consultation with the state or local public health department is recommended.	Symptomatic contacts of documented cases of group A streptococcal infection should be tested and treated if test results are positive.
Tuberculosis	Most children younger than 10 years are not considered contagious. For those with active disease, exclusion until determined to be noninfectious by physician or health department authority. No exclusion for latent tuberculosis infection.	Local health department personnel should be informed for contact investigation (see Tuberculosis, p 888).
Varicella (see Varicella-Zoster Infections, p 938)	Exclusion until all lesions have crusted or, in immunized people without crusts, until no new lesions appear within a 24-hour period.	For people without evidence of immunity, varicella vaccine should be administered ideally within 3 days but up to 5 days after exposure. If vaccine cannot be administered, varicella-zoster immune globulin or antiviral postexposure prophylaxis can be given (see Varicella-Zoster Virus, p 938). Varicella-zoster immune globulin should be administered up to 10 days after exposure, while valacyclovir or acyclovir should be administered beginning 7 days after exposure and continuing for 7 days.

[a] Many of these illnesses also require exclusion from school and other activities. Many of these diseases are reportable to local or state public health authorities, and reporting rules for local jurisdictions should be consulted. Public health authorities should be consulted if there are questions about exclusion criteria.

saliva, and in some cases, blood. Therefore, the application of Standard Precautions and appropriate hand hygiene, as recommended for children in group child care,[1] is the optimal means to prevent spread of infection from these exposures. Parents and students should be educated about the types of exposure that present a risk for school contacts. Although a student's right to privacy should be maintained, decisions about activities at school should be made by parents or guardians together with the child's physician, on a case-by-case basis, keeping the health needs of the infected student and the student's classmates in mind. School nurses are often helpful to consult, as they are familiar with the school landscape.

Although no prospective studies have been conducted to determine the risk of transmission of HIV, HBV, or HCV during contact sports among high school students, available evidence indicates that the transmission risk is low. Guidelines for management of bleeding injuries have been developed for college and professional athletes in recognition of the possibility of unidentified HIV, HBV, or HCV infection in any athlete. The following are recommendations for preventing transmission of HIV and other bloodborne pathogens in the athletic setting.

- Athletes infected with HIV, HBV, or HCV should be allowed to participate in competitive sports.
- Physicians should respect the rights of infected athletes to confidentiality. The infection status of patients should not be disclosed to other participants or the staff of athletic programs.
- Testing for bloodborne pathogens should not be mandatory for athletes or sports participants.
- Pediatricians are encouraged to counsel athletes who are infected with HIV, HBV, or HCV and to assure them that they have a low risk of infecting other competitors. Infected athletes should consider choosing a sport in which this transmission risk is minimal. This choice may be protective both for other participants and for the infected athletes themselves, decreasing their possible exposure to bloodborne pathogens other than the one(s) with which they are infected. Contact and collision sports such as wrestling and boxing have the greatest potential for contamination of injured skin by blood. The AAP opposes boxing as a sport for youth for other reasons.[2]
- Athletic programs should inform athletes and their parents that the program is operating under the policies of the aforementioned recommendations and that the athletes have a low risk of becoming infected with a bloodborne pathogen.
- Athletic programs should promote HBV immunization among all athletes, coaches, athletic trainers, equipment handlers, laundry personnel, janitorial staff, and other people who may be exposed to blood as an occupational hazard. HBV immunization is universally recommended for everyone aged 59 years and younger and for those who are older who have risk factors or who wish to be protected.
- Each coach and athletic trainer must receive training in first aid and emergency care.
- Coaches and members of the health care team should educate athletes that, in contrast to the assumed low risk of transmission during athletics, there are greater risks

---

[1] American Academy of Pediatrics. *Managing Infectious Diseases in Child Care and Schools: A Quick Reference Guide.* Shope TR, Hashikawa AN, eds. 6th ed. Itasca, IL: American Academy of Pediatrics; 2023

[2] American Academy of Pediatrics, Council on Sports Medicine and Fitness; Canadian Paediatric Society, Healthy Active Living and Sports Medicine Committee. Boxing participation by children and adolescents. *Pediatrics.* 2011;128(3):617–623 (Reaffirmed February 2015, March 2020)

of transmission of HIV and other bloodborne pathogens through sexual activity and needle sharing during the use of injection drugs, including anabolic steroids. Athletes should be told not to share personal items, such as razors, toothbrushes, and nail clippers, that might be contaminated with blood.

- Depending on the law in some states, schools may need to comply with Occupational Safety and Health Administration (OSHA) regulations (**www.osha. gov**) for prevention of bloodborne pathogens. The athletic program must determine which OSHA rules are applicable for their enterprise. Compliance with OSHA regulations is a reasonable and recommended precaution even if this is not required specifically by the state.
- The following precautions should be adopted in sports with direct body contact and other sports in which an athlete's blood or other body fluids visibly tinged with blood may contaminate the skin or mucous membranes of other participants or staff members of the athletic program. These precautions will not eliminate the risk that a participant or staff member may become infected with a bloodborne pathogen in the athletic setting but will reduce the risk substantially.
  - Athletes must cover existing cuts, abrasions, wounds, or other areas of broken skin with an occlusive dressing before and during participation. Caregivers should cover their own damaged skin to prevent transmission of infection to or from an injured athlete.
  - Disposable, waterproof gloves should be worn to avoid contact with blood or other body fluids visibly tinged with blood and any objects, such as equipment, bandages, or uniforms, contaminated with these fluids. Hands should be cleaned with soap and water or an alcohol-based antiseptic agent as soon as possible after gloves are removed.
  - Athletes with active bleeding should be removed from competition as soon as possible. Wounds should be cleaned with soap and water. Skin antiseptic agents may be used if soap and water are not available. Athletes may return to competition once bleeding has stopped, and cleansed wounds are covered with an occlusive dressing that will remain intact and not become soaked through during further play.
  - Athletes should be advised to report injuries and wounds in a timely fashion before or during competition.
  - Minor cuts or abrasions that are not bleeding do not require interruption of play but can be cleaned and covered during scheduled breaks. During these breaks, if an athlete's equipment or uniform fabric is wet with blood, the equipment should be cleaned and disinfected (see next bullet), or the uniform should be replaced.
  - Equipment and playing areas contaminated with blood must be cleaned using gloves and disposable absorbent material until all visible blood is gone and then disinfected with a product registered with the Environmental Protection Agency and applied in the manner and time recommended.[1] If the disinfecting product is bleach (1:80 dilution of household bleach), the decontaminated equipment or area should be in contact with the bleach solution for at least 30 seconds. The area then may be wiped with a disposable cloth after the minimum contact time or allowed to air dry.
  - Emergency care must not be delayed because gloves or other protective equipment are not available. If the responder does not have appropriate protective

---

[1] Centers for Disease Control and Prevention. Guidelines for environmental infection control in health-care facilities. Recommendations of CDC and the Healthcare Infection Control Practices Advisory Committee (HICPAC). *MMWR Recomm Rep.* 2003;52(RR-10):1–48 (updated July 2019)

equipment, a towel may be used to cover the wound until an off-the-field location is reached where gloves can be used during definitive treatment.

- Breathing bags (eg, Ambu manual resuscitators) and oropharyngeal airways should be available for use during resuscitation.
- Equipment handlers, laundry personnel, and janitorial staff must be educated in proper procedures for handling washable or disposable materials contaminated with blood.

OTHER INFECTIONS

Other common infections (Table 2.1, p 146) among children in group child care and schools may occur by direct contact with infected lesions, such as *Staphylococcus aureus*, group A *Streptococcus*, and herpes simplex virus. Shared fomites, such as towels, athletic equipment, and razors, have been implicated in the spread of methicillin-resistant *S aureus* (MRSA) within school settings. The AAP has guidance on control and prevention of MRSA and other infections in athletes and other school settings.[1] *Trichophyton tonsurans*, the predominant cause of tinea capitis (ringworm), remains viable for long periods on combs, hair brushes, furniture, and fabric. Tinea cruris (jock itch) and tinea pedis (athlete's foot) occur in adolescents and young adults. *Sarcoptes scabiei* (scabies) and *Pediculus capitis* (head lice) are transmitted primarily through person-to-person contact. In schools and group child care settings, transmission of scabies is unlikely without prolonged skin-to-skin contact; for lice, transmission occurs by direct head-to-head contact. Transmission of scabies and head lice through shared articles of clothing or hair accessories (combs, hair brushes, hats, and hair ornaments) is possible but uncommon. Cytomegalovirus (CMV) is common in children in child care settings and spreads via contact with infected bodily secretions; it is estimated that up to 70% of children 1 to 3 years of age who attend group child care may shed the virus in saliva or urine. CMV and parvovirus infections can have effects on the fetus of a pregnant child care worker, and those employed or volunteering in child care should discuss this occupational risk with their health care providers. Finally, human-animal contact involving family and classroom pets, animal displays, and petting zoos exposes children to pathogens harbored by these animals. Some animals are commonly colonized with *Salmonella* species, *Campylobacter* species, Shiga toxin-producing *E coli*, lymphocytic choriomeningitis virus, and other viruses that may be transmitted to children via contact (see Appendix VII, Diseases Transmitted by Animals [Zoonoses], p 1157). Detailed recommendations for management and exclusion and return-to-care or -school for these conditions are available in Table 2.2, Table 2.3, as well as the relevant disease-specific chapters in Section 3 and other references.[2,3]

---

[1] Davies HD, Jackson MA, Rice SG; American Academy of Pediatrics, Committee on Infectious Diseases, Council on Sports Medicine and Fitness. Infectious diseases associated with organized sports and outbreak control. *Pediatrics*. 2017;140(4):e20172477

[2] American Academy of Pediatrics. *Managing Infectious Diseases in Child Care and Schools: A Quick Reference Guide.* Shope TR, Hashikawa AN, eds. 6th ed. Itasca, IL: American Academy of Pediatrics; 2023

[3] American Academy of Pediatrics, American Public Health Association, National Resource Center for Health and Safety in Child Care and Early Education. *Caring for Our Children: National Health and Safety Performance Standards: Guidelines for Out-of-Home Child Care.* 4th ed. Itasca, IL: American Academy of Pediatrics; and Washington, DC: American Public Health Association; 2019

Management and Prevention of Infectious Diseases

There are 3 primary methods for reducing the transmission of infectious diseases in group child care and school settings: immunization, infection prevention and control, and exclusion and return-to-care or -school policies and practices.

IMMUNIZATION

Immunizations are by far the most effective means of preventing childhood infectious diseases. The United States relies on child care and school entry vaccination requirements to achieve and sustain high levels of vaccination coverage. Most states require vaccination of children entering child care programs, all states require vaccination of children at the time of entry into school, and many states have vaccination requirements for children throughout elementary school and high school and at the time of entry to college. Child care programs should require that all enrollees and staff members receive age-appropriate immunizations as recommended by the AAP and the Advisory Committee on Immunization Practices (ACIP) of the Centers for Disease Control and Prevention (CDC). Parents should be required to report their child's immunization status and programs should keep and review these records. Unless contraindications exist or children have recognized exemptions (as per state immunization laws), immunizations documented through vaccine cards or medical records should demonstrate complete immunization for age (**https://redbook. solutions.aap.org/SS/Immunization_Schedules.aspx**). The immunization mandates for children in child care and schools vary by state and can be found online (**www.immunize.org/laws**) and from the National Network for Immunization Information (**www.immunizationinfo.org/**). The AAP views nonmedical exemptions to child care- and school-required immunizations as inappropriate for individual, public health, and ethical reasons and advocates for their elimination.[1] State requirements often lag behind AAP and ACIP recommendations.

Children who have not received recommended age-appropriate immunizations before enrollment should be encouraged to be immunized as soon as possible, and the series should be completed according to the recommended childhood and adolescent immunization catch-up schedule as appropriate (**https://redbook.solutions. aap.org/SS/Immunization_Schedules.aspx**). Whether unimmunized or inadequately immunized children may attend child care or school will depend on state and local public health guidance. Parents need to be informed that if a vaccine-preventable disease occurs in a child care program or school, all unimmunized and underimmunized children will be excluded for the duration of possible exposure or until they have completed their immunizations. Local public health jurisdictions should be consulted for guidance.

All adults who work in a child care facility or school should receive all vaccines routinely recommended for adults (see adult immunization schedule at **www.cdc. gov/vaccines/schedules/hcp/adult.html**). By being fully immunized, child care providers and teachers protect not only themselves but also infants too young to

---

[1] American Academy of Pediatrics, Committee on Practice and Ambulatory Medicine, Committee on Infectious Diseases, Committee on State Government Affairs, Council on School Health, Section on Administration and Practice Management. Medical versus nonmedical immunization exemptions for child care and school attendance. *Pediatrics*. 2016;138(3):e20162145 (Reaffirmed February 2022)

receive or have completed their immunization series and children who have medical contraindications to immunizations. More detailed information about adult child care provider and teacher immunization requirements can be found in other references.[1,2]

INFECTION PREVENTION AND CONTROL

Group child care settings and schools both are rich environments for pathogens. However, group child care settings are much more problematic than schools, because young children are in close contact with each other, touching and sharing; they cough and sneeze without proper respiratory etiquette; and they need to be supervised or assisted with toileting and hand hygiene. As a result, viral, bacterial, fungal, and parasitic pathogens can be present in the air, on surfaces, in bodily secretions, and on the skin. Efforts to control the transmission of infectious diseases in child care settings are important but also difficult to implement effectively; as such, infection prevention and control in these settings requires a multifaceted approach. Programs should have written policies and training for staff to be sure they properly implement the best methods. These policies should include procedures for food and medication preparation; diaper changing; cleaning, sanitizing, and disinfecting surfaces; hand hygiene; respiratory etiquette; and other Standard Precautions.

It is difficult to decrease the spread of respiratory pathogens in group child care settings, with intensive education and infection control measures producing only modest reductions in incidence of respiratory illness, probably because respiratory pathogens are primarily spread by droplets expelled by sneezing and coughing. Young children have difficulty anticipating sneezing and coughing and do not effectively practice respiratory etiquette and hand hygiene. In addition, their social nature causes them to play in close proximity to each other, within the radius most contaminated large droplets may travel before contacting another child's mucous membranes. Nevertheless, immunization, hand hygiene, and respiratory etiquette are essential elements of infection control in child care settings, and it is important that staff practice these measures for themselves as well as educate and assist young children to properly do so. Aerosolized droplets that land on surfaces may contain microorganisms capable of causing infections. Therefore, surface cleaning, disinfecting, and sanitizing are important to prevent the spread of respiratory illness. In schools, however, efforts to improve hand hygiene and respiratory etiquette—covering mouth and nose with tissue when coughing or sneezing (if no tissue is available, use the upper arm or elbow area rather than hands)—to reduce transmission of respiratory infections such as influenza are more effective and should be taught and implemented. Recommendations about use of well-fitting face masks for children ≥2 years to prevent spread of COVID-19 were introduced during the COVID-19 pandemic (see COVID-19, p 324). Child care and schools should consult current public health recommendations for current guidance.

Infection control procedures in group child care settings are more effective in reducing diarrheal illness than respiratory illness. Adhering to diaper-changing procedures as

[1] American Academy of Pediatrics. *Managing Infectious Diseases in Child Care and Schools: A Quick Reference Guide.* Shope TR, Hashikawa AN, eds. 6th ed. Itasca, IL: American Academy of Pediatrics; 2023

[2] American Academy of Pediatrics, American Public Health Association, National Resource Center for Health and Safety in Child Care and Early Education. *Caring for Our Children: National Health and Safety Performance Standards: Guidelines for Out-of-Home Child Care.* 4th ed. Itasca, IL: American Academy of Pediatrics; and Washington, DC: American Public Health Association; 2019

recommended by the AAP[1] is a critical step to reduce fecal contamination and should be applied in child care settings as well as in schools that have diapered students with physical and intellectual disabilities. Surface cleaning, sanitizing, and disinfecting are especially important for reducing gastrointestinal tract illnesses. Cleaning removes visible soil to increase the effectiveness of sanitizing or disinfecting agents. Sanitizing reduces the amount of potential pathogens on food preparation surfaces, utensils, tables, countertops, and plastic toys. Disinfection requires stronger concentration or different agents than sanitizing and is used for areas with higher likelihood of pathogens, such as door handles, drinking fountains, and toilet and diaper changing areas.

As with respiratory tract infections, hand hygiene is essential to prevent the fecal-oral spread of gastrointestinal tract pathogens. Hand hygiene should occur for staff and children on arrival; when moving from one group to another; before and after contact with food or medication administration; after diaper changing, toileting, and contact with nasal or other body secretions, animals, or garbage; and after playing outside. Hand washing for 20 seconds with soap and water is the preferred method for hand hygiene, should be prioritized in child care and school settings, and is required whenever there is visible particulate matter. However, alcohol-based hand sanitizer may be substituted when soap and water is not available. Alcohol-based hand sanitizers have high alcohol content (60%–95%), which can be ingested or aerosolized; therefore, adult supervision is required. Hand hygiene using soap and water is preferred for *Cryptosporidium* species and norovirus because alcohol-based hand sanitizers are not as effective against these pathogens.

Other important environmental infection control and prevention measures for child care facilities include having adequate ventilation in the building (see **www.cdc. gov/coronavirus/2019-ncov/community/schools-childcare/ventilation. html** for ways to increase ventilation); providing enough physical space in the facility and between cots for naps (which may increase social distancing and reduce droplet spread); ensuring physical separation and separate personnel (if possible) involved in food preparation and diaper changing; requiring appropriate handling of animals (and excluding reptiles, turtles, amphibians, birds, primates, live poultry, ferrets, or rodents in the facility), with hand hygiene before and after contact; and adhering to recommended ratios of children to care providers.

Health departments should have plans for responding to reportable and non-reportable outbreaks of communicable diseases in child care programs and schools and should provide training, written information, and technical consultation when requested or alerted. In some instances, administration of appropriate antimicrobial therapy to a patient will limit further spread of infection (eg, *Shigella* species, streptococcal pharyngitis, pertussis). Antimicrobial prophylaxis administered to close contacts of children with infections caused by specific pathogens may be warranted in some circumstances (eg, meningococcal infection [see p 585], invasive *H influenzae* type a or type b [see p 400], and pertussis [see p 656]). Decisions about postexposure prophylaxis after an in-school exposure are best made in conjunction with local public health authorities and the primary care pediatrician. Temporary closure of classrooms or entire child care programs or schools can be used in limited circumstances: (1) to prevent spread of infection; (2) when an infection is expected to affect a large number of susceptible students and available control measures are considered inadequate;

---

[1] American Academy of Pediatrics. *Managing Infectious Diseases in Child Care and Schools: A Quick Reference Guide.* Shope TR, Hashikawa AN, eds. 6th ed. Itasca, IL: American Academy of Pediatrics; 2023

(3) when an infection affects a large number of staff and adequate staffing cannot be achieved; or (4) when an infection is expected to have a high rate of morbidity or mortality. Prolonged or frequent closures may result in unintended consequences for children and families including reduced learning and emotional and mental health impact. Collaborative efforts of public health officials, teachers, licensing agencies, child care providers, child care health consultants, physicians, nurses, parents, employers, and other members of the community are necessary to address problems of infection prevention and management in child care settings and schools. People involved with early education and child care and schools can use the published national standards[1] related to these topics to provide specific education and implementation measures.

EXCLUSION AND RETURN TO CARE OR SCHOOL

General recommendations for exclusion of children in group child care and schools are provided in Table 2.2 (p 148). Exclusions can put a significant economic strain on families, as parents may need to miss work to care for an ill child, and many exclusion decisions made by early child care and education professionals are not evidence-based and are inappropriate. No studies demonstrate that excluding children in group care and schools who are ill with common infectious diseases reduces the likelihood of spread to other children. However, to try to control environmental contamination and/or spread because the clinical consequences are significant, there are some infectious diseases for which exclusion is recommended (Table 2.2, p 148). Many children are infectious before developing symptoms. Asymptomatic infection, high carriage rates, and prolonged shedding of pathogens in body secretions are common and make it difficult to curb transmission by targeting only symptomatic children. Because mild illness is common among children and most minor illnesses do not constitute a reason for excluding a child from child care or school, decisions about exclusion should be primarily based on the child's behavior. A mildly ill child can remain in child care or school unless the illness prevents the child from participating in normal activities, as determined by the child care staff or teachers, or the illness requires a need for care that is greater than child care staff or teachers can provide.

Each day as the child enters the program or school, and throughout the day as needed, staff members and teachers should evaluate the well-being of the child and observe for signs of illness. Parents should be encouraged to share information with child care staff and teachers about their child's acute and chronic illnesses and medication use utilizing a formal care plan that is signed by the child's health care provider. Examples of illnesses and conditions that do not necessitate exclusion include:

- Common cold (however, because symptoms can be similar to COVID-19, during periods of high COVID-19 transmission, referral to public health guidance is recommended).
- Diarrhea, as long as stools are contained in the diaper (for infants), there are no accidents using the toilet (for older children), and stool frequency is no more than 2 stools above normal for that child.
- Rash without fever and without behavioral change.

---

[1] American Academy of Pediatrics, American Public Health Association, National Resource Center for Health and Safety in Child Care and Early Education. *Caring for Our Children: National Health and Safety Performance Standards: Guidelines for Out-of-Home Child Care.* 4th ed. Itasca, IL: American Academy of Pediatrics; and Washington, DC: American Public Health Association; 2019

- Hand-foot-and-mouth disease as long as children have no fever, have no uncontrolled drooling with mouth sores, and can participate normally in classroom activities. In some cases, particularly in cases of enterovirus A71, the health department may require children with hand-foot-and-mouth disease to stay home to control an outbreak.
- Lice. Children should not be excluded or sent home early from school or child care because of head lice, because head lice have a low contagion in these settings. "No-nit" policies requiring that children be free of nits before they return to a child care facility or school should be discouraged.[1]
- Ringworm and scabies (treatment can occur at the end of the day, with return the following day).
- Thrush.
- Fifth disease (parvovirus B19 infection) in an immunocompetent child.
- CMV infection.
- Herpes simplex virus (HSV) infection, as long as a child with HSV gingivostomatitis (ie, primary infection) has control of oral secretions. Exclusion of children with cold sores (ie, recurrent infection) from child care or school is not indicated.
- Chronic HBV infection (see p 437 for possible exceptions).
- Conjunctivitis without fever and without behavioral change.
- HIV infection (see p 489 for possible exceptions).
- Colonization with MRSA in children who do not have active lesions or illness that would otherwise require exclusion.

Asymptomatic children who excrete an enteropathogen usually do not need to be excluded (exceptions include children who are infected with Shiga toxin-producing *E coli*, *Shigella* species, or *Salmonella* serotype Typhi or Paratyphi).

Disease- or condition-specific recommendations for exclusion from child care and schools and management of contacts are shown in Table 2.3 (p 149). Despite the existence of national recommendations for exclusion since 1992,[2,3] states have been slow to adopt these. Each state has its own regulations pertaining to exclusion and return to care/school, and these may not be evidence based. Child care programs are required to follow these state-specific guidelines to maintain licensing, which can be found at **https://childcareta.acf.hhs.gov/licensing.** Exclusion and return to care guidelines for schools may be addressed by state departments of health or other public health agencies.

During outbreaks of certain diseases, the responsible local and state public health authorities are helpful for determining the benefits and risks of excluding children from their usual care program or school. All states have laws about reporting and isolation of people with specific communicable diseases. Local or state health departments should be contacted for information about these laws, and public health authorities in these areas should be notified about cases of nationally notifiable infectious diseases and unusual outbreaks of other illnesses involving children or adults in the child care

---

[1] Devore CD, Schutz GE; American Academy of Pediatrics, Council on School Health, Committee on Infectious Diseases. Head lice. *Pediatrics*. 2015;135(5):e1355-e1365 (Reaffirmed June 2020)

[2] American Academy of Pediatrics. *Managing Infectious Diseases in Child Care and Schools: A Quick Reference Guide.* Shope TR, Hashikawa AN, eds. 6th ed. Itasca, IL: American Academy of Pediatrics; 2023

[3] American Academy of Pediatrics, American Public Health Association, National Resource Center for Health and Safety in Child Care and Early Education. *Caring for Our Children: National Health and Safety Performance Standards: Guidelines for Out-of-Home Child Care.* 4th ed. Itasca, IL: American Academy of Pediatrics; and Washington, DC: American Public Health Association; 2019

environment or schools (see Appendix III, Nationally Notifiable Infectious Diseases in the United States, p 1141). For most outbreaks of vaccine-preventable illnesses, unvaccinated children should be excluded until they are vaccinated and the risk of transmission no longer exists. In circumstances requiring intervention to prevent spread of infection within the school setting, the privacy of children who are infected should be protected.

INFECTION PREVENTION AND CONTROL FOR HOSPITALIZED CHILDREN

Health care-associated infections (HAIs) are a threat to patient safety in hospitalized children. A comprehensive set of guidelines for preventing and controlling HAIs, including isolation precautions, occupational health recommendations, and guidelines for prevention of postoperative and device-related infections, can be found on the Centers for Disease Control and Prevention (CDC) website (**www.cdc.gov/infectioncontrol/guidelines/index.html**). Additional guidelines are available from the principal infection prevention and control societies in the United States (the Society for Healthcare Epidemiology of America and the Association for Professionals in Infection Control and Epidemiology), as well as other groups such as the Occupational Safety and Health Administration and the Cystic Fibrosis Foundation.[1] The investigation and control of outbreaks that occur in special pediatric settings (eg, hematopoietic stem cell transplant units, neonatal and surgical units) should always involve the infection prevention and control team in each facility. Accrediting organizations, such as The Joint Commission, have established infection prevention and control standards. Pediatricians and infection prevention and control professionals should be familiar with this increasingly complex array of guidelines, regulations, and standards. To accomplish this goal, infection prevention and control programs led by pediatric infectious diseases specialists are increasingly used in hospital settings. These programs require adequate institutional support to be sustainable over time. Ongoing infection prevention and control programs should include education, implementation, reinforcement, documentation, and evaluation of recommendations on a regular basis. Such activities should include conducting surveillance for high-risk HAIs, participating in improvement projects to reduce the incidence of HAIs, sharing data describing the incidence of specifically targeted HAIs, and measuring health care personnel compliance with key prevention activities, such as hand hygiene.

Infection preventionists should be familiar with the Targeted Assessment for Prevention (TAP) strategy developed by the CDC. This strategy targets health care facilities and specific units within facilities with a disproportionate burden of HAIs so that gaps in infection prevention in these locations can be addressed. The TAP report uses data in the National Healthcare Safety Network system to calculate a metric called the "cumulative attributable difference," which is the number of infections that must be prevented within a group, facility, or unit to achieve an HAI reduction goal (**www.cdc.gov/hai/prevent/tap.html**).

---

[1] Saiman L, Seigel JD, LiPuma JJ, et al. Infection prevention and control guideline for cystic fibrosis: 2013 update. *Infect Control Hosp Epidemiol.* 2014;35(Suppl 1): S1-S67; **www.cff.org/Care/Clinical-Care-Guidelines/Infection-Prevention-and-Control-Clinical-Care-Guidelines/Infection-Prevention-and-Control-Clinical-Care-Guidelines/**

Infection Prevention and Control Precautions

Infection prevention and control precautions are designed to protect hospitalized children, health care personnel, and visitors by limiting transmission of potential pathogens within the health care setting. The Healthcare Infection Control Practices Advisory Committee (HICPAC) of the CDC has recommended a core set of infection prevention and control practices that are required in all health care settings, regardless of the type of health care provided (**www.cdc.gov/infectioncontrol/ guidelines/core-practices/index.html**). These core practices represent fundamental standards of care that are not expected to change based on emerging evidence or to be regularly altered by changes in technology or practices. Additional evidence-based guidelines detailing transmission-based isolation precautions were published in 2007 (**www.cdc.gov/hicpac/pdf/isolation/Isolation2007.pdf**) with updates at **www.cdc.gov/infectioncontrol/guidelines/isolation/updates.html**. Adherence to this guidance, supplemented by health care facility policies and procedures for other aspects of infection and environmental control and occupational health, should reduce HAIs and result in safer patient care. Adaptations should be made according to the conditions and populations served by each facility, especially in the setting of an emerging infectious disease.

Routine and optimal performance of **Standard Precautions** is appropriate for care of *all* patients, regardless of diagnosis or suspected or confirmed infectious status. In addition to Standard Precautions, **Transmission-Based Precautions** are used when caring for patients who are infected or colonized with pathogens transmitted by airborne, droplet, or contact routes. Table 2.4 lists syndromes and conditions that are suggestive of contagious infection and require empiric isolation precautions pending identification of a specific pathogen. When the specific pathogen is known, isolation recommendations and duration of isolation are provided in the pathogen- or disease-specific chapters in Section 3 and can be found in the HICPAC guidelines (**www.cdc.gov/infectioncontrol/ guidelines/isolation/appendix/type-duration-precautions.html**).

In November 2023, HICPAC recommended changes to existing categories of transmission-based precautions. Contact precautions would continue to be recommended to interrupt transmission of pathogens spread by touch. Droplet and airborne precautions would be replaced by 3 new categories of transmission-based precautions to interrupt transmission of pathogens spread by air. These include Routine Air Precautions, Special Air Precautions, and Extended Air Precautions, and are intended to better address the continuum of respiratory pathogen transmission through air. If these recommendations are ultimately adopted by the CDC, HICPAC will update pathogen-specific recommendations.

STANDARD PRECAUTIONS

Standard Precautions are used for all patient care and during every patient encounter, regardless of diagnosis or concern for a transmissible infection. Standard Precautions are based on health care personnel's assessment of how to protect themselves from exposure and how to prevent the spread of pathogens from patient to patient. Standard Precautions include the following practices:

- **Respiratory hygiene/cough etiquette (www.cdc.gov/flu/professionals/ infectioncontrol/resphygiene.htm)** includes source containment of infectious respiratory tract secretions in symptomatic patients beginning at the initial point of

Table 2.4. Clinical Syndromes or Conditions Warranting Precautions in Addition to Standard Precautions to Prevent Transmission of Epidemiologically Important Pathogens Pending Confirmation of Diagnosis[a]

Clinical Syndrome or Condition[b]	Potential Pathogens[c]	Empiric Precautions[d]
Diarrhea		
Acute diarrhea with a likely infectious cause	Enteric pathogens[e]	Contact
Diarrhea in patient with a history of recent antimicrobial use	*Clostridioides difficile*	Contact; use soap and water for handwashing
Meningitis	*Neisseria meningitidis, Haemophilus influenzae* type b	Droplet
	Enteroviruses	Contact (and Droplet, if patient has respiratory symptoms)
Rash or exanthems, generalized, cause unknown		
Petechial or ecchymotic with fever	*Neisseria meningitidis*	Droplet
	Hemorrhagic fever viruses	Contact and Airborne
	Enteroviruses	Contact (and Droplet, if patient has respiratory symptoms)
Vesicular	Varicella-zoster virus	Contact and Airborne
Maculopapular with coryza and fever	Measles virus	Airborne
Respiratory tract infections		
Pulmonary cavitary disease	*Mycobacterium tuberculosis*	Airborne
Paroxysmal or severe persistent cough during periods of pertussis activity in the community	*Bordetella pertussis*	Droplet

Table 2.4. Clinical Syndromes or Conditions Warranting Precautions in Addition to Standard Precautions to Prevent Transmission of Epidemiologically Important Pathogens Pending Confirmation of Diagnosis,[a] continued

Clinical Syndrome or Condition[b]	Potential Pathogens[c]	Empiric Precautions[d]
Viral bronchiolitis and croup, in infants and young children	Respiratory viral pathogens	Contact and Droplet
Risk of multidrug-resistant microorganisms[f]		
Infection or colonization with a multidrug-resistant organism	Multi-drug resistant bacteria, *Candida auris*	Contact
Skin, wound, or urinary tract infection in a patient with a recent stay in a hospital or chronic care facility	Multi-drug resistant bacteria, *C auris*	Contact until resistant organism is excluded by cultures
Skin or wound infection		
Abscess or draining wound that cannot be covered	*Staphylococcus aureus*, group A *Streptococcus*	Contact

[a] Infection control professionals should modify or adapt this table according to local conditions. To ensure that appropriate empiric precautions are implemented, hospitals must have systems in place to evaluate patients routinely according to these criteria as part of their preadmission and admission care.

[b] Patients with the syndromes or conditions listed may have atypical signs or symptoms (eg, pertussis in neonates may present with apnea; paroxysmal or severe cough may be absent in pertussis in adults). The clinician's index of suspicion should be guided by the prevalence of specific conditions in the community and clinical judgment.

[c] The organisms listed in this column are not intended to represent the complete or even most likely diagnoses but, rather, possible causative agents that require additional precautions beyond **Standard Precautions** until a causative agent is identified or excluded.

[d] Duration of isolation precautions is not addressed in this table.

[e] These pathogens include Shiga toxin-producing *Escherichia coli* including *E coli* O157:H7, *Shigella* organisms, *Salmonella* organisms, *Campylobacter* organisms, hepatitis A virus, enteric viruses such as rotavirus, *Cryptosporidium* organisms, and *Giardia* organisms. Use masks when cleaning vomitus or stool during norovirus outbreak.

[f] Multidrug-resistant organisms should be defined by the infection control program on the basis of current state, regional, or national recommendations to be of special clinical or epidemiologic significance.

encounter (eg, emergency department triage and ambulatory clinic reception areas). Symptomatic children and their caregivers should cover their mouths/noses when sneezing/coughing, use tissues and dispose of them in no-touch receptacles, observe hand hygiene after soiling of hands with respiratory tract secretions, wear a disposable mask if tolerated, and maintain physical distancing as space permits.

- **Hand hygiene (www.cdc.gov/handhygiene/)** is necessary before and after all patient contact and after touching blood, body fluids, secretions, excretions, and contaminated items, including after removing (doffing) disposable gloves. Hand hygiene should also be performed after contact with the patient environment to ensure that health care personnel are not transmitting potential pathogens from contaminated surfaces that surround the patient. Hand hygiene should be performed either with soap and water or with alcohol-based agents. A helpful reference is the World Health Organization's Hand Hygiene: How, Why, and When document **(cdn.who.int/ media/docs/default-source/documents/health-topics/hand-hygiene-why-how-and-when-brochure.pdf).**

- When hands are visibly dirty or contaminated with blood or other body fluids, they should be washed with soap and water for at least 20 seconds (including wrists). During an outbreak, handwashing with soap and water is preferred over alcohol-based agents for preventing transmission of spores (eg, *Clostridioides difficile*) and some viruses like norovirus.

- **Gloves** (clean, nonsterile, single use) should be worn when touching blood, body fluids, secretions, excretions, and items contaminated with these fluids. Clean gloves should be used by health care personnel before touching mucous membranes and nonintact skin or when contact with body fluids is possible. Gloves should be changed after contact with potentially infectious material (eg, purulent drainage) and high-touch surfaces and between tasks and procedures on the same patient. Hand hygiene should be performed before donning gloves and after removing them.

- **Masks, eye protection, and face shields** should be worn to protect mucous membranes of the eyes, nose, and mouth whenever there is an expectation of possible exposure to blood, body fluids, secretions, or excretions.

- **Nonsterile gowns** that are fluid-resistant will protect skin and prevent soiling of clothing during procedures and patient care whenever there is an expectation of possible exposure to infectious material. Soiled gowns should be removed promptly and carefully to avoid contamination of clothing.

- **Cleaning and disinfection of multipatient care equipment (eg, stethoscopes) and instruments/devices** should be performed according to the manufacturer's recommendations to prevent pathogen transmission from contaminated items.

- **All used textiles (linens)** are considered contaminated and should be handled, transported, and processed in a manner that prevents aerosolization of microorganisms, skin and mucous membrane exposure, and contamination of clothing.

- **Care of the environment,** which includes shared toys and high-touch surfaces, requires that policies and procedures are established for routine and targeted cleaning of environmental surfaces as indicated by the level of patient contact and degree of soiling. A hospital disinfectant registered by the Environmental Protection Agency should be used.

- **Safe injection practices should be followed to prevent risks to patients and health care personnel.** Syringes should ***never*** be reused for more than one patient even if the needle is changed. Likewise, insulin pens and lancing devices must not be used for multiple patients. Do not use medications packaged as single-dose or single-use for more than one patient and do not enter a vial with a used syringe or needle. Limit the use of multidose vials and dedicate them to a single patient whenever possible. More information is available from the CDC at **www.cdc.gov/injectionsafety.** Bloodborne pathogen exposure of health care personnel should be avoided by taking precautions to prevent injuries caused by needles, scalpels, and other sharp instruments or devices during procedures; when handling sharp instruments after procedures; when cleaning used instruments; and during disposal of used needles. To prevent needlestick injuries, safety devices should be used whenever they are available. Needles should not be recapped, purposely bent or broken, removed from disposable syringes, or otherwise manipulated by hand. After use, disposable syringes and needles, scalpel blades, and other sharp items should be placed in puncture-resistant containers for disposal. These containers should be located as close as practicable to the usage area. Large-bore, reusable needles should be placed in a puncture-resistant container located close to the site of usage for easy transport to the reprocessing area to ensure maximal patient safety. Sharp devices with safety features are preferred whenever such devices have equivalent function to conventional sharp devices. Written policies and procedures relating to needlestick or sharp injuries are mandated by the Occupational Safety and Health Administration **(www.osha.gov/healthcare).**
- **During spinal procedures** (eg, lumbar puncture or placing a catheter), surgical masks should be worn to prevent contamination of the lumbar area with the health care personnel's respiratory flora and subsequent health care-associated meningitis or contaminated culture results.
- **Source control** refers to wearing respirators or well-fitting facemasks to cover a person's mouth and nose to prevent spread of respiratory secretions when they are breathing, talking, sneezing, or coughing. This infection prevention measure was initially recommended for all health care personnel by the CDC during the COVID-19 pandemic to prevent presymptomatic transmission of SARS-CoV-2 in health care settings and has been proven to be an effective means of limiting spread of respiratory viruses. See **www.cdc.gov/infectioncontrol/guidelines/isolation/index.html** for further information.

TRANSMISSION-BASED PRECAUTIONS

Transmission-Based Precautions are designed for patients documented or suspected to have colonization or infection with pathogens for which additional precautions beyond **Standard Precautions** are recommended to prevent transmission. The 3 types of transmission routes on which these precautions are based are airborne, droplet, and contact. Recent evidence suggests that airborne and droplet transmission are not discrete categories but exist on a continuum, influenced by many factors including their environment and their initial sizes.

- **Airborne transmission** occurs by dissemination of airborne droplet nuclei (small-particle residue [traditionally defined as ≤5 μm in size, although this definition has been challenged by data showing that droplets/aerosols 20 μm in size travel like aerosols from cough jets and air conditioning] of evaporated droplets containing microorganisms that remain suspended in the air for long periods) or small respirable particles containing the infectious agent or spores. Microorganisms transmitted by the airborne route can be dispersed widely by air currents and can be inhaled by a susceptible host within the same room or at a long distance from the source patient, depending on environmental factors. Special air handling and ventilation are required to prevent airborne transmission. Some examples of microorganisms transmitted by airborne droplet nuclei are *Mycobacterium tuberculosis*, measles virus, and varicella-zoster virus. Specific recommendations for **Airborne Precautions** are as follows:

- When possible, the patient should wear a mask while health care personnel are inside the room and during patient transport outside of the room.
- Contagious patients and care partners should be placed in a single-patient room (if unavailable, consult an infection preventionist), and the door should be kept closed at all times.
- The isolation room should provide at least 6 to 12 air changes per hour, air flow direction from the surrounding area to the room ("negative pressure"), and room air exhausted directly to the outside or recirculated through high-efficiency particulate air (HEPA) filters.
- Health care personnel should be trained to use respiratory protective devices appropriately, such as a fit-tested National Institute for Occupational Safety and Health-approved N95 or higher-level respirator, while inside the patient's room. The Centers for Disease Control and Prevention provides guidance on using respirators at **www.cdc.gov/coronavirus/2019-ncov/prevent-getting-sick/use-n95-respirator.html.**
- Susceptible health care personnel should not enter rooms of patients with known or suspected measles or varicella-zoster virus infections. If susceptible people must enter the room of a patient with measles or varicella infection or an immunocompromised patient with local or disseminated zoster infection, a respiratory protective device, such as a fit-tested N95 (or higher-level) respirator or a powered air-purifying respirator, should be worn.

- **Droplet transmission** occurs when respiratory droplets containing microorganisms are generated from an infected person, primarily during coughing, sneezing, or talking, and during the performance of certain procedures, such as suctioning and bronchoscopy, and are propelled a short distance (generally less than 3 feet, but in some cases more like aerosols) and deposited into the conjunctivae, nasal mucosa, or mouth of a susceptible person. Because these relatively large droplets do not remain suspended in air, special air handling and ventilation are not required to prevent droplet transmission. A few examples of the many microorganisms transmitted by droplets are *Bordetella pertussis*, group A *Streptococcus* species, rhinovirus, influenza virus, and *Neisseria meningitidis*. Specific recommendations for **Droplet Precautions** are as follows:

- When possible, the patient and care partners should wear a mask while health care personnel are inside the room and during patient transport outside of the room.
- The patient should be placed in a single-patient room, if possible. If unavailable, the facility may consider cohorting patients infected with the same organism. Spatial separation of more than 6 feet should be maintained between the bed of the infected patient and the beds of the other patients in multiple-bed rooms.

- A mask and eye protection or face shield should be worn on entry into the room or into the cubical space, and droplet precautions should be maintained when within 3 to 6 feet of the patient.
- Staff who enter the room of a patient with suspected of confirmed SARS-CoV-2 infection should use a fit-tested N95 (or higher-level) respirator.
- Masks and other personal protective equipment (PPE) should be removed before leaving the room or caring for another patient in the same room. Hand hygiene should be performed immediately after PPE removal.

- **Contact transmission** is the most common route of transmission of HAIs. *Direct contact* transmission involves the physical transfer of microorganisms from a person with infection or colonization to a susceptible host through direct contact with infectious agents, such as occurs when a health care professional examines a patient or performs other patient care activities that require direct personal contact. Direct contact transmission also can occur between 2 patients when one serves as the source of the infectious microorganisms and the other serves as a susceptible host. *Indirect contact* transmission involves contact of a susceptible host with a contaminated intermediate object ("fomite"), usually inanimate, such as contaminated instruments, needles, dressings, toys, or contaminated hands that are not cleansed or gloves that are not changed between patients. A few examples of the many microorganisms transmitted by contact include respiratory syncytial virus, *C difficile*, enterovirus, *Salmonella* species, *Shigella* species, and Shiga toxin-producing *Escherichia coli*. In addition, specific situations requiring **Contact Precautions** include the following:
  - Conjunctivitis (viral and hemorrhagic).
  - Colonization or infection with a specific multidrug-resistant organism (MDRO), as determined by the facility's infection prevention and control program based on current state, regional, or national recommendations to be of special clinical and epidemiologic significance (eg, carbapenemase-producing gram-negative bacilli, *Candida auris*, other MDROs), or another epidemiologically important organism (which may or may not be an MDRO). Information on the CDC containment strategy for responding to emerging antibiotic resistant threats is available on the CDC website (**www.cdc.gov/hai/containment/index.html**).

Specific recommendations for **Contact Precautions** are as follows:
- The patient and care partners should be placed in a single-patient room if possible. If unavailable, cohorting patients who are likely to be infected with the same organism and use of Standard and Contact Precautions is permissible.
- Gloves (clean, nonsterile, single use) should be used at all times.
- Gown and gloves should be used on entry into a patient room and during direct contact with a patient, environmental surfaces, or items in the patient room. Gown and gloves should be removed before leaving the patient's room or area, immediately followed by hand hygiene.
- When transport or movement outside of the room is necessary, infected or colonized areas of the patient's body should be covered and any potentially infectious drainage or secretions should be contained.
- Disposable noncritical patient-care equipment (eg, blood pressure cuffs) should be used, or patient-dedicated use of such equipment should be implemented. If common use of equipment for multiple patients is unavoidable, such equipment should be cleaned and disinfected per manufacturer's recommendations before use on another patient.

Airborne, Droplet, and **Contact Precautions** should be combined for diseases caused by organisms that have multiple routes of transmission. If available testing cannot differentiate between 2 organisms, the recommended precautions for each organism should be combined. When used alone or in combination, these **Transmission-Based Precautions** are always to be used in addition to **Standard Precautions,** which are recommended for all patients. The care of patients with a highly transmissible and highly lethal infection, such as Ebola virus, requires additional extensive infection prevention and control measures (**www.cdc.gov/vhf/ebola/clinicians/evd/infection-control.html**). Novel pathogens may also require additional infection prevention measures when the mode(s) of transmission are still unknown. Some pathogens, including SARS-CoV-2, may not be spread exclusively by distinct droplet versus airborne routes. Consultation with the facility's infection prevention department or public health authority is recommended.

PEDIATRIC CONSIDERATIONS

Unique differences in pediatric care necessitate modifications of these guidelines, including the following: (1) use of single-patient room isolation; (2) use of common areas, such as hospital waiting rooms, playrooms, and schoolrooms; and (3) family-centered care. More patients and their care partners or visitors with transmissible infections may be present in pediatric health care settings than in adult ones, especially during seasonal epidemics.

Single-patient rooms are recommended for all patients requiring **Transmission-Based Precautions** (ie, **Airborne, Droplet,** and **Contact**). Single-patient rooms can also be prioritized if the patient is at increased risk of acquiring infection or of developing an adverse outcome following infection. Patients placed on **Transmission-Based Precautions** and their caregivers or visitors should not leave their rooms to use common areas on the unit, such as playrooms, schoolrooms, or waiting areas, or elsewhere in the hospital, such as cafeteria or gift shop, except under special circumstances as defined by the facility's infection preventionist. The guidelines for **Standard Precautions** state that patients who cannot control body excretions should be in single-patient rooms. Because many young children are incontinent, this recommendation does not apply to routine care of uninfected, diapered children.

The Society for Healthcare Epidemiology of America has published infection prevention and control guidelines for residential facilities that serve pediatric patients and their families.[1] These types of facilities provide support services, including overnight lodging, for ill and injured children (including immune compromised hosts) and their families.

Strategies to Prevent Health Care-Associated Infections

HAIs in patients in acute care hospitals are associated with substantial morbidity. Important HAIs include central line-associated bloodstream infections, central nervous system shunt infections, surgical site infections, urinary catheter-associated urinary tract infections, ventilator-associated pneumonias, infections caused by viruses (eg, respiratory syncytial virus, rotavirus), and colitis attributable to *C difficile*. Infection

---

[1] Guzman-Cottrill J, Ravin K, Bryant K, Zerr D, Kociolek L, Siegel J. Infection prevention and control in residential facilities for pediatric patients and their families. *Infect Control Hosp Epidemiol*. 2013;34(10):1003-1041. doi:10.1086/673141 or **www.doi.org/10.1086/673141**

prevention strategies exist for each of these infections. Evidence-based protocols have been shown to reduce HAIs by using "bundled strategies" (when multiple prevention activities are implemented simultaneously) and with multidisciplinary participation from members of the health care team, including administrators, physicians, nurses, therapists, and housekeeping services. Studies in pediatrics have demonstrated bundles to be effective in reducing central line-associated bloodstream infections, surgical site infections, and ventilator-associated pneumonias. High-quality recommendations are available online (**www.solutionsforpatientsafety.org/s/CLABSI_Bundle_SPS.pdf** and **www.cdc.gov/infectioncontrol/guidelines/BSI/index.html**). Supporting the establishment and maintenance of breastfeeding and human milk feeding has also been shown to reduce rates of neonatal infections and sepsis.

Occupational Health

Transmission of infectious agents within health care settings is facilitated by close contact between patients and health care personnel and by lack of hygienic practices by infants and young children. Guidelines for infection control in health care personnel, including requirements for infrastructure and routine practices, are available at **www.cdc.gov/infectioncontrol/guidelines/healthcare-personnel/index.html.**

The consequences to pediatric patients of acquiring infections from adult health care personnel can be significant. Mild illnesses in adults, such as viral gastroenteritis, upper respiratory tract viral infection, pertussis, or herpes simplex virus infection, can cause life-threatening disease in infants and children. Patients at greatest risk are preterm infants, children who have chronic heart disease or pulmonary disease, and people who are immunocompromised. Health care personnel education, including understanding of hospital policies, is of paramount importance in infection prevention and preventing ill employees from reporting to work. Frequent educational sessions will reinforce safe techniques and the importance of infection prevention and control policies.

Standard Precautions and **Transmission-Based Precautions** are designed to prevent transmission of infectious agents in health care settings among patients and health care personnel. To further limit risks of transmission of organisms between children and health care personnel, health care facilities should have established occupational health policies and services. Specifically, personnel should be protected against vaccine-preventable diseases by establishing appropriate screening and immunization policies. Guidelines for immunization of health care personnel are available (**www.cdc.gov/vaccines/adults/rec-vac/hcw.html**).

For infections that are not vaccine-preventable, personnel should be counseled about exposures and the possible need for leave from work if they are exposed to, ill with, or a carrier of a specific pathogen, whether the exposure occurs in the home, community, or health care setting.

The frequency of and need for screening of health care personnel for tuberculosis should be determined by local epidemiologic data. The CDC has published guidance for the prevention of transmission of tuberculosis in health care settings (**www.cdc.gov/tb/topic/infectioncontrol/default.htm** and **www.cdc.gov/tb/publications/guidelines/infectioncontrol.htm**). People with commonly occurring infections, such as gastroenteritis, dermatitis, herpes simplex virus lesions on exposed skin, or upper respiratory tract infections, should be evaluated to determine the risk of transmission to patients or to other health care personnel.

Pregnant or lactating health care personnel who follow recommended precautions should not be at increased risk of most infections that have possible adverse effects on the fetus or infant (eg, parvovirus B19, cytomegalovirus, mpox, rubella, varicella, and Zika). Pregnant health care personnel should not care for patients with Ebola (**www.cdc.gov/niosh/topics/repro/infectious.html**). The CDC's National Institute for Occupational Safety and Health provides guidance for pregnant health care personnel and health care worker safety (**www.cdc.gov/niosh/topics/repro/healthcaresafetyresources.html**).

Health care personnel who are immunocompromised and at increased risk of severe infection (eg, *M tuberculosis,* measles virus, herpes simplex virus, and varicella-zoster virus) should seek advice from their primary health care professional.

Sibling Visitation

Sibling visits to birthing centers, postpartum rooms, pediatric wards, and intensive care units are encouraged, although some institutions restrict visitation of young children during times of peak respiratory viral activity because of their relatively high frequency of asymptomatic viral shedding and difficulties adhering to basic respiratory etiquette and hand hygiene practices.

Sibling visits may benefit hospitalized children. Neonatal intensive care often results in long hospital stays for the preterm or sick newborn infant, making family and caregiver visits important. Guidelines for sibling visits should be established to maximize opportunities for visiting while at the same time minimizing the risks of transmission of pathogens brought into the hospital setting by young visitors. Guidelines may need to be modified by local nursing, pediatric, obstetric, and infectious diseases staff members to address specific issues in their hospital settings and during outbreaks. Basic guidelines for sibling visits to pediatric patients are as follows:

- If a child has isolation precautions for a transmissible disease, visitation should be limited to parents and/or designated adult caregivers only, assuming that they do not have a similar isolation precaution for the same disease.
- Before the visit, a trained health care professional should interview the parent or guardian at a site outside the unit to assess the health of each sibling visitor. These interviews should be documented, and approval for each sibling visit should be noted. No child with fever or symptoms of an acute infection, including upper respiratory tract infection, gastroenteritis, or cellulitis, should be allowed to visit. Siblings who recently have been exposed to a person with a known communicable disease and are susceptible should not be allowed to visit.
- Siblings who are visiting should have received all recommended immunizations for their age. Before and during influenza season, siblings who visit should have received their annual influenza vaccine.
- The visiting sibling should visit only their sibling and be restricted from playrooms when other patients are present.
- Children should perform recommended hand hygiene before entry into the health care setting and before and after any patient contact, and as otherwise recommended (after using the toilet, before eating, etc).
- Throughout the visit, sibling activity should be supervised by a parent or responsible adult and limited to the patient room or other designated areas where other patients are not present.

- Whenever possible, special accommodations should be made for visitation of siblings who are currently breastfeeding when the mother is at the bedside of a hospitalized patient.

Adult Visitation

Guidelines should be established for adults who accompany hospitalized children. Guidelines may need to be modified by hospital staff to address specific issues and during outbreaks.
- People with fever or contagious illnesses should not visit.
- People who have had close contact with someone with SARS-CoV-2 infection or were in another situation that put them at risk for SARS-CoV-2 transmission should be counseled that it is safest to defer nonurgent in-person visitation until 10 days after their close contact, especially if they cannot wear respirators or well-fitting face masks to cover their mouth and nose (source control).
- If a child has isolation precautions for a contagious respiratory disease and a susceptible parent or guardian remains with the hospitalized child, the adult should follow source control precautions and wear a mask when health care personnel are inside the room.
- Medical and nursing staff should be vigilant about potential communicable diseases in parents and other adult visitors (eg, a relative with a cough who may have pertussis or tuberculosis; a parent with a cold visiting an immunosuppressed child). When identified, ill visitors should be asked to leave immediately.
- Before and during the winter respiratory virus season, all adult visitors should be encouraged to have received the annual influenza vaccine and COVID-19 vaccine, especially for oncology, hematopoietic stem cell transplant, and neonatal intensive care units.

Pet Visitation

- Pet visitation in the health care setting includes both visits by a child's personal pet and pet visitation as a part of child life therapeutic programs. Guidelines for pet visitation should be established to minimize risks of transmission of pathogens from pets to humans or injury from animals. The specific health care setting and the level of concern for zoonotic disease will influence establishment of pet visitation policies. The pet visitation policy should be developed in consultation with pediatricians, infection preventionists, nursing staff, the hospital epidemiologist, and veterinarians.[1]
- Patients having contact with pets must have approval from the patient's physician, nurse, and the facility's infection prevention and control program prior to the visit. For patients who are immunocompromised, including those receiving immunosuppressive therapy, the risks of exposure to the microflora of pets may outweigh the benefits of contact. Contact of children with pets should be considered for approval on a case-by-case basis.
- Personal pets other than dogs should be excluded from the hospital. Pets should be housebroken and at least 1 year of age. Exceptions may be made for end-of-life patients who are in single-patient rooms.

---

[1] Murthy R, Bearman G, Brown S, et al. SHEA Expert Guidance. Animals in healthcare facilities: recommendations to minimize potential risks. *Infect Control Hosp Epidemiol*. 2015;36(50):495-516. DOI: **http://dx.doi.org/10.1017/ice.2015.15**

- Visiting pets should have a certificate of immunization from a licensed veterinarian and verification that the pet is healthy. Some institutions require an assessment of temperament (eg, Canine Good Citizen certificate).
- The pet should be bathed and groomed for the visit.
- Pet visitation should be discouraged in an intensive care unit or hematology-oncology unit, but individual circumstances can be considered. Involvement with the infection control and prevention team is recommended.
- The visit of a pet should also be approved by an appropriate personnel member (eg, the director of the child life therapy program), who should observe the pet for temperament and general health at the time of visit. The pet should be free of obvious bacterial skin infections, infections caused by superficial dermatophytes, and ectoparasites (fleas and ticks).
- Pet visitation should be confined to designated areas. Contact should be confined to the petting and holding of animals, as appropriate. All contact should be supervised throughout the visit by appropriate personnel.
- Hand hygiene should be performed by the patient and all who have contact with the pet, both before and after pet visitation. Supervisors should be familiar with institutional policies for managing animal bites and cleaning pet urine, feces, or vomitus.
- Care should be taken to protect all indwelling devices, including catheter exit sites (eg, central venous catheters, peritoneal dialysis catheters). These sites should have semi-occlusive dressings whenever possible that will provide an effective barrier to pet contact, including licking, and be covered with clothing or gown. Concern for contamination of other body sites should be considered on a case-by-case basis. Specifically, wounds should be protected from animal contact.
- The pet policy should not apply to professionally trained service animals. These animals are not pets and separate policies should govern their uses and presence in the hospital, according to the requirements of the Americans with Disabilities Act.

INFECTION PREVENTION AND CONTROL IN AMBULATORY SETTINGS

Infection prevention and control is an integral part of pediatric practice in ambulatory care settings.[1] All health care personnel should be aware of the routes of transmission and techniques to prevent transmission of infectious agents. Written policies and procedures for infection prevention and control should be readily available, implemented, updated regularly, and adherence regularly assessed. Facilities should have ready access to an individual with training in infection prevention and control. **Standard Precautions,** as outlined for the hospitalized child (see Infection Prevention and Control for Hospitalized Children, p 163) and by the Centers for Disease Control and Prevention (CDC),[2] with a modification by the American Academy of Pediatrics

[1] Rathore MH, Jackson MA; American Academy of Pediatrics, Committee on Infectious Diseases. Infection prevention and control in pediatric ambulatory settings. *Pediatrics.* 2017;140(5):e20172857

[2] Centers for Disease Control and Prevention. Guideline for isolation precautions: preventing transmission of infectious agents in health care settings 2007. Recommendations of the Healthcare Infection Control Practices Advisory Committee. Atlanta, GA: Centers for Disease Control and Prevention; 2007. Available at: **www.cdc.gov/hicpac/2007IP/2007isolationPrecautions.html**

exempting the use of gloves for routine diaper changes and wiping a child's nose or eyes,[1] are appropriate and should be utilized for all patient encounters. Additional **Transmission-Based Precautions** may be indicated based on the symptoms of the child being evaluated (eg, gown, gloves, N95 [or higher-level] respirator and eye protection for the child with suspected SARS-CoV-2 infection). Universal source control (the use of respirators or well-fitting face masks to cover the mouth and nose of the patient and their caregivers to prevent spread of respiratory secretions when they are breathing, talking, sneezing, or coughing) may be indicated when community transmission of SARS-CoV-2 or other respiratory pathogens is high. The CDC has created a guideline and a checklist (**www.cdc.gov/infectioncontrol/pdf/outpatient/guide.pdf** and **www.cdc.gov/infectioncontrol/pdf/outpatient/guidechecklist.pdf**) that health care professionals can use to ensure that appropriate infection-control practices are being followed and, thus, reduce ambulatory health care-associated infections. Health care professionals should be familiar with the most current CDC infection prevention and control guidance for SARS-CoV-2 (**www.cdc.gov/coronavirus/2019-ncov/hcp/infection-control.html, www.cdc.gov/coronavirus/2019-ncov/hcp/facility-planning-operations.html,** and **www.cdc.gov/coronavirus/2019-ncov/hcp/facility-planning-operations.html**).

In November 2023, HICPAC recommended changes to existing categories of transmission-based precautions. Contact precautions would continue to be recommended to interrupt transmission of pathogens spread by touch. Droplet and airborne precautions would be replaced by 3 new categories of transmission-based precautions to interrupt transmission of pathogens spread by air. These include Routine Air Precautions, Special Air Precautions, and Extended Air Precautions, and are intended to better address the continuum of respiratory pathogen transmission through air. If these recommendations are ultimately adopted by the CDC, HICPAC will update pathogen-specific recommendations.

Key principles of infection prevention and control in an outpatient setting are as follows:

- Infection prevention and control should begin when the child's appointment is scheduled (eg, triage questions, such as travel, exposures, and symptoms, may guide additional precautions for when the patient arrives) and initiated when the child enters the office or clinic.
- **Standard Precautions** should be used when caring for all patients. **Standard Precautions** are supplemented by **Transmission-Based Precautions** and should include instructions to health care personnel on the proper donning (putting on) and doffing (removing) of personal protective equipment (gowns, face masks, protective eyewear [or face shield], and gloves). Patients known to be infected or colonized with highly resistant organisms (eg, *Candida auris*, carbapenemase-producing *Enterobacterales*) should be identified and placed on contact precautions during outpatient encounters. Any individual on the care team entering the room should follow the appropriate precautions, regardless of whether the patient is being examined. Contact between contagious children and uninfected children should be minimized. Children who are suspected of having highly contagious infections, such as varicella, measles, or COVID-19, should be promptly isolated. This may involve notification of clinic

[1] Rathore MH, Jackson MA; American Academy of Pediatrics, Committee on Infectious Diseases. Infection prevention and control in pediatric ambulatory settings. *Pediatrics*. 2017;140(5):e20172857

staff at the time of arrival so that the patient can be examined outside of the clinic or be routed directly to an examination room, minimizing wait times and/or bypassing the waiting room. Neonates and immunocompromised children should be promptly placed in a room and kept away from people with potentially contagious infections.

- In waiting rooms of ambulatory care facilities, respiratory hygiene/cough etiquette and use of masks should be implemented for patients with suspected respiratory tract infection as well as people accompanying them.[1]

  - It is recommended that patients with cystic fibrosis be taken directly to an examination room at the time of arrival, whenever possible.[2] If it is not feasible to use separate waiting areas to prevent contact between patients with cystic fibrosis, a minimum of 6 feet should be used to ensure their separation (this does not apply to members of the same household). Patients with cystic fibrosis who are in the waiting room should be masked (mask may be removed in the examination room). Health care providers should use contact precautions (gown and gloves) when caring for a patient with cystic fibrosis.

- All health care personnel should perform hand hygiene before and after each patient contact. In health care settings, alcohol-based hand products are preferred for decontaminating hands routinely. Soap and water are preferred when hands are visibly dirty or contaminated with proteinaceous material, such as blood or other body fluids, and after caring for a patient with known or suspected infectious diarrhea (eg, *Clostridioides difficile* or norovirus) even if gloves are worn. Parents and children should be taught the importance of hand hygiene. Guidelines on hand hygiene can be found on the CDC website (**www.cdc.gov/handhygiene/providers/guideline.html**).

- Health care personnel should receive influenza vaccination annually and stay current on vaccinations against other vaccine-preventable infections, including SARS-CoV-2, that can be transmitted in an ambulatory setting to patients or to other health care personnel. Recommended vaccines include influenza; COVID-19; tetanus toxoid, reduced diphtheria toxoid and acellular pertussis (Tdap); measles, mumps, and rubella (MMR); varicella; and hepatitis B. The latest recommendations can be found at **www.cdc.gov/vaccines/adults/rec-vac/hcw.html.** Health care personnel do not need to take additional action regarding measles vaccination if they have written documentation of 2 doses of MMR or laboratory-confirmed measles or laboratory evidence of immunity (positive immunoglobulin G [IgG] titers). Those who were born before 1957 are generally considered immune; however, if no other evidence of immunity exists, administering 2 doses of MMR should be considered and is recommended in an outbreak.

- Ambulatory facilities should implement sick leave options for health care personnel that encourage reporting of potentially infectious exposures and reduce presenteeism (working while sick).

- Depending on the setting where they work, health care personnel should be familiar with aseptic technique, particularly regarding insertion or manipulation of

---

[1] Centers for Disease Control and Prevention. Respiratory Hygiene/Cough Etiquette in Healthcare Settings. Available at: **www.cdc.gov/flu/professionals/infectioncontrol/resphygiene.htm**

[2] Saiman L, Seigel JD, LiPuma JJ, et al. Infection prevention and control guideline for cystic fibrosis: 2013 update. Infect Control Hosp Epidemiol. 2014;35(Suppl 1):S1-S67. Available at: **www.cff.org/Care/Clinical-Care-Guidelines/Infection-Prevention-and-Control-Clinical-Care-Guidelines/Infection-Prevention-and-Control-Clinical-Care-Guidelines/**

intravascular catheters, performance of other invasive procedures, and preparation and administration of parenteral medications. Aseptic technique includes selection and use of appropriate skin antiseptics. The preferred skin-preparation agent for immunization and venipuncture for routine blood collection is 70% isopropyl alcohol. For incision, suture, and collection of blood for culture, skin preparation with either 2% chlorhexidine gluconate (CHG) in 70% isopropyl alcohol–based solutions or iodine (1% or 2% tincture of iodine, 2% povidone-iodine) should be used.

- Medications should be drawn up in a designated clean medication preparation area that is not adjacent to potential sources of contamination, including sinks or other water sources or used items such as syringes, needles, intravenous tubing, or blood collection tubes. When administering medications, appropriate injection safety practices should be used (**www.cdc.gov/infectioncontrol/pdf/outpatient/guide.pdf**), including:
  - Cleansing the diaphragms of medication vials with alcohol before inserting a device into the vial.
  - Never administering medications from the same syringe to multiple patients, even if the needle is changed.
  - Never reusing a syringe to enter a medication vial or container.
  - Never administering medications from single-dose or single-use vials to more than one patient.
  - Dedicating multidose vials to a single patient whenever possible. If multidose vials will be used for more than one patient, they should be restricted to a centralized medication area and should not enter the immediate patient treatment area.
- Whenever available, medical devices designed to reduce the risk of needlesticks should be used. Sharps disposal containers that are impermeable and puncture resistant should be placed immediately adjacent to the areas where sharps are used (eg, areas where injections or venipunctures are performed). Sharps containers should be replaced when they are two-thirds full and kept out of reach of young children. Policies should be established for the removal and disposal of sharps containers consistent with state and local regulations. Guidance on safe injection practices is available on the CDC website (**www.cdc.gov/injectionsafety/**).
- Appropriate handling of medical waste should be outlined (**www.cdc.gov/infectioncontrol/pdf/outpatient/guide.pdf**).
- A written bloodborne pathogen exposure control plan that includes policies for management of exposures to blood and body fluids, such as through needlesticks and exposures of nonintact skin and mucous membranes, should be developed, readily available to all staff, and updated and reviewed with staff regularly (at least annually) (see Hepatitis B, p 437; Hepatitis C, p 458; Human Immunodeficiency Virus Infection, p 489; and **www.cdc.gov/niosh/topics/bbp/genres.html**).
- Manufacturer's guidelines for processing of medical devices and equipment, including cleaning, decontamination, disinfection, and sterilization, should be followed meticulously by personnel with training in the required reprocessing steps. Competency should be assessed periodically (at least annually). Once sterilized, devices and equipment should be kept in their sterile packaging until immediately prior to use.
- Cleaning of point-of-use equipment (eg, stethoscopes, otoscopes) should be performed after each patient encounter with Environmental Protection Agency (EPA)-registered disinfectants or detergents/disinfectants with label claims for use in health care.

- Policies and procedures should be established for cleaning and disinfection of environmental surfaces and general housekeeping. Supplies necessary for appropriate cleaning and disinfection procedures (eg, EPA-registered disinfectants) are available. Cleaners and disinfectants are used in accordance with manufacturer's instructions (eg, dilution, storage, shelf-life, contact time). Examination tables should be cleaned between use. Patients can be encouraged to bring their own toys. If toys are available in waiting areas, they should be disposable or able to be cleaned and disinfected or sanitized between each use.[1]
- Appropriate use of antimicrobial agents is essential to limit the emergence and spread of drug-resistant bacteria (see Antimicrobial Stewardship, p 981).
- Policies and procedures should be developed for communication with local and state health authorities about reportable diseases and suspected outbreaks (**www.cdc. gov/nndss/** and **www.cdc.gov/hai/outbreaks/**).
- Educational programs for health care personnel that encompass appropriate aspects of infection control should be implemented, reinforced, documented, and evaluated on a regular basis.
- Outpatient facilities and practices should have access to an individual with training in infection prevention who manages the infection prevention program (**www.cdc. gov/infectioncontrol/pdf/outpatient/guidechecklist.pdf**).
- Physicians should be aware of requirements of government agencies, such as the Occupational Safety and Health Administration (OSHA), as well as state and federal regulations that may apply to the operation of physicians' offices.

SEXUALLY TRANSMITTED INFECTIONS IN ADOLESCENTS AND CHILDREN

Physicians and other health care professionals perform a critical role in preventing and treating sexually transmitted infections (STIs) in the pediatric and adolescent population. STIs are a major problem for adolescents; an estimated 25% of adolescent females[2] will acquire an STI by 19 years of age. Although an STI in an infant or child early in life can be the result of vertical transmission, nonabusive horizontal transmission, or autoinoculation (particularly herpes simplex virus [HSV] and human papillomavirus [HPV]), STIs (eg, gonorrhea, syphilis, chlamydia, genital herpes, human immunodeficiency virus [HIV] infection, trichomoniasis, or anogenital warts) should raise suspicion of sexual abuse if acquired after the neonatal period. Whenever sexual abuse is suspected, appropriate social service and law enforcement agencies must be involved to evaluate the situation further, to ensure the child or adolescent's protection, and to provide appropriate counseling. When available, consultation with a child abuse pediatrician can help guide further evaluation, aid in decision making on reporting suspected abuse, and assist with rendering an opinion on the etiology of the STI.

---

[1] Rathore MH, Jackson MA; American Academy of Pediatrics, Committee on Infectious Diseases. Infection prevention and control in pediatric ambulatory settings. *Pediatrics*. 2017;140(5):e20172857

[2] In this chapter, the terms male, female, men, and women are used to mean sex assigned at birth.

STIs During Preventive Health Care of Adolescents

EPIDEMIOLOGY OF STIs IN ADOLESCENTS

Adolescents and young adults have the highest rates of several STIs when compared with any other age group. Adolescents are at greater risk of STIs because of their potentially high-risk sexual behaviors, inability to understand the risks of STIs, and increased biologic susceptibility. In addition, adolescents may face several potential obstacles in accessing comprehensive sexual health care services.[1] Young women, particularly women of color, young men who have sex with men (MSM), and transgender women are at particularly high risk of STIs, including HIV infection. Health care professionals frequently fail to confidentially ask adolescents and young adults about sexual behaviors, assess for STI risks, counsel about risk reduction, and screen for STIs.[2]

EVALUATION OF STIs IN ADOLESCENTS

At each health care visit, the health care provider should allow some private time, apart from the parent(s) or guardian(s), to speak with the adolescent confidentially.[3] In order to educate and prepare patients and families about the need for confidentiality as adolescence approaches, health care professionals should familiarize themselves with local statutes on minors' consent for HIV and STI services. Pediatricians should screen for STI risk by *routinely* asking all adolescent and young adult patients—apart from their parents—whether they ever have had any sexual encounters, are currently sexually active, or are planning to become sexually active, as well as about gender identity and sexual orientation. Pediatricians must be sure to clarify what is meant by the terms "sexual intercourse," "gender identity," "sexual orientation," and "sexually active," because these terms can have different meanings for adolescents. It is important that adolescents and young adults are educated to recognize that noncoital practices (oral/genital contact, anal intercourse, and hand/genital contact), as well as vaginal intercourse, put them at risk of STIs. If a patient indicates a history of sexual activity, the health care professional must further ascertain the types of sexual encounters, biological sex of the partner(s), and number of partners to determine what type(s) of STI testing to perform. More detailed recommendations for preventive health care for adolescents and young adults are available from the Centers for Disease Control and Prevention (CDC).[4]

---

[1] Centers for Disease Control and Prevention. *Sexually Transmitted Disease Surveillance 2021*. Available at: **www.cdc.gov/std/statistics/2021/**

[2] US Preventive Services Task Force. Behavioral counseling interventions to prevent sexually transmitted infections: US Preventive Services Task Force recommendation statement. *JAMA*. 2020;324(7):674-681

[3] The Society for Adolescent Health and Medicine and the American Academy of Pediatrics. Position paper: confidentiality protections for adolescents and young adults in the health care billing and insurance claims process. *J Adolesc Health*. 2016;58(3):374-377

[4] Centers for Disease Control and Prevention. Sexually transmitted infections treatment guidelines, 2021. *MMWR Recomm Rep*. 2021;70(RR-4):1-187. Available at: **www.cdc.gov/std/treatment-guidelines/default.htm**

TREATMENT OF STIs IN ADOLESCENTS

All 50 states allow minors to give their own consent for confidential STI testing and treatment. Pediatricians should consult their own state laws for further guidance. For specific STI treatment recommendations, see the disease-specific chapters in Section 3 and Tables 4.4 (p 1107) and 4.5 (p 1014). Single-dose therapies are available for many STIs, offering the advantage of high patient adherence; directly observed therapy should be provided where feasible. Patients and their partners treated for *Neisseria gonorrhoeae* infection, *Chlamydia trachomatis*, or *Trichomonas vaginalis* infection should be advised to refrain from sexual intercourse for at least 7 days after completion of appropriate treatment.

Partner treatment is essential, both from a public health perspective and to protect the infected patient from reinfection. Sexual partners during the past 60 days should be informed of exposure to the infection and encouraged to seek comprehensive STI evaluation and treatment. Health departments typically attempt to notify sex partners of patients infected with HIV or syphilis and arrange for treatment. Depending on health department resources, partner services may be offered for some gonorrhea cases and occasionally for chlamydia. If it appears unlikely that partners of patients treated for gonococcal, chlamydial, or trichomonas infections will seek care, pediatricians may consider providing expedited partner therapy (EPT) to patients in states where EPT is permissible.[1] EPT is the clinical practice of treating the sex partners of patients with diagnosed chlamydia or gonorrhea by providing prescriptions or medications to the patient to take to their partner without the health care professional first examining the partner. Information should include warning about the low risk of potential adverse events with EPT, with instructions to seek medical attention in the event that an adverse reaction occurs. Published studies suggest that in certain settings, >5% of MSM without previously diagnosed HIV infection will be diagnosed with HIV infection when evaluated as a partner of patients with gonorrhea or chlamydia. Considering limited data and the potential for other bacterial STIs among MSM partners, shared clinical decision-making regarding EPT is recommended among MSM. Guidance on the legal status of EPT by jurisdiction is available from the CDC (**www.cdc.gov/std/ept/legal/**).

PREVENTION OF STIs IN ADOLESCENTS

Pediatricians and other health care professionals can contribute to primary STI prevention by encouraging and supporting a teenager's decision to postpone sexual debut. For teenagers who become sexually active or are planning to be sexually active in the near future, pediatricians should discuss methods of protecting against STIs and pregnancies, including the correct and consistent use of external and internal condoms with all forms of sexual activity (vaginal, oral, and anal). Enhanced risk counseling should be targeted for teenagers who engage in illicit drug use or who are in juvenile detention or other state/county facilities, for whom consent abilities may be compromised or absent and risk of assault may be increased. Teenagers should be specifically counseled to consider the association between alcohol or drug use and failure to appropriately use barrier methods correctly when either partner is impaired. Health care

---

[1] Centers for Disease Control and Prevention. Sexually transmitted infections treatment guidelines, 2021. *MMWR Recomm Rep.* 2021;70(RR-4):1-187. Available at: **www.cdc.gov/std/treatment-guidelines/clinical-EPT.htm**

professionals should discuss other ways to decrease risk of acquiring STIs, including limiting the number of sex partners and choosing to abstain even if initiation of sexual intercourse already has occurred. Pediatricians should educate parents and adolescents how to recognize symptoms of STIs and to contact their provider for evaluation and treatment when symptoms occur. Adolescents and young adults who have not previously been vaccinated against HPV or hepatitis A or B viruses (HAV or HBV) should complete those immunization series.

Pediatricians should counsel their adolescent and young adult patients at substantial risk for HIV infection about preexposure prophylaxis (PrEP) as an effective strategy to prevent HIV infection. Three medications have been FDA approved for use as PrEP to help prevent an HIV-negative person from acquiring HIV from an HIV-positive sexual partner: emtricitabine with tenofovir disoproxil fumarate, emtricitabine with tenofovir alafenamide, and cabotegravir, which is the first long-acting injectable. The indications for PrEP, initial and follow-up prescribing, and laboratory testing recommendations are the same for adolescents and adults. Guidelines for PrEP are available from the US Public Health Service (**www.cdc.gov/hiv/pdf/risk/prep/cdc-hiv-prep-guidelines-2021.pdf**). When taken consistently, PrEP has been shown to significantly reduce the risk of HIV infection in people who are at risk. For sexual transmission, those considered at substantial risk for acquiring HIV include those who have engaged in anal or vaginal sex in the past 6 months AND IN ADDITION have 1 or more of the following: have an HIV-positive sexual partner; had a bacterial STI in the past 6 months; or report inconsistent or no condom use with sexual partner(s).

Sexual Assault and Abuse in Children and Adolescents/Young Adults

SUSPECTED SEXUAL ASSAULT

When the suspicion of sexual abuse or assault is raised, pediatricians should know how to respond to and evaluate the child or adolescent/young adult, when to refer the patient for evaluation by other professionals, when to report the case to the appropriate investigative agency, and how to counsel parents to decrease long-term deleterious effects of the abuse.[1,2] Factors to be considered in assessing the likelihood of sexual abuse in a child with an STI include the biological characteristics of the STI in question, the age and developmental status of the child or adolescent, and whether the child reports a history of sexual contact (see Table 2.5). Preferably, children with concerns about possible sexual abuse would be referred for evaluation and management to a specialized clinic or child advocacy center. In areas without specialized abuse-related services, pediatricians can educate themselves about childhood genital and anal examinations and about how to gather the medical history to make appropriate decisions about reporting to child protective service or law enforcement agencies, referring to

---

[1] Jenny C, Crawford-Jakubiak JE; American Academy of Pediatrics, Committee on Child Abuse and Neglect. The evaluation of children in the primary care setting when sexual abuse is suspected. *Pediatrics*. 2013;132(2):e558-e567 (Reaffirmed August 2018). Available at: **https://doi.org/10.1542/peds.2013-1741**

[2] Crawford-Jakubiak JE, Alderman EM, Leventhal JM; American Academy of Pediatrics, Committee on Child Abuse and Neglect; Committee on Adolescence. Care of the adolescent after an acute sexual assault. *Pediatrics*. 2017;139(3):e20164243. Available at: **https://doi.org/10.1542/peds.2017-0958**

Table 2.5. Implications of Commonly Encountered Sexually Transmitted (ST) or Sexually Associated (SA) Infections for Diagnosis and Reporting of Sexual Abuse Among Infants and Prepubertal Children

ST/SA Confirmed	Evidence for Sexual Abuse	Suggested Action
Neisseria gonorrhoeae[a]	Diagnostic	Report[b]
Syphilis[a]	Diagnostic	Report[b]
Human immunodeficiency virus[c]	Diagnostic	Report[b]
Chlamydia trachomatis[a]	Diagnostic	Report[b]
Trichomonas vaginalis[a]	Diagnostic	Report[b]
Anogenital herpes	Suspicious	Consider report[b,d]
Condylomata acuminata (anogenital warts)[a]	Suspicious	Consider report[b,d,e]
Anogenital molluscum contagiosum	Inconclusive	Medical follow-up
Bacterial vaginosis	Inconclusive	Medical follow-up

[a] If not likely to be perinatally acquired and rare vertical transmission is excluded.
[b] Reports should be made to the local or state agency mandated to receive reports of suspected child abuse or neglect.
[c] If not likely to be acquired perinatally or through transfusion.
[d] Unless a clear history of autoinoculation exists.
[e] Report if evidence exists to suspect abuse, including history, physical examination, or other identified infections. Lesions appearing for first time in child >5 years of age are more likely attributable to sexual transmission.

Table adapted from Kellogg N; American Academy of Pediatrics, Committee on Child Abuse and Neglect. The evaluation of sexual abuse in children. *Pediatrics.* 2005;116(2):506–512 (Updated 2013 clinical report [reaffirmed August 2018] available at **https://doi.org/10.1542/peds.2013-1741**) and Centers for Disease Control and Prevention. Sexually transmitted infections treatment guidelines, 2021. *MMWR Recomm Rep.* 2021;70(RR-4):1-187. Available at: **www.cdc.gov/std/treatment-guidelines/sexual-assault-children.htm.**

counseling facilities, or referring to pediatric clinics specializing in abuse evaluations. The AAP offers a variety of educational materials on child abuse to physicians.[1]

WHEN TO SCREEN FOR STIs AFTER POSSIBLE SEXUAL ASSAULT OF A PREPUBERTAL CHILD

Symptoms are uncommon even in children with proven STIs; therefore, testing all sites for all pathogens is standard of care in child abuse evaluations. Examinations and collection of genital specimens in prepubertal children should be performed by an experienced clinician. Factors that would lead clinicians to consider testing for STI include:

1. Child reports sexual abuse, regardless of the acts involved.
2. Child has a sibling, other relative, or another person in the household with an STI.
3. Child has signs or symptoms of STIs (eg, vaginal discharge or pain, genital itching or odor, urinary symptoms, or genital lesions or ulcers).
4. Child or parent requests STI testing.
5. Child is unable to verbalize details of assault.

---

[1] **www.aap.org/en-us/advocacy-and-policy/aap-health-initiatives/Child-Abuse-and-Neglect/Pages/Child-Abuse-and-Neglect.aspx**

STI EVALUATION AFTER SEXUAL ASSAULT OF A PREPUBERTAL CHILD

A chaperone who is not the parent or guardian of the child should be present at the time of evaluation. In the evaluation of prepubertal children for suspected sexual abuse/assault, the CDC offers the following recommendations[1]:

- Physical examination: Visually inspect the genital, perianal, and oropharyngeal areas for genital discharge, odor, bleeding, irritation, warts, and ulcerative lesions. In addition, if STI testing is indicated, then the following laboratory assessments should be performed.
  - Testing for *N gonorrhoeae* and *C trachomatis* should be performed with specimens collected from the pharynx and anus, as well as the vagina, and urine from the penile urethra. Cervical specimens are not recommended for prepubertal patients. For patients with a urethral discharge, a penile meatal specimen is an adequate substitute for an intraurethral swab specimen. Culture or a nucleic acid amplification test (NAAT) can be used to test for *N gonorrhoeae* and *C trachomatis*. Only an FDA-cleared NAAT should be used. Consultation with an expert is necessary before using a NAAT in this context, both to minimize the possibility of cross-reaction with nongonococcal *Neisseria* species and other commensals (eg, *Neisseria meningitidis*, *Neisseria sicca*, *Neisseria lactamica*, *Neisseria cinerea*, and *Moraxella catarrhalis*) and to ensure appropriate interpretation of results. If culture for isolation of *N gonorrhoeae* or *C trachomatis* is performed, only standard culture procedures should be performed. Specimens from the vagina, urethra, pharynx, or rectum should be streaked onto selective media for isolation of *N gonorrhoeae*, and all presumptive isolates of *N gonorrhoeae* should be identified definitively by at least 2 tests that involve different approaches (eg, biochemical, enzyme substrate, or molecular probes). Gram stains are inadequate to evaluate prepubertal children for gonorrhea and should not be used to diagnose or exclude gonorrhea. Every effort should be made to preserve specimens (either NAAT or culture including any isolates) obtained before treatment for further validation if needed. In the case of a positive specimen, the result should be confirmed either by retesting the original specimen or obtaining another. Given the overall low prevalence of *N gonorrhoeae* and *C trachomatis* in children, false-positive results may occur, and all specimens that are initially positive should be confirmed.
  - Testing for *Trichomonas vaginalis* should not be limited to patients with vaginal discharge if other indications for vaginal testing exist, because there is some evidence to indicate that asymptomatic sexually abused children could be infected with *T vaginalis* and might benefit from treatment. A NAAT can be used as an alternative or in addition to culture and wet mount, especially in situations in which culture and wet mount of vaginal swab specimens are not obtainable. Consultation with an expert is necessary before using a NAAT in this context to ensure appropriate interpretation of results. Because of the implications of a diagnosis of *T vaginalis* infection in a child, only a CLIA-validated, FDA-cleared NAAT should be used. Point-of-care tests for *T vaginalis* have not been validated for prepubertal children and should not be used. In the case of a positive specimen, the result should be

---

[1] Centers for Disease Control and Prevention. Sexually transmitted infection treatment guidelines, 2021. *MMWR Recomm Rep.* 2021;70(RR-4):1-187. Available at: **www.cdc.gov/std/treatment-guidelines/sexual-assault-children.htm**

confirmed either by retesting the original specimen or obtaining another. Given the overall low prevalence of *T vaginalis* in children, false-positive results may occur, and all specimens that are initially positive should be confirmed.

- Because herpes simplex virus (HSV) can be indicative of sexual abuse, specimens should be obtained from all vesicular or ulcerative genital or perianal lesions and then sent for NAAT or viral culture.
- Wet mount or NAAT of a vaginal swab specimen for bacterial vaginosis (BV) should be performed, if discharge is present.
- Serum samples should be collected to be evaluated, preserved for subsequent analysis, and used as a baseline for comparison with follow-up serologic tests. Sera can be tested for antibodies to *Treponema pallidum*, HIV, and HBV. Decisions regarding the infectious agents for which to perform serologic tests should be made on a case-by-case basis.

TESTING SEXUALLY ABUSED POSTPUBERTAL PATIENTS FOR STIs

In the evaluation of the sexual assault patient of **postpubertal** age, if a decision to perform STI testing is made, gonorrhea and chlamydia diagnostic evaluation from any sites of penetration or attempted penetration should be performed, per CDC guidance.[1] *C trachomatis* and *N gonorrhoeae* NAATs from specimens should be obtained at the sites of penetration as the preferred diagnostic evaluation of the **postpubertal** person who has been sexually assaulted (Table 2.6). Testing for *T vaginalis* should be offered using a provider-collected vaginal specimen or NAATs from that patient's urine. Point-of-care testing and/or wet mount with measurement of vaginal pH and KOH application for the whiff test from vaginal secretions should be performed for evidence of BV and candidiasis, especially if vaginal discharge, malodor, or itching is present. Screening for *C trachomatis* and *N gonorrhoeae* should be offered to MSM who report receptive oral or anal sex during the preceding year, regardless of whether there was sexual contact with these anatomic sites during the assault. Baseline and follow-up serum samples for evaluation for HIV infection, HBV, and syphilis should be obtained (Table. 2.7). In addition to STI testing, a pregnancy test should also be performed for patients capable of pregnancy, and the need for emergency contraception should be considered.

PROPHYLAXIS OF CHILDREN AND ADOLESCENTS AFTER SEXUAL ASSAULT

Antimicrobial therapy should be withheld until the STI diagnostic testing has been performed in cases of suspected sexual abuse/assault. Presumptive treatment for **prepubertal** children who have been sexually assaulted or abused is not recommended, because their incidence of STIs is low after abuse or assault, the risk of spread to the uterus, fallopian tubes, and ovaries is low, and follow-up usually can be ensured. If the result of an STI test is positive and confirmed with additional testing, treatment then should be given. Factors that may increase the likelihood of infection or that constitute an indication for prophylaxis are as listed under When to Screen for STIs After Possible Sexual Assault of a Prepubertal Child (p 183).

[1] Centers for Disease Control and Prevention. Sexually transmitted infections treatment guidelines, 2021. *MMWR Recomm Rep.* 2021;70(RR-4):1-187. Available at: **www.cdc.gov/std/treatment-guidelines/sexual-assault-children.htm**

Table 2.6. Sexually Transmitted Infection (STI) Testing[a] When Sexual Abuse or Assault Is Suspected

Organism/Syndrome	Specimens
Neisseria gonorrhoeae and *Chlamydia trachomatis*	Prepubertal: Culture or NAAT from pharynx, anus, urine from penile urethra, vagina. For patients with a urethral discharge, a penile meatal specimen is an adequate substitute for an intraurethral swab specimen.
	Postpubertal: NAAT from sites of penetration or attempted penetration. May include rectum, throat, urine, vagina or cervix, and penile urethra or meatus.
Syphilis	Darkfield examination (if available) of chancre fluid; nontreponemal and treponemal serologic tests at time of abuse and approximately 6 weeks and <3 months after the last suspected sexual exposure.
Human immunodeficiency virus	Fourth-generation HIV antibody/antigen testing of abuser (if possible); serologic testing of child at time of abuse and approximately 6 weeks and <3 months after the last suspected sexual exposure.
Hepatitis B virus	Serum hepatitis B surface antigen testing of abuser or hepatitis B surface antibody testing of child, unless the child has received 3 doses of hepatitis B vaccine. See Table 3.23 (p 456) for management.
Herpes simplex virus (HSV)	Culture or NAAT of lesion specimen; all virologic specimens should be typed (HSV-1 vs HSV-2).
Bacterial vaginosis (BV)	Prepubertal: Vaginal specimen wet mount or NAAT for BV, if discharge is present.
	Postpubertal: Vaginal point-of-care testing and/or wet mount or NAAT with measurement of vaginal pH and KOH application for the whiff test from vaginal secretions should be performed for evidence of BV, especially if vaginal discharge, malodor, or itching is present.
Human papillomavirus	Clinical examination, with biopsy of lesion specimen, if diagnosis unclear.
Trichomonas vaginalis	Prepubertal: Vaginal specimen NAAT and/or culture and wet mount. Testing for *T vaginalis* should not be limited to patients with vaginal discharge if other indications for vaginal testing exist.
	Postpubertal: Vaginal or urine NAAT.
Pediculosis pubis	Identification of eggs, nymphs, and lice with naked eye or using hand lens.

NAAT indicates nucleic acid amplification test.
[a] See text for examples of indications for testing for STIs.

Table 2.7. Prophylaxis After Sexual Victimization: Postpubertal Patients

Antimicrobial prophylaxis is recommended to include an empiric regimen to prevent chlamydia, gonorrhea, and trichomoniasis. Vaccination against hepatitis B and HPV is recommended if not fully immunized.	
For chlamydia, gonorrhea, and trichomoniasis	Ceftriaxone, 500 mg,[a] intramuscularly, in a single dose **PLUS** Doxycycline, 100 mg, orally, twice daily for 7 days **PLUS (IF FEMALE)** Metronidazole, 500 mg, orally, twice daily for 7 days
For hepatitis B virus infection	See Table 3.23, p 456
For human immunodeficiency virus (HIV) infection	See Fig 2.1 and text
For HPV	HPV vaccine series should be initiated at ≥9 y if not already begun or completed if not fully immunized (2 or 3 doses depending on age of initiation of vaccine)

HPV, human papillomavirus.
[a] For persons weighing ≥150 kg, 1 g of ceftriaxone should be administered.
Source: Centers for Disease Control and Prevention. Sexually transmitted infections treatment guidelines, 2021. *MMWR Recomm Rep*. 2021;70(RR-4):1-187. Available at: **www.cdc.gov/std/treatment-guidelines/sexual-assault-children.htm.**

In contrast, many experts believe that STI prophylaxis, after baseline testing has been performed, is warranted for **postpubertal** patients who seek care after an episode of sexual victimization. This is recommended in this population because of the greater possibility of a preexisting asymptomatic infection, the potential risk for acquisition of new infections with the assault, the substantial risk of pelvic inflammatory disease after untreated STIs in this age group, and established data demonstrating poor compliance with follow-up visits after sexual assault.[1] Regimens for prophylaxis are presented in Table 2.7. The need for emergency contraception should be considered as well.

Completion of the HPV, HBV, and HAV immunization series for children and adolescents 9 years and older should be documented. For more detailed diagnosis and treatment recommendations for specific STIs, see the disease-specific chapters in Section 3 and Tables 4.4 (p 1007) and 4.5 (p 1014).

HIV infection has been reported in children and adolescents for whom sexual abuse was the only known risk factor. Because of the demonstrated effectiveness of nonoccupational postexposure prophylaxis (PEP) to prevent HIV infection, the question arises whether HIV prophylaxis is warranted for children and adolescents after sexual assault (see Fig 2.1). The risk of HIV transmission from a single sexual assault that involves transfer of secretions and/or blood is low. Prophylaxis may be considered for patients who seek care within 72 hours after an assault if the assault

---

[1] Crawford-Jakubiak JE, Alderman EM, Leventhal JM; American Academy of Pediatrics, Committee on Child Abuse and Neglect; Committee on Adolescence. Care of the adolescent after an acute sexual assault. *Pediatrics*. 2017;139(3):e20164243. Available at: **https://doi.org/10.1542/peds.2016-4243**

Fig 2.1. Algorithm for Evaluation and Treatment of Possible Nonoccupational HIV Exposures[a]

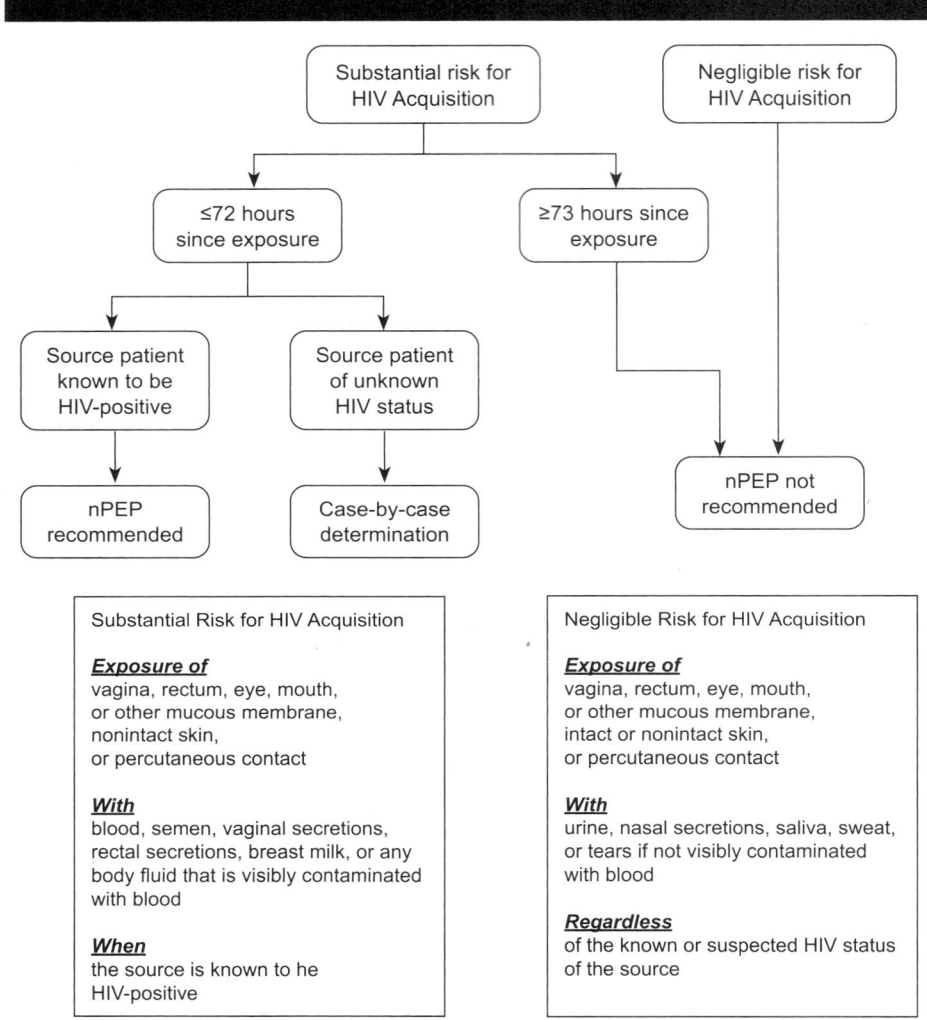

nPEP indicates nonoccupational postexposure prophylaxis.
[a]Dominguez, KL, Smith DK, Thomas V, Crepaz N, Lang KS, et al. Updated Guidelines for Antiretroviral Postexposure Prophylaxis After Sexual, Injection Drug Use, or Other Nonoccupational Exposures to HIV—United States, 2016. Atlanta, GA: Centers for Disease Control and Prevention; 2016. Available at: **https://stacks.cdc.gov/view/cdc/38856**

involved mucosal exposure to secretions; repeated abuse; multiple assailants; and oral, vaginal, and/or anal trauma and particularly if the alleged perpetrator(s) is known to have or is at high risk of having HIV infection (see Human Immunodeficiency Virus Infection, p 489).[1]

---

[1] Centers for Disease Control and Prevention. Preexposure prophylaxis for the prevention of HIV infection in the United States-2021 Update. Available at: **www.cdc.gov/hiv/pdf/risk/prep/cdc-hiv-prep-guidelines-2021.pdf**

The following are recommendations for postexposure HIV assessment within 72 hours of sexual assault[1]:

- Assess risk for HIV infection in the assailant, and test that person for HIV whenever possible.
- Use Fig 2.1 to evaluate the survivor for the need for HIV PEP.
- Consult with a specialist in HIV treatment if PEP is being considered.
- If the survivor appears to be at risk for acquiring HIV from the assault, discuss PEP, including benefits and risks.
- If the survivor chooses to start PEP, provide an initial course of 3 to 7 days of medication (ie, a starter pack) with a prescription for the remainder of the course, or provide a prescription for an entire 28-day course. Schedule an early follow-up visit to discuss test results and provide additional counseling.
- Before initiating PEP, order baseline serum creatinine, aspartate transaminase (AST), and alanine transaminase (ALT).
- Perform an HIV antibody test at original assessment; repeat at approximately 6 weeks and <3 months after the last suspected sexual exposure.
- Counsel individuals with ongoing risk of HIV acquisition about HIV PrEP and provide referrals to a PrEP provider.

Assistance with PEP-related decisions can be obtained by calling the National Clinician's Post Exposure Prophylaxis Hotline (PEP Line) (telephone: 888-448-4911).

A follow-up visit approximately 4 to 6 weeks after the most recent sexual exposure may include a repeat physical examination and collection of additional specimens. Additional follow-up visits at 3 and 6 months after the most recent sexual exposure may be necessary to obtain convalescent sera to test for HBV (if indicated), HCV (if indicated), syphilis, and HIV infection.

··

MEDICAL EVALUATION FOR INFECTIOUS DISEASES FOR INTERNATIONALLY ADOPTED, REFUGEE, AND OTHER IMMIGRANT CHILDREN[2,3]

Every year, thousands of children arrive in the United States from other countries. They arrive as immigrants, adoptees, refugees, asylum seekers, or as other migrants including undocumented children. The medical evaluation of these children is a challenging and important task and is influenced by multiple factors, including the child's

---

[1] Centers for Disease Control and Prevention. Sexually transmitted infections treatment guidelines, 2021. *MMWR Recomm Rep.* 2021;70(RR-4):1-187. Available at: **www.cdc.gov/std/treatment-guidelines/sexual-assault-children.htm**

[2] For additional information, see Canadian Paediatric Society (**www.kidsnewtocanada.ca**), the Centers for Disease Control and Prevention (**wwwnc.cdc.gov/travel/yellowbook/2024/family/international-adoption** and **wwwnc.cdc.gov/travel/yellowbook/2024/posttravel-evaluation/newly-arrived-immigrants-refugees-and-other-migrants**), and World Health Organization (**www.who.int**) websites.

[3] Information for parents can be found at **www.cdc.gov/immigrantrefugeehealth/adoption/index.html/**.

country of origin, socioeconomic status, and health history; availability of reliable health care in the country of origin; and the migration route, including type of travel (eg, by foot or by air), countries passed through, and the conditions during the journey.

Children arriving in the United States should be evaluated as soon as possible after arrival to begin medical assessment and preventive health services, including immunizations. Screening for infectious diseases is important to identify infections with a long latency period. Each of the groups mentioned previously has its own characteristics and special needs.

Internationally Adopted Children

There is a great deal of information available to guide management of children adopted internationally. Some health concerns may be addressed before adoption, although some are apparent to the adoptive family only after arrival. Many adoptive families interact with the health care system before the child arrives and make arrangements for the child to have health insurance at the time of arrival in the United States. There often are opportunities to provide advice to the family and to optimize immunizations that the family may need before traveling to receive their child and for family members and caregivers who will interact with the child after arrival. These immunizations serve to protect the child from diseases that might be transmitted from family and community members (eg, pertussis, influenza) and to protect the family and community from diseases that might be transmitted from the child (eg, hepatitis A, measles). Access to and quality of medical care for international adoptees before arrival in the United States can be variable. Internationally adopted children are required to have a medical examination performed by a physician designated by the US Department of State in their country of origin. This examination usually is limited to completing legal requirements for screening for certain communicable diseases of public health significance and to examine for serious physical or mental disorders that would prevent issuance of an immigrant visa. Such an evaluation is not a comprehensive assessment of the child's health. During preadoption visits, pediatricians should stress to prospective parents the importance of acquiring immunization and other health records. Parents who have not met with a physician before adoption should notify their physician when their child arrives so that a timely medical evaluation can be arranged. Guidance on comprehensive assessment of a newly adopted child is available from the American Academy of Pediatrics (AAP).[1]

Refugees

Refugees have legal status in the United States and are required to undergo medical examination before arrival. The Centers for Disease Control and Prevention (CDC) has issued recommendations for screening of refugees after arrival, and various states have different protocols for initial evaluation of refugees (**www.cdc. gov/immigrantrefugeehealth/guidelines/domestic-guidelines.html**). Immunizations are not required before travel for US-bound refugees, although most receive some age-appropriate vaccinations during the overseas medical examination.

---

[1] Jones VF, Schulte EE; American Academy of Pediatrics, Council on Foster Care, Adoption, and Kinship Care. Comprehensive health evaluation of the newly adopted child. *Pediatrics*. 2019;143(5):e20190657

Immigrants

Immigrant children and children in immigrant families represent the largest and most diverse group of new arrivals to the United States. Most pediatricians will encounter immigrant children in their practice. Evaluation is individual to each case, depending on whether the child is documented or has insurance coverage, the circumstances of immigration, country of origin and migration route, medical history, and socioeconomic status. Resources such as the toolkit developed by the AAP can guide the pediatrician in evaluating new immigrants. (**https://downloads.aap.org/AAP/PDF/ cocp_toolkit_full.pdf**).

Most immigrant children have received some immunizations but may have received them on schedules different from those used in the United States or may have missed essential immunizations. Written documentation of immunizations that includes month and year of administration is accepted as valid if the vaccinations conform to the US schedule. See Children Who Received Immunizations Outside the United States or Whose Immunization Status Is Unknown or Uncertain (p 119) for recommendations regarding immunizations.

Consideration for Testing for Infectious Agents

Infectious diseases are among the most common medical diagnoses identified in immigrant, refugee, and internationally adopted children after arrival in the United States, including diseases of long latency in asymptomatic children. Because of inconsistent use of the birth dose of hepatitis B vaccine (HepB); inconsistent perinatal screening for hepatitis B virus (HBV), syphilis, and human immunodeficiency virus (HIV); and the high prevalence of certain intestinal parasites and tuberculosis (TB), screening for these diseases should be considered for all immigrant children. Screening for other diseases can be considered on an individual basis, as discussed in the following paragraphs (see Table 2.8) and in the disease-specific chapters in Section 3.

HEPATITIS A

Hepatitis A virus (HAV) is endemic in most countries of origin of internationally adopted, refugee, and immigrant children. Some children may have acquired HAV infection early in life and may be immune, but others may be incubating HAV or remain susceptible at the time of entry into the United States. Serologic testing for acute infection (hepatitis A immunoglobulin [Ig] M) is appropriate for symptomatic children. Testing children 12 months of age and older for hepatitis A IgG antibody or total hepatitis A antibody (IgG plus IgM) can be considered at the initial visit to determine whether the child is immune and does not require immunization. Children 12 months of age and older without HAV immunity or documentation of 2 hepatitis A vaccine doses ≥6 months apart should receive HepA vaccine according to routine immunization schedules.

The preferred management strategy for the possibility of a child incubating HAV infection and transmitting the virus to others on arrival in the United States is to recommend hepatitis A vaccine (HepA) for all previously unvaccinated people who anticipate close personal contact (eg, household contact or other regular caregiver) with the child during the first 60 days after arrival from a country with high or intermediate HAV prevalence. Adoptive parents and accompanying family members traveling to adopt the child should ensure that they themselves are immunized or otherwise immune to HAV infection before traveling to a country of high or intermediate prevalence.

Table 2.8. Suggested Possible Screening Tests for Infectious Diseases in International Adoptees, Refugees, and Immigrants[a] (see text for detail)

Hepatitis B virus serologic testing:
Hepatitis B surface antigen (HBsAg), hepatitis B surface antibody (anti-HBs), and total hepatitis B core antibody (anti-HBc)[b]

Hepatitis C virus NAAT for children <18 mo, or serologic testing for children ≥18 mo, when indicated (see text)

Syphilis serologic testing:
Nontreponemal test (eg, RPR or VDRL)
Treponemal test (eg, EIA, CIA, TPPA, MHA-TP, or FTA-ABS)

Human immunodeficiency virus (HIV) 1 and 2 serologic testing; consider fourth-generation HIV antibody/antigen testing

Complete blood cell count with red blood cell indices and differential

Stool examination for ova and parasites (1–3 specimens) with specific request for *Giardia duodenalis* and *Cryptosporidium* species testing by direct fluorescent antibody or EIA testing

Interferon-gamma release assay (IGRA) or tuberculin skin test (TST)

In children from countries with endemic infection[c]:
Trypanosoma cruzi serologic testing

In children with eosinophilia (absolute eosinophil count exceeding 450 cells/mm^3) and negative stool ova and parasite examinations[d] can consider:
Toxocara canis serologic testing
Strongyloides species serologic testing[e]
Schistosoma species serologic testing for children from sub-Saharan African, Southeast Asian, and certain Latin American countries
Lymphatic filariasis serologic testing for children older than 2 years from countries with endemic infection

CIA indicates chemiluminescence assay; EIA, enzyme immunoassay; FTA-ABS, fluorescent treponemal antibody absorption; MHA-TP, microhemagglutination test for *Treponema pallidum;* NAAT, nucleic acid amplification test; RPR indicates rapid plasma reagin; TPPA, *T pallidum* particle agglutination; VDRL, Venereal Disease Research Laboratories.

[a] For evaluation of noninfectious disease conditions, see Linton JM, Green A; American Academy of Pediatrics, Council on Community Pediatrics. Providing care for children in immigrant families. *Pediatrics.* 2019;144(3):e20192077.

[b] Passively acquired maternal anti-HBc may be detected in infants born to HBV-infected mothers up to age 24 months.

[c] Argentina, Belize, Bolivia, Brazil, Chile, Colombia, Costa Rica, Ecuador, El Salvador, French Guiana, Guatemala, Guyana, Honduras, Mexico, Nicaragua, Panama, Paraguay, Peru, Suriname, Uruguay, and Venezuela.

[d] Some experts would perform serologic tests for schistosomiasis in children from areas with high endemicity regardless of eosinophil count because of its poor positive- and negative-predictive values.

[e] CDC recommends *Strongyloides* testing or presumptive treatment for all refugees.

HEPATITIS B

Studies conducted primarily during the 1990s identified prevalence of hepatitis B surface antigen (HBsAg) from 1% to 5% in internationally adopted children and from 4% to 7% in refugee children, depending on the country of origin and the year studied. HBV infection was associated with country of origin and was most common in children from Asia and Africa and from some countries of central and eastern Europe (eg, Romania, Bulgaria, Russia, and Ukraine). The number of countries with routine infant hepatitis B immunization programs has increased markedly in the past decade, and many countries have introduced a birth dose of hepatitis B vaccine (HepB).

Despite the number of countries that have added the birth dose of HepB, vaccination coverage among infants can be suboptimal. Even when a birth dose of HepB is administered, efficacy of postexposure prophylaxis is lower among infants whose birthing parent had a high HBV viral load and hepatitis B e antigen (HBeAg) positivity. All children who were born in or have lived in countries with intermediate (2%–7%) or high (≥8%) prevalence (see Fig 3.2, p 440) should be tested to identify cases of chronic infection, regardless of immunization status (see Hepatitis B, p 437). Even if a child has had HBV serologic tests performed before arrival in the United States, testing may be incomplete or children may become infected after testing, so testing should be repeated. Appropriate screening tests are those for hepatitis B surface antigen (HBsAg), hepatitis B surface antibody (anti-HBs), and total hepatitis B core antibody (anti-HBc). People with chronic HBV infection have circulating HBsAg and circulating total anti-HBc; in a minority of chronically infected individuals, anti-HBs also is present. Both anti-HBs and total anti-HBc are present in people with resolved infection, whereas anti-HBs alone is present in people immunized with hepatitis B vaccine. Antibody tests should be interpreted with caution for children in the first 1 to 2 years of life because of the potential for transplacentally transferred antibody. Unimmunized children with negative HBsAg and negative hepatitis B surface antibody (HBsAb) test results should be immunized according to the recommended childhood and adolescent immunization schedules (also see Children Who Received Immunizations Outside the United States or Whose Immunization Status Is Unknown or Uncertain, p 119).

Children testing positive for HBsAg should be evaluated further to distinguish between acute and chronic HBV infection. Persistence of HBsAg for at least 6 months indicates chronic HBV infection (**www.cdc.gov/hepatitis/hbv/ interpretationOfHepBSerologicResults.htm**; see Hepatitis B, p 437). Children with chronic HBV infection should be tested for biochemical evidence of liver disease and followed by a specialist who cares for patients with chronic HBV infection (see Hepatitis B, p 437). Transient presence of HBsAg can occur following hepatitis B immunization, from within the first 24 hours of immunization up to 3 weeks after immunization, so preimmunization assessment is important. All unimmunized household contacts of children with chronic HBV infection should be immunized (see Hepatitis B, p 437).

HEPATITIS C

Hepatitis C virus (HCV) screening for refugee and immigrant children is not recommended routinely during the new arrival medical examination unless individuals have risk factors, including a birthing parent with hepatitis C, overseas surgery, transfusion, major dental work, intravenous drug use, tattoos, sexual activity/abuse, female genital cutting, and other traditional cutting. Testing for HCV infection also can be considered for unaccompanied children and for internationally adopted children, given that most international adoptees in recent years have been adopted from countries with elevated prevalence (eg, China, Russia, southeast Asia) and because risk factors for infection rarely are known. An HCV antibody screen should be used as the initial screening test for children ≥18 months of age, with reflex testing for HCV RNA for positive antibody specimens.

A nucleic acid amplification test (NAAT) for HCV RNA detection can be performed, ideally from 2 through 6 months of age but also from 7 through 17 months of age if the child has not previously been tested by NAAT for HCV RNA. If the NAAT result at 2 through 17 months is negative, no further follow-up or additional testing is needed. If the child is 18 months of age or older, serologic testing should be performed for diagnosis (see Hepatitis C, p 458).

INTESTINAL PATHOGENS

Serial fecal examinations for ova and parasites tested in a laboratory experienced in parasitology will identify a pathogen in 15% to 35% of internationally adopted and refugee children. Gastrointestinal pathogen nucleic acid amplification testing (NAAT) is not recommended, because it does not detect the full array of parasites these children can have. Presence or absence of symptoms is not predictive of parasitosis. Prevalence of intestinal parasites varies by age of the child and by country of origin. For refugees, guidelines differ depending on whether the child received presumptive therapy before departure (**www.cdc.gov/immigrantrefugeehealth/ guidelines/overseas-guidelines.html**). The most common pathogens identified are *Giardia duodenalis, Dientamoeba fragilis, Hymenolepis* species, some *Schistosoma* species, *Strongyloides stercoralis,* and other soil-transmitted helminths including *Ascaris lumbricoides, Trichuris trichiura,* and hookworm *(Necator americanus). Entamoeba histolytica* and *Cryptosporidium* species are recovered less commonly. Regardless of nutritional status or presence of symptoms, 1 to 3 stool specimens collected on separate days (the CDC recommends 2 or more specimens for asymptomatic refugees from Asia, the Middle East, and Africa if they received no or incomplete predeparture treatment) may be examined for ova and parasites, and direct fluorescent antibody testing or enzyme immunoassay (EIA) may be performed for *Giardia* species and *Cryptosporidium* species.

Some clinicians prefer to administer albendazole for presumptive therapy for helminth infection. Therapy for intestinal parasites generally is successful, but complete eradication may not occur. Proof of eradication is not recommended for individuals who are asymptomatic following therapy. If symptoms persist after treatment, however, ova and parasite testing should be repeated to ensure successful elimination of parasites.

Children who fail to demonstrate adequate catch-up growth, who have unexplained anemia, or who have gastrointestinal tract symptoms or signs that occur or recur months or even years after arrival in the United States should be reevaluated for intestinal parasites. When newly arrived children have acute onset of bloody diarrhea, stool specimens should be tested for *Salmonella* species, *Shigella* species, *Campylobacter* species, Shiga toxin-producing *Escherichia coli* including *E coli* O157:H7, and *Entamoeba histolytica*. If a bacterial pathogen is detected by a nonculture method, confirmation with culture and antimicrobial susceptibility testing are helpful for informing decisions regarding possible treatment and public health measures.

TISSUE PARASITES/EOSINOPHILIA

Eosinophilia is commonly but not universally present in people with tissue parasites. Refugee children may have received presumptive treatment of intestinal helminths overseas before departure to the United States (**www.cdc.gov/ immigrantrefugeehealth/guidelines/overseas-guidelines.html#ipg**). In children who did not receive albendazole or ivermectin for presumptive therapy of intestinal helminths, who have negative stool ova and parasite test results, and in whom eosinophilia (absolute eosinophil count exceeding 450 cells/mm^3) is found on review of complete blood cell count, serologic testing for *Toxocara canis,* strongyloidiasis, schistosomiasis, and lymphatic filariasis should be considered, depending on country of birth and migration route (see Table 2.8). Although logistically attractive to perform all tests at the first encounter, predictive values of many serologic tests for parasites are suboptimal; therefore, common treatable causes of eosinophilia usually should be considered first. Because *T canis* is prevalent worldwide, screening is warranted in children who have no identified cause of eosinophilia. For all immigrant children with eosinophilia and no identified pathogen commonly associated with an increased eosinophil count, serologic testing for *S stercoralis* is reasonable regardless of country of origin, and testing for *Schistosoma* species should be performed for all children who are from sub-Saharan Africa, Southeast Asia, or areas of the Caribbean and South America where schistosomiasis is endemic. Serologic testing for lymphatic filariasis should be considered in children older than 2 years with eosinophilia who are from countries with endemic lymphatic filariasis (**www.cdc.gov/parasites/lymphaticfilariasis/index. html**). A positive serologic result should be confirmed by testing in a reference laboratory (CDC or National Institutes of Health) for release of drugs for treatment of lymphatic filariasis. Screening for loiasis should be performed for any child coming from a region of Africa with coendemic *Loa loa* before treatment for lymphatic filariasis or onchocerciasis, as there is a risk of encephalopathy resulting in death in children with *L loa* infection following treatment with diethylcarbamazine or ivermectin (**www.cdc. gov/parasites/loiasis/health_professionals/index.html**).

SEXUALLY TRANSMITTED INFECTIONS

Congenital syphilis, including with involvement of the central nervous system, may not have been diagnosed or may have been inadequately treated in children from some resource-limited countries. Individuals applying for US immigrant or refugee status or nonimmigrants required to have an overseas examination are required to have testing for syphilis if 18 through 44 years of age, and this group of individuals 18 through 24 years of age also are required to have testing for gonorrhea; people outside these age ranges (including children, as they are <18 years of age) are required to have testing only if there is reason to suspect or a history of syphilis (**www.cdc.gov/immigrantrefugeehealth/panel-physicians/ syphilis.html**) or gonorrhea (**www.cdc.gov/immigrantrefugeehealth/panel- physicians/gonorrhea.html**) infection (see Gonococcal Infections, p 394). Those who have positive test results are required to complete treatment before arrival in the United States (**www.cdc.gov/immigrantrefugeehealth/guidelines/domestic/ sexually-transmitted-diseases/index.html**).

Children adopted internationally and other immigrant children with risk factors should be tested for syphilis after arrival in the United States by reliable nontreponemal and treponemal serologic tests (see Syphilis, p 825). Children with positive nontreponemal or treponemal serologic test results should be evaluated by a health care professional with specific expertise to assess the differential diagnosis of pinta, yaws, and syphilis and to determine the stage of infection so that appropriate treatment can be administered (see Syphilis, p 825). Assessment for other STIs can be considered on the basis of sexual history, past medical history, history of sexual assault, and physical examination findings.

TUBERCULOSIS

Infection with an organism of the *Mycobacterium tuberculosis* complex commonly is encountered in immigrant and refugee children, although incidence rates of tuberculosis (TB) vary by country and by age within countries. Predeparture screening requirements for immigrants, adoptees, refugees, and other applicants depend on age and the TB burden in the country of birth and the migration route (**www.cdc. gov/immigrantrefugeehealth/guidelines/domestic/tuberculosis-guide-lines.html#fig-2**). For those from countries with tuberculosis incidence ≥20 cases per 100 000 population (**www.who.int/tb/publications/global_report/en/**) who are ≥15 years of age, screening and treatment requirements include: chest radiograph; 3 sputum smears and cultures for people with an abnormal chest radiograph, signs and symptoms of tuberculosis disease, or known HIV infection; drug susceptibility testing for people with positive cultures; and, for people with tuberculosis disease, treatment with a standard CDC-recommended regimen delivered as directly observed therapy to cure before travel to the United States. This treatment requirement may result in unanticipated delays in travel to the United States for adoptive children or refugee families. Refugees and immigrant children are screened with an interferon-gamma release assay (IGRA) if IGRA is licensed in the country. Children with a positive IGRA result are required to undergo chest radiography before departure. Children younger than 2 years are not tested unless it is brought to attention of screening physicians outside the United States that they are a known contact of an active case, have HIV infection, or have signs or symptoms suggestive of TB disease. Information about the screening and implementation requirements is available at **www.cdc.gov/immigrantrefugeehealth/panel-physicians/tuberculosis.html**.

Testing for *M tuberculosis* infection after arrival in the United States in immigrants, adoptees, and refugees is important, because TB can be more severe in young children and can reactivate in later years. Presence or absence of a bacille Calmette-Guérin (BCG) vaccine scar should be noted, but approximately 10% of children who received BCG vaccine as infants will not have a scar. BCG coverage in most countries where the vaccine is used is very high, but BCG vaccination has limitations. Efficacy of BCG vaccine against lethal forms of TB (eg, meningitis) in children is approximately 80%, but efficacy against pulmonary TB disease or TB infection is much lower. Receipt of BCG vaccine is not a contraindication to a tuberculin skin test (TST). Either TST or IGRA can be used for detection of *M tuberculosis* infection children of any age, but in children previously vaccinated with BCG, IGRA is preferred to avoid a false-positive TST result caused by a previous vaccination with BCG (see Tuberculosis, p 888, for further guidance). Some immigrants may be anergic initially because of malnutrition, stress, or untreated HIV infection, producing falsely negative TST results or indeterminant or falsely negative IGRA test results; repeat testing may be required. Routine chest radiography is not indicated in asymptomatic children in whom the IGRA or TST result is negative. In children with a positive IGRA or TST, further investigation, including chest radiography and a complete physical examination, is necessary to determine whether tuberculosis disease is present (see Tuberculosis, p 888). When tuberculosis disease is suspected in an immigrant child, efforts to isolate and test the organism for drug susceptibilities are imperative because of the high prevalence of drug resistance in many countries. TB disease, whether suspected or confirmed, is a reportable condition in all US jurisdictions regardless of a patient's immigration status; TB infection is reportable in some states. Physicians who are experts in the management of TB should be consulted when therapy for TB infection or disease is indicated for children from countries with prevalent isoniazid resistance (see Table 3.86, p 909, and **www.who.int/publications/i/item/9789240037021**).

HIV INFECTION

The risk of HIV infection in newly arrived children depends on the country of origin and on individual risk factors. Screening for HIV should be performed for all internationally adopted children, because adoptees may come from populations at high risk of infection and details of their history often are unknown. Although some children will have HIV test results documented in their referral information, test results from the child's country of origin may not be reliable.

Refugees and immigrants have not been required to have HIV testing routinely as part of the predeparture immigration medical assessment since 2010. HIV testing still is recommended for people who are diagnosed with TB disease as part of this medical assessment, and for any refugee diagnosed with another STI. HIV testing after arrival in the United States is recommended for refugees 13 through 64 years of age and is encouraged for refugees 12 years or younger and older than 64 years of age (**www.cdc.gov/immigrantrefugeehealth/guidelines/domestic/screening-hiv-infection-domestic.html**). The decision to screen immigrant children for HIV after arrival in the United States should depend on history and risk factors (eg, receipt of blood products, prenatal drug use), sexual activity (consensual or nonconsensual), physical examination findings, and prevalence of HIV infection in the child's country of origin. If there is a suspicion of HIV infection, testing should be performed before administration of live vaccines. Some experts believe HIV testing may be appropriate for most immigrant children. Repeat screening 3 to 6 months following resettlement is recommended for refugees with a recent exposure or high-risk activity to identify individuals who may be in the "window period" when they arrive in the United States.

CHAGAS DISEASE (AMERICAN TRYPANOSOMIASIS)

Chagas disease is found throughout much of Central and South America (see American Trypanosomiasis [Chagas Disease], p 884). Countries with endemic Chagas disease include Argentina, Belize, Bolivia, Brazil, Chile, Colombia, Costa Rica, Ecuador, El Salvador, French Guiana, Guatemala, Guyana, Honduras, Mexico, Nicaragua, Panama, Paraguay, Peru, Suriname, Uruguay, and Venezuela. Transmission within countries with endemic infection is focal, but if a child comes from, or received a blood transfusion in, a country with endemic Chagas disease, testing for *Trypanosoma cruzi* should be considered; see Fig 3.20 (p 886) and 3.21 (p 887). Treatment of children with Chagas disease is highly effective.

OTHER INFECTIOUS DISEASES

Skin infections that may occur in immigrant children include bacterial (eg, impetigo), fungal (eg, candidiasis and tinea corporis and capitis), and viral (molluscum contagiosum) infections, and ectoparasitic infestations (eg, scabies and pediculosis). New adoptive parents may need to be instructed on how to examine their child for signs of scabies, pediculosis, and tinea so that treatment can be initiated and transmission to others can be prevented (see Scabies, p 750, and Pediculosis chapters, p 644–652).

Diseases such as typhoid fever, leprosy, or melioidosis are encountered infrequently in immigrant children; routine screening for these diseases is not recommended. Findings of fever, splenomegaly, respiratory tract infection, anemia, or eosinophilia should prompt an appropriate evaluation on the basis of the epidemiology of infectious diseases that occur in the child's country of origin or along their migration route.

Routine screening for malaria is not recommended for immigrants, refugees, or internationally adopted children. Testing for malaria (thick and thin blood films) should be performed immediately for any febrile child who has arrived from an area with endemic malaria (see Malaria, p 561). Malaria also should be considered as a cause of asymptomatic splenomegaly in a child from an area with endemic malaria; evaluation should include nucleic acid amplification testing (NAAT) for malaria, because asymptomatic children with splenomegaly attributable to a history of repeated malaria infections may have a positive NAAT assay results but negative smears. If the malaria NAAT assay result is positive, the child should be treated with antimalarial drugs.

Refugee children from Sub-Saharan Africa may have received presumptive treatment for malaria before departure to the United States (**www.cdc.gov/immigrantrefugeehealth/guidelines/overseas-guidelines.html#malaria-guidance;** see Malaria, p 561). Refugees originating from Sub-Saharan Africa who have not received predeparture presumptive treatment should receive presumptive treatment or screening if seen within 3 months of arrival; pregnant people in the first trimester and infants weighing <5 kg should not receive presumptive treatment (**www.cdc.gov/immigrantrefugeehealth/guidelines/domestic/malaria-guidelines-domestic.html**).

In the United States, multiple outbreaks of measles have been reported in children adopted from China and in their US contacts. Measles transmission continues in many parts of the world. Prospective parents who are traveling internationally to adopt children, as well as their household contacts, should ensure that they have a history of measles disease or have been immunized adequately for measles according to US recommendations. If born in the United States after 1956, and in the absence of documented measles infection or contraindication to the vaccine, prospective parents and household contacts of adopted children should receive 2 doses of measles-containing vaccine after the age of 12 months and separated by at least 28 days (see Measles, p 570).

Although one of the major purposes of screening is to identify asymptomatic diseases with long latency, screening need not be performed for all such diseases; an example is neurocysticercosis, which may not be clinically apparent for many years.

For all immigrant children, establishing a medical home with a primary care provider is of prime importance. Country of birth and migration history will remain an important health determinant throughout the child's life.

Injuries From Needles Discarded in the Community

Contact with and injuries from hypodermic needles and syringes improperly discarded in public places pose a risk of transmission of bloodborne pathogens, including human immunodeficiency virus (HIV), hepatitis B virus (HBV), and hepatitis C virus (HCV). However, a review of 14 studies of children exposed to needlesticks in the community documented no transmissions with follow-up of 613 children for HIV, 575 children for HBV, and 394 children for HCV, although many of these children had received postexposure prophylaxis (PEP) for HIV and/or HBV. Infection risks and options for PEP vary depending on the virus and type and extent of exposure. Risk of infection also depends on the nature of the wound, the ability of the pathogens to survive on environmental surfaces, the volume of source material, the concentration of virus in the source material, infection prevalence rates among local injection drug users, the probability that the syringe and needle were used by a person with a substance use disorder, and the immunization status of the person with the needlestick. Although nonoccupational needlestick injuries may pose a lower risk of infection transmission than occupational needlestick injuries, a person injured by a needle in a nonoccupational setting should be evaluated and counseled and, in some cases, should receive PEP. A person who was injured by or exposed to a needlestick should be assessed even if the potential for the discarded syringe to contain a specific bloodborne pathogen is estimated to be low from the background prevalence rates of these infections in the local community.

Wound Care and Tetanus Prophylaxis

Management of people with needlestick injuries includes acute wound care and consideration of the need for antimicrobial prophylaxis. Standard wound care and cleansing with soap and water is indicated; such wounds rarely require closure. A tetanus toxoid-containing vaccine, with or without Tetanus Immune Globulin, should be considered as appropriate for the patient's age, severity of injury, immunization status, and potential for dirt or soil contamination of the needle (see Tetanus, p 848). Tetanus and diphtheria toxoids (Td) or tetanus toxoid, reduced diphtheria toxoid, and acellular pertussis vaccine (Tdap) may be used. If the patient's pertussis vaccination status is not current or is unknown, Tdap should be used (see Pertussis, p 656).

Bloodborne Pathogens

Bloodborne pathogens of primary concern in needlestick exposure are HIV, HBV, and HCV. Consideration of the need for PEP for HBV and HIV is the next step in exposure management; currently, there is no recommended PEP for HCV. Unlike an occupational blood or body fluid exposure, in which the status of the exposure source for HBV, HCV, and HIV often is known, these data usually are not available to help in the decision-making process in a nonoccupational exposure.

HEPATITIS B VIRUS

HBV retains infectivity when held at room temperature for at least 7 days after drying. Transmission to health care personnel with needlestick injury occurs at a rate of 23% to 62% from hepatitis B surface antigen (HBsAg)-positive and hepatitis B envelope antigen (HBeAg)-positive sources, and at a rate of 1% to 6% for HBsAg-positive and HBeAg-negative sources. Prompt and appropriate PEP intervention reduces this risk.[1] The effectiveness of PEP diminishes the longer it is delayed after exposure. Management following a needlestick is predicated on whether the source of the needle is known to be HBsAg-positive and on the HBV immunization status of the person receiving the needlestick and is detailed in Table 3.23 (p 456).

HUMAN IMMUNODEFICIENCY VIRUS

The risk of HIV transmission from a needle discarded in public is lower than the 0.3% risk of HIV transmission by needlestick from a person with known HIV infection to a health care worker, and no cases of HIV transmission by needlestick outside of health care settings have been reported in the United States. HIV is susceptible to drying. When HIV is exposed to air, the 50% tissue culture infective dose decreases by approximately 1 log every 9 hours. In injuries from discarded needles in public, viruses that may have been present have been exposed to drying and environmental temperatures. In addition, injury does not generally occur immediately after the needle was used, needles rarely contain fresh blood, and injuries are usually superficial.

Testing for HIV, if indicated, is performed at baseline and 4 to 6 weeks and again 3 months after the injury (see Human Immunodeficiency Virus Infection, p 489, **https://stacks.cdc.gov/view/cdc/38856,** and **https://nccc.ucsf.edu/ clinician-consultation/pep-post-exposure-prophylaxis/**). The decision to test for HIV does not compel the initiation of PEP, with treatment decisions based on a case-by-case consideration as detailed below. Because concurrent infection with HCV and HIV may be associated with delayed HIV seroconversion, a person whose HCV antibody test result is negative at baseline but seroconverts to positive after exposure should undergo an additional HIV test at 6 months. Testing also is indicated if an illness consistent with acute HIV-related syndrome develops before the 4- to 6-week testing and should include HIV RNA viral load. An alternative is to save a baseline serum specimen to be tested later for HIV if indicated. Counseling is necessary before and after testing (see Human Immunodeficiency Virus Infection, p 489). A positive initial test result in a pediatric patient requires further investigation of the cause, such as perinatal transmission, sexual abuse or activity, or drug use.

With needlestick injuries, a case-by-case assessment of risk of HIV transmission and of risks and benefits of PEP is indicated. In deciding whether or not to initiate PEP, higher-risk situations in which PEP should be recommended include the source being known to be living with HIV, detectable HIV viral load of the person living with HIV, the injury occurring in an area with a high prevalence of HIV infection and injection drug use (some sources suggest >15% prevalence as a threshold), the needle being a large lumen device with visible blood on it or in the syringe, or the injury involving deeper penetration of the needle or involving a mucosal membrane. In some lower-risk situations, it still may be appropriate to consider PEP on the basis of the specifics of a given case. Fig 2.1 (p 188) provides a framework for decision making on PEP utilization.

An HIV specialist should be consulted before deciding whether to initiate PEP. Other consultation services such as the National Clinical Consultation Center (PEP consultation line 888-448-4911; **https://nccc.ucsf.edu/about-the-center/history/**)

---

[1] Schillie S, Murphy TV, Sawyer M, et al. CDC guidance for evaluating health-care personnel for hepatitis B virus protection and for administering postexposure management. *MMWR Recomm Rep.* 2013;62(RR-10):1-19

or the New York City PEP Hotline (844-373-7692) are also available. For a needle-stick with high risk for HIV exposure, PEP should begin within 72 hours. If the needlestick is determined to warrant PEP, a 28-day combination antiretroviral regimen that is appropriate for the patient's age and medical conditions should be selected, and the recommended schedule of laboratory tests should be followed[1] (see Human Immunodeficiency Virus Infection, p 489). Testing the needle for HIV is not recommended.

HEPATITIS C VIRUS

HCV retains infectivity in blood in syringes for days to weeks, depending on syringe residual volume and ambient temperature. Although HCV transmission by sharing syringes and needles among injection drug users is efficient, the risk of transmission from a discarded needle or syringe is likely low. If testing is indicated, anti-HCV anti-body testing with reflex to HCV RNA viral load should be performed at baseline and 6 or more months after exposure. Anti-HCV antibody can be detected in 80% of newly infected patients within 15 weeks after exposure and in 97% by 6 months after exposure. Coinfection with HIV and HCV can delay HCV seroconversion. For earlier diagnosis, testing for HCV viral load may be performed at 3 to 6 weeks after exposure. However, a negative HCV viral load does not preclude the need for anti-HCV anti-body testing 6 months or later after exposure. To confirm infection, positive anti-HCV antibody results should be accompanied by HCV viral load (see Hepatitis C, p 458). Although treatment for hepatitis C infection is highly effective (**www.hcvguidelines. org/unique-populations/children),** there is no recommended PEP for HCV exposure. Immune globulin preparations for HCV are not available, because anti-HCV antibody-positive donors are excluded from the pool from which immune globulin products are prepared.

Preventing Needlestick Injuries

Needlestick injuries can be minimized by implementing public health programs on safe needle disposal and comprehensive syringe services programs including sterile needle access or exchange for used syringes and needles from people who inject drugs. Nearly 30 years of research has shown that comprehensive syringe services programs are safe, effective, and cost-saving; do not increase illegal drug use or crime; and play an important role in reducing the transmission of viral hepatitis, HIV, and other infections. On that basis, the American Academy of Pediatrics supports syringe service programs in conjunction with drug treatment and ongoing evaluation to ensure their effectiveness.

Children should be cautioned to avoid playing in areas known to be frequented by people who inject drugs and to notify a responsible adult parent, teacher, or other caregiver if a discarded syringe or needle is found. Adults should handle used injection paraphernalia with caution; guidance on safe disposal of discarded syringes and needles can be obtained from the local health department.

---

[1] Dominguez KL, Smith DK, Vasavi T, et al. Updated guidelines for antiretroviral postexposure prophylaxis after sexual, injection drug use, or other nonoccupational exposure to HIV—United States, 2016. Atlanta, GA: Centers for Disease Control and Prevention; 2016. Available at: **https://stacks.cdc.gov/view/cdc/38856**

BITE WOUNDS

An estimated 5 million human or animal bite wounds occur annually in the United States; dog bites account for approximately 90% of those wounds. The rate of infection after a bite varies but can be as high as 50% after a cat bite and 5% to 20% after a dog or human bite. Although postinjury rates of infection can be minimized through early administration of proper wound care, the bites of humans, wild animals, or nontraditional pets are potential sources of serious morbidity. Parents should teach children to avoid contact with wild animals and to secure garbage containers so that raccoons and other animals will not be attracted to the home and places where children play. Nontraditional pets, including ferrets, iguanas and other reptiles, and wild animals also pose infection and injury risks for children, and their ownership should be discouraged in households with young children. Health care professionals should be knowledgeable about and offer counseling to parents whose children will have animal contact at petting zoos and exotic animal summer camps. The Centers for Disease Control and Prevention (CDC) has websites that provide information on healthy interactions with pets and other animals.[1] Potential transmission of rabies is increased when a bite is from a wild animal (especially a bat or a carnivore) or from a domestic animal with uncertain immunization status that cannot be captured for adequate quarantine (see Rabies, p 702). Dead animals should be avoided because saliva from recently deceased mammals can contain active rabies virus, which can be transmitted via physical contact with virus-containing saliva.

Recommendations for bite wound management are provided in Table 2.9. Current guidelines from the Infectious Diseases Society of America (IDSA) state that primary wound closure is not recommended for most animal bite wounds.[2] Bite wounds on the face carry a relatively low rate of secondary infection, perhaps because of the generous vascular supply to the area or because these wounds likely receive prompt medical attention, and should be managed with copious irrigation, cautious debridement, and preemptive antibiotics; primary closure is acceptable. Cranial penetrating bite wounds to the scalp and skull sustained from large dogs or other large animals pose an increased risk for intracranial infection. Head imaging is recommended to examine possible skull penetration for these bite wounds. Reports of infection following primary closure on regions other than the face have major limitations including lack of a control group; lack of standardization of the type, severity, and location of the wound; and circumstances surrounding the injury. In addition, thorough wound cleansing before surgical closure has brought the rate of secondary infection of these wounds to well below 10%, no matter the species of animal that inflicted the wound. These factors combine to suggest that, although approximation of margins and closure by delayed primary or secondary intention is prudent for most infected nonfacial wounds, primary closure (or delayed primary closure following a brief antibiotic course) may be considered in some cases. High-pressure irrigation should be avoided because it might drive infectious agents into deeper tissue locations. Smaller, cosmetically unimportant

---

[1] **www.cdc.gov/healthypets/index.html**

[2] Stevens DL, Bisno AL, Chambers HF, et al. Practice guidelines for the diagnosis and management of skin and soft tissue infections: 2014 update by the Infectious Diseases Society of America. *Clin Infect Dis*. 2014;59(2):e10–e52

Table 2.9. Management of Human or Animal Bite Wounds

Category of Management	Management
Cleansing	Remove visible foreign material. Cleanse the wound surface with clean water or saline. Cleansers such as 1% povidone–iodine or 1% benzalkonium chloride can be used for particularly soiled wounds. Irrigate open wounds with a copious volume of sterile water or saline solution by moderate-pressure irrigation.[a] Avoid blind high-pressure irrigation of puncture wounds.
Wound culture	No, for fresh wounds,[b] unless signs of infection exist. Yes, for wounds that appear infected.[c]
Diagnostic imaging	Indicated for penetrating injuries overlying bones (including skull) or joints, for suspected fracture, or to assess foreign body inoculation.
Débridement	Remove superficial devitalized tissue and foreign material.
Operative débridement and exploration	Yes, if any of the following: • Extensive wounds with devitalized tissue or mechanical dysfunction. • Penetration of joints (eg, clenched fist injury) or cranium. • Plastic or other repairs requiring general anesthesia.
Assess mechanical function	Assess and address mechanical function of injured structures.
Wound closure	Yes, for selected (see text) fresh,[b] nonpuncture bite wounds.
Assess tetanus immunization status[d]	Yes, for all wounds.
Assess risk of rabies	Yes, if bite by any rabies-prone, unobservable wild or domestic animal with unknown immunization status.[e]
Assess risk of hepatitis B virus infection	Yes, for human bite wounds.[f]
Assess risk of human immunodeficiency virus (HIV) infection	Yes, for human bite wounds.[g] An HIV test in the person bitten or in the person who bit should be considered if bloody saliva from the biter came into contact with abraded or broken skin or if either person involved in the bite incident has HIV infection or is at risk for HIV infection. Guidance on initiating nonoccupational HIV postexposure prophylaxis (PEP) as soon as possible but no later than 72 hours after a potential HIV exposure is available.[h]

Table 2.9. Management of Human or Animal Bite Wounds, continued

Category of Management	Management
Initiate antimicrobial therapy[i]	Yes, for: • Moderate or severe bite wounds, especially if edema or crush injury is present. • Puncture wounds, especially if penetration of bone, tendon sheath, or joint has occurred. • Deep or surgically closed facial bite wounds. • Hand and foot bite wounds. • Genital area bite wounds. • Wounds in immunocompromised and asplenic people. • Wounds with signs of infection. • Cat bite wounds.
Follow-up	Inspect wound for signs of infection within 48 hours.

[a] Use of an 18-gauge needle with a large-volume syringe is effective. Antimicrobial or anti-infective solutions offer no advantage and may increase tissue irritation.

[b] Wounds less than 12 hours old.

[c] Both aerobic and anaerobic bacterial culture should be performed.

[d] See Tetanus, p 848.

[e] See Rabies, p 702.

[f] See Hepatitis B, p 437.

[g] See Human Immunodeficiency Virus Infection, p 489.

[h] Dominguez KL, Smith DK, Vasavi T, et al. Updated Guidelines for Antiretroviral Postexposure Prophylaxis After Sexual, Injection Drug Use, or Other Nonoccupational Exposure to HIV—United States, 2016. Atlanta, GA: Centers for Disease Control and Prevention; 2016. Available at: **https://stacks.cdc.gov/view/cdc/38856;** and National Clinician Consultation Center, University of California, San Francisco. PEP: Post-Exposure Prophylaxis. Available at: **https://nccc. ucsf.edu/clinician-consultation/pep-post-exposure-prophylaxis/.**

[i] See Table 2.10 (p 206) for suggested drug choices.

wounds can be cleansed and allowed to heal by secondary intention. Hand and foot wounds have a higher risk of infection. This is especially true of deeper wounds that penetrate multiple tissue planes and are more difficult to clean effectively. Injuries that are more complicated should be managed in consultation with an appropriate surgical specialist. To minimize infection risk, bite wounds should not be sealed with a tissue adhesive.

Most infected mammalian bite wound infections are polymicrobial, often involving a mixture of mouth flora from the biting animal and skin flora from the victim (gram-positive and gram-negative aerobes and anaerobes) (see Table 2.10). It usually takes at least 12 hours for signs of infection to manifest clinically. Patients with mild injuries in which the skin is abraded do not need to be treated with antimicrobial agents. For those injuries, cleansing is sufficient.

Specimens for both aerobic and anaerobic culture should be obtained from wounds that appear infected. Limited data exist to guide short-term antimicrobial therapy for patients with wounds that do not appear infected. Preemptive early antimicrobial therapy for 3 to 5 days is recommended for patients who (a) are immunocompromised; (b) are asplenic; (c) have advanced liver disease; (d) have preexisting or resultant edema of the affected area; (e) have moderate to severe injuries, especially to the hand or face; or (f) have injuries that may have penetrated the periosteum or joint capsule.[1] Antimicrobial therapy is recommended following cat bites, given the frequency of associated infection. In certain cases, postexposure prophylaxis for rabies may be indicated. Always assume that bats, skunks, raccoons, foxes, and woodchucks are rabid unless the geographic area is known to be rabies-free or until the animal tests negative (see Rabies, p 702). Tetanus toxoid should be administered to patients with animal bite wounds who have not had toxoid vaccination within the prior 5 years (see Tetanus, p 848). Humans exposed to macaque bites or secretions are at risk for B virus (*Cercopithecine herpesvirus* 1) infection and could be considered for postexposure antiviral prophylaxis (valacyclovir) in certain situations.[2] Routine antiviral prophylaxis following most animal bite wounds is not indicated, although risks for transmission of hepatitis B virus and human immunodeficiency virus (HIV) should be assessed in human bite injuries (see Table 2.9).

Suggestions for initial choice of antimicrobial therapy for human and animal bites are provided in Table 2.10. The treatment of choice following most bite wounds for which therapy is indicated is amoxicillin-clavulanic acid. For a child who cannot take penicillin, alternative options include oral or parenteral treatment with trimethoprim-sulfamethoxazole, which is effective against *Staphylococcus aureus* (including methicillin-resistant *S aureus* [MRSA]), *Pasteurella multocida*, and *Eikenella corrodens*, in conjunction with clindamycin, which is active in vitro against anaerobic bacteria, streptococci, and many strains of *S aureus*. Extended-spectrum cephalosporins, such as parenteral ceftriaxone or oral cefpodoxime, do not have good anaerobic activity but can be used in conjunction with clindamycin as alternative therapy for penicillin-allergic patients who can tolerate cephalosporins. Doxycycline is an alternative agent that has activity against *P multocida* and can be used regardless of patient age (see Antimicrobial Agents and Related Therapy, p 973). Azithromycin and fluoroquinolones display good in vitro activity against organisms that commonly cause bite wound infections, but clinical data are lacking. Carbapenems are also an option for children with penicillin allergy. A 5-day course of treatment usually is sufficient for soft tissue infections, but the duration of treatment for bite wound-associated bone infections is based on location, severity, and pathogens isolated.

In the child with a confirmed bite wound-associated infection, initial therapy should be optimized when culture results become available. MRSA is a potential but uncommon bite wound pathogen; empiric therapy may require modification in cases of known colonization, severe infections, or when MRSA is isolated from an infected wound (see *Staphylococcus aureus*, p 767).

Bites from some animals may lead to infections with unusual microbes such as *Salmonella* species (eg, many reptiles), *Aeromonas* species (eg, alligators), or *Vibrio* species (eg, sharks). *Bartonella henselae* infections may be a late manifestation of cat, and sometimes dog, bites.

[1] Stevens DL, Bisno AL, Chambers HF, et al. Practice guidelines for the diagnosis and management of skin and soft tissue infections: 2014 update by the Infectious Diseases Society of America. *Clin Infect Dis.* 2014;59(2):e10–e52

[2] Cohen JI, Davenport DS, Steward JA, et al. Recommendations for prevention of and therapy for exposure to B virus (*Cercopithecine herpesvirus* 1). *Clin Infect Dis.* 2002;35(10):1191–1203

Table 2.10. Antimicrobial Agents for Human or Animal Bite Wounds

Source of Bite	Organism(s) Likely to Cause Infection	First-Line Therapy[a]	Alternatives for Penicillin-Allergic Patients[a,b]
Dog, cat, or mammal[c]	*Pasteurella* species, *Staphylococcus aureus*, streptococci, anaerobes, *Capnocytophaga* species, *Moraxella* species, *Corynebacterium* species, *Neisseria* species	Amoxicillin-clavulanate (oral) OR Ampicillin-sulbactam (IV)	Oral or IV: Extended-spectrum cephalosporin or trimethoprim-sulfamethoxazole[d] PLUS Clindamycin
Reptile[e]	Enteric gram-negative bacteria (including *Salmonella* species), anaerobes	Amoxicillin-clavulanate (oral) OR Ampicillin-sulbactam (IV)	Oral: Extended-spectrum cephalosporin or trimethoprim-sulfamethoxazole[d] PLUS Clindamycin OR IV: Extended-spectrum cephalosporin or gentamicin or aztreonam or quinolone PLUS Clindamycin
Human	Streptococci, *S aureus*, *Eikenella corrodens*, *Haemophilus* species, anaerobes	Amoxicillin-clavulanate (oral) OR Ampicillin-sulbactam (IV)	Oral or IV: Extended-spectrum cephalosporin or trimethoprim-sulfamethoxazole[d] PLUS Clindamycin

[a] Coverage for methicillin-resistant *Staphylococcus aureus* (MRSA) can be considered for severe bite wounds. Note that neither amoxicillin-clavulanate nor ampicillin-sulbactam will provide MRSA coverage.

[b] For patients with history of suspected IgE-mediated allergy or severe drug reaction to penicillin, alternative drugs are recommended (see text).

[c] Data are lacking to guide antimicrobial use for bites that are not overtly infected from small mammals, such as guinea pigs and hamsters.

[d] Doxycycline provides alternative coverage for *Pasteurella multocida* and MRSA.

[e] The role of empirical antimicrobial use for noninfected snake bite wounds is not well-defined. Therapy should be chosen based on results of cultures from infected wounds.

PREVENTION OF MOSQUITO-BORNE AND TICK-BORNE INFECTIONS

Mosquito-borne diseases in the continental United States are caused by arboviruses (eg, West Nile, La Crosse, Jamestown Canyon, St. Louis encephalitis, and eastern equine encephalitis [see Arboviruses, p 237, and Table 2.11]). Several mosquito species in the *Culex* genus transmit West Nile and St. Louis encephalitis viruses to

Table 2.11. Diseases Transmitted by Mosquitoes and Ticks in the United States[a]

Organism/Disease	Primary Vector	Geographic Region
Mosquito-borne Infections		
West Nile virus	*Culex* species	Across continental United States
La Crosse encephalitis virus	*Aedes triseriatus*	Upper midwestern, mid-Atlantic, and southeastern states
Jamestown Canyon virus	Unknown	Upper midwestern states
St. Louis encephalitis virus	*Culex* species	Midwestern and western states
Eastern equine encephalitis virus	*Aedes, Coquillettidia,* and *Culex* species	Midwestern and eastern states
Dengue virus	*Aedes aegypti* and *Aedes albopictus*	US territories (Puerto Rico, US Virgin Islands, American Samoa)
Chikungunya virus	*A aegypti* and *A albopictus*	US territories (Puerto Rico, US Virgin Islands, American Samoa)
Zika virus	*A aegypti* and *A albopictus*	US territories (Puerto Rico, US Virgin Islands, American Samoa)
Tick-borne Infections		
Rickettsia rickettsii (Rocky Mountain spotted fever)	*Dermacentor variabilis* (American dog tick), *Dermacentor andersoni* (Rocky Mountain wood tick), *Rhipicephalus sanguineus* (brown dog tick)	Throughout the United States but most common in midwestern and southeastern states
Colorado tick fever	*Dermacentor andersoni*	Western states
Borrelia burgdorferi, Borrelia mayonii (Lyme disease)	*Ixodes scapularis, Ixodes pacificus*	Northeastern and upper midwestern states

Table 2.11. Diseases Transmitted by Mosquitoes and Ticks in the United States,[a] continued

Organism/Disease	Primary Vector	Geographic Region
Anaplasma phagocytophilum (anaplasmosis)	*I scapularis, I pacificus*	Northeastern and upper midwestern states
Babesia microti (babesiosis)	*Ixodes* species	Northeastern and midwestern states
Borrelia miyamotoi (hard tick relapsing fever)	*Ixodes* species	Upper midwestern, northeastern, and mid-Atlantic states
Powassan virus	*Ixodes* species	Northeastern and upper midwestern states
Ehrlichia muris eauclairensis	*Ixodes* species	Cases have been reported in Minnesota and Wisconsin
Ehrlichia chaffeensis, Ehrlichia ewingii (ehrlichiosis)	*Amblyomma americanum* (lone star tick)	Southeastern and south-central states
Heartland virus	*A americanum* (lone star tick)	Southeastern and south-central states
Southern tick-associated rash illness (STARI)	*A americanum* (lone star tick)	Southeastern and eastern states
Borrelia hermsii, Borrelia turicatae (tick-borne relapsing fever)	*Ornithodoros* species	Western mountainous states
Rickettsia parkeri (spotted fever)	*Amblyomma maculatum*	Southeastern states
Francisella tularensis (tularemia)	*D andersoni, D variabilis,* or *A americanum*	Reported in all states

[a]Mosquito-borne and tick-borne infections that are transmitted primarily in other countries are not included here (eg, malaria, yellow fever virus, Japanese encephalitis virus, tick-borne encephalitis virus).

humans (primarily *Culex pipiens, Culex quinquefasciatus,* and *Culex tarsalis*). Eastern equine encephalitis virus can be transmitted by *Aedes, Coquillettidia,* and *Culex* species. The main mosquito vector of La Crosse virus is the treehole-inhabiting species *Aedes triseriatus*. Primary vector species of Jamestown Canyon virus have not been identified. Local transmission of other mosquito-borne viruses (eg, dengue, chikungunya, and Zika viruses) occurs in US territories (eg, Puerto Rico, US Virgin Islands, American Samoa) and occasionally in the continental United States. Chikungunya, dengue, and Zika viruses are primarily transmitted by 2 container-inhabiting mosquito species, *Aedes aegypti* and *Aedes albopictus*. International travelers may encounter similar or different arboviruses (eg, yellow fever, Japanese encephalitis, tick-borne encephalitis) or other mosquito-borne infections (eg, malaria) during travel (also see disease-specific chapters in Section 3).

Tick-borne infectious diseases in the United States include those caused by bacteria (spirochetes and rickettsia), protozoa, and viruses. Different species of ticks transmit different infectious agents. *Dermacentor variabilis* (American dog tick), *Dermacentor andersoni* (Rocky Mountain wood tick), and *Rhipicephalus sanguineus* (brown dog tick) are the primary vectors of *Rickettsia rickettsii* (Rocky Mountain spotted fever). *Dermacentor andersoni* also transmits Colorado tick fever virus. *Ixodes scapularis* (deer or blacklegged tick) and *Ixodes pacificus* (western blacklegged tick) transmit *Borrelia burgdorferi* (Lyme disease) and *Anaplasma phagocytophilum* (anaplasmosis). *Ixodes* ticks also transmit *Babesia microti* (babesiosis), *Borrelia miyamotoi* (hard tick relapsing fever), *Borrelia mayonii* (Lyme disease), *Ehrlichia muris eauclairensis*, and Powassan virus. *Amblyomma americanum* (lone star tick) transmits *Ehrlichia chaffeensis*, *Ehrlichia ewingii* (ehrlichiosis), and Heartland virus, and is associated with southern tick-associated rash illness (STARI). *Francisella tularensis* (tularemia) can be transmitted by *D andersoni*, *D variabilis*, or *A americanum*. Soft-bodied ticks (*Ornithodoros* species) transmit *Borrelia hermsii* and *Borrelia turicatae* to cause tick-borne relapsing fever. *Amblyomma maculatum* (the Gulf Coast tick) can transmit *Rickettsia parkeri*, a form of spotted fever rickettsiosis.

Prevention of infection depends on avoiding known areas of disease, reducing arthropod habitats, using repellents and clothing to protect against biting arthropods, and limiting the amount of time that ticks are attached to the skin.

Vaccines for yellow fever, Japanese encephalitis, and tick-borne encephalitis are licensed and available in the United States for use in travelers. A dengue vaccine is approved in the United States for use in children 6 through 16 years of age with laboratory-confirmed previous dengue infection living in areas where dengue is endemic. Chemoprophylactic drugs are available to protect against malaria.

General Protective Measures

Pediatricians can educate patients and families to take the following measures to reduce exposures to vectorborne diseases:

- **Understand which arthropod-related infections are common in your area.** Physicians need to be aware of the burden of arthropod-related infections in their local areas. Local health departments can provide information about domestic disease risks and patterns. Travelers, to the extent possible, should avoid known areas of disease transmission. The Centers for Disease Control and Prevention (CDC) Travelers' Health website provides updates on regional disease transmission patterns and outbreaks **(wwwnc.cdc.gov/travel/)**. Climate change is affecting the geographic range of arthropod vectors.
- **Eliminate standing water sources that attract mosquitoes.** Mosquitoes lay eggs on or near standing water, and large numbers of mosquitoes can arise from sources of standing water at or near the home. Measures to limit places where mosquitoes can lay eggs around the home include drainage, cleaning, or removal of receptacles for standing water (eg, tires, toys, flower pots, cans, buckets, barrels, other containers that collect rain water); keeping swimming pools, decorative pools, and children's wading pools in working condition so that water does not become stagnant; replacing water in bird baths several times weekly; and clearing clogged rain gutters. Under certain circumstances, large-scale mosquito-control measures may be conducted by community or public health officials. These efforts include drainage of standing water, use of larvicides in waters that are sources of mosquitoes, and use of adulticides to control adult mosquitoes. More information on integrated pest management is available from the US Environmental Protection Agency (EPA) at **www.epa.gov/ipm/introduction-integrated-pest-management.**

- **Reduce exposure to mosquitoes.** Mosquitoes may bite at any time of day. Although different species of mosquitoes have different peak biting times, precautions should be taken anytime when outdoors. Peak biting time for vectors of malaria are from dusk to dawn, and peak biting times for vectors carrying West Nile, dengue, chikungunya, and Zika viruses are at dawn and dusk. Bed nets, screens, and nets tucked around strollers and other confined spaces where young children play are important barriers against mosquitoes. Mosquito traps, electrocutors (bug zappers), ultrasonic repellers, and other devices marketed to prevent mosquitoes from biting people should not be relied on to reduce mosquito bites.
- **Reduce exposure to ticks.** Ticks generally live in grassy, brushy, or wooded areas and on animals. People are more likely to come in contact with ticks while with animals or when camping, gardening, or hunting. The residential backyard is a primary environment where people are bitten by ticks that transmit pathogens that may cause disease. Tick-infested areas should be avoided whenever possible. When hiking, use the center of trails to reduce exposure to questing ticks on vegetation. Risk of exposure to some ticks can be reduced by locating play equipment in sunny, dry areas away from forest edges; creating a barrier of dry wood chips or gravel between recreation areas and forest; regularly mowing vegetation; and keeping leaves raked and underbrush cleared. The brown dog tick (*Rhipicephalus sanguineus*), a concern in the southwestern United States, can survive in more arid environments and can be introduced indoors where it may be found in cracks and crevices in the house; on walls, carpet, and furniture; or in animal housing or bedding. Control of tick populations in the community often is not practical but can be effective in more defined areas, such as around places where children play. Using acaricides (pesticides targeting ticks) on a property or on pets can reduce tick populations.
- **Wear appropriate protective clothing.** Whenever possible, clothing should be worn that covers the arms, legs, head, and other exposed skin areas when entering mosquito or tick habitats. Tucking in shirts and wearing closed-toe shoes instead of sandals may reduce opportunities for ticks to attach. Visualization of crawling arthropods is improved with light-colored clothing.
- **Consider treatment of clothing and gear.** Permethrin (a synthetic pyrethroid) is both a pesticide and a repellent that can be sprayed onto clothes and gear. Permethrin repels both mosquitoes and ticks. Clothing and gear should be treated with products containing 0.5% permethrin. Permethrin should not be sprayed directly onto skin, and treated clothing should be dried before wearing. The US EPA has registered the commercial sale of permethrin-treated outdoor clothing, hats, bed nets, and camping gear, which is safe for children and pregnant people when used according to the product label. Adverse reactions to permethrin are mild and transient and may include skin rash, burning, stinging, erythema, tingling, or numbness. Permethrin-treated clothing remains effective through multiple launderings but may need retreatment over time. Permethrin or repellents should not be used on clothing or mosquito nets where children may chew or suck on the material. More information on repellant treated clothing is available at **www.epa. gov/insect-repellents/repellent-treated-clothing** and **www.epa.gov/ mosquitocontrol/permethrin-resmethrin-d-phenothrin-sumithrinr- synthetic-pyrethroids-mosquito.**

Repellents for Use on Skin

The EPA regulates repellent products in the United States. The CDC, US Food and Drug Administration (FDA), and American Academy of Pediatrics (AAP) recommend that people use repellent products that have been registered by the EPA, which indicates that the materials have been reviewed for both efficacy and human safety when applied according to the instructions on the label.

Arthropods are attracted to people by body heat, odors on the skin, vibrations, and carbon dioxide and other volatile chemicals from the breath. The active ingredients in repellents, with the exception of permethrin-based repellents, help ward off mosquitoes or ticks but do not kill them. Repellents should be used during outdoor activities when mosquitoes or ticks are present and should always be used according to the label instructions. Protection times listed below generally are against mosquitoes; duration of protection generally is shorter against ticks. Protection also varies by type and concentration of active ingredient, product formulation, ambient temperatures, and types of activity (eg, protection time is reduced by perspiration, washing of skin, and involvement in water recreation). Product labels should be followed for application and reapplication recommendations. Repellents should not be reapplied more frequently than recommended on the label. More information on insect repellants is available from the EPA (**www.epa.gov/insect-repellents/ find-insect-repellent-right-you**).

EPA-REGISTERED REPELLENTS

Several types of EPA-registered products provide repellent activity sufficient to help people reduce the bites of disease-carrying mosquitoes and ticks (**www.epa. gov/insect-repellents** and **wwwnc.cdc.gov/travel/yellowbook/2024/ environmental-hazards-risks/mosquitoes-ticks-and-other-arthropods**). Products containing the following active ingredients typically provide reasonably long-lasting protection from mosquitoes and ticks when applied directly to the skin. More information about these ingredients can be found at **www.epa.gov/ insect-repellents/skin-applied-repellent-ingredients.**

DEET. Chemical name: N,N-diethyl-meta-toluamide or N,N-diethyl-3-methyl-benzamide. Commercial products registered for direct application to human skin contain from 5% to 99% DEET (**www.epa.gov/insect-repellents/deet**). DEET repels both mosquitoes and ticks. In general, higher concentrations of active ingredient provide longer duration of protection. Protection times for DEET against mosquitoes range from 1 to 2 hours for products containing 5% concentrations (which may not protect against ticks) to 10 hours or more for products containing 40% or more DEET. There does not appear to be a meaningful increase in protection time for products containing >50% DEET. Time-released DEET formulations are available that provide 11 to 12 hours of protection with concentrations of 20% to 30% DEET.

DEET does not present a health problem if used appropriately. Adverse effects related to DEET are rare and most often are associated with ingestions or chronic or excessive use and do not appear to be related to DEET concentration used. Although rare, encephalopathy has been reported after excessive skin application in children and after unintentional ingestion. Urticaria and contact dermatitis have been reported in a small number of people. DEET is irritating to eyes and mucous membranes and should not be applied to these areas. Highly concentrated formulations can damage plastic and certain synthetic fabrics.

PICARIDIN (KBR 3023). Chemical name: 2-(2-hydroxyethyl)-1-piperidinecarboxylic acid 1-methylpropyl ester. Picaridin has concentration-related efficacy and ages for use similar to DEET. Products containing 5% picaridin provide 3 to 4 hours of protection against mosquitoes and ticks, and products with 20% picaridin can provide protection for 8 to 12 hours. Although experience with this product is less than with DEET, no serious toxicity has been reported. Picaridin-containing compounds have been used as repellents for 2 decades in Europe and Australia and for more than 10 years in the United States as a 20% formulation with no serious toxicity reported.

OIL OF LEMON EUCALYPTUS. Chemical name: para-menthane-3,8-diol (PMD). PMD is the synthesized version of oil of lemon eucalyptus (OLE). Only EPA-registered repellent products containing the active ingredient OLE or PMD should be used. "Pure" oil of lemon eucalyptus has not been tested for safety and efficacy and is not registered with the EPA as an insect repellent. Products with 8% to 10% PMD protect for up to 2 hours, and products containing 30% to 40% OLE provide 6 hours of protection. These products should not be used on children younger than 3 years.

IR3535. Chemical name: 3-(N-butyl-N-acetyl)-aminopropionic acid. IR3535 is available in formulations ranging from 7.5% to 20%, with estimated protection times ranging from 2 hours to up to 10 hours depending on concentration.

2-UNDECANONE. Chemical name: methyl nonyl ketone. 2-undecanone is a synthetic version of an organic compound that can also be extracted from oil of rue, a perennial shrub. It can also be found naturally in wild-grown tomatoes, cloves, and other plant sources. 2-undecanone products contain 7.75% active ingredient and provides protection for up to 5 hours for mosquitoes and 2 hours for ticks.

NONREGISTERED PRODUCTS

Topical products based on citronella, catnip oil, and other essential plant oils provide minimal protection and are not recommended. Ingestion of garlic or vitamin B_1 and wearing devices that emit sounds or impregnated wristbands are ineffective.

APPLICATION OF REPELLENTS

The following are recommended precautions for use of repellents:
- Apply repellents only to exposed skin or clothing, as directed on the product label. Do not apply repellents under clothing.
- Never use repellents over cuts, wounds, or irritated skin.
- When using sprays, do not spray directly on face—spray on hands first and then apply to face. Do not apply repellents to eyes or mouth and apply sparingly around ears.
- Children should not handle repellents. Adults should apply repellents to their own hands first, and then gently spread on the child's exposed skin. Adults should avoid applying directly to children's hands, because children frequently put fingers and hands into their mouths. Children also may be exposed to the pesticides applied to their pets.
- Use just enough repellent to cover exposed skin or clothing.
- Sprays should not be applied in enclosed areas or near food.

- Wash hands after application to avoid accidental exposure to eyes or ingestion.
- Do not apply repellents for use on humans to pets.

REPELLENTS AND SUNSCREEN. Sunscreen should be applied first when using both products simultaneously. Repellents that are applied according to label instructions may be used with sunscreen with no reduction in repellent activity; limited data show a one-third decrease in the sun protection factor (SPF) of sunscreens when DEET-containing insect repellents are used after a sunscreen is applied. Reapplication of sunscreen or repellent may be needed depending on the duration of protection needed and type of activity. Products that combine sunscreen and repellent are not recommended.

Tick Inspection and Removal

Parents or caregivers should promptly inspect children's bodies, clothing, and equipment after possible tick exposure ("tick check"). When conducting tick checks, special attention should be given to the exposed regions of the body where ticks often attach, including the head, neck, around the ears, and inside the umbilicus, behind the knees, between the legs, and around the waist. Ticks also may attach at areas of tighter clothing (eg, sock line, belt line, axillae, groin). Timely tick checks at least daily increase the likelihood of finding and removing ticks before they can transmit an infectious agent. Longer periods of attachment significantly increase the probability of transmission of tick-borne pathogens, although certain pathogens (eg, Powassan virus) are believed to be transmitted in less than 15 minutes. It is important to remove clothes as soon as possible after potential tick exposure because they may harbor crawling ticks. Bathing or showering after coming indoors (preferably within 2 hours) can be an opportunity to locate attached or crawling ticks and has been shown to be an important personal protective measure against several tick-borne diseases. Unattached ticks can enter the home by hiding in clothing. Placing dry clothing in a dryer on high heat for at least 10 minutes (damp clothes can take up to 1 hour) has been used to kill unattached ticks on clothes.

TICK REMOVAL

Ticks should be removed from skin as soon as possible. Do not wait for the tick to detach itself from the skin by "painting" it with petroleum jelly or using heat. When possible, use fine-tipped forceps or tweezers to grasp the tick as close to the skin as possible and gently pull straight out without twisting motions. Be careful not to break mouthparts as the tick is removed. Tweezers should be cleaned of any potential tick body tissue or fluids that may have been left after pulling on the attached tick. Tweezers then can be used to remove mouthparts or cement (an adhesive secretion that anchors tick mouthparts to the skin) left on the skin. Avoid cutting or digging into skin to remove small remnants; if unable to remove the mouth parts easily, leave them alone and let the skin heal. If fingers are used to remove ticks, they should be protected with a barrier, such as tissue or plastic gloves, and washed after removal of the tick. The bite site should be washed with soap and water to reduce the risk of secondary skin infections.

TESTING TICKS

Testing ticks removed from animals or humans for infectious pathogens is unnecessary because it is not diagnostically informative.

Other Preventive Measures

PETS

Maintaining tick-free pets also will decrease tick exposure in and around the home. Daily inspection of pets, removal of ticks, and use of appropriate veterinary products to prevent ticks on pets are indicated. Consult a veterinarian for information on effective products. Apply recommended products as instructed.

CHEMOPROPHYLAXIS

In areas of high Lyme disease incidence, chemoprophylaxis with a single dose of doxycycline to prevent Lyme disease after an *Ixodes* tick bite may be considered under certain conditions (see **www.cdc.gov/lyme/resources/FS-Guidance-for-Clinicians-Patients-after-TickBite-508.pdf** and Lyme Disease, p 549). Doxycycline can be used regardless of patient age (see Antimicrobial Agents and Related Therapy, p 973). Chemoprophylaxis is not recommended for other tick-borne diseases, including those caused by rickettsiae. Following a tick bite, individuals should be on alert for signs or symptoms of tick-borne illnesses and consult a physician if a fever, rash, or other concerns develop.

Chemoprophylaxis is recommended for travelers to areas where malaria is endemic (see Malaria, p 561)

···

PREVENTION OF ILLNESSES ASSOCIATED WITH RECREATIONAL WATER USE

Recreational water-associated illness (RWI) can be caused by pathogens transmitted through ingestion, inhalation of aerosols, or contact with contaminated water in swimming pools, splash pads, water playgrounds, hot tubs, lakes, rivers, or oceans. RWI also can be caused by chemicals or toxins in recreational water via ingestion, inhalation, or contact. Illnesses associated with recreational water can involve the gastrointestinal tract, respiratory tract, central nervous system, skin, ears, or eyes. From 2015 through 2019, 208 outbreaks associated with treated recreational water (eg, in pools, splash pads, hot tubs) were reported to the Centers for Disease Control and Prevention (CDC).[1] These outbreaks resulted in more than 3600 cases of illness, including 13 deaths, and only represent a small fraction of the true disease burden as most RWI is unreported. The leading cause of these outbreaks was *Cryptosporidium* species. Cryptosporidiosis can cause life-threatening infection in immunocompromised persons (see Cryptosporidiosis, p 338). Another common cause in these outbreaks was *Legionella* species (see *Legionella pneumophila* Infections, p 531). Although not confirmed in this series, *Pseudomonas* species can cause folliculitis ("hot tub rash") or acute otitis externa ("swimmer's ear"). Among 140 outbreaks from 2000 to 2014 associated with untreated recreational water venues (eg, lakes, rivers),[2] common causes included norovirus (see Norovirus and Sapovirus

---

[1] Hlavsa MC, Aluko SA, Miller AD, et al. Outbreaks associated with treated recreational water—United States, 2015–2019. *MMWR Morb Mortal Wkly Rep.* 2021;70(20):733-738.

[2] Graciaa DS, Cope JR, Roberts VA, et al. Outbreaks associated with untreated recreational water—United States, 2000–2014. *MMWR Morb Mortal Wkly Rep.* 2018;67(25):701-706

Infections, p 622), pathogenic *Escherichia coli* (see *Escherichia coli* Diarrhea, p 376), *Shigella* species (see *Shigella* Infections, p 756), *Cryptosporidium* (see Cryptosporidiosis, p 338), avian schistosomes (cercarial dermatitis), and algal toxins associated with harmful algal blooms. Leptospirosis (see Leptospirosis, p 542), although less common, also caused outbreaks. Two deaths were attributed to primary amoebic meningoencephalitis (PAM) caused by *Naegleria fowleri* (see Amebic Meningoencephalitis and Keratitis, p 228), a free-living amoeba found in natural or ambient bodies of freshwater.

Although rare (0–8 infections per year), *N fowleri* infection is nearly always fatal (>97% fatality rate). Infection primarily affects healthy young males and can occur during swimming in warm, freshwater lakes, ponds, reservoirs, rivers, or streams. Cases have also been associated with inadequately chlorinated swimming pools, an artificial whitewater river, a manmade surf park, and splash pads. After the amebae enter the nasal cavity, they migrate to the brain via the olfactory nerve. Signs and symptoms of *N fowleri* infection are clinically similar to bacterial meningitis.

According to CDC's One Health Harmful Algal Bloom Surveillance System, during 2020, 13 states reported 227 harmful algal blooms that resulted in 95 human illnesses and 1170 animal illnesses.[1] Marine and freshwater organisms that cause blooms occur naturally; however, rapid growth can result in harmful blooms that sometimes release toxins. Warmer water temperatures and excess of nutrients are factors that can affect their growth. Blooms can appear as foam, scum, or mats on the surface of water, although not every bloom produces toxins. Some blooms might not be easily visible if they grow below the surface of the water. Cyanobacteria ("blue-green algae") are the most common cause of harmful freshwater blooms. Cyanobacteria produce toxins known as cyanotoxins (including microcystin and cylindrospermopsin) that cause a range of illnesses, from skin or eye irritation to respiratory, gastrointestinal, or neurologic symptoms depending on the type of toxin, the route of exposure, and the exposure dose.

Cyanotoxin exposures can also cause severe illness and deaths to pets and livestock from swimming or drinking in affected waterbodies. This can occur quickly and can be an early indicator that a water body contains a harmful cyanobacterial bloom.

In marine waters, harmful algal blooms are usually caused by microalgae called diatoms and dinoflagellates. The dinoflagellate *Karena brevis* can produce brevetoxin and is responsible for the red tide blooms observed in the Gulf Coast of the southeast United States. Inhalation or dermal exposure to brevetoxin in marine waters can result in respiratory tract, skin, or eye irritation. Additional information about harmful blooms and associated illnesses and outreach materials including fact sheets, communication resources and other media, is available from the CDC's harmful algal bloom-associated illnesses website (**www.cdc.gov/habs**).

During swimming, the water is shared among a few to thousands of people each day, depending on venue size. Fecal contamination of recreational water venues is a common occurrence because of the high incidence of diarrhea and fecal incontinence (particularly in young children [ie, age <5 years]) and the presence of residual fecal material on bodies of swimmers (up to 10 g on young children). Reported recreational water-associated outbreaks can disproportionally affect young children, usually occur during the summer months, and most frequently manifest as acute

---

[1] Vigar M, Thuneibat M, Gerdes M, Jacobi A, Roberts VA. Summary Report—One Health Harmful Algal Bloom System (OHHABS), United States, 2020. Atlanta, GA: Centers for Disease Control and Prevention; 2022. Available at: **www.cdc.gov/habs/data/2020-ohhabs-data-summary.html**

gastrointestinal illness. In addition to fecal contamination by swimmers, untreated recreational waters can be impacted by sewage treatment plant discharges, septic systems, or agricultural waste, which might contain a wide range of potentially infectious pathogens (eg, norovirus, *E coli*, *Shigella* species, *Cryptosporidium* species). Other microorganisms in untreated recreational waters might also cause infection (eg, *Vibrio vulnificus* and *Vibrio parahaemolyticus*, see Other *Vibrio* Infections p 955).

To help protect swimmers from infectious pathogens, water in treated recreational water venues is chlorinated. Maintaining pH and disinfectant concentration as recommended by the CDC (**www.cdc.gov/healthywater/swimming/**) is sufficient to inactivate most infectious pathogens within minutes. However, some infectious pathogens are moderately to extremely chlorine tolerant and can survive for extended periods of time, even in properly chlorinated pools (eg, *Giardia duodenalis* has been shown to survive for up to 45 minutes). *Legionella* and *Pseudomonas* species are effectively controlled by chlorination, but because they persist in biofilms, they can proliferate when proper disinfectant concentrations are not maintained. *Cryptosporidium* oocysts can survive for more than 7 days even in properly chlorinated pools, thus contributing to the role of *Cryptosporidium* as the leading cause of recreational water–associated outbreaks. Additional water treatments (eg, ultraviolet light, ozone) can more efficiently inactivate *Cryptosporidium* oocysts.

Recreational water use is a major route for *Cryptosporidium* transmission because of the organism's extreme chlorine tolerance, low infectious dose, immediate infectiousness upon excretion, and high pathogen excretion volume, in addition to poor swimmer hygiene (eg, swimming when ill with diarrhea) and swimmer behavior (eg, ingesting recreational water). One or more swimmers who are ill with diarrhea can contaminate large volumes of water and expose large numbers of swimmers to *Cryptosporidium* and, if pool disinfection is inadequate, other pathogens. Outbreaks associated with treated recreational water venues generally can be prevented and controlled through a combination of proper pH, adequate disinfectant concentration, and improved swimmer hygiene and behavior. Pediatricians and parents of young children can learn more about healthy swimming at **www.cdc.gov/healthywater/swimming/**. Over-the-counter test strips can be purchased to check the level of free chlorine (the active form of chlorine that inactivates pathogens) and pH of swimming pool or splash pad water. The CDC also publishes the Model Aquatic Health Code (**www.cdc.gov/mahc/editions/current.html**), which provides detailed and regularly updated guidance to reduce risk of RWI and injury through the design, construction, operation, and management of treated recreational water venues open to the public.

Control Measures

Swimming is generally a healthy and safe means of physical activity. Transmission of infectious pathogens that cause most RWIs can be prevented by reducing contamination of recreational water venues and limiting exposure to contaminated water. Pediatricians should counsel families as follows:

- Regularly test pools and splash pads to ensure that the water's free chlorine or bromine (another commonly used disinfectant) concentration and the pH are correct and safe:
  - Free chlorine concentration should be at least 1 part per million (ppm).
  - Bromine concentration should be at least 3 ppm.
  - pH should be 7.0 to 7.8.

- Do not go into recreational water when ill with diarrhea.
  - After complete cessation of symptoms, people who had diarrhea attributable to *Cryptosporidium* species also should avoid recreational water activities for an additional 2 weeks. This is because of prolonged excretion of infectious *Cryptosporidium* oocysts after complete cessation of symptoms, the potential for intermittent exacerbations of diarrhea, and the increased transmission potential in treated recreational water venues (eg, swimming pools) because of the organism's extreme chlorine tolerance.
  - After cessation of symptoms, children who had diarrhea attributable to other potential waterborne pathogens (eg, *Shigella* species) and who are incontinent should avoid recreational water activities for 1 additional week (or as advised by local public health authorities).
- Avoid ingestion of recreational water.
- Do not go into recreational water with open wounds (eg, from surgery or a piercing), because wounds can serve as portals of entry for pathogens.
- Stay out of the water in lakes, rivers, or oceans if:
  - Beaches are closed or an advisory is posted for high bacterial levels or other conditions, such as sewage spills or harmful algal blooms.
  - Recent heavy rainfall has occurred in the previous 48 to 72 hours (rain can wash contaminants from the land, like septic tank overflows or animal feces, into the water).
  - If discharge pipes are draining into or around the water.
  - Fish or other animals in or near the water are dead.
  - Water is discolored, malodorous, foamy, scummy, or cloudy (cloudier than usual).
- The only certain way to prevent *N fowleri* infection caused by swimming is to refrain from water-related activities in warm freshwater. To reduce exposure risk to *N fowleri:*
  - Use nose clips, hold nose shut, or keep head above water when taking part in water-related activities in bodies of warm freshwater.
  - Avoid putting your head under water in hot springs or other untreated thermal waters.
  - Avoid water-related activities in warm freshwater during periods of high temperature.
- To reduce exposure risk to harmful blooms caused by cyanobacteria or microalgae:
  - Check for local or state advisories (may be found on websites of local environmental or health departments; also see **www.epa.gov/cyanohabs/ state-habs-monitoring-programs-and-resources**).
  - Avoid water that contains algal blooms (when in doubt, stay out).
  - Keep children and pets from drinking or playing in discolored, malodorous, foamy, or scummy water.
  - Get out and rinse off with clean tap water as soon as possible after swimming in water that might contain a harmful bloom.
  - Rinse off pets, especially dogs, immediately if they swim in discolored, malodorous, foamy, or scummy water. Do not let pets lick the algae off their fur.
- Practice good swimmer hygiene:
  - Shower with soap and water for at least 1 minute before entering recreational water.
  - Instruct children not to urinate or defecate in the water.

- Take children to the bathroom every hour. Check diapered children every hour and change diapers in a bathroom or diaper changing area—not waterside—to help keep infectious agents, urine, and feces out of the water. Swim diapers and swim pants, although able to hold in some solid feces, do not prevent leakage of pathogens such as *Cryptosporidium* species into the water.
- Wash hands with soap and water after using the bathroom and changing diapers and before consumption of food and drink.

Healthy swimming promotion materials are available at **www.cdc.gov/ healthywater/swimming/materials/index.html.**

"Swimmer's Ear"/Acute Otitis Externa

Participation in recreational water activities can predispose children to infections of the external auditory canal. Acute otitis externa (AOE) or "swimmer's ear," one of the most common infections encountered by clinicians and responsible for an estimated 4.7 million illnesses annually in the United States,[1] is a diffuse inflammation of the external auditory canal and is usually attributable to bacterial infection. Recreational water activities, showering, and bathing can introduce water into the ear canal, wash away protective ear wax, increase the pH, and cause maceration of the thin skin of the ear canal, thus predisposing the ear canal to infection. AOE is most common among children 5 to 14 years of age but can occur in all age groups, including adults. A marked seasonality is observed, with cases peaking during the summer months. Warm, humid environments and frequent submersion of the head while swimming are risk factors for AOE.

Bacterial infections cause 90% of AOE cases. The 2 most common bacterial causes of AOE are *Pseudomonas aeruginosa* and *Staphylococcus aureus*. Many cases are polymicrobial. Fungal pathogens (eg, *Aspergillus* species and *Candida* species) are responsible for a minority (10%) of AOE cases. Cultures of swab specimens taken from the external ear canal in AOE may not be entirely diagnostic because these can reflect normal ear canal flora or pathogenic organisms.

AOE readily responds to treatment with topical antimicrobial agents with or without a topical steroid. Unless the infection has spread to surrounding tissues or the patient has complicating factors (eg, has diabetes or is immunocompromised), topical treatment alone should be sufficient, and systemic antimicrobials usually are not required. Polymyxin B sulfate/neomycin sulfate, gentamicin sulfate, and ciprofloxacin for 7 to 10 days are topical antibiotic agents used commonly. If clinical improvement is not noted by 48 to 72 hours, the patient should be reevaluated for possible foreign body obstruction of the canal, noncompliance with therapy, or alternate diagnoses, such as contact dermatitis or traumatic cellulitis. If delivery of topical antibiotics is being impeded by drainage obstructing the external auditory canal, placement of a cellulose wick or referral to an otolaryngologist for aural toilet should be considered. Topical agents that have the potential for ototoxicity (eg, gentamicin, neomycin, agents with a low pH, hydrocortisone-neomycin-polymyxin) should not be used in children with tympanostomy tubes or a perforated tympanic membrane. Patients with AOE should avoid submerging their head in water for 7 to 10 days, but competitive

---

[1] Collier SA, Deng L, Adam EA, et al. Estimate of burden and direct healthcare cost of infectious waterborne disease in the United States. *Emerg Infect Dis.* 2021;27(1):140-149

swimmers might be able to return to the pool if pain has resolved and they use well-fitting ear plugs.

All swimmers should be instructed to keep their ear canals as dry as possible. This can be accomplished by covering the opening of the external auditory canal with a bathing cap or by using ear plugs or molds. Following swimming or showering, the ears should be dried thoroughly using a towel or a hairdryer on the lowest heat and fan setting.

If a person experiences recurring episodes of AOE, consideration can be given to use of antimicrobial otic drops after recreational water exposure as an additional preventive measure. Commercial ear-drying agents are available for use as directed, or a 1:1 mixture of acetic acid (white vinegar) and isopropanol (rubbing alcohol) may be placed in the external ear canal after swimming or showering to restore the proper acidic pH to the ear canal and to dry residual water. Otic drying agents should not be used in the presence of tympanostomy tubes, tympanic membrane perforation, AOE infection, or ear drainage.

Additional information on prevention of otitis externa is available at **www.cdc. gov/healthywater/swimming/swimmers/rwi/ear-infections.html.**

Summaries of Infectious Diseases

Actinomycosis

CLINICAL MANIFESTATIONS: Actinomycosis results from pathogen introduction following a breakdown in mucocutaneous protective barriers. Spread within the host is by direct invasion of adjacent tissues, typically forming sinus tracts that cross tissue planes. The most common species causing human disease is *Actinomyces israelii.*

There are 3 common anatomic sites of infection. **Cervicofacial** is most common, often occurring after tooth extraction, oral surgery, or other oral/facial trauma or even from carious teeth. Localized pain and induration may progress to cervical abscess and "woody hard" nodular lesions ("lumpy jaw"), which can develop draining sinus tracts, usually at the angle of the jaw or in the submandibular region. Infection may contribute to recurrent or persistent tonsillitis. **Thoracic** disease most commonly is secondary to aspiration of oropharyngeal secretions but can be an extension of cervicofacial infection. It occurs rarely after esophageal disruption secondary to surgery or nonpenetrating trauma. Thoracic presentation includes pneumonia, which can be complicated by abscesses, empyema, and rarely, pleurodermal sinuses. Focal or multifocal mediastinal and pulmonary masses may be mistaken for tumors. **Abdominal** actinomycosis usually is attributable to penetrating trauma or intestinal perforation. The appendix and cecum are the most common sites; signs and symptoms can mimic appendicitis. Slowly developing masses may simulate abdominal or retroperitoneal neoplasms. Intra-abdominal abscesses and peritoneal-dermal draining sinuses occur eventually. Chronic localized disease often forms draining sinus tracts with purulent discharge. **Other sites** of infection include the liver, pelvis (in some cases, linked to use of intrauterine devices), heart, testicles, and brain (usually associated with a primary pulmonary focus). Noninvasive primary cutaneous actinomycosis has occurred. *Actinomyces* infections have been associated with adverse pregnancy outcomes and cases of neonatal bacteremia have been described.

ETIOLOGY: *A israelii* and at least 5 other *Actinomyces* species cause human disease. All are slow-growing, microaerophilic or facultative anaerobic, gram-positive, filamentous branching bacilli. They can be part of normal oral, gastrointestinal tract, or vaginal flora. *Actinomyces* species frequently are copathogens in tissues harboring multiple anaerobic and/or aerobic species. Isolation of *Aggregatibacter (Actinobacillus) actinomycetemcomitans,* frequently detected with *Actinomyces* species, may predict the presence of actinomycosis.

EPIDEMIOLOGY: *Actinomyces* species occur worldwide, being components of endogenous oral and gastrointestinal tract flora. *Actinomyces* species are opportunistic pathogens in the setting of disrupted mucosal barriers. Infection is uncommon in infants and children, with 80% of cases occurring in adults. The male-to-female ratio in children is 1.5:1. Although microbiologically confirmed infections caused by *Actinomyces* species now are less common, there are reports in patients who have undergone transplantation or are receiving biologics.

The **incubation period** varies from several days to several years.

DIAGNOSTIC TESTS: Microscopic demonstration of beaded, branched, gram-positive bacilli in purulent material or tissue specimens suggests the diagnosis. Only specimens from normally sterile sites should be submitted for culture. Specimens must be obtained, transported, and cultured anaerobically on semiselective (kanamycin/vancomycin) media such as the modified Thayer-Martin agar or buffered charcoal yeast extract (BCYE) agar. Acid-fast testing can distinguish *Actinomyces* species, which are acid-fast negative, from *Nocardia* species, which are variably acid-fast positive staining. Yellow "sulfur granules" visualized microscopically or macroscopically in drainage or loculations of purulent material suggest the diagnosis. A Gram stain of "sulfur granules" discloses a dense aggregate of bacterial filaments mixed with inflammatory debris. *A israelii* forms "spiderlike" microcolonies on culture medium after 48 hours. *Actinomyces* species can be identified in tissue specimens using a nucleic acid amplification test (NAAT), matrix-assisted laser desorption/ionization time-of-flight (MALDI-TOF) mass spectrometry, or sequencing of the 16s rRNA.

TREATMENT: Management of actinomycosis is informed exclusively by case reports, case series, and in vitro susceptibility testing. Initial therapy should include intravenous penicillin G or ampicillin for 4 to 6 weeks followed by high doses of oral penicillin (up to 2 g/day for adults), usually for a total of 6 to 12 months depending on the extent of disease and success of surgical management (when indicated). Surgical drainage often is a necessary adjunct to medical management and may shorten duration of antimicrobial therapy. Treatment for mild disease can be initiated with oral therapy and may not require as long a treatment duration. Amoxicillin and doxycycline are alternative choices. Amoxicillin/clavulanate, piperacillin/tazobactam, ceftriaxone, clarithromycin, linezolid, and imipenem/meropenem also show high activity in vitro but may be unnecessarily broad-spectrum. All *Actinomyces* species appear to be resistant to ciprofloxacin and metronidazole.

INFECTION PREVENTION AND CONTROL MEASURES IN HEALTH CARE SETTINGS: Standard precautions are recommended. Person-to-person spread does not occur.

CONTROL MEASURES: Appropriate oral hygiene, regular dental care, and careful cleansing of wounds, including human bite wounds, can prevent infection.

Adenovirus Infections

CLINICAL MANIFESTATIONS: Adenovirus infections of the upper respiratory tract are common and often subclinical; when symptomatic, adenoviruses may cause common cold symptoms, pharyngitis, tonsillitis, otitis media, or pharyngoconjunctival fever. Adenoviruses occasionally cause a pertussis-like syndrome, croup, bronchiolitis, influenza-like illness, exudative tonsillitis, severe hepatitis, and hemorrhagic cystitis. Ocular adenovirus infections may present as follicular conjunctivitis or as epidemic keratoconjunctivitis. Enteric adenoviruses are an important cause of childhood gastroenteritis. Life-threatening disseminated infection, lower respiratory infection (eg, severe pneumonia, bronchiolitis obliterans), hepatitis, meningitis, and encephalitis occur occasionally, especially among young infants and immunocompromised people.

ETIOLOGY: Adenoviruses are double-stranded, nonenveloped DNA viruses of the *Adenoviridae* family and *Mastadenovirus* genus, with more than 100 recognized types and multiple genetic variants divided into 7 species (A–G) that infect humans. Some adenovirus types are associated primarily with respiratory tract disease (types 1–5, 7, 14, 21, and 55), epidemic keratoconjunctivitis (types 8, 37, 53, 54, and 64 [previously 19a]), or gastroenteritis (types 40 and 41). Severe respiratory infections are often attributable to adenovirus types 3, 7, and 14.

EPIDEMIOLOGY: Infection in children can occur at any age. Adenoviruses causing respiratory tract infections usually are transmitted by respiratory tract secretions through person-to-person contact, airborne droplets, and fomites. Adenoviruses are hardy viruses, can survive on environmental surfaces for long periods, and are not easily inactivated by many disinfectants. Outbreaks of febrile respiratory tract illness attributable to adenoviruses can be a significant problem in military trainees, college students, children attending overnight camps, patients hospitalized in hematopoietic cell transplant units, and residents of long-term care facilities. Community outbreaks of adenovirus-associated pharyngoconjunctival fever have been attributed to water exposure from contaminated swimming pools and fomites, such as shared towels. Health care-associated transmission of adenoviral infections can occur in hospitals, residential institutions, and nursing homes from exposures to infected health care personnel, patients, or contaminated equipment. Adenovirus infections in solid organ transplant recipients can occur from donor tissues as well as endogenous reactivation. Epidemic keratoconjunctivitis commonly occurs by direct contact and has been associated with equipment used during eye examinations. Enteric strains of adenoviruses are transmitted by the fecal-oral route.

Adenoviruses do not demonstrate the marked seasonality of other respiratory tract viruses and instead circulate throughout the year. Enteric disease also occurs year-round and primarily affects children younger than 4 years. Adenovirus infections are most communicable during the first few days of an acute illness, but persistent and intermittent shedding for longer periods, even months, can occur, especially among people with weakened immune systems. In healthy people, infection with one adenovirus type should confer type-specific immunity or at least lessen symptoms associated with reinfection, which forms the basis of adenovirus vaccines used in military populations (see Control Measures).

The **incubation period** for respiratory tract infection varies from 2 to 14 days; for gastroenteritis, the **incubation period** is 3 to 10 days.

DIAGNOSTIC TESTS: Methods for diagnosis of adenovirus infection include molecular detection, isolation in cell culture, and antigen detection. Molecular assays (eg, nucleic acid amplification tests [NAATs]) are the preferred diagnostic method for detection of adenoviruses, and these assays are widely available. However, the persistent and intermittent shedding that commonly follows an acute adenoviral infection can complicate the clinical interpretation of a positive molecular test result. Quantitative adenovirus assays can be useful for management of immunocompromised patients, such as hematopoietic cell and solid organ transplant recipients. Adenoviruses associated with respiratory tract and ocular disease can be isolated by culture from respiratory specimens (eg, nasopharyngeal swab, oropharyngeal swab, nasal wash, sputum) and eye secretions in standard susceptible cell lines. Rapid antigen-detection techniques, including immunofluorescence and enzyme immunoassay, have been used to detect virus in respiratory tract secretions, conjunctival swab specimens, and stool, but these methods lack sensitivity. Adenovirus typing by molecular methods is available from some reference laboratories. Although its clinical utility is limited, typing can help establish an etiologic association with disease and to investigate clusters of adenovirus-associated illness. Serodiagnosis is used primarily for epidemiologic studies and has no clinical utility.

TREATMENT: Treatment of adenovirus infection is primarily supportive, with most adenoviral infections in otherwise healthy persons being self-limited. Symptomatic infection in immunocompromised patients, however, should be managed with reduced immunosuppression, when feasible, and consideration of use of antiviral agents, with options presented below. For immunocompromised patients with asymptomatic detection of adenovirus DNA in the blood, there is no consensus regarding optimal management. This scenario is often encountered in the transplant setting in which patients are monitored post-transplant with serial quantitative NAATs. The detection of defined thresholds of blood DNA in this setting might allow for risk-based preemptive treatment strategies including reduced immunosuppression, when appropriate, and antiviral agents.

There are no antivirals approved by the US Food and Drug Administration for the treatment of adenovirus infections. Intravenous cidofovir has emerged as the preferred antiviral agent for treatment of severe, progressive, or disseminated adenovirus diseases in immunocompromised hosts, but its utilization is limited by its associated nephrotoxicity and myelotoxicity and there is no consensus on the optimal dose. Brincidofovir, an oral prodrug of cidofovir, was evaluated in a randomized controlled trial of pediatric and adult hematopoietic cell transplant recipients, and although brincidofovir-treated subjects had a tendency to lower odds of treatment failure and all-cause mortality compared with the placebo recipients, the differences were not statistically significant. Ribavirin has shown inconsistent therapeutic benefit in case reports and a small cohort study.

There is some evidence that ganciclovir has inhibitory effects at concentrations achievable when applied topically against some adenovirus types causing keratoconjunctivitis, raising its potential role as a topical agent in this setting. For conjunctival disease, topical cidofovir has been shown to be effective in the eradication of actively replicating viruses and limiting the duration of symptoms. However, further study is needed to determine the long-term adverse effects of both topical ganciclovir and topical cidofovir.

Transplant patients with severe hypogammaglobulinemia at the time of active adenovirus infection might benefit from immune globulin administration. Adoptive transfer of adenovirus-specific T-lymphocytes is under investigation for the treatment of severe adenovirus diseases in hematopoietic cell transplant recipients, but there are limited data in solid organ transplant recipients and other populations.

INFECTION PREVENTION AND CONTROL MEASURES IN HEALTH CARE SETTINGS: In addition to standard precautions for young children with respiratory tract infections, contact and droplet precautions are indicated for the duration of hospitalization. In immunocompromised patients, contact and droplet precautions should be extended because of the likelihood of prolonged shedding of the virus. For patients with conjunctivitis and for diapered and incontinent children with adenoviral gastroenteritis, contact precautions are indicated for the duration of illness.

CONTROL MEASURES: Appropriate hand hygiene, respiratory hygiene, and cough etiquette should be followed. However, adenoviruses are difficult to inactivate with alcohol-based gels, and they may remain viable on skin, fomites, and environmental surfaces for extended periods. Thus, assiduous adherence to hand hygiene and use of disposable gloves when caring for infected patients are recommended.

Children who are in group child care, particularly children from 6 months through 2 years of age, are at increased risk of adenoviral respiratory tract infections and gastroenteritis. Effective measures for preventing spread of adenovirus infection in group child care settings have not been determined, but frequent hand hygiene is recommended. If 2 or more children in a group child care setting develop conjunctivitis in the same period of time, advice should be sought from the health consultant of the program or the state health department.

Adequate chlorination of swimming pools is recommended to prevent pharyngoconjunctival fever. Epidemic keratoconjunctivitis associated with ophthalmologic practice can be difficult to control and requires use of single-dose medication dispensing and strict attention to hand hygiene and instrument sterilization procedures. Health care professionals with known or suspected adenoviral conjunctivitis should avoid direct patient contact until symptoms have resolved.

A live, nonattenuated, oral adenovirus vaccine for types 4 and 7 (2 oral tablets, 1 for each of the 2 strains) is licensed by the US Food and Drug Administration for prevention of febrile acute respiratory tract disease among persons 17 through 50 years of age. The vaccine is currently only approved for use in the US military.

Amebiasis

CLINICAL MANIFESTATIONS: Most individuals infected with *Entamoeba histolytica* have asymptomatic noninvasive intestinal tract carriage. When present, symptoms associated with *E histolytica* infection generally include cramps, watery or bloody diarrhea, and weight loss. Occasionally, the parasite may spread to other organs, most commonly the liver (liver abscess), in which case fever and right upper quadrant pain are common. Disease is more severe in the very young, the elderly, malnourished people, pregnant individuals, and people who receive corticosteroids. People with symptomatic intestinal amebiasis generally have gradual onset of symptoms over 1 to 3 weeks. The mildest form of intestinal tract disease is nondysenteric colitis. Amebic dysentery is the most common clinical manifestation of amebiasis and generally includes diarrhea with either gross or microscopic blood or mucous in the stool, lower abdominal pain, and tenesmus. Weight loss is common because of the gradual onset, but fever occurs only in a minority of patients (8%–38%). Symptoms may be chronic, with periods of diarrhea and intestinal spasms alternating with periods of constipation. The presentation may mimic that of inflammatory bowel disease. Progressive involvement of the colon may produce toxic megacolon, fulminant colitis, ulceration of the colon and perianal area, and rarely, perforation. Colonic perforation may occur at multiple sites and has a high fatality rate. Progression may occur in patients treated inappropriately with corticosteroids or antimotility drugs. An amebic granuloma (ameboma) may form as an annular lesion of the colon and may present as a palpable mass on physical examination. Amebomas can occur in any area of the colon but are most common in the cecum and may be mistaken for colonic carcinoma. Amebomas usually resolve with antiamebic therapy and do not require surgery.

Extraintestinal disease occurs in a small proportion of patients. The liver is the most common extraintestinal site, and infection may spread from there to the pleural space, lungs, and pericardium. Liver abscess may be acute, with fever, abdominal pain, tachypnea, liver tenderness, and hepatomegaly, or may be chronic, with weight loss and vague abdominal symptoms. Liver abscess can also be asymptomatic and only discovered on abdominal imaging performed for other reasons. Rupture of abscesses into the abdomen or chest may lead to death. Infection also may spread directly from the colon to the genitourinary tract and the skin. The organism may spread hematogenously to the brain and other areas of the body. Evidence of recent or concurrent intestinal tract infection usually is absent in extraintestinal disease.

ETIOLOGY: The genus *Entamoeba* includes 6 species that live in the human intestine. Four of these species are identical morphologically: *E histolytica, Entamoeba dispar, Entamoeba moshkovskii,* and *Entamoeba bangladeshi. Dientamoeba fragilis* also can lead to asymptomatic infection and intraluminal intestinal disease. Not all *Entamoeba* species are virulent. *E dispar* and *Entamoeba coli* generally are recognized as commensals. Although *E moshkovskii* generally was believed to be nonpathogenic, it may be associated with diarrhea in infants. The pathogenic potential of *E bangladeshi* is not clear. *Entamoeba* and *Dientamoeba* organisms are excreted as cysts or trophozoites in stool of infected people.

EPIDEMIOLOGY: *E histolytica* can be found worldwide but is more prevalent in people of lower socioeconomic status who live in resource-limited countries, where prevalence of amebic infection may be as high as 50% in some communities. Groups at increased risk of infection in industrialized countries include immigrants from or long-term visitors to areas with endemic infection, institutionalized people, and men who have sex with men. Intestinal and asymptomatic infection are distributed equally across the sexes, but incidence of invasive disease, especially liver abscess, is significantly higher in male adults, possibly because of a male susceptibility to invasive disease.

E histolytica is transmitted via ingestion of infective amebic cysts, through fecally contaminated food or water, or oral-anal sexual practices. Transmission also can occur via direct rectal inoculation through colonic irrigation devices. Ingested cysts, which are unaffected by gastric acid, undergo excystation in the alkaline small intestine and produce trophozoites that can cause invasive disease in the colon. Cysts that develop subsequently are the source of transmission, especially from asymptomatic cyst excreters. Infected patients excrete cysts intermittently, sometimes for years if untreated. Cysts can remain viable in the environment for weeks to months and are relatively resistant to chlorine. Ingestion of a single cyst is sufficient to cause disease.

The **incubation period** is variable, ranging from a few days to months or years, but commonly is 2 to 4 weeks for colitis and longer for amebic liver abscess.

DIAGNOSTIC TESTS: Intestinal amebiasis can be diagnosed by molecular tests, direct microscopy, and antigen detection tests. Stool nucleic acid amplification tests (NAATs) have the highest sensitivity and specificity, are available in US Food and Drug Administration (FDA)-approved multiplex assays, and can differentiate *E histolytica* from other *Entamoeba* species. Traditionally, diagnosis of intestinal tract infection was made by identifying trophozoites or cysts in stool specimens, either on wet mount or after fixing and staining. This technique is still used in some laboratories, but it is labor intensive, its sensitivity is lower than for NAATs, and it requires review of multiple stool samples. Microscopy also does not differentiate between *E histolytica* and less pathogenic species, although trophozoites containing ingested red blood cells are more likely to be *E histolytica*. Antigen test kits are available in some clinical laboratories for testing of *E histolytica* directly from stool specimens. Examination of biopsy specimens, endoscopy scrapings (not swabs), and abscess aspirates using microscopy or antigen detection typically is not fruitful; a NAAT is preferred, when available but is only FDA approved for stool specimens. Some monoclonal antibody-based antigen detection assays also can differentiate *E histolytica* from other *Entamoeba* species. *D fragilis* is diagnosed by microscopy.

The indirect hemagglutination (IHA) test has been replaced by commercially available enzyme immunoassay (EIA) kits for routine serodiagnosis of amebiasis, especially in countries without endemic disease. The EIA detects antibody specific for *E histolytica* in ≥95% of patients with extraintestinal amebiasis, 70% of patients with active intestinal tract infection, and 10% of asymptomatic people who are passing cysts of *E histolytica*. Patients may continue to have positive serologic test results even after adequate therapy. In countries without endemic disease, diagnosis of an *E histolytica* liver abscess or other extraintestinal infections typically is made by a combination of serologic testing and radiologic evaluation, because stool testing by microscopy or NAAT is often negative.

Ultrasonography, computed tomography, and magnetic resonance imaging can identify liver abscesses presumptively; those caused by *E histolytica* typically are solitary, homogenous, and hypoechoic on ultrasonography. Imaging also can identify other extraintestinal sites of infection.

TREATMENT: Treatment should be provided to all patients with *E histolytica*, including those who are asymptomatic, given the propensity of this organism to spread among family members and other contacts and to cause invasive infection. In settings where tests to distinguish species are not available, treatment should be administered to symptomatic people based on positive results of microscopic examination. Corticosteroids and antimotility drugs should not be used, because they can worsen symptoms and aggravate the disease process. The following treatment regimens and follow-up are recommended:

- **Asymptomatic cyst excreters (intraluminal infections):** treat with an intraluminal amebicide alone (paromomycin, iodoquinol [also known as diiodohydroxyquinoline], or diloxanide furoate). (See Table 4.11, Drugs for Parasitic Infections, p 1068). Metronidazole and tinidazole are not effective against cysts and these agents are not necessary for asymptomatic excreters.
- **Patients with invasive colitis manifesting as mild, moderate, or severe intestinal tract symptoms or extraintestinal disease (including liver abscess):** treat with a tissue agent, metronidazole or tinidazole (See Table 4.11, Drugs for Parasitic Infections, p 1068), followed by an intraluminal amebicide at the same doses as for asymptomatic infection. Nitazoxanide or secnidazole also may be effective as tissue agents for mild to moderate intestinal amebiasis, although they are not approved by the FDA for this indication.
- **Additional considerations in patients with hepatic abscess, pleural or pericardial abscess, or other severe complications:** In most cases of liver abscess, drainage is not required and does not speed recovery. Percutaneous or surgical aspiration of large liver abscesses occasionally may be required when response of

the abscess to medical therapy is unsatisfactory or there is risk of rupture. Although patients typically improve symptomatically within days, it may take months for a liver abscess to resolve on ultrasonography. Rupture into the peritoneal or pleural space usually requires drainage. For patients who have peritonitis attributable to intestinal perforation, broad-spectrum antibacterial therapy should be used in addition to an amebicide. In cases with toxic megacolon, colectomy may be necessary.

Follow-up stool examination is recommended after completion of therapy for intestinal disease, because no pharmacologic regimen is completely effective in eradicating intestinal tract infection. Household members and other suspected contacts should have stool examinations performed and should be treated if results are positive for *E histolytica*.

E dispar and *Entamoeba coli* generally are considered nonpathogenic and do not necessarily require treatment. The pathogenic significance of *E moshkovskii* and *E bangladeshi* is unclear; treatment of symptomatic infection is reasonable. *D fragilis* is treated with iodoquinol, paromomycin, or metronidazole.

INFECTION PREVENTION AND CONTROL MEASURES IN HEALTH CARE SETTINGS: Standard precautions are considered adequate for hospitalized patients; health care-associated transmission is rare.

CONTROL MEASURES: Careful hand hygiene after defecation, sanitary disposal of fecal material, and treatment of drinking water will control spread of infection. Sexual transmission may be controlled by use of condoms and avoidance of sexual activity with those who have diarrhea or recently recovered from diarrhea. Because of the risk of shedding infectious cysts, people diagnosed with amebiasis should refrain from using recreational water venues (eg, swimming pools, water parks) until after their course of luminal chemotherapy is completed and diarrhea has resolved. Some states prohibit return to work or school for food handlers or children until symptoms have resolved.

Amebic Meningoencephalitis and Keratitis
(*Naegleria fowleri, Acanthamoeba* species, and *Balamuthia mandrillaris*)

CLINICAL MANIFESTATIONS: *Naegleria fowleri* can cause a rapidly progressive, almost always fatal, primary amebic meningoencephalitis (PAM). Early symptoms include fever, headache, nausea, and vomiting. The illness progresses rapidly to signs of meningoencephalitis, including nuchal rigidity, lethargy, confusion, personality changes, altered level of consciousness, and rarely, disturbances of smell and taste. Seizures are common, and death generally occurs within a week of onset of symptoms. No distinct clinical features differentiate this disease from fulminant bacterial meningitis other than history of freshwater exposure.

Granulomatous amebic encephalitis (GAE) caused by *Acanthamoeba* species and *Balamuthia mandrillaris* has a more insidious onset than PAM and develops as a subacute or chronic disease. In general, patients with GAE die several weeks to months after onset of symptoms. Signs and symptoms may include altered mental status, personality changes, seizures, headaches, ataxia, cranial nerve palsies, hemiparesis, and other focal neurologic deficits. Fever often is low grade and intermittent. The course may resemble that of a bacterial brain abscess or a brain tumor. Chronic granulomatous skin lesions (pustules, nodules, ulcers) may be present with or without central nervous system (CNS) involvement, particularly in patients who are immunocompromised. Lesions may be present for months before brain involvement in some cases. *Acanthamoeba* also can cause rhinosinusitis, which can present alone or with skin or CNS involvement.

The most common symptoms of amebic keratitis, a vision-threatening infection usually caused by *Acanthamoeba* species, are eye pain (often out of proportion to clinical signs), photophobia, tearing, and foreign body sensation. Characteristic clinical findings include radial keratoneuritis and stromal ring infiltrate. *Acanthamoeba* keratitis generally follows an indolent course and initially may resemble herpes simplex or bacterial keratitis; delay in diagnosis is associated with worse outcome.

ETIOLOGY: *N fowleri*, *Acanthamoeba* species, and *B mandrillaris* are free-living amebae that exist as motile, infectious trophozoites and environmentally hardy cysts.

EPIDEMIOLOGY: *N fowleri* is found in warm fresh water and moist soil. Most infections with *N fowleri* have been associated with swimming in natural bodies of warm fresh water, such as ponds, lakes, and hot springs, but other sources have included tap water from household plumbing systems and geothermal sources as well as poorly chlorinated swimming pools, splash pads, and municipal water. Disease has been reported worldwide but is uncommon. In the United States, infection occurs primarily in the summer and usually affects children and young adults. The recent northward extension of reported cases may be the result of climatic changes. Disease has followed use of tap water for ritual or therapeutic nasal irrigation or exposures related to recreational activities (eg, tap water used for a backyard waterslide). Trophozoites of the amebae invade the brain directly from the nose along the olfactory nerves via the cribriform plate.

Acanthamoeba species are distributed worldwide and have been found in soil; dust; cooling towers of electric and nuclear power plants; heating, ventilating, and air conditioning units; fresh and brackish water; whirlpool baths; and physiotherapy pools. The environmental niche of *B mandrillaris* is not delineated clearly, although it has been isolated from soil. CNS infection attributable to *Acanthamoeba* species occurs primarily in debilitated and immunocompromised people. Some patients, and nearly all reported children infected with *B mandrillaris*, have had no demonstrable underlying disease or defect. CNS infection by both amebae probably occurs most commonly by inhalation or direct contact with contaminated soil or water. The primary foci of these infections most likely are respiratory tract or skin, followed by hematogenous spread to the brain. *Acanthamoeba* rhinosinusitis and GAE have been associated with nasal rinsing with tap water. Fatal encephalitis caused by *Balamuthia* species transmitted by a donated organ has been reported.

Acanthamoeba keratitis occurs primarily in people who wear contact lenses,[1] although it also has been associated with corneal trauma. Poor contact lens hygiene and/or disinfection practices as well as swimming with contact lenses are risk factors.

The **incubation period** for *N fowleri* infection ranges from 1 to 9 days.

The **incubation periods** for *Acanthamoeba* and *Balamuthia* GAE are unknown. It is believed to take several weeks or months to develop the first symptoms of CNS disease following exposure to the amebae. Patients exposed to *Balamuthia* through solid organ transplantation can develop symptoms of *Balamuthia* GAE more quickly—within a few weeks.

The **incubation period** for *Acanthamoeba* keratitis is unknown but believed to range from several days to several weeks.

[1] Centers for Disease Control and Prevention. Contact lens–related corneal infections—United States, 2005–2015. *MMWR Morb Mortal Wkly Rep.* 2016;65(32):817–820

DIAGNOSTIC TESTS: In *N fowleri* infection, computed tomography scans of the head without contrast are unremarkable or show only cerebral edema but with contrast might show meningeal enhancement of the basilar cisterns and sulci. These changes, however, are not specific for amebic infection. Cerebrospinal fluid (CSF) pressure usually is elevated (300 to >600 mm water), and CSF indices may show a polymorphonuclear pleocytosis, red blood cells, an increased protein concentration, and a normal to very low glucose concentration. Motile trophozoites may be visualized by microscopic examination of CSF on a wet mount. If structures resembling trophozoites are seen but no motility is observed, smears of CSF should be stained with Giemsa, trichrome, or Wright stains to verify the trophozoites. Gram staining is unhelpful in *N fowleri* CNS infection, because heat fixation may destroy amebae. Trophozoites, but not cysts, can be visualized in sections of brain during autopsy. Microscopic images containing suspicious amebic structures can be evaluated by the morphology experts at the Centers for Disease Control and Prevention (CDC)'s DPDx (Laboratory Identification of Parasites of Public Health Concern; **www.cdc.gov/dpdx/index.html**). Nucleic acid amplification tests (NAATs) and immunofluorescence assays performed on CSF and biopsy material to identify the organism are available through the CDC, as are consultation services for diagnosis and management (email: **parasites@cdc.gov**; telephone: 404-718-4745; after hours: 770-488-7100).

In infection with *Acanthamoeba* species and *B mandrillaris*, computed tomography and magnetic resonance imaging of the head may show single or multiple space-occupying, ring-enhancing lesions that can mimic brain abscesses, neurocysticercosis, tumors, cerebrovascular accidents, or other diseases. In GAE infections, CSF indices often are nonspecific but may include a lymphocytic pleocytosis and an increased protein concentration with normal or low glucose. Trophozoites are seen rarely in CSF and can be identified with Giemsa stain. Trophozoites and cysts can be visualized in sections of brain, skin, and other organs; in cases of *Acanthamoeba* keratitis, they also can be visualized in corneal scrapings and by confocal microscopy in vivo in the cornea on examination by an expert ophthalmologist. NAATs and immunofluorescence assays can be performed on clinical specimens to identify *Acanthamoeba* species and *Balamuthia* species; these tests are available through the CDC, as are consultation services for diagnosis and management (email: **parasites@cdc.gov**; telephone: 404-718-4745; after hours: 770-488-7100).

TREATMENT: The most current guidance for treatment of PAM can be found on the CDC website (**www.cdc.gov/parasites/naegleria/treatment-hcp.html**) or by contacting the CDC (email: **parasites@cdc.gov**; telephone: 404-718-4745; after hours: 770-488-7100). Early diagnosis and institution of combination high-dose drug therapy is believed to be important for optimizing outcome. If meningoencephalitis possibly caused by *N fowleri* is suspected, treatment should not be withheld pending confirmation. Presence of amebic organisms in CSF is valuable for probable diagnosis, but confirmatory diagnostic tests should be performed. Although an effective treatment regimen for PAM has not been identified, amphotericin B deoxycholate is the drug of choice in combination with other agents. In vitro testing indicates that *N fowleri* is highly susceptible to amphotericin B. Miltefosine, which is approved for treatment of leishmaniasis, has been used successfully to treat PAM caused by *N fowleri*. The CDC no longer provides miltefosine for treatment of free-living ameba infections; miltefosine is available commercially in the United States (**impavido.com**). There have been 4 US survivors of PAM, and on the basis of most recent cases, treatment with the combination of amphotericin B, azithromycin, fluconazole, miltefosine, and rifampin is recommended. These patients also received dexamethasone to control cerebral edema.

Effective treatment for infections caused by *Acanthamoeba* species and *B mandrillaris* has not been established. Several patients with *Acanthamoeba* GAE and *Acanthamoeba* cutaneous infections without CNS involvement have been treated successfully with a multidrug regimen consisting of fluconazole or ketoconazole, trimethoprim-sulfamethoxazole, and rifampin. Metronidazole may be added to this combination. Miltefosine has in vitro activity against *Acanthamoeba* infections and also may be considered as part of combination drug therapy for *Acanthamoeba* GAE. Other drugs that have been used include various combinations of pentamidine, sulfadiazine, and flucytosine, often with one or more of the above drugs. Caspofungin has in vitro activity against *Acanthamoeba* species, but clinical data are limited for its use in this infection. Isolated *Acanthamoeba* skin lesions can be treated with topical application of ketoconazole and/or chlorhexidine gluconate, but skin lesions often represent disseminated disease, particularly in immunocompromised patients, which requires systemic therapy. For patients with *B mandrillaris* encephalitis, successful treatment typically has required multiple drugs in combination—for example, pentamidine, sulfadiazine, fluconazole, either azithromycin or clarithromycin, and flucytosine. Surgical resection of the CNS lesions, accompanied by antimicrobial therapy, also has been reported to be successful. Miltefosine has amebicidal activity against *B mandrillaris* in vitro.

Patients with *Acanthamoeba* keratitis should be evaluated and treated by an ophthalmologist. Early diagnosis and therapy are important for a good outcome.

INFECTION PREVENTION AND CONTROL MEASURES IN HEALTH CARE SETTINGS: Standard precautions are recommended.

CONTROL MEASURES: People should assume that there is always a slight risk of developing PAM caused by *N fowleri* when entering warm fresh water. Only avoidance of such water-related activities can prevent *Naegleria* infection, although the risk might be reduced by taking measures to limit water exposure through known routes of entry, such as getting water up the nose (eg, diving, swimming underwater, doing handstands in water). Using tap water for sinus rinses generally is discouraged, but when used should be either previously boiled or properly filtered or labeled as sterile or distilled (additional information available at **www.cdc.gov/naegleria**).

Presently, no clearly defined recommendations are available to prevent GAE attributable to *Acanthamoeba* species or *B mandrillaris*; avoiding nasal rinsing with tap water is recommended.

To prevent *Acanthamoeba* keratitis, steps should be taken to avoid corneal trauma, such as the use of protective eyewear during high-risk activities, and contact lens users should maintain good contact lens hygiene and disinfection practices, use only sterile solutions as applicable, change lens cases frequently, and avoid swimming and showering while wearing contact lenses. Advice for people who wear contact lenses can be found on the CDC website (**www.cdc.gov/contactlenses**).[1]

---

[1] Centers for Disease Control and Prevention. Estimated burden of keratitis—United States, 2010. *MMWR Morb Mortal Wkly Rep.* 2014;63(45):1027-1030

Anthrax[1]

CLINICAL MANIFESTATIONS: Anthrax resulting from wild-type infection or secondary to a bioterror event can occur in multiple forms, depending on the route of infection: cutaneous, inhalation, ingestion, or injection.

Manifestations of anthrax are mainly from the 2 primary toxins, lethal toxin and edema toxin. **Cutaneous** anthrax accounts for 95% of all human infections and begins as a pruritic papule or vesicle that progresses over 2 to 6 days to an ulcerated lesion with subsequent formation of a central black eschar. The lesion characteristically is painless and has surrounding edema and hyperemia; there can be associated regional lymphadenopathy and lymphangitis. Some patients may have fever, malaise, and headache. Up to 30% of adults with cutaneous anthrax will progress to invasive, systemic disease.

Inhalation anthrax is a frequently lethal form of the disease and is a medical emergency. The initial presentation is nonspecific and usually includes fever, malaise, and nonproductive cough. Many patients also complain of chest pain, headache, nausea, vomiting, and abdominal pain; sweating may be profuse. Illness usually progresses to the fulminant phase within 2 to 5 days. Illness has been noted to sometimes be biphasic, with a period of improvement between prodromal symptoms and overwhelming illness. Significant vital sign abnormalities are often present early, and fulminant manifestations include hypotension, dyspnea, hypoxia, cyanosis, and shock. Most patients with inhalation anthrax fulfill sepsis criteria, and up to half develop meningitis. Imaging abnormalities noted at presentation include pleural effusions in most, widened mediastinum in up to half, and pulmonary infiltrates in many.

Ingestion anthrax usually presents as one of 2 clinical syndromes: gastrointestinal or oropharyngeal. Patients with the gastrointestinal form often have nausea, anorexia, vomiting, and fever that progresses to severe abdominal pain, often accompanied by marked ascites. Vomiting and diarrhea, which are not always present, may be bloody. Although gastrointestinal tract involvement at multiple sites may occur following hematogenous spread, the cecum and terminal ileum often are involved when the disease is primary. Patients with oropharyngeal anthrax may have dysphagia accompanied by posterior oropharyngeal necrotic ulcers. There may be marked, often unilateral neck swelling, regional lymphadenopathy, fever, and sepsis. Evidence of coagulopathy is common.

Injection anthrax occurs primarily among adult injection drug users, associated with anthrax-contaminated heroin, and has not been reported in children. Smoking and snorting contaminated heroin also have been identified as exposure routes.

Any route of infection can lead to bacteremia and sepsis. Patients with inhalation, ingestion, or injection anthrax should be considered to have systemic illness. Patients with cutaneous anthrax should be considered to have systemic illness if they develop tachycardia, tachypnea, hypotension, hyperthermia, hypothermia, or leukocytosis or have lesions that involve the head, neck, or upper torso or that are large, bullous, multiple, or surrounded by edema. Anthrax meningitis or hemorrhagic meningoencephalitis can occur in any patient with systemic illness and in patients without another apparent route of infection. With appropriate treatment and supportive care, case fatality rates range from <2% for cutaneous anthrax to 45% for inhalation anthrax and 92% for anthrax meningitis.

---

[1] **www.cdc.gov/anthrax/index.html**

ETIOLOGY: *Bacillus anthracis* is an aerobic, gram-positive, encapsulated, spore-forming, nonhemolytic, nonmotile rod. *B anthracis* has 3 major virulence factors: an antiphagocytic capsule and 2 exotoxins, called lethal toxin and edema toxin. The toxins are responsible for most of the morbidity associated with anthrax and clinical manifestations of hemorrhage, edema, and necrosis.

EPIDEMIOLOGY: Anthrax is a zoonotic disease that most commonly affects domestic and wild herbivores and occurs in many rural regions of the world. *B anthracis* spores can remain viable in the soil for decades, representing a potential source of infection for livestock or wildlife through ingestion of spore-contaminated vegetation or water. In exposed susceptible hosts, spores germinate to become vegetative bacteria. Wild-type infection of humans occurs through contact with infected animals or contaminated animal products, including carcasses, hides, hair, wool, meat, and bone meal. Outbreaks of ingestion anthrax have occurred after consumption of meat from infected animals. Historically, more than 95% of anthrax cases in the United States were cutaneous infections among animal handlers or mill workers. The incidence of wild-type human anthrax decreased in the United States from an estimated 130 cases annually in the early 1900s to 0 to 2 cases per year from 1979 through 2011. Only 2 anthrax cases (both cutaneous) were confirmed in the United States from 2012–2021. Cases of inhalation, cutaneous, and ingestion (gastrointestinal) anthrax have occurred in drum makers working with animal hides contaminated with *B anthracis* spores and in people participating in events where spore-contaminated drums were played. Severe soft tissue infections among injection heroin users, including cases with disseminated systemic infection, have been reported in Europe.

B anthracis is one of the agents most likely to be used as a biological weapon, because (1) its spores are highly stable; (2) spores can infect via the respiratory route; and (3) the resulting disease, inhalation anthrax, has a high fatality rate, even with appropriate treatment. In 1979, an accidental release of *B anthracis* spores from a military microbiology facility in the former Soviet Union resulted in at least 68 deaths. In 2001, 22 cases of anthrax (11 inhalation, 11 cutaneous) were identified in the United States after intentional contamination of the mail; 5 (45%) of the inhalation anthrax cases were fatal. In addition to aerosolization, *B anthracis* spores introduced into food products or water supplies could theoretically pose a risk to the public's health. Use of *B anthracis* in a biological attack would require immediate response and mobilization of public health resources (**www.cdc.gov/anthrax/bioterrorism/index.html**).[1]

Although the **incubation periods** for both cutaneous and ingestion anthrax are typically less than 1 week, rare cases for both have been reported more than 2 weeks after exposure. Because of spore dormancy (persistence of viable spores that have not yet germinated) and slow clearance of spores from the lungs, the **incubation period** for inhalation anthrax may be prolonged and has been reported to range from 2 days to 6 weeks in humans and up to 2 months in experimental nonhuman primates. Discharge from cutaneous lesions is potentially infectious, but person-to-person transmission has only rarely been reported, and other forms of anthrax have not been associated with person-to person transmission. Both inhalation and cutaneous anthrax have occurred in laboratory workers.

---

[1] Centers for Disease Control and Prevention. Clinical framework and medical countermeasure use during an anthrax mass-casualty incident: CDC recommendations. *MMWR Recomm Rep.* 2015;64(RR-4):1-22

DIAGNOSTIC TESTS: *B anthracis* is readily isolated on routine agar media (eg, sheep's blood agar) used in clinical laboratories and can be presumptively identified through traditional microbiological methods. Depending on the clinical presentation, Gram stain and culture should be performed on blood, pleural fluid, cerebrospinal fluid (CSF), swabs from lesions, and other clinical specimens. Whenever possible, specimens for these tests should be obtained before initiating antimicrobial therapy, because previous treatment with antimicrobial agents lessens the sensitivity of isolation by culture and visualization of the organism by Gram stain.

B anthracis isolates can be definitively identified using tests such as a nucleic acid amplification test (NAAT) via the Laboratory Response Network (LRN) in each state, accessed through state and local health departments. Additional diagnostic tests for anthrax are available through state health departments and the Centers for Disease Control and Prevention (CDC), including bacterial DNA detection in specimens by NAAT, tissue immunohistochemistry, an enzyme immunoassay that measures immunoglobulin G antibodies against *B anthracis* protective antigen in paired sera, and a matrix-assisted laser desorption/ionization–time-of-flight (MALDI-TOF) mass spectrometry assay measuring lethal factor activity in acute sera (**www.cdc.gov/ anthrax/lab-testing/index.html**).

Clinical evaluation of patients with suspected inhalation anthrax should include a chest radiograph and/or computed tomography scan to evaluate for pleural effusion, widened mediastinum, and/or pulmonary infiltrates. Because hemorrhagic meningitis is a common complication of systemic anthrax, cranial imaging followed by lumbar punctures should be performed whenever feasible to guide therapy on systemically ill patients with any type of anthrax.

For mass-exposure bioterrorism events, the CDC will provide current information on diagnosis, susceptibility, and suggestions for management at **www.cdc.gov/ anthrax/bioterrorism/index.html.**

TREATMENT[1,2]: No controlled trials in humans have been performed to validate current treatment recommendations for anthrax. A high index of suspicion and rapid administration of appropriate antibiotic therapy to people suspected of being infected, along with access to critical care support, are essential for effective treatment of anthrax. Consultation with an expert in infectious diseases is recommended.

For localized cutaneous anthrax (ie, lacking systemic systems), monotherapy may be used with oral first-line agents including ciprofloxacin, levofloxacin, doxycycline, or minocycline. If the isolate is known to be penicillin susceptible, amoxicillin and penicillin VK are alternatives. If the strain is beta-lactamase positive, amoxicillin/ clavulanate may be used. Details on dosing, alternative antibiotics, and use of anti-toxins are available.[1] If the localized cutaneous disease was naturally acquired, the regimen should continue for 7 to 10 days or until the patient is clinically stable; following this, if an aerosol exposure might have occurred (eg, bioterrorism-related or drum-incident) then patients should transition to a postexposure prophylaxis (PEP)

[1] Bower WA, Yu Y, Person MK, et al. CDC guidelines for the prevention and treatment of anthrax, 2023. *MMWR Recomm Rep.* 2023;72(RR-6):1-47

[2] Bower WA, Schiffer J, Atmar RL, et al. Use of anthrax vaccine in the United States: recommendations of the Advisory Committee on Immunization Practices, 2019. *MMWR Recomm Rep.* 2019;68(4):1-14

regimen. The total duration of treatment plus PEP should be 42 to 60 days from illness onset, depending on the patient's age and anthrax vaccine status (see Control Measures).

First-line treatment for systemic anthrax with or without meningitis includes combination intravenous therapy with 2 first-line agents from different antibiotic classes plus a protein synthesis (preferred if available) or RNA synthesis inhibitor. Empiric regimens can include ciprofloxacin (or levofloxacin) plus meropenem plus either linezolid or minocycline; or ciprofloxacin (or levofloxacin) plus meropenem plus rifampin. If the isolate is known to be susceptible to penicillin, ampicillin or penicillin G may be used plus a protein synthesis inhibitor (eg, linezolid, minocycline, or doxycycline). These patients are at high risk for meningitis. However, if it has been determined that meningitis is not present, the regimen can be simplified to be a first-line agent (eg, meropenem or ciprofloxacin) plus a protein synthesis inhibitor (eg, linezolid or doxycycline). Additional details on regimens, including first-line antibiotics, alternative antibiotics, and recommendations in cases of antibiotic shortages, are available.[1] Because of intrinsic resistance, cephalosporins and trimethoprim-sulfamethoxazole should not be used.

An anthrax antitoxin should be added when available. There are 3 antitoxins approved by the US Food and Drug Administration (FDA): the monoclonal antibodies raxibacumab and obiltoxaximab, and polyclonal anthrax immune globulin intravenous (AIGIV).[1] When available, raxibacumab or obiltoxaximab is preferred over AIGIV. Consult with state or local public health authorities and the CDC to discuss antitoxin use and release from the strategic national stockpile.

Adjunctive corticosteroids should be considered for edema involving the head and neck, evidence of anthrax meningitis (started at the time of initial antibiotic therapy), and vasopressor-resistant shock.[2]

For patients with systemic disease, antibiotic therapy should continue for 14 days or longer. However, intravenous treatment may be transitioned to oral therapy on the basis of patient improvement and clinical judgment. Whether patients should receive PEP following treatment for systemic anthrax depends on whether there was an aerosol exposure and whether the patient is immunocompetent. PEP is not needed in patients with naturally acquired (not in a bioterror event) noninhalation anthrax. Following an aerosol exposure to *B anthracis* spores, immunocompetent patients will develop immunity, making PEP unnecessary. However, immunocompromised patients with aerosol exposures should transition to an oral PEP regimen and be vaccinated. The total duration of treatment plus PEP is 60 days from illness onset.

Anthrax can progress rapidly, making access to critical care essential for many patients. If pleural fluid or ascites is present, aggressive drainage may improve survival. The edema that may complicate cutaneous anthrax of the face or neck can obstruct the airway, and aggressive monitoring for airway compromise is indicated in these patients. Anthrax hemorrhagic meningoencephalitis management requires neurologic

---

[1] Bower WA, Yu Y, Person MK, et al. CDC guidelines for the prevention and treatment of anthrax, 2023. *MMWR Recomm Rep.* 2023;72(RR-6):1-47

[2] Hendricks KA, Wright ME, Shadomy SV, et al. Centers for Disease Control and Prevention expert panel meetings on prevention and treatment of anthrax in adults. *Emerg Infect Dis.* 2014;20(2).

critical care because of the profound brain injury, hemorrhage, and swelling documented in animal models and humans.

INFECTION PREVENTION AND CONTROL MEASURES IN HEALTH CARE SETTINGS: Standard precautions are recommended. In addition, contact precautions should be implemented when draining cutaneous lesions are present. Cutaneous lesions become sterile within 24 hours of starting appropriate antimicrobial therapy. Patients with cutaneous illness pose minimal risk for transmission if the wound is kept covered during the first day of antimicrobial therapy. Contaminated dressings and bedclothes should be incinerated or steam sterilized (121°C for 30 minutes) to destroy spores. Terminal cleaning of the patient's room can be accomplished with an Environmental Protection Agency-registered hospital-grade disinfectant and should follow standard facility practices typically used for all patients. Autopsies performed on patients with systemic anthrax require special precautions.

CONTROL MEASURES[1]: BioThrax (anthrax vaccine adsorbed [AVA]) and Cyfendus (AVA Adjuvanted) are the only anthrax vaccines currently licensed in the United States for use in humans. Both are non-live vaccines prepared from a cell-free culture filtrate. AVA's efficacy for prevention of anthrax is based on animal studies, a single placebo-controlled human trial of the alum-precipitated precursor of the current AVA, observational data from humans, and immunogenicity data from humans and other mammals. In a human trial in adult mill workers, the alum-precipitated precursor to AVA demonstrated 93% efficacy for preventing cutaneous and inhalation anthrax. AVA Adjuvanted was approved by the US Food and Drug Administration in July 2023 for postexposure prophylaxis. Multiple reviews and publications evaluating AVA safety have found adverse events usually are local injection site reactions, with rare systemic symptoms, including fever, chills, muscle aches, and hypersensitivity.

PEP for exposure to aerosolized *B anthracis* spores includes 2 components: antimicrobials and vaccine. Symptom monitoring and PEP are critical for preventing wild-type anthrax in people. Options for PEP antimicrobials include ciprofloxacin, levofloxacin, doxycycline, moxifloxacin, clindamycin, and for penicillin-susceptible strains, amoxicillin or penicillin. In the event of a bioterrorism event, information for health care professionals and the public relevant to that exposure will be posted on the CDC anthrax website (**www.cdc.gov/anthrax/index.html**).

PEP for previously unvaccinated people 18 years or older who have been exposed to aerosolized *B anthracis* spores consists of up to 60 days of appropriate antimicrobial prophylaxis combined with 3 subcutaneous doses of anthrax vaccine. The anthrax vaccines are not licensed for use in pregnant people; however, in a postevent setting that poses a high risk of exposure to aerosolized *B anthracis* spores, pregnancy is neither a precaution nor a contraindication to their use as PEP vaccination. Similarly, they are not licensed for use in pediatric populations and have not been studied prospectively in children. However, anthrax vaccine is likely to be made available for children at the time of an event as an investigational vaccine under an appropriate regulatory mechanism that will include informed consent. Information on the process required for use of anthrax vaccines in children will be available on the CDC website at the time of

[1] Bower WA, Schiffer J, Atmar RL, et al. Use of anthrax vaccine in the United States: recommendations of the Advisory Committee on Immunization Practices, 2019. *MMWR Recomm Rep*. 2019;68(4):1-14

an event (**www.cdc.gov/anthrax/index.html**) as well as through the American Academy of Pediatrics (AAP) and the FDA. All exposed children 6 weeks and older should receive anthrax vaccine postexposure in addition to 60 days of antimicrobial chemoprophylaxis. Children younger than 6 weeks of age should immediately begin antimicrobial prophylaxis, but initiation of the vaccine series should be delayed until they reach 6 weeks of age.

Until information becomes available about antimicrobial susceptibility of the implicated strain of *B anthracis*, oral ciprofloxacin, doxycycline, and levofloxacin are equivalent first-line antimicrobial agents for initial PEP for all people ≥1 month of age.[1] If the antimicrobial susceptibility profile of isolated strains demonstrates appropriate sensitivity to amoxicillin, public health authorities may recommend changing PEP antimicrobial therapy for children either to oral amoxicillin at 75 mg/kg per day, divided into 3 daily doses administered every 8 hours (each dose not to exceed 500 mg), or to penicillin VK at 50–75 mg/kg/day divided into 4 doses (each dose not to exceed 500 mg). Additional agents and dosing are available.[1] Because of intrinsic resistance, cephalosporins and trimethoprim-sulfamethoxazole should not be used for prophylaxis.

Public Health Reporting. Anthrax is a nationally and immediately notifiable condition, as specified by the US Council of State and Territorial Epidemiologists; therefore, every suspected case should be reported **immediately** to the state or local health department.

Arboviruses (also see Chikungunya, p 295, Dengue, p 352, West Nile Virus, p 957, and Zika, p 963)
(Including Cache Valley, Colorado Tick Fever, Eastern Equine Encephalitis, Heartland, Jamestown Canyon, Japanese Encephalitis, La Crosse, Powassan, St. Louis Encephalitis, Tick-borne Encephalitis, and Yellow Fever Viruses)

CLINICAL MANIFESTATIONS: Most infections with arthropod-borne viruses (arboviruses) are subclinical. Symptomatic illness usually manifests as 1 of 3 primary clinical syndromes: generalized febrile illness, neuroinvasive disease, or hemorrhagic fever (Table 3.1).

- **Generalized febrile illness.** Most arboviruses are capable of causing a nonspecific febrile illness that often includes headache, arthralgia, myalgia, and rash. Some arboviruses can cause more characteristic clinical manifestations, such as neuroinvasive disease (see West Nile Virus, p 957), severe polyarthralgia (see Chikungunya, p 295), thrombocytopenia and leukopenia (eg, Heartland virus), or jaundice (eg, yellow fever virus). With some arboviruses, fatigue, malaise, and weakness can linger for weeks following the initial infection.
- **Neuroinvasive disease.** Many arboviruses cause neuroinvasive disease, including aseptic meningitis, encephalitis, or myelitis. Less common neurologic manifestations (eg, Guillain-Barré syndrome) also can occur. Neurologic symptoms may be preceded by a prodrome similar to the generalized febrile illness, or neurologic findings may be the initial indication of infection. Specific symptoms vary by virus but can

---

[1] Bower WA, Yu Y, Person MK, et al. CDC guidelines for the prevention and treatment of anthrax, 2023. *MMWR Recomm Rep.* 2023;72(RR-6):1-47

Table 3.1. Clinical Manifestations for Selected Domestic and International Arboviral Diseases

Virus	Generalized Febrile Illness	Neuroinvasive Disease[a]	Hemorrhagic Fever
Domestic			
Cache Valley	Yes	Yes	No
Colorado tick fever	Yes	Rare	No
Eastern equine encephalitis	Yes	Yes	No
Heartland[b]	Yes	No	No
Jamestown Canyon	Yes	Yes	No
La Crosse	Yes	Yes	No
Powassan	Yes	Yes	No
St. Louis encephalitis	Yes	Yes	No
West Nile	Yes	Yes	No
International			
Chikungunya[c]	Yes	Rare	No
Dengue[c]	Yes	Rare	Yes
Japanese encephalitis	Yes	Yes	No
Tick-borne encephalitis	Yes	Yes	No
Yellow fever	Yes	No	Yes
Zika[c]	Yes	Yes	No

[a] Meningitis, encephalitis, or myelitis.

[b] As of 2021, no pediatric infections documented; however, testing of children has been limited.

[c] Endemic with periodic outbreaks in US territories (Puerto Rico, US Virgin Islands, American Samoa); local mosquito-borne transmission of chikungunya, dengue, and Zika viruses previously identified in Florida and Texas; local transmission of dengue virus also previously identified in Hawaii.

include vomiting, stiff neck, mental status changes, seizures, or focal neurologic deficits. Some viruses (eg, West Nile and Japanese encephalitis viruses) can cause a syndrome of acute flaccid paralysis, either in conjunction with meningoencephalitis or as an isolated finding. Severity and long-term outcome of the illness vary by etiologic agent and the underlying characteristics of the host, such as age, immune status, and preexisting medical conditions.

- **Hemorrhagic fever.** Hemorrhagic fever can be caused by some arboviruses, such as dengue (see Dengue, p 352) and yellow fever viruses. After several days of nonspecific febrile illness, the patient may develop overt signs of hemorrhage (eg, petechiae, ecchymoses, bleeding from the nose and gums, hematemesis, melena) and shock (eg, decreased peripheral circulation, azotemia, tachycardia, hypotension). Hemorrhagic fever and shock caused by yellow fever virus has a high mortality rate and may be confused with other viral hemorrhagic fevers that can occur in the same geographic areas (eg, Argentine hemorrhagic fever, Bolivian hemorrhagic fever, Ebola, Lassa fever, or Marburg). Although dengue may be associated with severe hemorrhage, the shock is attributable primarily to a capillary leak syndrome, which, if properly treated with fluids, has a good prognosis. For information on other potential infections causing hemorrhagic manifestations, see Dengue (p 352), Hemorrhagic Fevers Caused by Arenaviruses (p 417), Hemorrhagic Fevers Caused by Bunyaviruses (p 420), and Hemorrhagic Fevers Caused by Filoviruses: Ebola and Marburg (p 423).

ETIOLOGY: Arboviruses are RNA viruses that are transmitted to humans primarily through bites of infected arthropods (mosquitoes, ticks, sand flies, and biting midges). More than 100 arboviruses are known to cause human disease. The viral families responsible for most arboviral infections in humans are *Flaviviridae* (genus *Flavivirus*), *Togaviridae* (genus *Alphavirus*), *Peribunyaviridae* (genus *Orthobunyavirus*), and *Phenuiviridae* (genera *Phlebovirus* and *Bandavirus*). *Reoviridae* (genus *Coltivirus*) also are responsible for a smaller number of human arboviral infections (eg, Colorado tick fever) (Table 3.2).

EPIDEMIOLOGY: Most arboviruses maintain enzootic cycles of transmission between birds or small mammals and arthropod vectors. Humans and domestic animals usually are infected incidentally as "dead-end" hosts. Important exceptions are chikungunya, dengue, yellow fever, and Zika viruses, which can be spread from person-to-arthropod-to-person (anthroponotic transmission). For other arboviruses, humans usually do not develop a sustained or high enough level of viremia to infect biting arthropod vectors. Direct person-to-person spread of some arboviruses has been documented to occur through blood transfusion, organ transplantation, sexual transmission, intrauterine transmission, perinatal transmission, and human milk (see Breastfeeding and Human Milk, p 135). Transmission through percutaneous, mucosal, or aerosol exposure to some arboviruses has occurred rarely in laboratory and occupational settings.

Arboviral infections occur in the United States primarily from late spring through early fall, when mosquitoes and ticks are most active. The number of domestic or imported arboviral disease cases reported in the United States varies greatly by specific etiology and year. Underdiagnosis of milder disease makes accurate determination of the number of cases difficult.

In general, the risk of developing severe clinical disease for most arboviral infections in the United States is higher among adults than among children. One notable exception is La Crosse virus infection, for which children are at highest risk of severe neurologic disease and possible long-term sequelae. Eastern equine encephalitis virus causes a low incidence of disease but has a high case fatality rate (30%–40%) across all age groups.

The **incubation periods** for arboviral diseases typically range between 2 and 15 days. Longer incubation periods can occur in immunocompromised people and with tick-borne viruses, such as Colorado tick fever, Powassan, and tick-borne encephalitis viruses.

DIAGNOSTIC TESTS: Arboviral infections are confirmed most frequently by detection of virus-specific antibody in serum or cerebrospinal fluid (CSF). Acute-phase serum specimens should be tested for virus-specific immunoglobulin (Ig) M antibody. With clinical and epidemiologic correlation, a positive IgM test result has good diagnostic predictive value, but cross-reaction between related arboviruses from the same viral

Table 3.2. Genus, Geographic Location, and Vectors for Selected Domestic and International Arboviral Diseases

Virus	Genus	Predominant Geographic Locations		Vector
		United States	Non-United States	
Domestic				
Cache Valley	*Orthobunyavirus*	Widespread	Canada, Central America, and the Caribbean	Mosquitoes
Colorado tick fever	*Coltivirus*	Rocky Mountain and western states	Western Canada	Ticks
Eastern equine encephalitis	*Alphavirus*	Eastern, Midwest, and Gulf coast states	Americas	Mosquitoes
Heartland	*Bandavirus*	Central and Southeast	None	Ticks
Jamestown Canyon	*Orthobunyavirus*	Widespread	Canada	Mosquitoes
La Crosse	*Orthobunyavirus*	Midwest and Appalachia	Canada	Mosquitoes
Powassan	*Flavivirus*	Northeast and Midwest	Canada, Russia	Ticks
St. Louis encephalitis	*Flavivirus*	Widespread	Americas	Mosquitoes
West Nile	*Flavivirus*	Widespread	Americas, Europe, Africa, Asia	Mosquitoes
International				
Chikungunya	*Alphavirus*	Imported and periodic local transmission[a]	Worldwide in tropical and subtropical areas	Mosquitoes
Dengue	*Flavivirus*	Imported and periodic local transmission[a]	Worldwide in tropical and subtropical areas	Mosquitoes
Japanese encephalitis	*Flavivirus*	Imported only	Australia, and other limited parts of Asia	Mosquitoes
Tick-borne encephalitis	*Flavivirus*	Imported only	Europe, northern Asia	Ticks
Yellow fever	*Flavivirus*	Imported only	South America, Africa	Mosquitoes
Zika	*Flavivirus*	Imported and periodic local transmission[a]	Worldwide in tropical and subtropical areas	Mosquitoes

[a] Endemic with periodic outbreaks in US territories (Puerto Rico, US Virgin Islands, American Samoa); local mosquito-borne transmission of chikungunya, dengue, and Zika viruses previously identified in Florida and Texas; local transmission of dengue virus also previously identified in Hawaii.

family can occur (eg, West Nile and St. Louis encephalitis viruses, both flaviviruses). For most arboviral infections, IgM is detectable within a week after onset of illness and persists for 30 to 90 days, but longer persistence has been documented, especially with West Nile and Zika viruses. Therefore, a positive serum IgM test result occasionally can reflect a prior infection. Serum collected within 10 days of illness onset might not have detectable IgM, and the test should be repeated on a convalescent-phase serum sample. IgG antibody generally is detectable in serum shortly after IgM and persists for years. A plaque-reduction neutralization test can be performed to measure virus-specific neutralizing antibodies and to discriminate between cross-reacting antibodies in primary arboviral infections. Either seroconversion or a fourfold or greater increase in virus-specific neutralizing antibodies between acute- and convalescent-phase serum specimens collected 2 to 3 weeks apart is diagnostic of recent infection. In patients who have been immunized against or infected with another arbovirus from the same virus family in the past (ie, secondary infection), cross-reactive antibodies in both the IgM and neutralizing antibody assays might make it difficult to identify which arbovirus is causing the patient's current illness. For some arboviral infections (eg, Colorado tick fever or Heartland virus disease), the immune response may be delayed, with IgM antibodies not appearing until 2 to 3 weeks after onset of illness and neutralizing antibodies taking up to a month to develop. Patients with significant immunosuppression (eg, patients who have received a solid organ transplant, recent chemotherapy, or certain immunosuppressive therapies, such as rituximab) may have a delayed or blunted serologic response, and nucleic acid amplification tests (NAATs) may be indicated in these cases. Immunization and travel history, date of symptom onset, and information regarding other arboviruses known to circulate in the geographic area that may cross-react in serologic assays should be considered when interpreting results.

Viral culture and NAATs for RNA detection can be performed on acute-phase serum, CSF, or tissue specimens. Arboviruses that are more likely to be detected using culture or NAATs early in the illness include Colorado tick fever, dengue, Heartland, yellow fever, and Zika viruses. For other arboviruses, results of these tests often are negative even early in the clinical course because of the relatively short duration of viremia in immunocompetent persons. Immunohistochemical staining (IHC) can detect specific viral antigen in fixed tissue.

Antibody testing for common domestic arboviral diseases is performed in most state public health laboratories and many commercial laboratories. Confirmatory plaque reduction neutralization tests, viral culture, NAATs, immunohistochemical staining, and testing for less common domestic and international arboviruses are performed at the Centers for Disease Control and Prevention (CDC; telephone: 970-221-6400) and selected other reference laboratories. Confirmatory testing typically is arranged through local and state health departments.

TREATMENT: The primary treatment for all arboviral disease is supportive care. Although various antiviral and immunologic therapies have been evaluated for several arboviral diseases, none has shown clear benefit.

INFECTION PREVENTION AND CONTROL MEASURES IN HEALTH CARE SETTINGS: Standard precautions are recommended.

CONTROL MEASURES: Reduction of vectors in areas with endemic transmission is important to decrease risk of infection. Use of personal protective methods, such as insect repellent, wearing long pants and long-sleeved shirts while outdoors, conducting a full-body check for ticks after outdoor activities, staying in screened or air-conditioned dwellings, and limiting outdoor activities during peak vector feeding times, can help decrease risk of human infection (see Prevention of Mosquito-borne and Tick-borne Infections, p 207). Some arboviral infections also can be prevented through screening of blood donations or through immunization. The blood supply in the United States is screened routinely for West Nile virus. Some arboviruses can be transmitted through human milk, although transmission appears rare. Mothers should be encouraged to breastfeed even in areas of active arboviral transmission because benefits of breastfeeding seem to outweigh the low risk of illness in breastfeeding infants (see Breastfeeding and Human Milk, p 135). The CDC has issued guidance for prevention of sexual transmission (see Zika, p 963).

Vaccines available in the United States to protect against arbovirus disease include the following products.

Yellow Fever Vaccine.[1] Live attenuated (17D strain) yellow fever vaccine is available from state-approved clinics or immunization providers. Unless contraindicated, yellow fever immunization is recommended for all people 9 months or older living in or traveling to areas with endemic disease in South America and Africa and is required by international regulations for travel to and from certain countries (**wwwnc.cdc.gov/travel/**). Infants younger than 6 months should not be immunized with yellow fever vaccine, because they have an increased risk of vaccine-associated encephalitis. The decision to immunize infants between 6 and 9 months of age must balance the infant's risk of exposure with risk of vaccine-associated encephalitis.

Booster doses of yellow fever vaccine are no longer recommended for most travelers, because a single dose of yellow fever vaccine provides long-lasting protection. Additional doses are recommended for certain populations (ie, people initially vaccinated when they were pregnant, patients who received a hematopoietic cell transplant after their initial vaccination, and people infected with human immunodeficiency virus [HIV]; **www.cdc.gov/mmwr/preview/mmwrhtml/mm6423a5.htm#Box**), as they might not have a robust or sustained immune response to yellow fever vaccine compared with other recipients. Additional doses may be administered to certain groups believed to be at increased risk for yellow fever disease because of their itinerary and duration of travel or because of more consistent exposure to the virus (eg, laboratory workers).

Yellow fever vaccine is a live-virus vaccine produced in chicken eggs and, thus, is contraindicated in people who have a history of acute hypersensitivity to eggs or egg products and in people who are immunocompromised. Procedures for immunizing people with severe egg allergy are described in the vaccine package insert. Generally, people who are able to eat eggs or egg products may receive the vaccine.

Pregnancy and breastfeeding are precautions to yellow fever vaccine administration, because rare cases of transmission of the vaccine virus in utero or through breastfeeding have been documented (see Immunization in Pregnancy, p 89, and Breastfeeding and Human Milk, p 135). Whenever possible, pregnant and breastfeeding individuals should defer travel to areas where yellow fever is endemic. If travel to an area with endemic disease is unavoidable and risks for yellow fever virus exposure are believed to outweigh the vaccination risks, a pregnant or breastfeeding person

---

[1] Centers for Disease Control and Prevention. Yellow Fever ACIP Vaccine Recommendations. Available at: **www.cdc.gov/vaccines/hcp/acip-recs/vacc-specific/yf.html**

should be vaccinated. If risks of vaccination are believed to outweigh risks for yellow fever virus exposure, a pregnant or breastfeeding person should be excused from immunization and issued a medical waiver letter to fulfill health regulations. For more detailed information on the yellow fever vaccine, including adverse events, precautions, and contraindications, visit **wwwnc.cdc.gov/travel/** or **www.cdc.gov/yellowfever/healthcareproviders/vaccine-info.html** or see Travel-Related Immunizations (p 128).

Japanese Encephalitis Vaccine.[1] Risk of Japanese encephalitis for most travelers to Asia is very low but varies based on destination, duration of travel, season, activities, and accommodations. All travelers to countries with endemic Japanese encephalitis should be informed of the potential for infection and should use personal protective measures to reduce risk of mosquito bites. For some travelers who might be at increased risk for Japanese encephalitis, Japanese encephalitis vaccine can reduce the risk for infection further. Japanese encephalitis vaccine is recommended for those becoming residents of a country with endemic transmission, longer-term travelers (eg, a month or longer), and frequent travelers to areas with endemic disease (**www.cdc.gov/vaccines/hcp/acip-recs/vacc-specific/je.html**). Japanese encephalitis vaccine also should be considered for shorter-term travelers if they plan to travel outside of an urban area and have an itinerary or activities that will increase their risk of mosquito exposure in an area with endemic transmission. Information on the location of Japanese encephalitis virus transmission and detailed information on vaccine recommendations and adverse events can be obtained from the CDC (**www.cdc.gov/japaneseencephalitis/**).

The Japanese encephalitis vaccine licensed in the United States is non-live Vero cell culture-derived vaccine (Ixiaro [JE-VC]) available for use in adults and children 2 months and older. The primary vaccination series is 2 doses administered 28 days apart for those younger than 18 years or older than 65 years of age, and 7–28 days apart for those 18 to 65 years of age. The dose is 0.25 mL for children 2 months through 2 years of age and 0.5 mL for adults and children 3 years and older. For adults and children, a booster dose may be administered at 1 year or longer after the primary series if ongoing exposure or re-exposure is expected.

No safety concerns have been identified in passive postmarketing surveillance of more than 1 million doses of JE-VC distributed in the United States. Safety, immunogenicity, and efficacy of JE-VC have not been assessed in pregnant individuals.

Dengue Vaccine.[2] A recombinant live attenuated tetravalent dengue vaccine (Dengvaxia) is licensed in multiple countries in Asia, Latin America, and Europe. The US Food and Drug Administration has approved Dengvaxia in 2019 for use in people 6 through 16 years of age who have laboratory evidence of previous dengue virus infection and who live in areas with endemic infection (see Dengue, p 352). The vaccine is given as a 3-dose series with 6 months between doses. The Centers for Disease Control and Prevention (CDC) Advisory Committee on Immunization Practices (ACIP) currently recommends vaccination with the Dengvaxia vaccine for children 9 through 16 years of age who live in an area where dengue is endemic and have evidence of a previous dengue infection;

---

[1] Hills SL, Walter EB, Atmar RL, Fischer M. Japanese encephalitis vaccine: Recommendations of the Advisory Committee on Immunization Practices (ACIP). *MMWR Recomm Rep* 2019;68(RR-2):1–33.

[2] Paz-Bailey G, Adams L, Wong JM, et al. Dengue vaccine: recommendations of the Advisory Committee on Immunization Practices, United States, 2021. *MMWR Recomm Rep.* 2021;70(6):1-16

as of December 2023, the ACIP had not yet voted on recommending its lower age range align with the FDA's approved range. Recommendations for use of dengue vaccine in the United States were published in 2021, and vaccination in Puerto Rico began in 2022.

Tick-borne Encephalitis Vaccine.[1] A tick-borne encephalitis vaccine became available for the first time in the United States in August 2021. Risk for tick-borne encephalitis is very low for most travelers to the parts of Europe and Asia where the disease is endemic. Some people are at increased risk for infection based on their season and location of travel and their activities. Tick-borne encephalitis vaccine is recommended for people who are moving or traveling to an area with endemic infection and will have extensive exposure to ticks based on their planned outdoor activities and itinerary. It may be considered for others who might engage in outdoor activities in areas with endemic infection, with the decision to vaccinate based on assessment of their planned activities and itinerary, risk factors for a poorer medical outcome, and personal perception and tolerance of risk. Detailed information on the location of tick-borne encephalitis, risk factors for infection, and vaccine considerations can be found on the CDC website (**www.cdc.gov/tick-borne-encephalitis/index.html**).

The non-live tick-borne encephalitis vaccine can be used in adults and children 1 year and older. The 3-dose primary vaccination series for children and adolescents 1 through 15 years of age consists of 0.25-mL doses on day 0 (dose 1), at 1–3 months after the first vaccination (dose 2), and 5–12 months after the second vaccination (dose 3). The schedule for persons 16 years and older is similar, but dose 2 can be given as early as 14 days after dose 1. The vaccine dose recommended for people 16 years and older is 0.5 mL. A booster dose may be administered at least 3 years after completion of the primary series if ongoing exposure or re-exposure is expected.

The vaccine is contraindicated in any person with a history of a severe allergic reaction (eg, anaphylaxis) to any vaccine component, including chicken protein, neomycin, gentamicin, and protamine sulfate. A complete list of components is provided in the package insert.

Public Health Reporting. Most arboviral diseases are nationally notifiable conditions and should be reported to the appropriate local and state health authorities. Underdiagnosis of these diseases because of challenges with laboratory confirmation and lack of active surveillance is common, suggesting that the actual numbers of cases are likely significantly higher. For select arboviruses (eg, chikungunya, dengue, Zika, and yellow fever viruses), patients may remain viremic during their acute illness. Such patients pose a risk for further person-to-mosquito-to-person transmission, increasing the importance of timely reporting.

Arcanobacterium haemolyticum Infections

CLINICAL MANIFESTATIONS: Acute pharyngitis attributable to *Arcanobacterium haemolyticum* often is indistinguishable from group A streptococcal pharyngitis. *A haemolyticum* has been associated with fever, pharyngeal erythema and exudates, cervical lymphadenopathy, and rash, but palatal petechiae and strawberry tongue are typically absent. A morbilliform or scarlatiniform exanthem is present in half of cases, usually

---

[1] Hills SL, Poehling KA, Chen WH, Staples JE. Tick-borne encephalitis vaccine: recommendations of the Advisory Committee on Immunization Practices, United States, 2023. *MMWR Recomm Rep.* 2023;72(RR-5):1-29

beginning on extensor surfaces of the distal extremities, spreading to the torso, back, and neck, sparing the face, palms, and soles. Rash typically develops 1 to 4 days after onset of sore throat, although the rash may precede pharyngitis. Desquamation can occur. Respiratory tract infections that mimic diphtheria, including membranous pharyngitis, and peritonsillar and pharyngeal abscesses occasionally occur. Skin and soft tissue infections, including chronic ulcers, cellulitis, paronychia, and wound infection, have been attributed to *A haemolyticum*. Rarely, invasive infections have been reported, including Lemierre syndrome, bacteremia, sepsis, endocarditis, brain abscess, orbital cellulitis, and pyogenic arthritis.

ETIOLOGY: *A haemolyticum* is a catalase-negative, weakly acid-fast, facultatively anaerobic, hemolytic, gram-positive to gram-variable, slender, sometimes club-shaped bacillus.

EPIDEMIOLOGY: Humans are the primary reservoir of *A haemolyticum*. Household studies suggest that spread occurs from person to person, presumably via droplet respiratory secretions. Severe disease occurs almost exclusively among immunocompromised people; invasive cases have been reported rarely in previously healthy people. *Arcanobacterium* pharyngitis occurs primarily in adolescents and young adults and only rarely in young children. *A haemolyticum* accounts for approximately 0.5% of pharyngeal infections overall and up to 2.5% of pharyngeal infections in 15- to 25-year-olds. Isolation of the bacterium from the nasopharynx of asymptomatic people is rare.

The **incubation period** is unknown.

DIAGNOSTIC TESTS: *A haemolyticum* grows on blood-enriched agar, but colonies are small, have narrow bands of beta hemolysis, and may not be visible for 48 to 72 hours. The organism is not detected by rapid antigen tests for group A streptococci. Detection is enhanced by culture on rabbit or human blood agar, which yields larger colony size and wider zones of hemolysis compared with sheep blood agar. Presence of 5% carbon dioxide enhances growth, and pits characteristically form under colonies on blood agar plates. *A haemolyticum* may be missed in routine throat cultures on sheep blood agar if laboratory personnel are not trained specifically to identify the organism. Two biotypes of *A haemolyticum* have been identified: a rough biotype predominates in respiratory tract infections and a smooth biotype typically is found in skin and soft tissue infections.

TREATMENT: Optimal management of patients with *A haemolyticum* pharyngitis has not been determined, and symptoms can resolve without antibiotic treatment. Erythromycin and azithromycin are drugs of choice for *A haemolyticum* tonsillopharyngitis, but no controlled trials have been performed. *A haemolyticum* generally is susceptible in vitro to macrolides, clindamycin, cephalosporins, ciprofloxacin, vancomycin, and gentamicin. Treatment failures with penicillin despite predicted susceptibility from in vitro testing occur and may be attributable to tolerance. Resistance to trimethoprim-sulfamethoxazole is common. In rare cases of invasive infection, susceptibility tests should be performed, and treatment should be individualized. While awaiting results, initial empiric combination therapy can be initiated using a parenteral beta lactam agent, with or without gentamicin or a macrolide, and with consideration of metronidazole if *Fusobacterium* infection is suspected, such as in cases of Lemierre syndrome.

INFECTION PREVENTION AND CONTROL MEASURES IN HEALTH CARE SETTINGS: Standard precautions are recommended.

CONTROL MEASURES: None.

Ascaris lumbricoides Infections

CLINICAL MANIFESTATIONS: Most infections with *Ascaris lumbricoides* are asymptomatic, although moderate to heavy infections may lead to nonspecific gastrointestinal tract symptoms, malnutrition, and growth delay. During the larval migratory phase, an acute transient pneumonitis (Löffler syndrome) associated with cough, wheezing, substernal discomfort, shortness of breath, fever, and marked eosinophilia may occur. Acute intestinal obstruction has been associated with heavy infections. Children are prone to this complication because of the small diameter of the intestinal lumen and their propensity to acquire large worm burdens. Heavy worm burdens also can affect nutritional status, intellectual development, cognitive performance, and growth. Worm migration can cause peritonitis secondary to intestinal wall perforation as well as appendicitis or common bile duct obstruction resulting in biliary colic, cholangitis, or pancreatitis. Adult worms can be stimulated to migrate by stressful conditions (eg, fever, illness, or anesthesia) and by some anthelmintic drugs.

ETIOLOGY: After embryonated eggs are ingested, larvae hatch in the small intestine, penetrate the mucosa, and are transported passively by portal blood to the liver and lungs. After migrating from alveolar capillaries into the small airways, larvae ascend through the tracheobronchial tree to the pharynx, are swallowed, and mature into adults in the small intestine. Female worms produce approximately 200 000 eggs per day, which are excreted in stool and must incubate in soil to become infectious. Adult worms can live in the lumen of the small intestine for up to 18 months. Female worms are longer than male worms and can measure 40 cm in length and 6 mm in diameter.

EPIDEMIOLOGY: *A lumbricoides* is the most prevalent of all human intestinal nematodes (roundworms), with more than 800 million people infected worldwide. Infection is acquired by ingestion of *Ascaris* eggs in feces-contaminated food or dirt. Direct person-to-person transmission does not occur. Infection is most common in resource-limited countries, including rural and urban communities characterized by poor sanitation. *Ascaris suum*, a pig roundworm similar to *A lumbricoides*, also causes human disease. Sporadic clusters of ascariasis attributable to *A suum* associated with pig farming or use of pig stool for fertilizer have been reported in the United States.

The **incubation period** (interval between ingestion of eggs and development of egg-laying adults) is approximately 9 to 11 weeks.

DIAGNOSTIC TESTS: Ascariasis is diagnosed by examining a fresh or preserved stool specimen for eggs using light microscopy. Concentration techniques and examination of multiple specimens may be needed. Patients who harbor only male *Ascaris* worms will have negative test results on stool microscopy. Adult worms also may be passed from the rectum, through the nares, or from the mouth, usually in vomitus. Imaging of the gastrointestinal tract or biliary tree using computed tomography or ultrasonography may detect adult *Ascaris* worms, which can cause filling defects following administration of oral contrast.

TREATMENT: Albendazole and mebendazole are first-line agents for treatment of ascariasis, with cure rates from 90% to 100% with albendazole (see Drugs for Parasitic Infections, p 1068). Ivermectin, nitazoxanide, and pyrantel pamoate are alternative therapies. Albendazole, pyrantel pamoate, ivermectin, and nitazoxanide are not approved by the US Food and Drug Administration for treatment of ascariasis, although albendazole has become the drug of choice for most soil-transmitted nematode infections, including ascariasis. Reexamination of stool specimens may be performed at approximately 2 weeks after deworming to document cure and again at 2 to 3 months to account for migrating larvae present at the time of treatment that may now be mature adults, because these anthelmintic agents are not effective against larvae. Patients who remain infected should be retreated, preferably with albendazole or the multidose regimen of mebendazole, and the reasons for the repeated infections should be explored and addressed.

Conservative management of small bowel obstruction, including nasogastric suction, intravenous fluids, and repletion of electrolytes, may alleviate symptoms before administration of anthelmintic therapy. Diatrizoate meglumine and diatrizoate sodium solution or careful use of mineral oil (cases of lipoid pneumonia have been reported after this use), administered orally or by nasogastric tube, may cause relaxation of a bolus of worms. Endoscopic retrograde cholangiopancreatography has been used successfully for extraction of worms from the biliary tree. Surgical intervention (eg, laparotomy) is indicated for intestinal or biliary tract obstruction that does not resolve with conservative therapy or for patients with volvulus or peritonitis secondary to perforation.

INFECTION PREVENTION AND CONTROL MEASURES IN HEALTH CARE SETTINGS: Standard precautions are recommended.

CONTROL MEASURES: Sanitary disposal of human feces prevents transmission. Vegetables cultivated in areas where human feces are used as fertilizer must be washed thoroughly and cooked before eating.

Preventive chemotherapy (once or twice annually with albendazole or mebendazole) targeting high-risk groups, most notably preschool and school-aged children and pregnant people (after the first trimester), is recommended by the World Health Organization for control of *A lumbricoides* and other soil-transmitted nematodes in high prevalence communities. Reinfection is common in these areas, and additional public health measures, including improved sanitation, safe drinking water, and health education, likely will be required to eliminate these infections.

Aspergillosis

CLINICAL MANIFESTATIONS: Aspergillosis manifests as 5 principal clinical entities: invasive aspergillosis, aspergilloma, allergic bronchopulmonary aspergillosis, allergic sinusitis, and chronic pulmonary aspergillosis. Colonization of the respiratory tract is common. The clinical manifestations and severity depend on host immune status (either immunocompromised or atopic).

- Invasive aspergillosis occurs mostly in immunocompromised patients with prolonged neutropenia, graft-versus-host disease, or impaired phagocyte function (eg, chronic granulomatous disease) or those who have received T-lymphocyte immunosuppressive therapy (eg, corticosteroids, calcineurin inhibitors) or biologic agents (eg, tumor necrosis factor [TNF]-alpha inhibitors, small-molecule kinase inhibitors). Children at highest risk include those with new-onset acute myelogenous leukemia, relapse of hematologic malignancy, aplastic anemia, chronic granulomatous disease, and recipients of allogeneic hematopoietic cell and solid organ (eg, particularly lung) transplants. Invasive infection usually involves pulmonary, sinus, cerebral, or cutaneous sites. Rarely, endocarditis, osteomyelitis, meningitis, peritonitis, infection of the eye or orbit, and gastrointestinal tract involvement occur. The hallmark of invasive aspergillosis is angioinvasion with resulting thrombosis, dissemination to other organs, and occasionally erosion of the blood vessel wall with catastrophic hemorrhage. Invasive aspergillosis in patients with chronic granulomatous disease is unique in that it is more indolent and displays a general lack of angioinvasion. Invasive aspergillosis also has been described among patients in the intensive care unit with severe influenza and COVID-19 with or without underlying immunocompromise.

- Aspergillomas and otomycosis are 2 syndromes of nonallergic colonization by *Aspergillus* species in immunocompetent children. Aspergillomas ("fungal balls") grow in preexisting pulmonary cavities or bronchogenic cysts without invading pulmonary tissue; almost all patients have underlying lung disease, such as cystic fibrosis or tuberculosis. Patients with otomycosis have chronic otitis media with colonization of the external auditory canal by a fungal mat that produces a dark discharge.

- Allergic bronchopulmonary aspergillosis is a hypersensitivity lung disease that manifests as episodic wheezing, expectoration of brown mucus plugs, low-grade fever, eosinophilia, and transient pulmonary infiltrates. This form of aspergillosis occurs most commonly in immunocompetent children with asthma or cystic fibrosis and can be a trigger for asthmatic flares and acute pulmonary exacerbation in patients with cystic fibrosis.

- Allergic sinusitis is a far less common allergic response to colonization by *Aspergillus* species than is allergic bronchopulmonary aspergillosis. Allergic sinusitis occurs in children with nasal polyps or previous episodes of sinusitis or in children who have undergone sinus surgery. Allergic sinusitis is characterized by symptoms of chronic sinusitis with dark plugs of nasal discharge and is different from invasive *Aspergillus* sinusitis.

- Chronic aspergillosis typically affects patients who are not immunocompromised or are less immunocompromised, although exposure to corticosteroids is common, and patients often have underlying pulmonary conditions. Diagnosis of chronic aspergillosis requires at least 3 months of chronic pulmonary symptoms or chronic illness or progressive radiologic abnormalities, along with an elevated *Aspergillus* immunoglobulin (Ig) G concentration or other microbiological evidence. Because of the ubiquitous nature of *Aspergillus* species, a positive sputum culture alone is not diagnostic.

ETIOLOGY: *Aspergillus* species are molds that grow on decaying vegetation and in soil and are very common in the environment. *Aspergillus fumigatus* is the most common (>75%) cause of invasive aspergillosis, with *Aspergillus flavus* being the next most common. Several other major species, including *Aspergillus terreus, Aspergillus nidulans,* and *Aspergillus niger,* also cause invasive human infections. *A nidulans* is the second most encountered mold in patients with chronic granulomatous disease, causing almost exclusively invasive infections characterized by aggressive behavior including lung infection that invades the chest wall with contiguous osteomyelitis and chest wall abscesses. Of increasing concern are emerging *Aspergillus* species that are resistant to antifungals, such as *Aspergillus fumigatus,* which can harbor environmentally acquired resistance mutations to azole antifungals; *A terreus,* which is intrinsically resistant to amphotericin B; and *Aspergillus calidoustus,* which is often resistant to most antifungals including azole antifungals (see Table 4.7, p 1021).

EPIDEMIOLOGY: The principal route of transmission is inhalation of conidia (spores) originating from multiple environmental sources (eg, plants, vegetables, dust from construction or demolition), soil, and water supplies (eg, shower heads). Incidence of disease in hematopoietic cell transplant recipients is highest during periods of neutropenia or during treatment for graft-versus-host disease. In solid organ transplant recipients, the risk is highest approximately 6 months after transplantation or during periods of increased immunosuppression. Disease has followed use of contaminated marijuana in the immunocompromised host. Health care-associated outbreaks of invasive pulmonary aspergillosis in susceptible hosts have occurred in which the probable source of the fungus was a nearby construction site or faulty ventilation system, but the source of health care-associated aspergillosis frequently is not known. Cutaneous aspergillosis occurs less frequently and usually involves sites of skin injury, such as intravenous catheter sites (including in neonates), sites of traumatic inoculation, and sites associated with occlusive dressings, burns, or surgery. Transmission by direct inoculation of skin abrasions or wounds is less likely. Person-to-person spread does not occur.

The **incubation period** is unknown and may be variable.

DIAGNOSTIC TESTS: Dichotomously branched and septate hyphae, identified by microscopic examination of 10% potassium hydroxide wet preparations or of Gomori methenamine-silver nitrate stain of tissue or bronchoalveolar lavage specimens, are suggestive of the diagnosis. Isolation of *Aspergillus* species in culture from a sterile site or molecular testing with specific reagents is required for definitive diagnosis. The organism usually is not recoverable from blood (except some species like *A terreus*) but is isolated readily from lung, sinus, and skin biopsy specimens when cultured on Sabouraud dextrose agar or brain-heart infusion media (without cycloheximide). *Aspergillus* species can be associated with colonization or may be a laboratory contaminant, but when evaluating results from immunocompromised patients, recovery of this organism frequently indicates infection. Biopsy with histopathology can be used to establish the diagnosis, but *Aspergillus* hyphae are similar to other hyaline molds (eg, *Fusarium*). Care should be taken to distinguish aspergillosis from mucormycosis, which can appear similar by diagnostic imaging studies, but mucormycosis is pauci-septate (few septa) and requires a different treatment regimen.

An enzyme immunosorbent assay for detection of galactomannan, a molecule found in the cell wall of *Aspergillus* species, from serum or bronchoalveolar lavage (BAL) fluid is available commercially and may be useful in children and adults with hematologic malignancies or hematopoietic cell transplant recipients. A test result of ≥ 0.5 from the serum or ≥ 1.0 from BAL fluid supports a diagnosis of invasive aspergillosis. Measuring galactomannan during periods of highest risk (eg, neutropenia and active graft-versus-host disease) if the patient is not receiving mold-active antifungal prophylaxis may be useful for early detection of invasive aspergillosis in these patients. False-positive test results have been reported and can be related to consumption of food products containing galactomannan (eg, rice and pasta), other invasive fungal infections (eg, *Fusarium, Penicillium, Histoplasma capsulatum*), and colonization of the gut of neonates with *Bifidobacterium* species. Previous cross-reactivity with antimicrobial agents derived from fungi, especially piperacillin-tazobactam, no longer occurs because of manufacturing changes.

A negative galactomannan test result does not exclude diagnosis of invasive aspergillosis, and its greatest utility may be in monitoring response to disease rather than in its use as a diagnostic marker. False-negative galactomannan test results consistently occur in patients with chronic granulomatous disease, so the test should not be used in these patients. Galactomannan is not recommended for routine screening in patients receiving mold-active antifungal therapy or prophylaxis (see Table 4.7, p 1021). Galactomannan is not recommended for screening in solid organ transplant recipients because of very poor sensitivity.

Detection of *Aspergillus* DNA using a nucleic acid amplification test (NAAT) performed on 2 consecutive blood samples or 2 duplicate bronchoalveolar lavage fluid samples, or in 1 blood and one bronchoalveolar lavage sample, supports a diagnosis of invasive aspergillosis in high-risk adults with underlying hematologic malignancies and hematopoietic cell transplantation recipients; however, the clinical utility of the NAAT in children remains unknown. Some NAATs may also allow detection to the species level and identify mutations associated with triazole resistance.

Limited data suggest that testing for other nonspecific fungal biomarkers, such as 1,3-β-D glucan, may be useful in the diagnosis of aspergillosis. This test is not specific for aspergillosis, however, and specificity may be further limited in a variety of clinical settings, including exposure to certain antibiotics, hemodialysis, and coinfection with certain bacteria.

Unlike adults, children frequently do not manifest cavitation or the air crescent or halo signs on chest radiography, and lack of these characteristic signs does not exclude the diagnosis of invasive aspergillosis.

In allergic aspergillosis, diagnosis is suggested by a typical clinical syndrome with elevated total concentrations of IgE (≥1000 ng/mL) and *Aspergillus*-specific serum IgE, eosinophilia, and a positive result from a skin test for *Aspergillus* antigens. In people with cystic fibrosis, the diagnosis is more difficult because wheezing, eosinophilia, and a positive skin test result not associated with allergic bronchopulmonary aspergillosis often are present.

TREATMENT[1]: Voriconazole is the drug of choice for all clinical forms of invasive aspergillosis (see Antifungal Drugs for Systemic Fungal Infections, p 1017), except in neonates, for whom amphotericin B deoxycholate in high doses is recommended because of voriconazole's potential visual adverse effects. Voriconazole has been shown to be superior to amphotericin B in a large, randomized trial in adults. Immune reconstitution is paramount; decreasing immunosuppression, if possible (specifically corticosteroid dose), is critical to disease control. The diagnostic workup needs to be aggressive to confirm disease, but it should never delay antifungal therapy in the setting of true concern for invasive aspergillosis. Therapy is continued for a minimum of 6 to 12 weeks, but treatment duration should be individualized on the basis of degree and duration of immunosuppression. Response to therapy may be assessed by monitoring of serum galactomannan concentrations in those with significant elevation at onset, along with clinical and radiologic evaluation.

Close monitoring of voriconazole serum trough concentrations is critical for both efficacy and safety. Most experts agree that voriconazole trough concentrations should be measured on day 3 or later after initiating treatment and for children, therapeutic trough concentrations are 2 to 6 µg/mL. It is important to individualize dosing in

[1] Patterson TF, Thompson GR III, Denning DW. Practice guidelines for the diagnosis and management of aspergillosis: 2016 update by the Infectious Diseases Society of America. *Clin Infect Dis*. 2016;63(4):e1-e60

patients following initiation of voriconazole therapy, because there is high interpatient variability in metabolism.

Certain *Aspergillus* species (*A calidoustus*) are inherently resistant to azoles, and isolation of azole-resistant *A fumigatus* is increasing and may be related to environmental acquisition through use of agricultural fungicides in previously azole-naïve patients. Resistance can also develop in patients receiving long-term azole therapy.

Alternative therapies include liposomal amphotericin B, isavuconazole, posaconazole, or other lipid formulations of amphotericin B. Primary therapy with an echinocandin alone (caspofungin, micafungin) is not recommended, but an echinocandin can be used in settings in which an azole or amphotericin B are contraindicated. Posaconazole absorption is improved significantly with use of the extended-release tablet rather than the oral suspension; a new powder formulation for delayed-release oral suspension is available for children ≥2 years of age weighing ≤40 kg. Isavuconazole is noninferior to voriconazole for primary treatment of invasive aspergillosis, with fewer drug-related adverse events in adults, but has not been fully studied in children. Combination antifungal therapy with voriconazole and an echinocandin may be considered in select patients with documented invasive aspergillosis. In areas with high azole resistance, empiric therapy until antifungal susceptibilities are obtained should include voriconazole plus an echinocandin, or liposomal amphotericin B monotherapy.

If primary antifungal therapy fails, general strategies for salvage therapy include: (a) changing the class of antifungal; (b) tapering or reversal of underlying immunosuppression when feasible; (c) susceptibility testing of any *Aspergillus* isolates recovered; and (d) surgical resection of necrotic lesions in selected cases. In pulmonary disease, surgery is indicated when a mass is impinging on a great vessel.

Allergic bronchopulmonary aspergillosis is treated with antifungal therapy, usually with itraconazole or another mold-active azole; in addition, corticosteroids are a cornerstone of therapy for exacerbations. Itraconazole has a demonstrable corticosteroid-sparing effect. Guidelines specific to treatment of allergic bronchopulmonary aspergillosis in patients with cystic fibrosis are available (**www.cff.org/Care/Clinical-Care-Guidelines/Infection-Prevention-and-Control-Clinical-Care-Guidelines/Allergic-Bronchopulmonary-Aspergillosis-Clinical-Care-Guidelines/**).

Allergic sinus aspergillosis also is treated with corticosteroids, and surgery has been reported to be beneficial in many cases. Antifungal therapy has not been found to be useful but could be considered for refractory infection and/or relapsing disease. There may be an emerging role for immunotherapy.

INFECTION PREVENTION AND CONTROL MEASURES IN HEALTH CARE SETTINGS: Standard precautions are recommended.

CONTROL MEASURES: Outbreaks of invasive aspergillosis and *Aspergillus* colonization have occurred among hospitalized patients during construction in hospitals and at nearby sites. Environmental measures reported to be effective include erecting suitable barriers between patient care areas and construction sites, routine cleaning of air-handling systems, repair of faulty air flow, and replacement of contaminated air filters. High-efficiency particulate air filters and laminar flow rooms markedly decrease the risk of exposure to conidia in patient care areas. Plants and flowers may be reservoirs for *Aspergillus* and should be avoided in intensive care units and immunocompromised patient care settings. Use of high-efficiency respirators during transport away from protective environment rooms has been associated with reduced incidence of invasive pulmonary aspergillosis during hospital construction.

Posaconazole has been shown to be effective in 2 randomized controlled trials as prophylaxis against invasive aspergillosis for patients 13 years and older who have undergone hematopoietic cell transplantation and have graft-versus-host disease as well as in patients with hematologic malignancies with prolonged neutropenia, although breakthrough disease has been reported in those with gastrointestinal tract issues (eg, graft-versus-host disease) affecting drug bioavailability. Low-dose amphotericin B, itraconazole, voriconazole, or posaconazole prophylaxis have been reported for other high-risk patients, but controlled trials have not been completed in pediatric patients.

Patients at risk of invasive infection should avoid high environmental exposure (eg, gardening) following discharge from the hospital. People with allergic aspergillosis should take measures to reduce exposure to *Aspergillus* species in the home.

Astrovirus Infections

CLINICAL MANIFESTATIONS: Astrovirus illness most commonly manifests as 2 to 5 days of acute watery diarrhea accompanied by low-grade fever, malaise, and nausea, and less commonly, vomiting and mild dehydration. Illness in an immunocompetent host is self-limited, lasting a median of 5 to 6 days. Asymptomatic infections are common. Astrovirus infections also have been associated with respiratory illness, encephalitis, and meningitis, particularly in immunocompromised individuals.

ETIOLOGY: Members of the family *Astroviridae,* astroviruses are nonenveloped, single-stranded RNA viruses with viral particles having a characteristic star-like appearance when visualized by electron microscopy. Astroviruses are classified into 2 genera: *Mamastrovirus* (MAstV) and *Avastrovirus,* which infect mammals and birds, respectively. Four MAstV species have been identified in humans: MAstV 1, MAstV 6, MAstV 8, and MAstV 9. MAstV 1 includes the 8 antigenic types of classic human astroviruses (HAstV types 1–8), whereas MAstV 6, MAstV 8, and MAstV 9 are novel astroviruses that have been identified in recent years and include Melbourne (MLB) and Virginia/human-mink-ovine-like (VA/HMO) strains.

EPIDEMIOLOGY: Human astroviruses (HAstVs) have a worldwide distribution. Multiple antigenic types cocirculate in the same geographic region. HAstVs have been detected in as many as 5% to 17% of sporadic cases of nonbacterial gastroenteritis among young children in the community but appear to cause a lower proportion of cases of more severe childhood gastroenteritis requiring hospitalization (2.5%–9%). HAstV infections occur predominantly in children younger than 4 years and have a seasonal peak during the late winter and spring in the United States. Transmission is via the fecal-oral route through contaminated food or water, person-to-person contact, or contaminated surfaces. Outbreaks tend to occur in closed populations of the young and the elderly, particularly among hospitalized children (health care-associated infections) and children in child care centers (Table 2.1). In general, virus is shed 1 to 2 days before illness and lasts a median of 5 days after onset of symptoms, but asymptomatic excretion after illness can last for several weeks in healthy children. Persistent excretion may occur in immunocompromised hosts. MAstV 6, MAstV 8, and MAstV 9 have been detected sporadically in stool samples, blood, respiratory samples, cerebrospinal fluid, and brain tissue of immunocompromised patients with acute encephalitis.

The **incubation period** is 3 to 4 days.

DIAGNOSTIC TESTS: There are several US Food and Drug Administration (FDA) approved multiplex nucleic acid-based assays for the detection of gastrointestinal tract pathogens, at least 2 of which include astrovirus (MAstV 1). Similar to tests for other gastroenteritis viruses, interpretation of assay results may be complicated by the detection of multiple gastrointestinal tract pathogens in a single sample, particularly in young children.

A few research and reference laboratories test stool samples using nucleic acid amplification tests (NAATs). To link cases from different disease clusters, positive samples can be typed by amplification and sequencing of small regions of the astrovirus capsid gene.

TREATMENT: No specific antiviral therapy is available. Oral or parenteral fluids and electrolytes are given to prevent and correct dehydration.

INFECTION PREVENTION AND CONTROL MEASURES IN HEALTH CARE SETTINGS: In addition to standard precautions, contact precautions are recommended for diapered children or incontinent people for the duration of illness or to control institutional outbreaks.

CONTROL MEASURES: No specific control measures are available. The spread of infection in child care settings can be decreased by using general measures for control of diarrhea, such as training care providers in infection-control procedures, maintaining cleanliness of surfaces, keeping food preparation duties and areas separate from child care activities, exercising adequate hand hygiene, cohorting ill children, and excluding ill child care providers, food handlers, and children (see Children in Group Child Care and Schools, p 145).

Babesiosis

CLINICAL MANIFESTATIONS: *Babesia* infection in children and adolescents often is asymptomatic or associated with mild, nonspecific symptoms. The infection also can be severe and life-threatening, particularly in people who are immunocompromised, including those at the extremes of age (neonates and the elderly), those who lack a spleen, and those who have human immunodeficiency virus (HIV) infection/acquired immunodeficiency syndrome (AIDS) or cancer or are on immunosuppressive drugs. Babesiosis, like malaria, is characterized by the presence of fever and hemolytic anemia. Clinical manifestations can include malaise and fatigue, often followed by fever, chills, sweats, anorexia, myalgia, headache, arthralgia, and/or nausea. Severe babesiosis may require hospitalization for management of marked anemia, adult respiratory distress syndrome, disseminated intravascular coagulation, congestive heart failure, renal impairment, shock, or splenic rupture. Congenital infection with nonspecific manifestations suggestive of sepsis has been reported, as has persistent relapsing disease in highly immunocompromised hosts.

Babesiosis should be considered in a patient who resides in or traveled to an area with endemic infection and develops compatible symptoms and characteristic laboratory abnormalities, including anemia, thrombocytopenia, or evidence of intravascular hemolysis (abnormal aspartate aminotransferase [AST], alanine aminotransferase [ALT], alkaline phosphatase, lactate dehydrogenase [LDH], total and direct bilirubin concentrations, or reduced haptoglobin).

ETIOLOGY: *Babesia* species are intraerythrocytic protozoa that usually are transmitted by the bite of a hard-bodied tick. The etiologic agents of human babesiosis in the United States include *Babesia microti*, the most common cause of infection, *Babesia duncani*, and rarely, *Babesia divergens*.

EPIDEMIOLOGY: Babesiosis predominantly is a tick-borne zoonosis. *Babesia* parasites also can be transmitted via blood transfusion, via organ transplantation, and perinatally. The primary reservoir host for *B microti* in the United States is the white-footed mouse *(Peromyscus leucopus)*, and the primary tick vector is *Ixodes scapularis*, which can transmit other pathogens, such as *Borrelia burgdorferi*, the causative agent of Lyme disease, and *Anaplasma phagocytophilum*, the causative agent of human granulocytic anaplasmosis. A tick bite often is not noticed, in part because the nymphal stage of the tick is approximately the size of a poppy seed. White-tailed deer *(Odocoileus virginianus)* serve as hosts for tick procreation and a blood meal, but deer are not reservoir hosts of *B microti*. An increase in deer populations in the Northeast and northern Midwest during the past few decades is thought to be a major factor in the increase and spread of *I scapularis* ticks. Most cases of babesiosis in the United States have been reported from states on the East Coast (Connecticut, Massachusetts, New Jersey, New York, Rhode Island) and the northern Midwest (Minnesota, Wisconsin), where deer populations have increased (**www.cdc.gov/parasites/babesiosis/data-statistics/ maps/maps.html**). Over the last few years, increasing numbers of cases have been reported from neighboring states such as Maine, New Hampshire, and Vermont. Occasional human cases of babesiosis caused by *B duncani* have been described in California, Oregon, and Washington State, and single cases caused by *B divergens* have been reported in Arkansas, Kentucky, Michigan, Missouri, and Washington State. Most US vector-borne cases of babesiosis occur during late spring, summer, or fall; transfusion-associated cases can occur year-round. More than 2000 cases of babesiosis are reported annually to the Centers for Disease Control and Prevention, but the number of cases likely is higher.

The **incubation period** ranges from approximately 1 to 6 weeks after a tick bite. A study of transfusion-associated cases found a median incubation period following a contaminated blood transfusion of 37 days (range, 11 to 176 days), but it may be longer (eg, latent infection can become symptomatic after splenectomy).

DIAGNOSTIC TESTS[1]: Acute, symptomatic cases of babesiosis typically are diagnosed by microscopic identification of *Babesia* parasites on Giemsa- or Wright-stained blood smears. *Babesia* parasites may be confused with *Plasmodium falciparum*, but they can be distinguished by an experienced microscopist. The tetrad (Maltese-cross) form is pathognomonic for *Babesia* but often is not present.

In cases in which blood smear examination is negative but the index of suspicion for babesiosis remains high, molecular testing using a nucleic acid amplification test (NAAT) offers increased sensitivity in settings of low-level *B microti* parasitemia. NAAT results may remain positive for several months to more than a year after successful treatment. Some physicians may order a NAAT rather than a blood smear to confirm the diagnosis, especially if a skilled microscopist is not available. NAATs are

---

[1] Krause PJ, Auwaerter PG, Bannuru RR, et al. Clinical practice guidelines by the Infectious Diseases Society of America (IDSA): 2020 Guideline on diagnosis and management of babesiosis. *Clin Infect Dis.* 2021;72(2):e49-e64

species-specific, and most laboratories only offer *B microti* NAAT (**www.cdc.gov/ dpdx/babesiosis/index.html**).

A single serologic test for *Babesia* antibody detection should not be used to diagnose acute disease because of difficulty distinguishing acute disease from previous infection. In geographic areas where both *B microti* and *B burgdorferi* are endemic, between 2% and 20% of patients with early Lyme disease have been reported to experience concurrent babesiosis coinfection, and 10% to 50% of patients with babesiosis have been found to be coinfected with *B burgdorferi*. Other tick-borne coinfections, such as anaplasmosis, should be considered as well in patients with babesiosis and/or Lyme disease. When coinfection is documented, patients should receive therapies appropriate for each infection.

TREATMENT[1]: Atovaquone (administered orally) plus azithromycin (administered orally in ambulatory patients with mild to moderate disease and intravenously in hospitalized patients with severe disease) for 7 to 10 days is the regimen of choice (see Drugs for Parasitic Infections, p 1068). Oral or intravenous clindamycin plus oral quinine sulfate may be used for patients who do not respond to atovaquone and azithromycin, although quinine commonly causes serious adverse effects. Severe babesiosis can be life-threatening despite antimicrobial therapy. Limited data suggest exchange transfusion has potential benefits that may outweigh potential adverse effects, particularly in patients with high levels of parasitemia (>10%) or evidence of severe organ dysfunction. Treatment for at least 6 weeks or longer is recommended for severely immunocompromised patients experiencing persistent relapsing disease despite recommended antibiotic therapy, with negative blood smears for 2 weeks or longer before discontinuing therapy. Higher doses of azithromycin (500 to 1000 mg per day, orally, in adolescents/adults) should be considered when treating a highly immunocompromised patient (see Table 4.11, Drugs for Parasitic Infections, p 1068). Limited data are available for treatment of disease caused by *B duncani* or *B divergens*, but most reported patients have been treated with intravenous clindamycin plus oral quinine. Efficacy of atovaquone plus azithromycin in treating *B duncani* infection has not been evaluated.

Peripheral blood smears should be performed during acute illness to monitor *Babesia* parasitemia for all patients. Testing of immunocompromised patients should continue daily until parasitemia is less than 4% and then weekly until blood smear results are negative; a NAAT should be considered for those whose symptoms persist after the blood smear results have become negative. Immunocompetent persons do not require testing once symptoms have resolved; NAAT results may remain positive for months or years after appropriate treatment, and this does not indicate treatment failure.

INFECTION PREVENTION AND CONTROL MEASURES IN HEALTH CARE SETTINGS: Standard precautions are recommended.

CONTROL MEASURES: Recommendations for prevention of tick bites are similar to those for prevention of Lyme disease and other tick-borne infections (see Prevention of Mosquito-borne and Tick-borne Infections, p 207). People with a known history of *Babesia* infection are deferred indefinitely from donating blood. In 2019, the US Food and Drug Administration (FDA) issued guidance to industry for

---

[1] Krause PJ, Auwaerter PG, Bannuru RR, et al. Clinical practice guidelines by the Infectious Diseases Society of America (IDSA): 2020 Guideline on diagnosis and management of babesiosis. *Clin Infect Dis*. 2021;72(2):e49-e64

regional, year-round testing using a licensed NAAT for *Babesia* infection or use of an FDA-approved pathogen-reduction device in the 14 highest-risk states (**www.fda.gov/regulatory-information/search-fda-guidance-documents/recommendations-reducing-risk-transfusion-transmitted-babesiosis**).

Public Health Reporting. Babesiosis is a nationally notifiable disease. Please refer to the state or local health department for details on reporting cases.

Bacillus cereus Infections and Intoxications

CLINICAL MANIFESTATIONS: *Bacillus cereus* primarily causes 2 toxin-mediated foodborne illnesses, emetic and diarrheal, but it also can cause invasive extraintestinal infection. The **emetic syndrome** develops after a short incubation period, similar to staphylococcal foodborne illness. It is characterized by nausea, vomiting, and abdominal cramps, and diarrhea may follow in up to one third of patients. The **diarrheal syndrome** has a longer incubation period, is more severe, and resembles *Clostridium perfringens* foodborne illness. It is characterized by moderate to severe abdominal cramps and watery diarrhea, vomiting in approximately 25% of patients, and occasionally low-grade fever. Both illnesses usually are short-lived, about 24 hours, but the emetic toxin is occasionally associated with fulminant liver failure.

Invasive extraintestinal infection can be severe and includes wound and soft tissue infections; sepsis and bacteremia, including central line-associated bloodstream infection; endocarditis; osteomyelitis; purulent meningitis and ventricular shunt infection; pneumonia; and ocular infections (ie, endophthalmitis and keratitis). Infection can be acquired through use of contaminated blood products, especially platelets. *B cereus* is a leading cause of bacterial endophthalmitis following penetrating ocular trauma. Endogenous endophthalmitis can result from bacteremic seeding. Other ocular manifestations include an indolent keratitis related to corneal abrasions and may be seen in contact lens users or those who have undergone cataract surgery.

Rare infections attributable to *B cereus* strains that express anthrax toxin genes, which clinically resemble anthrax, have been reported.

ETIOLOGY: *B cereus* is an aerobic and facultative anaerobic, spore-forming, gram-positive or gram-variable bacillus.

EPIDEMIOLOGY: *B cereus* is ubiquitous in the environment because of the high resistance of its endospores to extreme conditions, including heat, cold, desiccation, salinity, and radiation, and commonly is present in small numbers in raw, dried, and processed foods and in the feces of healthy people. The organism is a common cause of foodborne illness in the United States but may be underrecognized because few people seek care for mild illness and health care providers and clinical laboratories do not routinely test for *B cereus*. Several confirmed outbreaks were reported to the Centers for Disease Control and Prevention (CDC) in recent years. A wide variety of food vehicles has been implicated.

Spores of *B cereus* are heat resistant and can survive pasteurization, brief cooking, boiling, and high saline concentrations. Spores germinate to vegetative forms that produce enterotoxins over a wide range of temperatures, both in foods and in the gastrointestinal tract.

The diarrheal syndrome is caused by several distinct toxins that are produced after spores germinate in the gastrointestinal tract. The diarrheal toxins are heat labile and can be destroyed by heating.

The emetic syndrome occurs after eating contaminated food containing a preformed toxin called cereulide. The best known association of the emetic syndrome is with ingestion of fried rice made from boiled rice stored at room temperature overnight, because *B cereus* can be present in uncooked rice. However, a wide variety of foods, especially starchy foods (including cereals), cheese products, meats, and vegetables, has been implicated. The toxin is elaborated by vegetative forms that germinate from spores when the food is reheated; it is heat stable and gastric acid resistant.

Risk factors for invasive disease attributable to *B cereus* include history of injection drug use, presence of indwelling intravascular catheters or implanted devices, neutropenia or immunosuppression, and preterm birth. *B cereus* endophthalmitis has occurred after penetrating ocular trauma and injection drug use. Hospital outbreaks have been associated with contaminated medical equipment, but pseudo-outbreaks are more common and refer to sharp increases in contamination rates of clinical specimens associated with common source contamination (eg, ethanol pads or solutions, linens, blood culture media).

Foodborne illness caused by *B cereus* is not transmissible from person to person. The **incubation period** for foodborne illness is 30 minutes to 6 hours for the emetic syndrome and 6 to 15 hours for the diarrheal syndrome (see Appendix VI, Clinical Syndromes Associated With Foodborne Diseases, p 1150).

DIAGNOSTIC TESTS: Diagnostic testing is not recommended for sporadic cases. For foodborne outbreaks, isolation of *B cereus* from the stool or vomitus of 2 or more ill people and not from control patients, or isolation of 10^5 colony-forming units/g or greater from epidemiologically implicated food, suggests that *B cereus* is the cause of the outbreak. Because the organism can be recovered from stool specimens from some well people, the presence of *B cereus* in feces or vomitus of ill people alone is not definitive evidence of infection. Food samples must be tested for both the emetic toxin and diarrheal enterotoxins, because either alone can cause illness. Although there currently is no commercial kit that detects the cereulide emetic toxin, *B cereus* colonies isolated from food or specimens of ill individuals may be identified using nucleic acid amplification tests (NAATs) for the emetic toxin gene in diagnostic laboratories.

In patients with risk factors for invasive disease (eg, preterm infants, people with immunosuppressing conditions), isolation of *B cereus* from wounds or from blood or other sterile body fluids is significant. The common perception of *Bacillus* species as "contaminants" may delay recognition and treatment of serious *B cereus* infections.

TREATMENT: *B cereus* foodborne illness usually requires only supportive care, including rehydration. Antimicrobial therapy is indicated for patients with invasive disease. Prompt removal of any potentially contaminated foreign bodies, such as central lines or implants, is essential. For intraocular infections, an ophthalmologist should be consulted regarding surgical management and use of intravitreal antimicrobial therapy in addition to systemic therapy. *B cereus* is usually resistant to beta-lactam antibiotics and often to clindamycin but is susceptible to vancomycin, which is the drug of choice. Alternative drugs, including linezolid, clindamycin, aminoglycosides, erythromycin, tetracyclines, and fluoroquinolones, may be considered depending on susceptibility results.

INFECTION PREVENTION AND CONTROL MEASURES IN HEALTH CARE SETTINGS: Standard precautions are recommended.

CONTROL MEASURES: Proper cooking and appropriate storage of foods will help prevent foodborne illness attributable to *B cereus*. For example, rice cooked for later use should be refrigerated and not stored at room temperature. Information on recommended safe food handling practices, including time and temperature requirements during cooking, storage, and reheating, can be found at **www.foodsafety.gov.** In health care settings, careful hand hygiene and strict aseptic technique are important in caring for immunocompromised patients or patients with indwelling intravascular catheters to minimize the risk of invasive disease. The organism can survive in high concentrations of ethanol, but careful hand washing and use of 2% chlorhexidine are effective preventive measures.

Bacterial Vaginosis

CLINICAL MANIFESTATIONS: Bacterial vaginosis (BV) is a vaginal dysbiosis characterized by changes in vaginal flora, with a replacement of normal hydrogen peroxide- and lactic-acid–producing *Lactobacillus* species with a diverse community of BV-associated bacteria. BV is diagnosed primarily in sexually active postpubertal female individuals.[1] Symptoms may include vaginal discharge and/or vaginal odor. However, studies have shown that up to 50% to 75% of people who meet microbiologic criteria for a diagnosis of BV are asymptomatic. Classic signs, when present, include a thin off-white, homogenous, adherent vaginal discharge with an unpleasant fishy odor. Symptoms of pruritus, dysuria, or abdominal pain are not typically associated with BV but can be suggestive of mixed vaginitis (symptoms attributable to more than 1 infectious cause). In pregnant people, BV has been associated with adverse outcomes, including intra-amniotic infection, premature rupture of membranes, preterm delivery, and postpartum endometritis.

Vaginitis and vulvitis in prepubertal female children rarely, if ever, are manifestations of BV. Vaginitis in prepubertal children frequently is nonspecific. Causes of vaginitis in this population include things that alter the vaginal flora, such as certain soaps, detergents, foreign bodies, and infections attributable to group A streptococci, *Escherichia coli*, herpes simplex virus, *Neisseria gonorrhoeae*, *Chlamydia trachomatis*, *Trichomonas vaginalis*, or enteric bacteria, including *Shigella* species. In any prepubertal female child who has symptoms of BV, a full history and workup should be considered to rule out sexual abuse and/or a sexually transmitted infection (STI [see Sexual Assault and Abuse in Children and Adolescents/Young Adults, p 182]). If sexual abuse is suspected, those who are mandated to report need to follow their state's regulations for immediate reporting.

ETIOLOGY: BV is a result of a change in the vaginal microbiota. Hydrogen peroxide-producing lactobacilli, which normally predominate and play a protective role by maintaining a low vaginal pH, are replaced by mostly anaerobic organisms. High concentrations of *Gardnerella vaginalis*, *Prevotella* species, *Atopobium vaginae*, *Porphyromonas* species, *Bacteroides* species, *Peptostreptococcus* species, *Mycoplasma hominis*, *Ureaplasma urealyticum*, and *Mobiluncus, Megasphaera, Sneathia, Clostridiales*, and *Fusobacterium* species have been identified in individuals with BV. These anaerobes produce large amounts of proteolytic enzymes, which break down vaginal peptides into a variety of malodorous amines, leading to the typical BV vaginal odor.

---

[1] The terms female and male refer to sex assigned at birth.

EPIDEMIOLOGY: BV is the most common cause of vaginal discharge in sexually active adolescents and adults. BV occurs more frequently in female individuals with multiple sexual partners (male or female), those with a new sexual partner, those who do not use condoms, and those who douche. BV rarely develops in a female person who has never been sexually active. BV can increase the risk of acquisition of other STIs, including human immunodeficiency virus (HIV), herpes simplex virus, *Mycoplasma genitalium*, *N gonorrhoeae*, *C trachomatis*, *T vaginalis*, and human papillomavirus (HPV), and increase the risk of infectious complications following gynecologic surgeries and complications of pregnancy. BV can also increase the risk of HIV transmission to male sexual partners.

DIAGNOSTIC TESTS: The Amsel criteria and the Nugent score are commonly used to clinically diagnose BV when microscopy is available. At least 3 of the Amsel criteria are required for a BV diagnosis:

- Homogenous, thin grey or white vaginal discharge that smoothly coats the vaginal walls;
- Vaginal fluid pH greater than 4.5;
- A fishy (amine) odor of vaginal discharge before or after addition of 10% potassium hydroxide (ie, the "whiff test"); or
- Presence of clue cells (squamous vaginal epithelial cells covered with bacteria, which cause a stippled or granular appearance and ragged "moth-eaten" borders) representing at least 20% of the total vaginal epithelial cells seen on microscopic evaluation of vaginal fluid.

The Nugent score is used as the gold standard for diagnosing BV in the research setting and is commonly a standard against which newer diagnostic tests for BV are measured. A Gram stain of the vaginal fluid is evaluated, and a numerical score is generated on the basis of the apparent quantity of lactobacilli relative to BV-associated bacteria (*G vaginalis* and *Mobiluncus* species). The score is interpreted as normal (0–3), intermediate (4–6), or BV (7–10).

With microscopy use declining, a wide variety of available commercial laboratory tests are increasingly used to diagnose BV, ranging from point-of-care tests to nucleic acid amplification tests (NAATs) performed in clinical labs. The NAATs are based on detection of specific BV-associated bacterial nucleic acids and have high sensitivity and specificity for specific BV-associated bacteria and certain lactobacilli. They can be performed on either clinician- or self-collected vaginal specimens, and results are usually available in less than 24 hours. BV NAATs should only be used to test symptomatic patients.

Despite the availability of BV NAATs, because of their lower cost and ability to provide a rapid diagnosis, traditional BV diagnostics methods, such as Amsel criteria, Nugent score, and DNA probe tests, remain useful for diagnosing BV in symptomatic patients.

No recommendations exist to screen asymptomatic female individuals for BV. Culture for *G vaginalis* is not recommended as a diagnostic tool, because it is not specific, and Papanicolaou (Pap) testing is not recommended because of its extremely low sensitivity.

Sexually active individuals with BV should be evaluated for STI coinfection, including chlamydia, gonorrhea, trichomoniasis, syphilis, and HIV infection. If the hepatitis B and HPV vaccine series have not been completed, these immunizations should be offered.

TREATMENT[1]: Symptomatic patients with BV should be treated. The goals of treatment are to relieve the symptoms and signs of infection and potentially to decrease the risk of acquiring other STIs. Treatment considerations should include patient preference for oral versus intravaginal treatment, possible adverse effects, and the presence of coinfections.

Nonpregnant people with BV may be treated orally with metronidazole or topically with metronidazole gel 0.75% or clindamycin cream 2% (see Table 4.4, p 1007, and Table 4.5, p 1014). Alternative regimens include oral tinidazole, oral clindamycin, oral secnidazole, or clindamycin intravaginal ovules. Patients should refrain from sexual intercourse or use condoms during treatment, keeping in mind that clindamycin cream is oil based and can weaken latex condoms and diaphragms for up to 5 days after completion of therapy. Douching may increase the risk for relapse, and no data support douching for treatment or symptom relief. There is no evidence that treatment of sexual partners affects treatment response or recurrence risk. Follow-up is not necessary if symptoms resolve.

Pregnant people with symptoms of BV should be treated, because they are at high risk of adverse pregnancy outcomes. Metronidazole crosses the placenta, but there are no studies showing any teratogenicity. Because oral therapy has not been shown to be superior to topical therapy for treating symptomatic BV, symptomatic pregnant people can be treated with either the oral or vaginal metronidazole or clindamycin regimens recommended for nonpregnant people. Tinidazole should be avoided during pregnancy, as animal studies have shown teratogenic effects. Data are insufficient regarding efficacy and adverse effects of secnidazole, clindamycin 2% vaginal cream, metronidazole 1.3% vaginal gel, and 750-mg vaginal metronidazole tablets during pregnancy, so their use should be avoided in pregnant people.

Breastfeeding people with symptoms of BV should be treated. Metronidazole is secreted in human milk. Multiple reported case series identified no evidence of metronidazole-associated adverse effects for breastfed infants. Clindamycin has the potential to cause adverse effects on the breastfed infant's gastrointestinal flora. Infant side effects are less likely with vaginal clindamycin than oral use, because only approximately 30% of a vaginal dose is systemically absorbed. Because safety information on tinidazole or secnidazole in breastfeeding people is limited, they should only be used in difficult to treat cases. Interruption of breastfeeding is recommended during treatment and for 3 days after the last dose of secnidazole and tinidazole.

Approximately 30% of appropriately treated people have a BV recurrence within 3 months. Retreatment with the same regimen or an alternative regimen are both reasonable options for treating persistent or recurrent BV after the first occurrence. For people with multiple recurrences (more than 3 in the previous 12 months), either 0.75% metronidazole gel or 750-mg metronidazole vaginal suppository twice weekly for at least 3 months has been shown to reduce recurrences, although this benefit does not persist when suppressive therapy is discontinued. Limited data suggest an oral nitroimidazole (metronidazole or tinidazole, 500 mg, twice daily for 7 days) followed by intravaginal boric acid (600 mg daily for 21 days) and suppressive 0.75% metronidazole gel (twice weekly for 4 to 6 months) might be an option for patients with

---

[1] Centers for Disease Control and Prevention. Sexually transmitted infections treatment guidelines, 2021. *MMWR Recomm Rep.* 2021;70(RR-4):1-187. Available at: **www.cdc.gov/std/treatment-guidelines/bv.htm**

multiple recurrences of BV. Boric acid can cause death if ingested orally; it should be stored in a secure place inaccessible to children. Boric acid should not be used in pregnancy. Monthly oral metronidazole, 2 g, administered with fluconazole, 150 mg, has also been evaluated as suppressive therapy; this regimen reduced the incidence of BV and promoted colonization with normal vaginal microbiota. Studies thus far do not support currently available *Lactobacillus* formulations or probiotics as an adjunctive or replacement therapy for BV management.

INFECTION PREVENTION AND CONTROL MEASURES IN HEALTH CARE SETTINGS: Standard precautions are recommended.

CONTROL MEASURES: None.

Bacteroides, Prevotella, and Other Anaerobic Gram-Negative Bacilli Infections

CLINICAL MANIFESTATIONS: *Bacteroides, Prevotella,* and other anaerobic gram-negative bacilli (AGNB) residing in the oral cavity have been associated with chronic sinusitis, chronic otitis media, parotitis, dental infection, peritonsillar abscess, cervical adenitis, retropharyngeal space infection, aspiration pneumonia, lung abscess, pleural empyema, or necrotizing pneumonia. Species residing in the gastrointestinal tract have been recovered in patients with peritonitis, intra-abdominal abscess, pelvic inflammatory disease, Bartholin cyst abscess, tubo-ovarian abscess, endometritis, acute and chronic prostatitis, prostatic and scrotal abscesses, scrotal gangrene, postoperative wound infection, and vulvovaginal and perianal infections. Invasion of the bloodstream from the oral cavity or gastrointestinal tract may result in brain abscess, meningitis, endocarditis, arthritis, or osteomyelitis. Skin and soft tissue infections include bacterial gangrene and necrotizing fasciitis; omphalitis in newborn infants; cellulitis at the site of fetal monitor probes, human bite wounds, or burns; infections adjacent to the oral cavity or rectum; and infected decubitus ulcers. Neonatal infections, including conjunctivitis, pneumonia, bacteremia, or meningitis, rarely occur. When *Bacteroides, Prevotella,* and other AGNB are implicated, infections are typically polymicrobial.

ETIOLOGY: Most *Bacteroides, Prevotella, Porphyromonas,* and *Fusobacterium* organisms associated with human disease are pleomorphic, non–spore-forming, facultatively anaerobic, gram-negative bacilli.

EPIDEMIOLOGY: *Bacteroides, Prevotella,* and other AGNB are part of the normal oral, gastrointestinal tract, and genital tract flora. The *Bacteroides fragilis* group predominates in gastrointestinal tract flora. Enterotoxigenic *B fragilis* may be associated with diarrhea. Members of the *Prevotella melaninogenica* (formerly *Bacteroides melaninogenicus*) and *Prevotella oralis* (formerly *Bacteroides oralis*) groups reside in the oral cavity. These species result in infections as opportunists, usually after an alteration in skin or mucosal membranes in conjunction with other endogenous species, and often are associated with chronic mucosal injury. Rates of upper respiratory tract, head, and neck infections associated with AGNB are higher in children than in adults. Endogenous infection results from aspiration, bowel perforation, or damage to mucosal surfaces from trauma, surgery, or chemotherapy. Mucosal injury or granulocytopenia predispose to infection. Except in infections resulting from human bites, no evidence of person-to-person transmission of AGNB exists. The prevalence of AGNB infections is likely underestimated because of preanalytical collection, transportation, and specimen cultivation issues.

The **incubation period** is variable and depends on the inoculum and the site of involvement but usually is 1 to 5 days.

DIAGNOSTIC TESTS: Anaerobic culture media are necessary for recovery of *Bacteroides, Prevotella,* and other AGNB. Because infections usually are polymicrobial, aerobic and anaerobic cultures should be obtained when AGNB species are suspected. A putrid odor, with or without gas in the infected site, suggests anaerobic infection. Use of an anaerobic transport tube or a sealed syringe is recommended for collection of clinical specimens.

TREATMENT: Abscesses should be drained when feasible; abscesses involving the brain, liver, and lungs may resolve with effective antimicrobial therapy alone. Necrotizing soft tissue lesions require surgical débridement and antimicrobial therapy.

The choice of antimicrobial agent(s) is based on anticipated or known in vitro susceptibility testing and local antimicrobial resistance patterns. Anaerobic infections of the oral and respiratory tracts generally are susceptible to penicillin G, ampicillin, and clindamycin. However, because some species of *Bacteroides* and almost 50% of *Prevotella* species produce beta-lactamase, and penicillin treatment failure has emerged, penicillin is not recommended for empiric coverage or for treatment of severe oropharyngeal or pleuropulmonary infections or for any abdominopelvic infections. A beta-lactam combined with a beta-lactamase inhibitor (ampicillin-sulbactam, amoxicillin-clavulanate, or piperacillin-tazobactam) can be used to treat these infections.

Anaerobic infections of the gastrointestinal tract are often caused by *B fragilis*, which is typically resistant to penicillin G but susceptible to metronidazole, beta-lactam plus beta-lactamase inhibitors, carbapenems, cefoxitin, and chloramphenicol. The emergence of clindamycin resistance in *B fragilis* now limits its use. Tigecycline has in vitro activity against *Prevotella* and *Bacteroides* species but limited pediatric dosing and safety data are available, particularly for children younger than 8 years. Tigecycline has a black box warning for an increase in all-cause mortality and should be reserved for situations in which alternative agents are not suitable. Moxifloxacin may be an alternative to treat anaerobic infections in children with severe beta-lactam allergies, although emerging resistance is a concern. Cefuroxime, cefotaxime, and ceftriaxone are not reliably effective.

INFECTION PREVENTION AND CONTROL MEASURES IN HEALTH CARE SETTINGS: Standard precautions are recommended.

CONTROL MEASURES: None.

Balantidium coli Infections
(Balantidiasis)

CLINICAL MANIFESTATIONS: Most human infections are asymptomatic. Symptomatic infection is characterized either by acute onset of bloody or watery mucoid diarrhea with abdominal pain or with chronic or intermittent episodes of diarrhea, anorexia, and weight loss. Inflammation of the gastrointestinal tract and local lymphatic vessels can result in bowel dilation, ulceration, perforation, and extraintestinal spread or secondary bacterial invasion. Colitis produced by *Balantidium coli* can mimic that of *Entamoeba histolytica* or noninfectious causes. Fulminant disease can occur in malnourished or otherwise debilitated or immunocompromised patients. Rare cases of appendicitis, pneumonia, and urinary tract infections have been reported.

ETIOLOGY: *B coli*, a ciliated protozoan, is the largest pathogenic protozoan known to infect humans.

EPIDEMIOLOGY: Pigs are the primary host reservoir of *B coli*, but the parasite has also been found in other mammals, especially primates and livestock. Infections have been reported in most areas of the world but are more common in tropical and subtropical areas or areas with poor sanitation systems. Cysts excreted in feces can be transmitted directly from hand to mouth or indirectly through fecally contaminated water or food. Excysted trophozoites infect the colon. A person is infectious as long as cysts are excreted in stool. Cysts may remain viable in the environment for months.

The **incubation period** is not established but may be several days.

DIAGNOSTIC TESTS: Diagnosis usually is made by demonstrating trophozoites (or less frequently, cysts) in stool, intestinal biopsy specimens, or ova and parasite examination of fluid aspirates from extraintestinal sites. Excretion of parasites can be intermittent, and repeated stool examinations over several days may be necessary. Trophozoites are more often identified in diarrheal stools, and cysts (40–60 μm in diameter) are more common in formed stools. Trophozoites exhibit characteristic spiraling motility on wet mount. Because trophozoites degenerate rapidly, fresh diarrheal stools require either prompt microscopic examination or placement in stool fixation medium. Stool studies may be negative in the rare cases of extraintestinal manifestations of disease.

TREATMENT: The drugs of choice are tetracycline and metronidazole (see Table 4.11, Drugs for Parasitic Infections, p 1068). Alternative drugs include iodoquinol and nitazoxanide.

INFECTION PREVENTION AND CONTROL MEASURES IN HEALTH CARE SETTINGS: Standard and contact precautions are recommended, because human-to-human transmission can occur rarely.

CONTROL MEASURES: Avoiding food or water that may be contaminated with feces (especially pig feces) is key to avoiding infection. Control measures include sanitary disposal of human and porcine feces and good handwashing. Cysts are resistant to the levels of chlorination used for drinking water, and waterborne outbreaks of disease have occurred despite chlorination. Fresh produce should be avoided in high-risk settings as washing alone may be insufficient to eliminate transmission.

Bartonella henselae (Cat-Scratch Disease)

CLINICAL MANIFESTATIONS: Cat scratch disease, the predominant clinical manifestation of *Bartonella henselae* infection, presents in 85% to 90% of children as a localized cutaneous and regional lymphadenopathy disorder. A skin papule or pustule develops within 12 days at the presumed site of inoculation in approximately two thirds of cases and usually precedes development of lymphadenopathy by 1 to 2 weeks (range, 7–60 days). Lymphadenopathy occurs in nodes that drain the site of inoculation, typically axillary, but cervical, submandibular, submental, epitrochlear, or inguinal nodes can be involved. Low-grade fever lasting several days develops in 30% of patients. The skin overlying affected lymph nodes can be normal or can be tender, warm, erythematous, and indurated, and approximately 10% to 20% of affected nodes suppurate. Typically, lymphadenopathy resolves spontaneously in 2 to 4 months.

Less common manifestations of *B henselae* infection likely reflect bloodborne disseminated disease and include culture-negative endocarditis, encephalopathy, osteolytic lesions, glomerulonephritis, pneumonia, thrombocytopenic purpura, erythema nodosum, and prolonged fever with granulomata in the liver and spleen. Chronic *Bartonella* infection in nonimmunocompromised children has not been substantiated scientifically.

Ocular manifestations occur in 5% to 10% of patients. The most classic and frequent presentation of ocular *B henselae* infection is Parinaud oculoglandular syndrome, which consists of follicular conjunctivitis and ipsilateral preauricular lymphadenopathy. Another occasional ocular manifestation is neuroretinitis, which is characterized by abrupt unilateral (and rarely bilateral) painless vision impairment, granulomatous optic disc swelling, and macular edema, with lipid exudates (macular star). Rare presentations include retinochoroiditis, anterior uveitis, vitritis, pars planitis, retinal vasculitis, retinitis, branch retinal arteriolar or venular occlusions, macular hole, or, very rarely, retinal detachments.

B henselae (as well as *Bartonella quintana*) can cause bacillary angiomatosis (vascular proliferative lesions of skin and subcutaneous tissue) and bacillary peliosis (reticuloendothelial lesions in visceral organs, primarily the liver). These are primarily reported in immunocompromised patients, including people with HIV, but can also occur in immunocompetent people.

ETIOLOGY: *B henselae* is a fastidious, slow-growing, gram-negative bacillus. Other *Bartonella* species, such as *Bartonella clarridgeiae*, also have been found to cause cat scratch disease (CSD). *B henselae* is related closely to *B quintana*, a louse-borne disease that causes a distinct febrile illness with relapsing fevers, shin pain, headache, and myalgia. This illness resulted in significant disease among troops during World War I, leading to its former name of "trench fever." People experiencing homelessness are at increased risk of *B quintana* infection because of lack of access to adequate sanitation and hygiene. *B quintana* also can cause bacillary angiomatosis and endocarditis.

EPIDEMIOLOGY: *B henselae* is a common cause of regional lymphadenopathy in children. The highest incidence is found in children 5 to 9 years of age; infections occur more often during the fall and winter. Cats are the natural reservoir for *B henselae*, with a seroprevalence of 30% to 40% in domestic and adopted shelter cats in the United States. Other animals, including dogs, can be infected and are rarely associated with human illness. Cat-to-cat transmission occurs via the cat flea *(Ctenocephalides felis)*, with feline infection resulting in bacteremia that usually is asymptomatic and lasts weeks to months. Fleas acquire the organism when feeding on a bacteremic cat and then shed infectious organisms in their feces. The bacteria are transmitted to humans by inoculation from cat saliva or flea feces through a scratch or wound from a cat. Most patients with CSD have a history of recent contact with apparently healthy cats, especially kittens. Kittens are nearly 5 times as likely to be bacteremic with *B henselae* than are older cats. Cats obtained from shelters or adopted as strays also have high rates of bacteremia. There is no convincing evidence that ticks can transmit *Bartonella* species to humans. No evidence of person-to-person transmission exists.

The **incubation period** from the time of the scratch to appearance of the primary cutaneous lesion is 3 to 12 days; the median period from the appearance of the primary lesion to the appearance of lymphadenopathy is 12 days (range, 7 to 60 days).

DIAGNOSTIC TESTS: Both enzyme immunoassay (EIA) and indirect immunofluorescent antibody (IFA) platforms for detection of IgM and IgG serum antibodies to antigens of *Bartonella* species are available for diagnosis of CSD. Both platforms have limitations in sensitivity and specificity. With both types of tests, cross-reactivity with other infectious agents (such as *Chlamydia pneumoniae, Coxiella burnetii,* and especially other *Bartonella* species) is common. Elevated immunoglobulin (Ig) M titers may suggest recent infection, but both false-positive and false-negative IgM test results occur. In adults, there is a high rate of anti-*B henselae* IgG seroprevalence in the general population attributable to prior exposure. Usually, if an IFA or EIA IgG titer is <1:64, the patient does not have acute infection. Titers between 1:64 and 1:256 may represent past or acute infection, and follow-up titers in 2 to 4 weeks should be considered. An IgG titer of ≥1:256 or a fourfold increase in IgG titer between acute and convalescent samples is consistent with acute infection.

Nucleic acid amplification tests (NAATs) are available in some commercial and research laboratories for testing of tissue or body fluids. *Bartonella* NAATs are highly specific and fairly sensitive for use on tissue, although some tests do not distinguish between the various *Bartonella* species. NAATs of valvular tissue can be important in cases of culture-negative endocarditis. The sensitivity of *Bartonella* NAATs is much lower for whole blood, and this specimen type is not generally recommended for NAATs but may be useful in select circumstances.

B henselae is a fastidious organism; recovery by routine culture requires prolonged incubation (>10 days) and rarely is successful unless performed in specialized laboratories with experienced staff.

If tissue (eg, lymph node) specimens are available, bacilli occasionally may be visualized using a silver stain (eg, Warthin-Starry or Steiner stain); however, these stains are not specific for *B henselae.* Early histologic changes in lymph node specimens consist of lymphocytic infiltration with epithelioid granuloma formation. Later changes consist of polymorphonuclear leukocyte infiltration with granulomas that become necrotic and resemble granulomas from patients with tularemia, brucellosis, or mycobacterial infections.

TREATMENT: Management of localized uncomplicated CSD primarily is aimed at relief of symptoms, because the disease is self-limited, resolving spontaneously in 2 to 4 months. No antibiotic regimen has been shown to be beneficial in improving the clinical cure rate, and in most cases, antibiotic therapy is not indicated. Painful suppurative nodes can be treated with needle aspiration for relief of symptoms. Incision and drainage should be avoided, because this may facilitate fistula formation; surgical excision generally is unnecessary.

Some experts recommend antimicrobial therapy in acutely or severely ill immunocompetent patients with systemic symptoms, particularly people with retinitis, hepatic or splenic involvement, osteomyelitis, or painful adenitis. Several antimicrobial agents (azithromycin, clarithromycin, ciprofloxacin, doxycycline, trimethoprim-sulfamethoxazole, ceftriaxone, gentamicin, and rifampin) have in vitro activity against *B henselae.* However, outcomes for most forms of CSD are generally excellent with or without antibiotic therapy.

Doxycycline plus rifampin are often used for treatment of patients with neuroretinitis. A duration of therapy of 4 to 6 weeks generally has been used on the basis of a small case series in young adults. Doxycycline may be used regardless of patient age.

Reports in the literature note that a large majority of such patients experience significant visual recovery to 20/40 or better. Corticosteroids should be considered in conjunction with ophthalmology consultation.

Antimicrobial therapy is recommended for all immunocompromised people, because treatment of bacillary angiomatosis and bacillary peliosis has been shown to be beneficial. Azithromycin or doxycycline is effective for treatment of these conditions; therapy should be administered for 3 months for bacillary angiomatosis and for 4 months for bacillary peliosis to prevent relapse. Consultation with an infectious disease specialist is recommended for treatment in immunocompromised people.

For pediatric patients with unusual manifestations of *Bartonella* infection (eg, endocarditis or endovascular infection, neuroretinitis, disease in immunocompromised patients), consultation with a pediatric infectious diseases expert is recommended.

INFECTION PREVENTION AND CONTROL MEASURES IN HEALTH CARE SETTINGS: Standard precautions are recommended.

CONTROL MEASURES: CSD is a preventable infection. All cats >8 weeks of age should be treated topically for fleas and ticks regularly. Effort should be undertaken to avoid scratches and bites from cats or kittens. Sites of cat scratches or bites should be washed immediately, and cats should not be allowed to lick open cuts or wounds. Immunocompromised people should avoid contact with cats younger than 1 year, stray cats, and cats that scratch or bite. Testing or treatment of cats for *Bartonella* infection is not recommended, nor is declawing or removal of the cat from the household.

Baylisascaris Infections

CLINICAL MANIFESTATIONS: Clinical signs of infection with *Baylisascaris procyonis,* the common raccoon roundworm, are likely dependent on inoculum size. Clinically evident infections usually present as acute onset of central nervous system (CNS) disease (neural larva migrans [NLM], eosinophilic meningoencephalitis), with sudden lethargy or somnolence, weakness, irritability, behavioral regression, and decreased awareness and interaction. There may be nuchal rigidity, decreased head control, torticollis, loss of fine motor skills, seizures, impaired vision or speech, ataxia, and difficulty sitting or standing without assistance. Once CNS onset has occurred, usually 2 to 4 weeks after infection, signs may worsen rapidly. NLM is typically accompanied by marked peripheral and/or cerebrospinal fluid (CSF) eosinophilia. Outcomes are related to the amount of inflammatory and mechanical damage occurring from the presence of larvae in the CNS and range from severe neurologic sequelae and death to milder sequelae and, in some cases, improvement with early and aggressive treatment. Other clinical presentations include visceral and ocular larva migrans (VLM, OLM); all 3 types (NLM, VLM, and OLM) may occur concomitantly. The nonspecific signs of VLM, such as rash, fever, abdominal pain, pneumonitis, and hepatomegaly, may be overshadowed by the manifestations of NLM. OLM can result in diffuse unilateral subacute neuroretinitis (DUSN), and direct visualization of a larva in the retina is sometimes possible. Similar to larva migrans caused by *Toxocara* species, subclinical and covert infections seem to be the most common outcome and are likely the result of incidental, low-level *Baylisascaris* infection.

ETIOLOGY: *B procyonis* is a 9- to 22-cm long roundworm (nematode) that infects raccoons, often subclinically, as its definitive host and a wide variety (>150 species) of mammals and birds as paratenic hosts, in which its larvae aggressively migrate throughout the body. Domestic dogs can also serve as definitive hosts, but less commonly. Some other carnivores (skunks, kinkajous, bears, etc) harbor related *Baylisascaris* species that are potential sources of infection, although no human cases with these animals as a source have been documented.

EPIDEMIOLOGY: *B procyonis* is widely but variably distributed throughout the United States and Canada and also is found in Europe and Japan. In areas where it is endemic, 20% to >80% of raccoons can harbor the parasite in their intestines. When infective eggs or an infected paratenic host is eaten by a raccoon, the larvae grow to maturity in the small intestine, where adult female worms shed millions of eggs per day in the feces. Eggs become infective only after 2 to 4 weeks in the environment and may persist long-term in the soil. Embryonated eggs containing infective larvae are ingested from the soil by raccoons and other animals, including humans, particularly children. Risk of human infection is greatest in areas where significant raccoon populations live in peridomestic settings. More than 30 cases of *Baylisascaris* CNS disease (including 22 in children), 25 cases of OLM-DUSN (including 10 in children), and 100 seropositive asymptomatic cases have been reported in the United States and Canada, and it is likely that cases may be undiagnosed and/or underreported.

The main risk factor for *Baylisascaris* infection is contact with raccoon latrines, which are communal defecation sites often found at or on the base of trees; raised flat surfaces such as tree stumps, logs, rocks, decks, and rooftops; or unsealed attics or garages. Other risk factors include geophagia/pica, age younger than 4 years, and in older children, developmental delay. Most reported cases of CNS disease have been in male individuals.[1]

Unlike *Toxocara* species, *Baylisascaris* larvae grow rapidly following infection, reaching considerable size (1400–1900 μm x 50–80 μm) by 10 to 15 days postinfection. They are aggressive migrators and may enter the brain of experimentally infected animals as early as 3 to 5 days postinfection. Only approximately 5% to 7% of larvae migrate into the CNS, but their size, numbers, aggressiveness, and metabolic products correlate with their high pathogenicity. In one fatal case in an 18-month-old, the brain alone contained an estimated >3200 larvae. Low-level infections, even those involving the CNS, can produce a spectrum of milder focal and/or nonspecific signs.

The **incubation period** in overt CNS cases is usually 2 to 4 weeks.

DIAGNOSTIC TESTS: *Baylisascaris* infection is confirmed by identification of larvae in biopsy specimens. A presumptive diagnosis of NLM can be made on the basis of clinical (meningoencephalitis, sometimes with concomitant VLM and/or OLM-DUSN), epidemiologic (raccoon exposure), and laboratory (blood and CSF eosinophilia) findings. Antibody detection in serum and CSF for patients with clinical symptoms is available at the Centers for Disease Control and Prevention as well as the National Reference Centre for Parasitology in Canada. Neuroimaging results can be normal initially, but as larvae migrate and cause damage to CNS tissues, diffuse or multifocal abnormalities typically develop symmetrically in deep periventricular white matter, the

---

[1] The term male refers to sex assigned at birth.

cerebellum, or elsewhere; these may progress to atrophic changes. In ocular disease, ophthalmologic examination can reveal chorioretinal lesions and rarely larvae. Stool examination is not helpful, because eggs are not shed in human feces.

TREATMENT: Early diagnostic consideration and treatment are critical. Albendazole, in conjunction with high-dose corticosteroids, has been advocated most widely on the basis of good CNS and CSF penetration and efficacy in experimental animals (see Drugs for Parasitic Infections, p 1068). If infection is suspected, treatment should be initiated promptly, even while the diagnostic evaluation is being completed. Empiric therapy with albendazole should be considered for children with a history of ingestion of soil known or potentially contaminated with raccoon feces; in controlled studies, experimentally infected animals given albendazole on days 1 to 10 postinfection did not develop CNS disease, whereas all untreated animals died. Treatment with albendazole and corticosteroids may not affect clinical outcome if severe CNS disease manifestations are evident. Limited data are available regarding safety and efficacy of alternate anthelmintic therapies in children, although mebendazole and ivermectin have been proposed as alternatives if albendazole is unavailable; both may show efficacy against somatic larvae especially early in infection, but because ivermectin does not cross the blood-brain barrier well, it has limited usefulness in clinical NLM. Larvae localized to the retina and away from sensitive areas can be killed by direct photocoagulation.

INFECTION PREVENTION AND CONTROL MEASURES IN HEALTH CARE SETTINGS: Standard precautions are recommended. The disease is not transmitted from person-to-person.

CONTROL MEASURES: *Baylisascaris* infections are prevented by avoiding ingestion of soil or other articles contaminated with the feces of infected animal reservoirs, primarily raccoons. People should be educated about the potential risks of this infection, and the keeping of raccoons and other wildlife as pets should be discouraged strongly. Children should be taught to recognize and avoid raccoon defecation sites (latrines) and other animal feces and to wash their hands after contact with soil, pets, or other animals. Raccoon visitation may be discouraged by limiting access to human or pet food sources; problematic animals can be trapped and removed by wildlife personnel. Raccoon latrines identified near homes, child care centers, and other facilities can be decontaminated by feces removal followed by treating the area with boiling water or a propane torch to kill residual eggs, in keeping with local fire safety regulations, or through proper removal if located within the home or other buildings (eg, attic, shed, garage).

Infections With *Blastocystis* Species

CLINICAL MANIFESTATIONS: The importance of *Blastocystis* species as a cause of gastrointestinal tract disease is controversial. The asymptomatic carrier state is well documented. Clinical symptoms reported include bloating, flatulence, acute or chronic watery diarrhea without fecal leukocytes or blood, constipation, abdominal pain, nausea, anorexia, weight loss, and poor growth; fever is generally absent. Some case series and reports have noted an association between infection with *Blastocystis* and chronic urticaria and irritable bowel syndrome. When *Blastocystis* organisms are identified in stool from symptomatic patients, other causes of this symptom complex, particularly

Giardia duodenalis and *Cryptosporidium parvum,* should be investigated before assuming that blastocystosis is the cause of the signs and symptoms. Nucleic acid amplification test (NAAT) fingerprinting suggests that some *Blastocystis* subtypes are disease associated and others are not. An emerging literature reflects increased interest in understanding the role of *Blastocystis* in the gastrointestinal tract microbiome.

ETIOLOGY: *Blastocystis* species (previously referred to as *Blastocystis hominis)* consists of multiple subtypes that reside in the gastrointestinal tracts of humans as well as other mammals, reptiles, amphibians, and fish. Some *Blastocystis* species believed to be specific to other animals are now recognized as being able to be transmitted to humans. Previously classified as a protozoan, more recent molecular studies have led the organism to be characterized as a stramenopile (a eukaryote). Multiple forms have been described: vacuolar, which is observed most commonly in clinical specimens; granular, which is seen rarely in fresh stools; ameboid; and cystic.

EPIDEMIOLOGY: *Blastocystis* infection (colonization) is observed commonly throughout the world, although prevalence among countries and communities varies. In general, prevalence is lower in high-income than lower-income countries, ranging from 1% in Japan to 100% in among school-aged children in countries without modern sanitation. Because transmission is believed to occur via the fecal-oral route, presence of the organism may be a marker for presence of other pathogens spread by fecal contamination. *Blastocystis* infection is more common among people with pets or living near farm animals, but exposure is not sufficient for infection as pathogenicity appears related to subtype, host immunocompetence, and other factors. Organisms may remain in the gastrointestinal tract for years.

The **incubation period** has not been established.

DIAGNOSTIC TESTS: Microscopy is used commonly for diagnosis. Trichome staining is more sensitive than wet mount staining with Lugol iodine. Because of irregular shedding of the parasite, multiple stool specimens should be obtained for evaluation. A variety of morphologies may be seen during microscopy; vacuolar and cystic forms are seen most commonly in stool specimens. The vacuolar form varies markedly in size from 2 to 200 μm and is characterized by a large central body (similar to large vacuole) surrounded by multiple nuclei. The cyst form is smaller, usually 3 to 5μm, and can be difficult to identify. The parasite may be present in varying numbers, and infections may be reported as light to heavy. The presence of 5 or more organisms per high-power (x400 magnification for wet mount and x1000 for oil immersion) field can indicate heavy infection, which to some experts suggests causation when other enteropathogens are absent. Other experts consider the presence of 10 or more organisms per 10 oil immersion fields (x1000 magnification) to represent heavy infection. Laboratory cultures may improve sensitivity, although slower growing subtypes may be missed in mixed infections.

A serum antibody test is available, but its diagnostic utility is still unclear. Molecular testing with a nucleic acid amplification test (NAAT), including multiplex platforms, detects the presence of *Blastocystis* in far more people than does microscopy alone. The clinical significance and utility of such detections remain unclear. Codetection with other potential pathogens is common.

TREATMENT: Indications for treatment are not established. Some experts recommend that treatment should be reserved for patients who have persistent symptoms and in whom no other pathogen or process is found to explain the gastrointestinal tract symptoms. Randomized controlled treatment trials with both metronidazole and nitazoxanide have demonstrated benefit in symptomatic patients, although microbiologic resolution does not always occur. Tinidazole is an alternative that may be tolerated better than metronidazole. Case series suggest high resolution of symptoms in symptomatic patients treated with trimethoprim-sulfamethoxazole but variable success in clearing the organism (see Table 4.11, Drugs for Parasitic Infections, p 1068). Case reports or small series indicate paromomycin, iodoquinol, and ketoconazole alone or in combination have varying success. Other experts believe that *Blastocystis* infection does not cause symptomatic disease and recommend only a careful search for other causes of symptoms. Apparent responses to therapy may reflect the natural courses of infection caused by other etiologies, or the therapeutic response of another, unrecognized causative organism by the drug selected to treat *Blastocystis*.

INFECTION PREVENTION AND CONTROL MEASURES IN HEALTH CARE SETTINGS: Standard precautions should be followed; contact precautions also are recommended for diapered or incontinent people.

CONTROL MEASURES: Personal hygiene measures, including hand washing with soap and warm water after using the toilet, after changing diapers, and before preparing food, should be practiced.

Blastomycosis

CLINICAL MANIFESTATIONS: Infections can be acute, chronic, or fulminant but are asymptomatic in up to 50% of infected people. The most common clinical manifestation of blastomycosis in children is cough (often productive) accompanying pulmonary disease, with fever, chest pain, and nonspecific symptoms such as fatigue and myalgia. Rarely, patients may develop acute respiratory distress syndrome (ARDS). Typical radiographic patterns include consolidation, patchy pneumonitis, a mass-like infiltrate, or nodules. Blastomycosis can be misdiagnosed as bacterial pneumonia, tuberculosis, sarcoidosis, or malignant neoplasm. Disseminated blastomycosis, which can occur in up to 25% of symptomatic cases, most commonly involves the skin and osteoarticular structures. Cutaneous manifestations can be verrucous, nodular, ulcerative, or pustular. Abscesses usually are subcutaneous but can involve any organ. Erythema nodosum, which is common in patients with histoplasmosis and coccidioidomycosis, is rare in blastomycosis. Central nervous system infection is less common, and intrauterine or congenital infection is rare.

ETIOLOGY: Blastomycosis is caused by *Blastomyces* species *(Blastomyces dermatitidis, Blastomyces gilchristii, Blastomyces helices, Blastomyces percursus,* and *Blastomyces emzantsi),* which are thermally dimorphic fungi existing in the yeast form at 37°C (98°F) in infected tissues and in a mycelial form at room temperature and in soil. Conidia, produced from hyphae of the mycelial form, are infectious.

EPIDEMIOLOGY: Infection is acquired through inhalation of conidia from the environment. Increased mortality rates for patients with pulmonary blastomycosis have been associated with advanced age, chronic obstructive pulmonary disease, cancer, and Black race. Person-to-person transmission does not occur. In the United States, blastomycosis is endemic in the central states, with most cases occurring in the Ohio and Mississippi river valleys, the southeastern states, and states that border the Great Lakes; however, sporadic cases have occurred outside these areas. *Blastomyces* species are found in moist soil and decomposing organic matter like wood and leaves. Similar to *Histoplasma capsulatum*, *Blastomyces* species can grow in bird and animal excreta. Occupational and recreational activities associated with infection often involve environmental disruption such as construction of homes or roads, boating and canoeing, tubing on a river, fishing, exploration of beaver dams and underground forts, and community compost piles.

The **incubation period** ranges from approximately 2 weeks to 3 months.

DIAGNOSTIC TESTS: Definitive diagnosis of blastomycosis is based on microscopic identification of characteristic thick-walled, broad-based, single budding yeast cells either by culture at 37°C or in histopathologic specimens. The organism may be seen in sputum, tracheal aspirates, cerebrospinal fluid, urine, or histopathologic specimens from lesions processed with 10% potassium hydroxide or a silver stain. Histopathology demonstrates granulomatous inflammation. Children with pneumonia who are unable to produce sputum may require bronchoalveolar lavage or open biopsy to establish the diagnosis. Bronchoalveolar lavage is high yield, including in patients with bone or skin manifestations. Organisms can be cultured on brain-heart infusion media and Sabouraud dextrose agar at 25°C to 30°C as a mold; identification can be confirmed by conversion to yeast phase at 37°C. Chemiluminescent DNA probes are available for identification of *B dermatitidis;* rare false-positive identification attributable to cross-reactivity with other endemic fungi has been reported. Nucleic acid amplification tests (NAATs) can be used directly on certain clinical specimens but are not widely performed.

Because serologic tests (immunodiffusion and complement fixation) lack adequate sensitivity, they are generally not useful for diagnosis. An enzyme immunoassay that detects *Blastomyces* antigen in urine and blood has replaced classic serologic studies and performs well for the diagnosis of disseminated and pulmonary disease as well as for monitoring response to antifungal therapy. Antigen testing in urine has higher sensitivity than antigen testing of serum, and antigen testing in bronchoalveolar lavage fluid or cerebrospinal fluid is also available. Cross-reactions may occur in patients with dimorphic fungal diseases (eg, coccidioidomycosis, histoplasmosis, paracoccidioidomycosis, sporotrichosis, *Emergomyces africanus* disease, and talaromycosis [formerly penicillosis]); clinical and epidemiologic distinctions aid in differentiating these entities.

TREATMENT[1,2]: Because of the high risk of dissemination, most experts recommend that all cases of blastomycosis in children should be treated. Amphotericin B deoxycholate or an amphotericin B lipid formulation is recommended for initial therapy of severe pulmonary disease for 1 to 2 weeks or until improvement, followed by 6 to 12 months of itraconazole therapy. Oral itraconazole is recommended for 6 to

[1] Chapman SW, Dismukes WE, Proia LA, et al. Clinical guidelines for the management of blastomycosis: 2008 update by the Infectious Diseases Society of America. *Clin Infect Dis.* 2008;46(12):1801–1812

[2] Thompson GR III, Le T, Chindamporn A, et al. Global guideline for the diagnosis and management of the endemic mycoses: an initiative of the European Confederation of Medical Mycology in cooperation with the International Society for Human and Animal Mycology [Erratum in: *Lancet Infect Dis.* 2021;21(11):e341]. *Lancet Infect Dis.* 2021;21(12):e364-e374

12 months for mild to moderate infection (see Table 4.7, p 1021). Some experts suggest 12 months of therapy for patients with osteoarticular disease. For central nervous system infection, a lipid formulation of amphotericin B is recommended for 4 to 6 weeks, followed by an azole for at least 12 months and until resolution of all cerebrospinal fluid and neuroimaging abnormalities. The optimal azole for prolonged central nervous system infection treatment is unknown, but voriconazole is suggested, given the limited central nervous system penetration of itraconazole. Itraconazole is indicated for treatment of non–life-threatening infection outside the central nervous system in adults and is recommended in children.

Serum trough concentrations of itraconazole should be 1 to 2 µg/mL. A trough level should be checked 10 days or later following initiation to ensure adequate drug exposure. When measured by high-pressure liquid chromatography, both itraconazole and its bioactive hydroxyitraconazole metabolite are reported, the sum of which should be considered in assessing the trough concentration. The itraconazole oral solution formulation is preferred over the capsule formulation because of improved absorption, and should be taken on an empty stomach. However, a super bioavailable (SUBA) itraconazole is now approved by the Food and Drug Administration for the treatment of pulmonary and extrapulmonary blastomycosis in individuals 18 years or older, with pharmacokinetic studies of this formulation demonstrating less variable absorption than conventional itraconazole capsules and a similar side effect profile; data in children are lacking.

INFECTION PREVENTION AND CONTROL MEASURES IN HEALTH CARE SETTINGS: Standard precautions are recommended.

CONTROL MEASURES: None. Immunocompromised individuals should avoid activities that disturb soil in areas where blastomycosis is common.

Bocavirus

CLINICAL MANIFESTATIONS: Human bocavirus (HBoV) was identified in 2005 from a cohort of children with acute respiratory tract symptoms. Pneumonia, bronchiolitis, exacerbations of asthma, upper respiratory tract infection, and acute otitis media have been attributed to HBoV. Rare cases of encephalitis, myocarditis, and disseminated infection have also been reported. Symptoms may include cough, rhinorrhea, wheezing, and fever. HBoV has been identified in up to 33% of children with acute respiratory tract infections in various settings (such as inpatients, outpatients, and group child care attendees). High rates of HBoV subclinical infections have been documented, complicating the etiologic association between HBoV detection and identification of disease. Confirming whether HBoV is a pathogen in human infection is further challenging because of frequent simultaneous detection of other viral pathogens. However, a number of lines of evidence support the role of HBoV as a pathogen, at least during primary infection. These include longitudinal cohort studies showing an association of primary infection with symptomatic illness and case-control studies showing associations of illness with monoinfection, high viral load, viremia, serologic evidence of new infection, and detection of HBoV mRNA. HBoV has been detected in stool samples from children with acute gastroenteritis; however, further studies are needed to better understand the role of HBoV in gastroenteritis.

ETIOLOGY: HBoV is a nonenveloped, single-stranded DNA virus classified in the family *Parvoviridae*, subfamily *Parvovirinae*, genus *Bocaparvovirus*, on the basis of its genetic similarity to the closely related **bo**vine parvovirus 1 and **ca**nine minute virus, from which the name "**boca**virus" was derived. Four distinct genotypes have been described (HBoV types 1–4). HBoV1 replicates in the respiratory tract and has been associated with upper and lower respiratory tract illness. HBoV2, HBoV3, and HBoV4 have been found predominantly in stool and are overall more likely to be detected among children with gastroenteritis than those without gastroenteritis.

EPIDEMIOLOGY: Detection of HBoV has been described only in humans. Transmission is believed to be mainly from respiratory tract secretions, although fecaloral transmission might also be possible.

The frequent codetection of other viral pathogens of the respiratory tract in association with HBoV has led to speculation about the pathologic role played by HBoV; however, evidence indicates that HBoV can act as either a harmless passenger or lead to illness. Codetection of HBoV with other respiratory viruses is more common when HBoV is present at lower viral loads ($\leq 10^4$ copies/mL). Extended and intermittent shedding of HBoV has been reported for up to a year after initial detection; approximately 15% of children remain positive for 3 or more weeks. HBoV circulates worldwide and throughout the year. In temperate climates, seasonal clustering in the spring associated with increased transmission of other respiratory tract viruses has been reported.

DIAGNOSTIC TESTS: Commercial molecular diagnostic assays for HBoV are available. HBoV quantitative nucleic acid amplification tests (NAATs) (respiratory and serum specimens), detection of HBoV mRNA in the respiratory tract, and detection of HBoV-specific immunoglobulin (Ig) M and IgG antibody also are used by research laboratories to detect the presence of virus and infection.

Because HBoV can be shed for long periods after primary infection, can possibly reactivate during subsequent viral infections, and has a high rate of detection in healthy people, clinical interpretation of HBoV detection is challenging. A positive test result is more likely to represent the cause of illness if no other pathogens are detected, there is viremia, or there is serologic evidence of new infection.

TREATMENT: No specific therapy is available.

INFECTION PREVENTION AND CONTROL MEASURES IN HEALTH CARE SETTINGS: Because of the presence of virus in respiratory tract secretions and stool, standard, contact, and droplet precautions should be initiated to limit the spread of infection for the duration of the symptomatic illness in infants and young children. Prolonged shedding of virus in respiratory tract secretions and in stool can occur after resolution of symptoms, particularly among immunocompromised children; longer duration of precautions might be considered in these situations.

CONTROL MEASURES: Respiratory precautions should be followed. Although possible health care-associated transmission of HBoV has been described, transmission of HBoV in health care settings seems to be rare. Appropriate hand hygiene is recommended, particularly when handling respiratory tract secretions or diapers of ill children. The presence of HBoV DNA in serum also raises the possibility of transmission by transfusion, although this mode of transmission has not been documented.

Borrelia Infections Other Than Lyme Disease
(Relapsing Fever)

CLINICAL MANIFESTATIONS: Several types of relapsing fever infections occur in humans: tick-borne relapsing fever spread by soft-bodied ticks, louse-borne relapsing fever, and *Borrelia miyamotoi* infection, or hard tick relapsing fever, spread by hard-bodied ticks. Tick-borne and louse-borne relapsing fevers have many clinical similarities; *B miyamotoi* can cause an acute febrile illness but its clinical features are less well described. Both tick-borne relapsing fever and louse-borne relapsing fever are characterized by sudden onset of high fever, shaking chills, sweats, headache, muscle and joint pain, altered sensorium, and nausea. A fleeting macular rash of the trunk and petechiae of the skin and mucous membranes sometimes occur but are not common. Findings and complications can differ between types of relapsing fever and include hepatosplenomegaly, jaundice, thrombocytopenia, iridocyclitis, cough with pleuritic pain, pneumonitis, Bell's palsy, meningitis, and myocarditis. Neurologic complications are more common with tick-borne relapsing fever and occur in 10% to 40% of cases. Mortality rates are 10% to 70% in untreated louse-borne relapsing fever (possibly related to comorbidities and outbreaks associated with war, famine, and forced migration) and 4% to 10% in untreated tick-borne relapsing fever. Infection during pregnancy can result in spontaneous abortion, preterm birth, stillbirth, or neonatal infection with high perinatal mortality, as well as death of the pregnant individual. Fatal cases occur predominantly in infants, older adults, and people with underlying illnesses. Early treatment reduces mortality to less than 5%. Untreated, an initial febrile period (typically lasting 2 to 7 days for tick-borne and up to 10 for louse-borne) terminates spontaneously and is followed by an afebrile period of several days to weeks, then by 1 relapse or more. Relapses are more common with tick-borne disease, with generally ≥2 relapses (range: 0–13), than for louse-borne disease, with generally <2 relapses (range: 1–5). Relapses typically become shorter and progressively milder as afebrile periods lengthen. Relapse is associated with expression of new borrelial antigens, and resolution of symptoms is associated with production of antibody specific to those new antigenic determinants.

B miyamotoi, the cause of hard tick relapsing fever, is phylogenetically similar to the agents of (soft) tick-borne and louse-borne relapsing fevers but appears to cause a wider spectrum of illness, varying from subclinical to severe. Symptoms are similar to those seen with *Anaplasma phagocytophilum* infection and include fever, chills, fatigue, myalgias, arthralgias, lymphadenopathy, and occasionally rash. Relapses can occur but are less common than in tick-borne and louse-borne relapsing fevers. Severe manifestations such as meningoencephalitis can occur and likely are more common in immunocompromised people.

ETIOLOGY: Worldwide, at least 14 *Borrelia* species cause tick-borne relapsing fever, including *Borrelia hermsii*, *Borrelia turicatae*, and (rarely) *Borrelia parkeri* in North America. Louse-borne relapsing fever is caused by *Borrelia recurrentis*. *B miyamotoi* is the only species known to cause hard tick relapsing fever.

EPIDEMIOLOGY: Because of differences in the distribution, life cycle, and feeding habits of their vector species, the epidemiology of tick-borne relapsing fever, louse-borne relapsing fever, and hard tick relapsing fever differ significantly. Tick-borne relapsing fever is transmitted through the bite of soft-bodied ticks (*Ornithodoros* species) and is distributed widely throughout the world. Soft-bodied ticks typically live within rodent nests. They become infected by feeding on rodents or other small mammals, and then transmit infection via their saliva during subsequent blood meals. They inflict painless bites and feed briefly (seconds to 30 minutes), usually at night, so that people often are unaware of having been bitten. In the United States, vector soft-bodied ticks are found most often in mountainous areas of the West. Human infection typically follows sleeping in rustic, rodent-infested cabins, although cases have been associated with primary residences and luxurious rental properties. Cases occur sporadically or in small clusters among families or cohabiting groups. Multistate outbreaks have been associated with travel to national parks, where numerous groups may cycle through an infested cabin. *B hermsii* is the most common cause of these infections. *B turicatae* infections occur less frequently; most cases have been reported from Texas and are associated with tick exposures in rodent-infested caves. Clinically apparent human infections with *B parkeri* in the United States are rare; the tick infected with this *Borrelia* species is associated with arid areas or grasslands in the western United States.

Louse-borne relapsing fever previously was widespread but currently is endemic in Ethiopia and occurs sporadically in surrounding countries; cases have been described in Western Europe in refugee and displaced populations originating from the horn of Africa. Epidemic transmission occurs when body lice *(Pediculus humanus)* become infected by feeding on humans with spirochetemia; infection is transmitted when infected lice are crushed and their body fluids contaminate a bite wound or skin abraded by scratching. No animal reservoir has been found for *B recurrentis*; human-to-human transmission occurs through infected lice.

The hard-bodied ticks *Ixodes scapularis* and *Ixodes pacificus* transmit *B miyamotoi* in North America. These ticks are better known as vectors of Lyme disease, anaplasmosis, and babesiosis; coinfections have been reported. Contact with *Ixodes* species that transmit *B miyamotoi* occurs through outdoor activity, especially in woody, brushy, or grassy areas in regions where Lyme disease is endemic. Unlike Lyme disease, *B miyamotoi* can be transmitted within the first 24 hours of tick attachment, and the probability of transmission increases with prolonged attachment. Most known cases of *B miyamotoi* infection have occurred in July or August, which is later than most Lyme disease cases. This suggests that *B miyamotoi* transmission occurs more often through the bite of larval, rather than nymphal, *Ixodes* ticks.

Unlike *B burgdorferi*, which must be acquired by feeding on an infected host, relapsing fever spirochetes can be transmitted transovarially in ticks; thus, larvae may be infected. Ticks in all stages of life may transmit *B miyamotoi* infection. The **incubation period** is about 7 days for tick-borne relapsing fever, 4 to 8 days (range, 2–15 days) for louse-borne relapsing fever, and 12 to 16 days for hard tick relapsing fever.

DIAGNOSTIC TESTS: Diagnostic testing differs for tick-borne relapsing fever, louse-borne relapsing fever, and hard tick relapsing fever. In tick-borne and louse-borne relapsing fevers, because of the high degree of spirochetemia during febrile episodes, spirochetes may be observed microscopically using dark-field technique and in Wright-, Giemsa-, or acridine orange-stained preparations of thick and thin smears. Organisms are visualized most easily in blood obtained during early febrile episodes before treatment. Direct detection using a nucleic acid amplification test (NAAT) is available at some commercial and reference laboratories and is more sensitive than microscopy, potentially allowing for detection during afebrile periods or in later relapses, when spirochetemia is lower. Serum antibodies to *Borrelia* species also can be detected by enzyme immunoassay or Western immunoblot analysis at some reference and commercial specialty laboratories. Serum tested early in infection may be negative, so it is important to obtain a serum sample for serologic testing during the convalescent period (at least 21 days after symptom onset); development of an immunoglobulin (Ig) G response in the convalescent sample is supportive of a tick-borne relapsing fever diagnosis.

Hard tick relapsing fever attributable to *B miyamotoi* can be diagnosed using a NAAT with blood or cerebrospinal fluid or serologic tests performed on acute and convalescent specimens. These are not available widely but may be ordered from a limited number of commercial and reference laboratories.

In interpreting serologic tests for *Borrelia* infections, it is important to note that early antibiotic treatment may limit antibody response. Antibody tests are not standardized and do not distinguish among relapsing fever species. Serologic cross-reactions can also occur with other spirochetes, including *B burgdorferi*, *Treponema pallidum*, and *Leptospira* species. Many NAATs also do not distinguish among relapsing fever species.

For inquiries about laboratory testing at the Centers for Disease Control and Prevention, visit **www.cdc.gov/laboratory/specimen-submission/list.html.**

TREATMENT: Treatment of tick-borne relapsing fever with a 10-day course of doxycycline typically results in prompt clearance of spirochetes and remission of symptoms. Doxycycline can be used regardless of patient age. Effective treatment with macrolide antibiotics, including erythromycin and azithromycin, also has been described. Intravenous beta-lactam antibiotics, such as penicillin or ceftriaxone, are preferred for treatment for pregnant people, when central nervous system involvement is present, in severe illness, or when oral therapy is not well tolerated.

Single-dose treatment using doxycycline or penicillin is effective for louse-borne relapsing fever in the majority of cases, but a longer treatment course is usually applied to minimize the probability of recurrence. Erythromycin or azithromycin may be considered as second-line agents.

Reports of successful treatment of hard tick relapsing fever using a 2-week course of doxycycline suggest this is adequate therapy. Amoxicillin, cefuroxime, and ceftriaxone also have been used or have shown in vitro susceptibility. Azithromycin also may be effective.

A Jarisch-Herxheimer reaction (an acute febrile reaction accompanied by headache, myalgia, respiratory distress in some cases, and a worsening of symptoms lasting less than 24 hours) can occur during the first few hours after initiating antimicrobial therapy for relapsing fever. Because this reaction sometimes is associated with transient hypotension attributable to decreased effective circulating blood volume, patients should be hospitalized and monitored closely, particularly during the first 4 hours of treatment.

INFECTION PREVENTION AND CONTROL MEASURES IN HEALTH CARE SETTINGS: Standard precautions are recommended. If louse infestation is present, contact precautions are indicated until delousing (see Pediculosis, p 644–650).

CONTROL MEASURES:
- Tick-borne relapsing fever: Soft-bodied ticks often can be found in rodent nests. Exposure is reduced most effectively by preventing rodent infestations of homes or

cabins by blocking rodent access to foundations and attics and using other forms of rodent control. Dwellings infested with soft ticks should be rodent-proofed and treated professionally with acaricides; rodent control without concurrent tick control may increase risk of infection transiently. In a single observational study from Israel, postexposure prophylaxis with single-dose doxycycline appeared to be effective in preventing tick-borne relapsing fever among 77 spelunkers, 10 of whom were children, following a high-risk exposure.

- Louse-borne relapsing fever: When in a louse-infested environment, body lice can be controlled by bathing, washing clothing at frequent intervals, and use of pediculicides (see Pediculosis, p 644–650).
- Hard tick relapsing fever: Hard-bodied tick exposure can be limited through awareness and avoidance of tick habitat, use of EPA-registered repellents, thorough and frequent tick checks of humans and pets, and bathing/showering soon after being outdoors. Attached ticks should be removed promptly (see Tick Inspection and Removal, p 213).

Reporting suspected cases of relapsing fever to health authorities is required in many states and is important for initiation of prompt investigation and institution of control measures.

Brucellosis

CLINICAL MANIFESTATIONS: Onset of brucellosis in children can be acute or insidious. Manifestations are nonspecific and include fever (often undulating or cyclical), night sweats, weakness, malaise, anorexia, weight loss, arthralgia, myalgia, back pain, abdominal pain, headache, or refusal to bear weight. Physical findings may include lymphadenopathy, hepatosplenomegaly, and arthritis. Abdominal pain and peripheral arthritis are reported more frequently in children than in adults. Meningitis, encephalitis, myelitis, radiculitis, neuropathies, and demyelinating syndromes have been reported. Diffuse hepatitis, hepatic granulomas, liver or spleen abscesses, epididymo-orchitis, pneumonia, lung nodules, pleural effusions, endocarditis, myocarditis, pericarditis, aortic aneurysms, uveitis, osteomyelitis, and cutaneous lesions have all been reported. Anemia, leukopenia, thrombocytopenia, or less frequently, pancytopenia and hemophagocytosis are hematologic findings that might suggest the diagnosis. The case fatality rate is less than 1%, and most deaths occur in children with endocarditis. A detailed history including travel, exposure to animals, food habits (including ingestion of unpasteurized milk or cheese), and occupational history should be obtained if brucellosis is considered. Chronic infection may last for years, and relapse following treatment of infection occurs in 5% to 15% of patients. Chronic disease is less common among children than among adults, although the rate of relapse has been found to be similar. Brucellosis in pregnancy is associated with risk of spontaneous abortion, stillbirth, or preterm delivery.

ETIOLOGY: *Brucella* bacteria are slow-growing, small, nonmotile, facultative intracellular gram-negative coccobacilli. The species that are commonly known to infect humans are *Brucella abortus*, *Brucella melitensis*, *Brucella suis*, and rarely, *Brucella canis*. However, human infections with *Brucella ceti*, *Brucella pinnipedialis*, *Brucella inopinata*, and *Brucella neotomae* also have been identified. *B abortus* strain RB51 is a live attenuated cattle vaccine strain that can be shed in milk and can cause infections in humans.

EPIDEMIOLOGY: Brucellosis is a zoonotic disease of wild and domestic animals. It is transmissible to humans by direct or indirect exposure to aborted fetuses, tissues, or fluids of infected animals. Transmission occurs by inoculation through mucous membranes or cuts and abrasions in the skin, inhalation of contaminated aerosols, ingestion of unpasteurized dairy products, or consumption of undercooked meats.[1] People in occupations such as farming, ranching, and veterinary medicine, as well as abattoir workers, meat inspectors, and laboratory personnel, are at increased risk. Clinicians should alert the laboratory if they anticipate *Brucella* organisms might grow from microbiologic specimens so that appropriate laboratory precautions can be taken. In the United States, approximately 80 to 120 cases of brucellosis are reported annually, and 3% to 10% of cases occur in people younger than 19 years. Human-to-human transmission is rare. Transplacental transmission and transmission via human milk are possible. Other less common modes of transmission include blood transfusion, hematopoietic cell transplant, and sexual transmission. The number of cases in the United States has decreased considerably with routine animal vaccination and pasteurization of milk products.

The **incubation period** varies from 3 days to 12 months, but most people become ill within 2 to 4 weeks of exposure.

DIAGNOSTIC TESTS: A definitive diagnosis is established by recovery of *Brucella* species from blood, bone marrow, or other tissue specimens. A variety of media will support growth of *Brucella* species, but the physician should contact laboratory personnel and ask that cultures be incubated for a minimum of 14 days. Newer blood culture systems can detect *Brucella* species within shorter periods. Caution should be taken with isolation of this organism because of the high risk of laboratory-acquired infection.

In patients with a clinically compatible illness, serologic testing using the serum agglutination test can confirm the diagnosis with a fourfold or greater increase in antibody titers between acute and convalescent phase serum specimens collected at least 2 weeks apart. The serum agglutination test, the gold standard test for serologic diagnosis, will detect antibodies against *B abortus, B suis,* and *B melitensis* but not against *B canis* or *B abortus* strain RB51. Although a single titer is not diagnostic, most patients with active infection in an area where brucellosis is not endemic will have a titer of 1:160 or greater within 2 to 4 weeks of clinical disease onset. Lower titers may be found early in the course of infection. Because of low sensitivity of some serologic assays, when results are negative but the clinical suspicion is high, testing should be repeated using a different assay. Enzyme immunoassay is a sensitive method for determining total or specific immunoglobulin (Ig) G, IgA, and IgM anti-*Brucella* antibody titers. The Centers for Disease Control and Prevention (CDC) recommends that positive enzyme immunoassay results be confirmed with an agglutination test.[2]

When interpreting serologic results, it is important to take into consideration exposure history, because a serologic response for *B canis* and *B abortus* strain RB51 will not be detected by commercially available tests. *Brucella* antibodies also cross-react with antibodies against other gram-negative bacteria, such as *Yersinia enterocolitica* serotype

---

[1] American Academy of Pediatrics, Committee on Infectious Diseases, Committee on Nutrition. Consumption of raw or unpasteurized milk and milk products by pregnant women and children. *Pediatrics.* 2014;133(1):175-179 (Reaffirmed November 2019)

[2] **www.cdc.gov/brucellosis/pdf/brucellosi-reference-guide.pdf**

09, *Francisella tularensis*, *Escherichia coli* O116 and O157, certain *Salmonella* species, *Vibrio cholerae*, *Xanthomonas maltophilia*, and *Afipia clevelandensis*. The timing of exposure and symptom development will assist in determining the classes of antibodies expected. IgM antibodies are produced within the first week, followed by a gradual increase in IgG antibodies. Low IgM titers may persist for months or years after initial infection. Increased concentrations of IgG agglutinins are found in acute infection, chronic infection, and relapse.

Nucleic acid amplification tests (NAATs) that can be performed on blood and body tissue samples have been developed and are available at the CDC. If a laboratory is not available to perform diagnostic testing for *Brucella* species, the physician should contact the local or state health department for assistance.

TREATMENT: Prolonged antimicrobial therapy is imperative for achieving a cure. Relapses generally are not associated with development of *Brucella* resistance but rather with premature discontinuation of therapy, localized infection, or monotherapy. Because monotherapy is associated with a high rate of relapse, combination therapy is recommended as standard treatment. Most combination regimens include oral doxycycline or trimethoprim-sulfamethoxazole plus rifampin.

Oral doxycycline is the drug of choice in persons 8 years of age and older, and should be administered together with oral rifampin for a minimum of 6 weeks. In children younger than 8 years, most data and experience support the use of trimethoprim-sulfamethoxazole administered together with oral rifampin for at least 6 weeks, although oral doxycycline plus rifampin is an alternative. An aminoglycoside can be used in place of rifampin (gentamicin for 7 days or streptomycin for 14 days), in combination with doxycycline or trimethoprim-sulfamethoxazole. See Table 4.3 (p 993) for antibiotic dosages. Failure to complete the full 6-week course of therapy may result in relapse.

For treatment of serious infections or complications, including endocarditis, meningitis, spondylitis, and osteomyelitis, a 3-drug regimen should be used, with gentamicin included for the first 7 days of therapy in addition to doxycycline (or trimethoprim-sulfamethoxazole if doxycycline is not used) and rifampin, for a minimum of 6 weeks. For life-threatening complications of brucellosis, such as meningitis or endocarditis, the duration of therapy often is extended for 4 to 6 months. Surgical intervention should be considered in patients with complications, such as deep tissue abscesses, endocarditis, mycotic aneurysm, and foreign body infections. Joint effusions may need to be drained.

Because of antibiotic resistance with *B abortus* strain RB51, rifampin and penicillin should not be used for treatment of infection caused by this cattle vaccine strain (see Control Measures).

The benefit of corticosteroids for people with neurobrucellosis is unproven. Occasionally, a Jarisch-Herxheimer-like reaction (an acute febrile reaction accompanied by headache, myalgia, respiratory distress in some cases, and a worsening of symptoms lasting less than 24 hours) occurs shortly after initiation of antimicrobial therapy, but this reaction rarely is severe enough to require corticosteroids.

INFECTION PREVENTION AND CONTROL MEASURES IN HEALTH CARE SETTINGS: In addition to standard precautions, contact precautions are indicated for patients with draining wounds. If aerosol-generating procedures are performed, respiratory protection (eg, use of N95 or higher respirators) also is indicated.

CONTROL MEASURES: The control of human brucellosis depends on control of transmission of *Brucella* species from cattle, goats, swine, elk, bison, and other animals. Vaccination of cattle, sheep, and goats can be effective but needs to be sustained over several years. Contact with infected animals should be avoided, especially female animals that have aborted or are giving birth.

Lactating parents with active brucellosis should not breastfeed their infants until their infection is cleared. Breastfeeding infants of a lactating parent who is diagnosed with brucellosis should be closely monitored for evidence of infection. Pasteurization of dairy products for human consumption as well as thorough cooking of meat are important for preventing infection. The certification of unpasteurized milk does not eliminate the risk of transmission of *Brucella* organisms.

B abortus strain RB51 is a live attenuated cattle vaccine strain that can be shed in milk and can cause infections in humans. People who have consumed raw milk or raw milk products that are potentially contaminated with the live attenuated cattle vaccine strain *B abortus* strain RB51 are at high risk for brucellosis. For these people, postexposure prophylaxis with doxycycline plus trimethoprim-sulfamethoxazole is recommended for 21 days, in addition to symptom monitoring for 6 months following the last exposure. Because of antibiotic resistance with *B abortus* strain RB51, rifampin and penicillin should not be used (see **https://emergency.cdc.gov/han/han00417. asp**). Cases of brucellosis should be reported to the local health department.

Burkholderia Infections

CLINICAL MANIFESTATIONS: Species within the *Burkholderia cepacia* complex have been primarily associated with infections in individuals with cystic fibrosis (CF) or chronic granulomatous disease (CGD). Airway infections of *B cepacia* complex in people with CF usually occur later in the course of disease, after respiratory epithelial damage and bronchiectasis have occurred. Patients with CF can become chronically infected with little change in the rate of pulmonary decompensation or can experience an accelerated decline in pulmonary function and/or a very rapid clinical deterioration that results in death. In patients with chronic granulomatous disease, pneumonia is the most common manifestation of *B cepacia* complex infection; lymphadenitis also occurs. Disease onset is insidious, with low-grade fever early in the course of illness and systemic effects occurring 3 to 4 weeks later. Pleural effusions are common, and lung abscesses can also occur. Infections have also been reported in people with hemoglobinopathies, malignant neoplasms, and in preterm infants. Health care-associated infections including wound infections, urinary tract infections, pneumonia, and bacteremia have been reported. Infections in immunocompetent and otherwise healthy people are rare.

Burkholderia pseudomallei is the cause of melioidosis. Melioidosis can be asymptomatic or can manifest as a localized infection or as fulminant septicemia with or without pneumonia. Approximately 50% of adults with melioidosis are bacteremic on admission to the hospital; bacteremia is less common in children. Pneumonia is the most commonly reported clinical manifestation of melioidosis in adults, whereas localized cutaneous disease is the most common presentation in immunocompetent children. Genitourinary tract infections including prostatic abscesses, septic arthritis and osteomyelitis, and central nervous system involvement, including brain abscesses, also occur. Acute suppurative parotitis is a manifestation that occurs frequently in children in Thailand and Cambodia but is less commonly seen in other areas with endemic infection. Necrotizing fasciitis has been reported with severe cutaneous infection. In disseminated infection, hepatic and splenic abscesses can occur, as can disseminated cutaneous abscesses. Relapses are common without prolonged therapy. Chronic melioidosis (presence of symptoms >2 months), which occurs in fewer than 10% of cases, presents most frequently as a subacute pulmonary disease, mimicking tuberculosis. The case fatality rate for melioidosis is 6% to 50%.

ETIOLOGY: The *Burkholderia* genus comprises more than 125 diverse species that are oxidase- and catalase-producing, non–lactose-fermenting, gram-negative bacilli. *B cepacia* complex comprises at least 22 species. Additional members of the complex continue to be identified but are rare human pathogens. Other clinically important species of *Burkholderia* include *B pseudomallei*, *Burkholderia mallei* (the agent responsible for glanders), *Burkholderia gladioli*, *Burkholderia thailandensis*, and *Burkholderia oklahomensis*.

EPIDEMIOLOGY: *Burkholderia* species are environmentally derived waterborne and soilborne organisms that can survive for prolonged periods in a moist environment, with the exception of *B mallei*, which is host-adapted and not known to persist in the environment. Depending on the species, transmission may occur from other people (person to person), from contact with contaminated fomites, and from exposure to environmental sources.

Epidemiologic studies of recreational camps and social events attended by people with CF from different geographic areas have documented person-to-person spread of *B cepacia* complex. The source of acquisition of *B cepacia* complex by patients with CGD has not been clearly identified, although environmental sources seem likely. *B cepacia* complex can persist in the environment and spread through lapses in infection control, including indirect contact via environmental surfaces. Health care-associated spread of *B cepacia* complex has been associated with contamination of disinfectant solutions used to clean reusable patient equipment, such as bronchoscopes and pressure transducers, or to disinfect skin. Its intrinsic resistance to preservatives enables the organism to contaminate many types of aqueous medical and personal care products, leading to large outbreaks. Contaminated mouthwash, liquid docusate sodium, nasal sprays, sublingual probes, prefilled saline flush syringes, ultrasonography gel, and inhaled medications have been identified as causes of multistate outbreaks of colonization and infection. *B gladioli* also is isolated from sputum of people with CF and may be mistaken for *B cepacia* complex. *B gladioli* may be associated with transient or more prolonged, chronic infection in patients with CF; poor outcomes have been noted in lung transplant recipients who have *B gladioli* infection.

The geographic range of *B pseudomallei* is expanding, and disease is known to be endemic in tropical and subtropical regions such as Southeast Asia, northern Australia, areas of the Indian Subcontinent, southern China, Hong Kong, Taiwan, several Pacific and Indian Ocean Islands, and some areas of South and Central America. The US Virgin Islands, Puerto Rico, the Gulf Coast region of Mississippi, and possibly areas in Texas have the organism present in soil. Melioidosis can occur in patients in the United States, usually among travelers returning from areas with endemic disease. A few US cases have been associated with exposure to imported products including freshwater tropical fish and an aromatherapy spray containing essential oils.

In areas of high endemicity, children may be exposed to *B pseudomallei* early in life, with the highest seroconversion rates occurring between 6 months and 4 years of age.

Melioidosis is seasonal in countries with endemic infection, with more than 75% of cases occurring during the rainy season. Disease can be acquired by direct inhalation of aerosolized organisms or dust particles containing organisms, by percutaneous or wound inoculation with contaminated soil or water, or by ingestion of contaminated soil, water, or food. People also can become infected through laboratory exposures when proper techniques and/or proper personal protective equipment guidelines are not followed. Symptomatic infection can occur in children 1 year or younger, with pneumonia and parotitis reported in infants as young as 8 months; in addition, human milk transmission from breastfeeding parents with mastitis has been reported.

Risk factors for melioidosis include frequent contact with soil and water as well as underlying chronic disease, such as diabetes mellitus, renal insufficiency, chronic pulmonary disease, thalassemia, and immunosuppression not related to human immunodeficiency virus (HIV) infection. *B pseudomallei* also has been reported to cause pulmonary infection in people with cystic fibrosis and septicemia in children with CGD.

The **incubation period** for melioidosis is 1 to 21 days, with a median of 9 days, but can be prolonged (years).

DIAGNOSTIC TESTS: Culture is the appropriate method to diagnose *B cepacia* complex infection. In CF airway infection, culture of sputum on selective agar is recommended to decrease the potential for overgrowth by mucoid *Pseudomonas aeruginosa*. Confirmation of identification of *B cepacia* complex species by matrix-assisted laser desorption/ionization-time of flight (MALDI-TOF) mass spectrometry or by nucleic acid amplification test (NAAT) is recommended.

Definitive diagnosis of melioidosis is made by isolation of *B pseudomallei* from blood or other specimens. The likelihood of successfully isolating the organism is increased by culture of sputum, throat, rectum, and ulcer or skin lesion specimens, in addition to blood. Serologic testing is not adequate for diagnosis in areas with endemic infection because of high background seropositivity. However, a positive result by the indirect hemagglutination assay for a traveler who has returned from an area with endemic infection may support the diagnosis of melioidosis; definitive diagnosis still requires isolation of *B pseudomallei* from blood or other specimens.

Suspected isolates of *B pseudomallei* and *B mallei* should be referred to local or state Public Health Laboratory Response Network Laboratories. Whenever there is clinical suspicion for melioidosis or glanders, the initial laboratory should be notified so that staff can take appropriate precautions, and if identified, the potential for occupational exposure should be evaluated.

TREATMENT: Drugs that may have activity against *B cepacia* complex include trimethoprim-sulfamethoxazole, ceftazidime, minocycline, fluoroquinolones, carbapenems, and newer beta-lactam/beta-lactamase inhibitor combinations. Some experts recommend combinations of antimicrobial agents that provide synergistic activity against *B cepacia* complex in vitro. The majority of *B cepacia* complex isolates are intrinsically resistant to aminoglycosides and polymyxins and are resistant to many beta lactam agents such as penicillin, ampicillin, carboxypenicillins, and first- and second-generation cephalosporins.

The drugs of choice for initial treatment of melioidosis depend on the type of clinical infection, susceptibility testing, and presence of comorbidities in the patient (eg, diabetes mellitus, liver or renal disease, cancer, hemoglobinopathies, cystic fibrosis).

Treatment of severe invasive infection should include meropenem or ceftazidime (rare resistance) for a minimum of 14 days, with prolonged therapy (at least 4–8 weeks) for deep-seated and complicated infections. After acute therapy is completed, oral eradication therapy with trimethoprim-sulfamethoxazole for 3 to 6 months is recommended to reduce recurrence. Amoxicillin clavulanate is considered a second-line oral agent and may be associated with a higher rate of relapse.

INFECTION PREVENTION AND CONTROL MEASURES IN HEALTH CARE SETTINGS: The Cystic Fibrosis Foundation recommends implementation of contact precautions in addition to standard precautions for care of all patients with CF in inpatient or ambulatory care settings, regardless of respiratory tract cultures. Human-to-human transmission is extremely rare for *B pseudomallei*, and standard precautions are recommended.

CONTROL MEASURES: Because some strains of *B cepacia* complex cause a highly virulent course in some patients with new acquisition, the Cystic Fibrosis Foundation recommends that all CF care centers limit contact between patients. This includes inpatient, outpatient, and social settings. When in a health care setting, patients with CF should wear a mask while outside of a clinic examination room or a hospital room. Education of patients and families about hand hygiene and appropriate personal hygiene is recommended.

Prevention of infection with *B pseudomallei* in areas with endemic disease can be difficult because contact with contaminated water and soil is common. People with diabetes mellitus, renal insufficiency, or general immunocompromising conditions should avoid contact with soil and standing water in areas suspected to be contaminated. Wearing boots and gloves during agricultural work in areas with endemic disease and thorough cleaning and protecting of skin wounds is recommended. Patients with CF and diabetes should be educated regarding their risk of infection when traveling to regions where *B pseudomallei* is endemic. A human vaccine is not available, but research is ongoing. Potential laboratory exposures with *B pseudomallei* or *B mallei* should be reviewed with public health authorities to determine management including indications for postexposure prophylaxis (generally with trimethoprim-sulfamethoxazole for 21 days or amoxicillin clavulanate for 21 days). Public health authorities may recommend postexposure prophylaxis to *B pseudomallei* in certain instances.

Public Health Reporting. Melioidosis is a nationally notifiable disease, and cases should be reported to local or state health departments.

Campylobacter Infections

CLINICAL MANIFESTATIONS: Predominant symptoms of *Campylobacter* infection include diarrhea, abdominal pain, malaise, and fever. Stools can contain visible or occult blood. In neonates and young infants, bloody diarrhea without fever can be the only manifestation of infection. Febrile seizures may precede gastrointestinal tract symptoms in young children. Abdominal pain resulting from campylobacteriosis can mimic appendicitis or intussusception. Mild infection lasts 1 or 2 days and resembles viral gastroenteritis. Most patients recover in less than 1 week, but 10% to 20% have a relapse or a prolonged or severe illness. Severe or persistent infection can mimic acute inflammatory bowel disease. Bacteremia is uncommon but can occur in patients with underlying conditions. Immunocompromised hosts can have prolonged, relapsing, or extraintestinal infections, especially with *Campylobacter fetus*. Immunoreactive complications, such as Guillain-Barré syndrome (occurring in 1:1000), Miller Fisher variant of Guillain-Barré syndrome (ophthalmoplegia, areflexia, ataxia), reactive arthritis (with the classic triad consisting of arthritis, urethritis, and bilateral conjunctivitis), myocarditis, pericarditis, and erythema nodosum, can occur during convalescence. Postinfectious irritable bowel syndrome can occur after campylobacteriosis.

ETIOLOGY: *Campylobacter* species are motile, comma-shaped, gram-negative bacilli that are associated with gastroenteritis. There are at least 25 species within the genus *Campylobacter*, but *Campylobacter jejuni* and *Campylobacter coli* are the species isolated most commonly from patients with diarrhea. *C fetus* is predominantly associated with systemic illness in neonates and debilitated hosts. Other *Campylobacter* species, including *Campylobacter lari*, *Campylobacter upsaliensis*, and *Campylobacter hyointestinalis*, can result in similar diarrheal or systemic illnesses in children.

EPIDEMIOLOGY: Although many cases go unidentified, *Campylobacter* species was associated with an estimated 19.5 laboratory-confirmed infections per 100 000 people in 2019, the highest incidence of bacterial foodborne infection in the United States. Although incidence decreased in the early 2000s, data from the Foodborne Diseases Active Surveillance Network (FoodNet) indicated that in recent years, the incidence of reported infections increased, likely resulting from the increased use and sensitivity of culture-independent diagnostic tests (CIDTs). The highest rates of infection occur in children younger than 5 years. Most *Campylobacter* infections are acquired domestically, but up to 1 in 5 cases result from international travel. As few as 500 *Campylobacter* organisms can result in infection.

The gastrointestinal tracts of domestic and wild birds and animals are reservoirs of the bacteria. *C jejuni* and *C coli* have been isolated from feces of 30% to 100% of healthy chickens, turkeys, and waterfowl. Poultry carcasses commonly are contaminated. Many farm animals, pets, and meat sources can harbor the organism and are potential sources of infection. Most cases of *Campylobacter* infection are associated with consumption of undercooked poultry, meat, and other food that has been contaminated. Outbreaks of *Campylobacter* infection have been associated with unpasteurized dairy products, contaminated water, improperly cooked poultry, and produce.[1] Transmission of *C jejuni* and *C coli* occurs by ingestion of contaminated food or water or by direct contact with fecal material from infected animals or people. *Campylobacter* infections usually are sporadic; outbreaks are rarely detected but have occurred among school age participants on field trips to dairy farms where they consumed unpasteurized milk, and among people who had contact with pet store puppies (**www.cdc. gov/campylobacter/outbreaks/outbreaks.html**). Person-to-person spread occurs occasionally, particularly among very young children, and risk is greatest during the acute phase of illness. Person-to-person transmission has occurred from infected birthing parents to neonates and has resulted in health care-associated outbreaks in nurseries. In perinatal infection, *C jejuni* and *C coli* usually cause neonatal gastroenteritis, whereas *C fetus* often causes neonatal septicemia or meningitis. Enteritis occurs

---

[1] American Academy of Pediatrics, Committee on Infectious Diseases, Committee on Nutrition. Consumption of raw or unpasteurized milk and milk products by pregnant women and children. *Pediatrics*. 2014;133(1):175-179 (Reaffirmed November 2019)

in people of all ages. Excretion of *Campylobacter* organisms typically lasts 2 to 3 weeks without antimicrobial treatment but can occur for 7 weeks.

The **incubation period** usually is 2 to 5 days but can be longer.

DIAGNOSTIC TESTS: *C jejuni* and *C coli* can be recovered from feces, and *Campylobacter* species, including *C fetus*, can be recovered from blood. Isolation of *C jejuni* and *C coli* from stool specimens requires selective media, microaerobic conditions, and an incubation temperature of 42°C. Additional methods may be necessary to isolate other species of *Campylobacter*, such as hydrogen-rich microaerobic conditions and filter plating on media without antibiotic supplements. Notably, not all clinical laboratories identify *Campylobacter* to the species level; clinicians can consult state public health laboratories for further identification. Molecular and antigen CIDTs can provide rapid diagnostic testing; however, these tests will not produce an isolate to provide antibiotic susceptibilities. False-positive results from antigen-based tests have been reported. Molecular tests that detect bacterial DNA may not reflect viable organisms; therefore, clinical correlation is needed. Additionally, some diagnostics may not distinguish between *C jejuni* and *C coli* and may not detect other *Campylobacter* species. Referral of isolates and CIDT-positive specimens to state public health laboratories is based on state requirements. Molecular analysis of isolates is important for national *Campylobacter* surveillance and outbreak monitoring.

TREATMENT: Rehydration is the mainstay of treatment for all children with diarrhea. Most patients with *Campylobacter* diarrhea do not require antimicrobial therapy. Antibiotics should be given in invasive cases of *Campylobacter* infection (eg, bacteremia) and can be considered in patients at risk for severe disease including the very young, elderly, or immunosuppressed. Macrolide antibiotics such as azithromycin and erythromycin shorten the duration of illness and excretion of the bacteria. Approximately 2% of *C jejuni* and 5% to 9% of *C coli* isolates are resistant to macrolides. Antimicrobials may prevent relapse when administered early in gastrointestinal tract infection. Treatment with azithromycin usually eradicates the organism from stool within 2 or 3 days. Fluoroquinolones, such as ciprofloxacin, may be effective, but throughout the world, resistance to ciprofloxacin is common (up to 35% of *C jejuni* and *C coli* isolates in 2019 from the United States; see also Fluoroquinolones, p 973). *C fetus* generally is susceptible to aminoglycosides, extended-spectrum cephalosporins, meropenem, imipenem, ampicillin, and erythromycin. Regularly updated resistance information for *C jejuni* and *C coli* based on CDC surveillance can be found at **wwwn.cdc.gov/narmsnow/**. Antimicrobial susceptibility testing of the isolate or epidemiologic data from the location of acquisition can help guide appropriate therapy. If antimicrobial therapy is administered for treatment of gastroenteritis, the recommended duration is 3 to 5 days. Antimotility agents are generally not recommended in children because of their limited benefit and reports of adverse outcomes in those who received these agents as monotherapy.

INFECTION PREVENTION AND CONTROL MEASURES IN HEALTH CARE SETTINGS: In addition to standard precautions, contact precautions are recommended for diapered and incontinent children for the duration of illness.

CONTROL MEASURES:

- Hand hygiene should be performed after handling raw poultry and cutting boards, and utensils should be washed with soap and hot water after contact with raw poultry. Food preparation areas and cutting boards used for raw poultry should be separate from all other foods, especially fruits and vegetables.

- Poultry should be cooked thoroughly.
- Hand hygiene should be performed after contact with feces of dogs, cats, and farm animals.
- People should not drink raw milk.[1] The certification of raw milk does not eliminate the risk of transmission of *Campylobacter* organisms.
- Chlorination of water supplies is important.
- People with diarrhea should be excluded from food handling, care of patients in hospitals, and care of people in custodial care and child care centers.
- Infected food handlers and hospital employees who are asymptomatic need not be excluded from work if proper personal hygiene measures, including hand hygiene, are maintained.
- People with diarrhea should not go into recreational water (see Prevention of Illnesses Associated With Recreational Water, p 214) and should abstain from recreational water for 1 week after resolution of symptoms (or as advised by local public health authorities).
- Outbreaks of campylobacteriosis are uncommon in child care centers. General measures for interrupting enteric transmission in child care centers are recommended (see Children in Group Child Care and Schools, p 145). Infants and children should be excluded from child care centers until either stools are contained in the diaper or, if the child is continent, when no longer having fecal accidents and stool frequency is no more than 2 stools above that child's normal frequency, even if the stools remain loose. Although antibiotics are not generally recommended, azithromycin or erythromycin treatment may reduce the potential for person-person transmission.
- Diagnostic testing of asymptomatic exposed children is not recommended.

Public Health Reporting. *Campylobacter* infection is a nationally notifiable disease, and cases should be reported to local or state health departments.

Candidiasis

CLINICAL MANIFESTATIONS: Mucocutaneous infection results in oral-pharyngeal (thrush)or vaginal or cervical candidiasis; intertriginous lesions of the gluteal folds, buttocks, neck, groin, and axilla; paronychia; and onychia. Dysfunction of T lymphocytes, other immunologic disorders, and endocrinologic diseases are associated with chronic mucocutaneous candidiasis. Chronic or recurrent oral candidiasis can be the presenting sign of human immunodeficiency virus (HIV) infection or primary immunodeficiency. Esophageal and laryngeal candidiasis can occur in immunocompromised patients. Candidemia can result from indwelling central vascular catheters, especially in patients receiving prolonged intravenous infusions with parenteral alimentation or lipids, or from translocation from the gastrointestinal tract, especially in the setting of neutropenia. End-organ involvement (ie, disseminated candidiasis) can present with or without candidemia. Disseminated candidiasis is more common in certain patient groups, such as extremely preterm neonates and immunocompromised or debilitated hosts, can involve virtually any organ or anatomic site, and can be fatal. Peritonitis can occur in patients undergoing peritoneal dialysis, especially in patients receiving

---

[1] American Academy of Pediatrics, Committee on Infectious Diseases, Committee on Nutrition. Consumption of raw or unpasteurized milk and milk products by pregnant women and children. *Pediatrics.* 2014;133(1):175-179 (Reaffirmed November 2019)

prolonged broad-spectrum antimicrobial therapy. Candiduria can occur in patients with indwelling urinary catheters, focal renal infection, or disseminated disease. Congenital cutaneous candidiasis involves the presence of a diffuse skin rash of major skin areas of the body, extremities, face, or scalp and/or funisitis presenting in the first week of life with identification of *Candida* species or yeast from culture or staining of the skin, placenta, or umbilical cord. Dermatologic findings include desquamation (scaling, peeling, flaking, or exfoliation), maculopapular, papulopustular, or erythematous rashes alone or in combination.

ETIOLOGY: *Candida* species are yeasts that reproduce by budding. *Candida albicans* and several other species form long chains of elongated yeast forms called pseudohyphae. *C albicans* is the most common species associated with candidiasis, but in some regions and patient populations, non-*albicans Candida* species now account for more than half of invasive infections. *Candida parapsilosis* is the most common non-*albicans* species in pediatric and neonatal populations. Numerous other non-*albicans* species, including but not limited to *Candida tropicalis, Candida glabrata, Candida krusei, Candida guilliermondii, Candida lusitaniae,* and *Candida dubliniensis,* can cause serious infections, especially in immunocompromised and debilitated hosts. *Candida auris* is a *Candida* species that is often multidrug resistant and generally acquired in health care settings.

EPIDEMIOLOGY: Mucocutaneous or invasive *Candida* infections occur endogenously from anatomical sites (eg, skin, mouth, intestinal tract, and vagina) colonized by *Candida* species. Vulvovaginal candidiasis is associated with pregnancy, and newborn infants can acquire the organism in utero, during passage through the vagina, or postnatally. Mild mucocutaneous infection is common in healthy infants. People with poorly controlled diabetes mellitus may also develop localized mucocutaneous infections. Invasive candidiasis typically occurs in those with impaired immunity. Factors such as extreme prematurity, neutropenia, or treatment with corticosteroids or cytotoxic chemotherapy increase the risk of invasive infection. People with neutrophil defects, such as chronic granulomatous disease or myeloperoxidase deficiency, also are at increased risk. People undergoing intravenous alimentation or receiving broad-spectrum antimicrobial agents, especially extended-spectrum cephalosporins, carbapenems, and vancomycin, or requiring long-term indwelling central venous or peritoneal dialysis catheters, have increased susceptibility to infection. Postsurgical patients can be at risk, particularly after cardiothoracic or abdominal procedures. Person-to-person transmission occurs rarely for most *Candida* species but can occur with *C auris*.

The **incubation period** is unknown.

DIAGNOSTIC TESTS: Presumptive diagnosis of mucocutaneous candidiasis in the oropharynx (thrush) and inguinal (diaper candidiasis) or vaginal (vulvovaginal candidiasis) sites usually can be made clinically, although other organisms can cause clinically similar lesions. Yeast cells and pseudohyphae can be found in infected tissue and are identifiable by microscopic examination of scrapings prepared with Gram, calcofluor white, or fluorescent antibody stains or in a 10% to 20% potassium hydroxide suspension. Endoscopy is useful for diagnosis of esophagitis. Although ophthalmologic examination can reveal typical retinal lesions attributable to hematogenous dissemination, the yield of routine ophthalmologic evaluation in patients with candidemia is low. Lesions in the brain, kidney, liver, heart, or spleen can be detected by ultrasonography, computed tomography (CT), or magnetic resonance imaging, but these lesions may not be detected by imaging early in the course of disease or during neutropenia.

A definitive diagnosis of invasive candidiasis requires isolation of the organism from a normally sterile body site (eg, blood, cerebrospinal fluid, bone marrow) or demonstration of organisms in a tissue biopsy specimen. Negative results of culture for *Candida* species do not exclude invasive infection; the sensitivity of blood culture is <50%. Special fungal culture media are not needed to grow *Candida* species. A presumptive species identification of *C albicans* can be made by demonstrating germ tube formation, and molecular fluorescence in situ hybridization testing can rapidly distinguish *Candida* species. Recovery of the organism is expedited using automated blood culture systems or a lysis-centrifugation method. Peptide nucleic acid fluorescent in situ hybridization (PNA FISH) probes cleared by the US Food and Drug Administration (FDA) and multiplex nucleic acid amplification tests (NAATs) have been developed for rapid detection of *Candida* species directly from positive blood culture bottles.

Because of its high resistance and transmissibility, it is important to distinguish *C auris* from other *Candida* species. *C auris* may be misidentified as another *Candida* species when using certain laboratory methods. Options for *C auris* diagnostic testing are expanding, but the current gold standards for identifying *C auris* isolates are matrix-assisted laser desorption/ionization–time-of-flight (MALDI-TOF) and whole genome sequencing.

Patients with suspected infection can have their serum tested using the assay for (1,3)-beta-D-glucan from fungal cell walls, but this biomarker has a number of limitations. It does not distinguish *Candida* species from other fungi. There are limited data from pediatric cohorts, there are a significant number of false-positive results, and the diagnostic cut-point for this assay is not well established in children. A molecular assay (T2Candida) cleared by the FDA uses magnetic resonance technology to identify 5 different *Candida* species from a whole blood specimen but data on the performance of this assay in children are limited.

Testing for azole susceptibility is recommended for all bloodstream and other clinically relevant *Candida* isolates. Testing for echinocandin susceptibility should be considered in patients who have had prior treatment with an echinocandin and among those who have infection with *C glabrata*, *C parapsilosis*, or *C auris*.

TREATMENT[1]:

Mucous Membrane and Skin Infections. Oral candidiasis in immunocompetent hosts is treated with oral nystatin suspension, clotrimazole troches applied to lesions, or miconazole mucoadhesive buccal tablets. Troches should not be used in infants. Fluconazole may be more effective than oral nystatin or clotrimazole troches and may be considered if other treatments fail. Fluconazole can be beneficial for immunocompromised patients with oropharyngeal candidiasis. For fluconazole-refractory disease, itraconazole, voriconazole, posaconazole, amphotericin B preparations, or intravenous echinocandins (caspofungin, micafungin) are alternatives.

Esophagitis caused by *Candida* species generally is treated with oral fluconazole. Intravenous fluconazole should be used for patients who cannot tolerate oral therapy. For disease refractory to fluconazole, itraconazole solution (because of improved absorption compared with capsules), voriconazole, posaconazole, or an echinocandin is recommended. The recommended duration of therapy is 14 to 21 days but depends

---

[1] Pappas PG, Kauffman CA, Andes DR, et al. Clinical practice guideline for the management of candidiasis: 2016 update by the Infectious Diseases Society of America. *Clin Infect Dis.* 2016;62(4):e1-e50

on severity of illness and patient factors, such as age and degree of immunocompromise. Changing from intravenous to oral therapy with fluconazole is recommended when the patient is able to tolerate oral intake. Suppressive therapy with fluconazole (3 times weekly) is recommended for recurrent infections.

Skin infections are treated with topical nystatin, miconazole, clotrimazole, naftifine, ketoconazole, econazole, or ciclopirox (see Topical Drugs for Superficial Fungal Infections, p 1037). Nystatin usually is effective and is the least expensive of these drugs.

Vulvovaginal candidiasis is treated effectively with many topical formulations, including clotrimazole or miconazole (available over the counter). Such topically applied azole drugs are more effective than nystatin. Oral azole agents also are effective and should be considered for recurrent or refractory cases (see Recommended Doses of Parenteral and Oral Antifungal Drugs, p 1026).

Nipple and ductal breast infections with candidiasis have been described with breastfeeding. Topical treatment as above may be adequate for nipple infection, but systemic treatment with fluconazole is often used in breast infections, with continuation of breastfeeding.

For chronic mucocutaneous candidiasis, fluconazole, itraconazole, and voriconazole are effective drugs. Relapses are common with any of these agents once therapy is terminated, and treatment should be viewed as a lifelong process that generally requires intermittent pulses of antifungal agents. Invasive infections in these patients with this condition are rare.

For management of asymptomatic candiduria, elimination of predisposing factors, such as indwelling bladder catheters, is strongly recommended. Antifungal treatment is not recommended unless patients are at high risk of candidemia, such as neutropenic patients and preterm infants. If candiduria occurs in a preterm infant, evaluation should be performed (blood cultures, cerebrospinal fluid evaluation, ophthalmologic examination, brain imaging, and abdominal ultrasonography) and treatment should be initiated.

For patients with symptomatic *Candida* cystitis, elimination of predisposing factors, such as indwelling bladder catheters, is strongly recommended, in addition to use of fluconazole for 2 weeks. Repeated bladder irrigations with amphotericin B (50 µg/mL of sterile water) have been used to treat patients with candidal cystitis. However, the comparative effectiveness of this procedure has not been established, and it does not treat disease beyond the bladder; for these reasons, it is not recommended routinely. Urinary catheters, if not able to be removed, should be replaced promptly in patients with candiduria. Echinocandins have poor urinary concentration.

Keratomycosis is treated with corneal baths of voriconazole (1%) and always in conjunction with systemic therapy. Vision-threatening infections (near the macula or into the vitreous) require intravitreal injection of antifungal agents, usually amphotericin B or voriconazole, with or without vitrectomy, in addition to systemic antifungal agents.

Invasive Disease

General Recommendations. The echinocandins (caspofungin, micafungin, and anidulafungin) are all active in vitro against most *Candida* species and are recommended first-line drugs for invasive *Candida* infections beyond the neonatal period (see Antifungal Drugs for Systemic Fungal Infections, p 1017). Most *Candida* species are susceptible to amphotericin B, although *C lusitaniae, C auris,* and some strains of *C glabrata* and *C krusei* exhibit decreased susceptibility or resistance (see Table 4.7, Fungal Species and Antifungal Drugs, p 1021). *C auris* is often resistant to fluconazole and amphotericin B, but most strains remain susceptible to echinocandins. Thus, echinocandins should be used as initial therapy for *C auris*, and susceptibility testing should be performed along with careful monitoring of patients for treatment effectiveness. Investigation for a deep focus of infection should be conducted for all patients with candidemia, regardless of species, when candidemia persists despite appropriate therapy.

Fluconazole resistance is seen in most *C krusei* isolates (which are intrinsically resistant), in more than 50% of *C glabrata* isolates, and approximately 90% of *C auris* isolates. Although voriconazole is effective against *C krusei*, it is often ineffective against *C glabrata* and *C auris*. Earlier studies suggested decreased susceptibility to echinocandins among *C parapsilosis*, but data now suggest echinocandin resistance is extremely rare. If an echinocandin is initiated empirically and *C parapsilosis* is isolated in a patient who is recovering, then the echinocandin can be continued. Removal of infected devices (eg, vascular or peritoneal catheters, ventriculostomy drains, shunts, nerve stimulators, prosthetic reconstructive devices) is absolutely necessary in addition to antifungal treatment. Breastfeeding may continue during treatment of the parent for candidiasis.

Neonatal Candidiasis. In extremely low birth weight infants, candidemia and candiduria have similar mortality of 28% and 26%, respectively, and mortality is 50% or greater with meningitis, peritonitis, and if multiple sites are involved. Comparatively, mortality is much lower (2%) for infants weighing >1000 g at birth. Infants are more likely than older children and adults to have meningitis as a manifestation of candidiasis. Although meningitis can occur in association with candidemia, approximately half of infants with *Candida* meningitis do not have a positive blood culture. Central nervous system disease in the infant typically manifests as meningoencephalitis and should be assumed to be present in the infant with candidemia and signs and symptoms of meningoencephalitis because of the high incidence of this complication.

All infants with cultures positive for *Candida* in the blood should have a lumbar puncture, brain imaging, echocardiography, dilated retinal examination, and ultrasonography (or other imaging) of the renal system, liver, and spleen during the first week after diagnosis. For term infants with candiduria alone, only ultrasonography of the renal system is needed.

Amphotericin B deoxycholate (first choice for infants), fluconazole, or an echinocandin (generally reserved for salvage therapy and once central nervous system infection is excluded), can be used in infants with systemic candidiasis. Amphotericin B deoxycholate is recommended for treatment at a dose of 1 mg/kg intravenously, daily, as the majority of neonatal infections are susceptible and resistance is rare. Fluconazole may be used for isolates susceptible to fluconazole in patients who are clinically stable. Therapy for candidemia without metastatic disease should continue for 2 weeks after documented clearance of *Candida* species from the blood by culture and resolution of signs attributable to candidemia. Congenital cutaneous candidiasis should receive systemic antifungal therapy for 2 weeks. Therapy for central nervous system infection is at least 3 weeks and should be continued until all signs, symptoms, and cerebrospinal fluid and imaging abnormalities, if present, have resolved. For central nervous system infections, end-organ dissemination, or prolonged candidemia >7 days, some experts recommend double coverage with a second antifungal agent until clinical improvement is achieved. Rescreening for end-organ dissemination should be performed if blood cultures are persistently positive for *Candida* species. For candidemia, antifungal therapy plus prompt removal/replacement of central venous catheters is recommended within 24 hours of diagnosis and decreases both mortality and dissemination.

Lipid formulations of amphotericin B should be used with caution in infants, particularly in infants with urinary tract involvement. Published reports in adults and anecdotal reports in preterm infants indicate that lipid-associated amphotericin B preparations have failed to eradicate renal candidiasis, because these large-molecule drugs may not penetrate well into the renal parenchyma. It is unclear whether this is the reason for the inferior outcomes reported with the lipid formulations. Dosing may also be a factor, and if used lipid amphotericin B formulation can be dosed at 5 mg/kg daily. Flucytosine is not recommended routinely for infants because of concerns regarding toxicity and lack of efficacy.

Older Children and Adolescents. In neutropenic or nonneutropenic children and adults, an echinocandin (caspofungin, micafungin, anidulafungin) is preferred treatment according to guidelines, but fluconazole may be considered in those who are considered clinically stable and also are unlikely to have a fluconazole-resistant isolate. Transition from an echinocandin to fluconazole (usually in 5 to 7 days) is indicated in patients who are clinically stable, have isolates that are susceptible to fluconazole, and have negative blood cultures following initiation of antifungal therapy. Amphotericin B deoxycholate or lipid formulations are alternative therapies (see Antifungal Drugs for Systemic Fungal Infections, p 1017). In nonneutropenic patients with candidemia and no metastatic complications, treatment should continue for 2 weeks after documented clearance of *Candida* organisms from the bloodstream and resolution of clinical manifestations associated with candidemia.

In patients who are not critically ill, fluconazole is the alternative treatment for patients who have not had recent azole exposure, but voriconazole can be considered in situations in which additional mold coverage is desired. Duration of treatment for candidemia without metastatic complications is 2 weeks after documented clearance of *Candida* organisms from the bloodstream and resolution of symptoms attributable to candidemia. Avoidance or reduction of systemic immunosuppression is advised when feasible.

For chronic disseminated candidiasis (eg, hepatosplenic infection), initial therapy with lipid formulation amphotericin B or an echinocandin for several weeks is recommended, followed by oral fluconazole (only for patients who are unlikely to have a fluconazole-resistant isolate). Duration of therapy will vary based on resolution of clinical and radiographic findings as well as immune system recovery.

Management of Indwelling Catheters. Prompt removal of any infected vascular or peritoneal catheters is strongly recommended, although this recommendation is weaker for neutropenic children, because the source of candidemia in these patients is more likely to be gastrointestinal and it is difficult to determine the relative contribution of the catheter. Immediate replacement of a catheter over a wire in the same catheter site is not recommended. Replacement can be attempted once the infection is controlled.

Additional Assessments. Nonneutropenic patients with candidemia should have a dilated ophthalmologic examination within the first week after diagnosis. In neutropenic patients, dilated fundoscopic examinations should be performed within the first week after counts have recovered, because ophthalmologic findings of choroidal and vitreal infection may not be apparent until recovery from neutropenia is achieved. Although there is emerging evidence that ophthalmologic evaluations may be low yield, they are recommended in guidelines from the Infectious Diseases Society of America.

INFECTION PREVENTION AND CONTROL MEASURES IN HEALTH CARE SETTINGS: Standard precautions are recommended for all *Candida* species except *C auris*, for which both Standard and Contact Precautions are recommended because of the high transmissibility of this species.

CONTROL MEASURES: Prolonged broad-spectrum antimicrobial therapy and use of systemic corticosteroids in susceptible patients promote overgrowth of *Candida* and predispose to invasive infection. Meticulous care of central intravascular catheters is recommended for any patient requiring long-term intravenous access.

Additional control measures are recommended for *C auris*, because this organism is spread easily in health care facilities. Patients with *C auris* should be placed in a single room whenever possible, with Standard and Contact Precautions implemented. Hand hygiene should be performed diligently, and the patient care environment and reusable equipment should be cleaned and disinfected thoroughly using products effective against *C auris*. Communication of the patient's *C auris* status should be clear to associated health care personnel and, if the patient is transferred, to the receiving health care facility. Surveillance and screening of other patients also should be considered to identify transmission so that infection control measures can be implemented for any other patients who may have *C auris*.

Chemoprophylaxis. Invasive candidiasis in infants is associated with prolonged hospitalization and neurodevelopmental impairment or death in almost 75% of affected infants with extremely low birth weight (less than 1000 g). The poor outcomes, despite prompt diagnosis and therapy, make prevention of invasive candidiasis in this population desirable. A number of randomized controlled trials of fungal prophylaxis in extremely preterm infants have demonstrated significant reduction of invasive candidiasis in patients with risk factors and at high risk for *Candida*-associated mortality and neurodevelopmental impairment. Risk factors for invasive candidiasis in infants include extreme prematurity, gastrointestinal pathology, presence of a central venous catheter, exposure to third- or fourth-generation cephalosporins or carbapenems, postnatal steroids, and H2 blockers. Adherence to optimal infection control practices, including "bundles" for intravascular catheter insertion and maintenance and antimicrobial stewardship, can diminish infection rates and should be optimized as standard practice in a neonatal intensive care unit. Fluconazole is the preferred agent for prophylaxis and is recommended for extremely low birth weight infants (<1000 g) with factors that place them at significant risk for invasive candidiasis or who are in NICUs with significant rates (5%–10% or higher) of invasive candidiasis. Some experts recommend using additional criteria tailored to individual infant risk factors (eg, presence of central venous catheter, receipt of third- or fourth-generation cephalosporins or carbapenems, parenteral nutrition, gastrointestinal tract disease) to recommend fluconazole prophylaxis. The recommended regimen for extremely low birth weight infants is to initiate fluconazole prophylaxis intravenously shortly after birth at a dose of 3 or 6 mg/kg and then to administer it twice a week while requiring intravenous access (central or peripheral) for up to 6 weeks. Once infants tolerate enteral feeds, fluconazole can be transitioned to enteral administration, because fluconazole oral absorption is good, even in preterm infants. This chemoprophylaxis dosage, dosing interval, and duration has not been associated with emergence of fluconazole-resistant *Candida* species in randomized trials.

Antifungal prophylaxis should be considered for children undergoing allogenic hematopoietic cell transplantation and other highly myelosuppressive chemotherapy during the period of neutropenia. However, in patients with prolonged neutropenia, an antifungal prophylaxis agent with antimold activity is often preferred (see Table 4.7, p 1021). Fluconazole prophylaxis is recommended in certain solid organ transplant scenarios (eg, after prolonged surgical procedure for a liver transplant). Prophylaxis is not recommended routinely for other immunocompromised children, including children with HIV infection. Fluconazole prophylaxis can decrease the risk of mucosal (eg, oropharyngeal and esophageal) candidiasis in patients with advanced HIV disease. Increased incidence of breakthrough *C krusei* or *C glabrata* infections, species with increased resistance to fluconazole, has been reported in some patient populations that are frequently prescribed fluconazole.

Chancroid and Cutaneous Ulcers

CLINICAL MANIFESTATIONS: Chancroid is an acute ulcerative disease of the genitalia that occurs primarily in sexually active adolescents and adults. A clinical presentation with a painful genital ulcer and tender suppurative inguinal lymphadenopathy should raise suspicion for chancroid. An ulcer begins as an erythematous papule that becomes pustular and erodes over several days, forming a sharply demarcated, somewhat superficial lesion with a serpiginous border. The base of the ulcer is friable and can be covered with a gray or yellow, purulent exudate. Single or multiple ulcers can be present. Unlike a syphilitic chancre, which is typically painless and indurated, the chancroidal ulcer often is painful and nonindurated and can be associated with painful inguinal suppurative adenitis (bubo) ipsilateral to the lesion. Without treatment, ulcer(s) can spontaneously resolve, cause extensive erosion of the genitalia, or lead to scarring and phimosis, a painful inability to retract the foreskin of the penis.

In most male patients, chancroid manifests as a genital ulcer with or without inguinal tenderness; edema of the prepuce is common.[1] In female patients, most lesions are at the vaginal introitus, and symptoms include dysuria, dyspareunia, and vaginal discharge. People with anal infection may have pain on defecation or anal bleeding. Constitutional symptoms are unusual.

ETIOLOGY: Chancroid and cutaneous ulcers are caused by *Haemophilus ducreyi*, a gram-negative coccobacillus.

EPIDEMIOLOGY: Chancroid is a sexually transmitted infection. Chancroid is prevalent in some parts of Africa and the tropics but is uncommon in the United States, and when it does occur, it is usually imported from areas with endemic infection. Thus, recent travel to or from an area with endemic infection should raise suspicion for this diagnosis. Coinfection with syphilis or herpes simplex virus (HSV) occurs in up to 20% of patients. Chancroid is a well-established cofactor for acquisition and transmission of human immunodeficiency virus (HIV).

Because sexual contact is the major route of transmission in the United States, the diagnosis of chancroid ulcers in infants and young children, especially in the genital or

---

[1] The terms male and female refer to sex assigned at birth.

perineal region, is highly suspicious of sexual abuse. However, *H ducreyi* is recognized as a cause of nonsexually transmitted cutaneous ulcers in children and young adults in some tropical regions and, specifically, in countries where the cutaneous ulcer disease yaws, caused by *Treponema pallidum* subspecies *pertenue*, is endemic. The acquisition of a lower extremity ulcer attributable to *H ducreyi* in a child without genital ulcers and reported travel to a region with endemic yaws should not be considered evidence of sexual abuse.

For both chancroid and cutaneous ulcers, the **incubation period** is 1 to 10 days.

DIAGNOSTIC TESTS: Chancroid usually is diagnosed on the basis of clinical findings and by excluding other genital ulcerative diseases, such as syphilis, HSV infection, or lymphogranuloma venereum. Cutaneous ulcers can be diagnosed on the basis of clinical findings described, but clinical findings overlap, and mixed infections with *H ducreyi* and *T pallidum* subspecies *pertenue* (the cause of yaws) are common. Confirmation is made by isolation of *H ducreyi* from an ulcer (specimen should be taken from the base of the ulcer) or lymph node aspirate, although culture sensitivity is less than 80%. Because special culture media and conditions are required for isolation, laboratory personnel should be informed of the suspicion of *H ducreyi*. Approximately 30% to 40% of lymph node aspirates are culture positive. Nucleic acid amplification tests (NAATs) can provide a specific diagnosis but are not widely available. There is no NAAT for *H ducreyi* approved or cleared by the US Food and Drug Administration available in the United States. Such testing can be performed by clinical laboratories that have developed their own NAAT and have conducted CLIA verification studies.

TREATMENT: Genital strains of *H ducreyi* have been uniformly susceptible only to third-generation cephalosporins, macrolides, and quinolones. The prevalence of antibiotic resistance is unknown because of syndromic management of genital ulcers and the lack of diagnostic testing. Recommended regimens include azithromycin orally in a single dose, ceftriaxone intramuscularly in a single dose, ciprofloxacin orally for 3 days, or erythromycin orally for 7 days(see Table 4.4, p 1007, and Table 4.5, p 1014). Patients with HIV infection and those with an uncircumcised penis may require repeated or longer courses of therapy. In syndromic management approaches to genital ulcer disease, treatment will typically include syphilis as well as chancroid.

Clinical improvement occurs 3 to 7 days after initiation of therapy, and healing is complete in approximately 2 weeks. Adenitis often is slow to resolve and can require needle aspiration or surgical incision. Patients should be reexamined 3 to 7 days after initiating therapy to verify healing. If healing has not begun, the diagnosis may be incorrect or the patient may have an additional sexually transmitted infection (both of which necessitate further testing), the treatment may not have been used as instructed, or the *H ducreyi* strain causing the infection may be resistant to the prescribed antimicrobial therapy. Slow clinical improvement and relapses can occur after therapy, especially in people with HIV infection. Close clinical follow-up is recommended; retreatment with the original regimen usually is effective in patients who experience a relapse. In advanced cases, genital scarring and rectal or urogenital fistulas from suppurative buboes can result despite successful therapy.

Patients with chancroid should be evaluated for other sexually transmitted infections, including syphilis, HSV, chlamydia, gonorrhea, mpox, and HIV infection, at the time of diagnosis. Because chancroid is a risk factor for HIV infection and facilitates HIV transmission, if the initial HIV test result is negative, it should be repeated

3 months after the diagnosis of chancroid. Because syphilis and *H ducreyi* are frequently cotransmitted, serologic testing for syphilis also should be repeated 3 months after the diagnosis of chancroid. If the hepatitis B and human papillomavirus vaccine series have not been completed, these immunizations should be offered if appropriate for age. All people who had sexual contact with patients with chancroid within 10 days before onset of the patient's symptoms need to be examined and treated, even if they are asymptomatic.

Penicillin has long been used as empiric therapy for cutaneous ulcers in the tropics, but several beta-lactamase–producing cutaneous *H ducreyi* strains have been recovered. Cutaneous ulcers, therefore, should be treated with single-dose azithromycin (30 mg/kg, maximum 2 g) to cover both *T pallidum* subspecies *pertenue* (the cause of yaws) and *H ducreyi*. Cutaneous ulcers attributable to *H ducreyi* respond to single-dose azithromycin within 14 days. Given the environmental sources, it is unclear whether contacts of people with leg ulcers should be treated.

INFECTION PREVENTION AND CONTROL MEASURES IN HEALTH CARE SETTINGS: Standard precautions are recommended.

CONTROL MEASURES: Identification, examination, and treatment of sexual partners of patients with chancroid are important control measures. Regular condom use may decrease transmission, and penile circumcision is believed to be partially protective.

Chikungunya

CLINICAL MANIFESTATIONS: Most people infected with chikungunya virus become symptomatic. The disease most often is characterized by acute onset of high fever (typically >39°C [102°F]) and polyarthralgia. Other symptoms may include widespread maculopapular rash, headache, generalized myalgia, back pain, severe fatigue, arthritis, conjunctivitis, photophobia, anorexia, nausea, vomiting, diarrhea, and abdominal pain. Hemorrhagic manifestations are rare. Fever typically lasts for several days to a week and can be biphasic. Rash usually occurs after onset of fever, can be pruritic, and typically involves the trunk and extremities, but the palms, soles, and face may be affected. Joint symptoms are often severe and debilitating, are usually bilateral and symmetric, and occur most commonly in the hands and feet but can affect more proximal joints. Young children present with arthralgia less frequently than older children and adults. The term chikungunya derives from a word in the Kimakonde language from southeast Tanzania and northern Mozambique meaning "to become contorted," in reference to the stooped appearance of affected people attributable to the joint pain. Clinical laboratory findings can include lymphopenia, thrombocytopenia, elevated creatinine, and elevated hepatic aminotransferases. Acute symptoms typically resolve within 7 to 10 days. Meningoencephalitis, myelitis, seizures, Guillain-Barré syndrome, and cranial nerve palsies occur rarely but appear to be the most common severe complications of chikungunya virus infection. Other rare complications include uveitis, retinitis, myocarditis, arrhythmias, pericarditis, pneumonia, respiratory failure, hepatitis, nephritis, bullous skin lesions, and hemorrhage. Perinatal infection may present with a sepsis-like syndrome. Acrocyanosis without hemodynamic instability, symmetrical vesicobullous lesions, generalized brown-to-black macular hyperpigmentation, and edema of the lower extremities may occur in newborn infants. People at risk for severe disease include neonates exposed perinatally, older adults (eg, >65 years), and people with underlying medical conditions (eg, hypertension; diabetes mellitus; cardiovascular, liver, and kidney disease; and alcohol use disorder). Some patients might have relapse of rheumatologic symptoms (polyarthralgia, polyarthritis, and tenosynovitis) in the months following acute illness. Arthralgia is the most frequent chronic symptom. Studies report variable proportions of patients with persistent joint pains for months to years. Chronic chikungunya arthritis closely mimics classic rheumatoid arthritis and can be erosive with autoantibody positivity in some patients. Risk factors for chronic arthralgia are age >50 years, arthritis during the acute phase, severe or prolonged initial infection, and high viral load. Mortality is rare.

The similar epidemiology and possible cocirculation of chikungunya virus with dengue and Zika viruses demonstrate the increasing need to consider these diagnoses in travelers returning from tropical and subtropical regions of the Americas presenting with an acute febrile illness. Patients with coinfections may have more severe manifestations.

ETIOLOGY: Chikungunya virus is a single-stranded RNA virus in the *Alphavirus* genus of the *Togaviridae* family.

EPIDEMIOLOGY: Chikungunya virus is transmitted to humans primarily through the bites of infected mosquitoes, predominantly *Aedes aegypti* and *Aedes albopictus*. Humans are the primary host of chikungunya virus during epidemic periods. Following an initial infection, a person is likely to be protected from future infections. Bloodborne transmission is possible; cases have been documented among laboratory personnel handling infected blood and in a health care worker drawing blood from an infected patient. To date, there are no known reports of virus transmission through blood transfusion. Rare in utero transmission has been documented, mostly during the second trimester. Intrapartum transmission also has been documented when the mother was viremic around the time of delivery. There are no reports of infants infected with chikungunya virus through breastfeeding.

Before 2013, outbreaks of chikungunya infection were reported from countries in Africa, Asia, Europe, and the Indian and Pacific Oceans. In 2013, chikungunya virus was found for the first time in the Americas on islands in the Caribbean. The virus then spread rapidly throughout the Americas, with local transmission reported from 44 countries and territories and more than 1 million suspected cases reported by the end of 2014. Chikungunya virus disease cases were reported among US travelers returning from affected areas in the Americas beginning in 2014, and local transmission was identified in Florida, Puerto Rico, Texas, and the US Virgin Islands. Reports of cases in the United States can be found at **www.cdc.gov/chikungunya/geo/index. html.**

The **incubation period** typically is between 3 and 7 days (range, 1–12 days).

DIAGNOSTIC TESTS: Preliminary diagnosis is based on the patient's clinical features, places and dates of travel, and activities. Laboratory diagnosis generally is accomplished by testing serum to detect virus, viral nucleic acid, or virus-specific immunoglobulin (Ig) M and neutralizing antibodies. During the first week after onset of symptoms, chikungunya virus infection often can be diagnosed by performing a nucleic acid amplification test (NAAT) on serum. Chikungunya virus-specific IgM and neutralizing antibodies normally develop toward the end of the first week of illness. IgM levels tend to peak between 4 and 20 days after symptom onset and usually persist for 30 to 90 days, but longer persistence has been documented. Therefore, a positive IgM test result on serum occasionally may reflect a past infection. A plaque-reduction neutralization test can be performed to quantitate virus-specific neutralizing antibodies and to discriminate between cross-reacting antibodies (eg, Mayaro, Ross River, and onyong nyong viruses). Immunohistochemical staining can detect specific viral antigen in fixed tissue.

Routine molecular and serologic testing for chikungunya virus is performed at commercial laboratories, several state health department laboratories, and Centers for Disease Control and Prevention (CDC) laboratories. Plaque-reduction neutralization tests and immunohistochemical staining are performed at the CDC and selected other reference laboratories.

TREATMENT: Although several therapeutic options have been or are being evaluated, including use of traditional antiviral compounds and monoclonal antibodies, currently there is no treatment available and approved for chikungunya. Management is supportive care and includes rest, fluids, analgesics, and antipyretics. In areas where dengue is endemic, acetaminophen is the preferred treatment for fever and joint pain. Nonsteroidal anti-inflammatory drugs should be avoided initially until a dengue diagnosis is ruled out to reduce the risk of hemorrhagic complications with dengue infection. Corticosteroids also should be avoided during the acute phase, because they can cause impairment in the natural recovery process and there is a risk of rebound effect after discontinuation. Patients with persistent joint pain may benefit during the chronic phase from the use of nonsteroidal anti-inflammatory drugs, corticosteroids, and physiotherapy. Disease-modifying antirheumatic drugs (DMARDs) such as methotrexate, sulfasalazine, chloroquine, and hydroxychloroquine, have been used in some patients with severe persistent arthritis.

INFECTION PREVENTION AND CONTROL MEASURES IN HEALTH CARE SETTINGS: Standard precautions are recommended.

CONTROL MEASURES: On November 9, 2023, the US Food and Drug Administration approved Ixchiq, the first chikungunya vaccine. Ixchiq is approved for individuals 18 years and older who are at increased risk of exposure to chikungunya virus. This live attenuated vaccine is administered as a single intramuscular dose. Recommendations for use of the vaccine by the CDC Advisory Committee on Immunization Practices are anticipated in 2024. Reduction of vectors in areas with endemic transmission is important to reduce risk of infection. Symptomatic febrile patients should be protected from mosquito bites to reduce further spread. Use of certain personal protective measures can help decrease risk of human infection, including using insect repellent, wearing long pants and long-sleeved shirts, staying in screened or air-conditioned dwellings, and limiting outdoor activities during peak vector feeding times (see Prevention of Mosquito-borne and Tick-borne Infections, p 207).

Breastfeeding. Chikungunya viral RNA has been documented in human milk during an acute chikungunya virus infection, but no infants have been found to be infected through breastfeeding.

Public Health Reporting. Chikungunya is a nationally notifiable disease. Health care professionals should report suspected chikungunya cases to their state or local health departments to facilitate diagnosis and mitigate risk of local transmission. State health departments should report laboratory-confirmed cases to the CDC through ArboNET, the national surveillance system for arboviral diseases.

CHLAMYDIAL INFECTIONS

Chlamydia pneumoniae

CLINICAL MANIFESTATIONS: Patients may be asymptomatic or mildly to moderately ill with a variety of respiratory tract diseases caused by *Chlamydia pneumoniae*, including pneumonia, acute bronchitis, prolonged cough, and less commonly, pharyngitis, laryngitis, otitis media, and sinusitis. A sore throat precedes the onset of cough by a week or more in some patients. The clinical course can be biphasic, culminating in atypical pneumonia. *C pneumoniae* can present as severe community-acquired pneumonia in immunocompromised hosts and has been associated with onset or acute exacerbation of respiratory symptoms in patients with asthma, cystic fibrosis, and sickle cell disease with acute chest syndrome. Rare cases of meningoencephalitis and myocarditis have been attributed to *C pneumoniae*.

Physical examination may reveal nonexudative pharyngitis, pulmonary rales, and bronchospasm. Chest radiography may reveal a variety of findings ranging from pleural effusion and bilateral infiltrates to a single patchy subsegmental infiltrate. Illness can be prolonged, and cough can persist for 2 to 6 weeks or longer.

ETIOLOGY: *C pneumoniae* is an obligate intracellular bacterium for which entry into mucosal epithelial cells is necessary for intracellular survival and growth. It exists in both an infectious nonreplicating extracellular form called an elementary body and a replicating intracellular form called a reticulate body. Reticulate bodies replicate within a protective intracellular membrane-bound vesicle called an inclusion.

EPIDEMIOLOGY: *C pneumoniae* infection is presumed to be transmitted from person to person via infected respiratory tract secretions. Infection typically peaks between 5 and 15 years of age but may occur earlier in life in tropical and resource-limited areas. In the United States, approximately 50% of adults have *C pneumoniae*-specific serum antibody by 20 years of age, indicating previous infection. Recurrent infection is common, especially in adults. Clusters of infection have been reported in groups of children and adults. There is no evidence of seasonality.

The mean **incubation period** is 21 days.

DIAGNOSTIC TESTS: Nucleic acid amplification tests (NAATs) are the preferred method for the diagnosis of an acute *C pneumoniae* infection because of their utility for rapid and accurate detection. Specimen types that can be assayed may vary according to the laboratory; thus, acceptable and preferred specimen types as well as storage and transport conditions should be confirmed with the laboratory prior to testing. Multiplex NAATs have been cleared by the US Food and Drug Administration for the diagnosis of *C pneumoniae* using nasopharyngeal swab samples. These tests have high sensitivity and specificity for acute infection. However, nasopharyngeal shedding can occur for months after acute disease, even with treatment.

C pneumoniae is difficult to culture but can be isolated from swab specimens obtained from the nasopharynx or oropharynx, from sputum or bronchoalveolar lavage fluid specimens, or from tissue biopsy specimens at specialized laboratories using cell cultures (**www.cdc.gov/pneumonia/atypical/cpneumoniae/hcp/diagnostic.html**). Immunohistochemistry, used to detect *C pneumoniae* in tissue specimens, requires control antibodies and tissues, in addition to skill in recognizing staining artifacts to avoid false-positive results.

Serologic testing for *C pneumoniae* is problematic. The microimmunofluorescent antibody test is the most sensitive and specific serologic test for acute infection, but it is technically complex and its interpretation is subjective. A fourfold increase in immunoglobulin (Ig) G titer between acute and convalescent sera provides evidence of acute infection. Use of a single IgG titer in diagnosis of acute infection is not recommended, because IgG antibody may not appear until 6 to 8 weeks after onset of illness during primary infection and increases within 1 to 2 weeks after reinfection. In primary infection, IgM antibody appears approximately 2 to 3 weeks after onset of illness, and an IgM titer of 1:16 or greater is supportive of an acute infection. However, caution is advised when interpreting a single IgM antibody titer for diagnosis, because a single result can be either falsely positive because of cross-reactivity with other *Chlamydia* species or falsely negative in cases of reinfection, when IgM may not appear. Early antimicrobial therapy may suppress antibody responses. Past exposure is indicated by a stable IgG titer of 1:16 or greater.

TREATMENT: Most respiratory tract infections believed to be caused by *C pneumoniae* are treated empirically. For suspected *C pneumoniae* infections, treatment with macrolides (eg, azithromycin, erythromycin, or clarithromycin) is recommended. Doxycycline can be used without regard to patient age, but tetracycline should not be administered routinely to children younger than 8 years (see Tetracyclines, p 975). Fluoroquinolones (levofloxacin and moxifloxacin) are additional alternative drugs for patients who are unable to tolerate macrolide antibiotic agents but generally should not be used as first-line treatment. In vitro data suggest that *C pneumoniae* is not susceptible to sulfonamides.

Duration of therapy typically is 10 to 14 days for erythromycin, clarithromycin, tetracycline, or doxycycline. With azithromycin, the treatment duration typically is 5 days. Duration of therapy for levofloxacin is 7 to 14 days and for moxifloxacin is 10 days. However, for all these antimicrobial agents, the optimal duration of therapy has not been established.

INFECTION PREVENTION AND CONTROL MEASURES IN HEALTH CARE SETTINGS: Standard precautions.

CONTROL MEASURES: Recommended prevention measures include employing respiratory hygiene (or cough etiquette), and frequent hand hygiene.

Chlamydia psittaci
(Psittacosis, Ornithosis, Parrot Fever)

CLINICAL MANIFESTATIONS: Psittacosis (ornithosis) is an acute respiratory tract infection with systemic symptoms that often include fever, nonproductive cough, dyspnea, headache, myalgia, chills, and malaise. Infection often presents as atypical pneumonia in young or middle-aged adults with abrupt fever onset, headache, and dry cough, although symptoms can also include pharyngitis, diarrhea, constipation, nausea and vomiting, abdominal pain, arthralgia, rash (Horder spots, which are macular rashes similar to the rose spots of typhoid fever), and altered mental status. Extensive interstitial pneumonia can occur, with radiographic changes characteristically more severe than would be expected from physical examination findings. Rarely, infection with *Chlamydia psittaci* has been reported to affect organ systems other than the respiratory tract, resulting in arthritis, endocarditis, myocarditis, pericarditis, dilated cardiomyopathy, thrombophlebitis, nephritis, hepatitis, cranial nerve palsy (including sensorineural hearing loss), transverse myelitis, meningitis, and encephalitis. Infection in pregnancy may be life-threatening to the pregnant person and cause fetal loss. Reports suggest a rare association of psittacosis with ocular adnexal marginal zone lymphomas involving orbital soft tissue, lacrimal glands, and conjunctiva.

ETIOLOGY: *C psittaci* is a gram-negative, obligate intracellular bacterial pathogen that exists in 2 forms. The extracellular form is called an elementary body and is infectious. The elementary body enters the epithelial host cell and then differentiates into a replicating reticulate body within a membrane-bound vesicle, or inclusion.

EPIDEMIOLOGY: Psittacosis is worldwide in distribution and tends to occur sporadically in any season. Birds are the major reservoir of *C psittaci*. The term psittacosis commonly is used, although the term ornithosis more accurately describes the potential for nearly all domestic and wild birds, not just psittacine birds (eg, parakeets, parrots, macaws, cockatoos), to spread this infection. In the United States, a variety of birds including psittacine birds, poultry birds (eg, chickens, ducks, turkeys, pheasants), and pigeons have been reported as sources of human disease. Infected birds, whether they appear healthy or ill, may transmit the organism. Infection usually is acquired by direct contact or inhaling aerosolized excrement or respiratory secretions from the eyes or beaks of infected birds. Once dry, the organism remains viable for months, particularly at room temperature. Importation and illegal trafficking of exotic birds may be associated with disease in humans, because shipping, crowding, and other stress factors may increase shedding of the organism among birds with latent infection. Handling of plumage and mouth-to-beak contact are the modes of exposure described most frequently, although transmission has been reported through exposure to aviaries, poultry slaughter plants, bird exhibits, and lawn mowing. Excretion of *C psittaci* from birds may be intermittent or continuous for weeks or months. Pet bird owners and breeders, veterinarians, and workers at poultry slaughter plants, poultry farms, and pet shops may be at increased risk of infection. Laboratory personnel working with *C psittaci* also are at risk. Human-to-human transmission may occur but is rare.

The **incubation period** usually is 5 to 14 days but may be longer.

DIAGNOSTIC TESTS: The diagnosis of *C psittaci* disease historically has been based on clinical presentation and a positive serologic test result using microimmunofluorescence (MIF) with paired sera. Although the MIF test generally is more sensitive and specific than complement fixation (CF) tests, MIF still displays cross-reactivity with other *Chlamydia* species in some instances. Because of this, a titer less than 1:128 should be interpreted with caution. Paired acute- and convalescent-phase serum specimens obtained at least 2 to 4 weeks apart should be obtained and performed simultaneously within a single laboratory to ensure consistency of results.[1] Treatment with antimicrobial agents may suppress the antibody response and, in such cases, a third serum sample obtained 4 to 6 weeks after the acute-phase sample may be useful in confirming the diagnosis. Although serologic testing is more commonly used and available than molecular testing, serologic test results can often be ambiguous, subjective in their interpretation, and misleading because of the inherent limitations of this approach. If possible,

---

[1] National Association of State Public Health Veterinarians. Compendium of measures to control *Chlamydia psittaci* infection among humans (psittacosis) and pet birds (avian chlamydiosis). *J Avian Med Surg.* 2017;31(3). Available at: **www.nasphv.org/Documents/PsittacosisCompendium.pdf**

serologic testing should be considered a supportive test that augments the findings of other more reliable assays, such as nucleic acid amplification tests (NAATs), which can distinguish *C psittaci* from other chlamydial species. NAATs are available within specialized laboratories (**www.cdc.gov/laboratory/specimen-submission/detail.html?CDCTestCode=CDC-10153**), but none are cleared by the US Food and Drug Administration for detection of *C psittaci* in clinical specimens. Commercial respiratory multiplex NAATs do not test for *C psittaci*. Because the organism is difficult to recover in culture and laboratory-acquired cases have been reported, culture generally is not recommended and should be attempted only by experienced personnel in laboratories in which strict containment measures to prevent spread of the organism are used. *C psittaci* currently is classified as an organism requiring biosafety level 3 biocontainment practices.

TREATMENT: Doxycycline is the drug of choice and can be used without regard to patient age. Erythromycin and azithromycin are alternative agents and are recommended for pregnant people. Therapy should continue for 10 to 14 days after fever abates. Most *C psittaci* infections are responsive to antimicrobial agents within 1 to 2 days. In patients with severe infection, intravenous doxycycline may be considered.

INFECTION PREVENTION AND CONTROL MEASURES IN HEALTH CARE SETTINGS: Standard precautions are recommended.

CONTROL MEASURES: All birds suspected to be the source of human infection should be seen by a veterinarian for evaluation and management. Birds with *C psittaci* infection should be isolated and treated with appropriate antimicrobial agents.[1] Birds suspected of dying from *C psittaci* infection should be transported to an animal diagnostic laboratory for testing as directed by the laboratory. Birds exposed to psittacosis should be also isolated and monitored by a veterinarian for signs of illness even if they do not appear ill. All potentially contaminated caging and housing areas should be disinfected thoroughly before reuse to eliminate any infectious organisms. People cleaning cages, handling birds confirmed with *C psittaci*, or handling birds exposed to those confirmed with *C psittaci* should wear personal protective equipment including a smock or coveralls, gloves, eyewear, designated footwear or shoe covers, a disposable hat, and a disposable N95 or higher respirator. *C psittaci* is susceptible to many but not all household disinfectants and detergents. Effective disinfectants include 1:1000 dilutions of quaternary ammonium compounds, freshly prepared 1:32 dilutions of household bleach (1/2 cup per gallon), or other oxidizing agents such as accelerated hydrogen peroxide-based disinfectants.

Public Health Reporting. Human psittacosis is a nationally notifiable disease. Please refer to the state or local health department for details on reporting cases.

Chlamydia trachomatis

CLINICAL MANIFESTATIONS: *Chlamydia trachomatis* is associated with a range of clinical manifestations, including neonatal conjunctivitis, nasopharyngitis, and pneumonia in young infants as well as genital tract infection, lymphogranuloma venereum (LGV), and trachoma in children, adolescents, and adults.

---

[1] National Association of State Public Health Veterinarians. Compendium of measures to control *Chlamydia psittaci* infection among humans (psittacosis) and pet birds (avian chlamydiosis). *J Avian Med Surg.* 2017;31(3). Available at: **www.nasphv.org/Documents/PsittacosisCompendium.pdf**

- **Neonatal chlamydial conjunctivitis** is characterized by ocular congestion, edema, and discharge developing a few days to several weeks after birth and lasting for 1 to 2 weeks and sometimes longer. In contrast to trachoma (described below), scars and pannus formation (vascularization of the normally avascular cornea) are rare.
- **Pneumonia** in young infants usually is an afebrile subacute illness typically occurring at age 1 to 3 months. A repetitive staccato cough, tachypnea, and rales in an afebrile 1-month-old infant are characteristic but not always present. Wheezing is uncommon. Hyperinflation usually accompanies infiltrates seen on chest radiographs. Nasal stuffiness and otitis media may occur. Untreated disease can linger or recur. Severe chlamydial pneumonia has occurred in infants and some immunocompromised adults.
- **Genitourinary tract** manifestations, such as vaginitis in prepubertal children; urethritis, cervicitis, endometritis, salpingitis, and pelvic inflammatory disease, with or without perihepatitis (Fitz-Hugh-Curtis syndrome) in postpubertal children and adolescents; urethritis and epididymitis; and reactive arthritis (with the classic triad, formerly known as Reiter syndrome, consisting of arthritis, urethritis, and bilateral conjunctivitis) can occur. Infection can persist for months to years. Reinfection is common. Infection often is asymptomatic.
- **Proctocolitis** may occur in individuals who engage in receptive anal intercourse. Symptoms can resemble those of inflammatory bowel disease, including mucoid or hemorrhagic rectal discharge, constipation, tenesmus, and/or anorectal pain. Stricture or fistula formation can follow severe or inadequately treated infection. Infection often is asymptomatic.
- **LGV** classically is an invasive lymphatic infection with an initial ulcerative lesion on the genitalia accompanied by tender, suppurative inguinal and/or femoral lymphadenopathy that typically is unilateral. The ulcerative lesion often resolves by the time the patient seeks care for the adenopathy.
- **Trachoma** is a chronic follicular keratoconjunctivitis with pannus formation that results from repeated and chronic infection. Blindness secondary to extensive local scarring and inflammation occurs in 1% to 15% of people with trachoma.

ETIOLOGY: *C trachomatis* is an obligate intracellular bacterial agent with at least 15 serologic variants (serovars) divided between the following biologic variants (biovars): oculogenital (serovars A–K) and LGV (serovars L1, L2, and L3). Trachoma usually is caused by serovars A through C, and genital and perinatal infections are caused by serovars B and D through K.

EPIDEMIOLOGY: *C trachomatis* is the most commonly reported notifiable condition in the United States, with highest rates among sexually active female[1] adolescents (ages 15–24 years). A significant proportion of these patients are asymptomatic, providing an ongoing reservoir for infection. Among sexually active 15- to 24-year-olds participating in the 2015–2018 cycles of the National Health and Nutrition Examination Survey, the estimated 2018 incidence was 8219 per 100 000 population among 15- to 24-year-old female individuals and 4122 per 100 000 among 15- to 24-year-old male individuals.[2] Among those tested for chlamydial infection through the STD

---

[1] The terms female, male, women, and men refer to sex assigned at birth.

[2] Kreisel KM, Weston EJ, St. Cyr SB, Spicknall IH. Estimates of the prevalence and incidence of chlamydia and gonorrhea among US men and women, 2018. *Sex Transm Dis.* 2021;48(4):222-231

Surveillance Network of the Centers for Disease Control and Prevention (CDC) in 2020, the highest proportion of patients testing positive were women 19 years and younger (27.6%) and men 19 years and younger who have sex with women only (35.2%).[1,2]

Oculogenital serovars of *C trachomatis* can be perinatally transmitted to neonates during birth. Acquisition occurs in approximately 50% of infants born vaginally to infected individuals and in some infants born by cesarean delivery with membranes intact. In infants who contract *C trachomatis*, the risk of conjunctivitis is 25% to 50% and the risk of pneumonia is 5% to 30%. The nasopharynx is the anatomic site most commonly infected. Asymptomatic infection of the nasopharynx, conjunctivae, vagina, and rectum can be acquired at birth, and cultures from these sites of perinatal infection may remain positive for 2 to 3 years. Infection at these sites is not known to be communicable among infants and children. The degree of contagiousness of pulmonary disease is unknown but seems to be low.

Genital tract infection in adolescents and adults is sexually transmitted. The possibility of sexual abuse always should be considered in prepubertal children beyond infancy who have vaginal, urethral, or rectal chlamydial infection (see Table 2.5, p 183). Health care professionals are mandated to report suspected sexual abuse to their state child protective services agency.

LGV biovars are worldwide in distribution but are particularly prevalent in tropical and subtropical areas. Although disease occurs rarely in the United States, reports of outbreaks of LGV proctocolitis have been increasing among men who have sex with men (MSM). Perinatal transmission is rare. LGV is infectious during active disease. Little is known about the prevalence or duration of asymptomatic carriage.

Although rarely observed in the United States since the 1950s, trachoma is the leading infectious cause of blindness worldwide, causing up to 3% of the world's blindness. Trachoma is transmitted by transfer of ocular discharge and is generally confined to poor populations in resource-limited nations in Africa, the Middle East, Asia, and Latin America; the Pacific Islands; and remote aboriginal communities in Australia.

The **incubation period** of chlamydial illness is variable, depending on the type of infection, but usually is at least 1 week.

DIAGNOSTIC TESTS: Among **postpubertal individuals,** *C trachomatis* nucleic acid amplification tests (NAATs) are the most sensitive tests and are recommended for laboratory diagnosis. Commercial NAATs have been cleared by the US Food and Drug Administration (FDA) for testing vaginal (provider or patient collected), endocervical, penile urethral, throat, and rectal swab specimens; first-catch urine specimens; and liquid cytology specimens. The CDC recommends that *C trachomatis* urogenital infection be diagnosed in female individuals by vaginal or cervical swab specimens or first-catch urine. Patient-collected vaginal swab specimens are equivalent in sensitivity

[1] Centers for Disease Control and Prevention. 2018 STD Surveillance Report. Atlanta, GA: US Department of Health and Human Services; 2019. Available at: **www.cdc.gov/nchhstp/newsroom/2019/2018-STD-surveillance-report.html**

[2] Centers for Disease Control and Prevention. Sexually transmitted infections treatment guidelines, 2021. *MMWR Recomm Rep.* 2021;70(RR-4):1-187. Available at: **www.cdc.gov/std/treatment-guidelines/chlamydia.htm**

and specificity to those collected by a clinician using NAATs. Diagnosis of *C trachomatis* penile urethral infection can be made by testing first-catch urine or a urethral swab specimen. Patient collection of a penile meatal swab for *C trachomatis* testing may be a reasonable approach for patients who are either unable to provide urine or prefer to collect their own meatal swab over providing urine. NAATs have been demonstrated to have improved sensitivity and specificity compared with culture for the detection of *C trachomatis* at rectal and oropharyngeal sites. Data indicate that performance of NAATs on self-collected rectal swab specimens is comparable to those with clinician-collected rectal swab specimens. Most people with *C trachomatis* detected at oropharyngeal sites do not have oropharyngeal symptoms, and the clinical significance of oropharyngeal *C trachomatis* infection is unclear.

Newer NAAT-based point of care (POC), CLIA-waived tests perform well and are commercially available. Chlamydia POC tests can expedite treatment of infected people and their sex partners and limit unnecessary presumptive treatment at the time of clinical diagnosis and, therefore, improve antimicrobial stewardship.

Specimen collection for diagnosis of **neonatal chlamydial ophthalmia** should be obtained from the everted eyelid using a Dacron-tipped swab or the swab specified by the manufacturer's test kit; for culture and direct fluorescent antibody (DFA) assay, specimens must contain conjunctival cells, not exudate alone. For diagnosing **infant pneumonia** caused by *C trachomatis,* specimens should be collected from the posterior nasopharynx. Sensitive and specific methods used for diagnosis of both **neonatal ophthalmia and infant pneumonia** include cell culture and nonculture tests (eg, DFA assay and NAAT). DFA assay is the only nonculture FDA cleared test for the detection of chlamydia from conjunctival and oropharyngeal swab specimens; NAATs are not FDA cleared for the detection of chlamydia from these sites, but clinical laboratories may offer such testing once they verify the procedure according to CLIA regulations.

For the **evaluation of prepubertal children for suspected sexual abuse,** see STI Evaluation After Sexual Assault of a Prepubertal Child, p 184. Diagnosis of genitourinary tract chlamydial disease in a child should prompt examination for **other STIs,** including syphilis, gonorrhea, trichomoniasis, human immunodeficiency virus (HIV), hepatitis B virus, and hepatitis C virus and necessitates investigation for sexual abuse.

Serologic testing has little, if any, value in diagnosing uncomplicated genital *C trachomatis* infection.

A definitive **diagnosis of LGV** can be made only with LGV-specific molecular testing (eg, NAAT-based genotyping). These tests can differentiate LGV from non-LGV *C trachomatis* in rectal swab specimens; however, they are not widely available. Genital or oral lesion, rectal swab, and lymph node specimens (ie, lesion swab or bubo aspirate) can be tested for *C trachomatis* by NAAT or culture. NAAT is the preferred approach to testing, because it can detect both LGV strains and non-LGV *C trachomatis* strains. *Chlamydia* serologic testing (complement fixation or microimmunofluorescence) should not be routinely used to make a diagnosis of LGV, because the diagnostic utility of these methods has not been established, interpretation has not been standardized, and validation for clinical proctitis presentation has not been performed.

Diagnosis of **ocular trachoma** usually is made clinically in countries with endemic infection.

TREATMENT[1]:

- **Neonates with chlamydial ophthalmia neonatorum** are treated with oral erythromycin base or ethylsuccinate (50 mg/kg/day in 4 divided doses daily) for 14 days. Data on azithromycin for treating neonatal chlamydial infection are limited; however, a short therapy course might be effective. Topical antibiotic therapy alone is inadequate for treating chlamydial ophthalmia neonatorum and is unnecessary when systemic treatment is administered.
- **Infants with chlamydial pneumonia** are treated with oral erythromycin base or ethylsuccinate (50 mg/kg/day in 4 divided doses daily) for 14 days or alternatively with azithromycin (20 mg/kg as a single daily dose) for 3 days.
- Because the efficacy of erythromycin treatment for ophthalmia neonatorum or infant pneumonia is approximately 80%, a second course of therapy might be required. Clinical follow-up of infants treated with either drug is recommended to determine whether initial treatment was effective. Neonates with documented chlamydial infection should be evaluated for possible gonococcal infection. An association between orally administered erythromycin and azithromycin and infantile hypertrophic pyloric stenosis (IHPS) has been reported in infants younger than 6 weeks. Infants treated with either of these antimicrobial agents should be followed for signs and symptoms of IHPS.
- Infants born to individuals known to have untreated chlamydial infection are at high risk of infection; however, prophylactic antimicrobial treatment is not indicated, because the efficacy of such treatment is unknown. Infants should be monitored clinically to ensure appropriate treatment if infection develops.
- For treatment of other **chlamydial infections in infants and children: For children who weigh <45 kg,** the recommended regimen is oral erythromycin base or ethylsuccinate, 50 mg/kg/day, divided into 4 doses daily for 14 days. Data are limited on the effectiveness and optimal dose of azithromycin for treatment of chlamydial infections in infants and children who weigh <45 kg. **For children who weigh ≥45 kg but who are younger than 8 years,** the recommended regimen is azithromycin, 1 g, orally, in a single dose. **For children 8 years and older,** the recommended regimen is azithromycin, 1 g, orally, in a single dose, or doxycycline, 100 mg, orally, twice a day for 7 days.
- For uncomplicated *C trachomatis* **anogenital tract infection in adolescents or adults,** oral doxycycline (100 mg, twice daily) for 7 days is recommended (see Table 4.4, p 1007). Alternatives include oral azithromycin in a single 1-g dose, or levofloxacin (500 mg orally, once daily) for 7 days. Doxycycline is more effective treatment for rectal *C trachomatis* infection, which cannot be predicted by reported sexual practices. Inadequately treated rectal *C trachomatis* infection among female individuals can increase risk for repeat urogenital *C trachomatis* infection through autoinoculation from the anorectal site. When nonadherence to a 7-day doxycycline regimen is a substantial concern, azithromycin, 1 g, is an alternative treatment option.
- **For pregnant people,** the recommended treatment is azithromycin (1 g, orally, as a single dose), with amoxicillin (500 mg, orally, 3 times/day for 7 days) as an alternative regimen.
- For **LGV,** doxycycline (100 mg, orally, twice daily for 21 days) is the preferred treatment. Azithromycin (1 g, once weekly for 3 weeks) and erythromycin (500 mg, orally, 4 times daily for 21 days) are alternative regimens. All persons who have been treated for LGV should be retested for chlamydia approximately 3 months after treatment.

[1]Centers for Disease Control and Prevention. Sexually transmitted infections treatment guidelines, 2021. *MMWR Recomm Rep.* 2021;70(RR-4):1-187. Available at: **www.cdc.gov/std/treatment-guidelines/chlamydia.htm**

- Treatment for **trachoma** is azithromycin, orally, as a single dose of 20 mg/kg (maximum dose of 1 g), as recommended by the World Health Organization for all people diagnosed with trachoma as well as for all of their household contacts.

Follow-up Testing. Test of cure immediately following treatment is not recommended for **nonpregnant adult or adolescent** patients treated for uncomplicated chlamydial infection unless compliance is in question, symptoms persist, or reinfection is suspected. Test of cure (preferably by NAAT) is recommended approximately 4 weeks after treatment of **pregnant people.** Reinfection is common after initial infection and treatment, and all infected adolescents and adults, including pregnant people, should be retested for *C trachomatis* approximately 3 months following initial treatment, regardless of whether patients believe their sex partners were treated. If retesting at 3 months is not possible, patients should be retested when they next present for health care in the 12 months after initial treatment.

INFECTION PREVENTION AND CONTROL MEASURES IN HEALTH CARE SETTINGS: Standard precautions are recommended.

CONTROL MEASURES:

Pregnancy. Identification and treatment of people with *C trachomatis* genital tract infection during pregnancy and before delivery can prevent peripartum acquisition of disease in the infant. The CDC and US Preventive Services Task Force (USPSTF) recommend that all pregnant people aged ≤24 years of age as well as those older than 24 years who are at increased risk for chlamydia (eg, those who have a new sex partner, more than one sex partner, a sex partner with concurrent partners, or a sex partner who has an STI) should be routinely screened for *C trachomatis* at the first prenatal visit. Pregnant people who remain at increased risk for chlamydial infection also should be retested during the third trimester to prevent postnatal complications in the birthing person and chlamydial infection in the neonate.

Neonatal Chlamydial Conjunctivitis. Recommended topical prophylaxis with erythromycin or tetracycline for all newborn infants for prevention of gonococcal ophthalmia will not prevent neonatal chlamydial conjunctivitis or extraocular infection (see Neonatal Ophthalmia Prevention, p 1129).

Contacts of Infants With C trachomatis Conjunctivitis or Pneumonia. Birthing parents of infected infants should be evaluated and presumptively treated for *C trachomatis,* as should their sex partners.

Routine Screening.[1-4] All sexually active female individuals (≤24 years) should be tested at least annually for chlamydial infection, even if no symptoms are present or barrier contraception is reported. Rectal chlamydial testing for female patients can be considered on the basis of reported sexual behaviors and exposure with shared clinical

[1] American Academy of Pediatrics, Committee on Adolescence; Society for Adolescent Health and Medicine. Screening for nonviral sexually transmitted infections in adolescents and young adults. *Pediatrics*. 2014;134(1):e302-e311

[2] US Preventive Services Task Force. Screening for chlamydia and gonorrhea: US Preventive Services Task Force recommendation statement. *JAMA*. 2021;326(10).949-956

[3] Centers for Disease Control and Prevention. Sexually transmitted infections treatment guidelines, 2021. *MMWR Recomm Rep*. 2021;70(RR-4):1-187. Available at: **www.cdc.gov/std/treatment-guidelines/chlamydia.htm.**

[4] **www.cdc.gov/std/treatment-guidelines/screening-recommendations.htm**

decision making between the patient and the provider. In addition, opt-out chlamydia screening (ie, the patient is notified that testing will be performed unless the patient declines, regardless of reported sexual activity) for adolescent and young female adults can be considered during clinical encounters. Opt-out chlamydia screening may substantially increase screening, be cost-saving, and identify infections among patients who do not disclose sexual behavior.

Although evidence is insufficient to recommend routine screening for *C trachomatis* in sexually active male individuals, annual screening should be considered in clinical settings serving populations of male young adults with high prevalence of chlamydia (eg, correctional facilities, military recruits, STI clinics, high school clinics, adolescent clinics) or in populations with high burden of infection. Sexually active young MSM should be screened at least annually for rectal and urethral chlamydia if they engaged in receptive or insertive anal intercourse, respectively (regardless of condom use during exposure). Screening practices may be suboptimal because of inadequate disclosure or inadequate sexual history taking; thus, testing may be considered at rectal or pharyngeal sites in those who do not report exposure at these sites. More frequent chlamydia screening every 3 to 6 months is recommended if risk behaviors persist or if they or their sex partners have multiple partners.

Postexposure Prophylaxis. Doxycycline, 200 mg, administered within 24 to 72 hours of condomless sex (doxy-PEP) has been shown in studies to reduce the incidence of syphilis, chlamydia, and gonorrhea among cisgender men who have sex with men (MSM) and transgender women with a recent history of these infections.

Management of Sex Partners.[1] All people with sexual contact in the 60 days preceding diagnosis or onset of symptoms of patients with *C trachomatis* infection (whether symptomatic or asymptomatic), nongonococcal urethritis, cervicitis, epididymitis, or pelvic inflammatory disease should be evaluated and treated for *C trachomatis* infection. The patient's last sex partner should be treated even if last sexual contact was more than 60 days before diagnosis in the index case. If concerns exist that sex partners who are referred for evaluation and treatment will not seek care, expedited partner therapy (EPT), which is the practice of the index patient delivering the prescriptions or medications to the patient's sex partner without the health care provider first examining the partner, can be considered. To clarify the legal status of EPT in each state, refer to the CDC website **(www.cdc.gov/std/ept/legal/).**

Efforts should be made to educate partners about symptoms of chlamydia and to encourage partners to seek clinical evaluation. MSM with chlamydia have a high risk for coexisting STIs, especially undiagnosed HIV, among partners, and data are limited regarding EPT effectiveness in reducing persistent or recurrent chlamydia among MSM. Thus, shared clinical decision making for MSM regarding EPT is recommended.

Patients and contacts should abstain from unprotected intercourse until treatment of both partners is complete (ie, after completion of a multiple-dose treatment or for 7 days after single-dose therapy).

LGV. Nonspecific preventive measures for LGV are the same as measures for STIs in general and include education, case reporting, condom use, and avoidance of sexual contact with infected people. Partners exposed to an LGV-infected person within the

---

[1] Centers for Disease Control and Prevention. Sexually transmitted infections treatment guidelines, 2021. *MMWR Recomm Rep.* 2021;70(RR-4):1-187. Available at: **www.cdc.gov/std/treatment-guidelines/chlamydia.htm**

60 days before the patient's symptom onset should be tested and presumptively treated for chlamydia with doxycycline, 100 mg, orally, 2 times/day for 7 days.

Trachoma. Prevention methods recommended by the World Health Organization for global elimination of blindness attributable to trachoma by 2030 include surgery, antimicrobial agents, face washing, and environmental improvement (SAFE). Azithromycin (20 mg/kg, maximum 1 g), once a year as a single oral dose, is used in mass drug administration campaigns for trachoma control.

Clostridial Infections

Botulism and Infant Botulism
(Clostridium botulinum)

CLINICAL MANIFESTATIONS: Botulism is a neuroparalytic disorder typically characterized by an acute, afebrile, symmetric, descending, flaccid paralysis that can progress to respiratory distress or failure. Paralysis is caused by blockade of neurotransmitter release at the voluntary motor and autonomic neuromuscular junctions. Four naturally occurring forms of human botulism exist: infant, foodborne, wound, and adult intestinal colonization. Cases of iatrogenic botulism, which result from injection of excess therapeutic or cosmetic botulinum toxin, have been reported, and botulinum neurotoxins are considered a potential agent of bioterrorism. Symptoms of botulism can occur abruptly, within hours of exposure, or evolve gradually over several days and may include diplopia, dysphagia, dysphonia, and dysarthria. Loss of facial expression and/or pooling of oropharyngeal secretions may be present. Cranial nerve palsies are followed by symmetric, descending, flaccid paralysis of somatic musculature in patients who remain fully alert. In children, dysphagia and dysarthria are the most frequent cranial nerve symptoms, and generalized weakness is reported more than paralysis in the early stage of illness.

Infant botulism, which occurs predominantly in infants younger than 6 months (range, 1 day–14 months), is preceded by or begins with constipation and manifests as decreased movement, loss of facial expression, poor feeding or poor suck, ptosis, weak cry, diminished gag reflex, ocular palsies, loss of head control, and progressive descending generalized weakness and hypotonia. Some reports suggest that sudden infant death could result from rapidly progressing infant botulism.

ETIOLOGY: Botulism occurs after absorption of botulinum toxin into the circulation from a mucosal (eg, gastrointestinal) or wound surface. Infant botulism results after ingested spores of *Clostridium botulinum* or when related neurotoxigenic clostridial species colonize the intestine and then germinate, multiply, and produce botulinum toxin. There are 7 classic antigenic toxin types (A–G) of *C botulinum*. Type H toxin is a hybrid of types A and F. Non-*botulinum* species of *Clostridium* may rarely produce these neurotoxins and cause disease. The most common botulinum toxin serotypes associated with naturally occurring illness are types A, B, E, and rarely F. Most cases of infant botulism result from toxin types A and B, but a few cases of types E and F have been caused by *Clostridium butyricum* (type E), *C botulinum* (type E), and *Clostridium baratii* (type F). *C botulinum* spores are ubiquitous in soils and dust worldwide and have been isolated from the home environment and vacuum cleaner dust of infant botulism cases.

EPIDEMIOLOGY: Infant botulism cases may occur in breastfed infants before or after the first introduction of nonhuman milk substances; the source of spores usually is not identified. Honey has been identified as an avoidable source of spores. No case of infant botulism has been proven to be caused by consumption of corn syrup. Rarely, intestinal botulism can occur in older children and adults, usually after intestinal surgery and exposure to antimicrobial agents (**www.cdc.gov/botulism/infant-botulism.html**).

Foodborne botulism results when food that carries spores of *C botulinum* is preserved or stored improperly under anaerobic conditions that permit germination, multiplication, and toxin production. Illness follows ingestion of the food containing preformed botulinum toxin. Home processing of foods (eg, home canning) and inadequate refrigeration of cooked foods are the most common causes of foodborne botulism in the United States, followed by rare outbreaks associated with commercially processed foods, restaurant-associated foods, and wine produced in prisons ("pruno" or "hooch").

Wound botulism results when *C botulinum* contaminates traumatized tissue, germinates, multiplies, and produces toxin. Gross trauma or crush injury can be a predisposing event. In recent years, "skin popping" and self-injection of drugs such as heroin (including black tar heroin) and rarely methamphetamines have been associated with most cases.

Immunity to botulinum toxin does not develop after infection. Botulism is not transmitted from person-to-person. The usual **incubation period** for foodborne botulism is 12 to 48 hours (range, 6 hours–10 days). In infant botulism, the **incubation period** is estimated at 3 to 30 days from the time of ingestion of spores. For wound botulism, the **incubation period** is 4 to 14 days from time of injury until onset of symptoms.

DIAGNOSTIC TESTS: Appropriate specimens for culture and botulinum toxin detection should be obtained as soon as a diagnosis of botulism is suspected. Because results of laboratory testing may require several days, treatment with antitoxin should be initiated urgently for all forms of botulism on the basis of clinical suspicion. To increase the likelihood of diagnosis in foodborne botulism, all suspect foods should be collected, and serum and stool or enema specimens should be obtained from all people with suspected illness. In foodborne cases, the length of time serum specimens may have detectable toxin varies, and in some cases can be longer than 10 days after illness onset.

Enriched selective media are required to isolate *C botulinum* from stool and foods. Laboratory confirmation of infant botulism is made by demonstrating botulinum toxin in serum or feces or botulinum toxin-producing organisms in feces or enema fluid. Wound botulism is confirmed by demonstrating botulinum toxin-producing organisms in the wound or tissue or toxin in the serum. Foodborne botulism is confirmed by demonstrating botulinum toxin in food, serum, or stool or botulinum toxin-producing organism in stool. Confirmation can also occur when a symptomatic patient consumed the same food as a laboratory-confirmed patient.

A toxin neutralization bioassay in mice (available only at specialized public health laboratories) and an in vitro mass spectrometry assay can be used to detect botulinum toxin in serum, stool, enema fluid, gastric aspirate, or suspect foods. A nucleic acid amplification test (NAAT) available at some reference laboratories can detect botulinum neurotoxin genes (*BoNT*) in clostridial species in cultures (**www.cdc.gov/mmwr/volumes/70/rr/rr7002a1.htm**). For additional information on testing for botulinum toxin, consult your state health department.

Although toxin can be demonstrated in serum in some infants with botulism (13% in 1 study), this requires a large volume of serum, ideally collected before administration of antitoxin. Stool is the best specimen for diagnosis; enema effluent also can be useful. If constipation makes obtaining a stool specimen difficult, an enema of sterile, nonbacteriostatic water should be administered promptly.

Ancillary testing can be helpful when evaluating children with suspected botulism. Cerebrospinal fluid findings are generally normal in botulism. Brain imaging may help to exclude strokes or some inflammatory conditions. Tensilon (edrophonium) testing, which yields positive results in myasthenia gravis, usually yields negative results in botulism. The most prominent electromyographic finding in botulism is an incremental increase of evoked muscle potentials at high-frequency nerve stimulation (20–50 Hz). In addition, a characteristic pattern of brief, small-amplitude, overly abundant motor action potentials may be seen after stimulation of muscle, but its absence does not exclude the diagnosis.

TREATMENT:

Involvement of Public Health Authorities. When botulism of any type is suspected, it should be reported to the state health department; all states maintain a 24-hour telephone service. The Centers for Disease Control and Prevention (CDC) Clinical Emergency Botulism Service can also be contacted at 770-488-7100. Public health agencies can provide guidance on collection, storage, and shipping requirements for all necessary clinical specimens (and possible food sources, when relevant).

Meticulous Supportive Care. Meticulous supportive care, in particular respiratory and nutritional support, constitutes a fundamental aspect of therapy in all forms of botulism. Recovery from botulism may take weeks to months.

Antitoxin for Infant Botulism. Immediate administration of antitoxin is the key to successful therapy, because antitoxin treatment ends the toxemia and stops further uptake of toxin. However, because botulinum neurotoxin becomes internalized in the nerve ending, administration of antitoxin does not reverse paralysis.

Human-derived antitoxin should be administered immediately. Human botulism immune globulin for intravenous use (BIG-IV, which goes by the brand name BabyBIG) is licensed by the US Food and Drug Administration (FDA) for treatment of infant botulism caused by *C botulinum* type A or type B. BabyBIG is produced and distributed by the California Department of Public Health (CDPH). If the patient's clinical findings are consistent with infant botulism, immediately contact the Infant Botulism Treatment and Prevention Program (IBTPP) of the CDPH to arrange for shipment of BabyBIG (24-hour telephone number: 510-231-7600; **www. infantbotulism.org**). BabyBIG significantly decreases days of mechanical ventilation, days of intensive care unit stay, and total length of hospital stay by almost 1 month and is cost-saving. BabyBIG is first-line therapy for infant botulism. As with other immune globulin intravenous preparations, routine live-virus vaccines should be delayed for 6 months after receipt of BabyBIG because of potential interference with immune responses (see Table 1.11, p 69).

Equine-derived heptavalent botulinum antitoxin (BAT; see below) was licensed by the FDA in 2013 for treatment of adult and pediatric botulism and is available through the CDC. BAT has been used, on a case by case basis, to treat patients with type F infant botulism, as this antitoxin is not contained in BabyBIG.

Antitoxin for Noninfant Forms of Botulism. BAT is the only botulinum antitoxin approved in the United States for treatment of noninfant botulism. BAT contains antitoxins against botulinum toxin types A–G and has been "despeciated" by enzymatic removal of the Fc immunoglobulin fragment, resulting in a product that is >90% Fab and F(ab')$_2$ immunoglobulin fragments. This reduces but does not fully eliminate allergic reactions. As a precaution, epinephrine and antihistamine treatments should be available for any patient receiving BAT. It is possible that an infant could develop botulism from a food source or wound infection ("botulism in an infant" rather than "infant botulism"), such that BAT may be the appropriate antitoxin preparation. BAT is provided by the CDC with the product information that includes specific, detailed instructions for intravenous administration of antitoxin. Additional information may be found on the CDC website (**www.cdc.gov/botulism/** and **www.cdc.gov/botulism/resources. html**).

Antimicrobial Agents. Antimicrobial therapy is not prescribed in infant botulism unless clearly indicated for a concurrent infection. Aminoglycoside agents can potentiate the paralytic effects of the toxin and should be avoided. Given theoretical concerns of toxin release from antibiotic-induced bacterial cell death, providers should consider delaying the use of antibiotics in wound botulism until after antitoxin is administered, depending on the clinical situation. The role for antimicrobial therapy in the adult intestinal colonization form of botulism, if any, has not been established.

INFECTION PREVENTION AND CONTROL MEASURES IN HEALTH CARE SETTINGS: Standard precautions are recommended.

CONTROL MEASURES:
- Honey should not be given to children younger than 12 months because of the possibility of contaminating *C botulinum* spores. Many foods and commercial products contain honey, and the honey is included in a variety of ways. Because the details of each manufacturing process vary, the California Department of Public Health is unable to comment on the likelihood that the honey-containing food product may contain viable *C botulinum* spores (**www.infantbotulism.org/general/ faq.php**). Prudence would dictate that these types of foods also should be avoided during the first 12 months of life. Botulism is not transmitted by human milk, and breastfeeding parents may consume honey.
- Prophylactic antitoxin is not recommended for asymptomatic people who have ingested a food known to contain botulinum toxin. Physicians treating a patient who has been exposed to toxin or is suspected of having any type of botulism should contact their state health department immediately. People exposed to toxin who are asymptomatic should have close medical observation in nonsolitary settings.
- Education regarding safe practices in food preparation and home-canning methods should be promoted. Use of a pressure cooker (at 116°C [240.8°F]) is necessary to kill spores of *C botulinum*. Bringing the internal temperature of foods to 85°C (185°F) for 10 minutes will destroy the toxin. Cooked and leftover foods should be refrigerated in order limit the opportunity for toxin production. Time, temperature, and pressure requirements vary with altitude and the product being heated. Food containers that appear to bulge may contain gas produced by *C botulinum* and should be discarded. Other foods that appear to have spoiled should not be eaten or tasted (**https://nchfp.uga.edu/publications/publications_usda.html**).

Public Health Reporting. Botulism is a nationally notifiable disease, and it is required by law to be reported immediately to local and state health departments. Immediate reporting of suspected cases is particularly important, because a single case could be the harbinger of many more cases, as with foodborne botulism, and because of possible use of botulinum toxin as a bioterrorism weapon.

Clostridial Myonecrosis
(Gas Gangrene)

CLINICAL MANIFESTATIONS: Disease onset is heralded by acute and progressive pain at the site of the wound, often initially out of proportion to the appearance of the affected area. Later, there is edema, increasing exquisite tenderness, and exudate. Systemic findings include tachycardia disproportionate to the degree of fever, pallor, and diaphoresis. Crepitus is suggestive but not pathognomonic of *Clostridium* infection and is not always present. Tense bullae containing thin, serosanguineous, or dark fluid develop in the overlying skin and areas of green-black cutaneous necrosis appear. Fluid in the bullae has a foul odor. Disease can progress rapidly with development of hypotension, renal failure, and alterations in mental status. Diagnosis is based on clinical manifestations, including the characteristic appearance of necrotic muscle at surgery. Untreated clostridial myonecrosis, also known as gas gangrene, can lead to disseminated myonecrosis, suppurative visceral infection, septicemia, and death within hours.

Nontraumatic gas gangrene usually is caused by *Clostridium septicum* and is a complication of bacteremia, which is the result of an occult gastrointestinal mucosal lesion (most commonly colon cancer) or a complication of neutropenic colitis, leukemia, or diabetes mellitus.

ETIOLOGY: Clostridial myonecrosis is caused by *Clostridium* species, most often *Clostridium perfringens.* Other *Clostridium* species (eg, *Clostridium sordellii, C septicum, Clostridium novyi*) have also been associated with myonecrosis. These organisms are large, gram-positive, spore-forming, anaerobic bacilli with blunt ends. Disease manifestations are caused by potent clostridial exotoxins. Mixed infection with other gram-positive and gram-negative bacteria is common.

EPIDEMIOLOGY: Clostridial myonecrosis usually results from contamination of deep open wounds. The sources of *Clostridium* species are soil, contaminated foreign bodies, and human and animal feces. Dirty surgical or traumatic wounds, particularly those with retained foreign bodies or significant amounts of devitalized tissue, predispose to disease. Cases have occurred in people who inject drugs, in association with contaminated black tar heroin. Rarely, nontraumatic gas gangrene occurs in immunocompromised people, most frequently in those with underlying malignancy, neutrophil dysfunction, or diseases associated with bowel ischemia.

The **incubation period** from the time of injury is 6 hours to 4 days.

DIAGNOSTIC TESTS: Anaerobic cultures of wound exudate, involved soft tissue and muscle, and blood should be performed. Matrix-assisted laser desorption/ionization–time-of-flight (MALDI-TOF) devices have an approved indication from the US Food and Drug Administration to identify *C perfringens.* Because *Clostridium* species are ubiquitous, their recovery from a wound is not diagnostic unless typical clinical manifestations are present. A Gram-stained smear of wound discharge demonstrating characteristic gram-positive bacilli and few, if any, polymorphonuclear leukocytes suggests clostridial infection. Tissue specimens (not swab specimens) for anaerobic culture must be obtained to confirm the diagnosis. Because some pathogenic *Clostridium* species are exquisitely sensitive to oxygen, care should be taken when collecting and processing a sample to optimize anaerobic growth conditions. A radiograph of the affected site might demonstrate gas in the tissue, but this is a nonspecific finding that is not always present. Occasionally, blood cultures are positive and are considered diagnostic.

TREATMENT:
- Prompt and complete surgical excision of necrotic tissue and removal of foreign material is essential. Repeated surgical débridement may be required to ensure complete removal of all infected tissue. Vacuum-assisted wound closure can be used following multiple débridements.
- Management of shock, fluid and electrolyte imbalance, hemolytic anemia, and other complications is crucial.
- High-dose penicillin G should be administered intravenously (see Table 4.3, p 993). Clindamycin, metronidazole, meropenem, ertapenem, and chloramphenicol are alternative drugs for patients with a serious penicillin allergy or for treatment of polymicrobial infections. The combination of penicillin G and clindamycin may be superior to penicillin alone because of the theoretical benefit of clindamycin inhibiting toxin synthesis.
- Hyperbaric oxygen may be beneficial, but efficacy data from adequately controlled clinical studies are not available.

INFECTION PREVENTION AND CONTROL MEASURES IN HEALTH CARE SETTINGS: Standard precautions are recommended.

CONTROL MEASURES: Prompt and careful débridement, copious lavage of contaminated wounds, and removal of foreign material should be performed.

Penicillin G (50 000 U/kg per day) or clindamycin (20–30 mg/kg per day) has been used for prophylaxis in patients with grossly contaminated wounds, but there are no data on recommended duration or the effectiveness of such preventative measures.

Clostridioides difficile (Formerly *Clostridium difficile*)

CLINICAL MANIFESTATIONS: *Clostridioides difficile* (formerly *Clostridium difficile*) is associated with a wide spectrum of gastrointestinal illness, ranging from asymptomatic colonization (common, especially in young infants) to severe and prolonged colitis with shock. In children, *C difficile* infections are rarely fatal. Mild to moderate illness is characterized by watery diarrhea, low-grade fever, and abdominal pain. In the past, hospital onset of symptoms was believed to be the most common presentation. However, recent studies have found that *C difficile* often is diagnosed in nonhospitalized children. Pseudomembranous colitis is characterized by diarrhea with mucus in feces, abdominal cramps and pain, fever, and systemic toxicity. Toxic megacolon (acute dilatation of the colon) should be considered in children who develop marked abdominal tenderness and distension with minimal diarrhea and may be associated with hemodynamic instability. Other complications of *C difficile* disease include intestinal perforation, hypotension, shock, and death. Complicated infections are less common in children than adults. Severe or fatal disease is more likely to occur in neutropenic children with leukemia, infants with Hirschsprung disease, and patients with inflammatory bowel disease. Extraintestinal manifestations of *C difficile* infection are uncommon but can include bacteremia, wound infections, and reactive arthritis. Clinical illness attributable to *C difficile* is considered very rare in children younger than 12 months.

C difficile colonization occurs when there are no attributable clinical symptoms but test results are positive for *C difficile* organism or its toxins. *C difficile* disease occurs when attributable clinical symptoms are present in the setting of tests which are positive for *C difficile* organisms or its toxins.

ETIOLOGY: *C difficile* is a spore-forming, obligate anaerobic, gram-positive bacillus. Some strains produce exotoxins (toxins A and B), which are responsible for the clinical manifestations of disease when there is overgrowth of *C difficile* in the intestine.

EPIDEMIOLOGY: *C difficile* is shed in feces. People can acquire infection from the stool of other colonized or infected people through the fecal-oral route. Any surface (including hands), device, or material that has become contaminated with feces may also transmit *C difficile* spores. Hospitals, nursing homes, and child care facilities are major reservoirs for *C difficile*. Risk factors for acquisition of the bacterium include prolonged hospitalization and exposure to an infected person either in the hospital or the community. Risk factors for *C difficile* disease include antimicrobial therapy, repeated enemas, proton pump inhibitor therapy, prolonged placement of feeding tubes (including nasogastric, gastrostomy, and jejunostomy tubes), underlying bowel disease, gastrointestinal tract surgery, renal insufficiency, and immunocompromised state. *C difficile* colitis has been associated with exposure to almost every antimicrobial agent; amoxicillin, clindamycin, cephalosporins, carbapenems, and fluoroquinolones are the agents most frequently associated with *C difficile* infection, particularly for recurrent *C difficile* disease and infections with epidemic strains. The ribotype 027 (formerly known as NAP-1/BI/027) strain is a virulent strain of *C difficile* because of increased toxin production and is associated with an increased risk of severe and recurrent disease. Ribotype 027 strains of *C difficile* have emerged as a cause of outbreaks among adults and are reported sporadically in children.

C difficile disease and associated hospitalizations among children ≥1 year of age and adults in the United States decreased 24% from 2011 to 2017, after adjustment for more sensitive diagnostic testing (nucleic acid amplification tests [NAATs]). The overall decrease was driven by a 36% decrease in health care-associated cases, while community-associated cases did not change. The incidence of pediatric community-associated *C difficile* disease may be twice as frequent as health care-associated disease.

Asymptomatic intestinal colonization with *C difficile* (including toxin-producing strains) is common in children younger than 2 years; up to 50% of healthy infants are colonized. Colonization rates drop to 5% to 12% in healthy children 5 to 18 years. The rate of asymptomatic colonization with *C difficile* in hospitalized adults ranges from 3% to 26%.

The **incubation period** is unknown; colitis usually develops 5 to 10 days after initiation of the causative antimicrobial therapy but can occur on the first day of treatment and up to 10 weeks after therapy cessation.

DIAGNOSTIC TESTS: Endoscopic findings of pseudomembranes (2- to 5-mm, raised yellowish plaques) and hyperemic, friable rectal mucosa suggesting pseudomembranous colitis are highly correlated with *C difficile* disease. More commonly, the diagnosis of *C difficile* disease is based on laboratory detection of *C difficile* toxin(s) or toxin gene(s) in a diarrheal stool specimen. In general, laboratory tests for *C difficile* should not be ordered for a patient who is having formed stools unless ileus or toxic megacolon is suspected. Similarly, *C difficile* tests should not be ordered on a patient who is receiving laxatives or stool softeners or has evidence suggestive of a viral or noninfectious cause of diarrhea. Notwithstanding the availability of several test methods, there currently is no generally agreed on gold standard laboratory test method for the diagnosis of *C difficile* disease.

Molecular assays using NAATs have become the most common diagnostic test for toxigenic strains of *C difficile* in both adult and pediatric hospitals. NAATs detect genes responsible for the production of toxins A and B, rather than free toxins A and B in the stool, which instead are detected by enzyme immunoassay (EIA). EIAs for the toxins are rapid, performed easily, and highly specific for diagnosis of *C difficile* disease, but their sensitivity is relatively low. The cell culture cytotoxicity assay, which also tests for toxin in stool, is more sensitive than the EIA but is labor intensive and has a long turnaround time, limiting its usefulness in the clinical setting.

NAATs combine excellent sensitivity and analytic specificity and provide results to clinicians in times comparable to EIAs. However, detecting toxin gene(s) in patients who are only colonized with *C difficile* is common and likely contributes to misdiagnosis of *C difficile* disease in children with other causes of diarrhea, leading to unnecessary antibiotic treatment for *C difficile*. Several steps can be taken to reduce the likelihood of misdiagnosis/overdiagnosis of *C difficile* disease related to use of highly sensitive NAATs. Age should be considered, because colonization with *C difficile* in infants younger than 12 months is common and symptomatic infection in this age group is not believed to occur; therefore, *C difficile* diagnostic testing on samples from children younger than 12 months is discouraged unless other infectious and noninfectious causes of diarrhea have been excluded and should be limited to infants with significant diarrhea and underlying Hirschsprung disease, other severe motility disorders, or evidence of pseudomembranous colitis or in an outbreak situation.

Likewise, testing should not be performed routinely in toddlers with diarrhea who are 12 through 23 months of age unless other infectious or noninfectious causes have been excluded. For children 24 months and older, testing is recommended if there is new onset of prolonged and worsening diarrhea and risk factors (eg, inflammatory bowel disease, immunocompromising condition) or a recent course of antibiotics or health care exposures. Because shedding of *C difficile* in the stool can persist for several months after treatment and symptom resolution, tests of cure should not be performed. Rather, response to therapy should be based on symptom resolution.

A 2- or 3-stage approach to testing for *C difficile* increases the positive predictive value compared with 1-stage testing. Multistep algorithms have been suggested by the Infectious Diseases Society of America guidelines[1] that incorporate testing for stool toxin (EIA); testing for glutamate dehydrogenase (GDH), an enzyme expressed by both toxigenic and nontoxigenic strains of *C difficile*; and NAAT depending on whether the laboratory has prespecified criteria for which stool samples to test (eg, diarrheal stool samples on patients who are not receiving laxatives). This approach could include a NAAT alone or EIA as part of a multistep algorithm (GDH plus EIA, GDH plus EIA

[1] McDonald LC, Gerding DN, Johnson S, et al. Clinical practice guidelines for *Clostridium difficile* infection in adults and children: 2017 update by the Infectious Diseases Society of America (IDSA) and Society for Healthcare Epidemiology of America (SHEA). *Clin Infect Dis*. 2018;66(7):e1-e48

arbitrated by NAAT, or NAAT plus toxin). If diagnostic stewardship is not performed, the testing would include EIA as part of a multistep algorithm as outlined above (and not NAAT alone).

TREATMENT: A central tenet to control *C difficile* disease is the discontinuation of precipitating antimicrobial therapy. Stopping these agents allows for reemergence of healthy commensal gut flora, which prevent *C difficile* infection. A variety of therapies are available; use of a particular treatment modality is dependent on severity of illness, the number of recurrences of infection, tolerability of adverse effects, and cost. Recommended therapies for first occurrence, first recurrence, and second recurrence are provided in Table 3.3. Drugs that decrease intestinal motility should not be administered. Asymptomatic patients should not be treated.

When using oral vancomycin, some experts recommend oral administration of the intravenous formulation of vancomycin to reduce costs and risk of recurrence. The intravenous formulation is less expensive than the product available for oral use. Intravenously administered vancomycin is not effective for *C difficile* disease.

Fidaxomicin is approved by the US Food and Drug Administration for treatment of *C difficile*-associated diarrhea in adults and children 6 months and older. Studies have demonstrated equivalent efficacy to oral vancomycin, although subjects with life-threatening and fulminant infection, hypotension, septic shock, peritoneal signs, significant dehydration, or toxic megacolon were excluded. Secondary outcomes from trials in both children and adults suggest a lower *C difficile* recurrence rate in individuals receiving fidaxomicin versus vancomycin. On the basis of these limited data in children, fidaxomicin may be considered for treatment of the initial *C difficile* episode. However, given equivalent efficacy to oral vancomycin and the significantly higher cost of fidaxomicin, many experts limit use of fidaxomicin for treatment of *C difficile* recurrences. No comparative data of fidaxomicin versus metronidazole are available.

Up to 20% of patients experience a recurrence after discontinuing therapy, but infection usually responds to a second course of the same treatment. Metronidazole should not be used for treatment of a second recurrence or for prolonged therapy, because neurotoxicity is possible. A variety of tapered or pulsed regimens of oral vancomycin have been used to treat recurrent disease (Table 3.3).

Fecal transplant (intestinal microbiota transplantation) appears to be safe and effective in adults as well as children. In a multicenter retrospective study of 335 children with a *C difficile* infection that had been unresponsive to antibiotic treatment, 81% had a successful outcome following a single fecal transplant. In 2022, the US Food and Drug Administration approved Rebyota, a fecal microbiota product, with the indication to prevent recurrent *C difficile* infections in individuals 18 years or older, following successful antibiotic treatment of *C difficile* infection. Rebyota is not indicated for the treatment of *C difficile* infection. Bezlotoxumab, a human monoclonal antibody that neutralizes *C difficile* toxin B, is approved to reduce the recurrence of infection in at-risk adults receiving *C difficile*-directed antibacterial treatment. Pharmacokinetic and safety data support a dose of 10 mg/kg dose in children 1 to <18 years of age, although pediatric efficacy data are not yet available. These or other therapies may be appropriate for third recurrences of disease in children, especially in consultation with an infectious disease or gastroenterology expert. Cholestyramine is not recommended. Other potential adjunctive therapies of unclear efficacy include immune globulin therapy and probiotics (particularly *Saccharomyces boulardii* and kefir).

INFECTION PREVENTION AND CONTROL MEASURES IN HEALTH CARE SETTINGS: In addition to standard precautions, contact precautions and a private room (if feasible) are recommended at the time that disease is suspected through resolution of diarrhea.

Table 3.3. Treatments for *Clostridioides difficile* Disease

Severity	Recommendation
First Occurrence	
Mild-moderate	Metronidazole, 30 mg/kg/day, PO, every 6 h (preferred), every 6 h for 10 days (maximum 500 mg/dose)
	OR
	Vancomycin, 40 mg/kg/day, PO, every 6 h for 10 days (maximum 125 mg/dose)
	For pregnant/breastfeeding or metronidazole-intolerant patients: Vancomycin, 40 mg/kg/day, PO, every 6 h for 10 days (maximum 125 mg/dose)
	In patients for whom oral therapy cannot reach colon:
	To above regimen, **ADD** vancomycin, 500 mg/100 mL normal saline enema, as needed every 8 h until improvement
Severe[a]	Vancomycin, 40 mg/kg/day, PO, every 6 h for 10 days (maximum 125 mg/dose)
Severe and complicated[b]	If no abdominal distension (use both for 10 days):
	Vancomycin, 40 mg/kg/day, PO, every 6 h (maximum 125 mg/dose)
	PLUS metronidazole, 30 mg/kg/day, IV, every 6 h (maximum 500 mg/dose)
	If complicated with ileus or toxic colitis and/or significant abdominal distension (use all for 10 days):
	Vancomycin, 40 mg/kg/day, PO, every 6 h (maximum 500 mg/dose)
	PLUS metronidazole, 30 mg/kg/day, IV, every 6 h (maximum 500 mg/dose)
	PLUS vancomycin, 500 mg/100 mL normal saline enema, as needed every 8 h until improvement
Severity	**Recommendation**
First Recurrence	
Mild-moderate	Same regimen as for first occurrence (see above)
Severe	Vancomycin, 40 mg/kg/day, PO, every 6 h (maximum 125 mg/dose)

Table 3.3. Treatments for *Clostridioides difficile* Disease, continued

Severity	Recommendation
Second (or Additional) Recurrence	
All	Vancomycin, PO, as pulsed or prolonged tapered dose with one of the following regimens:

- Vancomycin orally, 10 mg/kg/dose (maximum 125 mg/dose) 4 times a day for 7 days, then 3 times a day for 7 days, then twice a day for 7 days, then once daily for 7 days, then once every other day for 7 days, then every 72 hours for 7 days

OR

- Vancomycin, orally, 10 mg/kg/dose (maximum 125 mg/dose) 4 times a day for 14 days, then twice a day for 7 to 14 days, then once daily for 7 to 14 days, then every 2 to 3 days for 2 to 8 weeks

OR

- Vancomycin, orally, 10 mg/kg/dose (maximum 125 mg/dose) 4 times a day for 14 days, then rifaximin, orally, 400 mg, 3 times a day for 14 days (note that rifaximin dosing in pediatric patients is not well described; it is poorly water-soluble and minimally absorbed and should be avoided if the patient recently has received rifaximin for *C difficile* disease or another indication).

OR

Fidaxomicin[c] weight band dosing[d] twice daily for 10 days

OR

Fecal microbiota product or transplantation, in eligible patients

---

PO indicates orally; IV, intravenously.

[a]Severe: not well defined in children, but should be considered in the presence of leukocytosis, leukopenia, or worsening renal function.

[b]Severe and complicated: intensive care unit admission, hypotension or shock, pseudomembranous colitis by endoscopy, ileus, toxic megacolon.

[c]May be considered for treatment of the initial *C difficile* episode. However, given high cost and equivalent efficacy to oral vancomycin, many experts limit use to treatment of *C difficile* recurrences.

[d]Per dose: 4 kg to <7 kg, 80 mg; 7 kg to <9 kg, 120 mg; 9 kg to <12.5 kg, 160 mg; ≥12.5 kg, 200 mg.

CONTROL MEASURES: Exercising meticulous hand hygiene, properly handling contaminated waste (including diapers), disinfecting fomites, and limiting use of antimicrobial agents are the best available methods for control of *C difficile* infection. Gloves and gowns should be worn for all in-room care to prevent hand contamination and perform hand hygiene immediately after glove removal. Because no single method of hand hygiene will eliminate all *C difficile* spores, using gloves to prevent hand contamination remains critical for preventing *C difficile* transmission via the hands of health care personnel. During an outbreak, after contact with a *C difficile*-infected patient, optimal hand hygiene includes removing gloves and washing hands with soap and water instead of alcohol-based hand sanitizers. In nonoutbreak hospital settings, either handwashing with soap and water or use of alcohol-based hand sanitizers is adequate; this is supported by data showing hospitals relying on alcohol-based hand hygiene do not have more frequent *C difficile* outbreaks.

Thorough cleaning of hospital rooms and bathrooms of patients with *C difficile* disease, as well as disinfection of reusable equipment with which infected patients had contact, is essential. Because *C difficile* spores are difficult to kill with standard hospital disinfectants approved by the US Environmental Protection Agency, many health care facilities have instituted the use of disinfectants with sporicidal activity (eg, hypochlorite).

Children with *C difficile* diarrhea should be excluded from child care settings until stools are contained in the diaper, and for the child who is continent, until stool frequency is no more than 2 stools above that child's normal frequency.

Clostridium perfringens Foodborne Illness

CLINICAL MANIFESTATIONS: *Clostridium perfringens* foodborne illness is characterized by a sudden onset of watery diarrhea and moderate-to-severe crampy, mid-epigastric pain. Symptoms usually resolve within 24 hours. The shorter incubation period, shorter duration of illness, and absence of fever in most patients differentiate *C perfringens* foodborne disease from shigellosis and salmonellosis. As compared with foodborne illnesses associated with heavy metals, *Staphylococcus aureus* enterotoxins, *Bacillus cereus* emetic toxin, and fish and shellfish toxins, *C perfringens* foodborne illness is infrequently associated with vomiting. Diarrheal illness caused by *B cereus* diarrheal enterotoxins can be indistinguishable from that caused by *C perfringens* (see Appendix VI, Clinical Syndromes Associated With Foodborne Diseases, p 1150). Necrotizing colitis and death from constipation have been described in patients with disease attributable to *C perfringens* type A who received antidiarrheal medications. Enteritis necroticans (also known as pigbel) results from hemorrhagic necrosis of the midgut and is a cause of severe illness and death attributable to *C perfringens* infection caused by contamination with *Clostridium* strains carrying a β toxin. Rare cases have been reported in the highlands of Papua New Guinea and in Thailand; protein malnutrition is an important risk factor. Additionally, enteritis necroticans attributed to *C perfringens* type C has been reported in a child with poorly controlled diabetes in the United States who consumed chitterlings (pig intestine).

ETIOLOGY: Typical illness is caused by a heat-labile *C perfringens* enterotoxin, produced during sporulation in the small intestine. *C perfringens* type F (formerly *cpe*-positive type A), which produces α toxin and enterotoxin, commonly causes foodborne illness. Enteritis necroticans is caused by *C perfringens* type C, which produces a β toxin that causes necrotizing small bowel inflammation.

EPIDEMIOLOGY: *C perfringens* is a gram-positive, spore-forming bacillus that is ubiquitous in the environment and the intestinal tracts of humans and animals and is commonly present in raw meat and poultry. Spores of *C perfringens* that survive cooking can germinate and multiply rapidly during slow cooling, when stored at temperatures from 20°C to 60°C (68°F–140°F), and during inadequate reheating. At an optimum temperature, *C perfringens* has one of the fastest rates of growth of any bacterium. Illness results from consumption of food containing high numbers of vegetative organisms

($>10^5$ colony forming units [CFU]/g) that produce enterotoxin in the intestine of the consumer.

Ingestion of the organism is commonly associated with foods prepared by restaurants or caterers or in institutional settings (eg, schools and camps) where food is prepared in large quantities, cooled slowly, and may be stored inappropriately for prolonged periods. Beef, poultry, gravies, and dried or precooked foods are commonly implicated sources. Most outbreaks occur in November or December, often linked to consumption of popular holiday foods. Illness is not transmissible from person-to-person.

The **incubation period** is 6 to 24 hours, usually 8 to 12 hours.

DIAGNOSTIC TESTS: Because the fecal flora of healthy people commonly includes *C perfringens*, counts of *C perfringens* of 10^6 CFU/g of feces or greater obtained within 48 hours of onset of illness support the diagnosis in symptomatic people. The diagnosis also can be supported by detection of enterotoxin in stool. *C perfringens* can be confirmed as the source of an outbreak if 10^6 CFU/g are isolated from stool, enterotoxin is demonstrated in the stool of 2 or more ill people, or the concentration of organisms is at least 10^5 CFU/g in the implicated food. Although *C perfringens* is an anaerobe, special transport conditions are unnecessary. Whole stool, rather than rectal swab specimens, should be obtained, transported in ice packs, and tested within 24 hours. For enumeration and enterotoxin testing, obtaining stool specimens in bulk without added transport media is required.

TREATMENT: *C perfringens* foodborne illness is typically self-limited. Oral rehydration or, occasionally, intravenous fluid and electrolyte replacement may be indicated to prevent or treat dehydration. Antimicrobial agents are not indicated.

INFECTION PREVENTION AND CONTROL MEASURES IN HEALTH CARE SETTINGS: Standard precautions are recommended.

CONTROL MEASURES: Preventive measures depend on limiting proliferation of *C perfringens* in foods by cooking foods thoroughly and maintaining food at warmer than 60°C (140°F) or cooler than 7°C (45°F). Meat dishes should be served hot. Leftovers should be reheated to at least 74°C (165°F). Foods should never be held at room temperature to cool; they should be refrigerated in shallow containers after removal from warming devices or serving tables as soon as possible and within 2 hours of preparation. Information on recommended safe food handling practices, including time and temperature requirements during cooking, storage, and reheating, can be found at **www.foodsafety.gov.**

Coccidioidomycosis

CLINICAL MANIFESTATIONS: Coccidioidomycosis, also called Valley fever, is an infection caused by fungi of the genus *Coccidioides*. Primary pulmonary infection is acquired by inhaling fungal conidia and is asymptomatic or self-limited in 60% to 65% of infected children and adults. Constitutional symptoms, including extreme fatigue and weight loss, are common and can persist for weeks or months. Symptomatic disease can resemble community-acquired pneumonia or other respiratory illnesses, with malaise, fever, cough, myalgia, arthralgia, headache, and chest pain. Pleural effusion, empyema, and mediastinal involvement are more common in children.

Acute infection may be associated only with cutaneous abnormalities, such as erythema multiforme, an erythematous maculopapular rash, or erythema nodosum manifesting as bilateral symmetrical violaceous nodules usually overlying the shins. Chronic pulmonary lesions are rare, but approximately 5% of infected people develop asymptomatic pulmonary radiographic residua (eg, cysts, nodules, cavitary lesions, coin lesions).

Nonpulmonary primary infection is rare and usually follows trauma associated with contamination of wounds by arthroconidia. Cutaneous lesions and soft tissue infections often are accompanied by regional lymphadenitis.

Disseminated (extrapulmonary) infection occurs in less than 1% of infected people; common sites of dissemination include skin, bones, joints, and the central nervous system (CNS). Meningitis is invariably fatal if untreated. Congenital (transplacental) infection is rare but can occur, with resultant pulmonary coccidioidomycosis soon after birth.

ETIOLOGY: *Coccidioides* species are dimorphic fungi. In soil, *Coccidioides* organisms exist in the mycelial phase as mold that grows as branching, septate hyphae. Infectious arthroconidia (ie, spores) produced from hyphae become airborne, infecting the host after inhalation or, rarely, inoculation. In tissues, arthroconidia enlarge to form spherules; mature spherules release hundreds to thousands of endospores that develop into new spherules and continue the tissue cycle. Molecular studies have divided the genus *Coccidioides* into 2 species: *Coccidioides immitis,* confined mainly to California and Washington, and *Coccidioides posadasii*, encompassing the remaining areas of distribution of the fungus within certain deserts of the southwestern United States, northern Mexico, and areas of Central and South America.

EPIDEMIOLOGY: *Coccidioides* species are found mostly in soil in areas of the southwestern United States with endemic infection, including California, Arizona, New Mexico, west and south Texas, southern Nevada, and Utah; northern Mexico; and throughout certain parts of Central and South America. Areas of endemicity can extend beyond traditionally defined ranges, which are expanding because of climate change.

In areas with endemic coccidioidomycosis, clusters of cases can follow dust-generating events, such as storms, seismic events, archaeological digging, and recreational and construction activities, including building of solar farms. The majority of cases occur without a known preceding event.

Infection is believed to provide lifelong immunity. Person-to-person transmission of coccidioidomycosis does not occur except in rare instances of cutaneous infection with actively draining lesions, donor-derived transmission via an infected organ, or congenital infection following in utero exposure. People with impairment of T-lymphocyte–mediated immunity caused by a congenital immune defect or human immunodeficiency virus (HIV) infection, individuals with defects in the interleukin-12/interferon-γ and STAT3 pathways, or those receiving immune-modulating medications (eg, tumor necrosis factor [TNF] alpha antagonists) are at major risk for severe primary coccidioidomycosis, disseminated disease, or relapse of past infection. Higher rates of severe or disseminated disease have been reported in people of African or Filipino ancestry, individuals in the third trimester of pregnancy and those postpartum, and children younger than 1 year. Cases may occur in people who do not reside in regions with endemic infection but who previously have visited these areas, including months or even years previously. In regions without endemic infection, careful travel histories should be obtained from people with symptoms or findings compatible with coccidioidomycosis.

The **incubation period** typically is 1 to 3 weeks in primary infection. Disseminated infection may develop years after primary infection.

DIAGNOSTIC TESTS: Diagnosis of coccidioidomycosis is best established using serologic, histopathologic, and culture methods. Nucleic acid amplification tests (NAATs) have been developed; one is now FDA approved for use in lower respiratory tract specimens. Antigen tests have also been developed.

Serologic tests are useful in the diagnosis and management of infection. One approach is to test first with enzyme immunoassay (EIA), which is highly sensitive and provides relatively rapid results, and if EIA is positive to then perform the more specific immunodiffusion test. The immunoglobulin (Ig) M response can be detected by EIA or immunodiffusion methods. IgM is detected in the first and third weeks in approximately 50% and 90% of primary infections, respectively, but a positive EIA IgM result alone should be interpreted with caution because of the low specificity of this test. IgG response can be detected 4 to 8 weeks after symptom onset by EIA, immunodiffusion, or complement fixation (CF) tests. Immunodiffusion is considered more specific, whereas CF is more sensitive. A combination of both CF and immunodiffusion tests is often helpful in diagnosis, although both immunodiffusion and especially CF are known to cross-react with *Histoplasma* organisms. Serum antibodies detected by CF usually are of low titer and are transient if the disease is asymptomatic or mild; persistent high titers ($\geq$1:16) occur with severe disease and are almost always seen in disseminated infection. Cerebrospinal fluid (CSF) antibodies also are detectable by immunodiffusion or CF testing. Increasing serum and CSF titers indicate progressive disease, and decreasing titers usually suggest improvement. False-positive titers can occur in patients with cryptococcal meningitis. Antibody titers detected by CF may not be reliable in immunocompromised patients; low or nondetectable titers in immunocompromised patients should be interpreted with caution. Among infants whose birthing parent had active coccidioidomycosis during pregnancy, serologic testing of infants during the first 3 months of life is not recommended, and serologic test results should be interpreted with caution during the first year of life.

Spherules are as large as 80 µm in diameter and can be visualized with 100x to 400x magnification in infected body fluid specimens (eg, pleural fluid, bronchoalveolar lavage) and biopsy specimens of skin lesions or organs. Silver or period-acid Schiff staining can be performed on biopsy specimens. The presence of a mature spherule with endospores is pathognomonic of infection.

Isolation of *Coccidioides* species in culture establishes the diagnosis, even in patients with mild symptoms. When a specimen from a patient suspected of having coccidioidomycosis is sent for culture, the diagnostic laboratory should be alerted as biosafety level 3 facilities are required. Culture of organisms is possible on a variety of artificial media but is hazardous to laboratory personnel, because spherules can convert to arthroconidia-bearing mycelia on culture plates. Suspect cultures should be sealed and handled using appropriate safety equipment and procedures. A DNA probe can identify *Coccidioides* species in cultures.

At least 1 commercial laboratory offers an EIA test for urine, serum, plasma, CSF, or bronchoalveolar lavage fluid for detection of *Coccidioides* antigen. Antigen test results may be positive in patients with more severe forms of disease (sensitivity, 71%)

in a study of immunosuppressed patients. Cross-reactions may occur in patients with dimorphic fungal diseases (eg, coccidioidomycosis, histoplasmosis, paracoccidioidomycosis, sporotrichosis, *Emergomyces africanus* disease, and talaromycosis [formerly penicillosis]); clinical and epidemiologic distinctions aid in differentiating these entities. Using serologic and antigen testing together may improve sensitivity and early detection of infection in progressive coccidioidomycosis.

TREATMENT[1,2]: Antifungal therapy is not recommended routinely for uncomplicated asymptomatic primary infection in people without risk factors for severe disease. Although most mild cases will resolve without therapy, some experts believe that treatment may reduce illness duration or risk of severe complications. Most experts recommend treatment of coccidioidomycosis with fluconazole for 3 to 6 months for people at risk of severe disease or people with severe primary infection. During pregnancy, amphotericin B (including lipid formulations) is the treatment of choice over fluconazole and other azole antifungals, as fluconazole has been demonstrated to be a teratogen in early pregnancy. Dosing of antifungal medication is in Antifungal Drugs for Systemic Fungal Infections, p 1017. Follow-up every 1 to 3 months for up to 2 years, either to document radiographic resolution or to identify residual abnormalities or pulmonary or extrapulmonary complications, is recommended. For diffuse pneumonia, defined as bilateral reticulonodular or miliary infiltrates, amphotericin B or high-dose fluconazole is recommended. Amphotericin B is used more frequently in the presence of severe hypoxemia or rapid clinical deterioration. The total length of therapy for diffuse pneumonia is 1 year.

Oral fluconazole or itraconazole is the recommended initial therapy for disseminated infection not involving the CNS. Amphotericin B is recommended as alternative therapy if lesions are progressing or are in critical locations, such as the vertebral column, or in fulminant infections, because it is believed to result in more rapid improvement.

Consultation with a specialist for treatment of patients with CNS disease caused by *Coccidioides* species is recommended. High-dose oral fluconazole (adult dose: 400–1200 mg/day, see Antifungal Drugs for Systemic Fungal Infections, p 1017) is recommended for treatment of patients with CNS infection. Patients who respond to azole therapy should continue this treatment indefinitely (for the remainder of their lives). For CNS infections that are unresponsive to oral azoles or are associated with severe basilar inflammation, intrathecal amphotericin B deoxycholate therapy can be used to augment the azole therapy. A subcutaneous reservoir can facilitate administration into the cisternal space or lateral ventricle. Hydrocephalus is a common complication of coccidioidal meningitis and nearly always requires a shunt for decompression.

There are reports of success with voriconazole, posaconazole, and isavuconazole in treatment of coccidioidomycosis, but this has not been established in children. These newer agents may be administered in certain clinical settings, such as therapeutic failure in severe coccidioidal disease (eg, meningitis). When used, these newer azoles

---

[1] Galgiani JN, Ampel NM, Blair JE, et al. 2016 Infectious Diseases Society of America (IDSA) clinical practice guideline for the treatment of coccidioidomycosis. *Clin Infect Dis.* 2016;63(6):e112-e146

[2] Thompson GR III, Le T, Chindamporn A, et al. Global guideline for the diagnosis and management of the endemic mycoses: an initiative of the European Confederation of Medical Mycology in cooperation with the International Society for Human and Animal Mycology. *Lancet Infect Dis.* 2021;21(12):e364-e374

should be administered in consultation with experts experienced with their use in treatment of coccidioidomycosis.

The duration of antifungal therapy is variable and depends on the site(s) of involvement, clinical response, and mycologic and immunologic test results. In general, therapy is continued until clinical and laboratory evidence indicates that active infection has resolved. Treatment for disseminated coccidioidomycosis is at least 6 months but for some patients may be extended to 1 year or longer. The role of subsequent suppressive azole therapy is uncertain, except for patients with CNS infection, osteomyelitis, or underlying human immunodeficiency virus (HIV) infection or for solid organ transplant recipients. Coccidioidal meningitis requires lifelong therapy. The duration of suppressive therapy also may be lifelong for other high-risk groups.[1]

Surgical consultation for potential excision or débridement is recommended for patients with pulmonary cavitary lesions who do not respond to antifungal therapy, whose cavities persist >2 years, or who have rupture of infection into the plural space. Surgical débridement or excision of lesions in bone, pericardium, and other sites has been advocated for localized, symptomatic, persistent, resistant, or progressive lesions. In some localized infections with sinuses, fistulae, or abscesses, amphotericin B has been instilled locally or used for irrigation of wounds. Antifungal prophylaxis for solid organ transplant recipients may be considered if they reside in areas with endemicity and have prior serologic evidence or a history of coccidioidomycosis. Patients should be advised to avoid pregnancy while receiving fluconazole, which is known to be teratogenic. Breastfeeding while receiving fluconazole is considered likely safe for the infant.

INFECTION PREVENTION AND CONTROL MEASURES IN HEALTH CARE SETTINGS: Standard precautions are recommended. Care should be taken in handling, changing, and discarding dressings, casts, and similar materials through which arthroconidial contamination could occur.

CONTROL MEASURES: Coccidioidomycosis is a reportable disease in many states and some countries. Measures to control dust are recommended in areas with endemic infection, including construction sites, archaeological project sites, or other locations where activities cause excessive soil disturbance. Immunocompromised people residing in or traveling to areas with endemic infection should be counseled to avoid exposure to activities that may aerosolize spores in contaminated soil.

Coronavirus Disease 2019 (COVID-19)

CLINICAL MANIFESTATIONS: Children infected with severe acute respiratory syndrome coronavirus 2 (SARS-CoV-2) generally have mild disease or may be asymptomatic, although severe and even fatal infections occur. The most common presenting symptoms of acute coronavirus disease 2019 (COVID-19) in children are fever and cough; other symptoms include shortness of breath, sore throat, headache, myalgia, fatigue, congestion, and rhinorrhea. Gastrointestinal symptoms such as nausea, vomiting, diarrhea, and poor appetite may occur without respiratory symptoms. Loss

[1] Panel on Opportunistic Infections in HIV-Exposed and HIV-Infected Children. Guidelines for the Prevention and Treatment of Opportunistic Infections in Children With and Exposed to HIV. Department of Health and Human Services. Available at: **https://clinicalinfo.hiv.gov/en/guidelines/hiv-clinical-guidelines-pediatric-opportunistic-infections/whats-new**

of smell (anosmia) or taste (ageusia), when it occurs, tends to be more specific for COVID-19 as opposed to other causes of respiratory illness and is more common in adolescents and adults with COVID-19 than in younger children. Conjunctivitis and rashes have also been reported. Children who have obesity or medical comorbidities are at risk for more severe disease. Complications of COVID-19 include respiratory failure, acute respiratory distress syndrome (ARDS), myocarditis, acute kidney injury, shock, coagulopathy, multiorgan failure, and neurologic complications (eg, encephalitis, encephalopathy, seizures, stroke). Diabetic ketoacidosis and intussusception also have been reported. Laboratory findings may be normal (typically the case for uncomplicated COVID-19 in children) or may include lymphopenia, leukopenia, elevated C-reactive protein or procalcitonin, and elevated alanine aminotransferase and aspartate aminotransferase. Chest imaging may be normal or there may be unilateral or bilateral lung involvement with multiple areas of consolidation and ground glass opacities in children who have moderate to severe disease. After the acute illness, some children, including some who experienced mild disease, have a variety of ongoing physical, neurologic, and psychiatric symptoms, often termed "long COVID," post-acute sequelae of COVID-19 (PASC), or post-COVID conditions.

Multisystem inflammatory syndrome in children (MIS-C) is a severe postinfectious complication of SARS-CoV-2 infection that generally occurs 2 to 6 weeks following infection; preceding infections are often mild or asymptomatic. The Centers for Disease Control and Prevention (CDC) and the Council for State and Territorial Epidemiologists (CSTE) have developed a surveillance case definition for MIS-C (**https://cdn.ymaws.com/www.cste.org/resource/resmgr/ps/ps2022/22-ID-02_MISC.pdf**); note that a surveillance case definition is not meant to be a clinical case definition and is used for public health reporting. Children with MIS-C present with fever, clinical severity requiring hospitalization or resulting in death, evidence of systemic inflammation by C-reactive protein of ≥3.0 mg/dL, and new-onset manifestation in 2 or more of the following systems: cardiac, mucocutaneous, shock, gastrointestinal, or hematologic. Patients also have evidence of recent SARS-CoV-2 infection (ie, a positive SARS-CoV-2–specific molecular test or SARS-CoV-2–specific antigen, in a clinical specimen up to 60 days prior to or during hospitalization or in a postmortem specimen, or serologic evidence of SARS-CoV-2 associated with the current illness) or a history of close contact with a confirmed or probable case of COVID-19 in the 60 days prior to hospitalization. The symptoms of MIS-C overlap with other infectious and noninfectious etiologies, and alternative diagnoses should be ruled out as part of the diagnostic evaluation. Many of these children present with severe abdominal pain and many have Kawasaki disease-like features. A large proportion of children with MIS-C have echocardiographic abnormalities including diminished cardiac function and coronary artery abnormalities and many have elevated troponin, B-type natriuretic peptide (BNP), or proBNP.

ETIOLOGY: SARS-CoV-2, the virus that causes COVID-19, is an enveloped, non-segmented single stranded RNA virus of the coronavirus family. The spike proteins of coronaviruses project from the virion to resemble a corona (Latin for "crown") on electron microscopy. SARS-CoV-2 and SARS-CoV-1 (which circulated 2002-2004) are lineage B betacoronaviruses. SARS-CoV-2 has a high rate of mutations in the spike protein and multiple variants and subvariants have circulated since the pandemic began.

EPIDEMIOLOGY: SARS-CoV-2 emerged in late 2019 in Wuhan, China. Infection spread rapidly over the ensuing months around the world. The World Health Organization (WHO) declared a global pandemic on March 11, 2020. By December 20, 2022, 3 years after the outbreak in Wuhan was recognized, nearly 655 million cases were confirmed and approximately 6.7 million deaths were reported globally. In the United States, there were nearly 100 million COVID-19 cases, with 17% occurring in children younger than 18 years. By December 14, 2022, there were nearly 1.1 million deaths overall in the United States attributable to COVID-19, including at least 1575 children. By February 2022, the CDC estimated that approximately 75% of children had serologic evidence of previous infection with SARS-CoV-2. Current data on cases and deaths are available at **https://covid.cdc.gov/covid-data-tracker/#datatracker-home.**

The risk of COVID-19 infection, hospitalization, or death is increased for American Indian/Alaska Native people, Black people, and Hispanic people compared with white, non-Hispanic people.

MIS-C is a rare diagnosis; by January 30, 2023, 9344 cases were reported to CDC, including 76 deaths. The median age of patients with MIS-C in the United States was 9 years, 60% of cases were in male children, and 57% of cases occurred in Hispanic or Black children. Ninety-eight percent of MIS-C cases had laboratory-confirmed SARS-CoV-2 infection and 2% had a recent exposure to someone with COVID-19.

SARS-CoV-2 is transmitted efficiently between people, including from presymptomatic, symptomatic, and asymptomatic infected individuals. Transmission occurs primarily by respiratory droplets and fine particles that are inhaled or deposited on mucous membranes generally when within 6 feet of an infectious person, although transmission via aerosols can occur beyond that distance. A person can also self-inoculate eyes, nose, and mouth. The CDC provides information on factors that increase or decrease the risk of transmission (**www.cdc.gov/coronavirus/2019-ncov/your-health/risks-exposure.html**), taking into account the length of time, cough/heavy breathing, symptoms, use of N95 or higher respirators/high-quality masks, ventilation/filtration, and distance. Crowded, enclosed, and poorly ventilated spaces are particularly effective environments for the transmission of SARS-CoV-2. Infected people are believed to be infectious 2 days prior to symptom onset through 10 days after symptom onset, with the viral load highest earlier in the course of infection. The risk of transmission may be further impacted by the degree of symptomatology and severity of disease as well as immune status (eg, history of vaccination, previous infection) of the infected and/or exposed individual.

Health care-associated transmission occurs with SARS-CoV-2 and is a concern for health care personnel and patients. Adherence to infection prevention guidance is important. Outbreaks of SARS-CoV-2 infection occur readily in congregate settings (eg, long-term care facilities, group homes, prisons, shelters, congregate workplaces, dormitories) and households.

Perinatal transmission of SARS-CoV-2 is infrequent, occurring in approximately 2% of infants born to SARS-CoV-2 positive persons, increasing to approximately 20% if the pregnant person has evidence of acute COVID-19 infection at delivery. Perinatal transmission is believed to be driven primarily through transmission of respiratory droplets and fine particles in the postnatal period. Transplacental or intrapartum transmission appears possible but is extremely rare. Although SARS-CoV-2–specific antibodies have been detected in human milk, SARS-CoV-2 is not believed to be transmissible via human milk.

The **incubation period** is 2 to 14 days (median, 5 days for the original SARS-CoV-2 strain). The period may differ by variant (eg, median is 3 days for the Omicron variant).

DIAGNOSTIC TESTS: There are a variety of nucleic acid amplification tests (NAATs) and antigen detection tests for the diagnosis of acute SARS-CoV-2 infections from respiratory samples (which can include nasopharyngeal, nasal, oropharyngeal, saliva, or lower respiratory specimens depending on the specific NAAT). Some molecular assays for SARS-CoV-2 are part of a multiplex test. Antigen tests, which generally have decreased sensitivity relative to molecular tests (especially for asymptomatic persons), are typically faster and cheaper than NAATs and are frequently used in point-of-care testing (nasopharyngeal or nasal specimen). In addition, a variety of over-the-counter tests that have received emergency use authorization (EUA) or clearance from the US Food and Drug Administration (FDA) are available. Serologic testing for SARS-CoV-2 can be used to indicate history of infection and can support a diagnosis of MIS-C. Prior infection results in antibody production against anti-spike (anti-S) and anti-nucleocapsid (anti-N), while prior vaccination results in antibody production against anti-spike (anti-S) alone.

The CDC (**www.cdc.gov/coronavirus/2019-ncov/hcp/testing-overview.html** and **www.cdc.gov/coronavirus/2019-ncov/lab/resources/antigen-tests-guidelines.html**) and FDA (**www.fda.gov/medical-devices/covid-19-emergency-use-authorizations-medical-devices/in-vitro-diagnostics-euas**) websites have more information on SARS-CoV-2 assays, including information about performance and when a confirmatory test is recommended. The FDA provides updated information about whether a diagnostic test may fail to detect a particular variant of SARS-CoV-2 (**www.fda.gov/medical-devices/coronavirus-covid-19-and-medical-devices/sars-cov-2-viral-mutations-impact-covid-19-tests?utm_medium=email&utm_source=govdelivery**).

TREATMENT OF COVID-19: Treatment of COVID-19 has evolved rapidly across the pandemic. The Infectious Diseases Society of America provides updated information on treatment for COVID-19 (**www.idsociety.org/practice-guideline/covid-19-guideline-treatment-and-management/**). There are no placebo-controlled randomized trials in children and there are limited data from observational studies; treatment recommendations for children, therefore, are generally extrapolated from trials performed in adults.

Nirmatrelvir plus ritonavir, which goes by the brand name Paxlovid, is an oral antiviral medication combination that initially received EUA from the FDA for people 12 years or older (weighing ≥40 kg) who are at high risk for severe COVID-19. Full approval for use in adults was granted on May 25, 2023. Nirmatrelvir plus ritonavir reduces hospitalization and all-cause mortality in high-risk adults.

Remdesivir is an intravenous antiviral drug that is approved by the FDA for the treatment of COVID-19 in hospitalized or nonhospitalized adult and pediatric (28 days of age and older and weighing at least 3 kg) patients with mild to moderate COVID-19 symptoms and high risk for progression to severe COVID-19, including hospitalization or death. Some experts administer remdesivir to hospitalized children requiring supplemental oxygen, particularly early in the course of illness, and to children who are outpatients with mild-moderate COVID-19 who are at high risk for severe disease. The latter therapy is administered as a 3-day course and should be given within 7 days of symptom onset versus the 5-day course given to hospitalized patients.

Additional therapies have been used in hospitalized patients. Dexamethasone is recommended in the NIH treatment guidelines for children with COVID-19 who require high-flow oxygen, noninvasive ventilation, invasive mechanical ventilation, or extracorporeal membrane oxygenation (ECMO). Dexamethasone has not been evaluated in, and may be harmful to, profoundly immunocompromised children and should be considered only on a case-by-case basis. The FDA has issued an EUA for baricitinib in children 2 years or older and a full approval for the treatment of COVID-19 in hospitalized adults requiring supplemental oxygen, noninvasive or invasive mechanical ventilation, or ECMO. It is administered daily for 14 days or until hospital discharge, whichever comes first. The FDA also issued an EUA for tocilizumab for children 2 years or older and a full approval for the treatment of COVID-19 in hospitalized adults who are receiving systemic corticosteroids and require supplemental oxygen, noninvasive or invasive mechanical ventilation, or ECMO. Experience with these agents in children is limited, and consultation with an expert in the treatment of severe COVID-19 in children is recommended.

Anti–SARS-CoV-2 monoclonal therapies have been developed for use in patients who have mild to moderate COVID-19 and are at high risk for progression to severe COVID-19, are within 7 days of symptom onset, and meet the age criteria for the particular product. However, the high proportion of circulating variants and subvariants resistant to the therapies has precluded their use since the end of 2022. Additional monoclonal therapies may become available. The CDC COVID data tracker (**https://covid.cdc.gov/covid-data-tracker/#variant-proportions**) provides information on currently circulating variants.

The FDA also has issued an EUA for use of high-titer anti–SARS-CoV-2 convalescent plasma for the treatment of COVID-19 in ambulatory or hospitalized patients who have immunosuppressive disease or are on immunosuppressive therapy not associated with treatment of COVID-19. Safety and effectiveness of COVID-19 convalescent plasma in the pediatric population have not been evaluated.

TREATMENT OF MIS-C: The American College of Rheumatology provides guidance on the evaluation and treatment of MIS-C (**https://assets.contentstack.io/v3/assets/bltee37abb6b278ab2c/blt08209081de21d613/covid-19-clinical-guidance-pediatric-patients-mis-c.pdf**). Currently, there are no trials evaluating the efficacy of treatment options. A multidisciplinary approach with the involvement of pediatric specialists in cardiology, rheumatology, infectious disease, hematology, immunology, and critical care is recommended to guide individual management. In addition to supportive care, expert consensus recommendations include treating hospitalized patients with immune globulin intravenous (2 g/kg, based on ideal body weight, maximum 100 g; if patient has cardiac dysfunction, dose can be 1 g/kg per day for 2 days) and low-dose methylprednisolone (1–2 mg/kg/day). Therapeutic options for refractory cases include high-dose methylprednisolone (10–30 mg/kg/day) and immunomodulating agents (anakinra, infliximab). Most experts also treat patients with MIS-C with low-dose aspirin (3–5 mg/kg/day, maximum 81 mg). Higher-intensity anticoagulation in patients at high risk for thrombosis or with severe cardiac dysfunction should be considered on a case-by-case basis in consultation with relevant subspecialists. Patients with coronary artery aneurysms should be managed per the American Heart Association (AHA) guideline for Kawasaki disease (**https://doi.org/10.1161/CIR.0000000000000484**).

INFECTION PREVENTION AND CONTROL MEASURES IN HEALTH CARE SETTINGS: The CDC recommends standard, airborne, droplet, and contact precautions for health care providers caring for patients who are potentially infected with SARS-CoV-2. These precautions include N95 or higher respiratory protection, gown, gloves, and eye protection (face shield or goggles). Aerosol-generating procedures should be performed in an airborne infection isolation room. Caregivers providing delivery room care for newborn infants of infected pregnant persons should utilize all such precautions. Patients should wear a face mask for source control when other people are in the room, if they are 2 years or older and can tolerate the mask.

CONTROL MEASURES: Please refer to the latest CDC guidance for the most up-to-date recommendations.

Infected Persons in the Community. The CDC recommends an isolation period for people with SARS-CoV-2 infection of at least 5 days (with day 0 being the first day of symptoms or a positive test result for those who never develop symptoms) for those with asymptomatic infection or mild disease if they are afebrile for at least 24 hours by the end of that period without the use of fever-reducing medicine and their symptoms are improving, and if they can continue to wear a face mask through 10 days after symptom onset (**www.cdc.gov/coronavirus/2019-ncov/hcp/duration-isolation.html**). A test-based strategy may be used to cease face mask use sooner (**www.cdc.gov/coronavirus/2019-ncov/your-health/isolation.html**). Patients with moderate disease are advised to isolate for 10 days after symptom onset. Patients with severe disease or severe immunocompromise may shed viable virus longer (the CDC recommends extending transmission-based precautions to 20 days after symptom onset for these patients; some severely immunocompromised people may continue to shed well beyond this time period [some for months] and require testing to determine end of isolation).

Exposed Persons in the Community. For people in the community who have a known exposure to someone with COVID-19, the CDC recommends that they wear a well-fitting face mask for 10 days whenever they are around another person or are in public, watch for symptoms, and if they have no symptoms, test at day 6 (day of exposure is day 0). They should take care not to be around those who are at risk for severe disease. If they develop symptoms, they should immediately isolate and test (**www.cdc.gov/coronavirus/2019-ncov/your-health/if-you-were-exposed.html**).

Vaccines. The incidence of COVID-19, hospitalization, and death is higher in unvaccinated people than in vaccinated people. Studies have found that people have better protection when they are up to date on COVID-19 vaccination, even with a history of a prior infection, and vaccination is recommended for people who have previously had COVID-19 (once clinically improved and no longer in isolation), including people with PASC. COVID-19 vaccine is protective against MIS-C (**www.cdc.gov/mmwr/volumes/71/wr/mm7102e1.htm**).

COVID-19 vaccine authorization, approvals, and recommendation are updated frequently; refer to the CDC (**www.cdc.gov/vaccines/covid-19/clinical-considerations/covid-19-vaccines-us.html**) and FDA (**www.fda.**

gov/emergency-preparedness-and-response/coronavirus-disease-2019-covid-19/covid-19-vaccines) websites for the most up-to-date information and recommendations on vaccines and their recommended intervals for administration.

As of December 2023, 3 COVID-19 vaccines are available in the United States. Two are mRNA vaccines (Pfizer-BioNTech and Moderna) that can be used in persons 6 months and older, and one (Novavax) is an adjuvanted protein vaccine that can be used in persons 12 years and older. The CDC should be consulted for the latest recommendations (**www.cdc.gov/vaccines/covid-19/clinical-considerations/interim-considerations-us.html#table-01**). For information on interchangeability of mRNA COVID-19 vaccines, see **www.cdc.gov/vaccines/covid-19/clinical-considerations/interim-considerations-us-appendix.html#appendix-a.**

Pregnancy. The CDC, the American College of Obstetricians and Gynecologists, and the Society for Maternal-Fetal Medicine recommend COVID-19 vaccines for people who are pregnant, might become pregnant, were recently pregnant, or are currently breastfeeding. There is an increased risk of severe COVID-19 and death during pregnancy and an increased risk for adverse pregnancy and neonatal outcomes. Accumulating data have confirmed the safety and effectiveness of COVID-19 vaccination in people who are pregnant as well as conveyance of protection for the newborn infant.

Additional Doses for Immunocompromised Patients. People who are moderately or severely immunocompromised may require additional doses of COVID-19 vaccine (**www.cdc.gov/coronavirus/2019-ncov/vaccines/recommendations/immuno.html**). People eligible for additional doses include are those who are receiving active cancer treatment for tumors or cancers of the blood, those who received an organ transplant and are taking medicine to suppress the immune system, those who received a hematopoietic cell transplant within the last 2 years or are taking medicine to suppress the immune system, those with moderate or severe primary immunodeficiency (such as DiGeorge syndrome, Wiskott-Aldrich syndrome), those with advanced or untreated HIV infection, and those with active treatment with high-dose corticosteroids or other drugs that may suppress an immune response.

Adverse Events. The most common adverse events following COVID-19 vaccination observed in clinical trials and vaccine safety surveillance are local and systemic reactions that are generally mild and transient. Anaphylaxis has rarely been reported after COVID-19 vaccines. Appropriate medical treatment for severe allergic reactions must be immediately available at any site administering the vaccine. The CDC recommends an observation period after COVID-19 vaccination (**www.cdc.gov/vaccines/covid-19/clinical-considerations/managing-anaphylaxis.html**).

Rare cases of myocarditis and pericarditis have been reported in adolescents and young adults following receipt of mRNA vaccines, most often following the second dose. COVID-19 vaccination reduces the risk of myocarditis caused by SARS-CoV-2 infection. The risk of myocarditis is up to 6 times higher after SARS-CoV-2 infection than after mRNA vaccines. Postvaccine myocarditis is milder, requiring shorter hospital stays (1–2 days) compared with myocarditis caused by SARS-CoV-2 infection. Pediatricians should consider myocarditis and pericarditis in adolescents or young adults with acute chest pain, shortness of breath, or palpitations and report any suspected cases after COVID-19 vaccination to VAERS. In adolescents and adults, the risk of postvaccination myocarditis and pericarditis might be reduced with an interval longer than 4 weeks, but extending the interval beyond 8 weeks has not been shown to provide additional benefit. For more information see **www.cdc.gov/vaccines/ covid-19/clinical-considerations/myocarditis.html.**

Special Situations:

- COVID-19 infection: The primary series vaccination of people with current SARS-CoV-2 infection should be deferred until the person has recovered from the acute illness and no longer requires isolation.
- Patients with MIS-C: A multicenter study was published in early 2023 in which 185 children with MIS-C who received at least 1 dose of COVID-19 vaccine following MIS-C were followed, and no serious adverse effects including myocarditis or the return of MIS-C were detected. Many experts consider the benefits of vaccination (reduced risk of severe disease from COVID-19, including a potential recurrence of MIS-C after reinfection) to outweigh potential risks when clinical recovery from MIS-C has been achieved (including return to baseline cardiac function) and it has been at least 90 days since the diagnosis of MIS-C.
- Other vaccines: COVID-19 vaccines can be administered at the same time as other vaccines. Patients who receive mpox vaccine (JYNNEOS or ACAM2000) may consider waiting 4 weeks before getting a COVID-19 vaccine (see Mpox, p 606). Those who previously received COVID-19 vaccines can receive an mpox vaccine (when indicated) without a minimum interval between vaccines.

Preexposure Prophylaxis. Long-acting monoclonal antibody combinations available earlier in the pandemic no longer have activity against currently circulating variants of SARS-CoV-2. Additional products may be developed in the future, however.

Nonpharmaceutical Control Measures. Nonpharmaceutical measures that make up layered mitigation include use of well-fitting, high-quality face masks for anyone 2 years and older (**www.cdc.gov/coronavirus/2019-ncov/prevent-getting-sick/types-of-masks.html**); the CDC has guidance on when to use face masks depending on COVID-19 levels in the community (**www.cdc.gov/coronavirus/2019-ncov/your-health/covid-by-county.html**) or if exposed to or infected with COVID-19. Other nonpharmaceutical mitigation measures include avoiding crowds, improving ventilation, exercising hand hygiene, and following recommendations for testing and isolation. Local or state public health agencies also may provide guidance for specific locations on mitigation measures. Additional guidance can be found on the CDC website (**www.cdc.gov/ coronavirus/2019-ncov/prevent-getting-sick/prevention.html**).

Schools. For recommendations on exposed and infected children during the COVID-19 pandemic, refer to CDC (**www.cdc.gov/coronavirus/2019-ncov/community/ schools-childcare/child-care-guidance.html**), state, and local health department guidance.

Care of Exposed Newborn Infants. Infants born to SARS-CoV-2 positive people may room in during the birth hospitalization. The parent should perform hand hygiene and use a well-fitting, high-quality face mask when providing hands-on care to the infant for the duration of time the parent is infectious. Consideration may be given to testing the well newborn infant for SARS-CoV-2 before discharge from the birth hospital, to facilitate precautions and pediatric monitoring in the community. Infants born to parents with COVID-19 who require neonatal intensive care for any reason should be cared for with standard, airborne, droplet, and contact precautions. Testing at the beginning and end of the incubation period for COVID-19 may facilitate management of the exposed infant in the intensive care setting.

Breastfeeding. The CDC recommends breastfeeding even if the nursing parent has COVID-19. Precautions should be taken including washing hands with soap and water (or using 60% alcohol-based hand sanitizer) prior to breastfeeding or expressing milk and wearing a well-fitting, high-quality mask when in close proximity to the child. Breast pump equipment and all feeding items should be cleaned and sanitized between uses. The infant is considered exposed and should follow recommended precautions. For further information about COVID-19 and breastfeeding, see **www.cdc.gov/ breastfeeding/breastfeeding-special-circumstances/maternal-or-infant-illnesses/covid-19-and-breastfeeding.html.**

Public Health Reporting. COVID-19 is a nationally notifiable disease. Please refer to the state or local health department for details on reporting cases.

Coronaviruses, Including MERS-CoV and SARS-CoV-1

CLINICAL MANIFESTATIONS: Human coronaviruses (HCoVs) 229E, OC43, NL63, and HKU1 are associated most frequently with an upper respiratory tract infection characterized by rhinorrhea, nasal congestion, sore throat, sneezing, and cough; fever may also occur. Symptoms are generally self-limited and typically peak on day 3 or 4 of illness. HCoV infections also may be associated with acute otitis media, croup, or asthma exacerbations. Less frequently, HCoVs are associated with lower respiratory tract infections, including bronchiolitis and pneumonia, primarily in younger patients or in those who are immunocompromised. Asymptomatic infections can occur.

MERS-CoV, the virus associated with the Middle East respiratory syndrome (MERS) that emerged in 2012, can cause severe disease, but asymptomatic infections and mild disease may also occur. Most cases have been identified in male adults with comorbidities. Infections in children are uncommon and typically are milder than in adults. Patients initially present with fever, myalgia, and chills followed by a nonproductive cough and dyspnea a few days later. Approximately 25% of patients may experience vomiting, diarrhea, or abdominal pain. Rapid deterioration of oxygenation with respiratory distress and progressive unilateral or bilateral airspace infiltrates on chest imaging may follow and may further progress to respiratory failure requiring mechanical ventilation. Acute kidney injury can also occur. The case fatality rate for MERS is high, estimated at approximately 35%, although this may partially reflect surveillance bias for more severe disease. Laboratory abnormalities may include thrombocytopenia, lymphopenia, and increased lactate dehydrogenase (LDH) concentration, particularly among severely infected individuals.

Severe acute respiratory syndrome coronavirus 1 (SARS-CoV-1) was responsible for the 2002–2003 global outbreak of SARS, which was associated with severe respiratory symptoms, although a spectrum of disease including asymptomatic infections and mild disease also occurred. Infections in children were generally less severe than in adults and typically presented with fever, cough, and rhinorrhea. Adolescents with SARS had clinical courses more closely resembling those of adult disease, presenting with fever, myalgia, headache, and chills. No deaths in children from SARS-CoV-1 infection were documented. The overall case fatality rate was 10% but was generally higher in older adults.

ETIOLOGY: Coronaviruses are enveloped, nonsegmented, single-stranded, positive-sense RNA viruses named after their crown (or Latin "corona")-like surface projections observed on electron microscopy that correspond to spike proteins. Coronaviruses are classified in the subfamily *Orthocoronavirinae* of the *Coronaviridae* family. Coronaviruses are generally host specific and can infect humans as well as a variety of different animals. Four distinct genera in the subfamily *Orthocoronavirinae* have been described: *Alphacoronavirus, Betacoronavirus, Gammacoronavirus,* and *Deltacoronavirus.* HCoVs 229E and NL63 belong to the genus *Alphacoronavirus.* HCoVs OC43 and HKU1 belong to lineage A, SARS-CoV-1 and SARS-CoV-2 belong to lineage B, and MERS-CoV belongs to lineage C of the genus *Betacoronavirus.*

EPIDEMIOLOGY: HCoVs 229E, OC43, NL63, and HKU1 can be found worldwide. They typically cause disease in the winter and spring months in temperate climates. Seroprevalence data for these HCoVs suggest that exposure is common in early childhood, with approximately 90% of adults being seropositive for HCoVs 229E, OC43, and NL63 and 60% being seropositive for HCoV HKU1. The modes of transmission for HCoVs 229E, OC43, NL63, and HKU1 have not been well studied. However, on the basis of studies of other respiratory tract viruses, it is likely that transmission occurs primarily via a combination of droplet and direct and indirect contact spread. HCoVs 229E and OC43 are most likely to be transmitted during the first few days of illness, when symptoms and respiratory viral loads are at their highest.

MERS-CoV likely evolved from bat coronaviruses and infected dromedary camels in parts of the Middle East and Africa, where serologic and molecular detection of MERS-CoV have been reported. MERS-CoV cases in humans continue mostly in the Middle East, primarily linked to close contact with camels or an infected person. Human-to-human transmission generally occurs in health care settings and less frequently in household settings. Transmission is thought to occur most commonly through droplet and contact spread, although airborne spread may occur. Updated figures on global cases can be found on the World Health Organization website (**www.who.int/emergencies/mers-cov/en/**).

SARS-CoV-1 likely evolved from a natural reservoir of SARS-CoV-like viruses in horseshoe bats through civet cats or other intermediate animal hosts in wet markets in China. Public health interventions ultimately aborted the epidemic. Human SARS-CoV-1 infection was last reported in 2004.

The **incubation period** for HCoV-229E is 2 to 5 days (median, 3 days). Further study is needed to confirm the incubation periods for HCoVs OC43, NL63, and HKU1. The **incubation period** for MERS-CoV is estimated to be 2 to 14 days (median 5 days). The **incubation period** for SARS-CoV-1 is 2 to 14 days (typically 2–7 days).

DIAGNOSTIC TESTS: Multiplex assays for detection of respiratory pathogens by nucleic acid amplification are commercially available that include HCoVs 229E, OC43, NL63, HKU1, and SARS-CoV-2 as targets. Notably, multiple respiratory viruses can be detected concurrently in some patients and detection of HCoV does not always implicate it as the cause of a patient's symptoms. State public health departments should be contacted for evaluation of suspected cases of MERS-CoV using a nucleic acid amplification test (NAAT). Guidance regarding testing for MERS-CoV (including specimen collection, typically upper respiratory, lower respiratory, and serum) is available on the CDC MERS website (**www.cdc.gov/coronavirus/ mers/guidelines-clinical-specimens.html**). State public health departments should be consulted for suspect cases of SARS-CoV-1.

TREATMENT: Infections attributable to HCoVs HKU1, OC43, 229E, and NL63 are treated with supportive care. Investigational therapy for MERS includes anti-MERS monoclonal antibodies. A report of the combination of lopinavir-ritonavir plus subcutaneous interferon-beta-1b indicated clinical benefit, but further evaluation is needed. Remdesivir has activity against MERS-CoV and SARS-CoV-1 using in vitro systems and against SARS-CoV-1 in a mouse model. Remdesivir also has activity against SARS-CoV-2 (see Coronavirus Disease 2019 [COVID-19], p 324).

INFECTION PREVENTION AND CONTROL MEASURES IN HEALTH CARE SETTINGS: Airborne, droplet, and contact precautions are recommended for patients with suspected or known MERS-CoV infection (or SARS-CoV-1 infection if it reemerges). This includes eye protection (face shield or goggles), N95 or higher respirator (or medical mask if not available), gown, and gloves; for aerosol-generating procedures, an N95 or higher respirator should be used. Airborne infection isolation rooms should be prioritized for aerosol-generating procedures. A well-ventilated single-occupancy room with a closed door may be used if aerosol-generating procedures are not performed.

For other HCoV infections, in addition to standard precautions, health care professionals should use droplet and contact precautions when examining and caring for infants and young children.

CONTROL MEASURES: Practicing appropriate hand and respiratory hygiene can help curb spread of all respiratory tract viruses, including coronaviruses. Cleaning and disinfection of high-touch environmental surfaces using standard disinfectants should decrease the potential for indirect transmission of coronaviruses via fomites.

MERS-CoV transmission within hospitals and households can be averted with case identification and the use of infection control and public health measures, including contact tracing. However, preventing the transmission of MERS-CoV from camels to humans is more challenging, given the prevalent use of camels in some Middle East countries. Most experts believe that intermittent sporadic cases will continue because of zoonotic transmission. Several candidate vaccines are currently in trials for both humans and camels.

Public Health Reporting. Suspect cases of MERS or SARS-CoV-1 infection should be reported promptly to your state or local health department.

Cryptococcus neoformans and *Cryptococcus gattii* Infections (Cryptococcosis)

CLINICAL MANIFESTATIONS: Primary pulmonary infection is acquired by inhalation of aerosolized *Cryptococcus* fungal propagules found in contaminated soil or organic material (eg, trees, rotting wood, and bird guano), and infection often is asymptomatic or mild. When symptomatic, pulmonary disease is characterized by cough, chest pain, and constitutional symptoms. Chest radiographs may reveal solitary or multiple masses; patchy, segmental, or lobar consolidation, which often is multifocal; or a nodular or reticulonodular pattern with interstitial changes. Pulmonary cryptococcosis may present as acute respiratory distress syndrome (ARDS) and can mimic *Pneumocystis* pneumonia. Hematogenous dissemination occurs particularly to the central nervous system (CNS) but also to bones, skin, and other body sites. Disseminated cryptococcosis is generally rare in children and almost always occurs in children with defects in T-lymphocyte–mediated immunity, including children with leukemia or lymphoma, those taking corticosteroids, children with congenital immunodeficiency such as hyperimmunoglobulin M syndrome or severe combined immunodeficiency syndrome, those with acquired immunodeficiency syndrome (AIDS) from advanced human immunodeficiency virus (HIV) infection, or those who have undergone solid organ transplantation. Several anatomic sites usually are infected, but manifestations of involvement at one site predominate. Cryptococcal meningitis, the most common and serious form of cryptococcal disease in children, often follows an indolent course but symptoms can be more acute in severely immunosuppressed patients. Symptoms are often typical of those of meningitis, meningoencephalitis, or space-occupying lesions but sometimes manifest only as subtle, nonspecific findings such as fever, headache, or behavioral changes. Cryptococcal fungemia without apparent organ involvement occurs in patients with HIV infection but is rare in children.

ETIOLOGY: There are more than 30 species of *Cryptococcus*, but only 2, *Cryptococcus neoformans* species complex and *Cryptococcus gattii* species complex, are regarded as consistent human pathogens. These 2 species have been divided into approximately 10 genotypes or sibling species but clinically are referred to together as cryptococcosis. Further taxonomic studies and disease correlations are anticipated in the future to aid in understanding the clinical relevance of these groups.

EPIDEMIOLOGY: *C neoformans* species complex is isolated primarily from soil contaminated with pigeon or other bird droppings and causes most human infections, especially infections in immunocompromised hosts. *C neoformans* infects 5% to 10% of adults with AIDS, but cryptococcal disease is rare in HIV-infected and non–HIV-infected children. *C gattii* species complex is associated with certain trees and the surrounding soil and has emerged as disease manifesting as a respiratory syndrome with or without neurologic findings in individuals from British Columbia, Canada, and the Pacific Northwest region of the United States, but primarily as meningitis and meningoencephalitis in other regions of the United States. A high frequency of disease also has been reported in Aboriginal people in Australia and in the central province of Papua New Guinea. *C gattii* causes disease in both immunocompetent and immunocompromised individuals, and cases have been reported in children. Person-to-person transmission generally does not occur with cryptococcal species; although rare, transmission from donor organ and tissue grafts has been reported. The prevalence of cryptococcal disease is lower in children compared with adults and even less in children younger than 6 years compared with older children.

The **incubation period** for *C neoformans* is unknown but likely variable; dissemination often represents reactivation of latent disease acquired previously. The **incubation period** for *C gattii* is estimated at 8 weeks to 13 months based on outbreak investigations, but these figures also are imprecise.

DIAGNOSTIC TESTS: The cerebrospinal fluid (CSF) profile of cryptococcal meningoencephalitis is characterized by low cell counts, low glucose, and elevated protein. Opening pressure may be markedly elevated, especially in HIV-infected individuals.

Laboratory diagnosis of cryptococcal infection is best performed using cryptococcal antigen (CrAg) detection methods or by culture. The latex agglutination test, lateral flow immunoassay, and enzyme immunoassay for detection of cryptococcal capsular polysaccharide antigen (galactoxylomannan) in serum or CSF specimens are excellent rapid diagnostic tests in patients with suspected meningitis. CrAg is detected in CSF or serum specimens from more than 95% of patients with cryptococcal meningitis. Antigen test results can be falsely negative when antigen concentrations are very high (prozone effect), which can be addressed by dilution of samples. CrAg assays are less useful in following response to therapy than they are in diagnosis, because CrAg can remain high even after viable yeasts can no longer be detected. Accuracy, ease of use, and cost have made the lateral flow immunoassay, which shows good agreement with standard CrAg testing, a common test in both resource-abundant and resource-limited settings and has allowed preemptive management strategies for adults in areas with high incidence of HIV infection.

Definitive diagnosis requires isolation of the yeast from body fluid or tissue specimens. Encapsulated yeast cells can be visualized using India ink or other stains of CSF and bronchoalveolar lavage specimens, but this method has limited sensitivity and is not recommended as a stand-alone rapid test. CSF specimens may contain only a few yeast cells, and a large quantity of CSF may be needed to recover organisms in culture. Automated blood culture systems are acceptable for growing *Cryptococcus*. Sabouraud dextrose agar is useful for isolation of *Cryptococcus* organisms from sputum, bronchopulmonary lavage, tissue, or CSF specimens. Differentiation between *C neoformans* species complex and *C gattii* species complex can be made by the use of the selective medium L-canavanine, glycine, bromothymol blue (CGB) agar. A matrix-assisted laser desorption/ionization–time-of-flight (MALDI-TOF) mass spectrometer can identify yeasts to species complex level accurately and rapidly. Nucleic acid amplification tests (NAATs) are commercially available but may miss low burden cryptococcal central nervous system infections. Focal pulmonary or skin lesions can be biopsied for fungal staining and culture. Although there are CLIA standards for in vitro cryptococcal susceptibility testing, there are no break point minimum inhibitory concentration (MIC) interpretations; therefore, generally, a threefold increase in MIC from original to relapse isolate is evidence for direct resistance.

TREATMENT: Practice management guidelines for cryptococcal disease are available.[1–3] No pediatric trials have been performed, so optimal dosing and duration of therapy for children with cryptococcal infection have not been determined precisely. *C neoformans* and *C gattii* infections are treated similarly. Amphotericin B deoxycholate (1 mg/kg/day) or liposomal amphotericin B (5–6 mg/kg/day) are indicated in combination with oral flucytosine (25 mg/kg/dose, 4 times/day when renal function

---

[1] Perfect J, Dismukes WE, Dromer F, et al. Clinical practice guidelines for the management of cryptococcal disease: 2010 update by the Infectious Diseases Society of America. *Clin Infect Dis*. 2010;50(3):291-322

[2] Panel on Opportunistic Infections in HIV-Exposed and HIV-Infected Children. Guidelines for the Prevention and Treatment of Opportunistic Infections in Children with and Exposed to HIV. Available at: **https://clinicalinfo.hiv.gov/en/guidelines/hiv-clinical-guidelines-pediatric-opportunistic-infections/whats-new**

[3] World Health Organization. Guidelines for diagnosing, preventing, and managing cryptococcal disease among adults, adolescents and children living with HIV. Available at: **www.who.int/publications/i/item/9789240052178**

is normal) as first-line induction therapy for pediatric patients with meningeal and/or other serious cryptococcal infections (see Antifungal Drugs for Systemic Fungal Infections, p 1017). Among HIV-positive adults with cryptococcal meningitis, induction with a single high dose of parenteral liposomal amphotericin B (10 mg/kg) plus 14 days of oral flucytosine (100 mg/kg/day) and oral fluconazole (1200 mg/day) demonstrated noninferiority to parenteral amphotericin B deoxycholate (1 mg/kg/day) plus oral flucytosine (100 mg/kg/day) for 7 days, followed by oral fluconazole (1200 mg/day) for 7 days. Frequent monitoring of blood counts and/or serum peak flucytosine concentrations (with a target of 40 to 60 µg/mL 2 hours after the dose) are recommended to prevent neutropenia. If flucytosine cannot be administered, amphotericin B alone has been successfully used in pediatric cryptococcosis, or amphotericin B can be combined with fluconazole for the induction phase of therapy. Ideally, a lumbar puncture should be performed after 2 weeks of therapy to document microbiologic clearance. Patients in whom culture is positive after 2 weeks of therapy will require a more prolonged induction treatment course.

Patients with meningitis should receive induction combination therapy for at least 2 weeks and until a repeat CSF culture is negative, followed by consolidation therapy with fluconazole (10–12 mg/kg/day; maximum 800 mg per day) for a minimum of 8 weeks.

For any relapse, primary induction antifungal therapy should be restarted for 4 to 10 weeks, CSF cultures should be repeated every 2 weeks until sterile, and antifungal susceptibility of the relapse isolate should be determined and compared with the original isolate. Monitoring of serum CrAg is not useful to determine response to therapy in patients with cryptococcal meningitis.

Increased intracranial pressure occurs frequently despite microbiologic response and often is associated with clinical deterioration. Significant elevation of intracranial pressure is a major source of morbidity and should be managed with frequent repeated lumbar punctures or placement of a lumbar drain in those with high intracranial pressures and symptoms. Immune reconstitution inflammatory syndrome (IRIS) is described in children, and although there are no guidelines for specific management of IRIS in children, a patient should be monitored closely for signs and symptoms associated with symptomatic central nervous system IRIS and a steroid taper should be considered for management. In antiretroviral-naïve HIV-infected patients with newly diagnosed cryptococcal meningitis or disseminated disease, delay in potent antiretroviral therapy is recommended until the end of the first 2 weeks of induction therapy; further delays in initiating combined antiretroviral therapy, especially in resource-limited settings, should be individualized.[1]

Children with HIV infection who have completed initial therapy for cryptococcosis should receive long-term (at least 1 year) secondary prophylaxis therapy with fluconazole (6 mg/kg daily; maximum dose 200 mg). The safety of discontinuing secondary prophylaxis for cryptococcosis after immune reconstitution with combined antiretroviral therapy (ART) has not been studied in children. However, on the basis of adult data and experience, discontinuing suppressive/maintenance therapy for cryptococcosis

---

[1] Panel on Opportunistic Infections in HIV-Exposed and HIV-Infected Children. Guidelines for the Prevention and Treatment of Opportunistic Infections in Children with and Exposed to HIV. Available at: **https://clinicalinfo.hiv.gov/en/guidelines/hiv-clinical-guidelines-pediatric-opportunistic-infections/whats-new**

(after receiving secondary prophylaxis for at least 1 year) can be considered for asymptomatic children ≥6 years of age, with increase in their CD4+ T-lymphocyte counts to ≥100 cells/mm^3 and an undetectable viral load after receiving ART for ≥3 months.[1] Secondary prophylaxis therapy should be reinitiated if the CD4+ T-lymphocyte count decreases to <100 cells/mm^3. Most experts would not discontinue secondary prophylaxis for patients younger than age 6 years and thus individualized management plans need to be made.

Patients with less severe nonmeningeal disease (pulmonary disease) can be treated with fluconazole alone, but data on use of fluconazole for children with *C neoformans* infection are limited; itraconazole is a potential alternative. Another potential treatment option for patients in whom amphotericin B treatment is not possible is combination therapy with fluconazole and flucytosine; this combination has superior efficacy compared with fluconazole alone for severe disease. Echinocandins are not active against cryptococcal infections and should not be used.

INFECTION PREVENTION AND CONTROL MEASURES IN HEALTH CARE SETTINGS: Standard precautions are recommended.

CONTROL MEASURES: None.

Cryptosporidiosis

CLINICAL MANIFESTATIONS: Cryptosporidiosis commonly presents with frequent, nonbloody, watery diarrhea, although infection can be asymptomatic. Other symptoms include abdominal cramps, fatigue, fever, vomiting, anorexia, and weight loss. In an immunocompetent person, symptomatic cryptosporidiosis is self-limited, usually resolving within 2 to 3 weeks. *Cryptosporidium* infection is a common cause of moderate to severe diarrhea and poor growth among young children in resource-limited countries.

In an immunocompromised person, such as a child who has received a solid organ transplant or has advanced human immunodeficiency virus (HIV) disease, cryptosporidiosis can result in profuse diarrhea lasting weeks to months, which can lead to severe, even life-threatening dehydration, malnutrition, and wasting. The diagnosis of cryptosporidiosis should be considered in any immunocompromised person with diarrhea. Extraintestinal (eg, pulmonary or biliary tract) cryptosporidiosis has been reported in immunocompromised people and is associated with CD4+ T-lymphocyte counts less than 50/mm^3.

ETIOLOGY: Cryptosporidia are oocyst-forming coccidian protozoa. Approximately 20 *Cryptosporidium* species or genotypes have been reported to infect humans, but *Cryptosporidium hominis* and *Cryptosporidium parvum* cause more than 90% of cases of human cryptosporidiosis. Oocysts are excreted in feces of an infected host and as few as 10 oocysts can cause infection. *Cryptosporidium* oocysts can tolerate extreme

---

[1] Panel on Opportunistic Infections in HIV-Exposed and HIV-Infected Children. Guidelines for the Prevention and Treatment of Opportunistic Infections in Children with and Exposed to HIV. Available at: **https://clinicalinfo.hiv.gov/en/guidelines/hiv-clinical-guidelines-pediatric-opportunistic-infections/whats-new**

environmental conditions and can survive in water and soil for several months. Even in properly chlorinated pools, *Cryptosporidium* oocysts can survive for more than 7 days.

EPIDEMIOLOGY: *Cryptosporidium* organisms can be transmitted between humans and to humans via contaminated water or food or from infected animals. Extensive water-borne disease outbreaks have been associated with contamination of drinking water and recreational water (eg, pools, lakes, and splash pads). *Cryptosporidium* infection is the leading cause of outbreaks associated with treated recreational water venues (eg, swimming pools and splash pads), responsible for 76 (49%) of 155 US outbreaks during 2015–2019 for which an infectious cause was identified, and 84% of all cases from those 155 outbreaks.

In children, the incidence of cryptosporidiosis is greatest during summer and early fall, corresponding to the outdoor swimming season. The incidence of reported cryptosporidiosis is highest in children 1 through 4 years of age.

Foodborne transmission can occur; *Cryptosporidium* organisms have been detected on raw produce and in raw or unpasteurized apple cider and milk. People can acquire infections from pets, livestock, and from animals found in petting zoos, particularly preweaned bovine calves, lambs, and goat kids. *Cryptosporidium* organisms can spread by person-to-person transmission and result in outbreaks in child care settings and are a cause of travelers' diarrhea. (**www.cdc.gov/parasites/crypto/audience-travelers.html**).

The **incubation period** of *Cryptosporidium* species usually is 2 to 10 days. Recurrence of symptoms has been reported frequently. In immunocompetent people, oocyst shedding usually ceases within 2 weeks after symptoms completely abate. In immunocompromised people, the period of oocyst shedding can continue for months.

DIAGNOSTIC TESTS: Molecular methods are being used increasingly for diagnosis of cryptosporidiosis and are now the standard of care. Nucleic acid amplification tests (NAATs) that target multiple gastrointestinal tract pathogens in a single assay have a sensitivity of 97% and a specificity of 98% for *Cryptosporidium* organisms.

Nonmolecular testing, including direct fluorescent antibody (DFA) detection of oocysts in stool and enzyme immunoassays (EIAs) or rapid point-of-care lateral flow immunochromatographic tests targeting cryptosporidial antigens in stool, can provide rapid results, but their potential false-positive results and low positive predictive values still necessitate molecular confirmation. The detection of oocysts on microscopic examination of stool specimens can be accomplished by direct wet mount if concentration of the oocysts is high. Alternatively, the formalin ethyl acetate stool concentration method can be used followed by staining of the stool specimen with a modified Kinyoun acid-fast stain. Oocysts generally are small (4–6 µm in diameter) and can be missed in a rapid scan of a slide. At least 3 stool specimens collected on separate days should be examined before considering test results to be negative, because shedding can be intermittent. Organisms also can be identified in intestinal fluid, tissue samples, or biopsy specimens.

TREATMENT: Supportive therapy with volume and electrolyte repletion is recommended for all patients with cryptosporidiosis. Immunocompetent people might not need specific therapy. If treatment of diarrhea associated with cryptosporidiosis is indicated, a 3-day course of nitazoxanide oral suspension has been approved by the FDA for non–HIV-infected, immunocompetent people 1 year or older (see Table 4.11, Drugs for Parasitic Infections, p 1068).

In children with HIV infection, nitazoxanide alone in a 3-day course is generally ineffective in the treatment of *Cryptosporidium* diarrhea. Improvement in CD4+ T-lymphocyte count associated with antiretroviral therapy can lead to resolution of symptoms and cessation of oocyst shedding. For this reason, administration of combination antiretroviral therapy (ART) is the primary treatment for cryptosporidiosis in patients with HIV infection. Given the seriousness of cryptosporidiosis in immunocompromised people, a 14-day course of nitazoxanide can be considered in immunocompromised HIV-infected children in conjunction with immune restoration with ART.[1] In immunocompromised children, including some children with HIV infection, paromomycin or azithromycin have been used in case series with some success as single agents, in combination, or in combination with nitazoxanide (either agent or both). There are little data on the use of paromomycin or azithromycin in immunocompetent children with *Cryptosporidium* diarrhea, so they should be considered for use primarily in immunocompromised children, and should be used in immunocompetent children only if nitazoxanide has failed or is not available.

INFECTION PREVENTION AND CONTROL MEASURES IN HEALTH CARE SETTINGS: In addition to standard precautions, contact precautions are recommended for diapered or incontinent people for the duration of illness. Hydrogen peroxide is preferred over bleach for environmental cleaning because of the organism's extreme chlorine tolerance.

CONTROL MEASURES: Appropriate control and prevention measures should be implemented promptly to prevent pathogen transmission. In general, these measures include the following, and other measures might be indicated depending on suspected source and mode of transmission:

- Wash hands frequently with soap and water. Alcohol-based hand sanitizers are not effective against *Cryptosporidium* species.
- Do not swim or participate in recreational water activities if sick with diarrhea. If cryptosporidiosis is diagnosed, wait 2 weeks after diarrhea has stopped completely before participating in recreational water activities.
- Avoid swallowing recreational water. Additional information on healthy swimming can be found at **www.cdc.gov/healthyswimming.**
- Do not consume food or drink that might be contaminated, such as water from lakes or rivers; inadequately treated water (eg, while traveling in areas with unsafe water); fruits or vegetables washed in water that might be contaminated; or unpasteurized milk or apple cider.
- If immunocompromised, avoid contact with farm animals and their feces (see **www.cdc.gov/parasites/crypto/gen_info/prevent_ic.html**).

Public Health Reporting. Cryptosporidiosis cases are reportable to local, state, and territorial health departments.

---

[1] Panel on Opportunistic Infections in HIV-Exposed and HIV-Infected Children. Guidelines for the Prevention and Treatment of Opportunistic Infections in Children with and Exposed to HIV. Available at: **https://clinicalinfo.hiv.gov/en/guidelines/hiv-clinical-guidelines-pediatric-opportunistic-infections/whats-new**

Cutaneous Larva Migrans

CLINICAL MANIFESTATIONS: Cutaneous larva migrans refers to a classic skin rash caused by zoonotic hookworms. It is a clinical diagnosis based on advancing serpiginous tracks in the skin with associated intense pruritus. Certain zoonotic nematode larvae may penetrate intact skin and produce pruritic, reddish papules at the site of skin entry. Humans usually are "dead-end" hosts for these parasites, and the larvae are unable to progress beyond the skin and eventually die. As the larvae migrate through skin, advancing up to 20 millimeters per day, intensely pruritic serpiginous tracks are formed, a condition also referred to as creeping eruption. Bullae may develop later as a complication of the larval migration. Larval activity can continue for several weeks, but the infection typically is self-limiting. Rarely complications such as Loeffler (also spelled Löffler) syndrome (pulmonary infiltration with peripheral eosinophilia) have been reported.

ETIOLOGY: Infective larvae of cat and dog hookworms (most often *Ancylostoma braziliense*, also *Ancylostoma caninum*, *Ancylostoma ceylanicum*, and *Uncinaria stenocephala*) cause cutaneous larva migrans. Other skin-penetrating nematodes can cause similar pruritic serpiginous skin rashes (eg, larva currens caused by *Strongyloides* species and "ground itch" of *Necator americanus*).

EPIDEMIOLOGY: Cutaneous larva migrans is a disease of children, utility workers, gardeners, sunbathers, and others who come in contact with soil or sand contaminated with cat and dog feces. Locally acquired cases in the United States are mostly in the Southeast. Most US cases are not acquired locally but occur among travelers to tropical and subtropical regions, particularly those who have walked barefoot or have had unprotected skin contact on beaches.

The **incubation period** typically is short, with signs and symptoms developing several days after larval penetration of the skin. Rarely, onset may be weeks to months after exposure.

DIAGNOSTIC TESTS: The diagnosis is made clinically, and biopsies are not indicated. Biopsy specimens typically demonstrate an eosinophilic inflammatory infiltrate, but the migrating parasite is not visualized. Eosinophilia and increased immunoglobulin (Ig) E serum concentrations occur in some cases. Enzyme immunoassay or Western blot analysis using antigens of *A caninum* have been developed in research laboratories, but these assays are not available for routine diagnostic use.

TREATMENT: The disease usually is self-limited with spontaneous cure after several weeks, but treatment can decrease symptoms and hasten their resolution. Orally administered albendazole or ivermectin is the recommended therapy (see Drugs for Parasitic Infections, p 1068). Repeated application of topical 10% albendazole may be useful in young children who cannot take oral medication, but it is not available commercially and must be formulated at a pharmacy. Outside the United States, topical thiabendazole has also been used successfully for treatment of localized larvae.

INFECTION PREVENTION AND CONTROL MEASURES IN HEALTH CARE SETTINGS: Standard precautions are recommended.

CONTROL MEASURES: Skin contact with moist soil or sand contaminated with animal feces should be avoided. Beaches should be kept free of dog and cat feces. Regular veterinary care of dogs and cats is recommended.

Cyclosporiasis

CLINICAL MANIFESTATIONS: Watery diarrhea is the most common symptom of cyclosporiasis and can be profuse and protracted. Anorexia, nausea, substantial weight loss, flatulence, abdominal cramping and bloating, and prolonged fatigue can occur. Low-grade fever occurs in approximately 50% of patients and vomiting, body aches, headaches, and other influenza-like symptoms also may occur. Biliary tract disease has been reported. Infection usually is self-limited, but untreated people may have remitting, relapsing symptoms for weeks to months. Asymptomatic infection has been documented, most commonly in settings where cyclosporiasis is endemic.

ETIOLOGY: *Cyclospora cayetanensis* is a coccidian protozoan; oocysts (rather than cysts) are passed in stools and must then sporulate before they are infectious. In the laboratory, sporulation occurs at temperatures between 22°C and 32°C for 1 to 2 weeks; the exact conditions that support sporulation in the natural environment are unknown.

EPIDEMIOLOGY: *C cayetanensis* is endemic in many resource-limited countries and has been reported as a cause of travelers' diarrhea. Foodborne and waterborne outbreaks have been reported. Most outbreaks in the United States and Canada for which a food vehicle and its source have been identified have been associated with consumption of imported fresh produce (eg, basil, cilantro, raspberries, sugar snap peas, lettuce). There has been a trend in the United States of seasonal increases in reported cases from May through August in recent years; many cases occur among people without a history of international travel. Recent increases in case numbers reported in the United States might be attributable, in part, to increased use of commercially available molecular testing panels.

Humans are the only known hosts for *C cayetanensis*. Direct person-to-person transmission is unlikely because excreted oocysts take at least 1 to 2 weeks (estimated) under favorable environmental conditions to sporulate and become infective. Oocysts are resistant to most disinfectants used in food and water processing and can remain viable for prolonged periods in cool, moist environments.

The **incubation period** typically is 1 week but can range from 2 days to 2 weeks or more.

DIAGNOSTIC TESTS: Diagnosis is made by identification of oocysts (8–10 μm in diameter) in stool, intestinal fluid/aspirates, or intestinal biopsy specimens. Oocysts may be shed in low concentrations, even by people with profuse diarrhea. This constraint underscores the utility of repeated stool examinations, sensitive recovery methods (eg, concentration procedures including formalin-ethyl acetate sedimentation or sucrose centrifugal flotation), and detection methods that highlight the organism. Oocysts are autofluorescent and are variably acid fast after modified acid-fast staining of stool specimens. Molecular diagnostic assays (eg, nucleic acid amplification tests) are available commercially as part of a multiplex gastrointestinal panel and at the Centers for Disease Control and Prevention.

TREATMENT: Trimethoprim-sulfamethoxazole, typically for 7 to 10 days, is the drug of choice (see Table 4.11, Drugs for Parasitic Infections, p 1068); immunocompromised patients may need longer courses of therapy. No highly effective alternatives have been identified for people who cannot tolerate trimethoprim-sulfamethoxazole (**www.cdc. gov/parasites/cyclosporiasis/health_professionals/tx.html**), but case reports suggest that nitazoxanide might be an effective alternative for patients who cannot tolerate sulfa drugs. Data from patients with human immunodeficiency virus (HIV) infection in Haiti have suggested that ciprofloxacin also may be effective, but anecdotal reports among immunocompetent patients do not support its efficacy.

INFECTION PREVENTION AND CONTROL MEASURES IN HEALTH CARE SETTINGS: In addition to standard precautions, contact precautions are recommended for diapered or incontinent persons.

CONTROL MEASURES: Avoiding food or water that may be contaminated with feces is the best known way to prevent cyclosporiasis. Fresh produce should be avoided in high-risk settings or should be washed thoroughly before it is eaten, although this may not eliminate risk for transmission completely.

Public Health Reporting. Cyclosporiasis is a nationally notifiable disease. Please refer to the state or local health department for details on reporting cases.

Cystoisosporiasis (Formerly Isosporiasis)

CLINICAL MANIFESTATIONS: Watery, nonbloody diarrhea is the most common symptom of cystoisosporiasis; diarrhea can be profuse and protracted, even in immunocompetent people. Manifestations are similar to those caused by other enteric protozoa (eg, *Cryptosporidium* and *Cyclospora* species) and can include abdominal pain, cramping, flatulence, anorexia, nausea, vomiting, weight loss, and low-grade fever. Severity of infection ranges from self-limiting in immunocompetent hosts to chronic, debilitating, sometimes life-threatening diarrheal infection with wasting in immunocompromised patients, particularly but not exclusively among people infected with human immunodeficiency virus (HIV). Biliary tract disease (cholecystitis/cholangiopathy) and reactive arthritis also have been reported. Peripheral eosinophilia may occur.

ETIOLOGY: *Cystoisospora belli* (formerly *Isospora belli*) is a coccidian protozoan; oocysts (rather than cysts) are passed in stools.

EPIDEMIOLOGY: Infection occurs predominantly in tropical and subtropical regions of the world and results from ingestion of sporulated oocysts in food or water contaminated with human feces. Humans are the only known host for *C belli* and shed noninfective oocysts in feces. These oocysts must mature (sporulate) outside the host in the environment to become infective. Therefore, direct person-to-person transmission of *Cystoisospora* is unlikely. Under favorable conditions, sporulation can be completed in 1 to 2 days and perhaps more quickly in some settings. Oocysts probably are resistant to most disinfectants and can remain viable for prolonged periods in a cool, moist environment.

The **incubation period** averages 1 week but may range from several days to 2 or more weeks.

DIAGNOSTIC TESTS: Identification of oocysts in feces or in duodenal aspirates is diagnostic, as is finding developmental stages of the parasite in biopsy specimens (eg, of the small intestine). Oocysts in stool are elongate and ellipsoidal (length, 25 to 35 μm). Oocysts can be shed in low numbers, even by people with profuse diarrhea. This underscores the utility of repeated stool examinations, sensitive recovery methods (eg, concentration methods), and the need for detection methods that highlight the organism (eg, oocysts stain bright red with modified acid-fast staining techniques and autofluoresce when viewed by ultraviolet fluorescence microscopy). Nucleic acid amplification tests (NAATs) have been developed for detecting *Cystoisospora* DNA in feces but are not widely available. Like *Cryptosporidium* and *Cyclospora* species, *Cystoisospora* organisms usually are not detected by routine stool ova and parasite examination. Therefore, the laboratory should be notified specifically when any coccidian parasite is suspected on clinical grounds so that special microscopic methods are used in addition to traditional ova and parasite examination.

TREATMENT: Treatment has been studied predominantly in patients with HIV infection. In the immunocompetent host, treatment may not be necessary, as symptoms usually are self-limited. If symptoms do not begin to resolve by 5 to 7 days, and in immunocompromised patients, trimethoprim-sulfamethoxazole (TMP-SMX) is the drug of choice (see Table 4.11, Drugs for Parasitic Infections, p 1068). Immunocompromised patients may need higher doses and a longer duration of therapy. Pyrimethamine (plus leucovorin, to prevent myelosuppression) is an alternative for people who cannot tolerate (or whose infection does not respond to) trimethoprim-sulfamethoxazole. Ciprofloxacin is less effective than trimethoprim-sulfamethoxazole. Nitazoxanide has been reported to be effective, but data are limited.

In adolescents and adults coinfected with HIV with CD4+ T-lymphocyte counts of <200 cells/mm^3, secondary prophylaxis with TMP-SMX is recommended to prevent recurrent disease. In adults, secondary prophylaxis may be discontinued once the CD4+ T-lymphocyte count is >200 cells/mm^3 for >6 months as a result of antiretroviral therapy. In children, a reasonable time to discontinue secondary prophylaxis would be after sustained improvement (for >6 months) in CD4+ T-lymphocyte count or CD4+ T-lymphocyte percentage from CDC immunologic category 3 to category 1 or 2 in response to antiretroviral therapy (**https://clinicalinfo.hiv.gov/en/guidelines/pediatric-opportunistic-infection/isosporiasis-cystoisosporiasis** and **www.cdc.gov/mmwr/preview/mmwrhtml/rr6303a1.htm?s_cid=rr6303a1_e**). These individuals should be monitored closely for recurrent symptoms. Supportive treatment for dehydration and/or malnutrition associated with severe diarrheal illness may be required.

INFECTION PREVENTION AND CONTROL MEASURES IN HEALTH CARE SETTINGS: In addition to standard precautions, contact precautions are recommended for diapered and incontinent people.

CONTROL MEASURES: Preventive measures include avoiding fecal exposure (eg, food, water, skin, and fomites contaminated with stool), practicing hand and personal hygiene, and thorough washing of fruits and vegetables before eating.

Cytomegalovirus Infection

CLINICAL MANIFESTATIONS: Manifestations of acquired human cytomegalovirus (CMV) infection vary with age and immunocompetence of the host. Asymptomatic infections are the most common, particularly in children. An infectious mononucleosis-like syndrome with prolonged fever and mild hepatitis, occurring in the absence of heterophile antibody production ("monospot negative"), may occur in adolescents and adults. End-organ disease, including pneumonia, colitis, retinitis, meningoencephalitis, or transverse myelitis, or a CMV syndrome characterized by fever, thrombocytopenia, leukopenia, and mild hepatitis may occur in immunocompromised hosts, including people receiving treatment for malignant neoplasms, people infected with human immunodeficiency virus (HIV), and people receiving immunosuppressive therapy for solid organ or hematopoietic cell transplantation. Less commonly, patients treated with biologic response modifiers (see Biologic Response Modifying Drugs Used to Decrease Inflammation, p 104) can exhibit CMV end-organ disease, such as retinitis and hepatitis.

Congenital CMV infection has a spectrum of clinical manifestations but usually is not evident at birth (asymptomatic congenital CMV infection). Approximately 10% of infants with congenital CMV infection exhibit clinical findings that are evident at birth (symptomatic congenital CMV disease), with manifestations including jaundice attributable to direct hyperbilirubinemia, petechiae attributable to thrombocytopenia, purpura, hepatosplenomegaly, microcephaly, intracerebral (typically periventricular) calcifications, and retinitis. Developmental delays can occur among affected infants in later infancy and early childhood. Death attributable to congenital CMV is estimated to occur in 3% to 10% of infants with symptomatic disease or 0.3% to 1.0% of all infants with congenital CMV infection.

Congenital CMV infection is the leading nongenetic cause of sensorineural hearing loss (SNHL) in children in the United States. Approximately 20% of all hearing loss at birth and 25% of all hearing loss at 4 years of age is attributable to congenital CMV infection. SNHL is the most common sequela following congenital CMV infection, with SNHL occurring in up to 50% of children with congenital infections that are symptomatic at birth and up to 15% of those with asymptomatic infections. Approximately 40% of infected children who ultimately develop SNHL will not have hearing loss detectable within the first month of life, illustrating the risk of late-onset SNHL in these populations. Approximately 50% of children with CMV-associated SNHL continue to have further deterioration (progression) of their hearing loss over time.

Infection acquired during the intrapartum period from cervical secretions or in the postpartum period from human milk usually is not associated with clinical illness in term infants. In preterm infants, however, postpartum infection resulting from human milk or from transfusion from CMV-seropositive donors has been associated with hepatitis, interstitial pneumonitis, colitis, hematologic abnormalities including thrombocytopenia, neutropenia, leukopenia, and a viral sepsis syndrome.

ETIOLOGY: Human CMV, also known as human herpesvirus 5, is a member of the herpesvirus family *(Herpesviridae)*, the beta-herpesvirus subfamily *(Betaherpesvirinae)*, and the *Cytomegalovirus* genus. The viral genome contains double-stranded DNA that range in size from 196 000 to 240 000 bp encoding at least 166 proteins and is the largest of the human herpesvirus genomes.

EPIDEMIOLOGY: CMV is highly species-specific, and only human CMV has been shown to infect and cause disease in humans. The virus is ubiquitous, and CMV strains exhibit extensive genetic diversity. Transmission occurs horizontally (by direct person-to-person contact with virus-containing secretions), vertically (from mother to infant before, during, or after birth), and via transfusions of blood, platelets, and white blood cells from infected donors. CMV also can be transmitted with solid organ or hematopoietic cell transplantation. Infections have no seasonal predilection. CMV persists in leukocytes and tissue cells after a primary infection, with intermittent virus shedding; symptomatic reinfection can occur throughout the lifetime of the infected person, particularly under conditions of immunosuppression. Reinfection with other strains of CMV can occur in seropositive hosts, including pregnant people. In the

United States, there appears to be 3 periods in life when there is an increased incidence of CMV acquisition: early childhood, adolescence, and the childbearing years.

Horizontal transmission probably is the result of exposure to saliva, urine, or genital secretions from infected individuals. Spread of CMV in households and child care centers is well documented. Excretion rates from urine or saliva in children 1 to 3 years of age who attend child care centers usually range from 30% to 40% but can be as high as 70%. In addition, children who attend child care frequently excrete large quantities of virus for prolonged periods. Young children can transmit CMV to their parents, including those who may be pregnant, and other caregivers, including child care staff (see Children in Group Child Care and Schools, p 145). In adolescents and adults, sexual transmission occurs, as evidenced by detection of virus in seminal and cervical fluids. As such, CMV is considered to be a sexually transmitted infection (STI).

CMV-seropositive healthy people have latent CMV in their leukocytes and tissues; hence, blood transfusions and organ transplantation can result in transmission. Severe CMV disease following transfusion or solid organ transplantation is more likely to occur if the recipient is CMV seronegative before transplantation. In contrast, among nonautologous hematopoietic cell transplant (HCT) recipients, CMV-seropositive individuals who receive transplants from seronegative donors are at greatest risk of disease when exposed to CMV after transplantation, likely because of the failure of the transplanted graft to provide immunity to the recipient. Latent CMV may reactivate in immunosuppressed individuals and result in disease if immunosuppression is severe (eg, in patients with acquired immunodeficiency syndrome [AIDS] or solid organ or HCT recipients).

Vertical transmission of CMV to an infant occurs in one of the following time periods: (1) in utero (congenital), by transplacental passage of parental bloodborne virus; (2) at birth (perinatal), by passage through an infected genital tract; or (3) following birth (postnatal), via ingestion of CMV-positive human milk. Approximately 5 per 1000 live-born infants are infected in utero and excrete CMV at birth, making this the most common congenital viral infection in the United States. Significant racial and ethnic differences exist in the prevalence of congenital CMV, with the highest prevalence of CMV in Black newborn infants (9.5/1000 live births) and lower prevalence in non-Hispanic white infants (2.7/1000 live births) and Hispanic white infants (3.0/1000 live births). In utero fetal infection can occur in pregnant people with no preexisting CMV immunity (primary infection) or in pregnant people with preexisting antibodies to CMV (nonprimary infection) either by acquisition of a different viral strain during pregnancy or by reactivation of an existing infection. Congenital infection and associated sequelae can occur irrespective of the trimester when the pregnant person is infected, but severe sequelae are associated more commonly with infection acquired during the first trimester. Damaging fetal infections and sequelae can occur following both primary and nonprimary infections in the pregnant person. It is estimated that more than three quarters of infants with congenital CMV infection in the United States are born to a person with nonprimary infection; in nations with near-universal CMV seroprevalence, most damaging congenital CMV infections occur in infants born to people with nonprimary infection.

Among infants who acquire infection perinatally from cervical secretions or postnatally from human milk, preterm infants born before 32 weeks' gestation and with a birth weight less than 1500 g are at greater risk of developing CMV disease than are full-term infants. Most infants who acquire CMV from ingestion of human milk from a CMV-seropositive parent do not develop clinical illness or sequelae, likely because of the presence of passively transferred antibody.

The **incubation period** for horizontally transmitted CMV infections is highly variable. Infection usually manifests 3 to 12 weeks after blood transfusions and between 1 and 4 months after organ transplantation. For vertical transmission through human milk in preterm infants, the median time to onset of CMV viruria is 7 weeks (range, 3–24 weeks).

DIAGNOSTIC TESTS: The diagnosis of CMV disease is confounded by the ubiquity of the virus, the high rate of asymptomatic excretion, the frequency of reactivated infections, reinfection with different strains of CMV, the development of serum immunoglobulin (Ig) M CMV-specific antibodies in some episodes of reactivation and reinfection, and concurrent infection with other pathogens.

Viral DNA can be detected by nucleic acid amplification tests (NAATs) in tissues and some fluids, including cerebrospinal fluid (CSF), amniotic fluid, human milk, aqueous and vitreous humor fluids, urine, saliva and other respiratory secretions, and peripheral blood. Detection of CMV DNA by NAAT in blood does not necessarily indicate acute infection or disease, especially in immunocompetent people. Several quantitative NAATs for detection of CMV have been cleared by the US Food and Drug Administration (FDA). These assays are sensitive, use standardized international units for reporting, provide rapid results compared with culture, and generally are the preferred method for detecting CMV DNA. The same specimen type should always be used when testing any given patient over time. Antigenemia assays also have been cleared by the FDA, but they are labor intensive and require timely processing of specimens to obtain accurate results. Because of these drawbacks, molecular assays are preferred.

CMV can be isolated in conventional cell culture from urine, saliva, peripheral blood leukocytes, human milk, semen, cervical secretions, and other tissues and body fluids. Recovery of virus from a target organ provides supportive evidence that the disease is caused by CMV infection. Standard viral cultures must be maintained for more than 28 days before considering such cultures negative. Shell vial culture coupled with staining of cells using immunofluorescence antibody techniques for immediate early antigen provides results within 24 to 36 hours but is not available in many laboratories.

Various serologic assays, including immunofluorescence assays, latex agglutination assays, and enzyme immunoassays, are available for detecting both IgG and IgM CMV-specific antibodies. Single serum specimens for IgG antibody testing are useful in screening for past infection in individuals at risk for CMV reactivation or for screening potential organ transplant donors and recipients. For diagnosis of suspected recent infection, testing for CMV IgG in paired sera obtained at least 2 weeks apart and testing for IgM in a single serum specimen may be useful. Determination of low-avidity CMV IgG in the presence of CMV IgM in a pregnant person can suggest more recent infection.

Fetal CMV infection can be diagnosed by detection of CMV DNA in amniotic fluid. Congenital infection with CMV requires detection of CMV or CMV DNA in urine, saliva, blood, or CSF obtained within 3 weeks of birth; detection beyond this initial period of life could reflect postnatal acquisition of virus. NAATs of saliva swab specimens from neonates have been shown to be >95% sensitive for the identification of congenital CMV infection. Positive saliva swab specimen test results requires confirmation with testing of urine because of potential contamination of saliva with CMV in human milk. The analytical sensitivity of CMV NAAT of dried blood spots is lower, limiting use of this type of specimen for widespread screening for congenital CMV infection. A positive NAAT result from a neonatal dried blood spot confirms congenital infection, but a negative result does not rule out congenital infection. Differentiation between congenital and perinatal infection is difficult at later than 3 weeks of age unless clinical manifestations of the former, such as chorioretinitis or periventricular calcifications, are present. At least 1 commercial assay has been cleared by the FDA for detection of CMV DNA from saliva of neonates within the first 3 weeks of life. IgM serologic methods have reduced sensitivity and specificity and may yield false-positive results, making serologic diagnosis of congenital CMV infection unreliable.

Targeted CMV newborn screening, in which infants who do not pass their newborn hearing screening are tested for CMV in saliva or urine within the first 2 to 3 weeks of life, is mandated in several states, and many birth hospitals have implemented targeted screening programs as standard of care. Universal screening of all newborn infants for CMV has been undertaken in Ontario and Saskatchewan, Canada, beginning in 2019 and 2022, respectively, and in 2022 Minnesota became the first state to add congenital CMV to its newborn screening program.

TREATMENT: Intravenous ganciclovir (see Non-HIV Antiviral Drugs, p 1044) is approved for induction and maintenance treatment of retinitis caused by acquired or recurrent CMV infection in immunocompromised adult patients, including people living with HIV, and for prophylaxis and treatment of CMV disease in adult transplant recipients. Valganciclovir, the oral prodrug of ganciclovir, is approved for treatment (induction and maintenance) of CMV retinitis in immunocompromised adult patients, including people living with HIV, and for prevention of CMV disease in kidney, kidney-pancreas, or heart transplant recipients at high risk of CMV disease. Valganciclovir also is approved for prevention of CMV disease in pediatric kidney transplant patients 4 months and older and for pediatric heart transplant patients 1 month and older. Ganciclovir and valganciclovir are used to treat CMV infections of other sites (esophagus, colon, lungs) and for preemptive treatment of immunosuppressed adults with CMV antigenemia or viremia. Valganciclovir is available in both tablet and powder for oral solution formulations. Oral ganciclovir and ganciclovir ocular implants are no longer available in the United States.

Neonates with moderately to severely symptomatic congenital CMV disease with or without central nervous system (CNS) involvement have improved audiologic and neurodevelopmental outcomes at 2 years of age when treated with oral valganciclovir for 6 **months** (see Non-HIV Antiviral Drugs, p 1044). The dose should be adjusted each month to account for weight gain. Neonates with isolated SNHL have improved audiologic outcomes when treated with oral valganciclovir for 6 **weeks**, with treatment begun by 13 weeks following birth. Treatment of mildly symptomatic neonates has not been studied. Treatment recommendations by degree of symptomatology are provided in Table 3.4. Infants with asymptomatic congenital CMV infection should not receive antiviral treatment outside the confines of a research study.

Therapy can be accomplished using oral valganciclovir for the entire treatment course, because drug exposure following appropriate dosing of valganciclovir is the same as that achieved with intravenous ganciclovir. If an infant is unable to absorb medications reliably from the gastrointestinal tract (eg, because of necrotizing enterocolitis or other bowel disorders), intravenous ganciclovir can be used initially. Significant neutropenia occurs in approximately 20% of infants treated with oral

Table 3.4. Classification of Congenital Cytomegalovirus Disease Severity and Treatment Recommendations

CMV Disease Severity	Signs and Symptoms	Treatment
Moderately to severely symptomatic	One or more of the following: • Single severe or multiorgan disease (eg, significant liver enzyme abnormalities and marked hepatosplenomegaly) or life-threatening organ dysfunction • Multiple persistent (eg, ≥2 weeks) manifestations attributable to congenital CMV infection: thrombocytopenia, petechiae, hepatomegaly, splenomegaly, hepatitis (increased aminotransferases or direct bilirubin) • Central nervous system involvement such as microcephaly, radiographic abnormalities (ventriculomegaly, intracerebral calcifications, white matter changes, periventricular echogenicity, cortical or cerebellar malformations, migration abnormalities), abnormal cerebrospinal fluid indices for age, chorioretinitis, or the detection of CMV DNA in cerebrospinal fluid • Greater than 2 mild disease manifestations (see below)	Valganciclovir[a] (see Non-HIV Antiviral Drugs, p 1044) given orally for 6 **months;** treatment should be started within the first 13 weeks following birth[b]
Asymptomatic with isolated sensorineural hearing loss	No clinically apparent signs to suggest congenital CMV disease, but sensorineural hearing loss	Valganciclovir (see Non-HIV Antiviral Drugs, p 1044) may be offered and given orally for 6 **weeks;** treatment should be started within the first 13 weeks following birth[b]
Mildly symptomatic	Two or fewer transient (eg, <2 weeks) or clinically insignificant findings (eg, petechiae, mild hepatomegaly, thrombocytopenia, raised levels of alanine aminotransferase)	There are insufficient data to recommend routine treatment, but it may be considered on a case by case basis in consultation with a pediatric infectious diseases expert
Asymptomatic	No apparent signs to suggest congenital CMV disease, and normal hearing	Therapy not recommended outside of a research study

Modified from Rawlinson W, Boppana S, Fowler KB, et al. Congenital cytomegalovirus infection in pregnancy and the neonate: consensus recommendations for prevention, diagnosis, and therapy. *Lancet Infect Dis.* 2017;17(6):e177-e188; and Luck SE, Wieringa JW, Blázquez-Gamero D, et al. Congenital cytomegalovirus: a European expert consensus statement on diagnosis and management. *Pediatr Infect Dis J.* 2017;36(12):1205-1213.

[a] If an infant is unable to absorb medications reliably from the gastrointestinal tract (eg, because of necrotizing enterocolitis or other bowel disorders), intravenous ganciclovir can be used initially (see Non-HIV Antiviral Drugs, p 1044).

[b] Antiviral treatment can start from birth through 12 weeks 6 days following delivery.

valganciclovir and in approximately 65% of infants treated with parenteral ganciclovir. Absolute neutrophil counts should be measured weekly for 6 weeks, then at 8 weeks, then monthly for the duration of antiviral treatment; serum alanine aminotransferase concentration should be measured monthly during treatment. When it occurs, neutropenia is more common during the first 4 to 6 weeks of therapy; if the absolute neutrophil count reproducibly drops below 500 cells/mm^3, either treatment can be held until counts recover above 750 cells/mm^3, or granulocyte colony-stimulating factor can be administered once daily for 1 to 3 consecutive days.

Patients with symptomatic or asymptomatic congenital CMV infection should have serial audiologic assessments throughout childhood. The American Academy of Pediatrics *Bright Futures: Guidelines for Health Supervision of Infants, Children, and Adolescents*, 4th Edition, recommends hearing screening/assessment at 4, 6, 9, 12, 15, 18, 24, and 30 months of age for children with congenital CMV, in addition to the standard hearing testing recommended for all children at 4, 5, 6, 8, and 10 years of age.

Preterm infants with perinatally acquired CMV infection can have symptomatic, end organ disease (eg, pneumonitis, hepatitis, thrombocytopenia). Antiviral treatment has not been studied in this population. If such patients are treated with parenteral ganciclovir, a reasonable approach is to treat for 2 weeks and then reassess responsiveness to therapy. If clinical data suggest benefit of treatment, an additional 1 to 2 weeks of parenteral ganciclovir can be considered if symptoms and signs have not resolved. Valganciclovir generally is not a reasonable alternative in this setting, given the degree of illness these infants experience and the corresponding effect that this potentially could have on gastrointestinal tract absorption of valganciclovir and first-pass hepatic metabolism to ganciclovir.

In HCT recipients, the combination of immune globulin intravenous (IGIV) or CMV immune globulin intravenous (CMV-IGIV) and intravenous ganciclovir has been reported to be synergistic in treatment of CMV pneumonia. Unlike CMV-IGIV, IGIV products have varying anti-CMV antibody concentrations from lot to lot, are not tested routinely for their quantities of anti-CMV antibodies, and do not have a specified titer of antibodies to CMV that have correlated with efficacy.

Valganciclovir and foscarnet have been approved for treatment and maintenance therapy of CMV retinitis in adults with AIDS, and letermovir has been approved in adults for prophylaxis of CMV infection and disease in adult CMV-seropositive recipients of allogeneic HCT (see Non-HIV Antiviral Drugs, p 1044). Foscarnet is more toxic (with high rates of limiting nephrotoxicity) but may be advantageous for some people living with HIV infection, including people with disease caused by ganciclovir-resistant virus or people who are unable to tolerate ganciclovir. Cidofovir can be used for CMV retinitis in adults with AIDS when there is a need to avoid both ganciclovir and foscarnet, but it is associated with significant nephrotoxicity and increased risk of immune recovery uveitis, hypotony, and neutropenia. In November 2021, maribavir was approved as the first drug for treating adults and pediatric patients (12 years and older and weighing at least 35 kg) with post-transplant CMV infection or disease that does not respond (with or without genetic mutations that cause resistance) to available antiviral treatment for CMV (see Non-HIV Antiviral Drugs, p 1044).

CMV establishes lifelong persistent infection, and as such, it is not eliminated from the body with antiviral treatment of CMV disease. Until immune reconstitution is achieved with antiretroviral therapy, chronic suppressive therapy should be administered to people living with HIV with a history of CMV end-organ disease (eg, retinitis, colitis, pneumonitis) to prevent recurrence. Discontinuing prophylaxis may be considered for pediatric patients 6 years and older with CD4+ T-lymphocyte counts of >100 cells/mm^3 for >6 consecutive months and for children younger than 6 years with percentages of total CD4+ T-lymphocytes of >15% for >6 consecutive months. For immunocompromised children with CMV retinitis, such decisions should be made in close consultation with an ophthalmologist and should account for such factors as magnitude and duration of CD4+ T-lymphocyte cell increases, anatomic location of the retinal lesion, vision in the contralateral eye, and the feasibility of regular ophthalmologic monitoring. All patients who have had anti-CMV maintenance therapy discontinued should continue to undergo regular ophthalmologic monitoring at 3- to 6-month intervals for early detection of CMV relapse as well as immune reconstitution uveitis.[1]

INFECTION PREVENTION AND CONTROL MEASURES IN HEALTH CARE SETTINGS: Standard precautions are recommended.

CONTROL MEASURES:

Care of Exposed People. When caring for children, hand hygiene, particularly after changing diapers, is advised to decrease transmission of CMV. Because asymptomatic excretion of CMV is common in people of all ages, a child with congenital CMV infection should not be treated differently from other children.

Although unrecognized exposure to people who are shedding CMV likely is common, concern may arise when immunocompromised patients or pregnant people, including health care professionals, are exposed to patients with clinically recognizable CMV infection. Standard precautions should be sufficient to interrupt transmission of CMV (see Infection Prevention and Control for Hospitalized Children, p 163).

Child Care. Workers in child care centers capable of becoming pregnant should be aware of CMV and its potential risks and should have access to appropriate hand hygiene measures to minimize occupationally acquired infection (**www.cdc.gov/ cmv/index.html**).

Immunoprophylaxis. CMV-IGIV is generally not recommended for prophylaxis of CMV disease in solid organ transplant recipients. CMV-IGIV may be useful for prevention of CMV in high-risk heart, lung, and small bowel transplant recipients when used in combination with antiviral agents.[2,3] The use of CMV-IGIV in pregnant people to prevent CMV transmission to the fetus is not recommended because of lack of effectiveness in randomized controlled clinical trials. Evaluation of investigational vaccines

---

[1] Panel on Opportunistic Infections in HIV-Exposed and HIV-Infected Children. Guidelines for the Prevention and Treatment of Opportunistic Infections in Children with and Exposed to HIV. Available at: **https:// clinicalinfo.hiv.gov/en/guidelines/hiv-clinical-guidelines-pediatric-opportunistic-infections/ whats-new**

[2] Kotton CN, Kumar D, Caliendo AM, Huprikar S, Chou S, Danziger-Isakov L, Humar A; The Transplantation Society International CMV Consensus Group. The Third International Consensus Guidelines on the Management of Cytomegalovirus in Solid-organ Transplantation. *Transplantation.* 2018;102(6):900-931

[3] Razonable RR, Humar A. Cytomegalovirus in solid organ transplant recipients. Guidelines of the American Society of Transplantation Infectious Diseases Community of Practice. *Clin Transplant.* 2019;33(9):e13512

in healthy volunteers and renal transplant recipients is in progress, but to date, only inconsistent evidence of efficacy has been reported.

Prevention of Transmission by Blood Transfusion. Transmission of CMV by blood transfusion to newborn infants or other immune-compromised hosts has been virtually eliminated by use of CMV antibody-negative donors and the use of leukoreduced blood products.

Prevention of Transmission by Human Milk. Pasteurization of donated human milk can decrease the likelihood of CMV transmission. Holder pasteurization (62.5°C [144.5°F] for 30 minutes) and short-term pasteurization (72°C [161.6°F] for 15 seconds) of human milk appear to inactivate CMV; short-term pasteurization may be less harmful to the beneficial constituents of human milk. Freezing human milk at −20°C (−4°F) for the sole purpose of reducing CMV infectivity is not advised because, although it may reduce the viral load of CMV, it does not change the risk of CMV sepsis-like syndrome and freezing reduces the bioactivity of human milk. If fresh donated human milk is needed for infants born to CMV antibody-negative birthing parents, providing these infants with milk from only CMV antibody-negative donors should be considered. For infants already infected with CMV, either congenitally or postnatally, the benefits of human milk from their birthing parents outweigh any risk of additional CMV exposure. For further information on human milk banks, see Human Milk Banks (p 143).

Prevention of Transmission in Transplant Recipients. CMV-seronegative recipients of tissue from CMV-seropositive donors are at high risk of CMV disease. If such circumstances cannot be avoided, prophylactic administration of antiviral therapy or monitoring for viremia and administering preemptive antiviral therapy are options to decrease the incidence of CMV disease. Monitoring and preemptive therapy result in lower risk for drug associated toxicity. For solid organ transplant patients receiving antiviral prophylaxis, the risk of delayed-onset CMV disease is highest during the first 3 months after cessation of antiviral prophylaxis. Among CMV-negative recipients of a liver transplant from a CMV-positive donor, preemptive therapy recently has been shown to significantly reduce CMV disease compared with prophylaxis.

Dengue

CLINICAL MANIFESTATIONS: Dengue infection may be asymptomatic or, if symptomatic, may have a wide range of clinical presentations. The 2009 World Health Organization classification for dengue severity (**https://apps.who. int/iris/bitstream/handle/10665/44188/9789241547871_eng. pdf?sequence=1&isAllowed=y**) is divided into: (1) **Dengue without warning signs:** fever plus 2 of the following: nausea/vomiting, rash, aches and pains, leukopenia, or positive tourniquet test; (2) **Dengue with warning signs:** dengue as defined above plus any of the following: abdominal pain or tenderness, persistent vomiting, clinical fluid accumulation (ascites, pleural effusion), mucosal bleeding, lethargy, restlessness, liver enlargement >2 cm, or increase in hematocrit concurrent with rapid decrease in platelet count; and (3) **Severe dengue:** dengue with at least 1 of the following criteria: severe plasma leakage leading to shock or fluid accumulation with respiratory distress, severe bleeding as evaluated by a clinician, or severe organ involvement (eg, aspartate aminotransferase [AST] or alanine aminotransferase [ALT]

≥1000 IU/L, impaired consciousness, failure of heart and other organs). Less common clinical syndromes include myocarditis, pancreatitis, hepatitis, hemophagocytic lymphohistiocytosis, and neurologic disease, including acute meningoencephalitis and post-dengue acute disseminated encephalomyelitis (ADEM).

Dengue begins abruptly with a nonspecific, acute febrile illness lasting 2 to 7 days **(febrile phase)**, often accompanied by muscle, joint, or bone pain, headache, retro-orbital pain, facial erythema, injected oropharynx, macular or maculopapular rash, leukopenia, and petechiae or other minor bleeding manifestations. During defervescence, usually on days 3 through 7 of illness, an increase in vascular permeability in parallel with increasing hematocrit (hemoconcentration) may occur. The increased vascular permeability may result in plasma leakage. The period of clinically significant plasma leakage usually lasts 24 to 48 hours **(critical phase)**, followed by a **convalescent phase** with gradual improvement and stabilization of the hemodynamic status. Warning signs of progression to severe dengue occur in the late febrile phase and include persistent vomiting, severe abdominal pain, mucosal bleeding, difficulty breathing, early signs of shock, and a rapid decline in platelet count with an increase in hematocrit. Patients with nonsevere disease begin to improve during the critical phase, but people with clinically significant plasma leakage develop severe disease that may include pleural effusions, ascites, hypovolemic shock, and hemorrhage.

ETIOLOGY: Four related RNA viruses of the genus *Flavivirus* (see Arboviruses, p 237), dengue viruses 1, 2, 3, and 4, cause symptomatic (approximately 25%) and asymptomatic (approximately 75%) infections. Infection with one dengue virus serotype most often produces lifelong immunity against that serotype, and a period of cross-protection (often lasting 1 to 2 years) against infection with the other 3 serotypes can be observed. After this, infection with a different serotype may predispose to more severe disease. Because there are 4 serotypes, a person has a lifetime risk of up to 4 dengue virus infections.

EPIDEMIOLOGY: Dengue virus is transmitted to humans primarily through the bite of infected *Aedes aegypti* (and less commonly, *Aedes albopictus* or *Aedes polynesiensis*) mosquitoes. Humans are the main amplifying host of dengue virus and the main source of virus for *Aedes* mosquitoes. A sylvatic nonhuman primate dengue virus transmission cycle exists in parts of Africa and Southeast Asia but rarely crosses to humans. Other forms of transmission are relatively rare and include vertical transmission; transmission via breastfeeding, blood, or organ donation; and health care-associated transmission via needlestick or mucocutaneous exposure. The rate of vertical transmission is around 20% and is even higher when dengue occurs late in pregnancy near delivery. Sexual transmission is also possible but is considered a very rare route of infection.

Dengue is a major public health problem in the tropics and subtropics; about half the world's population is thought to be at risk of infection with dengue viruses and approximately 100 to 400 million dengue infections occur annually worldwide **(www.who.int/news-room/fact-sheets/detail/dengue-and-severe-dengue)**. Dengue is endemic in the United States territories and freely associated states of Puerto Rico, the US Virgin Islands, American Samoa, the Federated States of Micronesia, the Republic of Marshall Islands, and the Republic of Palau.

Approximately 90% of the population in these areas at risk for dengue live in Puerto Rico, and 95% of locally acquired dengue cases reported in the United States from 2010 to 2020 occurred in Puerto Rico.[1] Incidence rates vary significantly by geographic locale, affected by factors such as population density, elevation, and mosquito breeding and water supply patterns. Outbreaks with local dengue virus transmission have occurred in Texas, Hawaii, and Florida and in Mexican cities bordering Yuma, Arizona (San Luis Rio Colorado, Sonora), and Calexico, California (Mexicali, Baja California). Although up to 28 states now have *Ae aegypti* and 40 states have *Ae albopictus* mosquitoes, local dengue virus transmission is uncommon because of housing characteristics including air conditioning and screens that reduce contact between people and infected mosquitoes. Millions of US travelers are at risk; dengue is the leading cause of febrile illness among travelers returning from the Caribbean, Latin America, and Southeast Asia. Dengue occurs in people of all ages but occurs at higher rates in healthy adolescents and young adults and is most likely to cause severe disease in infants, pregnant people, and patients with chronic diseases (eg, asthma, sickle cell anemia, and diabetes mellitus). Severe dengue disease is most likely to occur with second, heterologous dengue serotype infections, although it can occur with a first dengue infection or postsecondary heterologous dengue serotype infections.

The **incubation period** for dengue virus replication in mosquitoes is 8 to 12 days (extrinsic incubation); mosquitoes remain infectious for the remainder of their life cycle. In humans, the **incubation period** is 3 to 14 days before symptom onset (intrinsic incubation). Infected people, both symptomatic and asymptomatic, can transmit dengue virus to mosquitoes 1 to 2 days before symptoms develop and throughout the approximately 7-day viremic period.

DIAGNOSTIC TESTS: Laboratory confirmation of dengue can be made on a single serum, plasma, or whole blood specimen obtained within the first 7 days after the onset of symptoms by nucleic acid amplification tests (NAATs) or detection of dengue virus nonstructural protein 1 (NS-1) antigen by immunoassay.

For patients with a negative NAAT or NS1 test or patients presenting more than 7 days after symptom onset, a positive anti-dengue virus (DENV) immunoglobulin (Ig) M suggests recent infection, although with less certainty than NAAT or NS1 testing because of cross-reactivity with other flaviviruses.

Anti-DENV IgM antibodies are detectable beginning 3 to 5 days after illness onset; 99% of patients have IgM antibodies by day 10. IgM concentrations peak after 2 weeks and then often decline to undetectable levels over 2 to 3 months; they can cross-react with IgM antibodies against Zika virus and other closely related flaviviruses. In patients from areas with ongoing transmission of another flavivirus (eg, Zika virus) and whose only evidence of dengue is a positive anti-DENV IgM test, plaque reduction neutralization tests (PRNT) quantifying virus-specific neutralizing antibody titers can distinguish DENV from other flaviviruses in some but not all cases. PRNT, however, is rarely available in clinical laboratories and results typically are not available within a timeframe that is meaningful for clinicians managing acute disease. PRNT may be valuable in circumstances where confirming the diagnosis may have important clinical implications, such as distinguishing dengue from a Zika virus infection in a pregnant

---

[1] Paz-Bailey G, Adams L, Wong JM, et al. Dengue vaccine: recommendations of the Advisory Committee on Immunization Practices, United States, 2021. *MMWR Recomm Rep.* 2021;70(RR-6):1–16

individual.[1,2] Anti-DENV IgG antibody remains elevated for life after dengue virus infection. Anti-DENV IgG antibody may be falsely positive in people with previous infection with or immunization against other flaviviruses (eg, West Nile, Japanese encephalitis, yellow fever, or Zika viruses). See Fig 3.23, p 966, for dengue and Zika virus testing recommendations for nonpregnant persons with a clinically compatible illness and risk for infection with both viruses. A fourfold or greater increase in anti-DENV IgG antibody titers between the acute (≤5 days after onset of symptoms) and convalescent (>15 days after onset of symptoms) samples is indicative of recent infection. Conventional serologic tests may be less reliable for diagnosis of acute dengue virus infection in individuals who have been vaccinated with a dengue vaccine within the previous several months. Dengue diagnostic testing is available through commercial reference laboratories and some state public health laboratories; reference testing is available from the Dengue Branch of the Centers for Disease Control and Prevention (**www.cdc.gov/dengue/**).

TREATMENT: No specific antiviral therapy exists for dengue. During the febrile phase, patients should stay well hydrated and avoid use of aspirin (acetylsalicylic acid), salicylate-containing drugs, and other nonsteroidal anti-inflammatory drugs (eg, ibuprofen) to minimize potential for bleeding. Additional supportive care is required if the patient becomes dehydrated or develops warning signs of severe disease at or around the time of defervescence.

Early recognition of shock and intensive supportive therapy can reduce risk of death from severe dengue from approximately 5% to 10% to less than 1%. During the critical phase, maintenance of fluid volume and hemodynamic status is crucial to management of severe cases. Patients should be monitored for early signs of shock, occult bleeding, and plasma leakage to avoid prolonged shock, end organ damage, and fluid overload. Patients with refractory shock may require intravenous colloids and/or blood or blood products after an initial trial of intravenous crystalloids. Reabsorption of extravascular fluid occurs during the convalescent phase with stabilization of hemodynamic status and diuresis. It is important to watch for signs of fluid overload, which may manifest as a decrease in the patient's hematocrit as a result of the dilutional effect of reabsorbed fluid.

INFECTION PREVENTION AND CONTROL MEASURES IN HEALTH CARE SETTINGS: Standard precautions are recommended, with attention to the potential for bloodborne transmission. When indicated, attention should be given to control of *Aedes* mosquitoes to prevent secondary transmission of dengue virus from infected patients to others.

CONTROL MEASURES: Vector control can reduce dengue transiently, when applied rigorously, but is limited by widespread insecticide resistance in areas where the virus is endemic. A recombinant live attenuated tetravalent dengue vaccine, CYD-TDV (chimeric yellow fever dengue-tetravalent dengue vaccine) (Dengvaxia) with a 3-dose schedule administered at 0, 6, and 12 months has been approved by the US Food and Drug Administration for use in individuals 6 through 16 years of age with laboratory-confirmed previous dengue infection and living in areas with endemic infection.

---

[1] Sharp TM, Fischer M, Muñoz-Jordán JL, et al. Dengue and Zika virus diagnostic testing for patients with a clinically compatible illness and risk for infection with both viruses. *MMWR Recomm Rep.* 2019;68(1):1–10

[2] Wong JM, Adams LE, Durbin AP, et al. Dengue: a growing problem with new interventions. *Pediatrics.* 2022;149(6):e2021055522

The Centers for Disease Control and Prevention (CDC) Advisory Committee on Immunization Practices (ACIP) currently recommends vaccination with the Dengvaxia vaccine for children aged 9 through 16 years of age who live in an area where dengue is endemic and have evidence of a previous dengue infection; as of December 2023, the ACIP had not yet voted on recommending its lower age range align with the FDA's approved range. Evidence of previous dengue infection, such as laboratory confirmation of a previous dengue infection or detection of anti-dengue virus IgG using a highly specific serodiagnostic test, is required for eligible children before vaccination. Dengvaxia is contraindicated in children with severe immunodeficiency or immunosuppression attributable to underlying disease or therapy, including children with symptomatic HIV infection or CD4+ T-lymphocyte count of <200/mm^3.

Analyses of data from clinical trials revealed an increased risk for severe dengue in seronegative vaccine recipients compared with seropositive vaccine recipients, while confirming efficacy in preventing dengue cases, severe dengue, and hospitalizations attributable to any serotype in seropositive individuals. For this reason, CYD-TDV is not approved for use in individuals not infected previously by any dengue virus serotype or for whom this information is unknown, because those not infected previously are at increased risk for severe dengue when vaccinated and subsequently infected with dengue virus. Previous dengue infection can be documented by providing history of a laboratory-confirmed dengue infection or a positive result of a highly accurate serodiagnostic screening test. Immunogenicity and safety of recombinant live attenuated dengue vaccine after administration of immune globulin intravenous (IGIV) and other immunoglobulin-containing products has not been studied. Clinicians considering dengue vaccine for people who recently received blood products (including IGIV) or other immunoglobulin-containing products should delay prevaccination testing and administration of vaccine doses by 12 months. Safety and effectiveness of CYD-TDV have not been established in individuals living in areas where dengue is not endemic but who travel to areas with endemic infection, and this vaccine is not recommended for travelers.

Another live attenuated tetravalent dengue vaccine (QDENGA), administered subcutaneously as a 0.5-mL dose in a 2-dose schedule (0 and 3 months), is approved for use in several countries outside of the United States in individuals 4 years or older regardless of previous dengue exposure. However, on July 11, 2023, Takeda voluntarily withdrew the QDENGA biologic license application from US FDA review, so no approval in the United States is anticipated.

People traveling to areas where dengue is endemic (**www.healthmap.org/dengue/**) are at risk of dengue and should take precautions to protect themselves from mosquito bites. Travelers should select accommodations that are air conditioned and/or have screened windows and doors and use a bed net to sleep, although this may have limited effect because the vector mosquitoes bite primarily during the day. Travelers should wear clothing that covers arms and legs completely whenever possible, especially during early morning and late afternoon, and use mosquito repellents registered by the US Environmental Protection Agency (see Prevention of Mosquito-borne and Tick-borne Infections, p 207).

Public Health Reporting. Dengue is a nationally notifiable disease, whether obtained locally in the United States or during travel. Suspected cases should be reported to the state or local health department.

Diphtheria

CLINICAL MANIFESTATIONS: Respiratory tract diphtheria usually presents as membranous nasopharyngitis, obstructive laryngotracheitis, or bloody nasal discharge. Local infections are associated with low-grade fever and gradual onset of manifestations over 1 to 2 days. Less commonly, diphtheria presents as cutaneous, vaginal, conjunctival, or otic infection. Cutaneous diphtheria is more common in tropical areas and among people in urban areas lacking housing; the disease is typically mild and associated with shallow, indistinct ulcers. With upper respiratory infection, extensive neck swelling with cervical lymphadenitis (bull neck) is a sign of severe disease. Life-threatening complications of respiratory diphtheria include upper airway obstruction caused by membrane formation; myocarditis with heart block; and cranial and peripheral neuropathies. Palatal palsy, noted by nasal speech, frequently occurs in pharyngeal diphtheria. Case fatality rates attributable to respiratory disease are 5% to 10% and up to 50% in untreated people.

ETIOLOGY: Diphtheria is caused by toxigenic strains of *Corynebacterium diphtheriae*. Toxigenic strains of 2 zoonotic strains, *Corynebacterium ulcerans* and *Corynebacterium pseudotuberculosis*, also have emerged as important causes of diphtheria-like illness. *C diphtheriae* is an irregularly staining, gram-positive, non–spore-forming, nonmotile, pleomorphic bacillus with 4 biotypes (*mitis, intermedius, gravis*, and *belfanti*). All biotypes of *C diphtheriae* may be toxigenic or nontoxigenic. Bacteria remain confined to superficial layers of skin or mucosal surfaces, inducing a local inflammatory reaction. Within several days of respiratory tract infection, a dense pseudomembrane forms, becoming adherent to tissue. Toxigenic strains produce an exotoxin that consists of an enzymatically active A domain and a binding B domain, which promotes the entry of the A toxin into the cell. The toxin, an ADP-ribosylase, inhibits protein synthesis in all cells, including myocardial, renal, and peripheral nerve cells, resulting in myocarditis, acute tubular necrosis, and delayed peripheral nerve conduction. Nontoxigenic strains of *C diphtheriae* can cause an exudative pharyngitis and also have been associated with invasive infections including endocarditis and osteomyelitis.

EPIDEMIOLOGY: Humans are believed to be the sole reservoir of *C diphtheriae*. Infection is spread by respiratory tract droplets and by contact with discharges from skin lesions. In untreated people, organisms can be present in discharges from the nose and throat and from eye and skin lesions for 2 to 6 weeks after infection. Patients treated with an appropriate antimicrobial agent usually are not infectious beginning 48 hours after treatment is initiated. Transmission results from close contact with patients or carriers. People traveling to areas with endemic diphtheria or people who come into contact with infected travelers from such areas are at increased risk of infection; rarely, fomites or milk products can serve as vehicles of transmission. Severe disease occurs more often in people who are unimmunized or inadequately immunized. Fully immunized people may be asymptomatic carriers or have mild sore throat.

Prior to 2019, respiratory disease caused by *C diphtheriae*, regardless of toxigenicity status, was nationally notifiable. From 2000 through 2018, 8 cases of respiratory diphtheria were reported in the United States; however, the last bacteriologically confirmed case caused by toxigenic *C diphtheriae* occurred in 1997. There has been increasing recognition of cutaneous diphtheria, with 4 toxigenic cases identified from 2015 to 2018 among travelers to areas with endemic diphtheria. Therefore, beginning in 2019, national notification requirements were changed to capture disease caused by toxigenic *C diphtheriae* originating from any anatomic (respiratory or nonrespiratory) site. In the years 2019–2020, there were 3 cases of nonrespiratory diphtheria (2 cutaneous infections and 1 bloodstream infection) reported in the United States.

The incidence of respiratory diphtheria is greatest during fall and winter, but summer epidemics may occur in warm climates where skin infections are prevalent. Globally, endemic diphtheria occurs in parts of Africa, Latin American, Asia, the Middle East, and Europe, where immunization coverage with diphtheria toxoid-containing vaccines is suboptimal. Since 2011, large outbreaks have been reported in Indonesia, Laos, Haiti, Venezuela, Yemen, and Bangladesh. In 2020, the World Health Organization reported 10 107 global cases of diphtheria; although this was a decline in the number of reported cases compared with previous years, reporting was likely impacted by the COVID-19 pandemic.

The **incubation period** usually is 2 to 5 days (range, 1–10 days).

DIAGNOSTIC TESTS: Laboratory personnel should be notified if *C diphtheriae* is suspected. Specimens for culture should be obtained from the nares and throat and from any mucosal or cutaneous lesion. Obtaining multiple samples from respiratory sites increases yield of culture. Material should be obtained for culture from beneath the membrane (if present) or a portion of the membrane. Specimens collected for culture can be placed in any transport medium or in a sterile container and transported at 4°C. All isolates of *C diphtheriae* should be sent through the state health department to the Centers for Disease Control and Prevention (CDC) to verify toxigenicity status.

TREATMENT:

Antitoxin. Because patients with respiratory diphtheria can deteriorate rapidly, a single dose of diphtheria (equine) antitoxin (DAT) should be administered on the basis of clinical presentation, history of travel, and vaccination status before culture results are available. DAT, its indications for use, suggested dosage, and instructions for administration are available through the CDC Emergency Operations Center (telephone: 770-488-7100 or **www.cdc.gov/diphtheria/dat.html**). DAT is not available from any commercial source. To neutralize toxin as rapidly as possible, intravenous administration of antitoxin is preferred. Before intravenous administration of antitoxin, tests for sensitivity to horse serum should be performed according to instructions provided with the material. Allergic reactions to horse serum varying from anaphylaxis to rash can be expected in 5% to 20% of patients. The dose of antitoxin depends on the site and size of the membrane, duration of illness, and degree of toxic effects, and specific recommendations are available from the CDC. DAT is generally not recommended in cases of nonrespiratory diphtheria.

Antimicrobial Therapy. 14 days of erythromycin administered orally or parenterally or penicillin administered orally, intravenously, or intramuscularly constitute acceptable therapy for respiratory and nonrespiratory *C diphtheriae* infections (regardless of toxigenicity status) (see Table 4.3, p 993). Parenteral therapy should be given if the patient has severe disease or is unable to swallow. In areas of the world where there is increasing resistance of *C diphtheriae* isolates to penicillin, erythromycin is preferred empiric treatment. Fluoroquinolones (see Fluoroquinolones, p 973), rifampin, clarithromycin, and azithromycin have demonstrated in vitro activity against *C diphtheriae*. Antimicrobial therapy is required to eradicate *C diphtheriae* organisms, stop toxin production, and prevent transmission but is not a substitute for antitoxin. Elimination of the toxigenic *C diphtheriae* should be documented 24 hours after completion of treatment by 2 consecutive negative cultures from specimens taken 24 hours apart for both respiratory and nonrespiratory infections. Follow-up testing to confirm elimination is not required for nontoxigenic *C diphtheriae* infections.

Immunization. Active immunization against diphtheria should be undertaken during convalescence from diphtheria, because disease does not necessarily confer immunity.

Cutaneous Diphtheria. Thorough cleansing of the lesion with soap and water and administration of an appropriate antimicrobial agent for 10 days are recommended.

Carriers. If not immunized, *C diphtheriae* carriers should receive active immunization promptly and measures should be taken to ensure completion of the immunization schedule. If a carrier has been immunized previously but has not received a booster of diphtheria toxoid within 5 years, a booster dose of age-appropriate vaccine containing diphtheria toxoid (DTaP, Tdap, or Td) should be administered. Note that as of 2023, DT is no longer available in the United States (**www.cdc.gov/vaccines/vpd/dtap-tdap-td/hcp/recommendations.html** and **www.cdc.gov/vaccines/vpd/dtap-tdap-td/hcp/td-offlabel.html**). Carriers should receive antibiotic treatment with any of the following regimens: oral erythromycin for 10 to 14 days, oral azithromycin for 5 days, or a single dose of intramuscularly administered penicillin G benzathine.[1] Data are limited on the use of oral penicillin to eradicate carriage. If a person is carrying a toxigenic *C diphtheriae* strain, 2 follow-up cultures should be performed after completing antimicrobial treatment to detect persistence of carriage, which occurs following erythromycin treatment in some cases. The first culture should be performed 24 hours after completing treatment. If results of either culture is positive, an additional 10-day course of oral erythromycin should be administered and follow-up cultures should be performed again. Erythromycin-resistant strains have been identified, but their epidemiologic significance is undetermined. Follow-up cultures are not required for nontoxigenic *C diphtheriae* carriers.

INFECTION PREVENTION AND CONTROL MEASURES IN HEALTH CARE SETTINGS: In addition to standard precautions, droplet precautions are recommended for patients and carriers with respiratory diphtheria until 2 cultures from both the nose and throat collected 24 hours or more after completing antimicrobial treatment are negative for *C diphtheriae*. Contact precautions are recommended for patients with cutaneous diphtheria until 2 cultures of skin lesions taken at least 24 hours apart and 24 hours after cessation of antimicrobial therapy are negative.

CONTROL MEASURES:

Care of Exposed People. Whenever respiratory diphtheria is suspected or proven, local public health officials should be notified promptly. Toxigenic *C diphtheriae* isolated from any anatomical site (respiratory or nonrespiratory) requires contact investigation and prophylaxis of close contacts. Cutaneous or respiratory disease caused by nontoxigenic strains of *C diphtheriae* do not require routine investigation or prophylaxis of contacts. Management of exposed people is based on individual circumstances, including immunization status and likelihood of adherence to follow-up and prophylaxis. Close

---

[1] UK Health Security Agency. Public health control and management of diphtheria in England. 2022 guidelines. Available at: **https://assets.publishing.service.gov.uk/government/uploads/system/uploads/attachment_data/file/1106302/diphtheria-guidelines-2022-v16.1-corrected.pdf**

contacts of a person with infection caused by toxigenic diphtheria should be identified, and the following are recommended:

- Contact tracing usually can be limited to household members and people with direct, habitual close contact with the index patient or health care personnel exposed to nasopharyngeal secretions, people sharing kitchen facilities, or people caring for infected children.
- For close contacts, *regardless of their immunization status,* the following measures should be taken: (1) surveillance for evidence of disease for 7 days from last exposure to an untreated patient; (2) culture for *C diphtheriae;* and (3) antimicrobial prophylaxis with oral erythromycin (40–50 mg/kg per day for 7 to 10 days, maximum 1 g/day) or a single intramuscular injection of penicillin G benzathine (600 000 U for children weighing <30 kg, and 1.2 million U for children weighing ≥30 kg and for adults). Follow-up cultures of nasal or oropharyngeal specimens should be performed after completion of therapy for contacts proven to be carriers. If cultures are positive, an additional 10-day course of erythromycin should be administered, and follow-up cultures of pharyngeal specimens should be repeated after completion of therapy.
- Asymptomatic, previously immunized close contacts should receive a booster dose of an age-appropriate diphtheria toxoid-containing vaccine (DTaP, Tdap, or Td) if they have not received a booster dose of a diphtheria toxoid-containing vaccine within 5 years.
- Asymptomatic close contacts who have had fewer than 3 doses of a diphtheria toxoid-containing vaccine, children younger than 7 years in need of their fourth dose of DTaP, or people whose immunization status is not known should be immunized with an age-appropriate diphtheria toxoid-containing vaccine (DTaP, Tdap, or Td), as indicated.
- Contacts who cannot be kept under surveillance should receive penicillin G benzathine rather than erythromycin, and if not fully immunized or if immunization status is not known, they should be immunized with DTaP, Tdap, or Td vaccine, as appropriate for age.
- Use of equine diphtheria antitoxin in unimmunized close contacts is not recommended, because there is no evidence that antitoxin provides additional benefit.

Immunization. Universal immunization with a diphtheria toxoid-containing vaccine is the only effective control measure. The schedules for immunization against diphtheria are presented in the childhood and adolescent (**https://publications.aap.org/redbook/pages/Immunization-Schedules**) and adult (**www.cdc.gov/vaccines**) immunization schedules.

Immunization of children from 2 months of age through 6 years of age (to the seventh birthday) routinely consists of 5 doses of diphtheria and tetanus toxoid-containing and acellular pertussis vaccines (DTaP). Regular booster injections of diphtheria toxoid as Td or Tdap are required every 10 years after completion of the initial immunization series. Immunization against diphtheria and tetanus for children younger than 7 years in whom pertussis immunization is contraindicated (see Pertussis, p 656) is complicated by the fact that DT is no longer available in the United States (**www.cdc.gov/vaccines/vpd/dtap-tdap-td/hcp/recommendations.html** and **www.cdc.gov/vaccines/vpd/dtap-tdap-td/hcp/td-offlabel.html**). For young children with a contraindication to pertussis-containing vaccines (see Contraindications and Precautions to DTaP Immunization in the Pertussis chapter, p 664), vaccine providers may administer Td for all recommended remaining doses in place of DTaP.

Td contains a lower dose (approximately 1/12th the amount) of diphtheria toxoid compared with DT. The impact of this lower dose on the protection provided against diphtheria in young children is uncertain. Available evidence suggests young children who receive Td in place of DTaP may have suboptimal protection against diphtheria. Other recommendations for diphtheria immunization, including recommendations for older children (7 through 18 years of age) and adults, can be found in Tetanus (p 848) as well as the childhood and adolescent and adult immunization schedules.

Travelers to countries with endemic or epidemic diphtheria should have their diphtheria immunization status reviewed and updated when necessary.

Pneumococcal and meningococcal conjugate vaccines containing non-live diphtheria toxoid or CRM_{197} protein, a nontoxic variant of diphtheria toxin, are not substitutes for diphtheria toxoid immunization.

Ehrlichia, Anaplasma, and Related Infections
(Human Ehrlichiosis, Anaplasmosis, and Related Infections Attributable to Bacteria in the Family *Anaplasmataceae*)

CLINICAL MANIFESTATIONS: Early signs and symptoms of infections by members of the bacterial family *Anaplasmataceae* can be nonspecific. All are acute febrile illnesses with common systemic manifestations including fever, headache, chills, rigors, malaise, myalgia, and nausea. More variable symptoms include rash, arthralgia, vomiting, diarrhea, anorexia, cough, and confusion. Severe manifestations of these diseases can include acute respiratory distress syndrome, encephalopathy, meningitis, disseminated intravascular coagulation, toxic shock-like or septic shock-like syndromes, spontaneous hemorrhage, hepatic failure, and renal failure. Symptoms typically last 1 to 2 weeks when untreated, but prompt treatment with doxycycline shortens duration of illness and reduces the risk of serious manifestations and sequelae. Fatigue can last several weeks, and neurologic sequelae have been reported in some children after severe disease, more commonly with *Ehrlichia* infections.

A maculopapular rash is seen in up to 60% of ***Ehrlichia chaffeensis* infections** in children but in less than 30% of adults. The rash typically begins 5 days after symptom onset (notably fever). In adults, skin rash is reported more often for *Ehrlichia* infections than for *Anaplasma* infections. Rash occurs in less than 10% of cases of anaplasmosis and may suggest coinfection with another pathogen. Severe disease and fatal outcome are more common in *E chaffeensis* infections (approximately 1%–3% case fatality) than in *Anaplasma phagocytophilum* infections.

Coinfections of ***Anaplasma*** with other tick-borne diseases, including babesiosis, Powassan virus, Lyme disease, and other *Borrelia* infections, can cause illness that is more severe or of longer duration than a single infection. Case fatality is uncommon (<1%).

Significant laboratory findings in **both *Anaplasma* and *Ehrlichia* infections** may include leukopenia with neutropenia (anaplasmosis) or lymphopenia (ehrlichiosis), thrombocytopenia, hyponatremia, and elevated serum hepatic aminotransferase concentrations. Cerebrospinal fluid abnormalities (eg, pleocytosis with a predominance of lymphocytes and increased total protein concentration) are common. Hemophagocytic lymphohistiocytosis (HLH) occurs in 10% to 15% of children hospitalized with ehrlichiosis. People with underlying immunosuppressive conditions are at greater risk of severe disease. Severe disease has been reported in people who initially received trimethoprim-sulfamethoxazole before a correct diagnosis was made.

Table 3.5. Taxonomy of *Rickettsiales* predominant in the United States

Order	*Rickettsiales*			
Family	*Rickettsiaceae*		*Anaplasmataceae*	
Genera	*Rickettsiae*		*Anaplasma*	*Ehrlichia*
Species	Spotted fever group (SFG): Rocky Mountain spotted fever, Mediterranean spotted fever, Japanese spotted fever, etc	Typhus group: endemic, epidemic	*Anaplasma phagocytophilum*	*Ehrlichia chaffeensis, Ehrlichia ewingii, Ehrlichia muris eauclairensis*

Because of the nonspecific presenting symptoms, Rocky Mountain spotted fever should be considered in the differential diagnosis in the United States. Heartland and Bourbon virus infections also manifest with similar clinical features and should be considered in patients without a more likely explanation who have tested negative for *Ehrlichia* and *Anaplasma* infection or have not responded to doxycycline therapy.

ETIOLOGY: *Ehrlichia* and *Anaplasma* species are obligate intracellular bacteria, which appear as gram-negative cocci that measure 0.5 to 1.5 μm in diameter. Although genetically distinct, *Anaplasma* and *Ehrlichia* infections often are grouped with rickettsia because of overlapping clinical presentation and their vector-borne spread (Table 3.5). Ehrlichiosis is the manifestation of (predominantly) *E chaffeensis*, although *Ehrlichia ewingii* and *Ehrlichia muris eauclairensis* also are found in the United States (Table 3.6). Anaplasmosis is predominantly caused by *A phagocytophilum* in the United States.

EPIDEMIOLOGY: Reported and suspected cases of ehrlichiosis and anaplasmosis are confined to geographic regions where their vectors are prevalent, although climate change is impacting the geographic range of these vectors. Increased incidence is observed with heightened tick activity (mostly warm summer months) as well as with human activities involving exposure to ticks. Infections can occur year-round in endemic areas. As in other tick-borne diseases, patients with *Ehrlichia* or *Anaplasma* infection often have no recollection of being bitten by a tick.

The reported incidence of ***E chaffeensis* infection** in the United States in 2019 was 6.4 cases per million population. Reported incidence of *E ewingii* infection in 2017 was 0.1 cases per million population, but the incidence is believed to be underreported because of nonspecific illness similar to *E chaffeensis* infections. Ehrlichiosis caused by *E chaffeensis* and *E ewingii* is reported most commonly from the south-central and south-eastern United States, from the East Coast extending westward to Texas. *E chaffeensis* and *E ewingii* are transmitted by the bite of the Lone Star tick *(Amblyomma americanum)* and are reported from states within its geographic range. Cases attributable to *E muris eauclairensis* have been reported only from Minnesota and Wisconsin and are transmitted by the blacklegged tick *(Ixodes scapularis)*. Cases of ehrlichiosis have occurred after blood transfusion or solid organ donation from asymptomatic donors.

There were 6617 provisional cases of ***Anaplasma* infections** reported in the United States in 2021. Cases of human anaplasmosis are reported most frequently from the northeastern and upper midwestern United States. Cases of anaplasmosis

Table 3.6. Human Ehrlichiosis, Anaplasmosis, and Related Infections in the United States

Disease	Causal Agent	Major Target Cell	Tick Vector	Geographic Distribution
Ehrlichiosis caused by *Ehrlichia chaffeensis*	*E chaffeensis*	Usually monocytes	Lone star tick (US) *(Amblyomma americanum)*	Predominantly southeast, south-central, from the East Coast extending westward to Texas; has been reported outside USA
Anaplasmosis	*Anaplasma phagocytophilum*	Usually granulocytes	Blacklegged tick *(Ixodes scapularis)* or western blacklegged tick *(Ixodes pacificus)* (US)	Northeastern and upper Midwestern states and northern California; Europe and Asia
Ehrlichiosis caused by *Ehrlichia ewingii*	*E ewingii*	Usually granulocytes	Lone star tick (US) *(A americanum)*	Southeastern, south-central, and Midwestern states; Africa, Asia
Ehrlichiosis caused by *Ehrlichia muris eauclairensis*	*E muris eauclairensis*	Unknown, suspected in monocytes	Blacklegged tick *(Ixodes scapularis)*	Minnesota, Wisconsin

also have been reported in northern California. In most of the United States, *A phagocytophilum* is transmitted by *Ixodes scapularis,* which also is the vector for ehrlichiosis caused by *E muris eauclairensis,* Lyme disease *(Borrelia burgdorferi* and *Borrelia mayoni),* tickborne relapsing fever *(Borrelia miyamotoi),* Powassan virus, and babesiosis *(Babesia microti).* In the western United States, the western blacklegged tick *(Ixodes pacificus)* is the main vector for *A phagocytophilum.* Cases of *Anaplasma* infection have occurred after blood transfusion or solid organ donation from asymptomatic donors. Possible perinatal transmission of *A phagocytophilum* has been reported.

The **incubation period** is 5 to 14 days for both *E chaffeensis* and *A phagocytophilum.*

DIAGNOSTIC TESTS: Treatment of suspected ehrlichiosis or anaplasmosis with doxycycline should not be delayed while awaiting confirmation of the diagnosis. Nucleic acid amplification tests (NAATs) of whole blood for the organism are most sensitive for anaplasmosis and ehrlichiosis in the first week of illness. A negative result does not rule out the diagnosis. Sensitivity of NAATs decreases rapidly following administration of doxycycline.

Tissue biopsies may be analyzed by NAAT or immunohistochemistry. Because of the hazardous nature of these organisms, tissues should be fixed in paraffin or formalin before testing. Tissue analysis is available at specialized laboratories.

Serologic testing may be used to demonstrate a fourfold change in specific immunoglobulin (Ig) G antibody titer by indirect immunofluorescent antibody (IFA) assay between paired acute and convalescent specimens taken 2 to 4 weeks apart. A single mildly elevated IgG titer may not be diagnostic, particularly in regions with higher prevalence. IgM serologic assays are prone to false-positive reactions, and specific IgM can remain elevated for lengthy periods of time, reducing its diagnostic utility. Serologic tests for *E chaffeensis* and *A phagocytophilum* infections are available, but cross-reactivity between species can make interpretation of results difficult in areas where geographic distributions overlap.

Occasionally, *Anaplasma* and *Ehrlichia* bacteria can be identified in Giemsa or Wright-stained peripheral blood smears or buffy coat leukocyte preparations in the first week of illness. Bacteria enter the host cell via phagocytosis, and these compartments provide a protective environment for bacterial replication. These bacterial collections appear as morulae observed within granulocytes (targeted by *Anaplasma*) or monocytes (targeted by *Ehrlichia*). Culture for isolation of these pathogens is not performed routinely given requirement for biosafety level 3 facilities to prevent accidental inoculation or aerosolization.

TREATMENT: Doxycycline is the treatment of choice for all tick-borne rickettsial diseases, including ehrlichiosis and anaplasmosis (see Table 4.3, p 993). Early initiation of therapy can minimize complications and should not be delayed awaiting laboratory confirmation. Treatment with doxycycline is recommended in patients of all ages when rickettsial diseases are being considered (see Tetracyclines, p 975). After doxycycline is initiated, fever generally subsides within 24 to 48 hours.

Patients with suspected **ehrlichiosis** should be treated with doxycycline until at least 3 days after defervescence and until evidence of clinical improvement, typically 5 to 7 days. Patients with suspected **anaplasmosis** should be treated with doxycycline for 10 to 14 days to provide appropriate length of therapy for possible concurrent *Borrelia burgdorferi* infection (Lyme disease).

Rifampin may provide an alternative to doxycycline in patients with anaplasmosis who demonstrate hypersensitivity to doxycycline. Rifampin has been used successfully in several pregnant people with anaplasmosis, and studies suggest that this drug appears effective against *A phagocytophilum*. Small numbers of young children have also been treated successfully for anaplasmosis with rifampin for 7 to 10 days. Rifampin is not an effective treatment when coinfection with Lyme disease is present, nor is it effective treatment for Rocky Mountain spotted fever, a disease with similar clinical manifestations. Rifampin has been shown to be effective against *E chaffeensis* in a laboratory setting but has not been evaluated as an alternative therapy in a clinical setting.

Administration of trimethoprim-sulfamethoxazole has been linked to more severe outcomes in ehrlichiosis and is contraindicated.

INFECTION PREVENTION AND CONTROL MEASURES IN HEALTH CARE SETTINGS: Standard precautions are recommended. Human-to-human transmission via direct contact has not been documented.

CONTROL MEASURES: Limiting exposures to ticks and tick bites is the primary means of prevention (see Prevention of Mosquito-borne and Tick-borne Infections, p 207).

Risk of transmission through blood transfusion or organ transplantation should be considered in areas with endemic infection. Prophylactic administration of doxycycline after a tick bite is not indicated because of the low risk of infection and lack of proven effectiveness. Instead, persons bitten by ticks should be counseled to watch for symptoms, including fever and rash, within 2 weeks of a tick bite. Additional information is available on the Centers for Disease Control and Prevention (CDC) website (**www.cdc.gov/ehrlichiosis, www.cdc.gov/anaplasmosis** and **www.cdc.gov/ticks**), including a collaborative report providing recommendations for the diagnosis and management of tick-borne rickettsial diseases.[1]

Public Health Reporting. Ehrlichiosis and anaplasmosis are nationally notifiable diseases in the United States and should be reported to the state or local health department.

Serious Neonatal Bacterial Infections Caused by *Enterobacterales*
(Including Septicemia and Meningitis)

CLINICAL MANIFESTATIONS: Neonatal septicemia or meningitis caused by *Escherichia coli* and other gram-negative bacilli cannot be differentiated clinically from septicemia or meningitis caused by other organisms. The early signs of sepsis can be subtle and similar to signs observed in noninfectious processes. Signs of septicemia include fever, temperature instability, heart rate abnormalities, grunting respirations, apnea, cyanosis, lethargy, irritability, anorexia, vomiting, jaundice, abdominal distention, cellulitis, and diarrhea. Meningitis, especially early in the course, can occur without overt signs suggesting central nervous system involvement. Some gram-negative bacilli, such as *Citrobacter koseri*, *Cronobacter* (formerly *Enterobacter*) *sakazakii*, *Serratia marcescens*, and *Salmonella* species, are associated with increased risk for brain abscesses in infants with meningitis caused by these organisms.

ETIOLOGY: *Enterobacterales* are a large family of gram-negative, facultatively anaerobic, rod-shaped bacteria that include *Escherichia* species, *Klebsiella* species, *Enterobacter* species, *Proteus* species, *Providencia* species, and *Serratia* species, among many others. *E coli* strains, often those with the K1 capsular polysaccharide antigen, are the most common cause of neonatal septicemia and meningitis by *Enterobacterales* species. Other important *Enterobacterales* species causing neonatal septicemia include *Klebsiella* species, *Enterobacter* species, *Proteus* species, *Citrobacter* species, *Salmonella* species, and *Serratia* species. *Elizabethkinga meningoseptica*, although not an *Enterobacterales* species, is another multidrug-resistant gram-negative organism that causes a similar spectrum of disease in neonates.

EPIDEMIOLOGY: The source of *E coli* and other *Enterobacterales* organisms in neonatal infections during the first days of life typically is the vaginal tract of the birthing parent. Reservoirs for gram-negative bacilli can also be present within the health care environment. Acquisition of gram-negative organisms can occur through person-to-person transmission from hospital nursery personnel as well as from

[1] Biggs HM, Behravesh CB, Bradley KK, et al. Diagnosis and management of tickborne rickettsial diseases: Rocky Mountain spotted fever and other spotted fever group rickettsioses, ehrlichioses, and anaplasmosis—United States. *MMWR Recomm Rep.* 2016;65(RR-2):1–44. Available at: **www.cdc.gov/mmwr/volumes/65/rr/rr6502a1.htm**

nursery environmental sites such as sinks, countertops, powdered infant formula, and respiratory therapy equipment, especially among very preterm infants who require prolonged neonatal intensive care management. Predisposing factors for neonatal gram-negative bacterial infections include intrapartum infection in the birthing parent, gestation less than 37 weeks, low birth weight, and prolonged rupture of membranes. Metabolic abnormalities (eg, galactosemia), fetal hypoxia, and acidosis have been implicated as predisposing factors. Neonates with defects in the integrity of skin or mucosa (eg, myelomeningocele) or abnormalities of gastrointestinal or genitourinary tracts are at increased risk of gram-negative bacterial infections. In neonatal intensive care units, systems for respiratory and metabolic support, invasive or surgical procedures, and indwelling vascular catheters are risk factors for infection. Frequent use of broad-spectrum antimicrobial agents enables selection and proliferation of strains of gram-negative bacilli that may be resistant to multiple antimicrobial agents.

Multiple mechanisms of resistance in gram-negative bacilli can be present simultaneously. Resistance resulting from production of plasmid-derived extended-spectrum beta-lactamases (ESBLs) and AmpC beta-lactamases occurs primarily in *E coli* and *Klebsiella* species and from production of chromosomally-encoded AmpC beta-lactamases in *Enterobacter* species, but these mechanisms have been reported in many other gram-negative species. Resistant gram-negative infections have been associated with nursery outbreaks, especially in very low birth weight infants. Risk factors for neonatal infection with ESBL-producing organisms include prolonged mechanical ventilation, extended hospital stay, use of invasive devices, and prior use of antimicrobial agents. Infants whose birthing parent is colonized with ESBL-producing *E coli* are themselves at an increased risk of becoming colonized with ESBL-producing *E coli* compared with infants whose birthing parent is noncolonized. Organisms that produce ESBLs typically are resistant to penicillins, cephalosporins, and monobactams and can be resistant to aminoglycosides. Carbapenem-resistant *Enterobacterales* (CRE) that produce carbapenemases have also emerged, especially among *Klebsiella pneumoniae*, *E coli*, and *Enterobacter cloacae*. ESBL- and carbapenemase-producing strains often carry additional plasmid-borne genes that encode for high-level resistance to aminoglycosides, fluoroquinolones, and trimethoprim-sulfamethoxazole.

The **incubation period** is variable; time of onset of infection ranges from birth to several weeks after birth or longer in very low birth weight, preterm infants with prolonged hospitalizations.

DIAGNOSTIC TESTS: Diagnosis is established by growth of *E coli* or other gram-negative bacilli from blood, cerebrospinal fluid (CSF), or other usually sterile sites. Isolates may be identified by traditional biochemical tests, commercially available biochemical test systems, mass spectrometry of bacterial cell components, or molecular methods. Multiplexed molecular tests capable of rapidly identifying a variety of gram-negative rods including *E coli* directly in positive blood culture bottles have been cleared by the US Food and Drug Administration. Special screening and confirmatory laboratory procedures are required to detect some multidrug-resistant gram-negative organisms. Molecular diagnostics can rapidly identify pathogens and some resistance genes from positive blood cultures but do not detect all phenotypic resistance; therefore, antimicrobial resistance testing should be performed on isolates.

TREATMENT[1,2]:

- Initial empiric treatment for suspected early-onset gram-negative sepsis in neonates should be based on local and regional antimicrobial susceptibility data. The proportion of *E coli* bloodstream infections with onset within 72 hours of life that are resistant to ampicillin is high (approximately two-thirds) among very low birth weight infants. These *E coli* infections almost invariably are susceptible to gentamicin, although monotherapy with an aminoglycoside is not recommended.

- Ampicillin and an aminoglycoside may be first-line therapy for neonatal sepsis in areas with low ampicillin resistance among *E coli*. An alternative regimen of ampicillin and an extended-spectrum cephalosporin (eg, cefotaxime, ceftazidime, cefepime) can be used, but rapid emergence of cephalosporin-resistant organisms and increased risk of colonization or infection with ESBL-producing *Enterobacterales* can occur when cephalosporin use is routine in a neonatal unit. The empiric addition of broader-spectrum antibiotic therapy may be considered until culture results are available if the patient is a severely ill infant at high risk for gram-negative sepsis (such as infants with very low birth weight born after prolonged premature rupture of membranes, infants exposed to prolonged courses of antepartum antibiotic therapy, or infants with prolonged neonatal intensive care unit [NICU] hospitalization and exposure to multiple medical devices and antimicrobials).

- When there is a concern for gram-negative meningitis, an extended-spectrum cephalosporin (eg, cefotaxime, ceftazidime, cefepime) should be used unless prior patient isolates or local resistance profiles increase the likelihood of a multidrug-resistant gram-negative organism, in which case a carbapenem is the preferred choice for empiric therapy.

- Once the causative agent and its in vitro antimicrobial susceptibility pattern are known, nonmeningeal infections should be treated with the narrowest-spectrum antibiotic to which the organism is susceptible.

- For meningitis caused by an ampicillin-susceptible *E coli*, meningitic dosing of ampicillin is the preferred treatment because it is effective and narrow-spectrum. Meningitis caused by an ampicillin-resistant isolate can be treated with an extended spectrum cephalosporin to which it is susceptible. Combination therapy of a beta-lactam with an aminoglycoside can be used until CSF is sterile in complicated meningitis associated with empyema, brain abscess, or other scenarios that may delay CSF sterility. Expert advice from a pediatric infectious diseases specialist is helpful for management of meningitis.

- For ESBL-producing *Enterobacterales* infections, a carbapenem is the drug of choice. Of the aminoglycosides, amikacin retains the most activity against ESBL-producing strains.

- For *Enterobacterales* isolates that contain AmpC beta-lactamase but not ESBLs, cefepime can be used if susceptible, because cefepime does not induce AmpC expression and it resists hydrolysis by AmpC β-lactamases.

[1] Puopolo KM, Benitz WE, Zaoutis TE; American Academy of Pediatrics, Committee on Fetus and Newborn; Committee on Infectious Diseases. Management of neonates born at ≤34 6/7 weeks' gestation with suspected or proven early-onset bacterial sepsis. *Pediatrics*. 2018;142(6):e20182896

[2] Puopolo KM, Benitz WE, Zaoutis TE; American Academy of Pediatrics, Committee on Fetus and Newborn; Committee on Infectious Diseases. Management of neonates born at ≥35 0/7 weeks' gestation with suspected or proven early-onset bacterial sepsis. *Pediatrics*. 2018;142(6):e20182894

- For CRE, treatment should be tailored to the susceptibility profile of the isolate and the type of carbapenemase. Combination antibiotic therapy is often used. Antibiotics that may have activity against CRE include amikacin, trimethoprim-sulfamethoxazole, fluroquinolones, tigecycline, colistin, and polymyxin B.[1] Tigecycline has a black box warning for an increase in all-cause mortality and should be reserved for situations in which alternative agents are not suitable. In neonates, there is limited experience using newer antibiotic agents with activity against CRE, like ceftazidime-avibactam, ceftolozane-tazobactam, imipenem-relebactam, or cefiderocol. Expert advice from a pediatric infectious disease specialist is recommended for management of infections caused by carbapenem-resistant organisms.
- All neonates with gram-negative meningitis should undergo repeat lumbar puncture to ensure sterility of the CSF after 48 to 72 hours of therapy. If CSF remains culture-positive, the choice and dose of antimicrobial agents should be reevaluated, and another lumbar puncture should be performed after an additional 48 to 72 hours.
- Duration of therapy is based on clinical and bacteriologic response of the patient and the site(s) of infection. The usual duration of therapy for uncomplicated gram-negative bacteremia in an infant who has had clearance of blood cultures and is clinically improving is 10 days. Infants with persistent bacteremia, prolonged clinical course, or other complications may require longer duration of therapy. The minimum treatment duration for gram-negative meningitis is 21 days; this may be extended if there are complications like brain abscess.
- All infants with gram-negative meningitis should undergo careful follow-up examinations, including testing for hearing loss, neurologic abnormalities, and developmental delay.
- Immune globulin intravenous (IGIV) therapy for newborn infants receiving antimicrobial agents for suspected or proven serious infection does not improve outcomes and is not recommended.

INFECTION PREVENTION AND CONTROL MEASURES IN HEALTH CARE SETTINGS: Standard precautions are recommended. Exceptions include hospital nursery epidemics, infants with *Salmonella* infection, and infants with infection caused by gram-negative bacilli that are resistant to multiple antimicrobial agents, including ESBL-producing strains and CRE; in these situations, contact precautions also are indicated.[2]

CONTROL MEASURES: Infection-control personnel should be aware of pathogens causing infections in infants so that clusters of infections are recognized and investigated appropriately. Several cases of infection caused by the same genus and species of bacteria occurring in infants in physical proximity or caused by an unusual pathogen indicate the need for an epidemiologic investigation and related infection prevention and control measures (see Infection Prevention and Control for Hospitalized Children, p 163). Periodic review of in vitro antimicrobial susceptibility patterns of clinically important bacterial isolates from newborn infants, especially infants in the neonatal intensive care unit, can provide useful epidemiologic and therapeutic information.

---

[1] Infectious Diseases Society of America. IDSA Guidance on the Treatment of Antimicrobial Resistant Gram-Negative Infections. Infectious Diseases Society of America; 2023. Available at: **www.idsociety. org/practice-guideline/amr-guidance/**

[2] Centers for Disease Control and Prevention. Facility Guidance for Control of Carbapenem Resistant Enterobacteriaceae (CRE) November 2015 Update. Available at: **www.cdc.gov/hai/pdfs/cre/CRE-guidance-508.pdf**

Enterovirus (Nonpoliovirus)
(Group A and B Coxsackieviruses, Echoviruses, Numbered Enteroviruses)

CLINICAL MANIFESTATIONS: Nonpolio enteroviruses are responsible for significant and frequent illnesses in infants and children and result in a variety of clinical manifestations. The most common manifestation is nonspecific febrile illness, which in young infants may lead to evaluation for bacterial sepsis. Other manifestations can include: (1) respiratory: coryza, pharyngitis, herpangina, stomatitis, parotitis, croup, bronchiolitis, pneumonia, pleurodynia, and bronchospasm; (2) skin: hand-foot-and-mouth disease (HFMD), onychomadesis (shedding of nails), and nonspecific exanthems (particularly associated with echoviruses); (3) neurologic: aseptic meningitis (with or without pleocytosis), encephalitis, and acute flaccid myelitis (AFM); (4) gastrointestinal/genitourinary: vomiting, diarrhea, abdominal pain, hepatitis, pancreatitis, and orchitis; (5) eye: acute hemorrhagic conjunctivitis and uveitis; (6) heart: myopericarditis; and (7) muscle: pleurodynia and other skeletal myositis. Neonates, especially those who acquire infection in the absence of type-specific transplacentally acquired antibody, are at risk of severe and life-threatening disease, including viral sepsis, meningoencephalitis, myocarditis, hepatitis, coagulopathy, and pneumonitis. AFM is an uncommon but serious neurologic illness caused by some enteroviruses that presents with acute onset of flaccid limb weakness and/or cranial nerve dysfunction, most often accompanied by cerebrospinal fluid pleocytosis and nonenhancing lesions predominantly affecting the gray matter of the spinal cord and/or brainstem on magnetic resonance imaging.

Infection with enterovirus A71 (EV-A71) is associated with HFMD, herpangina, and in a small proportion of cases, severe neurologic disease, including AFM and brainstem encephalitis associated with myoclonus, ataxia, and autonomic instability. Noncardiogenic pulmonary edema secondary to brainstem encephalitis can result in fatal cardiopulmonary collapse and sequelae among survivors.

Enterovirus D68 (EV-D68) is associated with mild to severe respiratory illness in infants, children, and teenagers and has been responsible for localized and large multinational outbreaks of respiratory disease. Disease is often characterized by exacerbation of preexisting asthma or new-onset wheezing in children without history of asthma, often requiring hospitalization and, in some patients, intensive supportive care. EV-D68 is also associated with AFM and is believed to have been a major contributor to the biennial AFM outbreaks in the United States between 2014 and 2018.

Other noteworthy but not exclusive clinical associations include coxsackieviruses (CV) A6, A10, and A16 with HFMD (including severe HFMD, "eczema coxsackium," and atypical cutaneous involvement with CVA6); coxsackievirus A24 variant and enterovirus D70 (EV-D70) with acute hemorrhagic conjunctivitis; and coxsackieviruses B1 through B5 with pleurodynia and myopericarditis.

Patients with humoral and combined immune deficiencies can develop persistent central nervous system infections, a dermatomyositis-like syndrome, arthritis, hepatitis, and/or disseminated infection. Severe and/or chronic neurologic or multisystem disease is reported in hematopoietic cell and solid organ transplant recipients, children with malignancies, and patients treated with anti-CD20 monoclonal antibody (eg, rituximab).

ETIOLOGY: The enteroviruses, along with the rhinoviruses, comprise a genus of small, nonenveloped, single-stranded, positive-sense RNA viruses in the *Picornaviridae* family.

The nonpolio enteroviruses include more than 110 distinct types formerly subclassified as group A coxsackieviruses, group B coxsackieviruses, echoviruses, and newer numbered enteroviruses. A more recent classification system groups the human enteroviruses into 4 species (enterovirus [EV] A, B, C, and D) on the basis of genetic similarity in the viral protein 1, which corresponds well with serotype.

EPIDEMIOLOGY: Humans are the principal reservoir for enteroviruses, although some primates can become infected. Enterovirus infections are common and are distributed worldwide; the majority of infections are asymptomatic. Enteroviruses are spread by fecal-oral and respiratory routes and from mother to infant prenatally, in the peripartum period, and rarely via breastfeeding. EV-D68 is believed to be spread primarily by respiratory transmission; EV-D70 and CVA24 are shed in tears and spread via fingers and fomites. Enteroviruses may survive on environmental surfaces for periods long enough to allow transmission from fomites, and transmission via contaminated water, including swimming pools, and food can occur. Hospital nursery and other institutional outbreaks may occur. Infection incidence, clinical attack rates, and disease severity typically are greatest in infants and young children, and infections occur more frequently in tropical areas and where poor sanitation, poor hygiene, and high population density are present.

Although circulation can occur year-round, most enterovirus infections in temperate climates occur in the summer and fall (approximately June through October in the northern hemisphere); seasonal patterns are less evident in the tropics. Fecal shedding of most enteroviruses can persist for several weeks or months (generally 2–8 weeks) after onset of infection, but respiratory tract shedding usually is limited to 1 to 3 weeks or less. Enterovirus transmission can occur in the absence of signs of clinical illness.

The usual **incubation period** for enterovirus infections is 3 to 6 days, except for acute hemorrhagic conjunctivitis, in which the **incubation period** is 24 to 72 hours. Onset of neurologic disease, such as AFM, can lag several days or even weeks after illness onset, following improvement or resolution of prodromal symptoms.

DIAGNOSTIC TESTS: Enteroviruses generally can be detected by nucleic acid amplification tests (NAATs) and culture from a variety of specimens, including stool, rectal swab, throat swab, nasopharyngeal aspirates, conjunctival swab, tracheal aspirates, vesicle fluid, blood, urine, tissue biopsy specimens, and cerebrospinal fluid (CSF). Prolonged viral shedding after illness occurs, particularly from the pharynx and gastrointestinal tract, so a positive test result may not indicate an etiologic role in an illness. NAATs are rapid and more sensitive than isolation of enteroviruses in cell culture and can detect all enteroviruses, including types that are difficult or impossible to cultivate in cell cultures. Commercial enterovirus NAATs will not detect parechoviruses (and vice versa), and many cannot reliably distinguish enteroviruses from rhinoviruses. Multiplex NAATs designed to detect a number of bacterial and viral agents of meningitis and encephalitis, including enteroviruses, in CSF are available.

Enterovirus type is determined though partial genomic sequencing. Typing may be indicated in cases of special clinical interest or for epidemiologic purposes (eg, for investigation of disease clusters or outbreaks) and is available at some local or state public health laboratories and at the Centers for Disease Control and Prevention Picornavirus Laboratory.

Patients with EV-A71 and EV-D68 neurologic disease often have negative results of a NAAT and culture of CSF (even in the presence of CSF pleocytosis) and blood.

For EV-A71, NAAT and culture of throat or stool/rectal swab and/or vesicle fluid specimens (in cases of HFMD) are more frequently positive. EV-D68 is demonstrated primarily in respiratory tract specimens obtained early in the course of disease. Most commercial multiplex respiratory NAATs can detect enteroviruses, including EV-D68, but do not distinguish enteroviruses from rhinoviruses. Definitive identification of EV-D68 requires partial genomic sequencing or amplification with an EV-D68-specific NAAT.

TREATMENT: No specific therapy is available for enteroviruses infections. Immune globulin intravenous (IGIV), administered intravenously or via intraventricular administration, may be beneficial for chronic enterovirus meningoencephalitis in immunodeficient patients. IGIV is not approved for intraventricular administration. IGIV also has been used for life-threatening neonatal enterovirus infections (convalescent plasma from the birthing parent also has been used), severe enterovirus infections in transplant recipients and people with malignancies, suspected viral myocarditis, EV-A71 neurologic disease, and AFM, but without proven clinical efficacy. The CDC has provided interim guidance on the clinical management of children with AFM (**www.cdc.gov/acute-flaccid-myelitis/hcp/clinical-management.html**). Interferons occasionally have been used for treatment of enterovirus-associated myocarditis and chronic enterovirus meningoencephalitis, without definitive proof of efficacy.

The antiviral drug pleconaril has in vitro activity against many enteroviruses but is not available commercially. Pocapavir, an antiviral drug that is being developed for the treatment of chronic poliovirus infection in immunodeficient patients, also has activity in vitro against some nonpolio enteroviruses. It is not commercially available but may be accessible under a compassionate use mechanism. Fluoxetine has in vitro activity against enterovirus species B and D (including EV-D68), but studies have not demonstrated clinical benefit.

INFECTION PREVENTION AND CONTROL MEASURES IN HEALTH CARE SETTINGS: In addition to standard precautions, contact precautions are indicated for infants and young children for the duration of enterovirus illness. Droplet precautions also are indicated if the patient has respiratory symptoms. Cohorting of infected neonates has been effective in controlling hospital nursery enterovirus outbreaks.

CONTROL MEASURES: Hand hygiene, especially after diaper changing, and respiratory hygiene are important in decreasing spread of enteroviruses within families, child care facilities, and other institutions. Other measures include avoidance of contaminated utensils and fomites, and disinfection of surfaces. Because HFMD is normally mild, children can continue in to go to child care and schools as long as: they have no fever, they have no uncontrolled drooling with mouth sores, and they are able to participate normally in classroom activities. In some cases, the local health department may require children with HFMD to stay home to control an outbreak (see Children in Group Child Care and Schools, p 145). Recommended chlorination treatment of drinking water and swimming pools may help prevent transmission.

Maintenance administration of IGIV in patients with severe deficits of B-lymphocyte function (eg, severe combined immunodeficiency syndrome, X-linked agammaglobulinemia) may prevent chronic enterovirus infection of the central nervous system. Prophylactic use of immune globulin has been used to help abort nursery epidemics. EV-A71 vaccines have been licensed in China and are being evaluated in other Asian countries where disease is prevalent; vaccines for other enterovirus serotypes associated with more severe disease also are under investigation.

Epstein-Barr Virus Infections
(Infectious Mononucleosis)

CLINICAL MANIFESTATIONS: Infectious mononucleosis is the most common presentation of primary symptomatic Epstein-Barr virus (EBV) infection. It manifests typically as fever, pharyngitis with or without petechiae and often with exudate, lymphadenopathy, and hepatosplenomegaly. Atypical lymphocytosis and elevated hepatic aminotransferase concentrations are frequently found on laboratory evaluation. The spectrum of disease is wide, ranging from asymptomatic to fatal infection. Infections are typically unrecognized or nonspecific in infants and young children. Rash can occur in up to 20% of patients and is more common in patients treated with antibiotics, most commonly ampicillin or amoxicillin as well as with other penicillins. Central nervous system (CNS) manifestations include aseptic meningitis, encephalitis, myelitis, optic neuritis, cranial nerve palsies, transverse myelitis, Alice in Wonderland syndrome, and Guillain-Barré syndrome. Hematologic complications include splenic rupture, thrombocytopenia, agranulocytosis, hemolytic anemia, and hemophagocytic lymphohistiocytosis (HLH, or hemophagocytic syndrome). Pneumonia, clinical hepatitis, tonsil or adenoid enlargement resulting in upper airway obstruction, genital ulcerations, orchitis, and myocarditis are observed infrequently. Early in the course of primary infection, 1% of circulating B lymphocytes are infected with EBV, and EBV-specific cytotoxic/suppressor T lymphocytes account for up to 50% of the CD8+ T lymphocytes in the blood. Replication of EBV in B lymphocytes results in T-lymphocyte proliferation and inhibition of B-lymphocyte proliferation by T-lymphocyte cytotoxic responses, natural killer (NK) cell activation, and the production of neutralizing antibodies. Fatal disseminated infection or B-lymphocyte, T-lymphocyte, or NK-cell lymphomas rarely occur in children with no detectable immunologic abnormality as well as in children with congenital or acquired cellular immune deficiencies.

EBV is associated with several other distinct disorders, including X-linked lymphoproliferative syndrome, post-transplantation lymphoproliferative disorders, Burkitt lymphoma, Hodgkin lymphoma, nasopharyngeal carcinoma, undifferentiated B- or T-lymphocyte lymphomas, and leiomyosarcoma. X-linked lymphoproliferative syndrome occurs most often in people with an inherited, maternally derived, recessive genetic defect in the SH2DIA or XIAP/BIRC4 genes, which are important in several lymphocyte signaling pathways. The syndrome is characterized by several phenotypes, including occurrence of fatal infectious mononucleosis early in life among boys; HLH; nodular B-lymphocyte lymphomas, often with CNS involvement; and profound pancytopenia. Similarly, X-linked immunodeficiency with magnesium defect, EBV infection, and neoplasia (XMEN) disease is characterized by loss-of-function mutations in the gene encoding magnesium transporter 1 (MAGT1), chronic high-level EBV DNAemia with increased EBV-infected B cells, and heightened susceptibility to EBV-associated lymphomas. Several other genetic mutations associated with the failure to control EBV infection because of changes in T-lymphocyte and NK cell function have also been described.

EBV-associated lymphoproliferative disorders can also occur in patients who are immunocompromised, such as transplant recipients or people infected with human immunodeficiency virus (HIV). EBV seronegative recipients of organs from EBV-seropositive donors are at highest risk for EBV-associated post-transplant lymphoproliferative disease (PTLD), with the highest incidence occurring in small intestine transplant recipients, followed by lung and heart transplant recipients, and lowest among liver and kidney transplant recipients. Proliferative states range from benign lymph node hypertrophy to monoclonal lymphomas. Other EBV-associated lymphoproliferative syndromes are of greater importance outside the United States, such as Burkitt lymphoma, which can be endemic or sporadic. EBV is present in virtually 100% of cases of endemic Burkitt lymphoma (a B-lymphocyte tumor predominantly found in the jaw or facial bones primarily in Central Africa) versus 20% of sporadic Burkitt lymphoma (a B-lymphocyte tumor of abdominal lymphoid tissue predominantly in North America and Europe). EBV is found in nearly 100% of nasopharyngeal carcinomas in Southeast Asia and the Inuit populations. EBV also has been associated with Hodgkin disease (a B-lymphocyte tumor), non-Hodgkin lymphomas (both B and T lymphocyte types), gastric carcinoma "lymphoepitheliomas," and a variety of other epithelial malignancies.

Chronic fatigue syndrome is not directly caused by EBV infection; however, fatigue lasting 6 months or more may follow approximately 10% of cases of classic infectious mononucleosis.

ETIOLOGY: EBV (also known as human herpesvirus 4) is a gamma herpesvirus of the *Lymphocryptovirus* genus and is the most common cause of infectious mononucleosis (>90% of cases).

EPIDEMIOLOGY: Humans are the only known reservoir of EBV, and approximately 90% of US adults have been infected. Close personal contact usually is required for transmission. The virus is viable in saliva for several hours outside the body; the role of fomites in transmission is unknown. EBV may be transmitted by blood transfusion or transplantation. Infection commonly is contracted early in life, particularly among members of lower socioeconomic groups, where crowding and intrafamilial spread is common. Endemic infectious mononucleosis is common in group settings of adolescents, such as in educational or military institutions. No seasonal pattern has been clearly documented. Intermittent excretion of EBV in saliva is lifelong after infection and likely explains viral spread and persistence in the population.

The **incubation period** of infectious mononucleosis is estimated to be 30 to 50 days.

DIAGNOSTIC TESTS: Infectious mononucleosis is primarily a clinical diagnosis. An absolute increase in atypical lymphocytes and mild elevations in hepatic aminotransferase concentrations during the second week of illness with infectious mononucleosis are additional characteristic but nonspecific findings. Confirmation of primary EBV infection depends on results of serologic testing. Nonspecific tests for heterophile antibody, including the Paul-Bunnell test and slide agglutination reaction test, are available but have several limitations, including false-positive and false-negative results. The heterophile antibody response primarily is immunoglobulin (Ig) M, which appears during the first 2 weeks of illness and usually disappears over 6 months but may persist for 1 year and may also be positive with other conditions, both infectious (eg, CMV, adenovirus, HIV) and noninfectious (eg, leukemia, lymphoma, systemic lupus erythematosus). In addition, the results of heterophile antibody tests often are negative during early EBV infection and in children younger than 4 years of age.

Multiple specific serologic antibody tests for EBV infection are available (see Table 3.7 and Fig 3.1). The most commonly performed test is for antibody against the viral capsid antigen (VCA) of EBV. Because IgG antibodies against VCA occur in high titer early in infection and persist for life at modest levels, testing of acute and convalescent serum specimens for IgG anti-VCA alone is not useful for establishing the presence of active infection. In contrast, testing for the presence of IgM anti-VCA antibody and the absence or very low titers of antibodies to Epstein-Barr nuclear antigen (EBNA) is useful for identifying active and recent infections. Because serum antibody against EBNA is not present until several weeks to months after onset of infection and rises with convalescence, a very elevated anti-EBNA antibody concentration typically excludes active primary infection. Testing for antibodies against early antigen (EA) is not usually required to assess EBV-associated mononucleosis. Typical patterns of antibody responses to EBV infection are illustrated in Table 3.7 and Fig 3.1.

Serologic testing for EBV is useful, particularly for evaluating patients younger than 4 years or in whom the infectious mononucleosis syndrome is not classic. Testing for other agents, especially cytomegalovirus, *Toxoplasma*, human herpesvirus 6, adenovirus, and HIV (in those with HIV risk factors), may be indicated for some patients. Diagnosis of the entire range of EBV-associated illness requires use of additional molecular and antibody techniques, particularly for patients with immune deficiencies and transplant recipients.

Nucleic acid amplification tests (NAATs) for detection of EBV DNA in serum, plasma, whole blood, and tissue, and NAATs or in situ hybridization for detection of EBV RNA in lymphoid cells, tissue, and/or body fluids, are available and can be useful in evaluation of immunocompromised patients and in complex clinical situations.

TREATMENT: There is no antiviral treatment approved for EBV infection. Patients suspected of having infectious mononucleosis should not receive ampicillin or amoxicillin, which may cause nonallergic morbilliform rashes in a proportion of patients with active EBV infection. Although therapy with short-course corticosteroids may have a beneficial effect on some acute symptoms, because of potential adverse effects their use is usually considered only for patients with marked tonsillar inflammation with impending airway obstruction, massive splenomegaly, myocarditis, hemolytic anemia, HLH, or severe thrombocytopenia. In those situations, the dosage of prednisone usually is 1 mg/kg per day, orally (maximum 60 mg/day), for 5 to 7 days, usually with tapering over 1 to 2 weeks. Life-threatening HLH has been treated with cytotoxic agents and immunomodulators, including etoposide, corticosteroids, and/or cyclosporine; emapalumab is approved for the treatment of progressive or refractory HLH. Although acyclovir and valacyclovir have in vitro antiviral activity against EBV and reduce viral replication, they produce no clinical benefit in infectious mononucleosis or in the prevention or treatment of EBV-associated PTLD. Decreasing immunosuppressive therapy often is beneficial as part of a preemptive strategy during EBV viral surveillance in response to increasing EBV DNAemia in transplant patients and for patients with EBV-induced PTLD. Rituximab, a monoclonal antibody directed against CD20+ B lymphocytes, is used both preemptively and for treatment of CD20+ PTLD in hematopoietic cell and solid organ transplant patients. Adoptive immunotherapy

Table 3.7. Serum Epstein-Barr Virus (EBV) Antibodies in EBV Infection

Infection	VCA IgG	VCA IgM	EA (D)	EBNA
No previous infection	−	−	−	−
Acute infection	+	+	+/−	−
Recent infection	+	+/−	+/−	+/−
Past infection	+	−	+/−	+

VCA IgG indicates immunoglobulin (Ig) G class antibody to viral capsid antigen; VCA IgM, IgM class antibody to VCA; EA (D), early antigen diffuse staining; and EBNA, EBV nuclear antigen.

with EBV-specific cytotoxic T-lymphocytes may be a treatment option in hematopoietic cell transplant recipients.

Strenuous activity and contact sports should be avoided for at least 21 days after onset of symptoms of infectious mononucleosis because of concern for splenic rupture. After 21 days, limited noncontact aerobic activity can be allowed if there are no symptoms and there is no overt splenomegaly. Clearance to participate in contact sports is appropriate after 4 to 7 weeks following the onset of symptoms if the athlete

FIG 3.1. SCHEMATIC REPRESENTATION OF THE EVOLUTION OF ANTIBODIES TO VARIOUS EPSTEIN-BARR VIRUS ANTIGENS IN PATIENTS WITH INFECTIOUS MONONUCLEOSIS

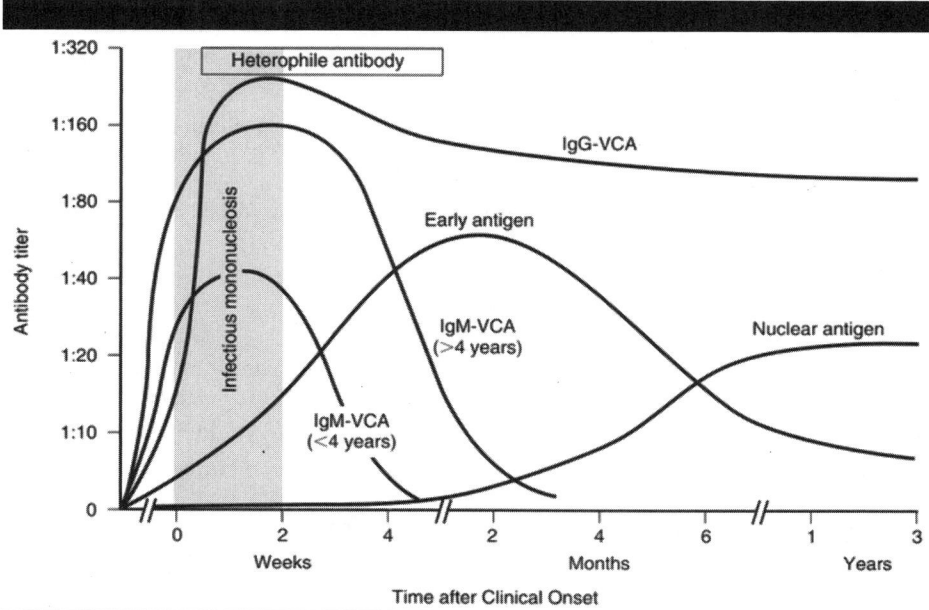

Source: *Manual of Clinical Laboratory Immunology*. Washington, DC: American Society for Microbiology; 1997:636. © 1997 American Society for Microbiology. Used with permission. No further reproduction or distribution is permitted without the prior written permission of American Society for Microbiology.

is asymptomatic and has no overt splenomegaly. Imaging modalities rarely are helpful in decisions about clearance to return to contact sports. Repeat EBV serologic testing is not useful in most clinical situations. It may take 3 to 6 months or longer following mononucleosis for an athlete to return to preillness fitness.

INFECTION PREVENTION AND CONTROL MEASURES IN HEALTH CARE SETTINGS: Standard precautions are recommended.

CONTROL MEASURES: None in the hospital or clinic. Avoid salivary exchange or sharing food or drink with someone who recently had infectious mononucleosis.

Escherichia coli Diarrhea
(Including Hemolytic-Uremic Syndrome)

CLINICAL MANIFESTATIONS: *Escherichia coli* is a common bacterial cause of diarrheal illness. At least 5 pathotypes of diarrhea-producing *E coli* strains have been identified. Clinical features of disease caused by each pathotype are summarized as follows (Table 3.8):

Table 3.8. Classification of *Escherichia coli* Associated With Diarrhea

Pathotype	Epidemiology	Type of Diarrhea	Mechanism of Pathogenesis
Shiga toxin-producing *E coli* (STEC)	Nonbloody and bloody diarrhea and hemolytic-uremic syndrome in all ages	Bloody or nonbloody	Shiga toxin production, large bowel adherence, coagulopathy
Enteropathogenic *E coli* (EPEC)	Acute and chronic endemic and epidemic diarrhea in infants in resource-limited countries; certain atypical strains in industrialized countries may cause disease	Watery	Small bowel adherence and effacement
Enterotoxigenic *E coli* (ETEC)	Infant diarrhea in resource-limited countries, travelers' diarrhea in all ages, and some cases in nontravelers	Watery	Heat stable and/or heat-labile enterotoxin production
Enteroinvasive *E coli* (EIEC)	Diarrhea with fever in all ages	Bloody or nonbloody; dysentery	Mucosal invasion and inflammation of large bowel
Enteroaggregative *E coli* (EAEC)	Acute and chronic diarrhea in all ages	Watery, occasionally bloody	Small and large bowel adherence, enterotoxin and cytotoxin production

- **Shiga toxin-producing *E coli* (STEC)** organisms are associated with diarrhea, hemorrhagic colitis, and hemolytic-uremic syndrome (HUS). STEC O157:H7 is the virulent STEC serotype most often implicated in outbreaks, but other serotypes are increasingly common causes of illness. STEC illness typically begins with nonbloody diarrhea. Stools usually become bloody after 2 or 3 days, representing the onset of hemorrhagic colitis. Severe abdominal pain typically is short lived, and low-grade fever is present in approximately one third of cases. Illness caused by *E coli* O157:H7 and other STEC organisms should be considered in people with presumptive diagnoses of intussusception, appendicitis, inflammatory bowel disease, and ischemic colitis. There are 2 types of Shiga toxin (Stx), Stx1 and Stx2, and several variants of each type. In the clinical setting, there is limited ability to differentiate between Stx variants.
- Diarrhea caused by **enteropathogenic *E coli* (EPEC)** is watery with prominent amounts of mucus but without gross blood. EPEC strains do not produce Shiga toxins and are distinguished from other diarrheagenic *E coli* by the distinctive attaching and effacing lesions they cause to the epithelium of the small intestine. Although usually mild, EPEC diarrhea can result in dehydration and death, particularly in resource-limited countries and immunocompromised patients. The diarrhea can be persistent and can result in wasting or growth restriction. Illness attributable to typical EPEC (caused by strains that harbor a virulence plasmid) occurs almost exclusively in children younger than 2 years and predominantly in resource-limited countries, either sporadically or in epidemics. Atypical EPEC (caused by strains which do not harbor a virulence plasmid) can cause diarrhea in all ages, including prolonged diarrhea.
- Diarrhea caused by **enterotoxigenic *E coli* (ETEC)** is a 1- to 5-day, self-limited illness of moderate severity, typically with watery stools and abdominal cramps. ETEC is common in infants in resource-limited countries and in travelers to those countries. ETEC is the leading cause of travelers' diarrhea. The prevalence of ETEC disease in the United States is unknown. With increasing use of culture-independent tests, ETEC infections may be detected more frequently especially in late summer into fall.
- Diarrhea caused by **enteroinvasive *E coli* (EIEC)** is similar clinically to diarrhea caused by *Shigella* species. Although dysentery can occur, diarrhea usually is watery without blood or mucus. Patients often are febrile, and stools can contain leukocytes. Severe cases of EIEC may require hospitalization.
- **Enteroaggregative *E coli* (EAEC)** organisms cause watery diarrhea and are common in people of all ages in industrialized as well as resource-limited countries. EAEC is a common cause of childhood diarrhea in resource-limited countries, acute travelers' diarrhea, and persistent diarrhea in children or human immunodeficiency virus (HIV)-infected people. EAEC has been associated with prolonged diarrhea (14 days or longer). Asymptomatic infection can be accompanied by subclinical inflammatory enteritis and may stunt a child's growth. With increasing use of culture-independent tests, EAEC is being identified more frequently in the United States, even among those without international travel history.

Sequelae of STEC Infection. HUS, manifested by varying degrees of hemolysis and uremia, is a serious sequela of STEC enteric infection believed to follow Stx-induced vasculitis and systemic complement cascade activation. STEC O157:H7 organisms are most commonly associated with HUS, which is defined by the triad of microangiopathic hemolytic anemia, thrombocytopenia, and acute renal dysfunction. HUS occurs more frequently in younger children; approximately 15% of children younger than 5 years develop HUS after *E coli* O157 infection as compared with approximately 6% among people of all ages. Non-O157 STEC infections also may cause HUS but at a much lower frequency (approximately 1%) than O157 infections. HUS typically develops 7 days (up to 2 weeks, and rarely 2–3 weeks) after onset of diarrhea. The risk of developing HUS is lower in children who have a longer interval between diarrhea onset and presentation to the emergency department. More than 50% of children with HUS require dialysis, and up to 5% die. Patients with HUS can develop neurologic complications (eg, seizures, coma, or cerebral vessel thrombosis). Children presenting with an increased white blood cell count ($>20 \times 10^9$/mL), neurologic complications, or need for dialysis are at higher risk of poor outcome, as are, seemingly paradoxically, children with hematocrit close to normal rather than low. There is increasing recognition of long-term risk for hypertension, proteinuria, and chronic kidney disease following HUS in children.

ETIOLOGY: The 5 pathotypes of diarrhea-producing *E coli* have been distinguished by genetic, pathogenic, and clinical characteristics. Each pathotype is defined by the presence of virulence-related genes, and each comprises characteristic serotypes, indicated by somatic (O) and flagellar (H) antigens. Diarrhea is caused by the direct effects of the pathogens in the intestine.

EPIDEMIOLOGY: Transmission of most diarrhea-associated *E coli* strains is through a fecal-oral mechanism.

STEC is shed in feces of cattle and, to a lesser extent, sheep, deer, and other ruminants. Human infection is acquired via contaminated food or water or via contact with an infected person, a fomite, or a carrier animal or its environment. Many foods have caused STEC outbreaks, including raw leafy vegetables, undercooked ground beef, cookie dough, raw flour, and unpasteurized milk and juice (see the *Red Book Online* outbreaks page for information on current outbreaks at **https://publications.aap.org/redbook/resources/17748**). Outbreak investigations have implicated petting zoos, drinking water, and ingestion of recreational water. The infectious dose of STEC is low; thus, person-to-person transmission is common in households and child care centers. The number of infections reported annually to the US laboratory-based enteric disease system of the Centers for Disease Control and Prevention (CDC) has increased in recent years because of the increasing use of culture-independent diagnostic tests.

The non-O157 STEC serogroups most commonly linked to illness in the United States are O26, O103, O111, O121, O145, and O45. Outbreaks from these serogroups are less common than those caused by serogroup O157 and are generally attributable to contaminated food or person-to-person transmission (often in a child care setting). There is a higher incidence of serogroup O157 infections in northern US states compared with other regions.

With the exception of EAEC, non-STEC pathotypes most commonly are associated with disease in resource-limited countries, where food and water supplies are commonly contaminated and facilities and supplies for hand hygiene are suboptimal. For young children in resource-limited countries, transmission of ETEC, EPEC, and other diarrheal pathogens via contaminated weaning foods (sometimes by use of untreated drinking water in the foods) is common. ETEC diarrhea occurs in people of all ages but is especially frequent and severe in infants in resource-limited countries and travelers from industrialized countries visiting resource-limited countries. Breastfeeding is protective in such settings.

The **incubation period** for most diarrhea-associated *E coli* strains is 10 hours to 6 days; for *E coli* O157:H7, the **incubation period** usually is 3 to 4 days (range, 1–10 days).

DIAGNOSTIC TESTS: Several US Food and Drug Administration (FDA)-approved multiplex nucleic acid amplification tests (NAATs) (usually offered as diagnostic panels) can detect a variety of enteric pathogens, including EAEC, EPEC, ETEC, and STEC. Some culture-independent tests include an *E coli* O157 specific marker to differentiate *E coli* O157 from non-O157 STEC serotypes. Using these newer culture-independent methods, EAEC, EPEC, and ETEC may be detected more frequently than in the past and may represent colonization. Therefore, the pretest probability of the disease and clinical context, including the presence of other potential pathogens, must be considered when interpreting results of these tests.

Several commercially available, rapid immunologic assays for Shiga toxins in stool or broth culture of stool, including enzyme immunoassays (EIA) and immunochromatographic assays, have been approved by the FDA. The Shiga toxin assays performed on broth enriched stool specimens (usually incubated 18–24 hours) generally are more sensitive than those that test stool directly.

Rapid diagnosis facilitates patient management. Hydration is the cornerstone of management for all diarrhea cases and may be particularly protective against the development of nephropathy associated with HUS. Most *E coli* O157 isolates can be identified presumptively when grown on sorbitol-containing selective media because they cannot ferment sorbitol within 24 hours. All presumptive *E coli* O157 isolates and all Shiga toxin-positive stool specimens that did not yield a presumptive *E coli* O157 isolate should be sent to a public health laboratory for further characterization, including identification of non-O157 serotype and determination of whole genome sequence.

Patients with postdiarrheal HUS should be presumed to have STEC infection, and STEC should be sought in stool specimens from all patients diagnosed with postdiarrheal HUS. However, the absence of STEC does not preclude the diagnosis of probable STEC-associated HUS, because HUS typically is diagnosed a week or more after onset of diarrhea, when the organism may not be detectable by conventional bacteriologic methods. In this setting, the selective enrichment of stool samples followed by immunomagnetic separation can markedly enhance the isolation of *E coli* O157 and other STEC for which immunomagnetic reagents are available. The test is available at some state public health laboratories and through requests to state health departments at the CDC. Serologic diagnosis using enzyme immunoassay to detect serum antibodies to *E coli* O157 and O111 lipopolysaccharides is available at the CDC for outbreak investigations and surveillance for patients with HUS; this testing can be arranged through state health departments.

TREATMENT: Treatment is primarily supportive for all diarrhea-producing *E coli*.[1] Orally administered electrolyte-containing solutions usually are adequate to prevent or treat dehydration and electrolyte abnormalities.[2] Antimotility agents should not be administered to children with inflammatory or bloody diarrhea. Many experts advocate intravenous volume expansion during the first 4 days of proven STEC infection to maintain renal perfusion and reduce the risk of renal injury. Careful monitoring of patients with hemorrhagic colitis (including complete blood cell count with smear, blood urea nitrogen, and creatinine concentrations) is recommended to detect changes suggestive of HUS. If patients have no laboratory evidence of hemolysis, thrombocytopenia, or nephropathy 3 days after resolution of diarrhea, their risk of developing HUS is low.

In resource-limited countries, nutritional rehabilitation, including supplemental zinc and vitamin A, should be provided as part of case management algorithms for diarrhea where feasible. Feeding, including breastfeeding, should be continued for young children with *E coli* enteric infection.

Bismuth subsalicylate has been approved by the FDA for use in children 12 years and older and may be used in mild cases of ETEC travelers' diarrhea. It can cause blackening of the tongue and stool, and patients should be advised to rinse their mouths after each dose. It contains salicylate and should not be used if there is concern for coinfection with varicella or influenza because of increased risk of Reye syndrome.

Antimicrobial Therapy. Antimicrobial therapy in patients with known or likely STEC infection remains controversial because of its association with an increased risk of developing HUS in some studies. A meta-analysis did not find that children with hemorrhagic colitis caused by STEC have a greater risk of developing HUS if treated with an antimicrobial agent. However, an association was found in analyses restricted to studies with low risk of bias and using the accepted HUS definition. Moreover, a controlled trial has not been performed, and a beneficial effect of antimicrobial treatment has not been proven. The most recently published observational studies found that treatment of diarrhea with at least some classes of antimicrobial agents was associated with HUS development. A large case-control study of 1308 US residents with *E coli* O157 infection found that people treated with a beta-lactam antibiotic had a 2.8-fold higher odds of developing HUS than those treated with other antibiotics. Most experts advise not prescribing antimicrobial therapy for children with *E coli* O157 enteritis or a clinical or epidemiologic presentation that strongly suggests STEC infection.

Antimicrobial therapy can be considered for travelers in resource-limited areas when diarrhea is moderate to severe or is associated with fever or bloody stools; however, the prevalence of antimicrobial resistance among enteric pathogens is increasing.[3] Several antimicrobial agents, such as azithromycin, fluoroquinolones (see Fluoroquinolones, p 973), and rifaximin can be effective in treatment of ETEC or

---

[1] Shane AL, Mody RK, Crump JA, et al. 2017 Infectious Diseases Society of America clinical practice guidelines for the diagnosis and management of infectious diarrhea. *Clin Infect Dis*. 2017;65(12):e45-e80. doi:10.1093/cid/cix669

[2] Centers for Disease Control and Prevention. Managing acute gastroenteritis among children: oral rehydration, maintenance, and nutritional therapy. *MMWR Recomm Rep*. 2003;52(RR-16):1–16

[3] **wwwnc.cdc.gov/travel/yellowbook/2024/preparing/travelers-diarrhea**

EAEC travelers' diarrhea. Treatment for no more than 3 days is advised. The choice of therapy depends on the pathogen and local antibiotic resistance patterns.

Patients with domestically acquired atypical EPEC (ie, as detected by molecular tests), EAEC, or ETEC will generally have self-limited diarrhea that does not require antimicrobial therapy. For patients with moderate or severe illness with persistent (>14 days) diarrhea attributable to diarrhea-producing *E coli* because they have no other pathogen detected, a treatment regimen similar to that used for ETEC or EAEC travelers' diarrhea (azithromycin, a fluoroquinolone, or rifaximin) may be used.

INFECTION PREVENTION AND CONTROL MEASURES IN HEALTH CARE SETTINGS:
In addition to standard precautions, contact precautions are indicated for diapered and incontinent patients with all types of *E coli* diarrhea for the duration of illness. Prolonged shedding has been noted in children younger than 5 years.

CONTROL MEASURES:

E coli *O157:H7 and Other STEC Infection.* All meat should be cooked thoroughly. Ground beef should be cooked to an internal temperature of 160°F (71°C) until no pink meat remains and the juices are clear. Raw milk should not be ingested, and the certification of raw milk does not eliminate the risk of transmission of *E coli* organisms.[1] Only pasteurized apple juice and cider products should be consumed. Care should be taken to prevent cross-contamination in areas of food preparation and good handwashing practices should be in place.

Outbreaks in Child Care Centers. If an outbreak of HUS or diarrhea attributable to STEC occurs in a child care center, immediate involvement of public health authorities is critical. Infection caused by STEC is notifiable, and rapid reporting of cases allows intervention to prevent further disease. Ill children with STEC O157 infection or virulent non-O157 STEC infection should not be permitted to reenter the child care center until all of the following: 2 stool cultures (obtained at least 48 hours after any antimicrobial therapy, if administered, has been discontinued) are negative, stools are contained in the diaper or the child is continent, stool frequency is no more than 2 stools above that child's normal frequency, and the health department agrees with the return to child care (see Table 2.3, p 149). Stool cultures should be performed for any symptomatic contacts, and these children should be excluded from child care centers while symptomatic and the evaluation is pending. In outbreak situations involving STEC strains, stool cultures of asymptomatic contacts may aid controlling spread; consultation with public health authorities is advised. Strict attention to hand hygiene is important but can be insufficient to prevent transmission. The child care center should be closed to new admissions during an outbreak, and care should be exercised to prevent transfer of exposed children to other centers.

Nursery and Other Institutional Outbreaks. Similar to child care institutional setting, strict attention to hand hygiene is essential for limiting spread. Ill patients should be separated from unexposed patients and their stool should be cultured as described above. Exposed patients should be observed closely.

[1] American Academy of Pediatrics, Committee on Infectious Diseases, Committee on Nutrition. Consumption of raw or unpasteurized milk and milk products by pregnant women and children. *Pediatrics.* 2014;133(1):175-179 (Reaffirmed November 2019)

Travelers' Diarrhea. Travelers' diarrhea usually is acquired by ingestion of contaminated food or water or contact with fomites and is a significant problem for people traveling in resource-limited countries. Diarrhea commonly is caused by ETEC and EAEC. Diarrhea attributable to non-O157 STEC infection is common among US residents who have traveled internationally in the previous week, but *E coli* O157 is rare. Travelers should be advised to drink only bottled or canned beverages and boiled or bottled water; travelers should avoid ice, raw produce, including salads, and fruit that they themselves have not peeled (only fruits with a thick peel, such as bananas and oranges, should be consumed). Cooked foods that have been left an ambient temperatures for prolonged periods should not be consumed. Hands should be washed carefully before preparing or eating food or feeding another person. Antimicrobial agents are not recommended for prevention of travelers' diarrhea in children. Rehydration is the mainstay of treatment. Packets of oral rehydration salts can be added to boiled or bottled water and ingested to help maintain fluid balance, and breastfeeding should be encouraged and continued for young children.

Recreational Water (eg, Swimming Pools, Water Slides). People should avoid ingesting recreational water. Because STEC has a low infectious dose and can be waterborne, people with proven or suspected STEC infection should not use recreational water venues when ill with diarrhea. As with other causes of diarrhea, children who have diarrhea attributable to STEC and who are incontinent should continue not to use recreational water venues until 1 week after symptoms resolve (or as advised by local or state public health authorities) (see Prevention of Illnesses Associated With Recreational Water Use, p 214). Showering before swimming, taking children to the restroom frequently, changing diapers at designated diapering stations, and then washing hands can limit transmission of diarrheal pathogens through recreational water.

Other Fungal Diseases

Uncommonly encountered fungi can cause infection in infants and children with immunosuppression or other underlying conditions. Fungi can cause invasive mold infections, such as mucormycosis, fusariosis, scedosporiosis, and the phaeohyphomycoses (black molds), as well as invasive yeast infections with organisms such as *Malazzesia, Trichosporon, Rhodotorula*, and many more (more common mycoses, including aspergillosis, blastomycosis, candidiasis, coccidioidomycosis, cryptococcosis, histoplasmosis, paracoccidioidomycosis, and sporotrichosis, are discussed in individual chapters of Section 3 of the *Red Book*). Children can acquire infection from these fungi through inhalation via the respiratory tract or direct inoculation after traumatic disruption of cutaneous barriers. A list of some of these fungi and the pertinent underlying host conditions, reservoirs or routes of entry, clinical manifestations, diagnostic laboratory tests, and treatments can be found in Table 3.9. Taken as a group, few in vitro antifungal susceptibility data are available on which to base treatment recommendations for these uncommon invasive fungal infections, especially in children; thus optimal treatments are not well established and antifungal choice may depend on the particular species (see Antifungal Drugs for Systemic Fungal Infections, p 1017, and Table 4.7, p 1021, which indicates in Footnote b which species are molds). In addition, attempts to achieve source control and improve the net state of immunosuppression, including reversing severity of neutropenia, are critical. Reduction of immunosuppression

Table 3.9. Additional Fungal Diseases

Disease and Agent	Underlying Host Condition(s)	Reservoir(s) or Route(s) of Entry	Common Clinical Manifestations	Diagnostic Laboratory Test(s)	First-Line Antifungal Treatment[a]
Hyalohyphomycosis					
Fusarium species	Granulocytopenia; hematopoietic cell transplantation; severe immunocompromise; severe neutropenia and/or T-lymphocyte immunodeficiency	Environment; respiratory tract; sinuses; skin; traumatic inoculation	Pulmonary infiltrates; cutaneous lesions (eg, ecthyma); sinusitis; keratitis; disseminated infection, onychomycosis	Culture of blood or tissue specimen, histopathologic examination of tissue	Voriconazole, or Voriconazole plus lipid amphotericin formulation[b]
Scedosporium apiospermum complex	None or trauma or immunosuppression; cystic fibrosis; chronic granulomatous disease; chronic glucocorticoid use; hematologic malignancy	Environment; respiratory tract; direct inoculation (eg, skin puncture)	Pneumonia; localized pulmonary process or disseminated infection; osteomyelitis or septic arthritis; mycetoma (immunocompetent patients); endocarditis; keratitis and endophthalmitis; brain abscesses; lesions of the skin, soft tissue, or bone	Culture and histopathologic examination of tissue	Voriconazole
Lomentospora (formerly *Scedosporium*) *prolificans*					Voriconazole plus terbinafine

Table 3.9. Additional Fungal Diseases, continued

Disease and Agent	Underlying Host Condition(s)	Reservoir(s) or Route(s) of Entry	Common Clinical Manifestations	Diagnostic Laboratory Test(s)	First-Line Antifungal Treatment[a]
Talaromycosis					
Talaromyces (Penicillium) marneffei	Human immunodeficiency virus infection; exposure to southeast Asia	Environment; respiratory tract	Pneumonitis; invasive dermatitis; disseminated infection	Culture of blood, bone marrow, or tissue; histopathologic examination of tissue	AMB; followed by itraconazole[c]
Phaeohyphomycosis					
Alternaria species	None, trauma, or immunosuppression	Environment; respiratory tract; skin	Sinusitis; cutaneous lesions	Culture and histopathologic examination of tissue	Azoles (voriconazole,[c] posaconazole,[c]) or AMB[b,d]
Cladophialophora species	None, trauma, or immunosuppression	Environment	Cerebral infection	Culture and histopathologic examination of tissue	Voriconazole,[c] with or without AMB[b] (posaconazole,[c] itraconazole,[c])

Table 3.9. Additional Fungal Diseases, continued

Disease and Agent	Underlying Host Condition(s)	Reservoir(s) or Route(s) of Entry	Common Clinical Manifestations	Diagnostic Laboratory Test(s)	First-Line Antifungal Treatment[a]
Curvularia species (including *Bipolaris*)	Immunosuppression; altered skin integrity; asthma or nasal polyps; chronic sinusitis	Environment	Allergic fungal sinusitis; invasive dermatitis; disseminated infection	Culture and histopathologic examination of tissue	Allergic fungal sinusitis: surgery and corticosteroids Invasive disease: azoles (voriconazole,[c] posaconazole,[c] itraconazole,[e]) or AMB,[d] alone or in combination with echinocandins[b]
Exophiala species, *Exserohilum* species	None, trauma, or immunosuppression	Environment	Sinusitis; cutaneous lesions; disseminated infection; meningitis associated with contaminated steroid for epidural use	Culture and histopathologic examination of tissue	Voriconazole,[c,f] itraconazole,[c,e] AMB[d]

Table 3.9. Additional Fungal Diseases, continued

Disease and Agent	Underlying Host Condition(s)	Reservoir(s) or Route(s) of Entry	Common Clinical Manifestations	Diagnostic Laboratory Test(s)	First-Line Antifungal Treatment[a]
Invasive Yeasts					
Trichosporon species	Immunosuppression; central venous catheter; urinary catheter; hematologic malignancy, often with neutropenia; acquired immunodeficiency syndrome; extensive burns; glucocorticoid treatment; heart valve surgery; exposure to tropical environments	Environment; normal flora of oral cavity, skin, and nails	Bloodstream infection; superficial skin lesions endocarditis; peritonitis; pneumonitis; disseminated infection	Blood culture; histopathologic examination of tissue or nodules; urine, sputum, and cerebrospinal cultures; bronchoscopy with alveolar lavage cultures	For invasive infections, voriconazole[f], posaconazole[c], itraconazole[e]; For superficial infections, shaving of the hair and application of a topical azole to the affected areas
Malassezia species	Immunosuppression; preterm birth; exposure to parenteral nutrition that includes fat emulsions	Skin	Pityriasis versicolor; seborrheic dermatitis; central line-associated bloodstream infection; interstitial pneumonitis; urinary tract infection; meningitis	Culture of blood, catheter tip, or tissue specimen (requires special laboratory handling)	AMB,[d] removal of catheters, and temporary cessation of lipid parenteral nutrition infusion

Table 3.9. Additional Fungal Diseases, continued

Disease and Agent	Underlying Host Condition(s)	Reservoir(s) or Route(s) of Entry	Common Clinical Manifestations	Diagnostic Laboratory Test(s)	First-Line Antifungal Treatment[a]
Mucormycosis (formerly Zygomycosis)					
Rhizopus; Mucor; Lichtheimia (formerly Absidia) species; *Rhizomucor* species; *Cunninghamella* species	Immunosuppression; hematologic malignant neoplasm; renal failure; diabetes mellitus; iron overload syndromes	Environment; respiratory tract; skin; ingestion	Rhinocerebral infection; pulmonary infection; disseminated infection; skin (traumatic wounds) and gastrointestinal tract (less commonly)	Histopathologic examination of tissue and culture	AMB[b,d] for initial therapy and consider posaconazole or isavuconazole for maintenance therapy

AMB indicates amphotericin B.

[a]Strongly or moderately recommended first line antifungal; additional details, including alternative first or second line antifungals available in the global guidelines:

  • Hoenigl M, Salmanton-García J, Walsh TJ, et al. Global guideline for the diagnosis and management of rare mould infections: an initiative of the European Confederation of Medical Mycology in cooperation with the International Society for Human and Animal Mycology and the American Society for Microbiology. *Lancet Infect Dis.* 2021;21(8):e246-e257;

  • Cornely O, Alastruey-Izquierdo A, Arenz D, et al. Global guideline for the diagnosis and management of mucormycosis: an initiative of the European Confederation of Medical Mycology in cooperation with the Mycoses Study Group Education and Research Consortium. *Lancet Infect Dis.* 2019;19(12):e405-e421

  • Chen SC-A, Perfect J, Colombo AL, et al. Global guidelines for the diagnosis and management of rare yeast infections: an initiative of the ECMM in cooperation with ISHAM and ASM. *Lancet Infect Dis.* 2021;21(12):e375-e386

[b]There are no definitive data to routinely recommend the use of antifungal combination therapy, although combination therapy may frequently be used particularly until final species identification is known to tailor therapy.

[c]No US Food and Drug Administration approval for this indication.

[d]Consider use of amphotericin B lipid formulations: liposomal amphotericin B is the preferred formulation; when lipid formulations are not available, deoxycholate amphotericin B may be an alternative.

[e]Itraconazole has been shown to be effective for cutaneous disease in adults, but safety and efficacy have not been established in children younger than 18 years.

[f]Voriconazole demonstrates activity in vitro, but no clinical data are available.

and surgical excision and débridement should always be considered in management of invasive fungal infections, if feasible. Physicians should consider consultation with a pediatric infectious disease specialist experienced in the diagnosis and treatment of invasive fungal infections when treating a child infected with one of these mycoses.

Fusobacterium Infections
(Including Lemierre Syndrome)

CLINICAL MANIFESTATIONS: *Fusobacterium* species, including *Fusobacterium necrophorum* and *Fusobacterium nucleatum,* can be isolated from oropharyngeal specimens in healthy people and are frequent components of human dental plaque with the potential to lead to periodontal disease. Invasive disease attributable to *Fusobacterium* species has been associated with otitis media, tonsillitis, gingivitis, and oropharyngeal trauma including dental and oropharyngeal surgery such as tonsillectomy. Ten percent of cases of invasive *Fusobacterium* infections are associated with concomitant Epstein-Barr virus infection.

Preceding oropharyngeal infection is the most frequent primary source for invasive infection. Invasive infections can be characterized by peritonsillar abscess, deep neck space infection, mastoiditis, and sinusitis that can be complicated by meningitis, cerebral abscess, dural sinus venous thrombosis, endocarditis, and pleural empyema. Otogenic and gynecologic sources of infection have also been reported.

Invasive infection following tonsillitis was described early in the 20th century and was referred to as postanginal sepsis or Lemierre syndrome. The classic syndrome starts with fever and sore throat that progresses to severe neck pain (anginal pain) that can be accompanied by unilateral neck swelling, trismus, dysphagia, and rigors associated with development of suppurative jugular venous thrombosis (JVT). Patients with classic Lemierre syndrome have a sepsis syndrome with metastatic complications from septic embolic phenomena associated with JVT. Patients with Lemierre syndrome may develop complications including multiple pulmonary septic emboli, pleural empyema, pyogenic arthritis, osteomyelitis, or disseminated intravascular coagulation. Laboratory abnormalities associated with Lemierre syndrome can include significantly elevated inflammatory markers, thrombocytopenia, elevated aminotransferases, hyperbilirubinemia, and elevated creatinine. Persistent headache or other neurologic signs may indicate the presence of cerebral venous sinus thrombosis (eg, cavernous sinus thrombosis), meningitis, or brain abscess. *Fusobacterium* species (most commonly *F necrophorum)* can be isolated from blood or other normally sterile sites and account for at least 60% to 80% of Lemierre syndrome cases. Lemierre-like syndromes have also been reported following infection with *Arcanobacterium haemolyticum*, *Bacteroides* species, *Klebsiella* species, anaerobic *Streptococcus* species, other anaerobic bacteria, and methicillin-susceptible and -resistant strains of *Staphylococcus aureus*.

With respect to thrombosis, the JVT can be completely vaso-occlusive. Some children with JVT associated with Lemierre syndrome have evidence of thrombophilia at diagnosis. These findings often resolve over several months and can indicate response to the inflammatory, prothrombotic process associated with infection, rather than an underlying hypercoagulable state.

Fusobacterium species have also been associated with intra-abdominal and pelvic infections including acute appendicitis, suppurative portomesenteric vein thrombosis, and suppurative thrombosis of the pelvic vasculature.

ETIOLOGY: *Fusobacterium* species are filamentous, anaerobic, non–spore-forming, gram-negative bacilli. Human infection usually results from *F necrophorum* subspecies *funduliforme*, but infections with other species including *F nucleatum, Fusobacterium gonidi-aformans, Fusobacterium naviforme, Fusobacterium mortiferum,* and *Fusobacterium varium* have been reported. Infection with *Fusobacterium* species, alone or in combination with other oral anaerobic bacteria, may result in Lemierre syndrome, but unlike other anaerobic infections, *Fusobacterium* species are frequently the only organisms identified in these infections.

EPIDEMIOLOGY: *Fusobacterium* species are commonly found in soil and in the respiratory tracts of animals, including cattle, dogs, fowl, goats, sheep, and horses, and can be isolated from the oropharynx of healthy people. *Fusobacterium* infections are most common in adolescents and young adults, but infections, including fatal cases of Lemierre syndrome, have been reported in infants and young children.

DIAGNOSTIC TESTS: *Fusobacterium* species can be isolated using conventional liquid anaerobic blood culture media. However, the organism grows best on semisolid media for fastidious anaerobic organisms or blood agar supplemented with vitamin K, hemin, menadione, and a reducing agent. Colonies generally are cream to yellow colored, smooth, and round and may show a narrow zone of alpha- or beta-hemolysis on blood agar, depending on the species of blood used in the medium; *F nucleatum* may appear as bread crumb-like colonies. Many strains fluoresce chartreuse green under ultraviolet light. Most *Fusobacterium* organisms are indole positive. On Gram stain, *F nucleatum* usually exhibits spindle-shaped cells with tapered ends, while *F necrophorum* and other species may be highly pleomorphic with swollen areas. The accurate identification of anaerobes to the species level has become important with the increasing incidence of microorganisms that are resistant to multiple drugs. Conventional and commercial culture-based biochemical test systems are reasonably accurate, at least to the genus level. Sequencing of the 16S rRNA gene and phylogenetic analysis or the use of mass spectrometry of bacterial cell components can accurately identify *Fusobacterium* species to the species level.

Currently, there are no commercially available tests for rapidly diagnosing *Fusobacterium* pharyngitis, although nucleic acid amplification tests (NAATs) have been used in dental settings to monitor bacterial species in saliva, including *Fusobacterium* species, in patients with periodontal disease. Routine throat cultures for beta-hemolytic streptococci do not generally include screening for the presence of *Fusobacterium* species. Researchers have used special media to grow *F necrophorum* from throat swab specimens or have used NAAT techniques to document and describe *F necrophorum* tonsillitis/pharyngitis and the frequency of *Fusobacterium* species colonization in pharyngeal specimens obtained from asymptomatic adolescents and young adults. A number of experimental multiplex NAAT panels and metagenomic sequencing platforms for the identification of pathogens in blood and other sterile sites are under development and may allow rapid identification of *Fusobacterium* infections in the future.

One should consider Lemierre syndrome in ill-appearing febrile children and especially adolescents having a sore throat with exquisite neck pain and swelling over the angle of the jaw, accompanied by rigors. Aerobic and anaerobic blood cultures should be performed to detect invasive *Fusobacterium* species and other possible pathogens. Imaging studies of the internal jugular veins should be obtained, but it is important to note that a significant proportion of patients with a diagnosis of Lemierre syndrome will not have a thrombus detected by imaging (thromboses may be missed or embolized prior to imaging). Computed tomography and magnetic resonance imaging are more sensitive than ultrasonography to document thrombosis and thrombophlebitis of the internal jugular vein early in the course of illness and to better identify thrombus extension beyond the areas visible by ultrasonography, including under the mandible and clavicle.

TREATMENT: Aggressive and prompt antimicrobial therapy is the mainstay of treatment. *Fusobacterium* species generally are susceptible to metronidazole, clindamycin, chloramphenicol, penicillin with beta-lactamase inhibitor combinations (ampicillin-sulbactam or piperacillin-tazobactam), carbapenems, cefoxitin, and ceftriaxone. Antimicrobial resistance has increased in anaerobic bacteria, and susceptibilities to particular antibiotic classes are less predictable. Therefore, susceptibility testing is indicated for all clinically significant anaerobic isolates, including *Fusobacterium* species. Combination therapy with metronidazole or clindamycin, in addition to a beta-lactam agent active against aerobic oral and respiratory tract pathogens (eg, cefotaxime, ceftriaxone, or cefuroxime), is recommended for patients with invasive infection caused by *Fusobacterium* species. Alternatively, some experts recommend monotherapy with a penicillin-beta-lactamase inhibitor combination (ampicillin-sulbactam or piperacillin-tazobactam) or a carbapenem (meropenem, imipenem, or ertapenem). Up to 50% of *F nucleatum* and 20% of *F necrophorum* isolates produce beta-lactamases, rendering them resistant to penicillin, ampicillin, and some cephalosporins. *Fusobacterium* species intrinsically are resistant to gentamicin, fluoroquinolone agents, and typically, macrolides. Tetracyclines have limited activity.

The duration of antimicrobial therapy depends on the anatomic location and severity of infection but usually is at least 6 weeks. Surgical intervention involving débridement or incision and drainage of abscesses may be necessary. Anticoagulation therapy has been used in both adults and children with JVT or cavernous sinus thrombosis. However, there is limited evidence for the impact of anticoagulation on patient outcomes.

INFECTION PREVENTION AND CONTROL MEASURES IN HEALTH CARE SETTINGS: Standard precautions are recommended. Person-to-person transmission of *Fusobacterium* species has not been documented.

CONTROL MEASURES: Proper oral hygiene and routine dental cleanings may reduce density of oral colonization with *Fusobacterium* species, prevent gingivitis and dental caries, and reduce the risk of invasive disease.

Giardia duodenalis (Formerly Giardia lamblia and Giardia intestinalis) Infections
(Giardiasis)

CLINICAL MANIFESTATIONS: Symptoms of *Giardia* infection are attributable to dysfunction of the small bowel caused by residing trophozoites and range from asymptomatic carriage to fulminant diarrhea and dehydration. Most infections are asymptomatic, but children are more often symptomatic than adults. Symptomatic patients are mildly to moderately ill and complain frequently of intermittent abdominal cramping, bloating, and foul-smelling flatus and stools. Chronic infection, often with weight loss, is common, similar to irritable bowel syndrome. A more fulminant presentation with acute and chronic diarrhea, malabsorption, failure to thrive, and weight loss may occur, but systemic symptoms other than malaise are uncommon and extraintestinal involvement (eg, arthritis, urticaria, retinal changes, and bile or pancreatic duct involvement) is unusual. Symptoms are also caused by lactose intolerance and malabsorption, which result in voluminous diarrhea often described as "greasy or fatty." Sometimes atypical upper gastrointestinal symptoms of belching, nausea, and vomiting predominate, causing a delay in diagnosis. Fever, mucus, and blood in stool are atypical and suggest infection with another agent(s). Duration of infection can be prolonged and may last years in immunosuppressed individuals. In children, development of immunity is poor and repeated infections are common. Patients with cystic fibrosis have an increased prevalence of *Giardia duodenalis* infection.

ETIOLOGY: *G duodenalis* (formerly called *Giardia lamblia* or *Giardia intestinalis)* is a flagellate protozoan that exists in trophozoite and cyst forms; the infective form is the cyst. *Giardia* organisms undergo a simple life cycle alternating between orally ingested, infectious, acid-resistant cysts and motile trophozoites that reside and multiply in the small intestine. Encystation occurs in the lower small bowel, and cysts are infectious when excreted. Infection is limited to the small intestine and biliary tract. *Giardia* cysts are infectious immediately after being excreted in feces and remain viable for 3 months in water at 4°C. A single freeze/thaw cycle kills most *Giardia* cysts; complete killing occurs after multiple freeze/thaw cycles. Heating, drying, and seawater are microcidal to cysts, depending on specific conditions.

EPIDEMIOLOGY: Giardiasis has a worldwide distribution and is the most common intestinal parasitic infection of humans identified in the United States and globally. The highest incidence of giardiasis in the United States is reported among children 1 through 9 years of age, adults 25 through 29 years of age, adults 55 through 59 years of age, and residents of northern states. Peak illness onset occurs from early summer through early fall. High infectivity is a result of the combination of enormous numbers of infectious cysts that may be excreted and the low infectious dose (as few as 10 to 100 cysts are able to cause infection). Giardiasis is communicable for as long as the infected person excretes cysts. Duration of cyst excretion is variable but can range from weeks to months. Transmission of *G duodenalis* is most likely to occur in situations in which exposure to feces with cysts is likely, including: (1) child care centers; (2) areas of the world with endemic disease; (3) close contact, including sexual contact, with infected people; (4) swallowing of contaminated drinking or recreational water; and (5) consumption of unfiltered or untreated water such as when camping or backpacking, including water downstream of beaver dams (leading to giardiasis being known as beaver fever). Although less common, outbreaks associated with food or food handlers have been reported. Among 63 outbreaks of giardiasis with an identified mode of transmission reported from 26 states between 2012 and 2017, waterborne outbreaks were the most common (46%), followed by person-to-person contact (44%) and contaminated food (9.5%). Most of the waterborne outbreaks were associated with drinking water, followed by exposure to recreational water. Surveys conducted in the United States have identified overall prevalence rates of *Giardia* organisms in stool specimens that range from 5% to 7%, with variations depending on age, geographic location, and season.

The **incubation period** usually is 1 to 3 weeks.

DIAGNOSTIC TESTS: *Giardia* cysts or trophozoites are not detected consistently in the stools of infected patients. Diagnostic sensitivity can be increased by examining up to 3 stool specimens over several days. New molecular enteric panel assays generally include *Giardia* organisms as a target pathogen. Diagnostic techniques include direct fluorescence antibody (DFA) assay with microscopy, rapid immunochromatographic cartridge assays, enzyme immunoassay (EIA), microscopy with trichrome staining, and molecular assays. If there is a suspicion of false-negative results, repeat testing should be performed, and use of a different methodology should be considered. Otherwise, retesting is only recommended if symptoms persist after treatment. Invasive testing of the duodenal contents or an intestinal biopsy is required only rarely. Molecular testing to identify the genetic assemblages and subtypes of *Giardia* is not helpful clinically. Giardiasis is not associated with eosinophilia.

TREATMENT: Some infections are self-limited, and treatment may not be required. Tinidazole, metronidazole, and nitazoxanide are the drugs of choice (see Table 4.11, p 1068). Although not approved by the US Food and Drug Administration (FDA) for treatment of *Giardia* infection, the use of metronidazole is widely accepted. It is the least expensive of these therapies but generally has poor palatability when compounded into a suspension. A 5- to 7-day course of metronidazole has an efficacy of 80% to 100% in pediatric patients. Tinidazole, approved by the FDA in 2004 for treatment of giardiasis for children 3 years and older, has high efficacy (about 90%), good tolerability, fewer adverse effects than metronidazole, and is provided as a single oral dose. A 3-day course of nitazoxanide oral suspension has similar efficacy as metronidazole and can also treat other intestinal parasites. Nitazoxanide is approved for use in children 1 year and older with *Giardia* infection. Paromomycin, a poorly absorbed aminoglycoside, is 50% to 70% effective and is the recommended treatment for pregnant persons with giardiasis. Metronidazole has been used in pregnancy, but data regarding safety in the first trimester are conflicting. Tinidazole should not be used during pregnancy.

Symptom recurrence after completing antimicrobial treatment can be attributable to reinfection or recurrence, post-*Giardia* irritable bowel, residual lactose intolerance (occurs in 20%–40% of patients), or symptoms attributable to another process or infection. Recurrences are associated with immunosuppression or poor immunity, insufficient treatment, drug resistance, or reexposure. Because new or residual symptoms are nonspecific, repeated testing should be performed. Options for retreatment include use of an alternative drug of a different class, a longer course of the first failed drug, or combination therapy with 2 different drug classes. One such combination is tinidazole plus quinacrine for at least 2 weeks, which is almost always curative.

Patients who are immunocompromised because of hypogammaglobulinemia or lymphoproliferative disease are at higher risk of giardiasis, and a cure is more difficult for these people. Among human immunodeficiency virus (HIV)-infected children and adults without acquired immunodeficiency syndrome (AIDS), effective combination antiretroviral therapy (ART) and antiparasitic therapy are the major initial treatments for these infections. Patients with AIDS often respond to standard therapy but in some cases additional treatment is required. If giardiasis is refractory to standard treatment among HIV-infected patients with AIDS, longer treatment duration or combination antiparasitic therapy (eg, tinidazole, nitazoxanide, or metronidazole plus one of the following: paromomycin, albendazole, or quinacrine) may be appropriate.

Treatment of asymptomatic carriers is controversial but is recommended in the United States and other areas of low prevalence to prevent infection within families or of other children, which is common. Treatment of children likely to be reinfected, such as those residing in areas of high prevalence, is not recommended unless medically indicated.

INFECTION PREVENTION AND CONTROL MEASURES IN HEALTH CARE SETTINGS: Standard precautions are recommended for most. Contact precautions for the duration of illness are recommended for diapered and incontinent children.

CONTROL MEASURES: Safe water, appropriate sanitation, and handwashing are the most important measures to avoid giardiasis. Avoid drinking and recreational water that may be contaminated. If the safety of drinking water is in doubt (eg, during travel to a location with poor sanitation or lack of water treatment systems), the following are recommended:

- Drink commercially bottled water from an unopened factory-sealed container.
- Disinfect tap water by heating it to a rolling boil for 1 minute.
- Use a filter that has been certified for cyst and oocyst reduction.

Boiling is the most reliable method to make water safe for drinking with required boiling time dependent on altitude (1 minute at sea level). Chemical disinfection with iodine is an alternative method of water treatment using either tincture of iodine or tetraglycine hydroperiodide tablets. Chlorine in various forms also has been used for chemical disinfection, but germicidal activity is dependent on several factors, including pH, temperature, and organic content of the water. Chlorination has low to moderate effectiveness in killing *Giardia*. Additional information about water purification, including a traveler's guide for buying water filters, can be found at. **www.cdc.gov/ healthywater/drinking/travel/index.html.**

Swallowing water during recreational activities in pools, hot tubs, interactive fountains, lakes, rivers, springs, ponds, streams, or the ocean, or drinking untreated water from lakes, rivers, springs, ponds, streams, or shallow wells, should be avoided.

Infected people and individuals at risk especially should adhere to strict hand-hygiene techniques after contact with feces. Use of gloves before handling infected feces or contaminated diapers is a more stringent approach. For additional prevention guidance, visit the CDC *Giardia* website **(www.cdc.gov/parasites/giardia).**

When an outbreak is suspected in a child care center (also see Children in Group Child Care and Schools, p 145), the local health department should be contacted and an epidemiologic investigation should be undertaken to identify and treat all symptomatic children, child care providers, and family members infected with *G duodenalis*. A directory of state and territorial, city and county, and tribal health departments can be found at **www.cdc.gov/publichealthgateway/healthdirectories/index. html.** Infected children should be excluded from child care until stools are contained in the diaper or the child is continent, stool frequency is no more than 2 stools above that child's normal frequency, and the health department agrees with the return to child care. Testing of asymptomatic individuals and treatment of asymptomatic carriers in a child care center outbreak are controversial.

People with diarrhea caused by *Giardia* species should not use recreational water venues (eg, swimming pools, water slides) while symptomatic. For additional information, see Prevention of Illnesses Associated With Recreational Water Use (p 214).

Public Health Reporting. Giardiasis is a nationally notifiable disease. Please refer to the state or local health department for details on reporting cases.

Gonococcal Infections

CLINICAL MANIFESTATIONS: Gonococcal infections are manifested by a spectrum of clinical presentations ranging from asymptomatic infection, to localized infections (usually mucosal), to disseminated disease, and should be considered in 3 distinct age groups: newborn infants, prepubertal children, and postpubertal sexually active adolescents and young adults. Multiple sites of infection can occur simultaneously in one person.

- **Asymptomatic infection** has been detected in the oropharynx of child sexual abuse survivors and in the urogenital tract of sexually active female (up to 80% are asymptomatic) and male (less than 10% can be asymptomatic) individuals.[1] In all age groups, most pharyngeal infections are asymptomatic. Likewise, most rectal infections are asymptomatic; rectal carriage can accompany 20% to 70% of urogenital infections in female individuals.

- **Localized disease** presents at the site of inoculation and includes (1) scalp abscess, which can be associated with fetal scalp monitoring; (2) ophthalmia neonatorum in newborn infants following exposure during birth, or conjunctivitis in any age group following eye inoculation with infected secretions (eg, through hand transfer from urogenital tract); (3) acute tonsillopharyngitis, accompanied by cervical adenopathy; (4) urethritis (with mucopurulent discharge, dysuria, and/or suprapubic pain) in any age group or sex; (5) genital disease such as vulvitis and/or vaginitis in prepubertal patients (with vaginal discharge and/or dysuria), bartholinitis and/or cervicitis in postpubertal patients (with mucopurulent discharge, intermenstrual bleeding, and/or dyspareunia), and penile abscess; and (6) proctitis (symptoms range from painless mucopurulent discharge and scant rectal bleeding to overt proctitis with associated rectal pain and tenesmus). Extension to the upper genital tract and beyond (less common in prepubertal children) can result in pelvic inflammatory disease (endometritis and/or salpingitis), perihepatitis (Fitz-Hugh-Curtis syndrome) in female individuals, and epididymitis, prostatitis, and/or seminal vesiculitis in male individuals, with resultant scarring, ectopic pregnancy, impairment of fertility, and chronic pelvic pain (particularly in female individuals; see Sexually Transmitted Infections in Adolescents and Children, p 179).

- **Disseminated gonococcal infection (DGI)** can occur in up to 3% of untreated people with mucosal gonorrhea. DGI can manifest as petechial or pustular skin lesions and as asymmetric polyarthralgia, tenosynovitis, or oligoarticular septic arthritis (arthritis-dermatitis syndrome). In neonates, DGI can present as sepsis, arthritis, or meningitis. Bacteremia can result in a maculopapular rash with necrosis, tenosynovitis, and migratory arthritis. Arthritis may be reactive (sterile) or septic in nature. Meningitis and endocarditis occur rarely.

ETIOLOGY: *Neisseria gonorrhoeae* is a gram-negative, oxidase-positive diplococcus.

EPIDEMIOLOGY: Gonococcal infections occur only in humans. The source of the organism is exudate and secretions from infected mucosal surfaces; *N gonorrhoeae* is communicable as long as a person harbors the organism. Transmission results from intimate contact, such as sexual acts and parturition. Sexual abuse is the most frequent cause of gonococcal infection in prepubertal children beyond the newborn period (see Sexual Assault and Abuse in Children and Adolescents/Young Adults, p 182).

---

[1] The terms female, male, women, and men refer to sex assigned at birth.

N gonorrhoeae infection is the second most commonly reported sexually transmitted infection (STI) in the United States, following *Chlamydia trachomatis* infection. Reported gonorrhea cases continued to be highest among adolescents and young adults. Rates of reported gonorrhea are highest in the southern United States and have significant racial/ethnic disparities. The rate of reported gonorrhea cases among Black people in the United States is significantly higher than among white people. These higher rates are not caused by ethnicity or genetic predisposition; rather, they are caused by social factors, such as poverty or inequities in education, which are more likely to affect minority groups. Disparities in gonorrhea rates also are identified in certain sexual networks. For example, surveillance networks that monitor trends in STI prevalence among men who have sex with men (MSM) have found very high proportions of positive gonorrhea pharyngeal, urethral, and rectal test results as well as coinfection with other STIs. Populations at greater risk for DGI include asymptomatic carriers; neonates; menstruating, pregnant, and postpartum people; MSM; and individuals with complement deficiency or taking eculizumab.

Gonorrhea can quickly develop resistance to antibiotics used to treat infection, and in 2019 more than half of all infections were estimated to be resistant to at least 1 antibiotic. Since 2010, almost all circulating strains in the United States, based on gonococcal isolates collected through sentinel surveillance in the Gonococcal Isolate Surveillance Project (GISP), remain susceptible to ceftriaxone, the primary treatment for gonorrhea; only 0.1% of isolates displayed elevated ceftriaxone minimum inhibitory concentrations (MICs) in 2020. In 2020, 4.8% of isolates had elevated azithromycin MICs; the proportion was higher among MSM versus men who have sex with women (9.2% vs 4.3%). In 2020, the prevalence of ciprofloxacin resistance was 34.8%.

Diagnosis of genitourinary tract gonorrhea infection should also prompt investigation for other STIs, including chlamydia, trichomoniasis, syphilis, and human immunodeficiency virus (HIV) infection. Concurrent infection with *C trachomatis* is common. People treated for gonococcal infection should also be treated with a regimen that is effective against *C trachomatis* if chlamydia infection has not been excluded.

The **incubation period** usually is 2 to 7 days.

DIAGNOSTIC TESTS[1-3]**:** Microscopic examination of Gram-stained smears of exudate from the conjunctivae, penile urethra, skin lesions, synovial fluid, and when clinically warranted, cerebrospinal fluid (CSF) may be useful in the initial evaluation. Identification of gram-negative intracellular diplococci in these smears can be helpful, particularly if the organism is not recovered in culture. However, because of low sensitivity, a negative smear result should not be considered sufficient for ruling out infection. Intracellular gram-negative diplococci identified on Gram stain of conjunctival exudate justify presumptive treatment for gonorrhea after appropriate cultures for *N gonorrhoeae* are performed.

[1] American Academy of Pediatrics, Committee on Adolescence; Society for Adolescent Health and Medicine. Screening for nonviral sexually transmitted infections in adolescents and young adults. *Pediatrics.* 2014;134(1):e302-e311

[2] Centers for Disease Control and Prevention. Recommendations for the laboratory-based detection of *Chlamydia trachomatis* and *Neisseria gonorrhoeae*—2014. *MMWR Recomm Rep.* 2014;63(RR-2):1-19

[3] Centers for Disease Control and Prevention. Sexually transmitted infections treatment guidelines, 2021. *MMWR Recomm Rep.* 2021;70(4):1-187. Available at **www.cdc.gov/std/treatment-guidelines/gonorrhea.htm**

N gonorrhoeae can be isolated from normally sterile sites, such as blood, CSF, or synovial fluid, using nonselective chocolate agar with incubation in 5% to 10% carbon dioxide. Selective media that inhibit normal flora and nonpathogenic *Neisseria* organisms are used for cultures from nonsterile sites, such as the cervix, vagina, rectum, urethra, and pharynx. Specimens for *N gonorrhoeae* culture from mucosal sites should be inoculated immediately onto appropriate agar because the organism is extremely sensitive to drying and temperature changes. Culture allows for antimicrobial susceptibility testing to aid in management if infection persists following initial therapy.

A nucleic acid amplification test (NAAT) is far superior in overall performance compared with other *N gonorrhoeae* culture and nonculture diagnostic methods to test genital and extragenital specimens. Many commercially available products now are cleared by the US Food and Drug Administration (FDA) for testing penile urethral meatal swab specimens, endocervical or vaginal swab specimens (provider or patient collected), urine specimens, oropharynx or rectal swab specimens (provider or patient collected), or liquid cytology specimens. Although NAATs are not FDA cleared for *N gonorrhoeae* testing on conjunctival swab specimens, they have been shown to be more sensitive compared with *N gonorrhoeae* culture. Product inserts for each NAAT manufacturer should be reviewed because approved collection methods and specimen types vary. For urogenital infections, the Centers for Disease Control and Prevention (CDC) recommends that optimal specimen types for gonorrhea screening using NAATs include first void urine for male patients and vaginal swab specimens for female patients. Patient-collected samples can be used in place of provider-collected samples in clinical settings when testing by NAAT for urine, penile urethral meatal, vaginal, rectal, and oropharyngeal swab specimens, and if appropriate instructions to patients have been provided. Certain NAAT platforms also permit combined testing of specimens for *N gonorrhoeae* and *C trachomatis*.

Infants and Children. Culture can be used to test urogenital and extragenital sites in infants and children. NAATs can be used to test for *N gonorrhoeae* from urine and vaginal specimens. Although data on NAATs from extragenital sites in children are more limited and performance is test dependent, no evidence suggests that performance of a NAAT for detection of *N gonorrhoeae* in children would differ from that in adults. Because of the implications of a diagnosis of *N gonorrhoeae* in a child, however, only validated, FDA-cleared NAATs should be used for extragenital specimens. Consultation with an expert is necessary before using a NAAT in this context, to minimize the possibility of cross-reaction with nongonococcal *Neisseria* species and other commensals. Gram stains are inadequate for evaluating prepubertal children for gonorrhea and should not be used to diagnose or exclude gonorrhea.

TREATMENT[1]**:** A single dose of intramuscular ceftriaxone is the recommended treatment for uncomplicated gonorrhea infections of the cervix, urethra, and rectum. If chlamydial infection has not been excluded, treatment for *C trachomatis* with either oral doxycycline, azithromycin, levofloxacin, or erythromycin, depending on weight of the child/adolescent. Treatment regimens for most syndromes caused by gonococcal infections, including urethritis, cervicitis, pelvic inflammatory disease, epididymitis, and

---

[1] Centers for Disease Control and Prevention. Sexually transmitted infections treatment guidelines, 2021. *MMWR Recomm Rep.* 2021;70(4):1-187. Available at **www.cdc.gov/std/treatment-guidelines/gonorrhea.htm.**

proctitis, are provided in the chapter on Sexually Transmitted Infections (Table 4.4, p 1007, and Table 4.5, p 1014). A single 500-mg dose of intramuscular ceftriaxone also is recommended for the treatment of uncomplicated gonococcal infections of the pharynx. Gonococcal infections of the pharynx are more difficult to eradicate than are infections at urogenital and anorectal sites.

Resistance to penicillin and tetracycline is widespread, and as of 2007, the CDC no longer recommends the use of fluoroquinolones for gonorrhea because of the increased prevalence of quinolone-resistant *N gonorrhoeae* in the United States. Over the past decade, the MIC for cefixime against *N gonorrhoeae* strains circulating in the United States and other countries has increased, and treatment failure following the use of cefixime has been described in North America, Europe, and Asia. Therefore, as of 2012, the CDC no longer recommends the use of cefixime as a first-line treatment for gonococcal infection. Only ceftriaxone is recommended currently for treatment of gonorrhea in the United States.

To maximize adherence with recommended therapies and reduce complications and transmission, medication for gonococcal infection should be provided on site and directly observed. If medications are not available when treatment is indicated, linkage to an STI treatment facility should be provided for same-day treatment. To minimize disease transmission, people treated for gonorrhea should be instructed to abstain from sexual activity for 7 days after treatment and until all sex partners are adequately treated (7 days after receiving treatment and resolution of symptoms, if present).

Neonatal Infection. Infants with clinical evidence of ophthalmia neonatorum or scalp abscess attributable to *N gonorrhoeae* should be hospitalized, managed in consultation with a pediatric infectious disease specialist, and evaluated for disseminated infection (sepsis, arthritis, meningitis).

One dose of ceftriaxone (25–50 mg/kg, intravenously [IV] or intramuscularly [IM]) is adequate therapy for gonococcal ophthalmia. For neonates who are unable to receive ceftriaxone because of simultaneous administration of intravenous calcium, 1 dose of cefotaxime (100 mg/kg, IV or IM) may be given. Topical antibiotic therapy alone is inadequate and unnecessary if systemic treatment is administered.

For gonococcal scalp abscesses and disseminated gonococcal infections in neonates, treatment is with ceftriaxone (25–50 mg/kg/day, IV, administered once daily) or cefotaxime (50 mg/kg/day in 2 divided daily doses, IV or IM) for 7 days, with a duration of 10 to 14 days if meningitis is documented.

INFECTION PREVENTION AND CONTROL MEASURES IN HEALTH CARE SETTINGS: Standard precautions are recommended, including for newborn infants with ophthalmia.

CONTROL MEASURES: Current control measures consist of counseling on the use of barrier protection during sexual intercourse, close follow-up of infected patients and their contacts, chemoprophylaxis recommended for specific clinical scenarios, routine screening in accordance with guidelines, and case reporting to public health authorities. There is no vaccine to prevent gonococcal infections.

Follow-up. A test-of-cure is not needed for people in whom uncomplicated urogenital or rectal gonorrhea is diagnosed who are treated with a single dose of ceftriaxone. Any person with pharyngeal gonorrhea should return between 7 to 14 days after initial treatment for a test-of cure using culture, NAAT, or both. If the NAAT result is positive, effort should be made to perform a confirmatory culture before retreatment, if a culture was not already collected. All positive cultures for test-of-cure should undergo antimicrobial susceptibility testing. People who have been treated for gonorrhea should be retested 3 months after treatment for the possibility of reinfection, regardless of whether they believe their sex partners were treated. If retesting at 3 months is not possible, clinicians should retest whenever people next present for medical care within 12 months following initial treatment. All people in whom gonorrhea is diagnosed should be tested for other STIs, including chlamydia, trichomoniasis (vaginal specimens), syphilis, and HIV infection.

Management of Sex Partners. Recent sex partners (ie, people having had sexual contact with the infected patient within the 60 days preceding onset of symptoms or gonorrhea diagnosis) should be referred for evaluation, testing, and presumptive treatment. If the patient's last potential sexual exposure was >60 days before onset of symptoms or diagnosis, the most recent sex partner should be treated. To avoid reinfection, sex partners should be instructed to abstain from condomless sexual intercourse for 7 days after they and their sexual partner(s) have completed treatment and after resolution of symptoms, if present.

For people with gonorrhea for whom health department partner-management strategies are impractical or unavailable and whose providers are concerned about partners' access to prompt clinical evaluation and treatment, expedited partner therapy (EPT) can be delivered to the partner by the patient, a disease investigation specialist, or a collaborating pharmacy, as permitted by law. Details are provided in the CDC STI Guidelines.[1]

Prophylaxis.

Neonatal Ophthalmia. If gonorrhea is prevalent in the region and prenatal treatment cannot be ensured, or where required by law, a prophylactic agent should be instilled into the eyes of all newborn infants (including those born by cesarean delivery) to prevent sight-threatening gonococcal ophthalmia (see Neonatal Ophthalmia Prevention, p 1129).

Newborn Infants Whose Birthing Parent Has Gonococcal Infection. A neonate whose birthing parent has untreated gonorrhea is at high risk for infection. These neonates should be tested for gonorrhea at exposed sites (eg, conjunctive, vaginal, rectal, and oropharynx) and treated presumptively for gonorrhea (see Neonatal Ophthalmia Prevention, p 1129).

Children and Adolescents With Sexual Exposure to a Patient Known to Have Gonorrhea. People sexually exposed within the 60 days preceding onset of symptoms or gonorrhea in the index case (or most recent sexual contact, if last potential sexual exposure was >60 days before onset of symptoms or gonorrhea) should undergo examination and culture and should receive the same treatment as do people known to have gonorrhea.

Postexposure Prophylaxis. Doxycycline, 200 mg, administered within 24 to 72 hours of condomless sex (doxy-PEP) has been shown in studies to reduce the incidence of syphilis, chlamydia, and gonorrhea among cisgender men who have sex with men (MSM) and transgender women with a recent history of these infections.

---

[1] Centers for Disease Control and Prevention. Sexually transmitted infections treatment guidelines, 2021. *MMWR Recomm Rep.* 2021;70(4):1-187. Available at **www.cdc.gov/std/treatment-guidelines/clinical-partnerServices.htm**

Routine Screening. Annual screening for *N gonorrhoeae* infection is recommended for all sexually active women younger than 25 years.[1] Additional risk factors for gonorrhea include inconsistent condom use among people who are not in mutually monogamous relationships, previous or coexisting STIs, and exchanging sex for money or drugs. Clinicians should consider the communities they serve and might opt to consult local public health authorities for guidance on identifying groups at increased risk. Gonococcal infection is concentrated in specific geographic locations and communities. MSM at high risk for gonorrhea infection (multiple anonymous partners, substance use) or those at risk for HIV acquisition should be screened at all sites of exposure every 3 to 6 months. At least annual screening is recommended for all MSM. A recent travel history with sexual contacts outside of the United States should be part of any gonorrhea evaluation.

All pregnant people younger than 25 years should be screened for gonorrhea at the first prenatal visit. Pregnant people 25 years and older should be screened if they are considered at risk (ie, a new sex partner, more than 1 sex partner, a sex partner with concurrent partners, or a sex partner who has an STI or lives in an area with a high rate of gonorrhea). A repeat screen in the third trimester is recommended for pregnant people at continued risk of gonococcal infection, including all patients younger than 25 years. Pregnant people with a diagnosis of gonorrhea should be treated immediately and rescreened within 3 months.

Public Health Reporting. All cases of gonorrhea must be reported to local public health officials (see Appendix III, Nationally Notifiable Infectious Diseases in the United States, p 1141). Cases in prepubertal children must be investigated to determine the source of infection (see Sexual Assault and Abuse in Children and Adolescents/Young Adults, p 182).

Granuloma Inguinale
(Donovanosis)

CLINICAL MANIFESTATIONS: Initial lesions of this sexually transmitted genital ulcerative disease are single or multiple painless subcutaneous nodules that gradually ulcerate. These nontender, granulomatous ulcers have raised, rolled margins, are beefy red and highly vascular, and bleed readily on contact. "Kissing" lesions may occur from auto-inoculation on adjacent skin. Lesions usually involve the genitalia or perineum without regional adenopathy; however, lesions at both the genitalia and inguinal region occur in 5% to 10% of patients. Subcutaneous granulomas extending into the inguinal area can mimic inguinal adenopathy (ie, "pseudobubo"). Extragenital lesions (eg, face, mouth) account for 6% of cases. Dissemination to intra-abdominal organs and bone is rare.

ETIOLOGY: The disease, donovanosis, is caused by *Klebsiella granulomatis* (formerly known as *Calymmatobacterium granulomatis*), an intracellular gram-negative bacillus.

EPIDEMIOLOGY: Indigenous granuloma inguinale occurs very rarely in the United States and most industrialized nations. Sporadic cases have been described in India, South America, and South Africa. The incidence of infection seems to correlate with sustained high temperatures and high relative humidity. Infection usually is acquired

---

[1] US Preventive Services Task Force. Final Recommendation Statement: Chlamydia and Gonorrhea: Screening. September 14, 2021. Available at: **www.uspreventiveservicestaskforce.org/uspstf/ recommendation/chlamydia-and-gonorrhea-screening**

by sexual contact, most commonly with a person with active infection. Young children and others can, less commonly, acquire infection by contact with infected secretions. The period of communicability extends throughout the duration of active lesions.

The **incubation period** is uncertain; a range of 1 to 360 days has been reported. Experimental production of typical donovanosis lesions was induced in humans 50 days after inoculation.

DIAGNOSTIC TESTS: The causative organism is difficult to culture, and diagnosis requires microscopic demonstration of dark-staining intracytoplasmic Donovan bodies on Wright, Leishman, or Giemsa staining of a crush preparation from subsurface scrapings of a lesion or tissue. The microorganism also can be detected by histologic examination of biopsy specimens. Culture of *K granulomatis* is difficult to perform and is not available routinely. No molecular tests exist that have been cleared by the US Food and Drug Administration for the detection of *K granulomatis*. Diagnosis by nucleic acid amplification test (NAAT) and serologic testing is only available in research laboratories.

TREATMENT[1]: The recommended treatment regimen is azithromycin (Table 4.4, p 1007) for at least 3 weeks and until all lesions have completely healed. Alternative treatment regimens include doxycycline, erythromycin, or trimethoprim-sulfamethoxazole. Pregnant and lactating people with granuloma inguinale should be treated with a macrolide regimen (azithromycin or erythromycin). Treatment has been shown to halt progression of lesions. Partial healing usually is noted within 7 days of initiation of therapy and typically proceeds inward from the ulcer margins. Prolonged therapy usually is required to permit granulation and re-epithelialization of the ulcers. Relapse can occur, especially if the antimicrobial agent is stopped before the primary lesion has healed completely. In addition, relapse can occur 6 to 18 months after apparently effective therapy. Complicated or long-standing infection can require surgical intervention.

Patients should be followed clinically until signs and symptoms have resolved. Patients should be evaluated for other sexually transmitted infections, including syphilis, HIV, gonorrhea, and chlamydia.

INFECTION PREVENTION AND CONTROL MEASURES IN HEALTH CARE SETTINGS: Standard precautions are recommended.

CONTROL MEASURES: People who have had sexual contact with a patient who has granuloma inguinale within the 60 days before onset of the patient's symptoms should be examined and offered therapy. However, the value of empiric therapy in the absence of clinical signs and symptoms has not been established.

Haemophilus influenzae Infections

CLINICAL MANIFESTATIONS: *Haemophilus influenzae* type b causes pneumonia, bacteremia, meningitis, epiglottitis, septic arthritis, cellulitis, otitis media, purulent pericarditis, and less commonly, endocarditis, endophthalmitis, osteomyelitis, peritonitis, and gangrene. Infections caused by encapsulated but non-type b *H influenzae* present in a similar manner to type b infections. Nonencapsulated strains more commonly cause infections of the respiratory tract (eg, otitis media, sinusitis, pneumonia, conjunctivitis),

---

[1] Centers for Disease Control and Prevention. Sexually transmitted infections treatment guidelines, 2021. *MMWR Recomm Rep*. 2021;70(RR-4). Available at: **www.cdc.gov/std/treatment-guidelines/donovanosis.htm**

but cases of bacteremia, meningitis, chorioamnionitis, and neonatal septicemia are well described.

ETIOLOGY: *H influenzae* is a pleomorphic gram-negative coccobacillus. Encapsulated strains express 1 of 6 antigenically distinct capsular polysaccharides (a through f); non-encapsulated strains lack complete capsule genes and are designated nontypeable.

EPIDEMIOLOGY[1]: The mode of transmission is person-to-person by inhalation of respiratory tract droplets or by direct contact with respiratory tract secretions. In neonates, infection is acquired intrapartum by aspiration of amniotic fluid or by contact with genital tract secretions containing the organism. Pharyngeal colonization by *H influenzae* is relatively common, especially with nontypeable strains. In the era before *H influenzae* type b (Hib) vaccines, the major reservoir of *H influenzae* type b was young infants and toddlers, who may asymptomatically carry the organism in their upper respiratory tracts.

Before introduction of effective Hib conjugate vaccines, *H influenzae* type b was the most common cause of bacterial meningitis in young children in the United States. The peak incidence of most invasive *H influenzae* type b infections occurred between 6 and 18 months of age, while the peak age for *H influenzae* type b epiglottitis was 2 to 4 years of age.

Unimmunized children younger than 5 years are at increased risk of invasive *H influenzae* type b disease. Other predisposing factors include sickle cell disease, asplenia, human immunodeficiency virus (HIV) infection, certain immunodeficiency syndromes, and chemotherapy for malignant neoplasms. Historically, invasive *H influenzae* type b infection was more common in child care attendees, children living in crowded conditions, and children who were not breastfed.

Since introduction of Hib conjugate vaccines in the United States, the incidence of invasive *H influenzae* type b disease has decreased by more than 99% in young children. In 2019, 18 cases of invasive *H influenzae* type b disease were reported in children younger than 5 years (0.09 cases per 100 000). In the United States, invasive *H influenzae* type b disease occurs primarily in underimmunized children and among infants too young to have completed the primary Hib immunization series; in addition, American Indian/Alaska Native (AI/AN) children continue to experience an elevated burden of disease. *H influenzae* type b remains an important pathogen in many resource-limited countries where Hib vaccine coverage is suboptimal.

The epidemiology of invasive *H influenzae* disease in the United States has shifted in the post-Hib vaccination era. Nontypeable *H influenzae* is now the most common cause of invasive *H influenzae* disease in all age groups. In 2019, the annual incidence of invasive nontypeable *H influenzae* disease was 1.7/100 000 in children younger than 5 years, and the rate was highest in children younger than 1 year (5.1/100 000). Among the cases in children younger than 1 year, approximately half were diagnosed within the first 2 weeks of life; many were in preterm neonates who had a positive culture on the day of birth. In addition to invasive disease, nontypeable *H influenzae* causes about 50% of episodes of acute otitis media and sinusitis in children and is a common cause of recurrent otitis media.

---

[1] Centers for Disease Control and Prevention. Prevention and control of *Haemophilus influenzae* type b disease: recommendations of the Advisory Committee on Immunization Practices (ACIP). *MMWR Recomm Rep.* 2014;63(RR-1):1–14

H influenzae type a has emerged as the most common encapsulated serotype causing invasive disease in children <5 years, with a clinical presentation similar to that of *H influenzae* type b. In some North American Indigenous populations (eg, Alaska Native children, northern Canadian Indigenous children), the rate of invasive *H influenzae* type a infection has been increasing and secondary cases have been reported. Although the incidence of invasive *H influenzae* type a is lower among the general population of US children, it has also been increasing in recent years, with a nearly 300% increase over the last 10 years among children younger than 1 year of age. Invasive disease may also be caused by the 4 other encapsulated non-type b strains (ie, c, d, e, and f).

The **incubation period** is unknown.

DIAGNOSTIC TESTS: The diagnosis of invasive disease is established by growth on appropriate media of *H influenzae* from cerebrospinal fluid (CSF), blood, synovial fluid, pleural fluid, or pericardial fluid. Because occult meningitis is known to occur in young children with invasive *H influenzae* type b disease, a lumbar puncture should be strongly considered in the presence of invasive disease, even in the absence of central nervous system signs and symptoms. Gram stain of an infected body fluid specimen can facilitate presumptive diagnosis. Antigen detection methods, which have historically been used on CSF, blood, and urine specimens, are not recommended because they lack sensitivity and specificity. Nucleic acid amplification tests (NAATs) available in multiplexed assays to detect *H influenzae* DNA directly in blood, CSF or pleural fluid, may be particularly useful in patients whose specimens are obtained after the initiation of antibiotics. Most of these assays do not determine the capsular polysaccharide type and, therefore, cannot identify the DNA amplicon as type b, type a, etc, and these tests do not provide antibiotic susceptibilities.

The capsular polysaccharide of *H influenzae* isolates associated with invasive infection should be determined. Molecular methods, such as NAATs of genes in the *cap* locus, are preferred over serotyping by slide agglutination for capsule typing. If typing is not available at the clinical laboratory, isolates should be submitted to the state health department or to a reference laboratory to be typed.

TREATMENT:
- Initial therapy for children with *H influenzae* meningitis is cefotaxime or ceftriaxone at meningitic doses (see Table 4.3, p 993). Intravenous ampicillin at meningitic doses may be substituted if the isolate is found to be susceptible. Beta-lactamase–negative, ampicillin-resistant strains of *H influenzae* have been described, and some experts recommend caution in using ampicillin when minimum inhibitory concentrations (MICs) of 1 to 2 µg/mL are found, especially in the setting of invasive infection or disease in immunocompromised hosts. Treatment of other invasive *H influenzae* infections is similar. Therapy is continued for 7 to 10 days by the intravenous route and longer in complicated infections.
- Dexamethasone is beneficial for treatment of infants and children with *H influenzae* type b meningitis to diminish the risk of hearing loss, if administered before or concurrently with the first dose of antimicrobial agent(s).
- Epiglottitis is a medical emergency. An airway must be established promptly via controlled intubation.
- Infected pleural or pericardial fluid should be drained.
- See the Systems-based Treatment Table (p 1) for discussion of other infections for which *H influenzae* may be a pathogen.

INFECTION PREVENTION AND CONTROL MEASURES IN HEALTH CARE SETTINGS:
In addition to standard precautions, in patients with invasive *H influenzae* type b disease, droplet precautions are recommended through 24 hours after initiation of effective antimicrobial therapy.

CONTROL MEASURES (FOR INVASIVE *H INFLUENZAE* TYPE B DISEASE):

Care of Exposed People. Secondary cases of *H influenzae* type b disease have occurred in unimmunized or incompletely immunized children exposed to invasive disease in a child care or household setting. Such children should be observed carefully for fever or other signs/symptoms of disease. Exposed young children in whom febrile illness develops should receive prompt medical evaluation.

Chemoprophylaxis.[1] The risk of invasive *H influenzae* type b disease is increased among unimmunized household contacts younger than 4 years. Rifampin eradicates *H influenzae* type b from the pharynx in approximately 95% of carriers and decreases the risk of secondary invasive illness in exposed household contacts. Child care center contacts also may be at increased risk of secondary disease when unimmunized or incompletely immunized children are attending, but secondary disease in child care contacts is rare when all contacts are older than 2 years. Indications and guidelines for chemoprophylaxis in different circumstances are summarized in Table 3.10.

- **Household.** See Table 3.10 for details regarding prophylaxis for household members of a person with invasive *H influenzae* type b disease, when at least 1 household member fits the listed criteria. Given that most secondary cases in households occur during the first week after hospitalization of the index case, prophylaxis should be initiated as soon as possible when it is indicated. Because some secondary cases occur later, initiation of prophylaxis 7 days or more after hospitalization of the index patient still may be of some benefit.
- **Child care and preschool.** When 2 or more cases of invasive *H influenzae* type b disease have occurred within 60 days and unimmunized or incompletely immunized children attend the child care facility or preschool, rifampin prophylaxis for all attendees (irrespective of their age and vaccine status) and child care providers should be considered. In addition to these recommendations for chemoprophylaxis, unimmunized or incompletely immunized children should receive a dose of Hib vaccine and should be scheduled for completion of the recommended age-specific immunization schedule **https://publications.aap.org/redbook/pages/Immunization-Schedules**). Data are insufficient on the risk of secondary transmission to recommend chemoprophylaxis for child care attendees and providers when a single case of invasive *H influenzae* type b disease occurs; the decision to provide chemoprophylaxis in this situation is at the discretion of the local or state health department.
- **Index case.** See Table 3.10.
- **Dosage.** For prophylaxis, rifampin should be administered orally, once a day for 4 days (20 mg/kg; maximum dose, 600 mg). The dose for infants younger than 1 month is not established; some experts recommend lowering the dose to 10 mg/kg. For adults, each dose is 600 mg. If rifampin is contraindicated, administering a

---

[1] Centers for Disease Control and Prevention. Prevention and control of *Haemophilus influenzae* type b disease: recommendations of the Advisory Committee on Immunization Practices (ACIP). *MMWR Recomm Rep.* 2014;63(RR-1):1–14

Table 3.10. Indications and Guidelines for Rifampin Chemoprophylaxis for Contacts of Index Cases of Invasive *Haemophilus influenzae* Type b Disease[a]

Chemoprophylaxis Recommended

- For all household contacts[b] in the following circumstances:

  - Household with at least 1 child younger than 4 years who is unimmunized or incompletely immunized[c]

  - Household with a child younger than 12 months who has not completed the primary *H influenzae* type b (Hib) vaccine series

  - Household with an immunocompromised child, regardless of that child's Hib immunization status or age

- For preschool and child care center contacts when 2 or more cases of *H influenzae* type b invasive disease have occurred within 60 days and unimmunized or incompletely immunized children attend the child care facility or preschool (see text)

- For index patient, if younger than 2 years or member of a household with a susceptible contact and treated with a regimen other than cefotaxime or ceftriaxone, chemoprophylaxis at the end of therapy for invasive infection

Chemoprophylaxis Not Recommended

- For occupants of households with no children younger than 4 years other than the index patient

- For occupants of households when all household contacts are immunocompetent, all household contacts 12 through 48 months of age have completed their Hib immunization series, and when household contacts younger than 12 months have completed their primary series of Hib immunizations

- For preschool and child care contacts of 1 index case

- For index patients over age 2 years or treated with a full course of cefotaxime or ceftriaxone for *H influenzae* type b invasive disease

- For pregnant people

[a]Similar criteria may be used for *H influenzae* type a; however, the criteria for Hib immunization are not applicable.
[b]Defined as people residing with the index patient or nonresidents who spent 4 or more hours with the index patient for at least 5 of the 7 days preceding the day of hospital admission of the index case.
[c]Complete immunization is defined as having had at least 1 dose of Hib conjugate vaccine at 15 months of age or older; 2 doses between 12 and 14 months of age; or the 2- or 3-dose primary series when younger than 12 months with a booster dose at 12 months of age or older.

single dose of ceftriaxone can be considered, although the durability of eradication using this approach has not been well established.

- **Invasive *H influenzae* type a disease.** Clinicians can consider chemoprophylaxis of household contacts of index cases of invasive *H influenzae* type a disease in those households with a child younger than 4 years or with an immunocompromised child. For these individuals and contacts, chemoprophylaxis recommendations for *H influenzae* type b listed in Table 3.10 may be followed; however, because there is not a licensed vaccine for *H influenzae* type a, the criteria regarding vaccination do not apply. A similar approach as *H influenzae* type b disease also may be considered for

Table 3.11. *Haemophilus influenzae* Type b (Hib) Conjugate Vaccines Licensed and Available for Use in Infants and Children in the United States[a]

Vaccine	Trade Name	Components	Manufacturer
PRP-T	ActHIB	PRP conjugated to tetanus toxoid	Sanofi Pasteur
PRP-T	Hiberix	PRP conjugated to tetanus toxoid	GlaxoSmithKline Biologicals
PRP-OMP	PedvaxHIB	PRP conjugated to OMP	Merck & Co, Inc
DTaP-IPV-Hib[b]	Pentacel	DTaP-IPV + PRP-T	Sanofi Pasteur
DTaP-IPV-Hib-HepB	Vaxelis	DTaP-IPV + PRP-OMP + HepB	Sanofi Pasteur and Merck & Co, Inc

PRP-T indicates polyribosylribotol phosphate-tetanus toxoid; OMP, outer membrane protein complex from *Neisseria meningitidis;* DTaP, diphtheria and tetanus toxoids and acellular pertussis; IPV, inactivated (non-live) poliovirus vaccine; HepB, hepatitis B vaccine.

[a] Hib conjugate vaccines may be administered in combination products or as reconstituted products, provided the combination or reconstituted vaccine is licensed by the US Food and Drug Administration (FDA) for the child's age and administration of the other vaccine component(s) also is justified.

[b] The DTaP-IPV liquid component is used to reconstitute a lyophilized ActHIB vaccine component to form Pentacel.

preschool and child care contacts in consultation with the local or state public health department.

Immunization.[1] Three single-antigen (monovalent) Hib conjugate vaccine products and 2 combination vaccine products that contain Hib conjugate are available in the United States (see Table 3.11). The Hib conjugate vaccine consists of the Hib capsular polysaccharide (polyribosylribotol phosphate [PRP]) covalently linked to a carrier protein. Protective antibodies are directed against PRP.

Depending on the vaccine, the recommended primary series consists of 3 doses administered at 2, 4, and 6 months of age or of 2 doses administered at 2 and 4 months of age (see Recommendations for Immunization, p 407, and Table 3.12). The regimens in Table 3.12 likely are to be equivalent in protection after completion of the recommended primary Hib series. For AI/AN children, administration of PRP-OMP (outer membrane protein complex) monovalent Hib vaccine (PedvaxHIB) is preferred, because this formulation elicits a protective immune response after dose 1 and this population historically experienced invasive *H influenzae* type b disease at a younger age compared with the general US population. Information on immunogenicity after dose 1 of new PRP-OMP–containing Hib vaccines is important for assessing their suitability for use in AI/AN children.

- **Combination Vaccines.** Two combination vaccines that contain Hib are licensed in the United States. DTaP-IPV-Hib (Pentacel) is administered as a 4-dose series at 2, 4, 6, and 15 through 18 months of age. DTaP-IPV-Hib-HepB (Vaxelis)

[1] Centers for Disease Control and Prevention. Prevention and control of *Haemophilus influenzae* type b disease: recommendations of the Advisory Committee on Immunization Practices (ACIP). *MMWR Recomm Rep.* 2014;63(RR-1):1–14

Table 3.12. Recommended Regimens for Routine *Haemophilus influenzae* Type b (Hib) Conjugate Immunization for Children Immunized at 2 Months Through 4 Years of Age[a]

Vaccine Product	Primary Series	Booster Dose	Catch-up Doses[b]
PRP-T (ActHIB, Sanofi Pasteur)	2, 4, 6 mo	12 through 15 mo	16 mo through 4 y
PRP-T (Hiberix, GlaxoSmithKline)	2, 4, 6 mo	12 through 15 mo	16 mo through 4 y
PRP-OMP (PedvaxHIB, Merck)[c,d]	2, 4 mo	12 through 15 mo	16 mo through 4 y
Combination vaccine			
DTaP-IPV-Hib (Pentacel, Sanofi Pasteur)	2, 4, 6 mo	12 through 15 mo	16 mo through 4 y
DTaP-IPV-Hib-HepB (Vaxelis, Sanofi Pasteur, Merck & Co, Inc)	2, 4, 6 mo	Use other Hib-containing vaccine for booster, at least 6 months after last priming dose	

PRP-T indicates polyribosylribotol phosphate-tetanus toxoid; OMP, outer membrane protein complex from *Neisseria meningitidis;* DTaP, diphtheria and tetanus toxoids and acellular pertussis; IPV, inactivated (non-live) poliovirus vaccine; Hep B, hepatitis B vaccine.

[a]See text and Table 3.11 (p 405) for further information about specific vaccines and Table 1.10 (p 65) for information about combination vaccines.

[b]See Catch-up Immunization Schedule (**https://publications.aap.org/redbook/pages/Immunization-Schedules**) for additional information.

[c]If a PRP-OMP(PedvaxHIB) vaccine is not administered as both doses in the primary series, a third dose of Hib conjugate vaccine is needed to complete the primary series.

[d]Preferred for American Indian/Alaska Native (AI/AN) children.

is administered as a 3-dose primary series at 2, 4, and 6 months of age; a Hib-containing vaccine other than Vaxelis should be administered for the booster dose at 15 to 18 months of age. Until information on the immunogenicity after the first dose of the PRP-OMP–containing combination vaccine (DTaP-IPV-Hib-HepB [Vaxelis]) is available, this vaccine does not have a preferential recommendation for use in AI/AN infants.

- **Vaccine Interchangeability.** Hib conjugate vaccines licensed within the age range for the primary vaccine series are considered interchangeable as long as recommendations for a total of 3 doses in the first year of life are followed (ie, if 2 doses of monovalent PRP-OMP are not administered, 3 doses of a Hib-containing vaccine are required). Data are not available on safety and effectiveness of interchangeability of some vaccines (see package inserts).
- **Dosage and Route of Administration.** The dose of each Hib conjugate vaccine is 0.5 mL, administered intramuscularly.
- **Children With Immunologic Impairment.** Children at increased risk of *H influenzae* type b disease may have impaired anti-PRP antibody responses to

conjugate vaccines. Examples include children with functional or anatomic asplenia, HIV infection, or immunoglobulin deficiency (including an isolated immunoglobulin [Ig] G2 subclass deficiency) or early component complement deficiency; recipients of hematopoietic cell transplants; and children undergoing chemotherapy for a malignant neoplasm. Some children with immunologic impairment may benefit from more doses of conjugate vaccine than usually indicated (see Recommendations for Immunization: Indications and Schedule).

- **Adverse Reactions.** Adverse reactions to Hib conjugate vaccines are uncommon. Pain, redness, and swelling at the injection site occur in approximately 25% of recipients, but these symptoms typically are mild and last fewer than 24 hours. Refer to the manufacturer package inserts for additional information.

Recommendations for Immunization
Indications and Schedule

- All children should be immunized with a Hib conjugate vaccine beginning at approximately 2 months of age (see Table 3.12). Other general recommendations are as follows:
  - Immunization can be initiated as early as 6 weeks of age.
  - Vaccine can be administered during visits for other childhood immunizations (see Simultaneous Administration of Multiple Vaccines, p 63).
- For routine immunization of children younger than 7 months, the following guidelines are recommended:
  - **Primary series.** Table 3.12 lists the options for the primary vaccination series. Doses are administered at approximately 2-month intervals. When sequential doses of different vaccine products are administered or uncertainty exists about which products previously were used, 3 doses of a conjugate vaccine are considered sufficient to complete the primary series, regardless of the regimen used (see package inserts; data are not available for some vaccines on interchangeability).
  - **Booster immunization at 12 through 15 months of age.** For children who have completed a primary series, an additional dose of conjugate vaccine is recommended at 12 through 15 months of age and at least 2 months after the last dose. Any monovalent or the pentavalent combination (Pentacel) Hib conjugate vaccine is acceptable for this dose. Vaxelis should not be used for the booster dose.
- Children younger than 5 years who did not receive Hib conjugate vaccine during the first 6 months of life should be immunized according to the recommended catch-up immunization schedule (see **https://publications.aap.org/redbook/pages/Immunization-Schedules** and Table 3.12). For accelerated immunization in infants younger than 12 months, a minimum of a 4-week interval between doses can be used.
- Children with invasive *H influenzae* type b infection who are younger than 24 months of age can remain at risk of developing a second episode of disease. These children should be immunized according to the age-appropriate schedule for unimmunized children as if they had received no previous Hib vaccine doses (see Table 3.12, and Table 1.10, p 65). Immunization should be initiated 1 month after onset of disease or as soon as possible thereafter.
- Immunologic evaluation should be performed in children who experience invasive *H influenzae* type b disease despite 2 to 3 doses of vaccine and in children with recurrent invasive disease attributable to type b strains.

- See Table 3.13 for special circumstances such as patients undergoing chemotherapy, radiation therapy, hematopoietic cell transplant, or splenectomy. Additional details are as follows:
  - **Lapsed immunizations.** Recommendations for children who have had a lapse in the schedule of immunizations are summarized in the annual immunization schedule (**https://publications.aap.org/redbook/pages/Immunization-Schedules**).
  - **Preterm infants.** For preterm infants who are medically stable, immunization should be based on chronologic age and should be initiated at 2 months following birth according to recommendations in Table 3.12.
  - **Functional/anatomic asplenia.** Children with decreased or absent splenic function who have received a primary series of Hib immunizations and a booster dose at 12 months or older need not be immunized further against *H influenzae* type b.

Table 3.13. Use of *Haemophilus influenzae* Type b (Hib) Conjugate Immunization in Special Populations

High-Risk Group	Vaccine Recommendations
Patient <12 mo	Follow routine Hib vaccination recommendations
Patients 12 through 59 mo	If unimmunized or received 0 or 1 dose before age 12 months: 2 doses 2 months apart
	If received 2 or more doses before age 12 months: 1 dose
	If completed a primary series and received a booster dose at age 12 months or older: no additional doses
Patients undergoing chemotherapy or radiation therapy, age <60 mo	If routine Hib doses administered 14 or more days before starting therapy: revaccination not required
	If dose administered within 14 days of starting therapy or during therapy: repeat doses starting at least 3 months following therapy completion of therapy
Patients undergoing elective splenectomy, age ≥15 mo	If unimmunized[a]: 1 dose, preferably at least 14 days prior to procedure
Asplenic patients ≥60 mo and adults	If unimmunized[a]: 1 dose[b]
HIV-infected children ≥60 mo	If unimmunized[a]: 1 dose[b]
HIV-infected adults	Hib vaccination is not recommended
Recipients of hematopoietic cell transplant, all ages	Regardless of Hib vaccination history: 3 doses (at least 1 month apart) beginning 6–12 mo after transplant[b]

[a] Patients who have not received a primary series and booster dose or at least 1 dose of Hib vaccine after 14 months of age are considered unimmunized.

[b] Recommended by the Centers for Disease Control and Prevention Advisory Committee on Immunizations Practices, although Hib vaccines are not licensed for individuals older than 5 years.

- **Other high-risk groups.** Children with HIV infection, IgG2 subclass deficiency, or early component complement deficiency are at increased risk of invasive *H influenzae* type b disease. Whether these children will benefit from additional doses after completion of the primary series of immunizations and the booster dose at 12 months or older is unknown.
- Catch-up immunization for high-risk groups (**https://publications.aap.org/redbook/pages/Immunization-Schedules**) (Table 3.13):
  - For children 12 through 59 months of age with an underlying condition predisposing to *H influenzae* type b disease (functional or anatomic asplenia, HIV infection, immunoglobulin deficiency, early component complement deficiency, or receipt of hematopoietic cell transplant or chemotherapy for a malignant neoplasm) who are not immunized or have received only 1 dose of conjugate vaccine before 12 months of age, 2 doses of any conjugate vaccine, separated by 2 months, are recommended. For children in this age group who received 2 or more doses before 12 months of age, 1 additional dose of conjugate vaccine is recommended.

Public Health Reporting. All cases of *H influenzae* invasive disease, including type b, non-type b, and nontypeable, should be reported to the local or state public health department.

Hantavirus Pulmonary Syndrome

CLINICAL MANIFESTATIONS: Hantaviruses cause 2 distinct clinical syndromes: (1) hantavirus pulmonary syndrome (HPS), also known as hantavirus cardiopulmonary syndrome (HCPS), characterized by noncardiogenic pulmonary edema, which is observed in the Americas; and (2) hemorrhagic fever with renal syndrome (HFRS), which occurs worldwide (see Hemorrhagic Fevers and Related Syndromes Caused by Bunyaviruses, p 420). After an incubation period of 1 to 8 weeks, the prodromal illness of HPS lasts 3 to 7 days and is characterized by fever, chills, headache, myalgia, nausea, vomiting, diarrhea, dizziness, and sometimes cough. Respiratory tract symptoms or signs usually do not occur during the first 3 to 7 days, but then pulmonary edema and severe hypoxemia appear abruptly and present as cough and dyspnea. The disease then progresses over hours. In severe cases, myocardial dysfunction causes hypotension, which is why the syndrome sometimes is called hantavirus cardiopulmonary syndrome.

Extensive bilateral interstitial and alveolar pulmonary edema with pleural effusions are attributable to diffuse pulmonary capillary leak. Intubation and assisted ventilation usually are required for only 2 to 4 days, with resolution heralded by onset of diuresis and rapid clinical improvement.

The severe myocardial depression is different from that of septic shock, with low cardiac indices and stroke volume index, normal pulmonary wedge pressure, and increased systemic vascular resistance. Poor prognostic indicators include persistent hypotension, marked hemoconcentration, a cardiac index of less than 2, and abrupt onset of lactic acidosis with a serum lactate concentration of >4 mmol/L (36 mg/dL).

The mortality rate for patients with HPS is between 30% and 40%; death usually occurs in the first 1 or 2 days of hospitalization. A disproportionate number of cases occurs in American Indian/Alaska Native (AI/AN) populations, and case fatality rates for these populations are higher than for non-Native populations. Milder forms of disease have been reported. Limited information suggests that clinical manifestations and prognosis are similar in adults and children. Serious sequelae are uncommon. There are typically 20 to 40 cases of HPS reported annually in the United States, with the majority (94%) of cases occurring west of the Mississippi River. Cases in children younger than 10 years are exceedingly rare. Children may be less likely to become infected than adults, because children are less likely to perform tasks that would place them at increased risk.

ETIOLOGY: Hantaviruses are RNA viruses of the *Hantaviridae* family. Sin Nombre virus (SNV) is the major cause of HPS in the western and central regions of the United States. Bayou virus, Black Creek Canal virus, Monongahela virus, and New York virus are responsible for sporadic cases in Louisiana, Texas, Florida, New York, and other areas of the eastern United States. Other hantaviruses, including Andes virus, Oran virus, Laguna Negra virus, and Choclo virus, are responsible for cases in South and Central America.

EPIDEMIOLOGY: Rodents are natural hosts for hantaviruses and acquire lifelong, asymptomatic, chronic infection with prolonged viruria and virus in saliva and feces. Humans acquire infection through direct contact with infected rodents, rodent droppings, or rodent nests or through the inhalation of aerosolized virus particles from rodent urine, droppings, or saliva. Rarely, infection may be acquired from rodent bites or contamination of broken skin with excreta. At-risk activities include handling or trapping rodents, cleaning or entering closed or rarely used rodent-infested structures, cleaning feed storage or animal shelter areas, hand plowing, and living in a home with an increased density of mice. For backpackers or campers, sleeping in a structure inhabited by rodents has been associated with HPS. Exceptionally heavy rainfall improves rodent food supplies, resulting in an increase in the rodent population with more frequent contact between humans and infected rodents, resulting in more human disease. Most cases occur during the spring and summer, with the geographic location determined by the habitat of the rodent carrier.

SNV is transmitted by the deer mouse, *Peromyscus maniculatus;* Black Creek Canal virus is transmitted by the cotton rat, *Sigmodon hispidus;* Bayou virus is transmitted by the rice rat, *Oryzomys palustris;* and the New York and Monongahela viruses are transmitted by the white-footed mouse, *Peromyscus leucopus* and *Peromyscus maniculatus.* Andes virus is transmitted by the long-tailed rice rat (*Oligoryzomys longicaudatus),* endemic in most of Argentina and Chile. Unlike all other hantaviruses, Andes virus can also be transmitted person to person.

DIAGNOSTIC TESTS: HPS should be considered when thrombocytopenia occurs with severe pneumonia clinically resembling acute respiratory distress syndrome in the proper epidemiologic setting. Other characteristic laboratory findings include neutrophilic leukocytosis with immature granulocytes, including more than 10% immunoblasts (basophilic cytoplasm, prominent nucleoli, and an increased nuclear:cytoplasmic ratio), increased hematocrit, and elevated lactate dehydrogenase. Increases in hepatic aminotransferases occur late. In areas where HPS is known to occur, use of a 5-point peripheral blood screen has aided in the early detection of patients with HPS. Elements of the screen are: (1) hemoglobin elevated for gender/age; (2) left shift of granulocytic series; (3) absence of toxic changes on the blood smear; (4) thrombocytopenia; and (5) immunoblasts and plasma cells >10% of lymphocytes. For cases fulfilling 4 of 5 criteria, the positive predictive value of the 5-point screen is >90%.

Hantavirus-specific immunoglobulin (Ig) M and IgG antibodies often are present at the onset of clinical disease, and serologic testing remains the method of choice for diagnosis. IgG may be negative in rapidly fatal cases. Although some commercial labs offer hantavirus serologies, any positive IgM test results are referred to state health departments or the Centers for Disease Control and Prevention (CDC) for confirmation. Molecular detection of virus has been described in peripheral blood mononuclear cells and other clinical specimens from the early phase of the disease but not usually in bronchoalveolar lavage fluids. Viral culture is not useful. Immunohistochemical staining of tissues (capillary endothelial cells of the lungs and almost every organ in the body) can establish the diagnosis at autopsy. Clinicians can contact the CDC Emergency Operations Center 770-488-7100 for assistance with diagnosis and management.

TREATMENT: Patients with suspected HPS should be transferred immediately to a tertiary care facility where supportive management of pulmonary edema, severe hypoxemia, and hypotension can occur during the first critical 24 to 48 hours.

In severe forms, early mechanical ventilation and inotropic and pressor support are necessary. Extracorporeal membrane oxygenation (ECMO) should be considered when pulmonary wedge pressure and cardiac indices have deteriorated and may provide short-term support for the severe capillary leak syndrome in the lungs.

There is no specific antiviral treatment for hantavirus infection. Ribavirin is active in vitro against hantaviruses, including SNV. However, 2 clinical studies of intravenous ribavirin (1 open-label study and 1 randomized, placebo-controlled, double-blind study) failed to show benefit in treatment of HPS in the cardiopulmonary stage.

Cytokine-blocking agents for HPS theoretically may have a role, but these agents have not been evaluated in a systematic fashion. Antibacterial agents do not provide benefit in this viral disease, but broad-spectrum antibiotic therapy often is administered until the diagnosis is established because bacterial shock is far more common than shock attributable to hantavirus.

INFECTION PREVENTION AND CONTROL MEASURES IN HEALTH CARE SETTINGS: Standard precautions are recommended. Health care-associated or person-to-person transmission has not been associated with HPS in the United States but has been rarely reported in Chile and Argentina with Andes virus.

CONTROL MEASURES:

Care of Exposed People. Serial clinical examinations should be used to monitor individuals at high risk of infection after exposure (see Epidemiology).

Environmental Control. Hantavirus infections of humans occur primarily in adults and are associated with domestic, occupational, or leisure activities facilitating contact with infected rodents, usually in a building in a rural setting. Eradicating the host reservoir is not feasible. Risk reduction includes practices that discourage rodents from colonizing the home and work environment and that minimize aerosolization and contact with rodent saliva and excreta. Tactics include eliminating food sources for rodents, reducing nesting sites by sealing holes, and using "snap traps" and rodenticides. Before entering areas with potential rodent infestations, doors and windows should be opened to ventilate the enclosure. Regionally and culturally appropriate educational materials should be used to direct prevention messages.

Hantaviruses, because of their lipid envelope, are susceptible to diluted bleach solutions, detergents, and most general household disinfectants. Dusty areas or articles should be moistened with 10% bleach or other disinfectant solution before being cleaned. Brooms and vacuum cleaners should not be used to clean rodent-infested areas. Use of a 10% bleach solution to disinfect dead rodents and wearing rubber gloves before handling trapped or dead rodents is recommended. Gloves and traps should be disinfected after use. The cleanup of areas potentially infested with hantavirus-infected rodents should be conducted by knowledgeable professionals using appropriate personal protective equipment. Potentially infected material should be handled according to local regulations for infectious waste.

Public Health Reporting. Possible hantavirus cases should be reported to local and state public health authorities. For state health department contact information, see **www. cdc.gov/hantavirus/surveillance/index.html.** HPS and nonpulmonary hantavirus infections are nationally notifiable diseases, reportable through the Nationally Notifiable Disease Surveillance System.

Helicobacter pylori Infections

CLINICAL MANIFESTATIONS: Most *Helicobacter pylori* infections in children are believed to be asymptomatic. *H pylori* may cause chronic active gastritis and may result in duodenal and, to a lesser extent, gastric ulcers. Persistent infection with *H pylori* also increases the risk for the development of gastric cancers including mucosal-associated lymphoid tissue (MALT) lymphoma and adenocarcinoma in adults. However, complications of infection are infrequent in children. In children, acute *H pylori* infection can result in gastroduodenal inflammation that can manifest as epigastric pain, nausea, vomiting, hematemesis, and guaiac-positive stools. If present, these symptoms usually are self-limited. There is no clear association between infection and recurrent abdominal pain in the absence of peptic ulcer disease. The presence of night-time wakening is associated with peptic ulcer disease rather than with chronic gastritis attributable to *H pylori* infection (for which night-time wakening rarely occurs). Endoscopic findings of *H pylori* infection include nodular gastritis, chronic gastritis, and rarely, the presence of gastric or duodenal erosions or ulcers. Extraintestinal conditions in children that have been associated with *H pylori* infection include treatment-refractory iron-deficiency anemia and chronic immune thrombocytopenia purpura.

ETIOLOGY: The *H pylori* bacterium is a gram-negative, spiral, curved, or U-shaped microaerobic bacillus that has single or multiple flagella at one end. The organism is positive for catalase, oxidase, and urease activity. The 2 main virulence factors associated with more severe disease include the cytotoxin associated gene (CagA) and the vacuolating cytotoxin (VacA).

EPIDEMIOLOGY: *H pylori* organisms have been isolated from humans and other primates. An animal reservoir for human transmission has not been demonstrated. Organisms are believed to be transmitted from infected humans by the fecal-oral, gastro-oral, and oral-oral routes. *H pylori* is estimated to have infected 70% of people living in resource-limited countries and 30% to 40% of people living in industrialized countries. Infection rates in children are low in resource-abundant, industrialized countries, except in children from lower socioeconomic groups, immigrants from resource-limited countries, and those living in poor hygienic conditions. Most infections are acquired in the first 8 years of life. The organism can persist in the stomach for years or for life.

Although all infected people have gastritis, over a lifetime, approximately 10% to 15% will develop peptic ulcer disease and less than 1% will develop gastric cancer.

The **incubation period** is unknown.

DIAGNOSTIC TESTS: Laboratory analysis of endoscopic specimens is the recommended approach for diagnosis in children. *H pylori* infection can be diagnosed by culture of gastric biopsy tissue on nonselective media (eg, chocolate agar, brucella agar, brain-heart infusion agar) or selective media (eg, Skirrow agar) at 37°C under microaerophilic conditions (decreased oxygen, increased carbon dioxide, and increased hydrogen concentrations) for 3 to 10 days. Colonies are small, smooth, and translucent and are positive for catalase, oxidase, and urease activity. Antimicrobial susceptibility testing of cultured isolates should be performed to guide therapy. Organisms can be visualized on histologic sections with Warthin-Starry silver, Steiner, Giemsa, or Genta staining. Presence of *H pylori* can be confirmed but not excluded on the basis of hematoxylin-eosin stains. Immunohistologic staining with specific *H pylori* antibodies may improve specificity. Because of production of high levels of urease by these organisms, urease testing of a gastric biopsy specimen can be used to detect the presence of *H pylori*. Urease hydrolyzes urea into ammonia and carbonate; the resulting increase in pH from the production of ammonia is detected in the assay.

Unlike in adults, noninvasive tests are not recommended for initial diagnosis of *H pylori* in children. Commercially available noninvasive tests include urea breath tests and stool antigen tests; these tests are designed for detection of active infection and have high sensitivity and specificity. Stool antigen tests by enzyme immunoassay monoclonal antibodies are available commercially and can be used for children of any age. The urea breath test detects labeled carbon dioxide in expired air after oral administration of isotope-labeled urea (^{13}C or ^{14}C). Although urea breath tests are expensive and are not useful in very young children, there is a test approved by the US Food and Drug Administration (FDA) for children 3 to 17 years of age.

H pylori can be detected by nucleic acid amplification tests (NAATs) or fluorescence in situ hybridization (FISH) of gastric biopsy tissue, and NAATs also have been used to detect the organism in stool specimens. However, none of these assays are currently cleared by the FDA for *H pylori* testing.

Serologic testing for *H pylori* infection by detection of immunoglobulin (Ig) G antibodies specific for *H pylori* should not be used in children for diagnosis or for confirming eradication.

Indications for H pylori *Testing.* Indications for testing for *H pylori* in children are not as broad as for adults, for whom there is stronger evidence for disease associations and lower risk of reinfection following treatment. Children with identified peptic ulcer disease may benefit from testing and treatment for *H pylori* infection. Patients with functional abdominal pain (absence of alarm symptoms by Rome criteria[1]) should not

---

[1] Hyams JS, Di Lorenzo C, Saps M, Shulman RJ, Staiano A, van Tilburg M. Functional disorders: children and adolescents. *Gastroenterology*. 2016;150(6):1456-1468

be tested, because there is a lack of evidence that treating *H pylori* infection provides relief. Testing is appropriate to confirm eradication of infection following completion of treatment.

The European Society for Paediatric Gastroenterology, Hepatology and Nutrition and the North American Society for Pediatric Gastroenterology, Hepatology & Nutrition (ESPGHAN/NASPGHAN) joint guideline recommends against a "test and treat" strategy for *H pylori* infection in children. Instead, they recommend the following[1]:

- The diagnosis of *H pylori* infection should be based on either (a) histopathology (*H pylori*–positive gastritis) plus at least 1 other positive biopsy-based test (eg, urease test or molecular-based assays including NAAT or fluorescent in situ hybridization) or (b) positive culture.
- When testing for *H pylori*, wait at least 2 weeks after stopping a proton pump inhibitor (PPI) and 4 weeks after stopping antimicrobial agents.
- Testing for *H pylori* should be performed in children with gastric or duodenal ulcers. If *H pylori* infection is identified, then treatment should be advised and eradication should be confirmed.
- Diagnostic testing for *H pylori* infection should not be performed as part of the initial investigation in children with iron-deficiency anemia. In children with refractory iron-deficiency anemia for which other causes have been ruled out, testing for *H pylori* during upper endoscopy may be considered.
- Diagnostic testing for *H pylori* infection should not be performed in children with functional abdominal pain (unless accompanied by alarm symptoms by Rome criteria[2]).
- Diagnostic testing for *H pylori* infection should not be performed when investigating causes of short stature.

The 2019 guideline from the American Society of Hematology (ASH) recommends against routine testing for *H pylori* in children with chronic immune thrombocytopenia purpura.[3]

Testing to confirm eradication of infection following completion of treatment is appropriate. Noninvasive tests may be used for this purpose.

TREATMENT[1]: Treatment options are detailed in Tables 3.14 and 3.15. Treatment is recommended for infected patients who have peptic ulcer disease, gastric mucosa-associated lymphoid tissue-type lymphoma, or early gastric cancer. Treatment of *H pylori* infection, if documented, may be considered for children who have unexplained and refractory iron-deficiency anemia. Additionally, the ESPGHAN/NASPGHAN

---

[1] Jones NL, Koletzko S, Goodman K, et al; European Society for Paediatric Gastroenterology, Hepatology and Nutrition and the North American Society for Pediatric Gastroenterology, Hepatology & Nutrition. Joint ESPGHAN/NASPGHAN guidelines for the management of *Helicobacter pylori* in children and adolescents (update 2016). *J Pediatr Gastroenterol Nutr*. 2017;64(6):991-1003. Available at: **https://naspghan. org/files/Joint_ESPGHAN_NASPGHAN_Guidelines_for_the.33.pdf**

[2] Hyams JS, Di Lorenzo C, Saps M, Shulman RJ, Staiano A, van Tilburg M. Functional disorders: children and adolescents. *Gastroenterology*. 2016;150(6):1456-1468

[3] Neunert C, Terrell DR, Arnold DM, et al The American Society of Hematology guidelines for immune thrombocytopenia. *Blood Adv*. 2019;3(23):3829-3866

Table 3.14. Recommended Options for First-Line Therapy for *Helicobacter pylori* Infection[a,b]

H pylori Antimicrobial Susceptibilities	Suggested First-Line Treatment
Susceptible to clarithromycin, susceptible to metronidazole	PPI + amoxicillin + clarithromycin for 14 days
Resistant to clarithromycin, susceptible to metronidazole	PPI + amoxicillin + metronidazole for 14 days OR Bismuth-based therapy as detailed in "Unknown" row below.
Susceptible to clarithromycin, resistant to metronidazole	PPI + amoxicillin + clarithromycin for 14 days
Resistant to clarithromycin, resistant to metronidazole ("double resistant")	<8 y of age: PPI + amoxicillin + metronidazole + bismuth for 14 days ≥8 y of age: PPI + tetracycline + metronidazole + bismuth for 14 days
Susceptibilities not known	<8 y of age: PPI + amoxicillin + metronidazole + bismuth for 14 days ≥8 y of age: PPI + tetracycline + metronidazole + bismuth for 14 days

PPI indicates proton pump inhibitor.

[a]Adapted from Jones NL, Koletzko S, Goodman K, et al; European Society for Paediatric Gastroenterology, Hepatology and Nutrition and the North American Society for Pediatric Gastroenterology, Hepatology & Nutrition. Joint ESPGHAN/NASPGHAN guidelines for the management of *Helicobacter pylori* in children and adolescents (update 2016). *J Pediatr Gastroenterol Nutr.* 2017;64(6):991-1003. Available at: **https://naspghan.org/files/Joint_ESPGHAN_NASPGHAN_ Guidelines_for_the.33.pdf.**
[b]Refer to joint ESPGHAN/NASPGHAN guidelines[a] for antibiotic dosing.

guideline recommends eradication if infection is associated with chronic immune thrombocytopenia purpura. For patients with *H pylori* infection in the absence of clinical or endoscopic evidence of peptic ulcer disease, treatment is not recommended unless the patient is within a risk group or region with high incidence of gastric cancer. Medication adherence is critical to the success of eradication.

The backbone of all recommended therapies includes a PPI and amoxicillin. Additions of metronidazole, clarithromycin, and/or bismuth are based on the patient's previous treatment experience or known susceptibilities to clarithromycin and metronidazole. Reports of increasing prevalence of antibiotic-resistant strains (particularly

Table 3.15. Rescue Therapies in Pediatric Patients Who Fail Therapy for *Helicobacter pylori*[a,b]

Initial Antibiotic Susceptibilities	Past Treatment Regimen	Suggested Rescue Treatment
Susceptible to clarithromycin, susceptible to metronidazole	PPI + amoxicillin + clarithromycin	PPI + amoxicillin + metronidazole
	PPI + amoxicillin + metronidazole	PPI + amoxicillin + clarithromycin
Susceptible to clarithromycin, susceptible to metronidazole	Sequential therapy[c]	Consider performing a second endoscopy and tissue culture and use cultured-directed treatment for 14 days OR Treat like double-resistant in Table 3.14
Resistant to clarithromycin	PPI + amoxicillin + metronidazole	Treat like double-resistant in Table 3.14
Resistant to metronidazole	PPI + amoxicillin + clarithromycin	Consider performing a second endoscopy and use a tailored treatment for 14 days OR Treat like double-resistant in Table 3.14
Susceptibilities not known	PPI + amoxicillin + clarithromycin OR PPI + amoxicillin + metronidazole OR Sequential therapy[c]	Consider performing a second endoscopy to assess secondary antimicrobial susceptibility OR Treat like double-resistant in Table 3.14

PPI indicates proton pump inhibitor.

[a] Adapted from Jones NL, Koletzko S, Goodman K, et al; European Society for Paediatric Gastroenterology, Hepatology and Nutrition and the North American Society for Pediatric Gastroenterology, Hepatology & Nutrition. Joint ESPGHAN/NASPGHAN guidelines for the management of *Helicobacter pylori* in children and adolescents (update 2016). *J Pediatr Gastroenterol Nutr*. 2017;64(6):991-1003. Available at **https://naspghan.org/files/Joint_ESPGHAN_NASPGHAN_ Guidelines_for_the.33.pdf.**

[b] Refer to joint ESPGHAN/NASPGHAN guidelines[a] for antibiotic dosing.

[c] Sequential therapy consists of PPI + amoxicillin for 5 days, followed by PPI + clarithromycin + metronidazole for 5 days.

clarithromycin resistance) as well as increasing failures of triple therapies suggest the need for bismuth-based quadruple therapy regimens (meaning 3 antibiotics and bismuth) and longer durations (14 days) for eradication of *H pylori*. A number of treatment regimens have been evaluated and are approved for use in adults; the safety and efficacy of these regimens in pediatric patients have not been firmly established. There is no current evidence to support the use of probiotics to reduce medication adverse effects or improve eradication of *H pylori*. Limited options exist for penicillin-allergic patients.

Initial Therapy

- In a treatment-naïve patient with *H pylori*, selection of therapeutic regimen is best guided by knowledge of the susceptibilities of that patient's organism.
- Treatment options are detailed in Table 3.14.
- A breath or stool test should be performed to document organism clearance 4 to 6 weeks after completion of initial therapy; relief of clinical symptoms is not an indicator of successful eradication.

Rescue Therapy

- Infection within the first 12 months following treatment is likely a relapse of the previous infection. In contrast to adults, reduced options exist for rescue therapy for children.
- Management and treatment options are detailed in Table 3.15.
- A breath or stool test should be performed to document organism eradication 4 to 6 weeks after completion of rescue therapy.

INFECTION PREVENTION AND CONTROL MEASURES IN HEALTH CARE SETTINGS: Standard precautions are recommended.

CONTROL MEASURES: Disinfection of gastroscopes prevents transmission of the organism between patients.

Hemorrhagic Fevers Caused by Arenaviruses[1]

CLINICAL MANIFESTATIONS: Arenaviruses are responsible for several hemorrhagic fever (HF) syndromes. Arenaviruses are divided into 2 groups: New World (Tacaribe complex, including Argentine HF, Bolivian HF, and Venezuelan HF), and Old World (including Lassa virus, lymphocytic choriomeningitis virus [LCMV], and Lujo virus) (see Etiology). LCMV is discussed in a separate chapter (p 559). Disease associated with arenaviruses ranges from asymptomatic or mild, acute, febrile infections to severe illnesses in which vascular leak, shock, and multiorgan dysfunction are prominent features. Fever, weakness, malaise, headache, arthralgia, and myalgia are common early symptoms. Patients may develop conjunctival suffusion, cough, retro-orbital pain, facial flushing, anorexia, vomiting, diarrhea, and abdominal pain after 3 to 4 days. Thrombocytopenia, leukopenia, petechiae, generalized lymphadenopathy, and encephalopathy usually are present in Argentine HF, Bolivian HF, and Venezuelan HF, and exudative pharyngitis often occurs in Lassa fever. Mucosal bleeding generally occurs in severe cases as a consequence of vascular damage, coagulopathy, thrombocytopenia, and platelet dysfunction. In Lassa fever, hemorrhagic manifestations occur in only one third

---

[1] Does not include lymphocytic choriomeningitis virus, which is reviewed on p 559.

of patients. Proteinuria is common; renal failure, although unusual overall, is seen frequently among hospitalized Lassa fever patients. Increased serum concentrations of aspartate aminotransferase (AST) can portend a severe or possibly fatal outcome of Lassa fever. Shock develops 7 to 9 days after onset of illness in more severely ill patients with these infections. Encephalopathic signs, such as tremor, alterations in consciousness, and seizures, can occur in South American HFs and in severe cases of Lassa fever. Transient or permanent deafness is reported in 30% of survivors of Lassa fever. The overall mortality rate in Lassa fever ranges from 1% to 20%, but is highest among hospitalized patients (15%–60%); for South American HFs, the mortality rate is 10% to 35%, and for Lujo virus HF, the mortality rate is 80% (estimated from a small number of patients). Pregnant people are at substantially higher risk of mortality (~80%) and spontaneous abortion, with 95% mortality in fetuses of infected people. Symptoms resolve 10 to 15 days after disease onset in surviving patients.

ETIOLOGY: Mammalian arenaviruses (mammarenaviruses) are enveloped, bisegmented, single-stranded RNA viruses. Old World arenaviruses include LCMV, which causes lymphocytic choriomeningitis, Lassa virus (Lassa HF), and Lujo virus (Lujo HF) in western and southern Africa. New World arenaviruses include Junín virus (Argentine HF), Machupo virus (Bolivian HF), Sabiá virus (Brazilian HF), Guanarito virus (Venezuelan HF), and Chapare virus (Chapare HF). Whitewater Arroyo virus is a rare cause of human disease in North America. Antibodies to Tamiami virus have been detected in people in North America, but clinical disease has not been confirmed. Several other arenaviruses are known only from their rodent reservoirs in the Old and New World.

EPIDEMIOLOGY: Arenaviruses are maintained in nature by association with specific rodent hosts, in which they produce chronic viremia and viruria. The principal routes of infection in humans are inhalation and direct contact of mucous membranes and skin (eg, through cuts, scratches, or abrasions) with urine and salivary secretions from these persistently infected rodents. Ingestion of food contaminated by rodent excrement also may cause disease transmission. All arenaviruses are infectious as aerosols, and human-to-human transmission may occur in community or hospital settings following unprotected contact or through droplets. Excretion of arenaviruses in urine and semen for several weeks after infection has been documented. Arenaviruses causing HF should be considered highly hazardous to people working with any of these viruses in the laboratory. Laboratory-acquired infections have been documented with Lassa, Machupo, Junín, and Sabiá viruses. The geographic distribution and habitats of the specific rodents that serve as reservoir hosts largely determine areas with endemic infection and populations at risk. Before a vaccine became available in Argentina, several hundred cases of Argentine HF occurred annually in agricultural workers and inhabitants of the Argentine pampas. Epidemics of Bolivian HF occurred in small towns between 1962 and 1964; sporadic disease activity in the countryside has continued since then. Venezuelan HF was first identified in 1989 and occurs in rural north-central Venezuela. Lassa fever is endemic in most of western Africa, where rodent hosts live in proximity to humans, causing thousands of infections annually. Lassa fever has been reported in the United States and Western Europe in people who have traveled to western Africa.

The **incubation periods** for these HF range from 6 to 21 days.

DIAGNOSTIC TESTS: Viral nucleic acid can be detected in acute disease by nucleic acid amplification tests (NAATs). Arenaviruses may be isolated from blood of acutely ill patients as well as from various tissues obtained postmortem, but isolation should be attempted only under biosafety level 4 (BSL-4) conditions. Virus antigen is detectable by enzyme immunoassay (EIA) in acute specimens and postmortem tissues. Virus-specific immunoglobulin (Ig) M antibodies, present in the serum during acute stages of illness, can be identified by immunofluorescent antibody or enzyme-linked immunosorbent assays but may be undetectable in rapidly fatal cases. The IgG antibody response is delayed. Diagnosis can be made retrospectively by immunohistochemical staining of formalin-fixed tissues obtained from autopsy.

If a viral HF is suspected, the state/local health department or Centers for Disease Control and Prevention (CDC; Viral Special Pathogens Branch: 404-639-1115) should be contacted to assist with case investigation, diagnosis, treatment, and control measures.

TREATMENT: Although not approved by the US Food and Drug Administration (FDA) for this purpose, intravenous ribavirin has been used as a therapeutic agent, together with supportive care, for treatment of acute Lassa fever infection for more than a quarter of a century. Use of intravenous ribavirin is based primarily on 1 clinical study, conducted about 40 years ago, which showed that ribavirin substantially decreased the mortality rate in patients with severe Lassa fever, particularly those treated early, during the first week of illness. Results of that study, however, have been questioned recently by other investigators. Early supportive care may improve survival.

Transfusion of immune plasma in defined doses of neutralizing antibodies is the standard specific treatment for Argentine HF and reduces mortality to 1% to 2% when administered during the first 8 days from onset of symptoms. Intravenous ribavirin has been used with success to abort a Sabiá laboratory infection and to treat Bolivian HF patients and the only known Lujo virus infection survivor. Ribavirin did not reduce mortality when initiated 8 days or more after onset of Argentine HF symptoms. Whether ribavirin treatment initiated early in the course of the disease has a role in the treatment of Argentine HF remains to be seen. Intravenous ribavirin is available only from the manufacturer through an emergency investigational new drug (eIND) application. Health care providers who need to obtain intravenous ribavirin should contact the FDA (**www.fda.gov/drugs/investigational-new-drug-ind-application/physicians-how-request-single-patient-expanded-access-compassionate-use**; 24-hour emergency lines: 866-300-4374 or 301-796-8240). Meticulous fluid and electrolyte balance is an important aspect of supportive care in each of the HFs.

INFECTION PREVENTION AND CONTROL MEASURES IN HEALTH CARE SETTINGS: In addition to standard precautions, contact and droplet precautions, including careful prevention of needlestick injuries and careful handling of clinical specimens for the duration of illness, are recommended for all HFs caused by arenaviruses. A negative-pressure ventilation room and airborne precautions are recommended for patients with suspected and confirmed infections who are undergoing aerosol-generating procedures. People entering the room should wear personal protective equipment including respirators and goggles. The CDC infection prevention recommendations for patients under investigation for Ebola virus disease in US hospitals are applicable.[1]

CONTROL MEASURES:

Care of Exposed People. No specific measures are warranted for exposed people unless direct contamination with blood, excretions, or secretions from an infected patient has occurred. If such contamination has occurred, recording body temperature twice daily for 21 days is recommended. Reporting of fever or of symptoms of infection is an indication for intravenous ribavirin treatment for Lassa fever, Bolivian HF, or Sabiá or Lujo virus infections. There is no evidence to support ribavirin for postexposure prophylaxis for Lassa fever.

Immunoprophylaxis. A live attenuated Junín vaccine protects against Argentine HF and probably against Bolivian HF. The vaccine is associated with minimal adverse effects in adults; similar findings have been obtained from limited safety studies in children 4 years and older. The vaccine is not licensed in the United States. Various vaccines for Lassa fever are currently in development and undergoing early phase clinical trials in western Africa.

Environmental. In town-based outbreaks of Bolivian HF, rodent control has proven successful. Area rodent control is not practical for control of Argentine HF or Venezuelan HF. Intensive rodent control efforts have decreased the rate of peridomestic Lassa virus infection, but rodents eventually reinvade human dwellings, and infection still occurs in rural settings.

Public Health Reporting. Because of the risk of health care-associated transmission, state health departments and the CDC should be contacted for specific advice about management and diagnosis of suspected cases. Lassa fever and New World arenavirus HFs are reportable in the United States according to guidelines of the US Council of State and Territorial Epidemiologists.

Hemorrhagic Fevers Caused by Bunyaviruses[2]

CLINICAL MANIFESTATIONS: Bunyaviruses are arthropod- or rodent-borne infections that often result in severe febrile disease with multisystem involvement and may be associated with high rates of morbidity and mortality.

Hemorrhagic fever with renal syndrome (HFRS) is a complex, multiphasic disease characterized by vascular instability and varying degrees of renal insufficiency. Fever, flushing, conjunctival injection, headache, blurred vision, abdominal pain, and lumbar pain are followed by hypotension, oliguria, and subsequently, polyuria. Petechiae are frequent, but more serious bleeding manifestations are rare. Shock and acute renal insufficiency may occur.

Crimean-Congo hemorrhagic fever (CCHF) is a multisystem disease characterized by hepatitis and hemorrhagic manifestations. Fever, headache, and myalgia are followed by signs of a diffuse capillary leak syndrome with facial suffusion,

[1] Centers for Disease Control and Prevention. Infection Prevention and Control Recommendations for Hospitalized Patients Under Investigation (PUIs) for Ebola Virus Disease (EVD) in U.S. Hospitals. Atlanta, GA: Centers for Disease Control and Prevention; 2018. Available at: **www.cdc.gov/vhf/ebola/clinicians/evd/infection-control.html**

[2] Does not include hantavirus pulmonary syndrome, which is reviewed on p 409.

conjunctivitis, icteric hepatitis, proteinuria, and disseminated intravascular coagulation associated with petechiae and purpura on the skin and mucous membranes. A hypotensive crisis often occurs after the appearance of frank hemorrhage from the gastrointestinal tract, nose, mouth, or uterus.

Rift Valley fever (RVF), in most cases, is a self-limited undifferentiated febrile illness. In 8% to 10% of cases, however, hemorrhagic fever with shock and icteric hepatitis, encephalitis, or retinitis develops.

ETIOLOGY: The order *Bunyavirales* includes segmented, single-stranded RNA viruses with different geographic distributions depending on their vector or reservoir. Hemorrhagic fever syndromes are associated with viruses from 3 families: *Hantaviridae* (Old World Hantaviruses), *Nairoviridae* (CCHF virus), and *Phenuiviridae* (RVF virus). Old World hantaviruses (Hantaan, Seoul, Dobrava, and Puumala viruses) cause HFRS, and New World hantaviruses (Sin Nombre and related viruses) cause hantavirus pulmonary syndrome (see Hantavirus Pulmonary Syndrome, p 409).

EPIDEMIOLOGY: The epidemiology of these diseases is a function of the distribution and behavior of their reservoirs and vectors. All families except *Hantaviridae* are associated with arthropod vectors. Hantavirus infections are transmitted via contact with virus shed in rodent urine, saliva, or droppings; inhalation of virus in dust from contaminated nesting materials; or being bitten by an infected rodent.

Classic HFRS occurs throughout much of Asia and Europe, with up to 100 000 cases per year. The most severe form of the disease is caused by the prototype Hantaan and Dobrava viruses in rural Asia and Europe, respectively; Puumala virus is associated with milder disease (nephropathia epidemica) in Western Europe. Seoul virus is distributed worldwide in association with brown Norway rat (*Rattus* species) and causes a disease of variable severity. Cases have been reported in the United States among rat fanciers. Person-to-person transmission has never been reported with HFRS. Fatal outcome is seen in 1% to 15% of cases, depending on the species of virus and the level of care.

CCHF occurs in much of sub-Saharan Africa, the Middle East, northwestern China, part of the Indian subcontinent, Ukraine, Russia, Georgia, Armenia, Central Asia, and Southeast Europe. CCHF virus is transmitted by hard ticks and occasionally by contact with viremic livestock and wild animals at slaughter. Health care-associated transmission of CCHF is a serious hazard. Fatal outcome is seen in 9% to 50% of hospitalized patients.

Large outbreaks of RVF have occurred throughout sub-Saharan Africa, Egypt, Saudi Arabia, and Yemen. The virus is mosquito-borne and also can also be transmitted directly from domestic livestock to humans via contact with infected abortuses or freshly slaughtered animal carcasses. Person-to-person transmission has not been reported, but laboratory-acquired cases are well documented. Overall fatal outcome occurs in 1% to 2% of cases but has been reported to be up to 30% in hospitalized patients.

The **incubation periods** for CCHF and RVF range from 2 to 10 days; for HFRS, the **incubation period** usually is longer, ranging from 7 to 42 days.

DIAGNOSTIC TESTS: Acute-phase quantitative nucleic acid amplification tests (NAATs) and serologic testing are the most common diagnostic tests (Table 3.16). Viral culture of blood and/or tissue is available in specialized laboratories. Immunoglobulin

Table 3.16. Diagnostic Tests for Hemorrhagic Fevers Caused by Bunyaviruses

Diagnostic Testing	HFRS	CCHF	RVF
Acute phase virus NAAT	Yes, but not routinely done	Yes	Yes
IgM and IgG serology	Yes (at time of illness onset or within 48 h)	Yes (detectable in early convalescence, but could be absent in fatal cases)	Yes (detectable in early convalescence)
Virus culture of blood or tissue	No (usually not detected at time of illness)	Yes (in biosafety level 4 [BSL-4] conditions)	Yes (in biosafety level 4 [BSL-4] conditions)

CCHF indicates Crimean-Congo hemorrhagic fever; HFRS, hemorrhagic fever with renal syndrome; IgG, immunoglobulin G; IgM, immunoglobulin M; NAAT, nucleic acid amplification testing; RVF, Rift Valley fever.

(Ig) M antibodies or increasing IgG titers in paired serum specimens, as demonstrated by enzyme immunoassay (EIA), are diagnostic; neutralizing antibody tests provide greater virus-strain specificity but rarely are used. Serum IgM and IgG virus-specific antibodies typically develop early in convalescence in CCHF and RVF but can be absent in rapidly fatal cases of CCHF. In HFRS, IgM and IgG antibodies usually are detectable at the time of onset of illness or within 48 hours, when it is too late for virus isolation and NAAT. Diagnosis can be made retrospectively by immunohistochemical staining of formalin-fixed tissues. Although some commercial labs offer hantavirus serologies, any positive IgM results are referred to the Centers for Disease Control and Prevention (CDC) for confirmation. CCHF and RVF testing are only available at the CDC. Referrals are made through the state health department.

TREATMENT: Currently, there are no drugs approved by the US Food and Drug Administration (FDA) for prophylaxis or treatment of HFRS, CCHF, or RVF. Ribavirin, administered intravenously to patients with HFRS within the first 4 days of illness, may be effective in decreasing renal dysfunction, vascular instability, and mortality. Intravenous ribavirin is not available commercially in the United States and is available only from the manufacturer through an emergency investigational new drug (eIND) application. Health care providers who need to obtain intravenous ribavirin should contact the FDA (**www.fda.gov/drugs/investigational-new-drug-ind-application/physicians-how-request-single-patient-expanded-access-compassionate-use**; 24-hour emergency lines: 866-300-4374 or 301-796-8240). Supportive therapy for HFRS should include: (1) treatment of shock; (2) monitoring of fluid balance; (3) dialysis for complications of renal failure; (4) control of hypertension during the oliguric phase; and (5) early recognition of possible myocardial failure with appropriate therapy.

Oral and intravenous ribavirin, when administered early in the course of CCHF, have been associated with milder disease, although no controlled studies have been performed. Ribavirin also may be efficacious as postexposure prophylaxis of CCHF.

During the RVF outbreak in Saudi Arabia in 2000, a clinical trial of ribavirin in patients with confirmed disease was halted because of an increased observation of encephalitis in patients receiving ribavirin (more than expected in RVF patients). Experimental data in hamster, mice, and rats reported the same type of observation when treatment was delayed. Therefore, ribavirin should be avoided in RVF.

INFECTION PREVENTION AND CONTROL MEASURES IN HEALTH CARE SETTINGS: In addition to standard precautions, contact and droplet precautions, including careful prevention of needlestick injuries and management of clinical specimens, are indicated for patients with CCHF for the duration for illness. Airborne isolation may be required in certain circumstances when patients undergo procedures that stimulate coughing and promote generation of aerosols. Standard precautions should be followed with RVF and HFRS.

CONTROL MEASURES:

Care of Exposed People. People having direct contact with blood or other secretions from patients with CCHF should be observed closely for 14 days with daily monitoring for fever. Immediate therapy with intravenous ribavirin should be considered at the first sign of disease. Ribavirin also may be efficacious as postexposure prophylaxis of CCHF.

Environmental.

Hemorrhagic Fever With Renal Syndrome. Monitoring of laboratory rat colonies, community pet rat colonies, and urban rodent control may be effective for rat-borne HFRS.

Crimean-Congo Hemorrhagic Fever. In countries with endemic CCHF, arachnicides for tick control generally have limited benefit but should be used in stockyard settings. Personal protective measures (eg, physical tick removal and protective clothing with permethrin sprays) may be effective for people at-risk (farmers, veterinarians, abattoir workers). See Prevention of Mosquito-borne and Tick-borne Infections, p 207.

Rift Valley Fever. Regular immunization of domestic animals should have an effect on limiting or preventing RVF outbreaks and protecting humans. Some livestock vaccines are currently in use in endemic areas. Personal protective clothing (with permethrin sprays) and insect repellants may be effective for people at risk (farmers, veterinarians, abattoir workers). Mosquito control measures are difficult to implement. See Prevention of Mosquito-borne and Tick-borne Infections, p 207.

Immunoprophylaxis. No vaccines currently are approved in Europe or the United States for use in humans against HFs caused by Bunyaviruses. Non-live vaccines are in use for HFRS and CCHF in some Asian countries and Eastern Europe, respectively.

Public Health Reporting. State health departments and the CDC should be contacted about any suspected diagnosis of viral hemorrhagic fever because of the risk of health care-associated transmission and diagnostic confusion with other hemorrhagic illnesses.

Hemorrhagic Fevers Caused by Filoviruses: Ebola and Marburg

CLINICAL MANIFESTATIONS: More is known about Ebola virus disease (EVD) than Marburg virus disease, although the same principles generally apply to the 2 filoviruses known to cause human disease. Historically, the overall incidence of EVD infections is lower in children compared with adults, but pediatric mortality is high, with the youngest children having the highest case fatality rates. Symptomatic disease ranges from mild to severe; case fatality rates for severely affected people range from 25% to 90%. Rarely, household contacts (particularly adolescents) of cases with Ebola virus disease may contract asymptomatic infections. After a mean incubation period of 6 to 10 days (range, 2–21 days), disease in children and adults begins with nonspecific signs and symptoms including fever, severe headache, myalgia, arthralgia, fatigue, abdominal pain, and weakness followed a few days later by nausea, vomiting, dysphagia, and diarrhea. Unexplained bleeding or bruising may occur late in the course of illness in a minority of children, whereas hemorrhage occurs in up to 50% of adults. The most common hemorrhagic manifestations consist of bleeding from the gastrointestinal tract, sometimes with oozing from the mucous membranes or venipuncture sites. Data from the 2014–2016 Ebola outbreak in West Africa, the largest since the virus was identified in 1976, indicate that children may have shorter incubation periods than adults and 20% of infected children have no fever at presentation. Respiratory symptoms are more common and central nervous system manifestations less common in children than in adults. A transient erythematous maculopapular rash may be seen on the torso or face after approximately 4 to 5 days of illness. Hiccups and conjunctival injection or subconjunctival hemorrhage also may occur. Leukopenia, frequently with lymphopenia, is followed later by elevated neutrophils, a left shift, and thrombocytopenia. Hepatic dysfunction and myositis commonly lead to elevations in aspartate aminotransferase (AST) and alanine aminotransferase (ALT). Metabolic derangements, including hypokalemia, hyponatremia, hypocalcemia, and hypomagnesemia, are common. In the most severe cases, disseminated intravascular coagulation, increased vascular permeability, and circulatory instability ensue around the end of the first week of disease.

Central nervous system manifestations and renal failure are frequent in end-stage disease. In fatal cases, death typically occurs 7 to 10 days after symptom onset, usually resulting from viral- or bacterial-induced septic shock and multiorgan failure. Factors associated with pediatric Ebola deaths in the 2014–2016 outbreak were age <5 years, bleeding at any time during hospitalization, and high Ebola viral load.

Approximately 30% of pregnant people with EVD present with spontaneous abortion and vaginal bleeding. Mortality in pregnant people approaches 90% when infection occurs during the third trimester. Ebola virus can cross the placenta, and pregnant people infected with the virus will likely transmit the virus to the fetus. In infants whose birthing parent is infected, Ebola virus RNA has been detected in amniotic fluid, fetal meconium, umbilical cord, and buccal swab specimens. There has been only 1 report of survival of a neonate whose birthing parent had active EVD. The neonate was treated with monoclonal antibodies, a buffy coat transfusion from an Ebola survivor, and the antiviral drug remdesivir shortly after birth. The exact mechanism of neonatal death is unknown, but high viral loads of Ebola virus have been documented in amniotic fluid, placental tissue, and fetal tissues of stillborn neonates.

In September 2022, Sudan ebolavirus caused an outbreak in Uganda with 25% of confirmed cases in children younger than 10 years and a high overall mortality rate.

EVD survivors are at risk for post-Ebola syndrome, which consists of persistent musculoskeletal, neurologic, ocular, and other symptoms, as well as reactivation of disease in immune-privileged sites, such as the eye, testicles, or the central nervous system. Disease reactivation is believed to be a rare event. EVD relapse and long-term shedding of virus in semen have been implicated in the origin of several clusters of EVD in West Africa.

ETIOLOGY: Filoviruses (from the Latin filo meaning thread, referring to their filamentous shape) are single-stranded, negative-sense RNA viruses. There are 6 genera in the family *Filoviridae*, but only 2, *Marburgvirus* and *Ebolavirus,* cause disease in humans, including 4 of the 6 viruses within the genus *Ebolavirus* and both known viruses within the genus *Marburgvirus*. These filoviruses are zoonotic pathogens endemic only in Africa.

EPIDEMIOLOGY: Fruit bats are believed to be the animal reservoir for most filoviruses. Human infection is believed to occur from inadvertent exposure to infected bat excreta or saliva following entry into roosting areas in caves, mines, and forests. Nonhuman primates, especially gorillas and chimpanzees, and other wild animals (eg, rodents, small antelopes) may become infected from bat contact and serve as amplifying hosts that transmit filoviruses to humans through contact with their blood and bodily fluids, usually associated with hunting and butchering (see Control Measures, Environmental).

Molecular epidemiologic evidence shows that most outbreaks result from a single point introduction (or very few) into humans from wild animals, followed by human-to-human transmission, almost invariably fueled by health care-associated transmission in areas with inadequate infection-control equipment and resources. Filoviruses are the most transmissible of all hemorrhagic fever viruses. The secondary attack rate in households is generally between 10% to 20% in African communities. Risk to household contacts is associated with direct physical contact, with little to no transmission observed otherwise. Human-to-human transmission usually occurs through oral, mucous membrane, or nonintact skin exposure to blood or bodily fluids of a symptomatic person with filovirus disease or by exposure to objects contaminated with infected blood or bodily fluids, most often in the context of providing care to a sick family or community member (community transmission) or patient (health care-associated transmission). Funeral rituals that involve the touching of the corpse also have been implicated. Sexual transmission has been documented and implicated in several clusters of disease. Ebola virus has been detected in human milk; genomic analysis of Ebola viruses from infants with fatal Ebola virus disease strongly suggests virus transmission through human milk (see Control Measures, Pregnancy and Breastfeeding). Respiratory spread of virus does not occur. Infection through fomites rarely may occur. Health care-associated transmission is highly unlikely if rigorous infection-control practices are in place in health care facilities (see Infection Prevention and Control Measures in Health Care Settings). Filoviruses are not spread through the air, by water, or in general by food (with the exception of bushmeat; see Control Measures, Environmental).

Children may be less likely to become infected from intrafamilial spread than adults when a primary case occurs in a household, possibly because they are not typically primary caregivers of sick individuals and are less likely to take part in funeral rituals that involve touching and washing of the deceased person's body. Underreporting of Ebola cases in children to health officials also is possible.

The degree of viremia correlates with the clinical state. People are most infectious late in the course of severe disease, especially when copious vomiting, diarrhea, and/or bleeding are present. Disease transmission does not occur during the incubation period, when the person is asymptomatic. Virus may persist in a few sites for several weeks to months after clinical recovery, including in testicles/semen, where it has been detected years after clinical recovery; vaginal fluid; placenta; amniotic fluid; human milk; saliva; the central nervous system (particularly cerebrospinal fluid); joints; conjunctivae; and the chambers of the eye (resulting in transient uveitis and other ocular problems). Because of the proven risk of transmission attributable to persistent virus in semen, abstinence or use of condoms is recommended for at least 12 months after infection or until the semen has tested negative on 2 separate occasions. Immunocompromising disorders, such as HIV infection, also may result in viral persistence. Guidance for the management of survivors of EVD can be found at **www.cdc.gov/vhf/ebola/clinicians/evaluating-patients/guidance-for-management-of-survivors-ebola.html.**

Updated information on identification, current management of people traveling from areas of transmission or with contact with a person with Ebola virus infection, and communicating with children about Ebola can be found on the Centers for Disease Control and Prevention (CDC) website (**www.cdc.gov/vhf/ebola/** and **www.cdc.gov/vhf/ebola/pdf/how-talk-children-about-ebola.pdf**) and the American Academy of Pediatrics (AAP) website (**www.healthychildren.org/English/health-issues/conditions/infections/Pages/Ebola.aspx**).

The **incubation period** for Ebola virus disease is typically 6 to 10 days (range, 2–21 days).

DIAGNOSTIC TESTS: The diagnosis of filovirus infection should be considered in a person who develops a fever within 21 days of travel to an area with endemic infection or a current outbreak. Because initial clinical manifestations are difficult to distinguish from those of more common febrile diseases, prompt laboratory testing is imperative in a suspected case. Malaria, measles, typhoid fever, Lassa fever, dengue, hepatitis A, influenza, and COVID-19 should be included in the differential diagnosis of a symptomatic person returning from Africa within 21 days and are much more likely than a filovirus to be the cause of fever. Filovirus disease can be diagnosed by testing of blood with a nucleic acid amplification test (NAAT), enzyme-linked immunosorbent assay (ELISA) for viral antigens or immunoglobulin (Ig) M, and virus isolation early in the disease course, with the latter being attempted only under biosafety level 4 (BSL-4) conditions. Viral RNA generally is detectable by NAAT 3 days after onset of symptoms. If blood is obtained within 3 days of symptom onset, 2 negative NAAT results at least 48 hours apart are required to rule out disease. IgM and IgG antibodies may be used later in the disease course or after recovery. Postmortem diagnosis can be made via immunohistochemical staining of skin or liver or spleen tissue. Testing generally is not performed routinely in clinical laboratories. Local and state public health department officials must be contacted and can facilitate testing at a regional certified laboratory or at the CDC. Current information on the most appropriate diagnostic testing for EVD is available on the CDC website (**www.cdc.gov/vhf/ebola/diagnosis/index.html**).

In October 2019, the US Food and Drug Administration (FDA) authorized marketing of the OraQuick Ebola Rapid Antigen Test under the De Novo premarket review pathway. This test is a rapid diagnostic test (RDT) for detecting Ebola virus in both symptomatic patients and recently deceased people and is the first Ebola RDT available through FDA authorization in the United States. The RDT should be used only in cases in which more sensitive molecular testing is not available. All OraQuick Ebola Rapid Antigen Test results are presumptive; all test results (positive and negative) must be verified through a NAAT at a Laboratory Response Network (LRN) laboratory located in 49 states and at the CDC.

TREATMENT: People suspected of having filovirus infection should be placed in strict isolation immediately, and public health officials should be notified. Early initiation of management in patients with filovirus disease is important for improving outcomes. Patient care is primarily supportive, including oral or intravenous fluids with electrolyte repletion, vasopressors, blood products, oxygen, nutritional support, antiemetics, analgesics, antipyretics, antimalarial and antimicrobial medications when coinfections are suspected or confirmed, and psychological support (**www.cdc.gov/vhf/ebola/ treatment/index.html**). Volume losses can be enormous (10 L/day in adults), and some centers in the United States report better results with repletion using lactated Ringer solution rather than normal saline solution in management of adult patients. When antimicrobial agents are used to treat sepsis, the medications should have coverage for intestinal microbiota based on limited evidence of translocation of gut bacteria into the blood of patients with filovirus disease. Use of needles and aerosol-generating procedures should be limited as much as possible.

On October 14, 2020, the FDA approved the first treatment for Zaire ebolavirus infection in adult and pediatric patients. Under the brand name Inmazeb, it consists of a mixture of 3 monoclonal antibodies: atoltivimab, maftivimab, and odesivimab-ebgn (**www.accessdata.fda.gov/drugsatfda_docs/label/2020/761169s000lbl. pdf**). On December 21, 2020, a second monoclonal antibody therapy, ansuvimab-zykl, which goes by the brand name Ebanga, received FDA approval, also for use in adult and pediatric patients (**www.accessdata.fda.gov/drugsatfda_docs/ label/2020/761172s000lbl.pdf**). There currently are no specific therapies approved by the FDA for other filovirus infections, including those caused by Sudan ebolavirus and Marburg virus. Because therapeutic options are likely to change following results from numerous ongoing clinical trials, it would be appropriate to consult with the CDC to determine the most current treatment guidelines (**www.cdc.gov/ vhf/ebola/treatment/index.html**).

INFECTION PREVENTION AND CONTROL MEASURES IN HEALTH CARE SETTINGS: Standard, contact, and droplet precautions are recommended for management of hospitalized patients with known or suspected EVD. Although it is prudent to place the patient in a negative-pressure room as an extra precaution, availability of such a resource should not prevent care, because there is no evidence for natural aerosol transmission between humans. A negative-pressure room should be used when aerosol-generating procedures are conducted, such as intubation or airway suctioning. Access to the patient should be limited to a small number of designated staff and family members with specific instructions and training on filovirus infection control and on the use of personal protective equipment (PPE). Although experience suggests that standard universal and contact precautions usually are protective, viral hemorrhagic fever precautions consisting of at least 2 pairs of gloves, fit-tested N95 (or higher) or particulate respirator, impermeable or fluid-resistant gown, face shield over N95 or higher respirator or powered air purifying respirator (PAPR) with face shield, protective apron, and shoe covers or rubber boots are recommended when filovirus infection is confirmed or suspected. Health care workers should have no skin exposed, and a buddy system should be used for supervision of donning and doffing PPE. All health care workers should be knowledgeable with and proficient in donning and doffing PPE before participating in management of a patient, as detailed on the CDC website (**www.cdc.gov/vhf/ebola/healthcare-us/ppe/guidance.html**). Particulate respirators are recommended when aerosol-generating procedures, such as endotracheal intubation, are performed. The duration of precautions should be determined in consultation with state and federal public health authorities.

The AAP has published a clinical report[1] that provides guidance to health care providers and hospitals on options to consider regarding parental presence at the bedside while caring for a child with suspected or proven EVD or other highly consequential infections.

CONTROL MEASURES:

Contact Tracing. Monitoring and movement of people with potential Ebola virus exposure currently is based on the degree of possible risk. At a minimum, asymptomatic people with any level of risk should self-monitor for fever and other symptoms of Ebola for 21 days. The individual should notify the public health authority immediately if fever or other symptoms develop. A full description of recommended management for people with consistent signs or symptoms and risk factors for EVD including neonates who are at risk can be found on the following CDC websites: **www.cdc.gov/vhf/ebola/clinicians/evaluating-patients/index.html** and **www.cdc.gov/vhf/ebola/clinicians/evd/neonatal-care.html.** Hospitalization of asymptomatic contacts is not warranted, but contacts who develop fever or other manifestations of filovirus disease should be isolated immediately until the diagnosis can be ruled out.

Ebola Vaccine. On December 19, 2019, the FDA approved the world's first Ebola vaccine, ERVEBO, for the prevention of EVD following conditional marketing approval from the European Medicines Agency (EMA) and prequalification by the World Health Organization. This live attenuated recombinant vesicular stomatitis virus platform-based (rVSV-ZEBOV-GP) vaccine has been used under an expanded access protocol in the 2018–2020 outbreak in the Democratic Republic of Congo in a ring vaccination trial of first responders, health care workers, burial providers, and close contacts of cases. The CDC Advisory Committee on Immunization Practices recommends its use for preexposure vaccination of adults 18 years or older in the United States who are at potential risk of exposure to Ebola virus (species Zaire ebolavirus) as a result of responding to an outbreak of Ebola virus disease, working as health care personnel at federal or state designated Ebola treatment centers in the United States, or working as laboratorians or other staff at biosafety level 4 facilities.[2] A number of experimental vaccines and passively transferred immunoglobulins have been shown to be efficacious in nonhuman primate models when administered before or after exposure.

---

[1] American Academy of Pediatrics, Committee on Infectious Diseases. Parental presence during treatment of Ebola or other highly consequential infection. *Pediatrics.* 2016;138(3):e20161891

[2] Choi MJ, Cossaboom CM, Whitesell AN, et al. Use of Ebola vaccine: recommendations of the Advisory Committee on Immunization Practices, United States, 2020. *MMWR Recomm Rep.* 2021;70(RR-1):1–12. DOI: **http://dx.doi.org/10.15585/mmwr.rr7001a1**

Currently there are no FDA-approved vaccines for Sudan ebolavirus, but several candidate vaccines have been developed and efforts are in place to test them.

Pregnancy and Breastfeeding. Limited human data from clinical trials with Ebola vaccines have not identified vaccine-associated risks during pregnancy. The decision regarding whether to vaccinate a pregnant person should consider the risk for exposure to Ebola virus. Live virus has been cultured from human milk up to 15 days after disease onset, and at least 2 fatal cases associated with breastfeeding have been reported. Given what is known about transmission of Ebola virus, regardless of breastfeeding status, infants whose lactating parent is acutely infected with Ebola virus already are at high risk of acquiring Ebola virus infection through close contact with the parent and are at high risk of death overall. Therefore, lactating parents with probable or confirmed Ebola virus infection should not have close contact with their infants and should substitute breastfeeding with an acceptable and safe alternative unless none is available (see Breastfeeding and Human Milk, p 135). Viral RNA has been detected in human milk for up to 16 months after illness onset but there is not enough evidence to provide guidance on when it is safe to resume breastfeeding after a parent's recovery. If feasible, milk should be tested for Ebola virus before resuming breastfeeding.

Travelers. Nonessential travel to areas where Ebola outbreaks are occurring is not recommended. Travelers to an area affected by an Ebola outbreak should practice careful hygiene (eg, wash hands with soap and water or a 9:1 water to bleach solution, use an alcohol-based hand sanitizer, and avoid contact with blood and body fluids). Travelers should not handle items that may have come in contact with an infected person's blood or body fluids, such as clothes, bedding, needles, and medical equipment. Funeral or burial rituals that require handling the body of someone who has died from Ebola should be avoided. Travelers should avoid hospitals where Ebola patients are being treated in areas of Africa with endemic disease; the US Embassy or consulate often is able to provide advice on facilities that should be avoided. Following return to the United States, travelers should monitor their health closely for 21 days and seek medical care immediately if they develop symptoms of Ebola (see Control Measures, Environmental). State laws mandating confinement or quarantine may apply. Current travel information for countries affected by Ebola can be found on the CDC website (**www.cdc.gov/vhf/ebola/travelers/index.html**).

Environmental. Avoiding contact with bats, primarily by avoiding entry into caves and mines in areas with endemic disease, is a key preventive measure for filoviruses. People also should avoid exposure to blood, bodily fluids, or meat of wild animals (bushmeat), especially nonhuman primates but also bats, porcupines, duikers (a type of antelope), and other mammals, in areas with endemic filovirus disease. In health care settings, detailed guidance for infection control is available at **www.cdc.gov/vhf/ebola/clinicians/cleaning/hospitals.html**. Disinfectants with a label claim for a non-enveloped virus should be used.

Public Health Reporting. Because of the risk of health care-associated transmission, state/local health departments and the CDC should be contacted immediately for specific advice about confirmation and management of suspected cases. In the United States, Ebola and Marburg hemorrhagic fevers are reportable by guidelines of the Council of State and Territorial Epidemiologists. If a filoviral hemorrhagic fever is suspected, the state/local health department or CDC Emergency Operations Center (telephone: 770-488-7100) should be contacted to assist with case investigation, diagnosis, management, and control measures.

Hepatitis A

CLINICAL MANIFESTATIONS: Hepatitis A is an acute, self-limited illness associated with fever, malaise, jaundice, anorexia, and nausea that typically lasts less than 2 months, although 10% to 15% of symptomatic people have prolonged or relapsing disease that lasts as long as 6 months. Symptomatic hepatitis A virus (HAV) infection occurs in approximately 30% of infected children younger than 6 years of age, but few of these children will have jaundice. Among older children and adults, infection usually is symptomatic, with jaundice occurring in 70% or more of cases. Fulminant hepatitis is rare but is more common in people with underlying liver disease. Chronic infection does not occur.

ETIOLOGY: HAV is a small, nonenveloped, positive-sense RNA virus with an icosahedral capsid and classified as a member of the family *Picornaviridae*, genus *Hepatovirus*.

EPIDEMIOLOGY: The most common mode of transmission is person-to-person, from fecal contamination and oral ingestion (ie, the fecal-oral route). In resource-limited countries where infection is endemic, most people are infected during the first decade of life. In the United States, rates of HAV infection decreased by 95% from 1996 to 2011 following implementation of universal infant vaccination in 2006. Since 2016, however, the United States has been in the midst of a widespread surge of person-to-person hepatitis A outbreaks unprecedented since introduction of the hepatitis A vaccine (HepA). Outbreaks, primarily among people who use drugs and people lacking housing, have occurred in 37 states; higher rates have been observed in impoverished counties. An estimated 37 700 infections occurred in 2019, a more than tenfold increase since 2015. The number of estimated cases decreased to 19 900 in 2020, possibly because of underreporting during the COVID-19 pandemic. Most HAV infection cases in the United States now are in adults 20 years and older.

Recognized risk groups for HAV infection include people who have close personal contact with a person infected with HAV, people with chronic liver disease, people with human immunodeficiency virus (HIV) infection, men who have sex with men, people who use injection or noninjection drugs, people who lack housing, people traveling to or working in countries that have highly or intermediately endemic HAV, people who have close contact with an adoptee from a country with high or intermediate HAV endemicity during the first 60 days following arrival, and people who work with HAV-infected primates or with HAV in a research laboratory setting. HAV infections and outbreaks associated with food-service establishments and food handlers, health care institutions, institutions for people with developmental disabilities, schools, and child care facilities typically reflect transmission in the community.

Outbreaks have been associated with consumption of raw produce (eg, green onions), fruits (eg, strawberries), oysters, and mussels. Waterborne outbreaks are rare and typically are associated with sewage-contaminated or inadequately treated water.

People with HAV infection are most infectious during the 1 to 2 weeks before onset of jaundice or elevation of liver enzymes, when concentration of virus in the stool is highest. Risk of transmission subsequently diminishes and is minimal by 1 week after onset of jaundice. HAV can be detected in stool for longer periods, especially in neonates and young children.

The **incubation period** is 15 to 50 days, with an average of 28 days.

DIAGNOSTIC TESTS: Serologic tests for HAV-specific total antibody (ie, immunoglobulin [Ig] G plus IgM), IgG-only anti-HAV, and IgM-only anti-HAV are available commercially, primarily in enzyme immunoassay format. Presence of serum IgM anti-HAV indicates current or recent infection, although false-positive results may occur, particularly if the pretest probability of infection is low. IgM anti-HAV is included in most acute hepatitis serologic test panels offered by hospital or reference laboratories. IgM anti-HAV is detectable in up to 20% of HepA vaccine recipients when measured 2 weeks after vaccination. In infected people, serum IgM anti-HAV becomes detectable 5 to 10 days before onset of symptoms and usually declines to undetectable concentrations within 6 months after infection, although positive test results for IgM anti-HAV more than 1 year after infection have been reported. IgG anti-HAV is detectable shortly after appearance of IgM. A positive IgG anti-HAV or total anti-HAV (IgM and IgG) test result with a negative IgM anti-HAV test result indicates immunity from past infection or vaccination. Nucleic acid amplification tests (NAATs) for hepatitis A are available but not currently licensed by the US Food and Drug Administration (FDA). NAAT may be considered for detection of very early infections and to assist with interpretation of questionable IgM anti-HAV results.

TREATMENT: Supportive and management of complications.

INFECTION PREVENTION AND CONTROL MEASURES IN HEALTH CARE SETTINGS: Contact precautions should be practiced in addition to standard precautions for diapered and incontinent patients for at least 1 week after onset of symptoms.

CONTROL MEASURES[1]:

General Measures. The major methods of prevention of HAV infections are improved sanitation (eg, in food preparation and of water sources) and personal hygiene (eg, hand hygiene after toilet use and diaper changes). HepA vaccine or immune globulin (IG) is effective in preventing infection when administered within 14 days of exposure (see Table 3.17).

Schools, Child Care, and Work. Children and adults with acute HAV infection who work as food handlers or attend or work in child care settings should be excluded for 1 week after onset of the illness (see Table 2.3, p 149).

Hepatitis A Vaccine. Two non-live single-antigen HepA vaccines, Havrix and Vaqta, are available in the United States. The vaccines are prepared from cell culture-adapted HAV, which is propagated in human fibroblasts, purified from cell lysates, formalin inactivated, and adsorbed to an aluminum hydroxide adjuvant. Vaqta contains no preservative. The hepatitis A and hepatitis B combination vaccine (HepA-HepB), Twinrix, can also be used for people 18 years and older.

Administration, Dosages, and Schedules (see Table 3.18). Both single-antigen HepA vaccines are licensed for people 12 months and older and have pediatric and adult

[1] Nelson NP, Weng MK, Hofmeister MG, et al. Prevention of hepatitis A virus infection in the United States: recommendations of the Advisory Committee on Immunization Practices, 2020. *MMWR Recomm Rep.* 2020;69(RR-5):1-38

Table 3.17. Recommendations for Postexposure Prophylaxis of Hepatitis A Virus (HAV)

Time Since Exposure	Age	Recommended
≤2 wk	<12 mo	IGIM (0.1mL/kg)[a]
	12 mo–40 y	HepA vaccine[b,c,d]
	>40 y	HepA vaccine[c,d]; consider IGIM
>2 wk	<12 mo	No prophylaxis
	≥12 mo	No prophylaxis, but HepA vaccine may be indicated for ongoing exposure

IGIM indicates immune globulin intramuscular; HepA indicates hepatitis A vaccine.
[a] Measles, mumps, and rubella vaccine (MMR) should not be administered for at least 6 months after receipt of IGIM.
[b] People with immunocompromising conditions or chronic liver disease should also receive IGIM.
[c] Although 1 dose of HepA vaccine is needed for postexposure prophylaxis, the 2-dose series should be completed according to the recommended schedule.
[d] People with severe allergy to HepA vaccine or its components should receive IGIM (0.1 mL/kg) but not HepA vaccine.

formulations that are administered in a 2-dose schedule. Pediatric formulations are available for ages 12 months through 18 years, and adult formulations are available for people 19 years and older. HepA-HepB vaccine can be used for people 18 years and older and can be administered in a standard 3-dose schedule or an accelerated 3-dose schedule plus a booster dose 12 months later. HepA and HepA-HepB vaccines are administered intramuscularly. Recommended doses and schedules for these vaccines are listed in Table 3.18.

Immunogenicity. HepA vaccines are highly immunogenic. At least 95% of healthy children, adolescents, and adults have protective antibody concentrations when measured 1 month after receipt of the first dose. One month after a second dose, more than 99% of healthy children, adolescents, and adults have protective antibody concentrations.

Antibody concentrations are lower in infants with transplacentally acquired anti-HAV in comparison with vaccine recipients lacking anti-HAV. Transplacentally acquired anti-HAV antibody is not detectable in most infants by 12 months of age. HepA vaccine is highly immunogenic for children who begin immunization at 12 months or older, regardless of anti-HAV status of the birthing parent.

Efficacy. In double-blind, controlled, randomized trials, the protective efficacy in preventing clinical HAV infection was 94% to 100%.

Duration of Protection. Detectable antibody persists for at least 25 years after completion of a 2-dose series of HepA vaccine. Kinetic models of antibody decline indicate that protective levels of anti-HAV could be present for at least up to 50 years. Booster doses beyond the 2-dose primary immunization series are not recommended.

Vaccine in Immunocompromised People. Because HepA vaccine is non-live, no special precautions need to be taken when vaccinating immunocompromised people. The immune response in immunocompromised people, including people with HIV infection, may be suboptimal based on the level of immunosuppression at the time of vaccine administration.

Table 3.18. Recommended Doses and Schedules for Non-Live Hepatitis A Virus Vaccines

Age	Vaccine	Hepatitis A Antigen Dose	Volume per Dose, mL	No. of Doses	Schedule
6–11 mo, traveling to area with endemic hepatitis A[a]	Havrix or Vaqta	720 ELU/25 U	0.5	1	One dose for infants traveling to areas with endemic hepatitis A; this dose does not count toward completing the immunization requirement; 2 doses needed at the routine schedule after 12 mo of age
12 mo–18 y	Havrix	720 ELU	0.5	2	Initial and 6–12 mo later
12 mo–18 y	Vaqta	25 U	0.5	2	Initial and 6–18 mo later
≥19 y	Havrix	1440 ELU	1.0	2	Initial and 6–12 mo later
≥19 y	Vaqta	50 U	1.0	2	Initial and 6–18 mo later
≥18 y	Twinrix[b]	720 ELU	1.0	3 or 4	3-dose series: Initial, 1 mo, and 6 mo 4-dose series: Initial, 7 days, 21–30 days, and 12 mo

ELU indicates enzyme-linked immunosorbent assay units.

[a] Nelson NP, Link-Gelles R, Hofmeister MG, et al. Update: Recommendations of the Advisory Committee on Immunization Practices for use of hepatitis A vaccine for postexposure and for preexposure prophylaxis for international travel. *MMWR Morb Mortl Wkly Rep*. 2018;67(43):1216-1220.

[b] A combination of hepatitis B (Engerix-B, 20 µg) and hepatitis A (Havrix, 720 ELU) vaccine (Twinrix) is licensed for use in people age ≥18 years in 3-dose and 4-dose schedules. For pre- and postexposure hepatitis A prophylaxis, the use of single-antigen hepatitis A vaccine (ie, Havrix or Vaqta) is recommended.

Vaccine Interchangeability. The 2 single-antigen HepA vaccines have similar effectiveness when administered as recommended. Completion of the immunization regimen with the same product is preferable, although interchangeability of products is acceptable if the same product is not available. Studies among adults have found no difference in the immunogenicity of a vaccine series consisting of both compared with using the same vaccine throughout the licensed schedule.

Administration With Other Vaccines. HepA vaccine may be administered concurrently with other vaccines. Vaccines should be administered in a separate syringe and at a separate injection site (see Simultaneous Administration of Multiple Vaccines, p 63).

Adverse Events. No serious adverse events attributed definitively to HepA vaccine have been reported. Adverse reactions are mild and include local pain and, less commonly, induration at the injection site. The vaccine can be administered either in the thigh or the arm; the site of injection does not affect the incidence of local reactions.

Precautions and Contraindications to Immunization. The vaccine should not be administered to people with hypersensitivity to any of the vaccine components. A retrospective cohort study published in 2019 of Vaccine Safety Datalink (VSD) data from 2004 through 2015 did not identify any concerning pattern of adverse events in pregnant people or their infants following hepatitis A immunizations during pregnancy. Risk to the fetus is considered to be low or nonexistent because the vaccine contains inactivated, purified virus particles. Hepatitis A vaccination is recommended during pregnancy for people at risk for HAV infection.

Preimmunization Serologic Testing. Preimmunization testing for anti-HAV generally is not recommended for children (see Table 1.19, p 122). Testing may be cost-effective for people who have a high likelihood of hepatitis A immunity from previous infection, including people whose childhood was in a country with high endemicity and people with a history of jaundice potentially caused by HAV.

Postimmunization Serologic Testing. Postimmunization testing for anti-HAV generally is not indicated because of the high seroconversion rates in adults and children. Some commercially available anti-HAV tests may not detect low but protective concentrations of antibody among immunized people.

Immune Globulin. Postexposure prophylaxis (PEP) with immune globulin intramuscular (IGIM), when administered within 2 weeks after exposure to HAV, is more than 85% effective in preventing symptomatic infection. When administered as preexposure prophylaxis (PrEP), a dose of 0.1 mL/kg confers protection against hepatitis A for up to 1 month, and a dose of 0.2 mL/kg protects for up to 2 months. Recommended PrEP and PEP IGIM doses and duration of protection are provided in Tables 3.19 and 3.17, respectively.

PREVENTION MEASURES:

PrEP Against HAV Infection (see Tables 3.19, p 435, and 3.18, p 433). HepA vaccine is recommended routinely for children age 12 through 23 months of age and children and adolescents age 2 to 18 years of age who have not received HepA vaccine previously. HepA vaccine is recommended for people 18 years or older who are at increased risk of infection or severe disease and during outbreaks. The routine childhood immunization schedule (**https://publications.aap.org/redbook/pages/Immunization-Schedules**) and Table 3.18 (p 433) include HepA-containing vaccines licensed by the FDA, their doses, and schedules.

People at Increased Risk of HAV Infection or its Consequences Who Should Be Immunized.

- **People with chronic liver disease.** Susceptible people with chronic liver disease (including, but not limited to, those with hepatitis C virus [HCV] and/or hepatitis B virus [HBV] infection, cirrhosis, fatty liver disease, alcoholic liver disease, autoimmune hepatitis, or an alanine aminotransferase [ALT] or aspartate aminotransferase [AST] concentrations greater than twice the upper limit of normal) and people who are unvaccinated and awaiting or have received liver transplants should be immunized.
- **People who use drugs.** The United States has been experiencing widespread person-to-person hepatitis A outbreaks since 2016, primarily affecting people who use drugs and people lacking housing. All people who use injection or noninjection drugs should be immunized against HAV.

Table 3.19. Recommendations for Preexposure Prophylaxis of Hepatitis A Virus (HAV) for Travelers to Countries With High or Intermediate Endemic Rates of Hepatitis A[a]

Age	Recommended	Notes
<6 mo	IGIM[b]	For travel lasting up to 1 mo, 0.1 mL/kg; up to 2 mo, 0.2 mL/kg (repeat 0.2 mL/kg every 2 mo thereafter if risk remains).[c]
6–11 mo	HepA vaccine	This dose does not count toward the routine 2-dose series. Start the hepatitis A vaccination series at age 12 mo.
12 mo–40 y	HepA vaccine	Those with immunocompromising conditions, chronic liver disease, or other chronic medical conditions may also receive IGIM.[b,d]
>40 y	HepA vaccine, consider IGIM	If departure is within 2 wk, may also receive IGIM[d]; those with immunocompromising conditions, or chronic liver disease may also receive IGIM.

HepA indicates hepatitis A vaccine; IGIM indicates immune globulin intramuscular.

[a] People age 12 months or older should receive HepA vaccine routinely; those who have a severe allergy to HepA or its components should receive IGIM.

[b] Measles, mumps, and rubella vaccine (MMR) should not be administered for at least 6 months after receipt of IGIM (see Table 1.11, p 69).

[c] Nelson NP, Link-Gelles R, Hofmeister MG, et al. Update: Recommendations of the Advisory Committee on Immunization Practices for use of hepatitis A vaccine for postexposure and for preexposure prophylaxis for international travel. *MMWR Morb Mortal Wkly Rep.* 2018;67(43):1216-1220.

[d] HepA vaccine and IGIM should be administered at the same time at different limbs.

- **People experiencing homelessness.** People 1 year or older experiencing homelessness should be immunized.
- **People who travel to or work in countries that have high or intermediate endemic hepatitis A** (parts of Africa and Asia, Central and South America, and Eastern Europe) should be protected against HAV infection before departure (see Table 3.19) as follows:
  - Infants age 6 through 11 months should receive a dose of HepA vaccine. This travel-related dose does not count toward the routine 2-dose series that should begin at age 12 months. HepA vaccine does not interfere with response to measles, mumps, and rubella vaccine (MMR), which is also is recommended for international travelers 6 months or older.
  - Healthy people 12 months through 40 years of age should receive a dose of HepA as soon as travel is considered and complete the 2-dose series according to the routine schedule.
  - Infants younger than 6 months and travelers for whom vaccine is contraindicated or who choose not to receive vaccine should receive IGIM before travel when protection against HAV is recommended. For travel duration up to 1 month, 1 dose of IGIM at 0.1 mL/kg is recommended; for travel up to 2 months, 1 dose of IGIM at 0.2 mL/kg is recommended, and for travel of ≥2 months, a 0.2-mL/kg dose of IG

should be repeated every 2 months for the duration of travel or until HepA vaccine is administered (ie, for infants at age $\geq$6 months) (see Table 3.19).

♦ People older than 40 years, people with immunocompromising conditions, and people with chronic liver disease should receive a single dose of HepA vaccine as soon as travel is considered. People traveling in <2 weeks should receive the initial dose of HepA vaccine and simultaneously may receive IGIM in a different anatomic injection site. The HepA vaccine series should be completed according to the routine schedule.

- **Close contacts of newly arriving international adoptees.**[1,2] Data from a study conducted at 3 adoption clinics in the United States indicate that 1% to 6% of newly arrived international adoptees have acute HAV infection. Risk of HAV infection among close personal contacts of international adoptees is estimated at 106 (range, 90–819) per 100 000 household contacts of international adoptees within the first 60 days of their arrival in the United States. HepA vaccine should be administered to all unvaccinated people who anticipate close personal contact (eg, household contact or regular babysitting) with a child adopted internationally from a country with high or intermediate endemic rates of hepatitis A during the first 60 days following arrival of the child in the United States. The first dose of the 2-dose HepA vaccine series should be administered as soon as adoption is planned, ideally 2 or more weeks before the arrival of the child.

- **Men who have sex with men.** Cyclic outbreaks of hepatitis A among men who have sex with men have been reported often, including in urban areas in the United States, Canada, and Australia. Therefore, men (adolescents and adults) who have sex with men should be immunized. Preimmunization serologic testing may be cost-effective for older people in this group.

- **People at risk of occupational exposure (eg, handle nonhuman primates infected with HAV or work with HAV in a research laboratory).** Outbreaks of HAV infection have been reported among people who work with nonhuman primates infected with HAV. People working with HAV-infected nonhuman primates or HAV in a research laboratory should receive HepA vaccine.

Postexposure Prophylaxis (PEP) (see Table 3.17, p 432). Use of HepA vaccine for PEP provides several advantages compared with IGIM, including induction of active immunity, much longer duration of protection, ease of administration, and greater acceptability and availability. IGIM (0.1 mL/kg) should be used for people who cannot receive HepA vaccine because they are too young or have a severe allergy to the vaccine or its components. Situations in which HepA vaccine and/or IGIM can be considered include the following:

- In general, **healthy people age 12 months and older** who previously have not received HepA vaccine and have been exposed to HAV should receive a dose of single-antigen HepA vaccine as soon as possible within 14 days of exposure (see Table 3.17, p 432, for prophylaxis guidance and dosages). The 2-dose series should be completed according to the recommended schedule.

[1] Centers for Disease Control and Prevention. Updated recommendations from the Advisory Committee on Immunization Practices (ACIP) for use of hepatitis A vaccine in close contacts of newly arriving international adoptees. *MMWR Morb Mortal Wkly Rep.* 2009;58(36):1006–1007

[2] American Academy of Pediatrics, Committee on Infectious Diseases. Recommendations for administering hepatitis A vaccine to contacts of international adoptees. *Pediatrics.* 2011;128(4):803–804

- In addition to HepA vaccine, IGIM (0.1 mL/kg) may be administered to **people 40 years or older**, depending on the provider's risk assessment.
- **People who are immunocompromised or have chronic liver disease** should receive a dose of HepA and IGIM (0.1 mL/kg) at different limbs at the same time and complete the 2-dose HepA series according to the recommended schedule. Efficacy of HepA vaccine or IGIM for PEP when administered more than 2 weeks after exposure has not been established.
- **Newborn infants born to HAV-infected people** may receive IGIM (0.1 mL/kg) if the birthing parent's HAV infection symptoms began between 2 weeks before and 1 week after delivery. Efficacy in this circumstance has not been established.
- Hepatitis outbreaks in **child care centers** now are rare following widespread adoption of universal childhood immunization. In facilities with diapered children, if 1 or more cases confirmed in child or staff attendees or 2 or more cases in households of staff or attendees, hepatitis A vaccine (HepA) or immune globulin intramuscular (IGIM), depending on age, should be administered within 14 days of exposure to all unimmunized staff and attendees. In centers without diapered children, HepA or IGIM should be administered only to unimmunized classroom contacts to an index case with hepatitis A (see Table 2.3, p 149).
- In **school and non-health care work settings**, HAV exposure generally does not pose a risk of infection. If multiple cases occur among children at a school, a common source of infection should be investigated. PEP is not indicated when a single case occurs in a school and the source of infection is outside the school or work setting.
- **Hospitals and other health care settings.** Health care-associated transmission of HAV is uncommon when recommended infection control practices are followed. PEP within the health care setting may be considered on a case-by-case basis depending on risk of transmission. Health care workers do not have increased prevalence of HAV infection.
- **Common-source food exposure and food handlers.** Food handlers are not at increased risk for hepatitis A infection based on their occupation. Most food handlers with HAV infection do not transmit HAV to others, but PEP can be considered based on risk of transmission.

Hepatitis B

CLINICAL MANIFESTATIONS: People acutely infected with hepatitis B virus (HBV) may be asymptomatic or symptomatic. The likelihood of developing symptoms increases with age: less than 1% of infants younger than 1 year, 5% to 15% of children 1 through 5 years, and 30% to 50% of people 6 through 30 years of age are symptomatic. Few data are available for adults older than 30 years. Acute HBV infection cannot be distinguished from other forms of acute viral hepatitis on the basis of clinical signs and symptoms or nonspecific laboratory findings. The spectrum of signs and symptoms varies and includes subacute illness with nonspecific symptoms (eg, anorexia, nausea, or malaise), clinical hepatitis with jaundice, or fulminant hepatitis. Extrahepatic manifestations associated with circulating immune complexes that have been reported in HBV-infected children include arthralgias, arthritis, polyarteritis nodosa, thrombocytopenia, and glomerulonephritis. Gianotti-Crosti syndrome (papular acrodermatitis), urticaria, macular rash, or purpuric lesions may be seen in acute HBV infection.

Chronic HBV infection is defined as persistence in serum for at least 6 months of any one of the following: hepatitis B surface antigen (HBsAg), HBV DNA, or hepatitis B envelope antigen (HBeAg). Chronic HBV infection is likely in the presence of HBsAg, HBV DNA, or HBeAg in serum from a person who tests negative for immunoglobulin (Ig) M antibody to hepatitis B core antigen (IgM anti-HBc).

Age at the time of infection is the primary determinant of risk of progressing to chronic infection. Up to 90% of infants infected perinatally or in the first year of life will develop chronic HBV infection. Between 25% and 50% of children infected between 1 and 5 years of age become chronically infected, whereas 5% to 10% of infected older children and adults develop chronic HBV infection. Patients who become infected with HBV while immunosuppressed or with an underlying chronic illness (eg, end-stage renal disease) have an increased risk of developing chronic infection. Without treatment, up to 25% of infants and children who acquire chronic HBV infection will die prematurely from HBV-related hepatocellular carcinoma (HCC) or cirrhosis.

The clinical course of untreated chronic HBV infection varies according to the population studied, reflecting differences in age at acquisition, rate of loss of HBeAg, and possibly HBV genotype. Most children have asymptomatic infection. For years to decades after initial infection, perinatally infected children are in an "immune tolerant" phase with normal or minimally elevated alanine aminotransferase (ALT) concentrations, minimal or mild liver histologic abnormalities, detectable HBeAg, and high HBV DNA concentrations (≥20 000 IU/mL). Some children with chronic HBV infection may exhibit growth impairment. Chronic HBV infection acquired during later childhood or adolescence usually is accompanied by more active liver disease and increased serum aminotransferase concentrations. Patients with detectable HBeAg (*HBeAg-positive chronic hepatitis B*) usually have high concentrations of HBV DNA and HBsAg in serum and are more likely to transmit infection. Over time (years to decades), HBeAg becomes undetectable in many chronically infected people. This transition often is accompanied by development of antibody to HBeAg (anti-HBe) and decreases in serum HBV DNA and serum aminotransferase concentrations and may be preceded by a temporary exacerbation of liver disease. These patients have *inactive chronic infection* but still may experience episodes of reactivation, manifested by increases in serum HBV DNA and aminotransferase concentrations. This may occur spontaneously or when these patients become immunosuppressed, receive anti-tumor necrosis factor agents or disease-modifying anti-rheumatic drugs, or have chronic hepatitis C virus (HCV) infection being treated with direct acting antiviral agents.

Because HBV-associated liver injury is believed to be immune-mediated, in people coinfected with human immunodeficiency virus (HIV) and HBV, the return of immune competence with antiretroviral treatment of HIV infection may lead to a reactivation of HBV-related liver inflammation and damage.

Some patients who lose HBeAg may continue to have ongoing histologic evidence of liver damage and moderate to high concentrations of HBV DNA (*HBeAg-negative chronic hepatitis B*). Patients with histologic evidence of chronic HBV infection, regardless of HBeAg status, remain at higher risk of death attributable to liver failure compared with HBV-infected people with no histologic evidence of liver inflammation and fibrosis. Chronically infected adults clear HBsAg without treatment at the rate of approximately 1% annually; for chronically infected children, however, the annual clearance rate is less than 1%.

ETIOLOGY: HBV has a partially double-stranded DNA genome contained within a 42-nm-diameter enveloped virion and belongs in the family *Hepadnaviridae*. Important components of the viral particle include an outer lipoprotein envelope containing HBsAg, an inner nucleocapsid consisting of hepatitis B core antigen (HBcAg), and the viral polymerase attached to the viral genome.

EPIDEMIOLOGY: HBV is transmitted through infected blood or body fluids. Although HBsAg has been detected in multiple body fluids including human milk, saliva, and tears, the most potentially infectious fluids include blood, serum, semen, vaginal secretions, and cerebrospinal, synovial, pleural, pericardial, peritoneal, and amniotic fluids. People with chronic HBV infection are the primary reservoirs for infection. Common modes of transmission include perinatal exposure to an infected birthing parent; percutaneous and permucosal exposure to infectious body fluids; sharing or using non-sterilized needles, syringes, or glucose monitoring equipment or devices; sexual contact with an infected person; and household exposure to a person with chronic HBV infection. Risks of HBV acquisition when a susceptible child bites a child who has chronic HBV infection or when a susceptible child is bitten by a child with chronic HBV infection are unknown (see Bite Wounds, p 202, and Table 2.9, p 203). A theoretical risk exists if HBsAg-positive blood enters the oral cavity of the biter, but transmission by this route has not been reported. Transmission by transfusion of contaminated blood or blood products is rare in the United States because of routine screening of blood donors and viral inactivation of certain blood products before administration.

Perinatal transmission of HBV is highly efficient and usually occurs from blood exposures during labor and delivery. In utero transmission accounts for less than 2% of all vertically transmitted HBV infections in most studies. Without postexposure prophylaxis, the risk of an infant acquiring HBV from an infected mother as a result of perinatal exposure is 70% to 90% for infants whose birthing parent is HBsAg and HBeAg positive; the risk is 5% to 20% for infants whose birthing parent is HBsAg positive but HBeAg negative. Infants whose birthing parent has very high HBV DNA levels (>200 000 IU/mL) are at high risk of breakthrough infection despite receipt of postexposure prophylaxis with antibody and vaccine at birth.

Prevalence of HBV infection and patterns of transmission vary markedly throughout the world (see Fig 3.2). Approximately 80% of people worldwide live in regions of intermediate to high HBV endemicity, defined as prevalence of chronic HBV infection of 2% or greater. Historically, most new HBV infections occurred as a result of perinatal or early childhood infections in regions of high HBV endemicity, defined as prevalence of HBV infection of 8% or greater. Infant immunization programs in some of these countries have reduced seroprevalence of HBsAg greatly, but many countries with endemic HBV have yet to implement widespread routine birth-dose and/or childhood hepatitis B immunization programs. In regions of intermediate HBV prevalence (2% to 7%), multiple modes of transmission occur (eg, perinatal, household, sexual, injection drug use, and health care associated). In countries with low prevalence (<2%) and where routine immunization has been adopted, new infections occur most often in age groups where routine immunization is not conducted.

FIG 3.2. MAP OF HEPATITIS B PREVALENCE GLOBALLY

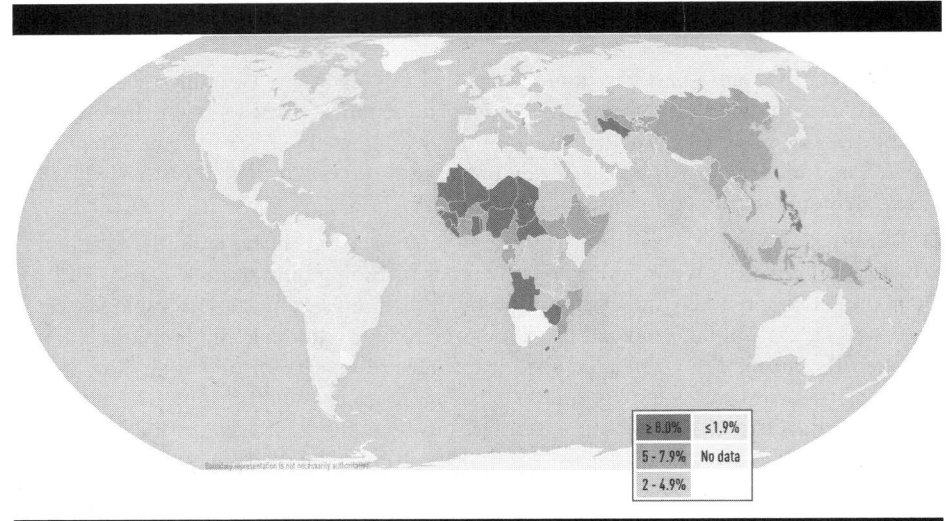

≥ 8.0%	≤1.9%
5 - 7.9%	No data
2 - 4.9%	

Reproduced from **https://wwwnc.cdc.gov/travel/yellowbook/2024/infections-diseases/hepatitis-b.** Data source: 2021 estimates of hepatitis B virus disease burden. CDA Foundation Polaris Observatory. Available from: **https://cdafound.org/polaris-countries-distribution/.**

In regions of the world with high prevalence of chronic HBV infection, transmission between children in household settings may account for a substantial amount of transmission. Precise mechanisms of transmission from child-to-child are unknown, but frequent interpersonal contact of nonintact skin or mucous membranes with blood-containing secretions, open skin lesions, or blood-containing saliva are potential means of transmission. Transmission from sharing inanimate objects, such as razors or toothbrushes, also may occur. HBV can survive in the environment for 7 or more days but is inactivated by commonly used disinfectants, including household bleach diluted 1:10 with water. HBV is not transmitted by the fecal-oral route.

The **incubation period** for acute HBV infection is 45 to 160 days, with an average of 90 days.

DIAGNOSTIC TESTS: Serologic protein antigen tests are available commercially to detect HBsAg and HBeAg. Serologic antibody assays also are available for detection of anti-HBs, total anti-HBc, IgM anti-HBc, and anti-HBe (see Table 3.20, Fig 3.3, and Fig 3.4). Most laboratories now use nucleic acid amplification tests (NAATs) for analysis of HBV DNA, with very high sensitivity at low levels and broad dynamic range for quantitation.

HBsAg is detectable during acute and chronic infection. If HBV infection is self-limited, HBsAg disappears in most patients within a few weeks to several months after infection, followed by appearance of anti-HBs. The time between disappearance of HBsAg and appearance of anti-HBs is termed the *window period* of infection. During the window period, the only marker of acute infection is IgM anti-HBc. IgM anti-HBc usually is not present in infants infected perinatally. People with chronic HBV infection have circulating HBsAg and circulating total anti-HBc (Fig 3.4); in a minority of chronically infected individuals, anti-HBs also is present. Both anti-HBs and total

Table 3.20. Diagnostic Tests for Hepatitis B Virus (HBV) Antigens, Antibodies, and DNA

Factors To Be Tested	HBV Antigen or Antibody	Use
HBsAg	Hepatitis B surface antigen	Detection of acutely or chronically infected people; antigen used in hepatitis B vaccine; rarely can be detected for up to 3 weeks after a dose of hepatitis B vaccine
Anti-HBs	Antibody to HBsAg	Identification of people who have resolved infections with HBV; determination of immunity after immunization
HBeAg	Hepatitis B envelope antigen	Identification of infected people with high serum HBV DNA concentrations at increased risk of transmitting HBV
Anti-HBe	Antibody to HBeAg	Identification of infected people with low to moderate serum HBV DNA concentrations at lower risk of transmitting HBV
Anti-HBc (total)	IgM + IgG antibody to HBcAg[a]	Identification of people with acute, resolved, or chronic HBV infection (not present after immunization); transplacentally acquired anti-HBc is detectable for as long as 24 months among infants born to HBsAg-positive birthing parent
IgM anti-HBc	IgM antibody to HBcAg[a]	Identification of people with acute or recent HBV infections (including HBsAg-negative people during the "window" phase of infection; unreliable for detecting perinatal HBV infection)
HBV DNA	N/A	Inform use of antiviral therapy, including in pregnant people (to decrease risk of perinatal transmission)

HBcAg indicates hepatitis B core antigen; IgM, immunoglobulin M.

[a] No test is available commercially to measure HBcAg or isolated IgG antibody to HBcAg (without also measuring IgM antibody to HBcAg, as total anti-HBc does).

anti-HBc are present in people with resolved infection, whereas anti-HBs alone is present in people immunized with hepatitis B (HepB) vaccine. The presence of HBeAg in serum correlates with higher concentrations of HBV DNA and greater infectivity. Tests for HBeAg and HBV DNA are necessary in selection of candidates to receive antiviral therapy and to monitor response to therapy.

Transient presence of HBsAg can occur following receipt of HepB vaccine, with (vaccine-derived) HBsAg being detected as early as 24 hours after and up to 3 weeks following administration of the vaccine.

TREATMENT: No therapy for uncomplicated *acute* HBV infection is recommended. Treatment with a nucleoside or nucleotide analogue is indicated if there is concern for

FIG 3.3. TYPICAL SEROLOGIC COURSE OF ACUTE HEPATITIS B VIRUS INFECTION WITH RECOVERY

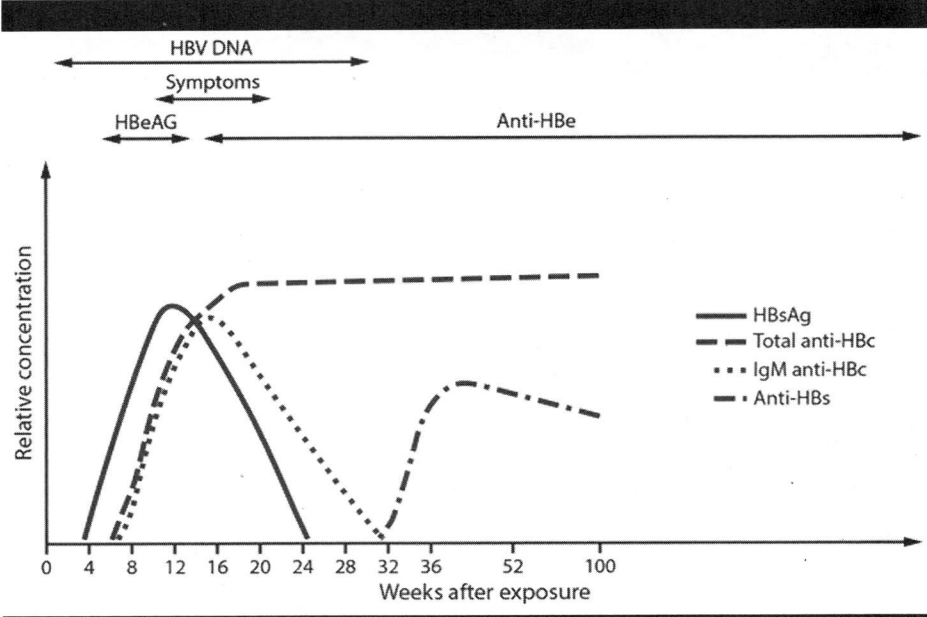

anti-HBc indicates antibody to hepatitis B core antigen; anti-HBe, antibody to hepatitis B e antigen; anti-HBs, antibody to hepatitis B surface antigen; HBeAg, hepatitis B e antigen; HBsAg, hepatitis B surface antigen; HBV, hepatitis B virus; IgM, immunoglobulin M.

From Conners EE, Panagiotakopoulos L, Hofmeister MG, et al. Screening and testing for hepatitis B virus infection: CDC recommendations – United States, 2023. *MMWR Recomm Rep.* 2023;72(RR-1):1-25. Available at: **http://dx.doi.org/10.15585/mmwr.rr7201a1**

severe infection with acute liver failure. Acute HBV infection may be difficult to distinguish from reactivation of HBV. If reactivation is a possibility, referral to a hepatitis specialist would be warranted. Hepatitis B immune globulin (HBIG) and corticosteroids are not effective treatment for acute or chronic disease.

The goal of treatment in chronic HBV infection is to prevent progression to cirrhosis, hepatic failure, and hepatocellular carcinoma, with antibody to HBeAg (anti-HBe) seroconversion, normalization of serum aminotransferase, and suppression of detectable serum HBV DNA concentrations as surrogate endpoints. Current indications for treatment of chronic HBV infection include evidence of ongoing HBV viral replication, as indicated by the presence for longer than 6 months of either serum HBV DNA greater than 20 000 IU/mL with HBeAg or greater than 2000 IU/mL without HBeAg, AND elevated serum ALT concentrations for longer than 6 months or evidence of chronic hepatitis on liver biopsy. Children without necroinflammatory liver disease and children in the immunotolerant phase (ie, normal ALT concentrations despite presence of HBV DNA) do not warrant antiviral therapy. Treatment response is measured by biochemical, serologic, virologic, and histologic response. The American Association for the Study of Liver Diseases and the Centers for Disease Control and Prevention (CDC) recommend that pregnant people with viral

FIG 3.4. TYPICAL SEROLOGIC COURSE OF ACUTE HEPATITIS B VIRUS (HBV) INFECTION WITH PROGRESSION TO CHRONIC HBV INFECTION

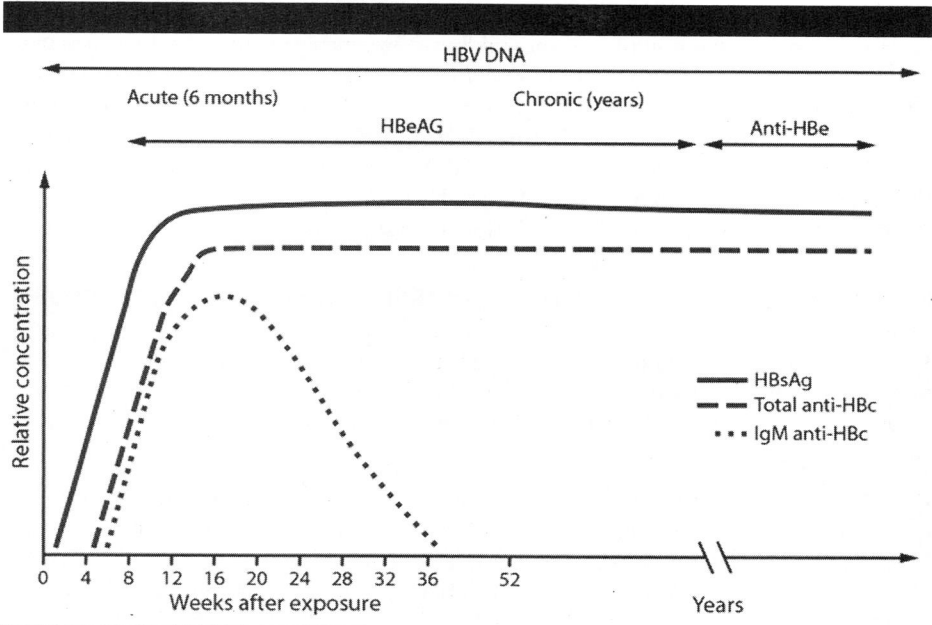

anti-HBc indicates antibody to hepatitis B core antigen; anti-HBe, antibody to hepatitis B e antigen; anti-HBs, antibody to hepatitis B surface antigen; HBeAg, hepatitis B e antigen; HBsAg, hepatitis B surface antigen; HBV, hepatitis B virus; IgM, immunoglobulin M.

From Conners EE, Panagiotakopoulos L, Hofmeister MG, et al. Screening and testing for hepatitis B virus infection: CDC recommendations—United States, 2023. *MMWR Recomm Rep.* 2023;72(RR-1):1-25

loads >200 000 IU/mL be offered antiviral therapy to prevent transmission to their newborn.[1,2]

The US Food and Drug Administration (FDA) has approved 3 nucleoside analogues (entecavir, lamivudine, and telbivudine), 3 nucleotide analogues (tenofovir disoproxil fumarate, tenofovir alafenamide fumarate, and adefovir), and 2 interferon-alfa drugs (interferon alfa-2b and pegylated interferon alfa-2a) for treatment of chronic HBV infection in adults. All are available in the United States except telbivudine, which has been discontinued. An important consideration in choice of treatment is to avoid selection of antiviral resistance mutations. Entecavir, tenofovir disoproxil fumarate, tenofovir alafenamide fumarate, and pegylated interferon alfa-2a are preferred in adults as first-line therapy because of lower likelihood of developing antiviral resistance mutations over long-term therapy. FDA licensure in the pediatric population

[1] Terrault NA, Lok ASF, McMahon BJ, et al. Update on prevention, diagnosis, and treatment of chronic hepatitis B: AASLD 2018 hepatitis B guidance. *Hepatology.* 2018;67(4):1560-1599

[2] Schillie S, Vellozzi C, Reingold A, et al. Prevention of hepatitis B Virus Infection in the United States: recommendations of the Advisory Committee on Immunization Practices. *MMWR Recomm Rep.* 2018;67(RR-1):1–31

is as follows: interferon alfa-2b, ≥ 1 year of age; entecavir, ≥ 2 years of age; tenofovir disoproxil fumarate, ≥ 2 years of age; and telbivudine, ≥ 16 years of age, although this drug is no longer available in the United States (see Non-HIV Antiviral Drugs, p 1044). Pegylated interferon alfa-2a is not approved for treatment of children with chronic hepatitis B but is approved for children ≥ 5 years of age to treat chronic hepatitis C virus infection. Developments in antiviral therapies of HBV and updated practice guidelines may be found on the American Association for the Study of Liver Diseases website (**www.aasld.org/practice-guidelines/chronic-hepatitis-b**). Specific therapy guidelines for children coinfected with HIV and HBV can be accessed online (**https://clinicalinfo.hiv.gov/en/guidelines**).

Consultation with health care professionals with expertise in treating chronic hepatitis B in children is recommended.

INFECTION PREVENTION AND CONTROL MEASURES IN HEALTH CARE SETTINGS: Standard precautions are indicated for patients with acute or chronic HBV infection. For infants whose birthing parent is HBsAg positive, no special care in addition to standard precautions, as described under Control Measures, is needed, other than removal of birthing parent's blood by a gloved attendant.

CONTROL MEASURES:

Hepatitis B Immune Globulin.[1] HBIG provides short-term protection (3–6 months) and is indicated in specific postexposure circumstances (see Care of Exposed People [Postexposure Immunoprophylaxis], p 455). HBIG is prepared from the plasma of donors with high concentrations of anti-HBs, with an anti-HBs titer of at least 1:100 000 by radioimmunoassay. Standard immune globulin is not effective for postexposure prophylaxis against HBV infection, because concentrations of anti-HBs are too low.

Hepatitis B Vaccine. HepB vaccine is used for preexposure and postexposure prophylaxis and provides long-term protection. Preexposure immunization with HepB vaccine is the most effective means to prevent HBV infections. Highly effective and safe HepB vaccines produced by recombinant DNA technology are licensed in the United States in non-live single-antigen formulations and as components of combination vaccines. Recombinant vaccines contain 5 to 40 µg of HBsAg protein/mL, and a completed vaccine series results in production of anti-HBs of at least 10 mIU/mL in most people, which provides long-term protection for immunocompetent recipients. Single-dose formulations, including all pediatric formulations, contain no thimerosal as a preservative. Although the concentration of recombinant HBsAg protein differs among vaccine products, rates of seroprotection are equivalent when administered to immunocompetent infants, children, adolescents, or young adults in the doses recommended (see Table 3.21). A 2-dose single-antigen hepatitis B vaccine with a novel adjuvant (HepB-CpG [Heplisav-B]) and a 3-dose, 3-antigen vaccine (S, pre-S2, and pre-S1 [PreHevbrio]) are available for people 18 years and older.

High seroconversion rates and protective concentrations of anti-HBs (10 mIU/mL or greater) are achieved when HepB vaccine is administered in any of

---

[1] Dosages recommended for postexposure prophylaxis are for products licensed in the United States. Because concentration of anti-HBs in other products may vary, different dosages may be recommended in other countries.

Table 3.21. Recommended Dosages of Hepatitis B Vaccines

Patients	Single-Dose Vaccines[a]			Multiple-Antigen Vaccines[e]	Combination Vaccines		
	RecombivaxHB[b] Dose, µg (mL)	Engerix-B[c] Dose, µg (mL)	Heplisav-B[d] Dose, µg (mL)	PreHevbrio Dose, µg (mL)	Pediarix[f] Dose, µg/mL	Twinrix Dose, µg (mL)[g]	Vaxelis[h] Dose, µg (mL)
Infants, children, and adolescents younger than 20 y (except as noted)	5 (0.5)	10 (0.5)	Not applicable	Not applicable	10 µg HBsAg (0.5) (ages 6 wk through 6 y only)	Not applicable	10 µg HBsAg (0.5) (ages 6 wk through 4 y only)
Adolescents 11–15 y of age[b]	10 (1)	Not approved for 2-dose schedule	Not applicable	Not applicable	Not applicable	Not applicable	Not applicable
Adults 18 y or older			20 (0.5)	10 (S, pre-S1, and pre-S2) (1)		20 (1)	
Adults 20 y or older	10 (1)	20 (1)			Not applicable	20 (1)	Not applicable
Adults undergoing dialysis	40 (1)[i,j]	40 (2)[j,k]	Not applicable	Not applicable	Not applicable	Not applicable	Not applicable

HBsAg, hepatitis B surface antigen.

[a] Recombivax and Engerix-B vaccines are administered in a 3-dose schedule at 0, 1, and 6 months; 4 doses may be administered if a combination vaccine is used (at 2, 4, and 6 months) to complete the series. Only single-antigen hepatitis B vaccine can be used for the birth dose. Single-antigen or combination vaccine containing hepatitis B vaccine may be used to complete the series. See text for management of infants whose birthing parent is HBsAg positive or HBsAg unknown.

[b] Available from Merck & Co Inc. A 2-dose schedule, administered at 0 months and then 4 to 6 months later, is licensed for adolescents 11 through 15 years of age using the adult formulation of Recombivax HB (10 µg).

Table 3.21. Recommended Dosages of Hepatitis B Vaccines, continued

[c] Available from GlaxoSmithKline Biologicals. The US Food and Drug Administration also has licensed this vaccine for use in an optional 4-dose (0.5-mL/dose for ages birth through 10 years and 1.0 mL/dose for ages 11-19 years) schedule at 0, 1, 2, and 12 months for all age groups. A 0-, 12-, and 24-month schedule is licensed for children 5 through 10 years of age at a 0.5-mL dose and for children 11 through 16 years of age at a 1.0-mL dose for whom an extended administration schedule is appropriate on the basis of risk of exposure.

[d] Available from Dynavax Technologies Corporation. A 2-dose schedule administered at 0 and 1 month for use in people ≥18 years of age; safety and effectiveness of Heplisav-B have not been established in adults on hemodialysis.

[e] Available from VBI Vaccines Inc. A 3-dose schedule administered at 0, 1, and 6 months for use in people ≥18 years of age; safety and effectiveness of PreHevbrio have not been established in adults on hemodialysis.

[f] Combination of diphtheria and tetanus toxoids and acellular pertussis (DTaP), inactivated (non-live) poliovirus (IPV), and hepatitis B (Engerix-B 10 µg) is approved for use at 2, 4, and 6 months of age (Pediarix [GlaxoSmithKline]). This vaccine should not be administered at birth, before 6 weeks of age, or at 7 years of age or older. For additional information, see Pertussis (p 656).

[g] A combination of hepatitis B (Engerix-B, 20 µg) and hepatitis A (Havrix, 720 enzyme-linked immunosorbent assay units [ELU]) vaccine; Twinrix is licensed for use in people 18 years of age and older in a 3-dose schedule at 0, 1, and 6 months. Alternately, a 4-dose schedule at days 0, 7, and 21 to 30, followed by a booster dose at 12 months, may be used.

[h] Combination of DTaP, IPV, Haemophilus influenzae type b conjugate, and hepatitis B recombinant vaccines approved for use at 2, 4, and 6 months of age to be used from 6 weeks of age through age 4. Not to be used for the birth dose or for children 5 years and older.

[i] Special formulation for adult dialysis patients administered at 0, 1, and 6 months.

[j] When administered to these populations, follow-up serologic testing is recommended 1–2 months after completion of 2-dose series.

[k] Two 1-mL doses administered in 1 or 2 injections in a 4-dose schedule at 0, 1, 2, and 6 months of age.

the recommended schedules, including schedules begun soon after birth in term infants (see Table 3.21). Only single-antigen HepB vaccine can be used for doses administered between birth and 6 weeks of age. Single-antigen or combination vaccine may be used to complete the series; 4 doses of vaccine may be administered if a birth dose is administered and a combination vaccine containing a hepatitis B component is used to complete the series. For minimum scheduling times between vaccine doses for infants, see Minimum Ages and Minimum Intervals Between Vaccine Doses (p 61).

Recommended schedules for routine and catch-up hepatitis B immunization are available annually from the CDC and American Academy of Pediatrics (**www.cdc. gov/vaccines/schedules/index.html** and **https://publications.aap.org/ redbook/pages/Immunization-Schedules**). Alternate administration schedules are available and licensed by the FDA (see Table 3.21, p 445). These alternate dosage and administration schedules result in equivalent immunogenicity and can be used when acceptable on the basis of low risk of exposure and to facilitate adherence.

HepB vaccine can be administered concurrently with other vaccines (see Simultaneous Administration of Multiple Vaccines, p 63).

Vaccine Interchangeability. In general, the various brands of age-appropriate HepB vaccines are interchangeable within an immunization series. Vaccination should not be deferred when the manufacturer of the previously administered vaccine is unknown or when the vaccine from the same manufacturer is unavailable. Adolescent patients who start their hepatitis B schedule with the adult formulation of Recombivax HB are not candidates to complete their series with the adult formulation of Engerix-B. Similarly, people 18 years or older who start their hepatitis B series with Heplisav-B should complete it with the same product. Of note, data are limited on safety and immunogenicity when PreHevbrio is interchanged with HepB vaccines from other manufacturers.

Routes of Administration. Vaccine is administered intramuscularly in the anterolateral thigh for infants or deltoid area for children and adults (see Vaccine Administration, p 52). Administration in the buttocks or by the intradermal route is not recommended at any age.

Efficacy and Duration of Protection. HepB vaccines licensed in the United States have a 90% to 95% efficacy for preventing HBV infection and clinical HBV disease among susceptible children and adults. Immunocompetent people who achieve anti-HBs concentration ≥ 10 mIU/mL after preexposure vaccination have virtually complete protection against infection with HBV. Long-term studies of immunocompetent adults and children indicate that immune memory remains intact for at least 3 decades and protects against symptomatic acute and chronic HBV infection, even though anti-HBs concentrations may become low or undetectable over time.

Booster Doses. Routine booster doses of HepB vaccine are not recommended for children and adults with normal immune status. For patients undergoing hemodialysis who are at continued risk of infection, immunity should be assessed by annual anti-HBs testing, and a booster dose should be administered when the anti-HBs concentration is <10 mIU/mL. Annual anti-HBs testing and booster doses when anti-HBs concentrations decrease to <10 mIU/mL should be considered for immunocompromised people (eg, people with HIV, hematopoietic cell transplant recipients, and people receiving chemotherapy) if they have an ongoing risk for HBV exposure. Similar consideration may be given to children with cystic fibrosis, liver disease, or celiac disease if there is an ongoing risk for HBV exposure. Children with HIV and celiac disease may not respond as well to HepB vaccine.

Adverse Events. Adverse effects reported in adults and children are pain at the injection site, fever, reported more commonly in children than adults, and fatigue, reported more commonly in adults. Anaphylaxis is uncommon, occurring in less than 1 in 1.3 million recipients. Large, controlled epidemiologic studies and review by the National Academy of Medicine[1] (NAM [see Understanding Vaccine Evaluation and Safety as an Approach to Addressing Parental Concerns, p 27]) found no evidence of an association between HepB vaccine and sudden infant death syndrome, type 1 diabetes mellitus, seizures, encephalitis, or autoimmune (eg, vasculitis) or demyelinating disease, including multiple sclerosis.

Immunization During Pregnancy or Lactation. No adverse effect on the developing fetus has been observed after immunization during pregnancy. Pregnancy and lactation are not contraindications to immunization. Data are not available to assess the safety of Heplisav-B or PreHevbrio during pregnancy, during breastfeeding, or on milk production and excretion. Thus, providers should vaccinate pregnant people needing HepB vaccination with Engerix-B, Recombivax HB, or Twinrix.

Serologic Testing.[2] Susceptibility testing before immunization is not indicated routinely for children or adolescents (Table 1.19, p 122). Screening with a triple panel (HBsAg, anti-HBs, and total anti-HBc) is recommended for all adults 18 years and older at least once in their lifetime. People at increased risk for hepatitis B infection, regardless of age, and anyone who requests HBV testing also should be screened. Testing of pregnant individuals for hepatitis B infection is recommended during each pregnancy (see Serologic Screening of Pregnant People, below). Infants whose birthing parent is HBsAg positive should have postvaccination serologic testing for HBsAg and anti-HBs at 9 to 12 months of age. Anti-HBs testing of health care personnel and others at increased or ongoing risk of hepatitis B exposure (see Booster Doses, p 447, and Postimmunization Testing for Anti-HBs, p 455) may be performed to document presence of protective antibody.

Preexposure Universal Immunization. Immunization with HepB vaccine is recommended for all infants, children, adolescents, and adults through 59 years of age (**www.cdc. gov/vaccines/schedules/hcp/imz/catchup.html, https://publications. aap.org/redbook/pages/Immunization-Schedules,** and **www.cdc.gov/ mmwr/volumes/71/wr/mm7113a1.htm**). Age-specific vaccine dosages are provided in Table 3.21 (p 445).

Newborn Immunization, Including Management Based on HBsAg Status of the Birthing Parent
Serologic Screening of Pregnant People.[2] Testing of all pregnant individuals is recommended to identify newborn infants who require immediate postexposure prophylaxis. Testing with HBsAg is recommended during each pregnancy, regardless of vaccination status or history of testing; a triple panel (HBsAg, anti-HBs, and total

[1] Institute of Medicine. *Adverse Effects of Vaccines: Evidence and Causality.* Washington, DC: National Academies Press; 2011

[2] Conners EE, Panagiotakopoulos L, Hofmeister MG, et al. Screening and testing for hepatitis B virus infection: CDC recommendations – United States, 2023. *MMWR Recomm Rep.* 2023;72(RR-1):1-25

anti-HBc) may be offered to those who have not had this performed previously. All pregnant individuals should be tested during an early prenatal visit and testing should be repeated at the time of admission to the hospital for delivery for HBsAg-negative people who are at high risk of HBV infection or who have had clinical hepatitis. Individuals who are HBsAg positive also should be tested for hepatitis B virus deoxyribonucleic acid (HBV DNA) and referred to appropriate specialists to assess need for treatment and to ensure follow-up of their infants and immunization of sexual and household contacts.

Birth Dose of Hepatitis B Vaccine and Use of HBIG.[1] The strategy for preventing hepatitis B in newborn infants, based on birth weight and birthing parent's HBsAg status, involves providing a birth dose of hepatitis B vaccine to all infants and, for some infants, HBIG. Starting vaccination at birth for all infants serves as a safety net in case a birthing parent's HBsAg-positive status was not identified at birth, such as if results were not obtained, were misinterpreted, were falsely negative, were transcribed or reported to the infant care team inaccurately, or were not communicated to the nursery. The strategy acknowledges and accounts for risk factors that may not have been reported and high-risk birthing parents who may not have been retested around the time of delivery.

HepB vaccine should be administered to all infants born to HBsAg-negative birth parents within 24 hours of birth for infants with birth weight ≥2000 g, and at hospital discharge or 1 month of age (whichever is first) for infants with birth weight <2000 g. HepB vaccine plus HBIG should be administered within 12 hours of birth to all newborn infants whose birthing parent is HBsAg positive. Appropriate management at birth of these infants and those whose birthing parent's HBsAg status is unknown is described below and in Fig 3.5.

Subsequent Immunization of Newborns Whose Birthing Parent is HBsAg Negative and Those Whose HBsAg Was Unknown at Birth But is Subsequently Confirmed as Negative (Tables 3.21, p 445, and 3.22, p 451). Infants whose birthing parent is HBsAg negative and those whose birthing parent's initial HBsAg status was unknown but subsequently is confirmed as negative should complete hepatitis B immunization according to routine immunization schedules with either single-antigen (at ages 1–2 months and 6–18 months) or combination hepatitis B-containing (ages 2, 4, and 6 months) vaccine. Minimum intervals of 4 weeks (28 days) should occur between doses 1 and 2, and 8 weeks between doses 2 and 3, with a minimum of 16 weeks between doses 1 and 3; when 4 doses are administered, substitute "dose 4" for "dose 3" in these calculations (**www.cdc. gov/vaccines/schedules/hcp/imz/child-adolescent.html** and **https:// publications.aap.org/redbook/pages/Immunization-Schedules**). Infants whose birthing parent's HBsAg is unknown and remains unknown are managed as infants whose birthing parent is HBsAg positive (see below).

Management of Infants Born to HBsAg-Positive People. All infants born to HBsAg-positive people, including infants weighing less than 2000 g, should receive the initial dose of HepB vaccine within 12 hours of birth (see Table 3.22, p 451, for appropriate dosages), and HBIG (0.5 mL) should be administered concurrently but at different

---

[1] American Academy of Pediatrics, Committee on Infectious Diseases. Elimination of perinatal hepatitis B: providing the first vaccine dose within 24 hours of birth. *Pediatrics*. 2017;140(3):e20171870

FIG 3.5. ADMINISTRATION OF BIRTH DOSE OF HEPATITIS B VACCINE BY BIRTH WEIGHT AND HBsAg STATUS OF BIRTHING PARENT

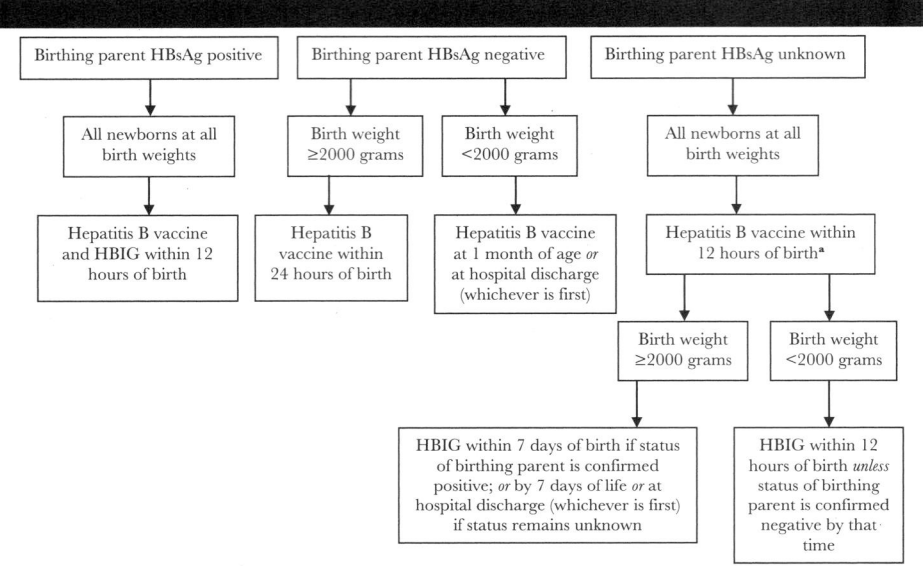

Modified from American Academy of Pediatrics, Committee on Infectious Diseases, Committee on Fetus and Newborn. Elimination of perinatal hepatitis b: providing the first vaccine dose within 24 hours of birth. *Pediatrics.* 2017;140(3):e20171870
[a] For newborn infants with birth weight <2000 g, this dose will not count toward total doses in series.

anatomic sites (eg, different extremities) (Fig 3.5). Infants whose birthing parent has other evidence suggestive of HBV infection (eg, presence of HBV DNA, HBeAg positive, or known to be chronically infected with HBV) should be managed this way as well. Effectiveness of HBIG diminishes the longer after exposure it is initiated. The interval of effectiveness is unlikely to exceed 7 days. Subsequent doses of vaccine should be administered as recommended in Table 3.22 (p 451). For infants who weigh <2000 g at birth, the initial vaccine dose should not be counted in the required 3-dose schedule (a total of 4 doses of HepB vaccine should be administered), and the subsequent 3 doses should be administered at months 1, 2 to 3, and 6 months for single-antigen products and months 2, 4, and 6 for hepatitis B-containing combination vaccines (Table 3.22, p 451). By the chronologic age of 1 month, all medically stable preterm infants, regardless of initial birth weight or gestational age, are as likely to respond to HepB immunization as are term and larger infants.

Breastfeeding of an infant by an HBsAg-positive parent poses no additional risk of acquisition of HBV infection by the infant with appropriate administration of HepB vaccine and HBIG (see Breastfeeding and Human Milk, p 135).

FOLLOW-UP MANAGEMENT OF INFANTS WHOSE BIRTHING PARENT IS HBsAg POSITIVE. Infants whose birthing parent is HBsAg positive should be tested for anti-HBs and HBsAg at 9 to 12 months of age, at least 1 to 2 months after completion of

Table 3.22. Hepatitis B Vaccine Schedules for Infants by Hepatitis B Surface Antigen (HBsAg) Status of Birthing Parent and Birth Weight

HBsAg Status of Birthing Parent	Single-Antigen Vaccine		Single-Antigen + Combination (Pediarix or Vaxelis)	
	Dose	Age	Dose	Age
Positive	1[a]	Birth (12 h or less)	1[a]	Birth (12 h or less) (combination vaccine should not be used for birth dose)
	HBIG[b]	Birth (12 h or less)	HBIG[b]	Birth (12 h or less)
	2	1 through 2 mo for BW ≥2000 g; 1 mo for BW <2000 g	2	2 mo
	3[c]	6 mo for BW ≥2000 g; 2–3 mo for BW <2000 g	3	4 mo
	4 Only if BW <2000 g	6 mo	4[d]	6 mo
Unknown[e]	1[a]	Birth (12 h or less) BW <2000 g HBIG at birth (12 h or less)	1[a]	Birth (12 h or less) (Combination vaccine should not be used for birth dose) BW <2000 g HBIG at birth (12 h or less)
	2	1 through 2 mo for BW ≥2000 g; 1 mo for BW <2000 g if status of birthing parent remains unknown	2	2 mo
	3[d]	6 mo for BW ≥2000 g; 2–3 mo for BW <2000 g if status of birthing parent remains unknown	3	4 mo
	4 Only if BW <2000 g AND status of birthing parent remains unknown	6 mo	4[d]	6 mo

Table 3.22. Hepatitis B Vaccine Schedules for Infants by Hepatitis B Surface Antigen (HBsAg) Status of Birthing Parent and Birth Weight, continued

HBsAg Status of Birthing Parent	Single-Antigen Vaccine		Single-Antigen + Combination (Pediarix or Vaxelis)	
	Dose	Age	Dose	Age
Negative	1[a]	Birth (24 h or less) for BW ≥2000 g; hospital discharge or age 1 mo for BW <2000 g	1[a]	Birth (24 h or less) for BW ≥2000 g; hospital discharge or age 1 mo for BW <2000 g (combination vaccine should not be used for birth dose)
	2	1 through 2 mo	2	2 mo
	3[d]	6 through 18 mo	3	4 mo
	4	Not applicable	4[d]	6 mo

BW indicates birth weight; HBIG, hepatitis B immune globulin.

[a] Recombivax HB or Engerix-B should be used for the birth dose. Pediarix and Vaxelis should not be administered at birth or before 6 weeks of age.

[b] HBIG (0.5 mL) administered intramuscularly in a separate site from vaccine.

[c] Birthing parents should have blood drawn and tested for HBsAg as soon as possible after admission for delivery. Infants with birth weight <2000 g should receive HBIG by 12 hours; for infants with birth weight ≥2000 g if the birthing parent is found to be HBsAg positive, the infant should receive HBIG as soon as possible but no later than 7 days of age.

[d] The final dose in the vaccine series should not be administered before 24 weeks (164 days) of age.

Source: Schillie S, Vellozzi C, Reingold A, et al. Prevention of hepatitis B virus infection in the United States: recommendations of the Advisory Committee on Immunization Practices. *MMWR Recomm Rep*. 2018;67(RR-1):1-31.

the immunization series).[1,2] Testing should not be performed before 9 months of age to maximize likelihood of detecting late onset of HBV infections. Immunized infants with anti-HBs concentrations ≥10 mIU/mL and who are HBsAg negative are considered not to be infected and to have adequate vaccine-associated immune protection. Infants with anti-HBs concentrations <10 mIU/mL and who are HBsAg negative following a 3-dose hepatitis B vaccine series should receive 1 additional dose of hepatitis B vaccine followed by testing for anti-HBs and HBsAg 1 to 2 months after the fourth dose. Infants with anti-HBs concentrations ≥10 mIU/mL and who are HBsAg negative after the fourth dose are considered not to be infected and to have adequate vaccine-associated immune protection. Infants with anti-HBs concentrations <10 mIU/mL and who are HBsAg negative after the fourth dose should receive 2 additional doses of vaccine, separated by at least 8 weeks, followed by testing for anti-HBs and HBsAg 1 to 2 months after the sixth dose. An alternate approach for children who have completed a 3-dose series of HepB vaccine but did not achieve anti-HBs titers ≥10 mIU/mL is to give 3 additional doses of HepB vaccine at the same dosing intervals as the first series and then retest for anti-HBs titers 1 to 2 months after the third dose of this second

[1] Schillie S, Murphy TV, Fenlon N, et al. Update: shortened interval for postvaccination serologic testing of infants born to hepatitis B-infected mothers. *MMWR Morb Mortal Wkly Rep*. 2015;64(30):1118-1120

[2] American Academy of Pediatrics, Committee on Infectious Diseases. Elimination of perinatal hepatitis B: providing the first vaccine dose within 24 hours of birth. *Pediatrics*. 2017;140(3):e20171870

series. Subsequent doses of hepatitis B vaccine when anti-HBs concentrations are <10 mIU/mL after the sixth dose are not indicated.

Management of Infants Whose Birthing Parent's HBsAg Status is Unknown or Whose Birthing Parent Was Not Tested for HBsAg During Pregnancy.

TERM INFANTS (WEIGHING ≥2000 g AT BIRTH). Pregnant people whose HBsAg status is unknown at delivery should undergo blood testing as soon as possible to determine their HBsAg status. While awaiting results, the infant should receive the first HepB vaccine dose within 12 hours of birth, as recommended for infants whose birthing parent is HBsAg positive (see Table 3.22, p 451, and Fig 3.5, p 450). Routine nursery procedures, such as skin-to-skin care, delayed bathing, and breastfeeding within the first hour, may continue as recommended by the facility. If the birthing parent is found to be HBsAg positive, term infants should receive HBIG (0.5 mL) as soon as possible, but within 7 days of birth, and should complete the HepB immunization series as recommended (see Tables 3.21, p 445, and 3.22, p 451). If the birthing parent is found to be HBsAg negative, HepB immunization in the dose and schedule recommended for term infants whose birthing parent is HBsAg negative should be completed (see Table 3.21, p 445). If the birthing parent's HBsAg status remains unknown, it is appropriate to administer HBIG within 7 days of birth and complete the HepB immunization series as recommended for infants whose birthing parent is HBsAg positive (Table 3.22, p 451, and Fig 3.5, p 450).

INFANTS WEIGHING LESS THAN 2000 g. HBsAg status of the birthing parent should be determined as soon as possible. Infants weighing <2000 g whose birthing parent's HBsAg status is unknown should receive HepB vaccine within the first 12 hours of life (Table 3.22, p 451, and Fig 3.5, p 450). Because of the potentially decreased immunogenicity of the HepB vaccine in infants weighing <2000 g at birth, these infants should also receive HBIG (0.5 mL) within 12 hours of birth if the birthing parent's HBsAg status cannot be determined by that time (Table 3.22, p 451, and Fig 3.5, p 450). The initial vaccine dose should not be counted toward the 3 doses of hepatitis B vaccine required to complete the immunization series, and the subsequent 3 doses (for a total of 4 doses) are administered according to the HBsAg status of the birthing parent. If the birthing parent is HBsAg positive or the parent's status remains unknown, the infant would receive the subsequent 3 doses administered at months 1, 2 to 3, and 6 months for single-antigen HepB products, and months 2, 4, and 6 for HepB-containing combination vaccines (Tables 3.21, p 445, and 3.22, p 451). Serologic testing for both of these groups of infants should be performed as described above for infants whose birthing parent is HBsAg positive and revaccination performed if necessary (p 448).

Routine Immunization of Infants, Children, and Adolescents Who Did Not Begin Immunization at Birth. Serologic testing to identify HBV infection (with a triple panel of HBsAg, anti-HBs, and total anti-HBc) should be performed for people in risk groups with high rates of infection, including people born in countries with intermediate or high HBV endemicity (even if immunized, because the series may have been started after the infection was acquired), children born in the United States who were not vaccinated as infants whose parents were born in a country with high HBV endemicity, current or past users of injection drugs, men who have sex with men, people with HIV or HCV infection, people currently or formerly incarcerated, people with STIs or multiple sexual partners, people on dialysis, household and sexual contacts of HBsAg-positive people, people with elevated ALT or AST levels of unknown origin, and anyone who requests

HBV testing. The first dose of vaccine may be given at the time of testing so that immunization is not delayed. Children identified as HBsAg positive should be referred for management and monitoring of hepatitis B infection. Those who are HBsAg negative and anti-HBs negative should be immunized according to doses and schedules noted in Table 3.21 (p 445). Routine postimmunization testing is not recommended.

Lapsed Immunizations. For infants, children, adolescents, and adults with lapsed immunizations (ie, the interval between doses is longer than that in one of the recommended schedules), the vaccine series should be completed without repeating doses, as long as minimum dosing intervals between the remaining doses necessary to complete the series are heeded (see Lapsed Immunizations, p 66).

Negative Anti-HBs in Previously Immunized Children. Providers may be asked to manage children tested for anti-HBs following receipt of hepatitis B immunization given at age-appropriate doses and intervals and found to have anti-HBs <10 mIU/mL. Serologic testing following routine immunization of children is not recommended routinely. If confirming response to vaccine is desired, such as after a needlestick injury, a single dose of vaccine may be administered, followed by testing for anti-HBs 1 to 2 months later. Children with anti-HBs ≥10 mIU/mL can be considered to have adequate vaccine-associated immune protection. Those with anti-HBs <10 mIU/mL may be given 2 more doses of hepatitis B with testing for anti-HBs 1 to 2 months after the last dose. A vaccine nonresponder is defined as a person with anti-HBs <10 mIU/mL after 2 complete series of HepB vaccine.

SPECIAL CONSIDERATIONS:

Considerations for High-Risk Groups:

Patients Undergoing Hemodialysis. Immunization is recommended for susceptible patients undergoing hemodialysis. Immunization early in the course of renal disease is encouraged, because response is better than in advanced disease. Specific dosage recommendations have not been made for children undergoing hemodialysis. Some experts recommend increased doses of HepB vaccine for children receiving hemodialysis to increase immunogenicity.

People Born in Countries Where the Prevalence of Chronic HBV Infection Is 2% or Greater. Foreign-born people (including immigrants, refugees, asylum seekers, and internationally adopted children) from countries where prevalence of chronic HBV infection is 2% or greater (see Fig 3.2) should be screened for HBsAg regardless of immunization status (see Medical Evaluation for Infectious Diseases for Internationally Adopted, Refugee, and Other Immigrant Children, p 189). Previously unimmunized family members and other household contacts should be immunized if a household member is found to be HBsAg positive. Positive HBsAg test results are nationally notifiable (see Nationally Notifiable Infectious Diseases in the United States, p 1141), and people with positive HBsAg test results should be referred for medical management to reduce their risk of complications from chronic HBV infection and to reduce risk of transmission.

Inmates in Juvenile Detention and Other Correctional Facilities. Unimmunized or underimmunized people in juvenile and adult correctional facilities should be immunized. If the length of stay is not sufficient to complete the immunization series, the series should be initiated, and follow-up mechanisms with a health care facility should be established to ensure completion of the series.

International Travelers. People traveling to areas where prevalence of chronic HBV infection is 2% or greater (see Fig 3.2, p 440) should be immunized. Ideally, HepB vaccination should be administered ≥6 months before travel so that a 3-dose regimen can be completed (see Preexposure Universal Immunization, p 448). If fewer than 4 months are available before departure, the alternative 4-dose schedule of 0, 1, 2, and 12 months, licensed for one vaccine (see Table 3.21, p 445), might provide opportunity for more rapid development of protection. Individual health care providers may choose to use an accelerated schedule (eg, doses at days 0, 7, and 21–30, with a booster at 12 months) for travelers who will depart before an approved immunization schedule can be completed. People who receive immunization on an accelerated schedule that is not licensed by the FDA also should receive a dose at 12 months after initiation of the series to promote long-term immunity. For people 18 years and older, the 2-dose regimen of Heplisav-B can be completed in 1 month and offers greater flexibility before travel.

Postimmunization Testing for Anti-HBs. Routine postimmunization testing for anti-HBs is not necessary after routine vaccination of healthy people but is recommended 1 to 2 months after the final vaccine dose for the following specific groups: (1) hemodialysis patients (and other people who might require outpatient hemodialysis); (2) people with HIV infection; (3) other immunocompromised patients (eg, hematopoietic cell transplant recipients or people receiving chemotherapy); (4) people at occupational risk of exposure from percutaneous injuries or mucosal or nonintact skin exposures (eg, certain health care and public safety workers); (5) sexual partners of HBsAg-positive people, and (6) infants whose birthing parent is HBsAg positive and infants whose birthing parent's HBsAg status remains unknown (testing should consist of HBsAg and anti-HBs).

Management of Nonresponders. Vaccine recipients who do not develop a serum anti-HBs response (≥10 mIU/mL) after a primary vaccine series should be tested for HBsAg to rule out the possibility of a chronic infection as an explanation of failure to respond to the vaccine. If the HBsAg test result is negative, a single dose of HepB vaccine can be administered followed by testing for anti-HBs in 1 to 2 months. If anti-HBs is ≥10 mIU/mL, no further testing is required. If anti-HBs is <10 mIU/mL, additional doses should be administered to complete the second vaccine series, with testing for anti-HBs 1 to 2 months after the last dose. For the 3-dose vaccine series using Engerix-B or Recombivax HB, this would require 2 additional doses of vaccine, and for the 2-dose series using Heplisav-B (licensed only in adults), this would require 1 additional dose. For very recently vaccinated HCP with anti-HBs <10 mIU/mL, in whom the low antibody concentration is more likely to reflect a failure to respond rather than waning antibody concentration, it may be more practical to revaccinate with an entire second series (3 doses of Engerix-B or Recombivax HB; 2 doses of Heplisav-B or PreHevbrio) followed by anti-HBs testing 1 to 2 months after the last dose. Heplisav-B may be used for revaccination following an initial HepB vaccine series that consisted of doses from a different manufacturer. A vaccine nonresponder is defined as a person with anti-HBs <10 mIU/mL after 2 complete series of HepB vaccine.

Care of Exposed People (Postexposure Immunoprophylaxis).

Household Contacts and Sexual Partners of HBsAg-Positive People. Household and sexual contacts of HBsAg-positive people (with acute or chronic HBV infection) identified through prenatal screening, blood donor screening, or diagnostic or other serologic testing should be screened for HBV infection with a triple panel (HBsAg, anti-HBs, and total anti-HBc). Unvaccinated and uninfected people should be immunized. The first dose of vaccine should be administered after the blood for serologic tests is obtained and while waiting for the results. People with chronic HBV should be referred for medical evaluation to prevent complications of the infection.

Prophylaxis with HBIG for other unimmunized household contacts of HBsAg-positive people is not indicated unless they have a discrete, identifiable exposure to the index patient (see next paragraph).

Postexposure Prophylaxis for People with Discrete Identifiable Exposures to Blood or Body Fluids. Management of people with a discrete, identifiable percutaneous (eg, needle stick, laceration, bite that breaks the skin), mucosal (eg, ocular or mucous membrane), or sexual exposure to blood or body fluids includes consideration of whether the HBsAg status of the person who was the source of exposure and the hepatitis B immunization and response status of the exposed person are known (also see Table 3.23). If possible, a blood specimen from the person who was the source of the exposure should be tested for HBsAg, and appropriate prophylaxis should be administered according to the hepatitis B immunization status and anti-HBs response status (if known) of the exposed person (see Table 3.23). Detailed guidelines for management of health care personnel and other people exposed to blood that is or might be HBsAg positive

Table 3.23. Guidelines for Postexposure Prophylaxis[a] of People With Nonoccupational Exposures[b] to Blood or Body Fluids That Contain Blood, by Exposure Type and Vaccination Status

Exposure	Treatment	
	Unvaccinated Person[c]	Previously Vaccinated Person[d]
HBsAg-positive source		
Household member	Consider testing if significant exposure; if negative administer hepatitis B vaccine series	Ensure completion of vaccine series
Percutaneous (eg, bite or needlestick) or mucosal exposure to HBsAg-positive blood or body fluids	Administer hepatitis B vaccine series and hepatitis B immune globulin (HBIG)	Administer hepatitis B vaccine booster dose
Sexual or needle-sharing contact of an HBsAg-positive person	Administer hepatitis B vaccine series and HBIG	Administer hepatitis B vaccine booster dose
Person who has been sexually assaulted or abused by a perpetrator who is HBsAg positive	Administer hepatitis B vaccine series and HBIG	Administer hepatitis B vaccine booster dose

Table 3.23. Guidelines for Postexposure Prophylaxis[a] of People With Nonoccupational Exposures[b] to Blood or Body Fluids That Contain Blood, by Exposure Type and Vaccination Status, continued

Exposure	Treatment	
	Unvaccinated Person[c]	Previously Vaccinated Person[d]
Source with unknown HBsAg status		
Person who has been sexually assaulted or abused by a perpetrator with unknown HBsAg status	Administer hepatitis B vaccine series	No treatment
Percutaneous (eg, bite or needlestick) or mucosal exposure to potentially infectious blood or body fluids from a source with unknown HBsAg status	Administer hepatitis B vaccine series	No treatment
Sexual or needle-sharing contact of person with unknown HBsAg status	Administer hepatitis B vaccine series	No treatment

HBsAg indicates hepatitis B surface antigen.

[a] When indicated, immunoprophylaxis should be initiated as soon as possible, preferably within 24 hours. Studies are limited on the maximum interval after exposure during which postexposure prophylaxis is effective, but the interval is unlikely to exceed 7 days for percutaneous exposures or 14 days for sexual exposures. The hepatitis B vaccine series should be completed.

[b] These guidelines apply to nonoccupational exposures. Guidelines for occupational exposures can be found in Schillie S, Murphy TV, Sawyer M, et al. CDC guidance for evaluating health-care personnel for hepatitis B virus protection and for administering post exposure management. *MMWR Recomm Rep.* 2013;62(RR-10):1–19.

[c] A person who is in the process of being vaccinated but who has not completed the vaccine series should complete the series and receive treatment as indicated.

[d] A person who has written documentation of a complete hepatitis B vaccine series and who did not receive postvaccination testing.

Source: Schillie S, Vellozzi C, Reingold A, et al. Prevention of hepatitis B virus infection in the United States: recommendations of the Advisory Committee on Immunization Practices. *MMWR Recomm Rep.* 2018;67(1):1–31.

are provided in the recommendations of the Advisory Committee on Immunization Practices of the CDC.[1]

Child Care.

Children who are HBsAg positive and who have no behavioral or medical risk factors, such as unusually aggressive behavior (eg, frequent biting), generalized dermatitis, or a bleeding problem, should be admitted to child care without restrictions. Under these circumstances, the risk of HBV transmission in child care settings is negligible, and routine screening for HBsAg is not warranted. Admission of HBsAg-positive children with behavioral or medical risk factors should be assessed on an individual basis by the child's physician, in consultation with the child care staff. A susceptible child who bites another child or adult who is HBsAg-positive should initiate or complete the hepatitis B vaccine series; HBIG is not recommended in this circumstance (see Bite Wounds, p 202).

---

[1] Schillie S, Murphy TV, Sawyer M, et al. CDC guidance for evaluating health-care personnel for hepatitis B virus protection and for administering post exposure management. *MMWR Recomm Rep.* 2013;62(RR-10):1–19

Hepatitis C

CLINICAL MANIFESTATIONS: Signs and symptoms of hepatitis C virus (HCV) infection are indistinguishable from those of hepatitis A (HAV) or hepatitis B virus (HBV) infections. Acute disease tends to be mild and insidious in onset, and most infections are asymptomatic. Jaundice occurs in less than 20% of patients with HCV infection, and abnormalities in serum alanine aminotransferase concentrations generally are less pronounced than in patients with HBV infection. Rates of spontaneous viral clearance vary, but roughly 20% or more of children with perinatal infection clear the virus by 2 years of age, with upwards of 65% clearing the virus by 5 years of age. Most children with chronic infection are asymptomatic and may not show biochemical evidence of liver disease initially. Liver failure secondary to HCV infection is one of the leading indications for liver transplantation among adults in the United States. Limited data indicate that cirrhosis and hepatocellular carcinoma occur less commonly in children than in adults, but because fibrosis increases with disease duration, individuals who are perinatally infected are at risk of developing severe disease in adolescence or as young adults.

ETIOLOGY: HCV is a small, single-stranded, positive-sense RNA virus and is a member of the family *Flaviviridae* in the genus *Hepacivirus*. At least 7 HCV genotypes exist and more than 60 subtypes have been described to date. Distribution of genotypes and subtypes varies by geographic location; genotype 1a is the most common genotype in the United States.

EPIDEMIOLOGY: Prevalence of HCV infection in the general population of the United States is estimated at 1.0%, equating to an estimated 2.4 (2.0–2.8) million people in the United States with chronic HCV infection. Incidence of HCV infection decreased markedly in the United States in all age groups from the 1990s to reach its lowest incidence in 2006–2010. Since 2010, however, there has been an increase in reported cases of acute HCV infection in the United States, largely related to injection drug use. The highest incidence of acute hepatitis C infection is in people 20 through 39 years of age, leading to an increase in the number of infants exposed prenatally to HCV **(www.cdc.gov/hepatitis/statistics/SurveillanceRpts.htm).** Worldwide, the prevalence of chronic HCV infection is highest in eastern Europe, central Asia, northern Africa, and the Middle East.

HCV is transmitted primarily through percutaneous (parenteral) exposures to infectious blood that can result from injection drug use, needlestick injuries, and inadequate infection control in health care settings. The most common risk factors for adults are injection drug use and multiple sexual partners. The most common route of infection for children is from birthing parent to infant transmission. The current risk of HCV infection after blood transfusion in the United States is estimated to be less than 1 per 2 million units transfused because of exclusion of high-risk donors and of HCV-positive units after antibody testing as well as screening of blood units by nucleic acid amplification tests (NAATs). All intravenous and intramuscular immune globulin and plasma products now available commercially in the United States undergo an inactivation procedure for HCV or are documented to have undetectable HCV RNA before release.

Of acute hepatitis C cases reported to public health authorities with available risk factor information, two-thirds are in people who acknowledge they inject drugs. Data from recent multicenter, population-based cohort studies indicate that approximately one third of people who inject drugs 18 to 30 years of age are infected with HCV.

People with sporadic percutaneous exposures, such as health care professionals, may be infected; per exposure risk of HCV transmission from needlestick is estimated at 0.2%. Health care–associated outbreaks have been documented, especially in nonhospital settings with inadequate infection control and injection safety procedures. Prevalence of HCV is higher among people with frequent direct percutaneous exposures, such as patients receiving hemodialysis (7%).

Sexual transmission of HCV between monogamous heterosexual partners is extremely rare. Transmission can occur in men who have sex with men, especially in association with sexual practices that result in mucosal trauma, presence of concurrent anogenital ulcerative disease, human immunodeficiency virus (HIV)-positive serostatus, or sex while using methamphetamines. HCV has been identified in semen and rectal and vaginal fluids, especially in those coinfected with HIV.

Transmission among family contacts could occur from direct or inapparent percutaneous or mucosal exposure to blood (eg, sharing toothbrushes or razors), but this is extremely uncommon.

Seroprevalence among pregnant people in the United States is estimated at 1% to 2% but is higher in some areas. Risk of perinatal transmission is approximately 6% to 7% among HIV-negative pregnant people with hepatitis C. The exact timing of vertical HCV transmission is not established. Recent guidelines from the Centers for Disease Control and Prevention (CDC) recommend testing of all pregnant people for HCV with each pregnancy. Factors that may increase risk of perinatal transmission include invasive prenatal diagnostic testing (eg, chorionic villus sampling), internal fetal monitoring, vaginal lacerations, and prolonged rupture of membranes (>6 hours). Method of delivery has no effect on perinatal infection risk. Coinfection in the pregnant person with poorly controlled HIV is associated with increased risk of perinatal transmission of HCV (twofold greater). Early and sustained control of HIV viremia with antiretroviral therapy (ART) may reduce risk of HCV transmission to infants.

All people with detectable HCV RNA in their blood are considered infectious.

The **incubation period** for HCV infection averages 6 to 7 weeks, with a range of 2 weeks to 6 months. The time from exposure to development of viremia generally is 1 to 3 weeks.

DIAGNOSTIC TESTS[1,2]**:** Diagnostic assays for the detection of anti-HCV antibody are available in various formats, which include enzyme immunoassays (EIA), chemiluminescent immunoassays (CIA), and immunochromatographic or rapid tests. NAATs for detection and quantitation of HCV RNA are used for diagnosis of current HCV infection and for monitoring response to antiviral therapy. Screening for HCV infection usually is accomplished by serologic testing for anti-HCV with reflex testing of reactive samples with NAAT to diagnose current infection. Third-generation anti-HCV assays cleared by the US Food and Drug Administration (FDA) are at least 97% sensitive and more than 99% specific. Anti-HCV antibodies can be detected approximately 8 to 11 weeks after exposure. In clinical settings where exposure to HCV is considered likely, testing for HCV RNA should be performed regardless of the anti-HCV

---

[1] Centers for Disease Control and Prevention. Testing for HCV Infection: an update of guidance for clinicians and laboratorians. *MMWR Morb Mortal Wkly Rep.* 2013;62(18):362-365

[2] Panagiotakopoulos L, Sandul AL, Conners EE, Foster MA, Nelson NP, Wester C. CDC recommendations for hepatitis C testing among perinatally exposed infants and children—United States, 2023. *MMWR Recomm Rep.* 2023;72(RR-4):1-19

result. Transplacentally acquired antibody may persist for up to 18 months in infants born to anti-HCV–positive mothers.

FDA-cleared NAATs for detection of HCV RNA are available commercially and are recommended in the 2013 CDC HCV testing algorithm as reflex tests for patients with anti-HCV reactive test results. HCV RNA can be detected in serum or plasma within 1 to 3 weeks after exposure to the virus and weeks before onset of liver enzyme abnormalities or appearance of anti-HCV antibody. Assays for detection of HCV RNA are used commonly in clinical practice to: (1) detect HCV infection after needle-stick or transfusion and before seroconversion; (2) identify current infection in anti-HCV–positive patients; (3) identify infection in infants early in life (ie, from perinatal transmission) when transplacentally acquired antibody interferes with ability to detect antibody produced by the infant; (4) identify HCV infection in severely immunocompromised or hemodialysis patients in whom there may be delayed seroconversion to anti-HCV; (5) detect a recent or acute infection when the HCV antibody is negative; and (6) monitor patients receiving antiviral therapy. False-positive and false-negative results of NAATs can occur from improper handling, storage, and contamination of test specimens. HCV genotyping is still needed for determining which direct-acting antiviral (DAA) agents should be used in individual patients, but as pan-genotypic antiviral drugs become available more widely, genotype testing may become less relevant.

Infants exposed perinatally should be tested by NAAT for HCV RNA at age 2 through 6 months to identify children who might go on to develop chronic HCV infection if not treated. Similarly, infants and children aged 7 through 17 months of age who are perinatally exposed to HCV and have not previously been tested should have a NAAT for HCV RNA performed. Infants with detectable HCV RNA should be managed in consultation with a health care provider with expertise in pediatric hepatitis C management. Infants with an undetectable HCV RNA result do not require further follow-up unless clinically warranted. Children aged ≥18 months who are perinatally exposed to HCV and have not previously been tested should be tested serologically for anti-HCV immunoglobulin (Ig) G (Fig 3.6).

TREATMENT: Two interferon-free, pan-genotypic antiviral drug regimens have been approved by the FDA for children as young as 3 years: sofosbuvir/velpatasvir and glecaprevir/pibrentasvir (see Non-HIV Antiviral Drugs, p 1044). Two additional antiviral drug therapies, sofosbuvir and ledipasvir/sofosbuvir, have activity against some but not all HCV genotypes and are approved for use in people 3 years or older. All HCV-infected children 3 years or older should be treated in line with public health goals of viral hepatitis elimination. Children with a diagnosis of current HCV infection should be cared for in consultation with a provider with expertise in pediatric hepatitis C for clinical monitoring and consideration for treatment. The American Association for the Study of Liver Disease (AASLD) and the Infectious Diseases Society of America (IDSA) summarize recommended antiviral drug treatment for adults (**www.hcvguidelines.org**) and children (**www.hcvguidelines.org/unique-populations/children**).

Management of Chronic HCV Infection. Because of the very high rate of severe hepatitis in patients with HCV-associated chronic liver disease, all patients with chronic HCV infection should be immunized against HAV and HBV. Risk of liver-related morbidity and mortality, including cirrhosis and primary hepatocellular carcinoma, increases with advancing age in individuals with chronic HCV infection. Among

FIG 3.6. TESTING OF CHILDREN PERINATALLY EXPOSED TO HCV

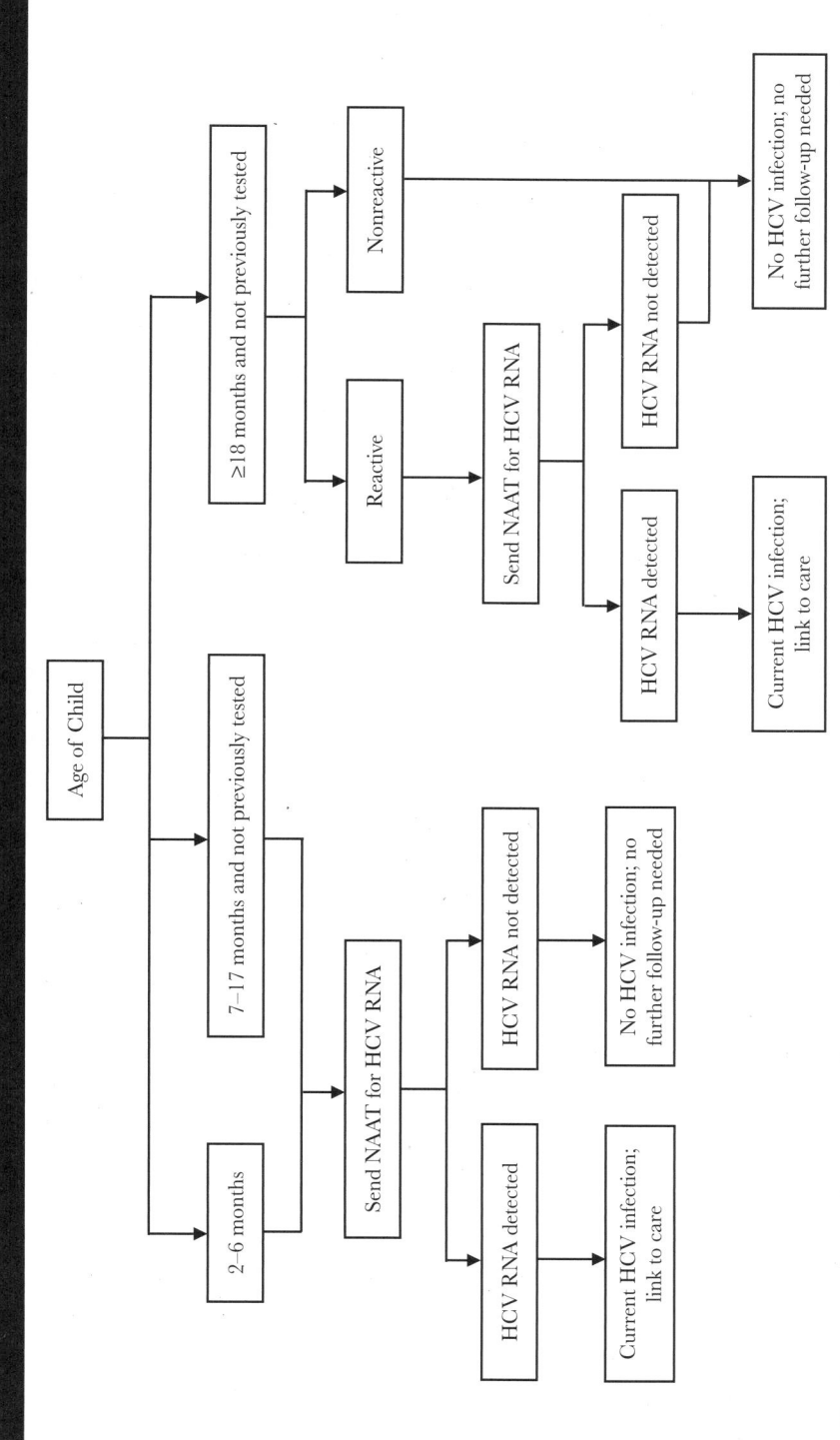

Modified from Conners EE, Panagiotakopoulos L, Hofmeister MG, et al. Screening and testing for hepatitis B virus infection: CDC Recommendations—United States, 2023. *MMWR Recomm Rep.* 2023;72(RR-1):1–25.

children, progression of liver disease appears to be accelerated when comorbid conditions, including HIV, childhood cancer, iron overload, or thalassemia, are present. Pediatricians should be alert for conditions that may worsen liver disease in patients with HCV infection, such as concomitant infections, and alcohol use. After assessment of risks and benefits, hepatotoxic drugs should be used with caution in children with chronic HCV infection. Notably, corticosteroids, cytotoxic chemotherapy, and therapeutic doses of acetaminophen are not contraindicated in children with chronic HCV infection, and acetaminophen is safe and effective in this population when dosed appropriately. Children with chronic infection should be followed closely, including sequential monitoring of serum alanine aminotransferase concentrations, because of the potential for chronic liver disease. Evidence-based, consensus recommendations from the IDSA, the AASLD, and the International Antiviral Society–USA for screening, treatment, and management of patients with HCV infection, including children and pregnant people, can be found online (**www.hcvguidelines.org**).

INFECTION PREVENTION AND CONTROL MEASURES IN HEALTH CARE SETTINGS: Standard precautions are recommended.

CONTROL MEASURES:

Care of Exposed People.

Immunoprophylaxis. Use of immune globulin for postexposure prophylaxis against HCV infection is not recommended based on lack of clinical efficacy in humans and data from animal studies. Potential donors of immune globulin are screened for antibody to HCV and excluded from donation if positive, so immune globulin preparations are devoid of anti-HCV antibody.

Pregnancy and Breastfeeding.[1,2] All pregnant people should be tested for HCV during each pregnancy. Pregnant persons with detectable HCV RNA are considered to have current HCV infection; if no HCV test is available from that pregnancy and the most recent NAAT indicated detectable HCV RNA in the absence of treatment, they also are considered to have current HCV infection. If anti-HCV testing is reactive and HCV RNA results are not available, pregnant persons are considered to have probable HCV infection; similarly, if no HCV test is available from pregnancy and the most recent anti-HCV test is reactive in the absence of an undetectable RNA or treatment, they also are considered to have probable HCV infection.

Transmission of HCV by breastfeeding has not been documented. Antibody to HCV (anti-HCV) and HCV RNA have been detected in colostrum, but risk of HCV transmission is similar in breastfed and formula-fed infants. According to current guidelines of the AASLD and IDSA, HCV infection in the parent is not a contraindication to breastfeeding (**www.hcvguidelines.org/unique-populations/pregnancy**). Breastfeeding parents who are HCV infected should interrupt breastfeeding temporarily if their nipples are bleeding or cracked and can consider expressing and discarding their milk until the nipples are healed. Once the nipples no longer are cracked or bleeding, breastfeeding may resume.

[1] Panagiotakopoulos L, Sandul AL, et al. CDC recommendations for hepatitis C testing among perinatally exposed infants and children—United States, 2023. *MMWR Recomm Rep.* 2023;72(RR-4):1-19

[2] Schillie S, Wester C, Osborne M, Wesolowski L, Ryerson AB. CDC recommendations for hepatitis C screening among adults—United States, 2020. *MMWR Recomm Rep.* 2020;69(RR-2):1-17

Child Care. Exclusion of children with HCV infection from out-of-home child care is not indicated.

Serologic Testing for HCV Infection.

Universal Screening Recommendations.

- Individuals 18 years or older should be tested at least once in their lifetime, except in settings where the prevalence of HCV infection is <0.1%.
- Pregnant people of any age (during each pregnancy).

People Who Have Risk Factors for HCV Infection.

In addition to the universal screening recommendations above, HCV testing is recommended for anyone at increased risk for HCV infection and other populations, including[1]:

- Children whose birthing parent has HCV infection;
- People who have ever injected drugs, including those who injected only once many years ago;
- Recipients of clotting factor concentrates made before 1987;
- Recipients of blood transfusions or solid organ transplants before July 1992;
- Patients who have ever received long-term hemodialysis treatment;
- People with known exposures to HCV, such as
  - Health care workers after needlesticks, sharps, or mucosal exposures involving HCV-positive blood;
  - Recipients of blood from a donor who later tested HCV-positive;
- All people with HIV infection;
- Patients with persistently abnormal liver enzyme test results; and
- Any person who requests hepatitis C testing, regardless of disclosure of risk, because many people might be reluctant to disclose stigmatizing risks.

Professional organizations have additional testing recommendations for specific populations, including those on PrEP, those in correctional or detention facilities, those who have had organ transplant, and those with end-stage renal disease).

Children Whose Birthing Parent Has HCV Infection.
Children whose birthing parent has HCV infection should be tested for HCV infection, because 5% to 7% of these children will acquire infection, and the risk of transmission is higher if the parent is coinfected with uncontrolled HIV.

Adoptees.
See Medical Evaluation for Infectious Diseases for Internationally Adopted, Refugee, and Other Immigrant Children (p 189) for specific situations when serologic testing is warranted.

Counseling of Patients With HCV Infection.
All people with HCV infection should be considered infectious, should be informed of the possibility of transmission to others, and should refrain from donating blood, organs, tissues, or semen and from sharing toothbrushes and razors.

Infected people should be counseled to avoid hepatotoxic agents, including medications, and should be informed of the risks of excessive alcohol ingestion. All patients with chronic HCV infection should be immunized against HAV and HBV.

Changes in sexual practices of infected people with a long-term, monogamous partner are not recommended, although these couples should be informed of possible

---

[1] Centers for Disease Control and Prevention. Recommendations for Hepatitis C Screening among adults- United States 2020. *MMWR Recomm Rep.* 2020;69(2):1-17. Available at: **www.cdc.gov/mmwr/volumes/69/rr/rr6902a1.htm**

risks and use of precautions to prevent transmission. People with multiple sexual partners should be advised to decrease number of partners and to use condoms to prevent transmission. No data exist to support counseling a person of childbearing age against pregnancy. Currently, HCV antiviral therapy is not recommended during pregnancy, but early phase clinical studies and anecdotal reports suggest this is safe and effective. People who become pregnant while receiving antiviral therapy should discuss risk and benefits of continuing treatment with their physician. The Coalition for Global Hepatitis Elimination has established a registry to track outcomes for any patient who is or becomes pregnant while receiving antiviral treatment. (**www.globalhep.org/ evidence-base/treatment-pregnancy-hepatitis-c-tip-hepc-registry**).

The CDC Division of Viral Hepatitis maintains a website (**www.cdc.gov/ hepatitis/HCV**) with information on hepatitis for health care professionals and the public. Information also can be obtained from the National Institutes of Health Web site (**www.niddk.nih.gov/health-information/liver-disease/ viral-hepatitis/hepatitis-c**).

Hepatitis D

CLINICAL MANIFESTATIONS: Hepatitis D virus (HDV) causes infection only in people with hepatitis B virus (HBV) infection. HDV requires hepatitis B surface antigen (HBsAg) for virion assembly and secretion. The importance of HDV infection lies in its ability to convert an asymptomatic or mild chronic HBV infection into more severe or rapidly progressive disease. HDV infection can be acquired either simultaneously with HBV infection (coinfection) or subsequent to HBV infection (superinfection). Coinfection is indistinguishable from acute hepatitis B and usually is transient and self-limited, whereas superinfection often results in chronic infection. Acute infection with HDV usually causes an illness indistinguishable from other viral hepatitis infections, except that the likelihood of fulminant hepatitis can be as high as 5%.

ETIOLOGY: HDV is the only species in the *Deltavirus* genus and possesses the smallest genome of any human pathogen. HDV has a circular, negative sense ssRNA genome and approximately 70 copies of hepatitis delta antigen, all of which is coated with HBsAg.

EPIDEMIOLOGY: HDV infection is present worldwide, in all age groups. Over the past 20 years, HDV prevalence has varied geographically, with decreases in some regions attributable to long-standing hepatitis B vaccination programs and increases in others related to changing migration patterns. High-prevalence areas include the Mediterranean basin, parts of Eastern Europe, the Amazon basin of South America, West and Central Africa, West and Central Asia, and the Middle East, although considerable heterogeneity exists within specific countries. Distribution does not necessarily parallel that of hepatitis B. HDV infection is found in the United States most commonly in people who inject drugs and people who have emigrated from areas with endemic HDV infection. At least 8 genotypes of HDV have been described, each with a typical geographic pattern, with genotype 1 being found worldwide. Acquisition of HDV is by parenteral transmission from infected blood or body fluids, such as through injection drug use or sexual contact. Transmission from birthing parent to newborn infant is uncommon. Intrafamilial spread can occur among people with chronic HBV infection.

The **incubation period** for HDV superinfection is approximately 2 to 8 weeks. When HBV and HDV viruses infect simultaneously, the incubation period is similar to that of HBV (45 to 160 days; average 90 days).

DIAGNOSTIC TESTS: Because of the dependence of HDV on HBV, diagnosis of hepatitis D cannot be made in the absence of markers of HBV infection. Testing for HDV should be considered, at a minimum, for patients with unusually severe or protracted hepatitis and for patients with positive HBsAg and specific risk factors, such as emigration from a region with endemic disease, injection drug use, men who have sex with men, coinfection with hepatitis C virus (HCV) or human immunodeficiency virus (HIV), or high-risk sexual practices. Abnormal aminotransferase concentrations with low or undetectable HBV DNA levels in patients with HBV infection is suspicious for HDV infection. Testing for immunoglobulin G antibodies against HDV (IgG anti-HDV) using a commercially available test can be performed as an initial screening test. Tests for IgM anti-HDV are of lesser utility because of low sensitivity and specificity. Anti-HDV becomes detectable several weeks after illness onset. Acute HDV super-infection and chronic HDV infection can be distinguished from acute HBV/HDV coinfection by the absence of immunoglobulin (Ig) M hepatitis B core antibody (IgM anti-HBc). Because IgG anti-HDV is detectable during acute, chronic, and resolved phases of infection, HDV RNA testing is required for diagnosing current HDV infection and for monitoring antiviral therapy. Patients with circulating HDV RNA should be staged for severity of liver disease, have surveillance for development of hepatocellular carcinoma, and be considered for treatment.

TREATMENT: HDV has proven difficult to treat, and there are no therapies approved by the US Food and Drug Administration. Data suggest 48 weeks of pegylated interferon-alfa may result in virologic response in up to 40% of patients but is associated with considerable side effects and late virologic relapse in approximately half of patients. Novel therapies under investigation in adults include viral entry inhibitors, prenylation inhibitors, and nucleic acid polymers. The viral entry inhibitor bulevirtide is available in the European Union for the treatment of adults with chronic HDV infection. The farnesyltransferase inhibitor lonafarnib, which is approved for treatment of progeria, has been found in a phase 3 study to decrease HDV RNA and normalize alanine aminotransferase (ALT) at the end of 48 weeks of treatment compared with placebo. Liver transplantation is used in certain individuals with liver failure attributable to HBV/HDV infection.

INFECTION PREVENTION AND CONTROL MEASURES IN HEALTH CARE SETTINGS: Standard precautions are recommended.

CONTROL MEASURES: The same control and preventive measures used for HBV infection are indicated. HBV immunization protects against HDV infection. People with chronic HBV infection should take care to avoid exposure to HDV. Harm reduction services, including access to sterile needles and syringes, are an important control measure for people who inject drugs.

Hepatitis E

CLINICAL MANIFESTATIONS: Hepatitis E virus (HEV) infection can be asymptomatic or can cause an acute illness with symptoms including jaundice, malaise, anorexia, fever, abdominal pain, arthralgia, and neurologic complications. Disease is more common among young adults and is more severe in pregnant people, in whom mortality rates can reach 10% to 25% if infection occurs during the third trimester. Chronic HEV infection is rare and, to date, has been reported only in high-income countries. Some recipients of solid organ transplants who acquire HEV after the transplant appear to be at higher risk of chronic infection.

ETIOLOGY: HEV is a spherical, nonenveloped, positive-sense, single-stranded RNA virus. HEV is classified in the genus *Paslahepevirus* of the family *Hepeviridae*. Members of the species *Paslahepevirus balayani* include 8 genotypes (based on phylogenetic analyses); these may infect humans (HEV-1, -2, -3, -4, and -7), pigs (HEV-3 and -4), rabbits (HEV-3), wild boars (HEV-3, -4, -5, and -6), mongooses (HEV-3), deer (HEV-3), yaks (HEV-4), and camels (HEV-7 and -8). There also are reports of human infection caused by the species *Rocahepevirus ratti* (rat HEV), which is usually found in rats and ferrets. Genotype prevalence varies across geographic regions.

EPIDEMIOLOGY: An estimated 20 million HEV infections occur each year worldwide, resulting in 3.4 million cases of acute hepatitis. A recent World Health Organization estimate suggested that there were 55 000 deaths attributable to hepatitis E in 2016. Most HEV infections occur in resource-limited countries (highest prevalence is in Asia and Africa); ingestion of fecally contaminated water is the most common route of HEV transmission, and large waterborne outbreaks occur frequently. HEV infection has been reported throughout the world, including Europe and North America. Foodborne infection with HEV-3 and, less frequently, HEV-4 has occurred sporadically in higher-income countries following consumption of uncooked or undercooked pork, deer meat, sausage, and shellfish. Person-to-person transmission appears to be much less efficient than with hepatitis A virus but occurs sporadically and in outbreak settings. There is limited information on vertical transmission of HEV; it can occur and can account for substantial fetal loss and perinatal mortality, but its contribution to overall disease burden appears to be small. It is unclear whether breastfeeding is a potential route of HEV transmission (see Control Measures).

HEV also is transmitted through blood and blood products. Transfusion-transmitted hepatitis E occurs primarily in countries with endemic disease and also is reported in areas without endemic infection. Serologic studies demonstrated that during 2009-2010 approximately 6% of the population of the United States had immunoglobulin (Ig) G antibodies against HEV, but symptomatic HEV infection in the United States is uncommon and generally occurs in people who acquire HEV-1 infection while traveling in countries with endemic HEV transmission. A number of people without a travel history have been diagnosed with acute hepatitis E, and evidence for the infection should be sought in patients with acute hepatitis of unknown etiology. Hepatitis E may masquerade as drug-induced liver injury.

The **incubation period** is 2 to 8 weeks, with an average of 6 weeks.

DIAGNOSTIC TESTS: HEV infection should be considered in any person with symptoms of viral hepatitis who has traveled to or from a region with endemic hepatitis E or a region where an outbreak of hepatitis E has been identified and in persons with signs and symptoms of viral hepatitis who test negative for serologic markers of hepatitis A, B, and C and other hepatotropic viruses. Testing for anti-HEV IgM and IgG is available through some commercial laboratories. Because anti-HEV assays are not approved by the US Food and Drug Administration and their performance characteristics are not well defined, results should be interpreted with caution, particularly in cases lacking a discrete onset of illness associated with jaundice or with no recent history of travel to a country with endemic HEV transmission. Definitive diagnosis can be made by demonstrating viral RNA in serum or stool samples by means of a nucleic acid amplification test (NAAT), which is available at a limited number of commercial laboratories and with prior approval through the Centers for Disease Control and Prevention. Because virus circulates in the body for a relatively short period, the inability to detect HEV in serum or stool does not eliminate the possibility that the person was infected with HEV.

TREATMENT: Management is supportive. Some case reports and case series have indicated that reduction of immunosuppression and/or use of antiviral drugs, such as ribavirin, with or without interferon-alpha, may result in viral clearance in immunocompromised patients with chronic hepatitis E, but no randomized controlled clinical trials have been performed.

INFECTION PREVENTION AND CONTROL MEASURES IN HEALTH CARE SETTINGS: In addition to standard precautions, contact precautions are recommended for diapered and incontinent patients for the duration of illness.

CONTROL MEASURES: Provision of safe water and improved hygiene practices are the most effective prevention measures. Travelers to regions where HEV is endemic (eg, Asia, Africa, the Middle East, and Central America) should follow precautions used for the prevention of travelers' diarrhea, avoiding food from street vendors, raw or undercooked seafood, meat or pork products, and raw vegetables. Travelers to Europe also should avoid uncooked or undercooked pork/boar sausage or other wild animal meats (eg, rabbit) that have not been heated properly. Until more data are available, breastfeeding among people with confirmed acute HEV infection is discouraged. A recombinant HEV vaccine is licensed in China but is not approved for use in the United States.

Herpes Simplex

CLINICAL MANIFESTATIONS:

Neonatal. In newborn infants with herpes simplex virus (HSV), infection can manifest as: (1) disseminated disease involving multiple organs, most prominently liver and lungs, and in 60% to 75% of cases also involving the central nervous system (CNS); (2) localized CNS disease, with or without skin, eye, or mouth involvement (CNS disease); or (3) disease localized to the skin, eyes, and/or mouth (SEM disease). Approximately 25% of cases of neonatal HSV manifest as disseminated disease, 30% manifest as CNS disease, and 45% manifest as SEM disease. Both HSV type 1 (HSV-1) and type 2 (HSV-2) can cause any of these manifestations of neonatal HSV disease. In the absence of characteristic skin lesions, the diagnosis of neonatal HSV infection is challenging and requires a high index of suspicion. More than 80% of neonates with SEM disease have skin vesicles; those without vesicles have infection limited to the eyes and/or oral mucosa. Approximately two thirds of neonates with disseminated or CNS disease have skin vesicles, but these lesions may not be present at the time of onset of symptoms. Disseminated infection should be considered in neonates with sepsis syndrome with negative bacteriologic culture results, severe liver dysfunction, consumptive coagulopathy, or suspected viral pneumonia, especially hemorrhagic pneumonia. HSV should be considered as a causative agent in neonates with fever (especially within the first 3 weeks of life), hypothermia, a vesicular rash, or abnormal cerebrospinal fluid (CSF) findings (especially in the presence of seizures or during a time of year when enteroviruses are not circulating in the community). Although asymptomatic HSV infection is common in older children, it rarely, if ever, occurs in neonates. Recurrent skin lesions are common in surviving infants, occurring in approximately 50% of survivors, often within 1 to 2 weeks of completing the initial treatment course of parenteral acyclovir or the longer-term suppressive course of oral acyclovir.

Initial signs of HSV infection can occur anytime between birth and approximately 6 weeks of age, although almost all infected infants develop clinical disease within the first month of life. Infants with disseminated disease and SEM disease have an earlier age of onset, typically presenting between the first and second weeks of life; infants with CNS disease usually present with illness between the second and third weeks of life.

Children Beyond the Neonatal Period and Adolescents. Most primary HSV childhood infections beyond the neonatal period are asymptomatic. Gingivostomatitis, which is the most common clinical manifestation of HSV during childhood, is almost exclusively caused by HSV-1 and is characterized by fever, irritability, tender submandibular adenopathy, and an ulcerative enanthem involving the gingiva and mucous membranes of the mouth, often with perioral vesicular lesions.

Genital herpes is characterized by vesicular or ulcerative lesions of the male or female genitalia, perineum, or perianal areas.[1] Until the last 2 decades, genital herpes most often was caused by HSV-2, but likely because of oral sexual practices, HSV-1 now accounts for more than half of all genital herpes cases in the United States. Most cases of primary genital herpes infection are asymptomatic, so they are not recognized by the infected person or diagnosed by a health care professional. When present, symptoms and signs of the initial episode may include fever, fatigue, myalgias, and inguinal lymphadenopathy.

In immunocompromised patients, severe local lesions and, less commonly, disseminated HSV infection with generalized vesicular skin lesions and visceral involvement can occur.

After primary infection, HSV persists for life in a latent form. Reactivation of latent virus most commonly is asymptomatic. When symptomatic, recurrent HSV-1 herpes labialis manifests as single or grouped vesicles in the perioral region, usually on the vermilion border of the lips (typically called "cold sores" or "fever blisters"). Symptomatic recurrent genital herpes manifests as vesicular lesions on the penis, scrotum, vulva, cervix, buttocks, perianal areas, thighs, or back. Among immunocompromised patients, genital HSV-2 recurrences are more frequent and of longer duration. Recurrences may be heralded by a prodrome of burning or itching at the site of an incipient recurrence, identification of which can be useful in instituting early antiviral therapy.

Ocular manifestations of HSV include conjunctivitis and keratitis that can result from primary or recurrent HSV infection. In addition, HSV can cause acute retinal necrosis and uveitis.

---

[1] The terms male and female refer to sex assigned at birth.

Eczema herpeticum can develop in patients with atopic dermatitis who are infected with HSV and can be difficult to distinguish from poorly controlled atopic dermatitis. Examination may reveal skin with punched-out erosions, hemorrhagic crusts, and/or vesicular lesions. Pustular lesions attributable to bacterial superinfection also may occur. Herpetic whitlow consists of single or multiple vesicular lesions on the distal parts of fingers. Wrestlers and other contact sports athletes can develop herpes gladiatorum, a cutaneous skin infection that usually is caused by HSV-1 but occasionally by HSV-2. In wrestling, 70% of herpes outbreaks involve the face. HSV infection can be a precipitating factor of other cutaneous manifestations, such as erythema multiforme. Recurrent erythema multiforme often is caused by symptomatic or asymptomatic HSV recurrences.

HSV encephalitis (HSE) occurs in children beyond the neonatal period, in adolescents, and in adults and can result from primary or recurrent HSV-1 infection. One fifth of HSE cases occur in the pediatric age group. Symptoms and signs usually include fever, alterations in the state of consciousness, personality changes, seizures, and focal neurologic findings. Encephalitis commonly has an acute onset with a fulminant course, leading to coma and death in untreated patients. HSE usually involves the temporal lobe, and magnetic resonance imaging is the most sensitive imaging modality. CSF pleocytosis with a predominance of lymphocytes is typical. Historically, erythrocytes in the CSF were considered suggestive of HSE, but with earlier diagnosis (prior to development of a hemorrhagic encephalitis), this finding is rare today.

HSV infection also can manifest as mild, self-limited aseptic meningitis, usually associated with primary genital HSV-2 infection. Unusual CNS manifestations of HSV include Bell's palsy, atypical pain syndromes, trigeminal neuralgia, ascending myelitis, transverse myelitis, postinfectious encephalomyelitis, and recurrent (Mollaret) meningitis.

ETIOLOGY: HSVs are large, enveloped, double-stranded DNA viruses. They are members of the family *Herpesviridae* and, along with varicella-zoster virus (human herpesvirus 3), are in the subfamily *Alphaherpesviridae*. Two distinct HSV types exist: HSV-1 and HSV-2. Infections with HSV-1 traditionally involve the face and skin above the waist; however, an increasing number of genital herpes cases are attributable to HSV-1. Infections with HSV-2 usually involve the genitalia and skin below the waist in sexually active adolescents and adults. Both HSV-1 and HSV-2 cause herpetic disease in neonates. HSV-1 and HSV-2 establish latency in sensory neurons following primary infection, with periodic reactivation causing recurrent symptomatic disease or asymptomatic viral shedding. Genital HSV-2 infection is more likely to recur than is genital HSV-1 infection.

EPIDEMIOLOGY: HSV infections can be transmitted from people who are symptomatic or asymptomatic with primary or recurrent infections.

Neonatal. The incidence of neonatal HSV infection in the United States has increased over the past 2 decades to approximately 1 in 2000 live births. HSV is transmitted to a neonate most often during birth through an infected genital tract but can be caused by an ascending infection through ruptured or apparently intact amniotic membranes. Other less common sources of neonatal infection include postnatal transmission from a parent, sibling, or other caregiver, most often from a nongenital infection (eg, mouth or hands), transmission from the mouth of a religious circumciser ("mohel") to the infant penis during ritual Jewish circumcisions that include direct orogenital suction (metzitzah b'peh), and intrauterine infection causing congenital malformations.

The risk of transmission to a neonate born to a person who acquires primary genital HSV infection near the time of delivery is estimated to be 25% to 60%. In contrast, the risk to a neonate born to a person shedding HSV as a result of reactivation of infection acquired during the first half of pregnancy or earlier is less than 2%. More than three quarters of infants who contract HSV infection are born to a person with no history or clinical findings suggestive of genital HSV infection during or preceding pregnancy. Therefore, a lack of history of genital HSV infection in the birthing parent does not preclude a diagnosis of neonatal HSV disease.

Children Beyond the Neonatal Period and Adolescents. Patients with primary gingivostomatitis or genital herpes usually shed virus for at least 1 week and occasionally for several weeks. Patients with symptomatic recurrences shed virus for a shorter period, typically 3 to 4 days. Intermittent asymptomatic reactivation of oral and genital herpes is common and likely occurs throughout the remainder of a person's life. The greatest concentration of virus is shed during symptomatic primary infections and the lowest during asymptomatic reactivation.

Several single gene defects have been reported that predispose to HSE. The ones characterized so far are mainly involved in the toll-like receptor 3 (TLR3) pathway, including deficiencies of TLR3 itself or in downstream signal transduction pathways (UNC93B1, TRIF/TICAM1, TRAF, TBK1) or deficiencies in innate/type 1 interferon pathways (IFN-alpha/-beta, IFN-lamba, STAT1, IRF3).

The **incubation period** for HSV infection occurring beyond the neonatal period ranges from 2 days to 2 weeks, with an average of 4 days.

DIAGNOSTIC TESTS: A nucleic acid amplification test (NAAT) usually can detect HSV DNA in CSF from neonates with CNS infection (neonatal HSV CNS disease) and from older children and adults with HSE and is the diagnostic method of choice for CNS HSV involvement. A NAAT of CSF can yield negative results in cases of HSE, especially early in the disease course. In difficult cases in which HSV CNS disease is expected but repeated CSF NAAT results are negative, histologic examination and viral culture of a brain tissue biopsy specimen is the most definitive method of confirming the diagnosis of HSE. Detection of intrathecal antibody against HSV also can assist in the diagnosis but may not be specific because of alterations in the blood-brain barrier. Viral cultures of CSF from a patient with HSE usually are negative.

HSV grows readily in traditional cell culture. Special transport media are available that allow transport to local or regional laboratories for culture. Cytopathogenic effects typical of HSV infection usually are observed 1 to 3 days after inoculation. Methods of culture confirmation include fluorescent antibody staining, enzyme immunoassays (EIAs), and monolayer culture with typing. Cultures that are negative on day 5 likely will remain negative. A viral isolate by culture is required if phenotypic antiviral susceptibility studies are to be performed.

For diagnosis of neonatal HSV infection, all of the following specimens should be obtained for each patient: (1) swab specimens from the conjunctivae, mouth, nasopharynx, and anus ("surface specimens") for HSV culture (if available) or NAAT (can use a separate swab for each site, or a single swab starting with the conjunctivae); (2) specimens of skin vesicles for HSV culture (if available) or NAAT; (3) CSF sample for

HSV NAAT; (4) whole blood sample for HSV NAAT; and (5) whole blood sample for measuring alanine aminotransferase (ALT). The performance characteristics of NAAT on skin and mucosal specimens from neonates has not been studied. Positive cultures obtained from any of the surface sites more than 12 to 24 hours after birth indicate viral replication and are, therefore, suggestive of infant infection, and therefore risk of progression to neonatal HSV disease, rather than merely contamination after intrapartum exposure. As with any NAAT, false-negative and false-positive results can occur. Any of the 3 manifestations of neonatal HSV disease (disseminated, CNS, SEM) can have associated viremia, so a positive whole blood NAAT result does not define an infant as having disseminated HSV and, therefore, should not be used to determine extent of disease and duration of treatment. Likewise, no data exist to support use of serial blood NAAT to monitor response to therapy. Rapid diagnostic techniques are available, such as direct fluorescent antibody staining of vesicle scrapings or EIA detection of HSV antigens. These techniques are as specific but less sensitive than culture.

HSV NAAT is the preferred method for detecting HSV in genital lesions. The sensitivity of viral culture is low, especially for recurrent lesions, and declines rapidly as lesions begin to heal. NAATs for HSV DNA are more sensitive and are widely available. Failure to detect HSV in genital lesions by culture or NAAT does not rule out HSV infection, because viral shedding is intermittent.

Type-specific antibodies to HSV develop during the first several weeks after infection and persist indefinitely. Approximately 20% of patients with a first episode of HSV-2 seroconvert for type-specific IgG antibody by 10 days, and the median time to seroconversion is 21 days with a type-specific enzyme-linked immunosorbent assay (ELISA); more than 95% of people seroconvert by 12 weeks following infection. Although type-specific HSV-2 antibody usually indicates previous anogenital infection, the presence of HSV-1 antibody does not distinguish anogenital from orolabial infection reliably because a substantial proportion of initial genital infections and virtually all initial orolabial infections are caused by HSV-1. Serologic testing is not useful in neonates. IgM testing for HSV-1 or HSV-2 is not useful because of the lack of a reliable commercially available IgM assay.

TREATMENT: For recommended antiviral dosages and duration of therapy with systemically administered acyclovir, valacyclovir, and famciclovir for different HSV infections, see Non-HIV Antiviral Drugs (p 1044). In pediatric patients who cannot swallow large pills, instructions for preparing a compounded liquid suspension of valacyclovir with a 28-day refrigerated shelf-life are provided in the drug's package insert.

Neonatal. Parenteral acyclovir is the treatment for neonatal HSV infections. The dosage of acyclovir is 60 mg/kg per day in 3 divided doses (20 mg/kg/dose), administered intravenously for 14 days in SEM disease and for a minimum of 21 days in CNS disease or disseminated disease. All infants with CNS involvement should have a repeat lumbar puncture performed near the end of therapy to document that the CSF is negative for HSV DNA on NAAT; in the unlikely event that the NAAT result remains positive near the end of a 21-day treatment course, intravenous acyclovir should be administered for another week, with repeat CSF NAAT performed near the end of the extended treatment period and another week of parenteral therapy if the result remains positive. Parenteral antiviral therapy should not be stopped until the CSF NAAT result for HSV DNA is negative. Consultation with a pediatric infectious diseases specialist is warranted in these cases.

Infants surviving neonatal HSV disease of any classification (disseminated, CNS, or SEM) should receive oral acyclovir suppression at 300 mg/m^2/dose, administered 3 times daily for 6 months after the completion of parenteral therapy for acute disease; the dose should be adjusted monthly to account for growth. Absolute neutrophil counts should be assessed at 2 and 4 weeks after initiating suppressive acyclovir therapy and then monthly during the treatment period. Longer durations or higher doses of antiviral suppression do not further improve neurodevelopmental outcomes. Valacyclovir has not been studied for longer than 5 days in young infants, so it should not be used routinely for antiviral suppression in this age group.

All infants with neonatal HSV disease, regardless of disease classification, should have an ophthalmologic examination and neuroimaging to establish baseline brain anatomy; magnetic resonance imaging is the most sensitive imaging modality but may require sedation, so computed tomography or ultrasonography of the head are acceptable alternatives. Topical ophthalmic drug (1% trifluridine or 0.15% ganciclovir), in addition to parenteral antiviral therapy, may be indicated in infants with ocular involvement attributable to HSV infection, including a positive virologic test result from a conjunctival swab sample, and an ophthalmologist should be involved in the management and treatment of acute neonatal ocular HSV disease. The older topical antiviral agents vidarabine and iododeoxyuridine are no longer available in the United States.

Genital Infection.

Primary. Oral acyclovir therapy shortens the duration of illness and viral shedding. Valacyclovir and famciclovir are not more effective than acyclovir but offer the advantage of less frequent dosing. Intravenous acyclovir is indicated for patients with a severe or complicated primary infection that requires hospitalization. Treatment of primary herpetic lesions does not affect the subsequent frequency or severity of recurrences. Antiviral drug dosages for primary genital HSV infection are found on p 1046 in Table 4.10, Non-HIV Antiviral Drugs.

Recurrent. Antiviral therapy for recurrent genital herpes can be administered either episodically to ameliorate or shorten the duration of lesions or continuously as suppressive therapy to decrease the frequency of recurrences. Many patients benefit from antiviral therapy, and treatment options should be discussed with patients with recurrent disease. Acyclovir, valacyclovir, and famciclovir have been approved for suppression of genital herpes in immunocompetent adults. Acyclovir and valacyclovir are most commonly used in pregnant people with first-episode genital herpes or severe recurrent herpes, and acyclovir should be administered intravenously to pregnant people with severe HSV infection. Antiviral drug dosages for episodic and suppressive treatment of recurrent genital HSV infection are found on p 1046 in Table 4.10, Non-HIV Antiviral Drugs.

Mucocutaneous.

Immunocompromised Hosts. Intravenous acyclovir is effective for treatment of mucocutaneous HSV infections. Acyclovir-resistant strains of HSV have been isolated from immunocompromised people receiving prolonged treatment with acyclovir. Because these strains will also be resistant to valacyclovir, and most are also resistant to famciclovir, foscarnet is the drug of choice for acyclovir-resistant HSV isolates.

Immunocompetent Hosts. Limited data are available on effects of acyclovir on the course of primary or recurrent nongenital mucocutaneous HSV infections in immuno-competent hosts. Therapeutic benefit has been noted in a limited number of children with primary gingivostomatitis treated with oral acyclovir. A small therapeutic benefit of oral acyclovir therapy has been demonstrated among adults with recurrent herpes labialis. Famciclovir or valacyclovir also can be considered. Topical acyclovir is not therapeutic. Antiviral drug dosages for acyclovir, famciclovir, and valacyclovir for episodic and suppressive treatment of recurrent orolabial HSV infection are found on p 1046, p 1050, and p 1062–1063, respectively, in Table 4.10, Non-HIV Antiviral Drugs.

Other HSV Infections.

Central Nervous System. Patients with HSE should be treated for 21 days with intravenous acyclovir. Use of concomitant corticosteroids has not been adequately studied in people and is not routinely recommended.

Ocular. Treatment of eye lesions should be undertaken in consultation with an ophthalmologist. Several topical drugs, such as 1% trifluridine and 0.15% ganciclovir, have proven efficacy for superficial keratitis. Topical corticosteroids administered without concomitant antiviral therapy are contraindicated in suspected HSV conjunctivitis; however, ophthalmologists may choose to use corticosteroids in conjunction with antiviral drugs to treat locally invasive infections. For children with recurrent ocular lesions, oral suppressive therapy with acyclovir may be of benefit and may be indicated for months or even years.

INFECTION PREVENTION AND CONTROL MEASURES IN HEALTH CARE SETTINGS: In addition to standard precautions, the following recommendations should be followed.

Neonates With HSV Infection. Neonates with HSV infection should be hospitalized and managed with contact precautions if mucocutaneous lesions are present.

Neonates Exposed to HSV During Delivery. An infant born to a person with active genital HSV lesions should be managed with contact precautions during the incubation period. The risk of HSV infection in an infant born to a person with a history of recurrent genital herpes who has no genital lesions at delivery is low, so special precautions are not necessary. Specific management options for neonates born to people with active genital HSV lesions are detailed in "Prevention of Neonatal Infection."

Postpartum Persons With HSV Infection. People with active HSV lesions should be instructed about the importance of careful hand hygiene before and after caring for their infants. A parent or caregiver with herpes labialis or stomatitis should wear a disposable surgical mask when touching the newborn infant until the lesions have crusted. The caregiver should not kiss or nuzzle the newborn infant until lesions have resolved. Herpetic lesions on other skin sites should be covered.

Breastfeeding is acceptable if no lesions are present on the breasts and if active lesions elsewhere on the caregiver are covered (see Breastfeeding and Human Milk, p 135).

Children With Mucocutaneous HSV Infection. Contact precautions are recommended for patients with severe mucocutaneous HSV infection. Patients with localized recurrent lesions should be managed with standard precautions.

Table 3.24. Infection Classification by Genital HSV Viral Type and Type-Specific Serologic Test Results From the Birthing Parent[a]

Classification of Infection in Birthing Parent	NAAT/Culture From Genital Lesion	HSV-1 and HSV-2 IgG Type-Specific Antibody Status of Birthing Parent
Documented first-episode primary infection	Positive, either virus	Both negative
Documented first-episode nonprimary infection	Positive for HSV-1	Positive for HSV-2 **AND** negative for HSV-1
	Positive for HSV-2	Positive for HSV-1 **AND** negative for HSV-2
Assumed first-episode (primary or nonprimary) infection	Positive for HSV-1 **OR** HSV-2	Not available
	Negative **OR** not available[b]	Negative for HSV-1 and/or HSV-2, **OR** not available
Recurrent infection	Positive for HSV-1	Positive for HSV-1
	Positive for HSV-2	Positive for HSV-2

HSV indicates herpes simplex virus; NAAT, nucleic acid amplification test; IgG, immunoglobulin G.
[a]To be used for people without a clinical history of genital herpes.
[b]When a genital lesion is strongly suspicious for HSV, clinical judgment should supersede the virologic test results for the conservative purposes of this neonatal management algorithm. Conversely, if, in retrospect, the genital lesion was not likely to be caused by HSV and the NAAT result/culture is negative, departure from the evaluation and management in this conservative algorithm may be warranted.

Patients With HSV Infection of the CNS. Standard precautions are recommended for patients with infection limited to the CNS.

CONTROL MEASURES:

Prevention of Neonatal Infection.

During Pregnancy. The American College of Obstetricians and Gynecologists recommends that people with a primary or nonprimary first-episode outbreak (defined in Table 3.24) in pregnancy, as well as those with a clinical history of genital herpes, be offered suppressive antiviral therapy at or beyond 36 weeks of gestation. However, cases of neonatal HSV disease have occurred among infants born to people who received such antiviral prophylaxis. First-episode primary and nonprimary genital infections can result in shedding of HSV in the genital tract for several weeks even after lesions resolve.

Care of Newborn Infants Whose Birthing Parent Has Active Genital Lesions at Delivery. Neonates exposed to active HSV genital lesions at delivery should not have delayed bathing.[1] The risk of transmitting HSV to the newborn infant during delivery is influenced directly by the classification of HSV infection of the birthing individual (Table 3.24); those with primary genital HSV infections who are shedding HSV at delivery are

---

[1] Nolt D, O'Leary ST, Aucott SW; American Academy of Pediatrics, Committee on Infectious Diseases, Committee on Fetus and Newborn. Risks of infectious diseases in newborns exposed to alternative perinatal practices. *Pediatrics.* 2022;149(2):e2021055554

10 to 30 times more likely to transmit the virus to their newborn infants, compared with those with a recurrent genital infection. With the commercial availability of serologic tests that can reliably distinguish type-specific HSV antibodies, the means to further refine management of asymptomatic neonates delivered to people with active genital HSV lesions now is possible. The American Academy of Pediatrics developed algorithms (Fig 3.7 and 3.8) addressing evaluation and management of asymptomatic neonates following vaginal or cesarean delivery to people with active genital HSV lesions.[1] The algorithms are intended to outline one approach to the management of these neonates and may not be feasible in settings with limited access to NAATs for HSV DNA or to type-specific serologic tests. If, at any point during the evaluation outlined in the evaluation algorithm (Fig 3.7), an infant develops symptoms that could indicate neonatal HSV disease (eg, fever, hypothermia, lethargy, irritability, vesicular rash, seizures, etc), a full diagnostic evaluation should be undertaken and intravenous acyclovir therapy should be initiated. In applying this algorithm, obstetric and pediatric providers will need to work closely with their diagnostic laboratories to ensure that serologic and virologic testing is available and turnaround times are acceptable. In situations in which this is not possible, the approach detailed in the algorithm will have limited, and perhaps no, applicability.

Care of Newborn Infants Whose Birthing Parent Has a History of Genital Herpes But No Active Genital Lesions at Delivery. Most infants whose birthing parent has a history of genital herpes but no genital lesions at delivery should be observed for signs of infection (eg, vesicular lesions of the skin, respiratory distress, seizures, or signs of sepsis) but should not have specimens for surface cultures for HSV obtained at 12 to 24 hours of life and should not receive empiric parenteral acyclovir. The exception are infants born to persons with documented first-episode primary or nonprimary infections (defined in Table 3.24) during the third trimester but who have no genital lesions at delivery. These infants should have HSV surface cultures, if available, and NAATs and HSV blood NAAT obtained at ~24 hours of age, regardless of mode of delivery or birthing parent's receipt of antiviral suppressive therapy. Results of these tests should be responded to as outlined in the right side of Fig 3.7. The rationale for this recommendation is that the American College of Obstetricians and Gynecologists states that cesarean delivery may be offered to people with documented first-episode infections during the third trimester because of the possibility of prolonged viral shedding.[2] Education of parents and caregivers about the signs and symptoms of neonatal HSV infection during the first 6 weeks of life is prudent.

Infected Health Care Professionals. Health care professionals with cold sores who have contact with infants should cover and not touch their lesions and should comply with hand hygiene policies. Transmission of HSV infection from health care professionals with genital lesions is not likely as long as they comply with hand hygiene policies. Health care professionals with an active herpetic whitlow should not have responsibility for direct care of neonates or immunocompromised patients and should wear gloves and use hand hygiene during direct care of other patients.

[1] Kimberlin DW, Baley J; American Academy of Pediatrics, Committee on Infectious Diseases. Guidance on management of asymptomatic neonates born to women with active genital herpes lesions. *Pediatrics.* 2013;131(2):e635-e646

[2] American College of Obstetricians and Gynecologists. Management of genital herpes in pregnancy. ACOG Practice Bulletin No. 220. *Obstet Gynecol.* 2020;135(5):e193-202

Fig 3.7. Algorithm for the <u>Evaluation</u> of Asymptomatic Neonates Following Vaginal or Cesarean Delivery to People with Active Genital Herpes Lesions

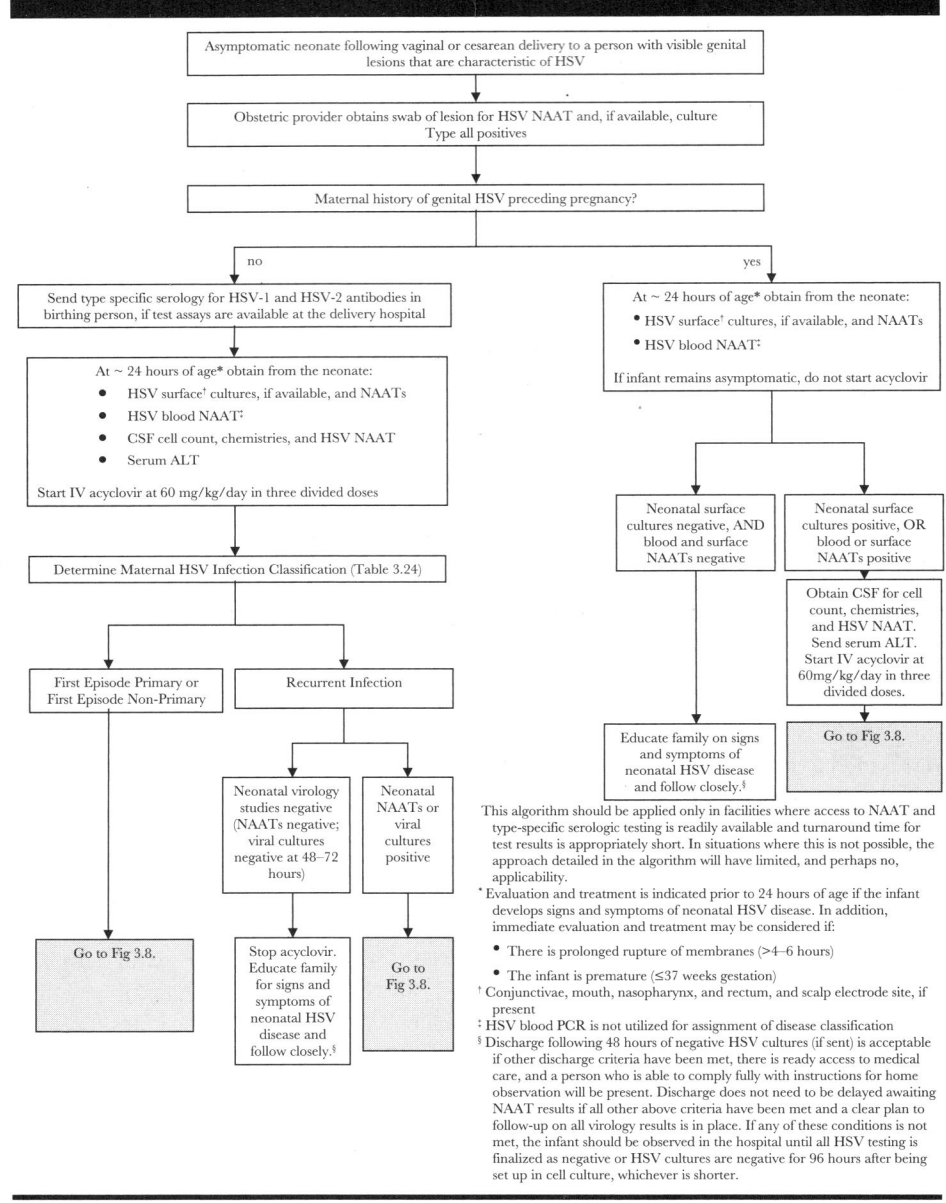

Adapted from Kimberlin DW, Baley J; American Academy of Pediatrics, Committee on Infectious Diseases. Guidance on management of asymptomatic neonates born to women with active genital herpes lesions. *Pediatrics.* 2013;131(2):e635-e646

Fig 3.8. Algorithm for the <u>Treatment</u> of Asymptomatic Neonates Following Vaginal or Cesarean Delivery to People with Active Genital Herpes Lesions

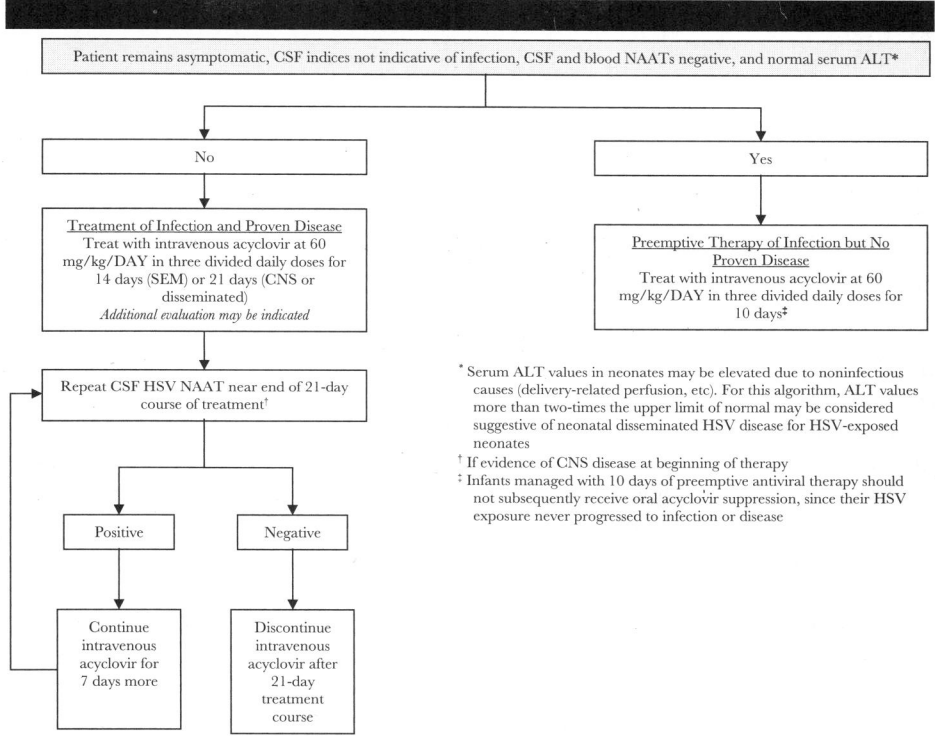

Patient remains asymptomatic, CSF indices not indicative of infection, CSF and blood NAATs negative, and normal serum ALT*

No

Treatment of Infection and Proven Disease
Treat with intravenous acyclovir at 60 mg/kg/DAY in three divided daily doses for 14 days (SEM) or 21 days (CNS or disseminated)
Additional evaluation may be indicated

Repeat CSF HSV NAAT near end of 21-day course of treatment†

Positive → Continue intravenous acyclovir for 7 days more

Negative → Discontinue intravenous acyclovir after 21-day treatment course

Yes

Preemptive Therapy of Infection but No Proven Disease
Treat with intravenous acyclovir at 60 mg/kg/DAY in three divided daily doses for 10 days‡

* Serum ALT values in neonates may be elevated due to noninfectious causes (delivery-related perfusion, etc). For this algorithm, ALT values more than two-times the upper limit of normal may be considered suggestive of neonatal disseminated HSV disease for HSV-exposed neonates
† If evidence of CNS disease at beginning of therapy
‡ Infants managed with 10 days of preemptive antiviral therapy should not subsequently receive oral acyclovir suppression, since their HSV exposure never progressed to infection or disease

Adapted from Kimberlin DW, Baley J; American Academy of Pediatrics, Committee on Infectious Diseases. Guidance on management of asymptomatic neonates born to women with active genital herpes lesions. *Pediatrics.* 2013;131(2):e635-e646

Infected Household, Family, and Other Close Contacts of Newborn Infants. Household members with herpetic skin or mouth lesions (eg, stomatitis, herpes labialis, or herpetic whitlow) should be counseled about the risk of transmission and should avoid contact of their lesions with neonates by taking the same measures as recommended for infected health care professionals, as well as avoiding kissing and nuzzling the infant while they have active lip/mouth lesions or touching the neonate while they have a herpetic whitlow.

Care of People With Extensive Dermatitis. Patients with dermatitis should not have oral contact with people with cold sores or touched by people with herpetic whitlow.

Care of Children With Mucocutaneous Infections Who Attend Child Care or School. Oral HSV infections are common among children who attend child care or school. Most of these infections are asymptomatic, with shedding of virus in saliva occurring in the absence of clinical disease. See Table 2.3 (Children in Group Child Care and Schools, p 145) for recommendations on exclusion from schools and group child care.

HSV Infections Among Wrestlers and Rugby Players.[1] HSV-1 has been identified as a cause of outbreak of skin infections among wrestlers (herpes gladiatorum) and rugby players (herpes rugbiorum) on numerous occasions, affecting up to 2.6% of high school and 7.6% of college wrestlers in the United States. During outbreaks, up to 34% of all high school wrestlers have been documented to be infected. The primary risk factor is direct skin-to-skin exposure to opponents with cutaneous lesions.

Athletes with active herpes gladiatorum or rugbiorum infections should be excluded from competition and contact practice. Prior to return to competition, skin lesions must have a firm adherent crust, athletes must have no evidence of secondary bacterial infection, and any systemic symptoms must have resolved. In addition, the athlete must have developed no new skin lesions for 72 hours and have been on appropriate antiviral therapy for at least 120 hours. When given within 24 hours of symptoms onset, valacyclovir has been shown to shorten the duration of time to HSV NAAT negativity from lesions of adolescent and adult wrestlers with recurrent herpes gladiatorum. Wrestlers receiving valacyclovir should be advised about the importance of good hydration to minimize the likelihood of nephrotoxicity. Efforts to reduce transmission should include: (1) examination of wrestlers and rugby players for vesicular or ulcerative lesions on exposed areas of their bodies and around their mouths or eyes before practice or competition by a person familiar with the appearance of mucocutaneous infections (including HSV, herpes zoster, and impetigo); (2) excluding athletes with these lesions from competition until all lesions are fully crusted or production of a physician's written statement indicating that their condition is noninfectious; and (3) cleaning of wrestling mats with a freshly prepared solution of household bleach (one quarter cup of bleach in 1 gallon of water), applied for a minimum contact time of 15 seconds at least daily, and preferably, between matches. Athletes with a history of *recurrent* herpes gladiatorum, herpes rugbiorum, or herpes labialis should be considered for suppressive antiviral therapy, again with cautionary guidance about the importance of maintaining good hydration to avoid the likelihood of nephrotoxicity. There is strong evidence that using prophylactic antiviral therapy can be useful in preventing both primary and secondary herpes outbreaks in high-risk environments, such as large wrestling camps.

Histoplasmosis

CLINICAL MANIFESTATIONS: *Histoplasma capsulatum* causes symptoms in fewer than 5% of infected people. Clinical manifestations are classified according to site (pulmonary or disseminated), duration (acute, subacute, or chronic), and pattern (primary or reactivation) of infection. Most symptomatic patients have acute pulmonary histoplasmosis, a brief, self-limited illness characterized by fever, chills, nonproductive cough, and malaise. Radiographic findings may consist of hilar or mediastinal adenopathy, diffuse interstitial or reticulonodular pulmonary infiltrates, or pulmonary nodules. Most patients recover without treatment 2 to 3 weeks after onset of symptoms.

Exposure to a large inoculum of conidia can cause severe pulmonary infection associated with high fevers, hypoxemia, diffuse reticulonodular infiltrates, and acute respiratory distress syndrome (ARDS). Mediastinal involvement, a rare complication

---

[1] Davies HD, Jackson MA; American Academy of Pediatrics, Committee on Infectious Diseases. Infectious diseases associated with organized sports and outbreak control. *Pediatrics*. 2017;140(4):e20172477

of pulmonary histoplasmosis, includes mediastinal lymphadenitis, which can cause airway encroachment in young children. Inflammatory syndromes (pericarditis and rheumatologic syndromes) can develop; erythema nodosum can occur in adolescents and adults. Primary cutaneous infections after trauma are uncommon. Chronic cavitary pulmonary histoplasmosis is extremely rare in children.

Progressive disseminated histoplasmosis (PDH) may occur in otherwise healthy infants and children younger than 2 years or in older children with primary or acquired cellular immune dysfunction. It can be a rapidly progressive illness following acute infection or can be a more chronic, slowly progressive disease. Early manifestations of PDH in children include prolonged fever, failure to thrive, and hepatosplenomegaly; if untreated, malnutrition, diffuse adenopathy, pneumonitis, mucosal ulceration, pancytopenia, disseminated intravascular coagulopathy, and gastrointestinal tract bleeding can ensue. PDH in older children and adults occurs most often in people with underlying immune deficiency (eg, human immunodeficiency virus/acquired immunodeficiency syndrome, solid organ transplant, hematologic malignancy, and biologic response modifiers including tumor necrosis factor antagonists). Central nervous system involvement occurs in 5% to 10% of patients with disseminated disease. Manifestations include chronic meningitis, focal brain or spinal cord lesions, encephalitis, stroke, and hydrocephalus. Chronic PDH generally occurs in adults with immune suppression and is characterized by prolonged fever, night sweats, weight loss, and fatigue; signs include hepatosplenomegaly, mucosal ulcerations, adrenal insufficiency, and pancytopenia. Clinicians should be alert to the risk of disseminated endemic mycoses in patients receiving tumor necrosis factor-alpha antagonists and disease-modifying antirheumatic drugs.

ETIOLOGY: *Histoplasma* strains, which may be classified into at least 8 distinct clades, are thermally dimorphic, endemic fungi that grow in the environment as a spore-bearing mold but convert to the yeast phase at 37°C.

EPIDEMIOLOGY: *H capsulatum* is highly endemic in the central and eastern United States, particularly the Mississippi, Ohio, and Missouri River valleys; Central America; the northernmost part of South America; and Argentina, but it can be found in most parts of the world (including Africa, the Americas, Asia, and Europe). *H capsulatum* case distribution may be affected by a warming climate. *H capsulatum* var *duboisii* is found only in central and western Africa.

Infection is acquired following inhalation of conidia that are aerosolized by disturbance of soil, especially when contaminated with bat guano or bird droppings. Infections occur sporadically or rarely in point-source epidemics after exposure to activities that disturb contaminated sites. In regions with endemic disease, recreational activities, such as playing in hollow trees and caving, and occupational activities, such as construction, excavation, demolition, farming, and cleaning of contaminated buildings, have been associated with outbreaks. Person-to-person transmission may occur via transplantation of infected organs, vertical transmission, and possibly through exposure to cutaneous lesions. Prior infection confers partial immunity; reinfection can occur but may require a larger inoculum.

The **incubation period** is variable but usually is 3 to 17 days.

DIAGNOSTIC TESTS: Detection of *H capsulatum* polysaccharide antigen in serum, urine, bronchoalveolar lavage fluid, or cerebrospinal fluid using a quantitative enzyme immunoassay is the preferred method of testing. Antigen detection is most sensitive for progressive disseminated infections. Combining both urine and serum antigen testing increases the likelihood of antigen detection. Results often are transiently positive early in the course of acute, self-limited pulmonary infections. A negative test result does not exclude infection. If the result initially is positive, the antigen test also is useful for monitoring treatment response and, thereafter, identifying relapse or reinfection. Cross-reactions may occur in patients with dimorphic fungal diseases (eg, blastomycosis, coccidioidomycosis, paracoccidioidomycosis, sporotrichosis, *Emergomyces africanus* disease, and talaromycosis [formerly penicillosis]); clinical and epidemiologic distinctions aid in differentiating these entities.

Antibody detection testing is available and is most useful in patients with subacute or chronic pulmonary disease and central nervous system involvement. Enzyme immunoassay, complement fixation and immunodiffusion are available. A fourfold increase in mycelial-phase complement fixation titers or a single titer of ≥1:32 in either test is strong presumptive evidence of active or recent infection in patients exposed to or residing within endemic regions. Cross-reacting antibodies can result most commonly from *Blastomyces* and *Coccidioides* species. The immunodiffusion test is a qualitative method that is more specific, but slightly less sensitive than the complement fixation test. It commonly is used in conjunction with the complement fixation test and detects the H and M glycoproteins of *H capsulatum* found in histoplasmin. The M band develops with acute infection, generally by 6 weeks after infection, is often present in chronic forms of histoplasmosis, and persists for months to years after the infection has resolved. The H band is much less common; is rarely, if ever, found without an M band; and is indicative of chronic or severe acute forms of histoplasmosis.

Culture is the definitive method of diagnosis. *H capsulatum* organisms from bone marrow, blood, sputum, and tissue specimens grow in the mycelia (mold) phase on standard mycologic media, including Sabouraud dextrose or potato dextrose agar incubated at 25°C to 30°C in 1 to 6 weeks. The yeast phase of the organism can be recovered on primary culture using enriched media, such as brain-heart infusion agar with blood (BHIB) incubated at 35°C to 37°C. Mycelial-phase organisms in culture can be confirmed as *H capsulatum* by conversion to yeast-phase organisms by repeated passage on BHIB at 35°C to 37°C. The lysis-centrifugation method is preferred for blood and bone marrow cultures. A DNA probe for *H capsulatum* permits rapid identification of cultured isolates. Care should be taken in working with the organism in the laboratory, because mold-phase growth may release large numbers of infectious microconidia into the air.

Demonstration of typical intracellular yeast forms by examination with Wright or Giemsa stains of blood, bone marrow, or bronchoalveolar lavage specimens strongly supports the diagnosis of histoplasmosis when clinical, epidemiologic, and other laboratory studies are compatible.

TREATMENT[1]: Immunocompetent children with uncomplicated or mild-to-moderate acute pulmonary histoplasmosis may not require antifungal therapy, because infection

[1] Thompson GR III, Le T, Chindamporn A, et al. Global guideline for the diagnosis and management of the endemic mycoses: an initiative of the European Confederation of Medical Mycology in cooperation with the International Society for Human and Animal Mycology [Erratum in: *Lancet Infect Dis.* 2021;21(11):e341]. *Lancet Infect Dis.* 2021;21(12):e364-e374

usually is self-limited. If the patient does not improve within 4 weeks, itraconazole should be given for 6 to 12 weeks.

Treatment is imperative for all forms of disseminated histoplasmosis, which can be either an acute (rapid onset and progression, usually in an immunocompromised patient) or chronic (slower evolution, usually in an immunocompetent patient) illness. Treatment with a lipid formulation of amphotericin B is recommended for severe acute pulmonary infection (see Table 4.7, p 1021). Methylprednisolone during the first 1 to 2 weeks of therapy may be considered if severe respiratory complications develop but should be used only in conjunction with antifungals.

After clinical improvement occurs in 1 to 2 weeks, itraconazole is recommended for an additional 12 weeks. Itraconazole is preferred over other mold-active azoles by most experts; when used in adults, itraconazole is more effective, has fewer adverse effects, and is less likely to induce resistance than is fluconazole. Serum trough concentrations of itraconazole should be 1 to 2 µg/mL. A trough level should be checked 10 days or later following initiation to ensure adequate drug exposure. When measured by high-pressure liquid chromatography, both itraconazole and its bioactive hydroxyitraconazole metabolite are reported, the sum of which should be considered in assessing the trough concentration. The itraconazole oral solution formulation is preferred over the capsule formulation because of improved absorption and should be taken on an empty stomach. However, a super bioavailable (SUBA) itraconazole is now approved by the US Food and Drug Administration for the treatment of pulmonary and extrapulmonary blastomycosis in individuals 18 years or older, with pharmacokinetic studies of this formulation demonstrating less variable absorption than conventional itraconazole capsules and a similar side effect profile; data in children are lacking.

All patients with chronic pulmonary histoplasmosis (eg, progressive cavitation of the lungs) should be treated. Mild to moderate cases should be treated with itraconazole for 1 to 2 years. Severe cases should be treated initially with a lipid formulation amphotericin B followed by itraconazole for the same duration.

Mediastinal and inflammatory manifestations of infection generally do not need to be treated with antifungal agents. Mediastinal adenitis that causes obstruction of a bronchus, the esophagus, or another mediastinal structure may improve with a brief course of corticosteroids. In these instances, itraconazole should be used concurrently and continued for 6 to 12 weeks thereafter. Dense fibrosis of mediastinal structures without an associated granulomatous inflammatory component does not respond to antifungal therapy, and surgical intervention may be necessary for severe cases. Pericarditis and rheumatologic syndromes may respond to treatment with nonsteroidal anti-inflammatory agents (indomethacin).

For treatment of moderately severe to severe progressive disseminated histoplasmosis (PDH) in an infant or child, a lipid formulation of amphotericin B is the drug of choice and usually is given for a minimum of 2 weeks. When the child has demonstrated substantial clinical improvement and a decline in the serum concentration of *Histoplasma* antigen, oral itraconazole is administered for a total of at least 12 months. Lifelong suppressive therapy with itraconazole may be required for patients with primary immunodeficiency syndromes, acquired immunodeficiency that cannot be reversed, or patients who relapse despite appropriate therapy. For those with mild to moderate PDH, itraconazole for at least 12 months is recommended. After completion of treatment for PDH, urine antigen concentrations should be monitored for 12 months. Stable, low, and decreasing concentrations that are unaccompanied by signs of active infection may not necessarily require prolongation or resumption of treatment.

INFECTION PREVENTION AND CONTROL MEASURES IN HEALTH CARE SETTINGS: Standard precautions are recommended.

CONTROL MEASURES: Histoplasmosis is a reportable disease in some states. Investigation for a common source of infection is indicated in outbreaks. Exposure to soil and dust from areas with significant accumulations of bird and bat droppings should be avoided, especially by immunocompromised individuals, including those receiving tumor necrosis factor inhibitors or disease-modifying antirheumatic drugs. If exposure is unavoidable, it should be minimized through use of respiratory protection (eg, N95 or higher respirator), gloves, and disposable clothing. Although an N95 or higher respirator is adequate in most circumstances, in environments with extremely high inoculum, powered air purifying respirators (PAPRs) with high-efficiency particulate air (HEPA) filters are recommended.

Areas suspected of being contaminated with *Histoplasma* species should be remediated. Old or abandoned structures likely to have been contaminated with bird or bat droppings should be saturated with water to reduce aerosolization of spores during demolition. Guidelines for preventing histoplasmosis have been designed for health and safety professionals, environmental consultants, and people supervising workers involved in activities in which contaminated materials are disturbed. Additional information about these guidelines is available from the National Institute for Occupational Safety and Health at **www.cdc.gov/niosh/topics/histoplasmosis/default. html.**

Hookworm Infections
(*Necator americanus* and *Ancylostoma* species)

CLINICAL MANIFESTATIONS: Early manifestations of hookworm infection may relate to skin penetration (stinging, burning, pruritus ["ground itch"], rash), migration through the lungs (Löffler-like pneumonitis), and early infection in the intestines (colicky abdominal pain, nausea, diarrhea). Wakana syndrome, characterized by pharyngeal itching, hoarseness, nausea, vomiting, cough, and dyspnea, may develop after ingestion of *Ancylostoma duodenale* larvae. These early features are usually mild. Individuals who are chronically infected may also have mild nonspecific or no symptoms. However, the most common clinical manifestation from chronic infection is iron deficiency anemia resulting from direct blood loss at the site where adult worms attach to the mucosa of the small intestine. Blood loss secondary to hookworm infection begins 5 to 8 weeks after initial infection. Chronic hookworm infection is a common cause of moderate and severe hypochromic, microcytic anemia in people living in resource-limited tropical countries, and heavy infection can also cause hypoproteinemia with edema. Chronic infection in children may lead to physical growth delay, deficits in cognition, and developmental delay.

ETIOLOGY: Hookworms are intestinal parasites that are included in the group of nematode pathogens infecting millions of people worldwide called soil-transmitted helminths (STHs). The anthropophilic species infecting humans include *Necator americanus* and *Ancylostoma duodenale*. A third species, *Ancylostoma ceylanicum*, is known to infect dogs and cats but is also highly prevalent among humans in focal areas across the globe. Several other zoonotic hookworms that can cause human disease *(Ancylostoma braziliense, Ancylostoma caninum, Uncinaria stenocephala)* mainly are responsible for causing cutaneous larva migrans when filariform larvae penetrate the skin and migrate in the upper dermis, causing an intensely pruritic track. *A caninum* rarely can migrate to the intestine and cause eosinophilic enteritis.

EPIDEMIOLOGY: Hookworm is the third most common human STH infection following ascariasis and trichuriasis. It has worldwide distribution but is most prominent in rural, tropical, and subtropical areas where soil is conducive to organism development and where contamination with human feces is common. *N americanus* is the most widespread and prevalent human hookworm. Human hookworm infections occur in the Americas, Africa, Asia, Australia, on a number of Pacific islands, and in the Mediterranean region. Hookworm larvae and eggs survive in loose, sandy, moist, shady, well-aerated, warm soil (optimal temperature 23°C–33°C [73°F–91°F]). Hookworm eggs from stool hatch in soil in 1 to 2 days as rhabditiform larvae. These larvae develop into infective filariform larvae in soil within 5 to 10 days and can survive for 3 to 4 weeks. *N americanus* and *Ancylostoma* transmission occur via skin penetration. *A duodenale* infection can also occur via oral ingestion of third-stage larvae, including from human milk. Untreated infected patients can remain colonized with *A duodenale* for approximately 1 year and can remain colonized with *N americanus* for approximately 3 to 5 years.

The **incubation period** from exposure to development of noncutaneous symptoms is 4 to 12 weeks. Eggs appear in feces approximately 5 to 8 weeks from the time of infection.

DIAGNOSTIC TESTS: Microscopy of stool to identify eggs morphologically is the most common method for diagnosing hookworm infections. Microscopy can be performed on fresh or frozen stool samples, with direct smears or stools preserved with fixatives such as formalin; preserving stool decreases sensitivity. There are several concentrating methods that can improve sensitivity and estimation of burden of disease through egg counting (formalin-ether concentration, Kato-Katz method, McMaster technique, FLOTAC, and mini-FLOTAC). Most commercial laboratories in the United States rely on preserved stool samples and use the formalin-ether concentration method or a variation thereof. Multiple samples may be needed to detect infection; some experts recommend examining at least 3 consecutive samples using concentration techniques when index of suspicion of infection is high. Molecular techniques include qualitative or quantitative nucleic acid amplification tests (NAATs) and multiplex polymerase chain reaction (PCR) assays, but these are only available in the United States through research laboratories.

Nonspecific laboratory tests may include those for peripheral eosinophilia, anemia, and hypoproteinemia. Cutaneous larva migrans attributable to transient cutaneous infection with dog or cat hookworms is diagnosed clinically.

TREATMENT: Albendazole and mebendazole are recommended, and pyrantel pamoate is an effective alternative in the treatment of hookworm infection; only mebendazole is approved by the US Food and Drug Administration for this indication (see Drugs for Parasitic Infections, p 1068). Albendazole should be taken with food; a fatty meal increases oral bioavailability. Pyrantel pamoate suspension can be mixed with milk or fruit juice. Studies in children as young as 1 year of age suggest that albendazole can be administered safely to this population. Retreatment is indicated for persistent or recurrent infection. Nutritional supplementation, including iron, is important when addressing associated iron deficiency anemia. Severely affected children may require blood transfusion.

INFECTION PREVENTION AND CONTROL MEASURES IN HEALTH CARE SETTINGS: Standard precautions are recommended. Direct person-to-person transmission does not occur.

CONTROL MEASURES: Sanitary disposal of feces to prevent contamination of soil is necessary in areas with endemic infection. Treatment of all known infected people and screening of high-risk groups (ie, children and agricultural workers) in areas with endemic infection may help decrease environmental contamination. Wearing shoes protects against hookworm infection, although infection risk remains if other body surfaces are in contact with the soil. Periodic deworming treatments targeting preschool-aged and school-aged children have been advocated to prevent morbidity associated with heavy intestinal helminth infections. Certain populations immigrating to the United States (eg, refugees) receive presumptive albendazole treatment for STHs, including hookworm, before departure for the United States.

Human Herpesvirus 6 (Including Roseola) and 7

CLINICAL MANIFESTATIONS: Human herpesvirus 6 comprises 2 distinct viral species, HHV-6B and HHV-6A. Clinical manifestations of primary infection with human herpesvirus 6B (HHV-6B) commonly include fever, fussiness, and rhinorrhea; generalized rash occurs in almost one-third of children and roseola (exanthem subitum) occurs in 20% to 25%. Acute HHV-6B infection may also be accompanied by cervical and characteristic postoccipital lymphadenopathy, gastrointestinal tract or respiratory tract signs, and inflamed tympanic membranes. Fever may be high (temperature >39.5°C [103.0°F]) and persist for 3 to 7 days. Approximately 20% of all emergency department visits for febrile children 6 through 12 months of age are attributable to HHV-6B. Roseola is distinguished by an erythematous maculopapular rash that typically appears once fever resolves and can last hours to days. Febrile seizures, sometimes leading to status epilepticus, are the most common complication and reason for hospitalization among children with primary HHV-6B infection. Primary HHV-6B infection has been shown to account for 20% to 30% of first-time febrile seizures in young children evaluated in emergency care settings. Other reported neurologic manifestations include a bulging fontanelle and encephalopathy or rarely, encephalitis; the latter more commonly noted in infants in Japan than in the United States or Europe. Hepatitis has been reported as a rare manifestation of primary HHV-6B infection. In contrast to HHV-6B, primary infection with HHV-6A has not been associated with any recognized disease. Congenital infection with HHV-6B and HHV-6A, which occurs in approximately 1% of newborn infants, has not been linked to any clinical disease, and most cases have been shown to be attributable to inherited chromosomally integrated HHV-6 (iciHHV-6).

The clinical manifestations occurring with human herpesvirus 7 (HHV-7) infection are less clear than with HHV-6B. Most primary infections with HHV-7 presumably are asymptomatic or mild and not distinctive. Some initial infections can present as typical roseola and may account for second or recurrent cases of roseola. Febrile illnesses associated with seizures also have been documented to occur during primary HHV-7 infection.

Following infection, HHV-6B, HHV-6A, and HHV-7 remain in a latent state and may reactivate. The clinical circumstances and manifestations of reactivation in healthy people are unclear. Illness associated with HHV-6B reactivation has been described primarily among recipients of solid organ and hematopoietic cell transplants. Clinical findings associated with HHV-6B reactivation include fever, rash, hepatitis, bone marrow suppression, acute graft-versus-host disease, graft rejection, pneumonia, delirium, and encephalitis. The best characterized of these is post-transplantation acute limbic encephalitis (PALE), a specific syndrome associated with HHV-6B reactivation in the central nervous system characterized by anterograde amnesia, seizures, insomnia, confusion, and the syndrome of inappropriate antidiuretic hormone secretion. It is estimated that approximately 2% of allogeneic hematopoietic cell transplant recipients will experience HHV-6B encephalitis, with cord blood transplant recipients being at highest risk. Significant morbidity and mortality has been attributed to this complication. A few cases of central nervous system symptoms have been reported in association with HHV-7 reactivation in immunocompromised hosts, but clinical findings generally have been reported much less frequently with HHV-7 than with HHV-6B reactivation.

ETIOLOGY: HHV-6B, HHV-6A, and HHV-7 are lymphotropic viruses that are closely related members of the *Herpesviridae* family, subfamily *Betaherpesvirinae*. As betaherpesviruses, HHV-6B, HHV-6A, and HHV-7 are most closely related to cytomegalovirus. As with all human herpesviruses, they establish lifelong latency after initial acquisition. In 2012, HHV-6A and HHV-6B were recognized as distinct species rather than as variants of the same species. This increased the number of known human herpesviruses to 9.

EPIDEMIOLOGY: HHV-6B and HHV-7 cause ubiquitous infections in children worldwide. Humans are the only known natural host. Nearly all children acquire HHV-6B infection within the first 2 years of life, probably from contact with asymptomatically shed infectious virus from upper respiratory secretions of a healthy family member or other close contact. Virus-specific antibody in pregnant people, which is present uniformly in the sera of infants at birth, provides transient partial protection. As transplacentally acquired antibody concentration decreases during the first year of life, the infection rate increases rapidly, peaking between 6 and 24 months of age. During the acute phase of primary infection, HHV-6B and HHV-7 can be isolated from peripheral blood mononuclear cells and HHV-7 from saliva of some children. Viral DNA subsequently may be detected throughout life by a nucleic acid amplification test (NAAT) in multiple body sites, including blood mononuclear cells, saliva, and salivary glands. Infections occur throughout the year without a seasonal pattern. Secondary cases rarely are identified. Occasional outbreaks of roseola have been reported.

Several genetic mutations have been associated with severe central nervous system disease during primary HHV-6B infection. These include RandBP2, POLG, and carnitine palmitoyl-transferase 2 gene mutations.

Congenital infection occurs in approximately 1% of newborn infants, as determined by the presence of HHV-6A or HHV-6B DNA in cord blood. Most congenital infections appear to result from the germline passage of inherited chromosomally integrated HHV-6 (iciHHV-6) from either parent, a unique mechanism of transmission of human viral congenital infection. Transplacental HHV-6 infection also may occur from reinfection or reactivation of HHV-6 in the pregnant person or possibly from reactivated iciHHV-6 in the pregnant person. HHV-6 has not been identified in human milk. Congenital infection typically is asymptomatic, and the clinical implications of iciHHV-6 are not fully known. However, reactivation of iciHHV-6 in severely immunocompromised hosts is possible and can be associated with disease.

HHV-7 infection usually occurs later in childhood than HHV-6B infection. By adulthood, the seroprevalence of HHV-7 is approximately 85%. Infectious HHV-7 is present in more than 75% of saliva specimens obtained from healthy adults. Acquisition of virus via infected respiratory tract secretions of healthy contacts is the probable mode of transmission of HHV-7 to young children. HHV-7 DNA has been detected in human milk, peripheral blood mononuclear cells, cervical secretions, and other body sites. Congenital HHV-7 infection has not been demonstrated.

The mean **incubation period** for HHV-6B is 9 to 10 days. For HHV-7, the **incubation period** is not known.

DIAGNOSTIC TESTS: Multiple assays for detection of HHV-6 and HHV-7 DNA have been developed; some are available commercially, but because laboratory diagnosis of HHV-6 or HHV-7 usually does not influence clinical management (infections among the severely immunocompromised are an exception), these tests have limited utility in clinical practice.

Reference laboratories offer diagnostic testing for HHV-6B, HHV-6A, and HHV-7 infections by detection of viral DNA by NAAT in blood, cerebrospinal fluid (CSF), other body fluids, or tissue specimens. However, detection of HHV-6A, HHV-6B, or HHV-7 DNA by NAAT might not differentiate between new infection, persistence or reactivation of virus from past infection, or iciHHV-6. At least 1 multiplexed NAAT diagnostic panel designed to detect agents of meningitis and encephalitis in CSF containing HHV-6 as one of its target pathogens has been cleared by the US Food and Drug Administration; however, given the prevalence of iciHHV-6 (1%), which yields a positive CSF NAAT result, a positive test result should be interpreted with caution in a patient with no underlying risk factors and no findings to suggest encephalitis. Quantitative NAATs have been used for monitoring the effectiveness of antiviral treatment in immunocompromised patients with viral reactivation.

Inherited chromosomal integration of HHV-6 is suggested when NAAT results are consistently positive for HHV-6 DNA in whole blood, tissue, or other fluids, often with high viral loads (eg, 1×10^6 copies in whole blood, which with a normal white blood cell count is approximately 1 copy of HHV-6 DNA per nucleated cell). Droplet digital polymerase chain reaction (PCR) or quantitative comparison of viral DNA copies to human cell number copies in whole blood samples may also be used to identify ici-HHV-6. iciHHV-6 can be suggested by testing whole blood from both parents to see if one of them has a high viral load and can be confirmed by detection of HHV-6 DNA in hair follicles in research settings. HHV-6 viral loads in acellular fluids, such as plasma and CSF, are variable in people with iciHHV-6 because of unpredictable degrees of contamination with cell contents and cannot be used to infer chromosomal integration.

Serologic tests including immunofluorescent antibody assay, virus neutralization, immunoblot, and enzyme immunoassay (EIA) are often difficult to interpret. A fourfold increase in serum antibody concentration alone does not necessarily indicate new infection, because an increase in titer may occur with reactivation and in association with other infections, especially other betaherpesvirus infections. However, documented seroconversion is considered evidence of recent primary infection in infants and young children, and serologic tests may be useful for epidemiologic studies. Detection of specific immunoglobulin (Ig) M antibody is not reliable for diagnosing new infection, because IgM antibodies to HHV-6 and HHV-7 are not always detectable in children with primary infection and also may be present in asymptomatic previously infected people. These antibody assays do not differentiate HHV-6A from HHV-6B infections. Detection of low-avidity HHV-6 or HHV-7 antibody with subsequent maturation to high-avidity antibody has been used in such situations to identify recent primary infection.

TREATMENT: Management is supportive. The use of ganciclovir (and, therefore, valganciclovir) or foscarnet may be beneficial for immunocompromised patients with HHV-6B or HHV-7 disease and is recommended for treatment of HHV-6B encephalitis in hematopoietic cell and solid organ transplant patients. Antiviral resistance may occur. Routine monitoring of HHV-6 and HHV-7 DNA concentrations in blood during transplantation is not recommended. HHV-6 and HHV-7 have been reported as associated with various additional clinical syndromes in immunocompetent hosts, including multiple sclerosis, drug hypersensitivity, and uterine infection leading to infertility. None of these associations are generally accepted as etiologic, and treatment of HHV-6 or HHV-7 in association with these syndromes is not recommended.

INFECTION PREVENTION AND CONTROL MEASURES IN HEALTH CARE SETTINGS: Standard precautions are recommended.

CONTROL MEASURES: None.

Human Herpesvirus 8

CLINICAL MANIFESTATIONS: Human herpesvirus (HHV-8), also known as Kaposi sarcoma-associated herpesvirus (KSHV), is the cause of Kaposi sarcoma (KS), primary effusion lymphoma, multicentric Castleman disease (MCD), and the Kaposi sarcoma herpesvirus-associated inflammatory cytokine syndrome (KICS). HHV-8 also is a potential trigger of hemophagocytic lymphohistiocytosis (HLH). In regions of the world with endemic HHV-8, a nonspecific primary infection syndrome in immunocompetent children consists of fever and a maculopapular rash, often accompanied by upper respiratory tract symptoms. Primary infection among immunocompromised people tends to present with more severe manifestations including pancytopenia, fever, rash, lymphadenopathy, splenomegaly, diarrhea, arthralgia, disseminated disease, and/or KS. In parts of Africa where HHV-8 is endemic, KS is a frequent, aggressive malignancy among children both with and without human immunodeficiency virus (HIV) infection. Clinical presentations can vary, but younger children most often present with prominent (>2 cm), firm, nontender lymphadenopathy, associated cytopenias (significant anemia and thrombocytopenia), and frequently without the characteristic cutaneous lesions or "woody" edema more commonly seen in adults. In the United States, KS is rare in children and occurs primarily in adults with poorly controlled HIV infection. Immune reconstitution inflammatory syndrome (IRIS)-KS can occur, most notably among HIV-positive children adopted from countries with endemic HHV-8. Among solid organ and, less often, hematopoietic cell transplant recipients, KS is an important cause of cancer-related deaths. Primary effusion lymphoma is rare among children. MCD has been described in immunosuppressed and immunocompetent children, but the proportion of cases attributable to infection with HHV-8 is unknown.

ETIOLOGY: HHV-8 is a member of the family *Herpesviridae*, the *Gammaherpesvirinae* subfamily, and the *Rhadinovirus* genus, and is a DNA virus closely related to Epstein-Barr virus and to herpesvirus saimiri of monkeys.

EPIDEMIOLOGY: In areas of Africa, the Amazon basin, the Mediterranean, and the Middle East with endemic HHV-8, seroprevalence ranges from approximately 30% to 80%. Low rates of seroprevalence, generally less than 5%, have been reported in the United States, Northern and Central Europe, and most areas of Asia. Higher rates, however, occur in specific geographic regions, among adolescents and adults with or at high risk of acquiring HIV infection, injection drug users, and children adopted from endemic regions including some Eastern European countries.

Acquisition of HHV-8 in areas with endemic infection frequently occurs before puberty, likely by exposure to saliva of close contacts. Virus is shed frequently in saliva of infected people and becomes latent for life in peripheral blood mononuclear cells and lymphoid tissue. In areas where infection is not endemic, sexual transmission appears to be the major route of infection, especially among men who have sex with men. Studies from areas with endemic infection have suggested transmission may occur by blood transfusion, but in the United States, evidence for this is lacking. Transplantation of infected donor organs has been documented to result in HHV-8 infection in the recipient. HHV-8 DNA has been detected in blood drawn at birth from infants born to HHV-8 seropositive people, but vertical transmission seems to be rare. Viral DNA has also been detected in human milk, but transmission via human milk is yet to be proven.

The **incubation period** of HHV-8 is unknown.

DIAGNOSTIC TESTS: Nucleic acid amplification tests (NAATs) and serologic assays for HHV-8 are available. NAATs may be used on peripheral blood, fluid from body cavity effusions, and tissue biopsy specimens. When KS is suspected, biopsy with histologic confirmation is the gold standard. Detection of HHV-8 in peripheral blood specimens by NAAT also has been used to identify exacerbations of other HHV-8-associated diseases, primarily MCD and KICS (especially at high copy number in these 2 diseases); however, HHV-8 DNA can be detected in the peripheral blood of asymptomatically infected people, and conversely HHV-8 infected people may not have active viremia.

Currently available serologic assays measuring antibodies to HHV-8 include immunofluorescence antibody (IFA) assay, enzyme immunoassays (EIAs), and Western blot assays using recombinant HHV-8 proteins. These serologic assays detect both latent and lytic infection, but each has challenges with accuracy or convenience, with resulting limitations on their use in the diagnosis and management of acute clinical disease.

TREATMENT: Epidemic KS (KS in children with HIV) should be treated with both antiretroviral therapy plus chemotherapy based on clinical staging. Retrospective cohort studies and in vitro assays suggest that antiretroviral therapy may inhibit

HHV-8 replication. In acquired immunodeficiency syndrome (AIDS)-associated KS, for participants receiving highly active antiretroviral therapy, monotherapy with either paclitaxel or pegylated liposomal doxorubicin are preferred agents. For clinically significant disease with tissue or fluid (primary effusion lymphoma) burden, the most widely used treatment modality is chemotherapy. Treatment of transplant KS may benefit from reduction in immunosuppressive therapy and use of sirolimus in lieu of tacrolimus as the suppressive agent.

Several antiviral agents have in vitro activity against HHV-8. Valganciclovir has been shown to inhibit HHV-8 replication in the only randomized trial of an antiviral drug for this infection. Case reports document an effect of ganciclovir, valganciclovir, ganciclovir combined with zidovudine, cidofovir, and foscarnet. Valacyclovir and famciclovir more modestly reduce HHV-8 replication. Antiviral therapy may play a more significant role in the treatment of diseases associated with active, lytic HHV-8 replication, specifically MCD and KICS, but this remains to be well established.

INFECTION PREVENTION AND CONTROL MEASURES IN HEALTH CARE SETTINGS: Standard precautions are recommended.

CONTROL MEASURES: Although there are no standard guidelines on preventing HHV-8 transmission, avoidance of behavioral practices that lead to exposure to saliva might be effective.

Human Immunodeficiency Virus Infection[1]

CLINICAL MANIFESTATIONS: Human immunodeficiency virus (HIV) infection results in a wide array of clinical manifestations. HIV type 1 (HIV-1) is much more common in the United States than HIV type 2 (HIV-2). Unless otherwise specified, this chapter addresses HIV-1 infection. Acquired immunodeficiency syndrome (AIDS) is the name given to an advanced stage of HIV infection based on specific criteria for children, adolescents, and adults that are established by the Centers for Disease Control and Prevention (CDC).

Acute retroviral syndrome is estimated to develop in 40% to 90% of adolescents and adults within the first few weeks after they become infected with HIV and is characterized by nonspecific mononucleosis-like symptoms, including fever, malaise, lymphadenopathy, and skin rash.

Clinical manifestations of untreated pediatric HIV infection include unexplained fevers, generalized lymphadenopathy, hepatomegaly, splenomegaly, failure to thrive, persistent oral and diaper candidiasis, recurrent diarrhea, parotitis, hepatitis, central nervous system (CNS) disease (eg, encephalopathy, hyperreflexia, hypertonia, floppiness, developmental delay), lymphoid interstitial pneumonia, recurrent invasive bacterial infections, and viral, parasitic, and fungal opportunistic infections (OIs).[2]

---

[1] For a complete listing of current policy statements from the American Academy of Pediatrics regarding human immunodeficiency virus and acquired immunodeficiency syndrome, see **https://publications.aap.org/pediatrics/collection/537/Committee-on-Pediatric-and-Adolescent-HIV**.

[2] Panel on Opportunistic Infections in Children with and Exposed to HIV. Guidelines for the Prevention and Treatment of Opportunistic Infections in Children With and Exposed to HIV. Department of Health and Human Services. Available at: **https://clinicalinfo.hiv.gov/en/guidelines/hiv-clinical-guidelines-pediatric-opportunistic-infections/whats-new**

In the era of antiretroviral therapy (ART), there has been a substantial decrease in frequency of all OIs. In the pre-ART era, the most common OIs observed among children in the United States were infections caused by invasive encapsulated bacteria, *Pneumocystis jirovecii* (previously called *Pneumocystis carinii*, hence the still-used acronym PCP for *Pneumocystis carinii* pneumonia), varicella-zoster virus, cytomegalovirus, herpes simplex virus, *Mycobacterium avium* complex, *Cryptococcus neoformans*, and *Candida* species. Less commonly observed opportunistic pathogens included Epstein-Barr virus (EBV), *Mycobacterium tuberculosis, Cryptosporidium* species, *Cystoisospora* (formerly *Isospora*) species, other enteric pathogens, *Aspergillus* species, and *Toxoplasma gondii.*

Immune reconstitution inflammatory syndrome (IRIS) is a paradoxical clinical deterioration often seen in severely immunosuppressed individuals that occurs shortly after the initiation of ART. Local and/or systemic symptoms develop secondary to an inflammatory response as cell-mediated immunity is restored. IRIS is observed in patients with previous infections with mycobacteria (including *Mycobacterium tuberculosis*), bacille Calmette-Guérin (BCG) vaccine, herpesviruses, and fungi (including *Cryptococcus* species).

Malignant neoplasms in children living with HIV infection are relatively uncommon, but leiomyosarcomas and non-Hodgkin B-cell lymphomas of the Burkitt type (including those in the CNS) occur more commonly in children living with HIV infection than in immunocompetent children. Kaposi sarcoma, caused by human herpesvirus 8, is rare in children in the United States but has been documented in children living with HIV who have emigrated from sub-Saharan African countries. The incidence of malignant neoplasms in children living with HIV has decreased during the ART era.

ETIOLOGY: HIV-1 and HIV- are cytopathic lentiviruses *(*genus *Lentivirus)* belonging to the family *Retroviridae.* Four distinct genetic groups of HIV exist: M, N, O, and P. Group M viruses are the most prevalent worldwide and comprise 10 genetic subtypes, or clades, known as A, B, C, D, F, G, H, J, K, and L, each of which has a distinct geographic distribution.

HIV-2, the second AIDS-causing virus, is found predominantly in West Africa. Nine HIV-2 groups (A through I) have been documented, of which groups A and D are presently circulating. HIV-2 has a milder disease course with a longer time to development of AIDS than HIV-1. Accurate diagnosis of HIV-2 is important clinically, because HIV-2 is intrinsically resistant to nonnucleoside reverse transcriptase inhibitors (NNRTIs) and the fusion inhibitor enfuvirtide.

EPIDEMIOLOGY: Humans are the only known reservoir for HIV-1 and HIV-2. Latent virus persists in peripheral blood mononuclear cells and in cells of the brain, bone marrow, and genital tract even when plasma viral load is undetectable. Only blood, semen, preseminal fluid, rectal fluids, cervicovaginal secretions, and human milk have been implicated in transmission of infection.

Established modes of HIV transmission include: (1) sexual contact (vaginal, anal, or orogenital); (2) percutaneous blood exposure (from contaminated needles or other sharp materials); (3) mucous membrane exposure to contaminated blood or other body fluids; (4) perinatal transmission during prepartum, intrapartum, and postpartum periods, including breastfeeding postnatally; and (5) transfusion with contaminated blood products. Cases of HIV transmission from caregivers living with HIV to children through feeding blood-contaminated premasticated food and from contact of nonintact skin with blood-containing body fluids have been reported in the United States. As a result of highly effective screening assays and protocols, transfusion of blood, blood components, and clotting factors has virtually been eliminated as a cause of HIV transmission in the United States since 1985. Since the mid-1990s, the number of reported pediatric AIDS cases has decreased significantly, primarily because of effective measures to prevent perinatal transmission of HIV and the widespread availability of ART for children living with HIV.

In the absence of breastfeeding, the risk of HIV infection for infants born to untreated people living with HIV (PWH) in the United States is approximately 25%, with most transmission occurring near the time of delivery. Viral load of the birthing person is the most critical determinant of perinatal transmission of HIV, although transmission has been observed across the entire range of viral loads. Current US guidelines recommend cesarean section before labor and before rupture of membranes at 38 completed weeks of gestation for PWH with HIV RNA >1000 copies/mL (irrespective of antiretroviral [ARV] use in pregnancy) or unknown HIV RNA near time of delivery (within 4 weeks of delivery) to minimize perinatal transmission of HIV. Cesarean delivery is not needed for reduction of HIV perinatal transmission risk in people receiving ART with HIV RNA ≤1000 copies/mL near time of delivery and should not be performed unless otherwise indicated. (**https://clinicalinfo.hiv.gov/en/guidelines/perinatal/ intrapartum-care-for-people-with-hiv?view=full**).

The rate of acquisition of HIV infection among infants has decreased significantly in the United States. The rate of new HIV infections among adolescents and young adults aged 13 to 24 years overall also is decreasing but is increasing among young men who have sex with men (MSM) in this age group. HIV infection in adolescents occurs disproportionately among youth from racial or ethnic minority groups and is attributable primarily to sexual exposure.

INCUBATION PERIOD: The usual age of onset of symptoms is approximately 12 to 18 months of age[1] for untreated infants and children in the United States who acquire HIV infection through perinatal transmission. However, some children living with HIV become ill in the first few months of life, whereas others remain relatively asymptomatic for more than 5 years and, rarely, until early adolescence.

Acute retroviral syndrome occurring in adolescents and adults following HIV acquisition occurs 7 to 14 days following viral acquisition and lasts for 5 to 7 days. Only a minority of patients are ill enough to seek medical care for acute retroviral syndrome, although more may recall a prior viral illness when queried later.

DIAGNOSTIC TESTS:

Serologic Assays. Immunoassays are used widely as the initial test for serum HIV antibody or for p24 antigen (see below) and HIV antibody. Serologic assays that are cleared by the US Food and Drug Administration (FDA) for the diagnosis of HIV include:

---

[1] Centers for Disease Control and Prevention. HIV Surveillance Report, 2017. Vol 29. Centers for Disease Control and Prevention; November 2018. Available at: **www.cdc.gov/hiv/pdf/library/reports/ surveillance/cdc-hiv-surveillance-report-2017-vol-29.pdf**

- Antigen/antibody combination immunoassays (fourth-generation tests) that detect HIV-1/HIV-2 antibodies as well as HIV-1 p24 antigen (see below): recommended for initial testing
- HIV-1/HIV-2 immunoassays that detect both IgG and IgM (third-generation antibody tests): alternative for initial testing
- HIV-1/HIV-2 antibody differentiation immunoassay that differentiates HIV-1 antibodies from HIV-2 antibodies (HIV-1/HIV-2 test): recommended for supplemental testing to confirm the results from the initial test
- HIV-1 and HIV-2 antibodies (separate results for each) as well as p24 antigen (fifth-generation test): FDA cleared for initial HIV screening but not as a confirmatory test

The 2018 CDC HIV laboratory testing algorithm (**https://stacks.cdc.gov/view/cdc/50872**) recommends an initial FDA-approved HIV-1/HIV-2 antigen/antibody combination immunoassay (fourth-generation assay). Specimens with a reactive antigen/antibody immunoassay result should be tested with an FDA-approved HIV-1/HIV-2 antibody differentiation immunoassay. Specimens that are reactive on the initial antigen/antibody immunoassay and nonreactive or indeterminate on the HIV-1/HIV-2 antibody differentiation immunoassay should be tested with an FDA-approved HIV-1 nucleic acid amplification test (NAAT). If acute HIV infection or previously undiagnosed HIV with end-stage AIDS is suspected, virologic testing may be indicated because of false-negative antibody assay results in these populations.

Nucleic Acid Amplification Tests. Plasma HIV DNA or RNA assays have been used to diagnose HIV infection. DNA nucleic acid amplification tests (NAATs) can detect 1 to 10 DNA copies of proviral DNA in peripheral blood mononuclear cells and are used qualitatively to diagnose HIV infection. Quantitative RNA NAATs (viral load) cleared by the FDA provide results that serve as a predictor of disease progression and are useful in monitoring changes in plasma HIV RNA levels during treatment with ART.

Reprogramming of T lymphocytes using gammaretroviral or lentiviral vectors in chimeric antigen receptor T cell (CAR-T cell) and lentiviral-based gene therapy may interfere with long terminal repeat (LTR) genomes in HIV NAATs, resulting in false-positive result. Laboratories should have appropriate alternate HIV-1 NAAT testing platforms made available for this emerging patient population.

HIV-2 Detection. Most HIV immunoassays currently approved by the FDA detect but do not routinely differentiate between HIV-1 and HIV-2 antibodies. It is important to notify the laboratory when ordering serologic tests for a patient in whom HIV-2 infection is a possibility so that FDA-approved HIV-1/HIV-2 antibody differentiation immunoassays can be used. There is at least 1 FDA approved qualitative diagnostic RNA test that detects and can confirm HIV-2 infection.

Diagnosis of Perinatally and Postnatally Acquired Infection. Because children born to PWH passively acquire antibodies from the birthing parent, antibody assays are not informative for the diagnosis of infection in children younger than 18 months unless assay results are negative. Therefore, laboratory diagnosis of HIV infection during the first 18 months of life is based on HIV NAATs (Table 3.25). In children 18 to 24 months and older, HIV antibody assays can be used for diagnosis. Most children serorevert by 18 months of age; however, delayed seroreversion beyond 18 months of age can occur. In one study, seroreversion occurred at a median age of 13.9 months, but 14%

Table 3.25. Laboratory Diagnosis of HIV Infection[a]

Test	Comment
HIV DNA NAAT or RNA NAAT	Preferred tests to diagnose HIV infection in infants and children younger than 18–24 months; highly sensitive and specific by 2 weeks of age and available; DNA test performed on peripheral blood mononuclear cells; RNA test performed on plasma.
HIV p24 Ag	Less sensitive, false-positive results during first month of life, variable results; not recommended.
ICD p24 Ag	Negative test result does not rule out infection; not recommended.
HIV culture	Expensive, not readily available, requires up to 4 weeks for results; not recommended.

Ag indicates antigen; HIV, human immunodeficiency virus; ICD, immune complex dissociated; NAAT, nucleic acid amplification test.

[a] Adapted from Read JS; American Academy of Pediatrics, Committee on Pediatric AIDS. Diagnosis of HIV-1 infection in children younger than 18 months in the United States, *Pediatrics*. 2007;120(6):e1547–e1562 (Reaffirmed April 2010, February 2015)

of infants remained seropositive after 18 months, 4.3% remained seropositive after 21 months, and 1.2% remained seropositive after 24 months.

HIV-1 RNA or DNA NAATs for diagnosis of infection in infants are equally recommended in current diagnostic guidelines (**https://clinicalinfo.hiv.gov/en/guidelines/perinatal/whats-new-guidelines**). Because DNA NAAT detects proviral DNA in cells while HIV RNA tests measure viral RNA in plasma, there is the potential for DNA testing to be more sensitive in infants with very low viral loads. However, studies have shown that RNA and DNA NAATs for the diagnosis of HIV-1 infection in infants produce comparable results, leading to the current recommendation that either assay can be used in this setting. HIV-1 RNA assays will identify 25% to 58% of infants infected with HIV in the first week of life, 89% by 1 month of age, and 90% to 100% by 2 to 3 months of age. An HIV RNA assay result with only a low HIV RNA copy number in an HIV-exposed infant may indicate a false-positive result. Repeat testing is recommended, and consultation with a pediatric HIV expert should be considered in these circumstances.

In HIV-exposed infants, diagnostic testing with HIV DNA or RNA assays is recommended at 14 to 21 days of age and, if results are negative, again at 1 to 2 months of age and at 4 to 6 months of age (Fig 3.9). An infant is considered infected if 2 samples from 2 different time points have positive results by DNA or RNA NAAT. For infants at higher risk of perinatal HIV transmission, additional virologic diagnostic testing is recommended at birth and at 8 to 10 weeks of life (which is 2 to 4 weeks after cessation of antiretroviral prophylaxis) (Fig 3.9). If testing is performed shortly after birth, umbilical cord blood should not be used because of possible contamination with the birthing parent's blood. Infants in whom HIV infection is diagnosed should promptly be transitioned from neonatal ARV prophylaxis to antiretroviral treatment (ART) if not already on presumptive HIV therapy for high-risk infants as per perinatal guidelines (**https://clinicalinfo.hiv.gov/en/guidelines/perinatal/antiretroviral-management-newborns-perinatal-hiv-exposure-or-hiv-infection?view=full**).

FIG 3.9. RECOMMENDED VIROLOGIC TESTING SCHEDULES FOR INFANTS EXPOSED TO HIV BY PERINATAL HIV TRANSMISSION RISK

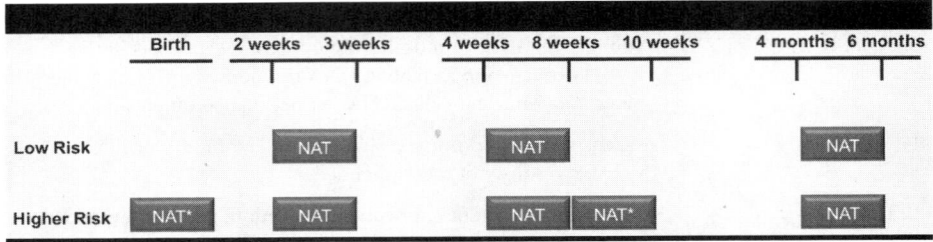

NAT indicates nucleic acid amplification test (referred to as NAAT in this chapter).

Low Risk: Infants born to people who received standard antiretroviral therapy (ART) during pregnancy with sustained viral suppression (usually defined as confirmed HIV RNA level below the lower limits of detection of an ultrasensitive assay) and no concerns related to adherence.

Higher Risk: Infants born to people with HIV infection who did not receive prenatal care, did not receive antepartum or intrapartum antiretrovirals (ARVs), received intrapartum ARV drugs only, initiated ART late in pregnancy (late second or third trimester), received a diagnosis of acute HIV infection during pregnancy, or had detectable HIV viral loads close to the time of delivery, including those who received ARV drugs and did not have sustained viral suppression.

*For higher-risk infants, additional virologic diagnostic testing should be considered at birth and 2 to 4 weeks after cessation of ARV prophylaxis (ie, at 8–10 weeks of life).

Reproduced with permission from Spach DH. Preventing Perinatal HIV Transmission. Seattle, WA: National HIV Curriculum, Infectious Diseases Education and Assessment, University of Washington. Available at: **www.hiv.uw.edu/go/ prevention/preventing-perinatal-transmission/core-concept/all.**

No additional HIV testing of any kind (HIV RNA, DNA NAAT, HIV antibody, HIV antigen/antibody) is routinely needed for nonbreastfed infants who meet the criteria for definitive exclusion of HIV and who have had no known or suspected HIV exposure after birth. Definitive exclusion of HIV infection in nonbreastfed infants is based on 2 or more negative virologic test results with 1 negative test result obtained at age ≥1 month and 1 at age ≥4 months, or 2 negative HIV antibody test results from separate specimens that were obtained at age ≥6 months (**https://clinicalinfo.hiv.gov/en/guidelines/perinatal/ diagnosis-hiv-infection-infants-and-children?view=full**).

Adolescents and HIV Testing. The American Academy of Pediatrics (AAP) recommends that routine HIV antibody screening be offered to all youth 15 years or older at least once in health care settings. Following initial screening, youth at increased risk, including those who are sexually active, should be rescreened at least annually, potentially as frequently as every 3 to 6 months if at very high risk (MSM, active injection drug users, transgender youth; having sexual partners with known HIV infection; exchanging sex for drugs or money; or those who have had a diagnosis of or request testing for other sexually transmitted infections [STIs], including mpox).[1,2] Use of any FDA-

---

[1] Hsu KK, Rakhmanina NY; American Academy of Pediatrics, Committee on Pediatric AIDS. Clinical report. Adolescents and young adults: the pediatrician's role in HIV testing and pre- and post-exposure HIV prophylaxis. *Pediatrics*. 2022;149(1):e2021055207

[2] Curran KG, Eberly K, Russell OO, et al. HIV and sexually transmitted infections among persons with monkeypox—eight U.S. jurisdictions, May 17-July 22, 2022. *MMWR Morb Mortal Wkly Rep.* 2022;71(36):1141-1147

cleared HIV antibody test is appropriate, except in youth with recent or ongoing antiretroviral prophylaxis use, such as HIV-1 preexposure prophylaxis (PrEP) and post-exposure prophylaxis (PEP). Recent data have shown that performance of HIV tests in persons who acquire HIV infection while taking ARV medications for such indications may be suboptimal compared with persons not exposed to these medications at or after the time of HIV acquisition because of inhibition of early viral replication that can affect the timing of the antibody development. In youth who have taken oral PrEP or PEP in the past 3 months or have received a long-acting PrEP injection in the past 12 months, an HIV antigen/antibody test **and** a qualitative or quantitative HIV-1 RNA test should be used. For any positive test result, immediate referral to an HIV specialist is appropriate to confirm diagnosis and initiate management. HIV testing is recommended and should be routine for all patients in STI clinics and those seeking treatment for STIs in other clinical settings.

Suspicion of acute retroviral syndrome should prompt urgent assessment with an antigen/antibody immunoassay or HIV RNA NAAT in conjunction with an antibody test. If the immunoassay result is negative or indeterminate, then testing for HIV RNA using a NAAT should follow. Clinicians should not assume that a laboratory report of a negative HIV antibody test result indicates that the necessary RNA screening for acute HIV infection has been conducted. HIV self-testing kits only detect HIV anti-bodies and, therefore, will not detect acute HIV infection.

TREATMENT:

Antiretroviral Therapy. Consultation with an expert in pediatric HIV infection is recom-mended in the care of infants, children, and adolescents living with HIV. Current treatment recommendations for HIV-infected infants and children (**https://clinicalinfo.hiv.gov/en/guidelines/pediatric-arv/whats-new-guidelines; https://nccc.ucsf.edu/clinician-consultation/hiv-aids-management/**) as well as adolescents (**https://clinicalinfo.hiv.gov/en/guidelines/adult-and-adolescent-arv/whats-new-guidelines**) are available online. Whenever possible, enrollment of infants, children, and adolescents living with HIV in clinical trials should be encouraged. Information about clinical trials for infants, children, and adolescents living with HIV can be obtained by contacting the AIDS Clinical Trials Information Service (**www.actis.org/**).

ART is indicated all for pediatric patients living with HIV and should be initi-ated as soon as possible after diagnosis of HIV infection is established. Initiation of treatment of adolescents generally follows guidelines for adults and is recom-mended strongly for all adolescents or adults living with HIV regardless of CD4+ T-lymphocyte count if medication adherence readiness is apparent. In general, ART with at least 3 active drugs is recommended for all individuals requiring ARV therapy. ARV resistance testing (viral genotyping) is recommended before starting treatment, but ART can be initiated prior to results in most cases. Sustained suppression of virus to undetectable levels is the desired goal. A change in ART should be considered if there is evidence of disease progression (virologic, immunologic, or clinical), drug tox-icity or intolerance, development of drug resistance, or availability of data suggesting the possibility of a superior or simpler regimen.

Opportunistic Infections. Guidelines for prevention and treatment of OIs in children (**https://clinicalinfo.hiv.gov/en/guidelines/pediatric-opportunistic-**

infection/whats-new) and adolescents and adults (https://clinicalinfo.hiv.gov/en/guidelines/adult-and-adolescent-opportunistic-infection/whats-new-guidelines) provide indications for administration of drugs for prevention, as well as treatment, of infection with *P jirovecii*, *M avium* complex, cytomegalovirus, *T gondii*, and other organisms.

Immunization Recommendations (also see Immunization in Special Clinical Circumstances, p 87, and Table 1.17, p 94).[1] All recommended childhood immunizations should be administered to HIV-exposed infants. If HIV infection is confirmed, guidelines for children living with HIV should be followed. Children and adolescents living with HIV should be immunized as soon as is age appropriate with all non-live and mRNA vaccines. Inactivated (non-live) influenza vaccine (IIV) should be administered annually according to the most current recommendations. The 3-dose series of human papillomavirus vaccine is indicated in adolescents living with HIV (https://redbook.solutions.aap.org/SS/Immunization_Schedules.aspx).

The live-virus measles, mumps, and rubella (MMR) vaccine and monovalent varicella vaccine can be administered to children and adolescents living with HIV without severe immunosuppression. Severely immunocompromised infants, children, adolescents, and young adults living with HIV (for people ≤5 years of age, defined as a CD4+ T-lymphocyte percentage <15%; for people >5 years of age, defined as a CD4+ T-lymphocyte percentage <15% **or** a CD4+ T-lymphocyte count <200 lymphocytes/mm³) should not receive measles virus-containing vaccine, because vaccine-related pneumonia has been reported. The quadrivalent measles, mumps, rubella, and varicella (MMRV) vaccine should not be administered to any infant or child living with HIV, regardless of degree of immunosuppression, because of lack of safety data in this group.

Rotavirus vaccine should be administered to all infants exposed to or infected with HIV irrespective of CD4+ T-lymphocyte percentage or count.

All children living with HIV should receive a dose of 23-valent polysaccharide pneumococcal vaccine after turning 24 months of age if at least 8 weeks have passed since the last 13-valent or 15-valent pneumococcal conjugate vaccine and they have not previously received at least 1 dose of 20-valent pneumococcal conjugate vaccine (see *Streptococcus pneumoniae* [Pneumococcal] Infections, p 810).

Children living with HIV who are 5 years and older and have not received *Haemophilus influenzae* type b (Hib) vaccine should receive 1 dose of Hib vaccine (see Table 3.13, p 408).

Children and adolescents living with HIV should receive COVID-19 vaccine, if authorized or approved by the FDA for their age group. Preliminary data in individuals living with HIV who have received COVID-19 vaccines indicate good humoral responses in those with well-controlled infection on ART with normal CD4+ T-lymphocyte counts. However, diminished responses were noted in individuals with advanced or untreated HIV infection.

Infants and children 2 months or older living with HIV infection should receive an age-appropriate series of the meningococcal ACWY conjugate vaccine (MenACWY)

---

[1] Rubin LG, Levin MJ, Ljungman P, et al. 2013 IDSA clinical practice guideline for vaccination of the immunocompromised host. *Clin Infect Dis*. 2014;58(3):309-318

(see Meningococcal Infections, p 585).[1] The same vaccine product should be used for all doses. However, if the product used for previous doses is unknown or unavailable, the vaccination series may be completed with any age- and formulation-appropriate meningococcal ACWY conjugate vaccine. Although no data on interchangeability of meningococcal conjugate vaccines in people living with HIV are available, limited data from a postlicensure study in healthy adolescents suggests safety and immunogenicity of MenACWY-CRM are not adversely affected by prior immunization with MenACWY-D. For children living with HIV 2 through 23 months of age, only MenACWY-CRM (Menveo) should be used, because interference with the immune response to pneumococcal conjugate vaccine occurs with MenACWY-D (Menactra), and MenACWY-TT (MenQuadfi) is not licensed for use in children younger than 2 years.

Children Who Are HIV Uninfected Residing in the Household of a Person Living With HIV.
Members of households in which an adult or child has HIV infection can receive MMR vaccine, because these vaccine viruses are not transmitted from person to person. To decrease the risk of transmission of influenza to patients with symptomatic HIV infection, all household members 6 months or older should receive yearly influenza immunization (see Influenza, p 511). Live attenuated influenza vaccine (LAIV) may be administered to healthy household and other close contacts of people with altered immunocompetence (see Household Members of Immunocompromised Patients, p 103). Likewise, all household members should receive a COVID-19 vaccine if authorized or approved by the FDA for their age group. Siblings and susceptible adult caregivers of patients living with HIV should be immunized with varicella vaccine to prevent acquisition of wild-type varicella-zoster virus infection, which can cause severe disease in immunocompromised hosts. Although the risk of transmission is low, immunocompromised patients should avoid contact with people who develop skin lesions after receipt of varicella vaccine until the lesions clear (see Household Members of Immunocompromised Patients, p 103).

Postexposure Passive Immunization of Children Living With HIV.
Measles (see Measles, p 570).[2] Children living with HIV who are exposed to measles require prophylaxis based on immune status and measles vaccine history. Children living with HIV with no to moderate immunosuppression who have evidence of immunity (eg, serologic evidence of immunity to measles or who received 2 doses of measles vaccine after initiation of ART) do not require any additional measures to prevent measles following an exposure. Mildly or moderately immunocompromised people living with HIV without evidence of immunity to measles (eg, no serologic evidence of immunity to measles and who have not received 2 doses of measles vaccine after initiation of ART) should receive immune globulin intramuscular (IGIM) at a dose of 0.5 mL/kg (maximum 15 mL). Severely immunocompromised hosts (for people ≤5 years of age, defined as a CD4+ T-lymphocyte percentage <15%; for people >5 years of age, defined as a CD4+ T-lymphocyte percentage <15% **or** a CD4+ T-lymphocyte count <200 lymphocytes/mm³) who are exposed to measles should receive immune

---

[1] Centers for Disease Control and Prevention. Recommendations for use of meningococcal conjugate vaccines in HIV-infected persons—Advisory Committee on Immunization Practices, 2016. *MMWR Morb Mortal Wkly Rep.* 2016;65(43):1189–1194

[2] Centers for Disease Control and Prevention. Prevention of measles, rubella, congenital rubella syndrome, and mumps, 2013 summary: recommendations of the Advisory Committee on Immunization Practices (ACIP). *MMWR Recomm Rep.* 2013;62(RR-4):1-34

globulin intravenous (IGIV) prophylaxis, 400 mg/kg, after exposure to measles, regardless of prior vaccination status, because they may not be protected by the vaccine. Children living with HIV who have received IGIV within 3 weeks of exposure do not require additional passive immunization.

Tetanus. Children living with HIV with severe immune suppression (for people ≤5 years of age, defined as a CD4+ T-lymphocyte percentage <15%; for people >5 years of age, defined as a CD4+ T-lymphocyte percentage <15% **or** a CD4+ T-lymphocyte count <200 lymphocytes/mm^3) who sustain wounds classified as tetanus prone (see Tetanus, p 848) should receive tetanus immune globulin regardless of immunization status.

Varicella. Children living with HIV who lack evidence of immunity to varicella (eg, serologic evidence of immunity to varicella, or documentation of receipt of 2 doses of varicella vaccine after initiation of ART, or health care provider-confirmed clinical diagnosis of varicella), or who have severe immune suppression (for people ≤5 years of age, defined as a CD4+ T-lymphocyte percentage <15%; for people >5 years of age, defined as a CD4+ T-lymphocyte percentage <15% **or** a CD4+ T-lymphocyte count <200 lymphocytes/mm^3) should receive varicella zoster immune globulin, if available, ideally within 96 hours but potentially beneficial up to 10 days, after close contact with a person who has chickenpox or shingles (see Varicella-Zoster Infections, p 938). An alternative to varicella-zoster immune globulin for passive immunization is oral valacyclovir or acyclovir beginning 7 days after exposure, and if this is not available then IGIV, 400 mg/kg, administered once within 10 days after exposure (see Fig 3.22, p 945). Children who have received IGIV for other reasons within 3 weeks of exposure do not require additional passive immunization.

Hepatitis A.[1] All people with HIV who experience high-risk exposure to a person with hepatitis A infection, regardless of the exposed person's hepatitis A vaccination history or current degree of HIV-associated immunosuppression, should receive IGIM at a dose of 0.1 mL/kg.

INFECTION PREVENTION AND CONTROL MEASURES IN HEALTH CARE SETTINGS: Standard precautions should be followed by all health care professionals regardless of suspected or confirmed HIV infection status of the patient.

CONTROL MEASURES:

Perinatal Transmission Prophylaxis.

Management of Infected Pregnant Person. Pregnant PWH should receive ART regimens, both for treatment of HIV infection and for prevention of perinatal transmission of HIV. Sustained virologic suppression is the goal both during pregnancy and following delivery. Detailed recommendations for use of ARVs in pregnant PWH can be found online **(https://clinicalinfo.hiv.gov/en/guidelines/perinatal/whats-new-guidelines).** Ideally, PWH initiating such a regimen during pregnancy should be tested for the presence of ARV resistance. However, initiation of ART should not be delayed pending results of resistance testing, especially if decisions are being made late in pregnancy. Intrapartum intravenous (IV) zidovudine should be given to PWH who present in labor or at least 3 hours prior to scheduled cesarean delivery with HIV RNA >1000 copies/

---

[1] Brennan J, Moore K, Sizemore L, et al. Notes from the field: acute hepatitis A virus infection among previously vaccinated persons with HIV infection—Tennessee, 2018. *MMWR Morb Mortal Wkly Rep.* 2019;68(14):328–329

mL near the time of delivery, unknown HIV RNA, known or suspected ART nonadherence since last HIV RNA result, or positive rapid antigen/antibody HIV result obtained around time of delivery in a person without a previous diagnosis of HIV. Intrapartum IV zidovudine may be considered on a case-by-case basis for PWH with HIV RNA ≥50 copies/mL and ≤1000 copies/mL within 4 weeks of delivery, but data are insufficient to determine whether IV zidovudine provides any additional protection against perinatal transmission in such cases (**https://clinicalinfo.hiv.gov/en/guidelines/perinatal/intrapartum-care-for-people-with-hiv?view=full**). In situations in which IV administration is not possible, oral administration can be considered.

Management of Exposed Infant. The newborn infant should be bathed and cleaned of secretions (especially bloody secretions) immediately after birth[1] and should begin ARV prophylaxis as soon as possible to the time of birth, preferably within 6 hours. Management options for evaluation and prophylactic therapy of newborn infants in the United States at low risk are presented in Fig 3.10. Presumptive therapy recommendations for newborn infants at higher risk of perinatal transmission are presented in Fig 3.11. Duration of ARV prophylaxis in the neonate is 2 to 6 weeks for low-risk perinatal HIV exposure (Fig 3.10), and the duration of presumptive therapy for high-risk perinatal HIV exposure is 6 weeks (Fig 3.11).

The newborn infant's physician should obtain the birthing parent's HIV infection status so appropriate care and follow-up of the infant can be accomplished. Infants born to people who (1) did not have HIV testing during pregnancy; (2) did not have third trimester HIV testing in areas where third trimester testing is recommended by the CDC; or (3) were diagnosed with other STIs during pregnancy (particularly syphilis) but were not tested for HIV should be tested with a rapid HIV antibody test as soon as possible after delivery. A positive antibody test would not be diagnostic for the infant, but would identify an undiagnosed HIV infection in the parent which in turn would necessitate presumptive HIV treatment and an HIV NAAT at birth in the infant. Whenever possible, PWH and their infants should be referred to a facility that provides HIV-related services for both the birthing parent and the baby.

Breastfeeding (Also See Breastfeeding and Human Milk, p 135).[2] Transmission of HIV by breastfeeding accounted for one third to one half of perinatal transmission of HIV worldwide in the pre-ART era. Transmission is more likely among pregnant people who acquire HIV infection late in pregnancy or during the postpartum period. In resource-limited settings, the World Health Organization recommends that people living with HIV breastfeed their infants exclusively for the first 6 months of life, because infant morbidity associated with formula feeding is unacceptably high and safe alternatives to human milk may not be readily available.

Replacement (formula) feeding is recommended for all infants born to people living with HIV infection in the United States, since this is the option that eliminates risk of transmission of HIV to the infant.[3] Replacement feeding should be recommended

---

[1] Nolt D, O'Leary ST, Aucott SW; American Academy of Pediatrics, Committee on Infectious Diseases, Committee on Fetus and Newborn. Risks of infectious diseases in newborns exposed to alternative perinatal practices. *Pediatrics.* 2022;149(2):e2021055554

[2] American Academy of Pediatrics, Committee on Pediatrics AIDS, Section on Breastfeeding. Policy statement: infant feeding for persons living with HIV in the United States. *Pediatrics.* 2023; in press

[3] Meek JY, Noble L; American Academy of Pediatrics, Section on Breastfeeding. Technical report. Breastfeeding and the use of human milk. *Pediatrics.* 2022;150(1):e2022057989

FIG 3.10. NEWBORN TESTING AND PROPHYLAXIS RECOMMENDATIONS FOLLOWING LOW-RISK PERINATAL HIV EXPOSURE*

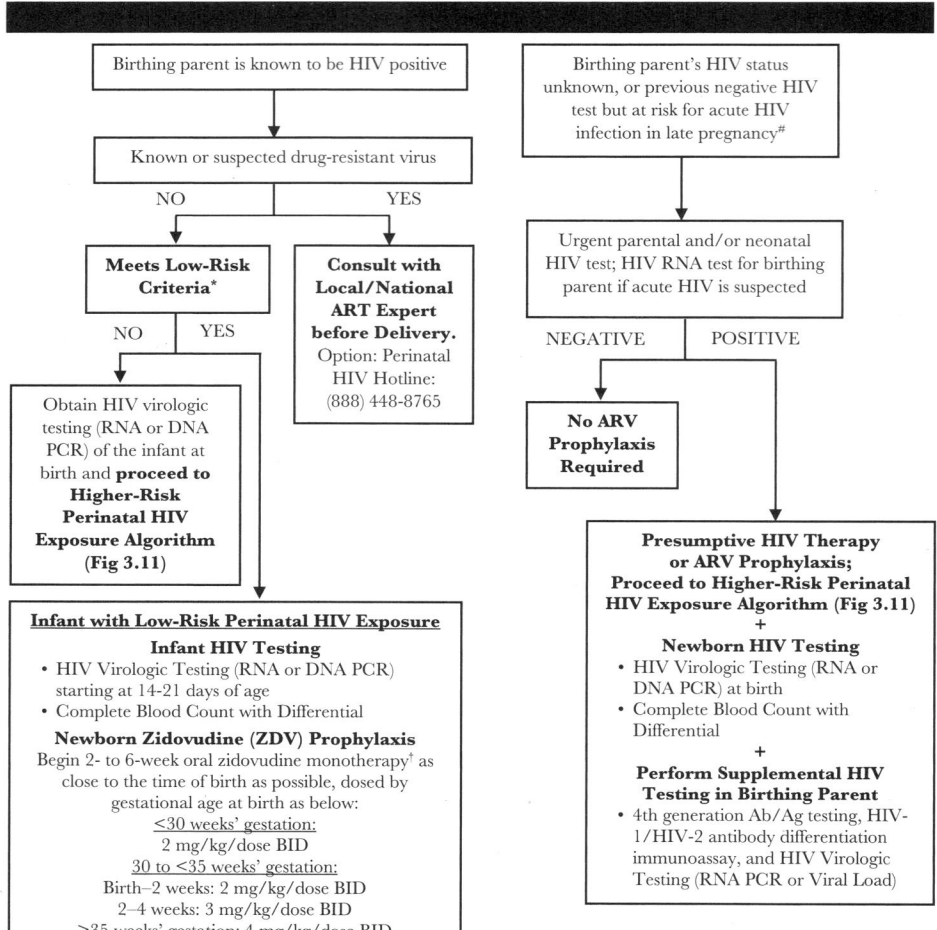

ART indicates antiretroviral therapy.

*Low-risk criteria: (1) person with HIV who received ART throughout pregnancy or from the early 1st/2nd trimester; **AND** (2) confirmed HIV RNA <50 copies/mL near delivery (within 4 weeks); **AND** (3) no concerns regarding ART adherence; **AND** (4) person did not have primary or acute HIV infection during pregnancy.

#Birthing people with previous negative HIV test at risk for seroconversion in late pregnancy are those with: documented STI, unprotected sex, partner with HIV, multiple partners, or IV drug use.

†If birthing parent has been on ART for at least 10 consecutive weeks during pregnancy and has maintained viral suppression (defined as at least 2 consecutive viral load measurements of <50 copies/mL at least 4 weeks apart), the infant can receive 2 weeks of ZDV. All other infants, and all infants <37 weeks' gestational age, should receive 4–6 weeks of ZDV.

Algorithm adapted by Paul Spearman, Rana Chakraborty and Athena Kourtis from Management of Infants Born to Women with HIV Infection, in Recommendations for the Use of Antiretroviral Drugs in Pregnant Women with HIV Infection and Interventions to Reduce Perinatal HIV Transmission in the United States, **clinicalinfo.hiv.gov**.

FIG 3.11. NEWBORN TESTING AND PROPHYLAXIS RECOMMENDATIONS FOLLOWING HIGHER-RISK PERINATAL HIV EXPOSURE*

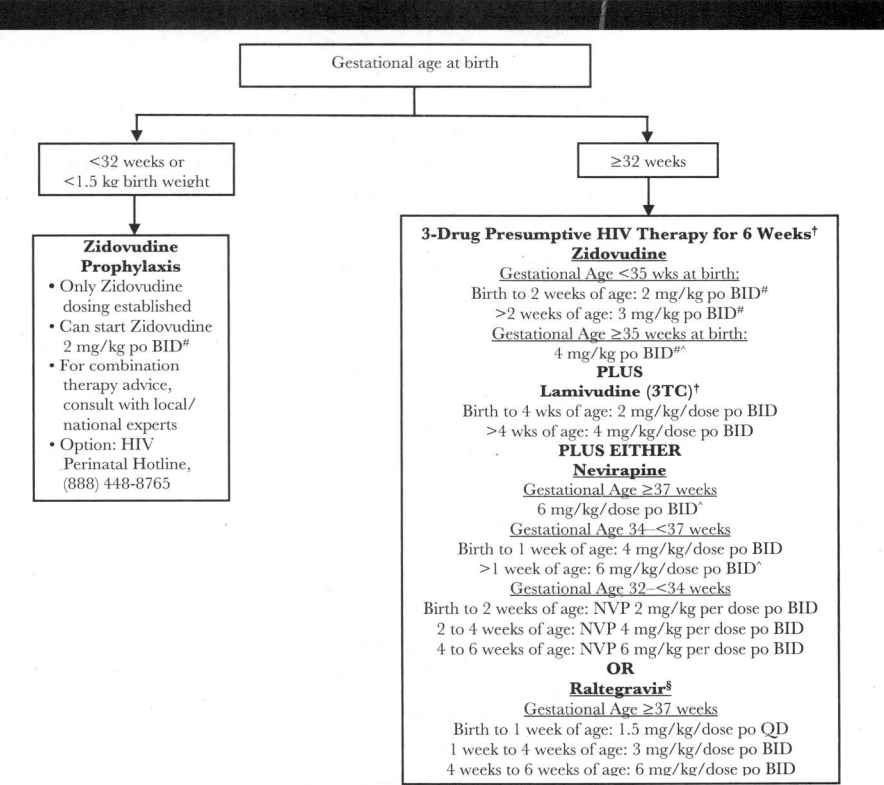

* Higher-risk criteria: birthing parents (1) who received neither antepartum nor intrapartum ARVs; **OR** (2) who received only intrapartum ARVs; **OR** (3) who received ante- and intrapartum ARVs but who do not have viral suppression (HIV RNA <50 copies/mL) near delivery, particularly if delivery was vaginal; **OR** (4) with acute or primary HIV infection during pregnancy or breastfeeding, in which case, the person should discontinue breastfeeding.

For newborns who are unable to tolerate oral agents, the IV dose of zidovudine is 75% of the oral dose, while maintaining the same dosing interval.

† All infants at higher risk of perinatal HIV exposure should be tested by HIV RNA or DNA PCR at birth. If birth HIV virologic testing in newborn is negative, some experts would discontinue lamivudine and nevirapine after 2 weeks and complete 6 weeks of prophylaxis with zidovudine alone.

^ ARV doses (such as ZDV and nevirapine) may need to be changed and the ARV regimen may need to be optimized if the infant has confirmed HIV infection. See **clinicalinfo.hiv.gov** for full dosing guidelines for infants with confirmed HIV infection.

§ If the birthing person has taken raltegravir 2–24 hours prior to delivery, the neonate's first dose of raltegravir should be delayed until 24–48 hours after birth; additional ARV drugs should be started as soon as possible. Do not use raltegravir if gestational age <37 weeks.

Algorithm adapted by Paul Spearman, Rana Chakraborty and Athena Kourtis from Management of Infants Born to Women with HIV Infection, in Recommendations for the Use of Antiretroviral Drugs in Pregnant Women with HIV Infection and Interventions to Reduce Perinatal HIV Transmission in the United States, **clinicalinfo.hiv.gov**.

if the birth parent is not receiving ART, or is not adherent and has a detectable viral load. Parents with HIV infection with fully suppressed viral load and who are adherent with ART who wish to breastfeed should be supported in their decision to do so. If a parent chooses to breastfeed, an appropriate plan of management can be developed, including encouraging adherence with ART during breastfeeding, use of antiretrovirals in the infant as prophylaxis while breastfeeding, exclusive breastfeeding for 6 months followed by weaning and introduction of complementary foods, lactation counseling, frequent viral load monitoring in the breastfeeding parent, and frequent infant testing for HIV infection (**https://clinicalinfo.hiv.gov/en/guidelines/perinatal/counseling-and-managing-women-living-hiv-united-states-who-desire-breastfeed**).

Prewarming or Premastication. Probable transmission of HIV by caregivers who prewarmed in their mouth or premasticated food for infants has been described in the United States. The CDC recommends that caregivers living with HIV be asked about whether they practice premastication and counseled not to prewarm or premasticate food for infants.

HIV in the Athletic Setting. Athletes and staff of athletic programs can be exposed to blood during certain athletic activities. Recommendations have been developed by the AAP for prevention of transmission of HIV and other bloodborne pathogens in the athletic setting (see Children in Group Child Care and Schools, Bloodborne Infections, p 148).

Sexual Abuse. In cases of proven or suspected sexual abuse, the child should be tested with an HIV antibody test at the original assessment, with testing repeated at approximately 6 weeks and <3 months (see Sexual Assault and Abuse in Children and Adolescents/Young Adults, p 182). Serologic evaluation for HIV infection of the perpetrator should be attempted as soon after the incident as possible. Counseling of the child and family needs to be provided (**https://stacks.cdc.gov/view/cdc/38856**).

Prevention of HIV Transmission Through Sexual Activity. Abstinence from sexual activity is the only certain way to prevent sexual transmission of HIV. Safer sex practices, including use of condoms for all sexual encounters (vaginal, anal, and oral sex) can reduce HIV transmission significantly by reducing exposure to body fluids containing HIV. Sustained HIV RNA to blood levels <200 copies/mL with ART eliminates the risk of HIV sexual transmission in discordant couples.

PrEP with ARVs (eg, tenofovir plus emtricitabine; cabotegravir) reduces the risk of HIV acquisition from sex by 99% when taken consistently. Among people who inject drugs, PrEP reduces the risk of acquiring HIV infection by at least 74% when taken consistently. PrEP is much less effective if it is not taken consistently. PrEP is FDA approved for adolescents and adults weighing at least 35 kg (77 lb). The AAP recommends that youth at substantial risk for HIV acquisition be routinely offered HIV PrEP.[1] Detailed guidance is available from CDC at **www.cdc.gov/hiv/risk/prep/index.html** and **www.cdc.gov/hiv/pdf/risk/prep/cdc-hiv-prep-guidelines-2021.pdf.** If advice is needed, clinicians may consult the National Clinician Consultation Center PrEP Line at 1-855-448-7737 (9:00 AM–8:00 PM Eastern Time).

---

[1] Hsu KK, Rakhmanina NY; American Academy of Pediatrics, Committee on Pediatric AIDS. Clinical report. Adolescents and young adults: the pediatrician's role in HIV testing and pre- and post-exposure HIV prophylaxis. *Pediatrics.* 2022;149(1):e2021055207

ARV-based vaginal microbicides and ARV-coated vaginal rings have reduced HIV acquisition in uninfected women. Data from clinical trials conducted in African countries also provide evidence that medical penile circumcision can reduce HIV acquisition in heterosexual male individuals by 38% to 66% over 24 months.

Postexposure Prophylaxis for Possible Sexual or Other Nonoccupational Exposure to HIV. Decisions to provide ARVs after possible nonoccupational (ie, community) exposure to HIV must balance the potential benefits and risks. Decisions regarding the need for ARV prophylaxis in such instances are predicated on the probability that the source is infected or contaminated with HIV, the likelihood of transmission by the particular exposure, and the interval between exposure and initiation of therapy, balanced against expected adverse effects associated with the regimen.

The risk of transmission of HIV from a puncture wound attributable to a needle found in the community likely is much lower than 0.3%, which is the estimated probability of HIV transmission from a puncture wound involving a known HIV-contaminated needle in a health care setting. The actual risks of HIV infection in an infant or child after a needlestick injury or sexual abuse are unknown, but to date there are no confirmed transmissions of HIV from accidental nonoccupational needlestick injuries (needles found in the community). The estimated risk of HIV transmission from receptive penile-anal sexual exposure is 138 per 10 000 exposures. The estimated risk per episode of receptive vaginal exposure is 8 per 10 000 exposures.

ARVs generally should not be used if the risk of transmission is low (eg, trivial needlestick injury with a drug needle from an unknown nonoccupational source) or if care is sought more than 72 hours after the reported exposure (see Injuries From Needles Discarded in the Community, p 198). The benefits of PEP are greatest when risk of infection is high, intervention is prompt, and adherence is likely. Consultation with an experienced pediatric HIV health care professional is essential. Detailed guidelines for PEP for children can be found at **https://stacks.cdc.gov/view/cdc/38856** and **https://nccc.ucsf.edu/clinician-consultation/pep-post-exposure-prophylaxis/.** The AAP recommends that youth be offered HIV PEP following high-risk sexual exposures.[1]

Postexposure Prophylaxis for Occupational Exposure to HIV. Guidelines for use of occupational PEP have been published by CDC and should be started as soon as possible after the exposure but within 72 hours for maximal effectiveness **(https://stacks.cdc.gov/view/cdc/38856).** In addition, the National Clinician Consultation Center at 1-888-448-4911 provides guidance seven days a week between 9 AM and 9 PM Eastern Time and can provide valuable support to providers.

Public Health Reporting. HIV infection is a nationally notifiable disease in the United States.

Human Papillomaviruses

CLINICAL MANIFESTATIONS: Most human papillomavirus (HPV) infections are subclinical, and 90% spontaneously become undetectable within 2 years. However, persistent HPV infection can cause benign epithelial proliferation (warts) of the

---

[1] Hsu KK, Rakhmanina NY; American Academy of Pediatrics, Committee on Pediatric AIDS. Clinical report. Adolescents and young adults: the pediatrician's role in HIV testing and pre- and post-exposure HIV prophylaxis. *Pediatrics.* 2022;149(1):e2021055207

skin and mucous membranes as well as cancers of the lower anogenital tract and the oropharynx. HPV types can be grouped into cutaneous and mucosal types. The cutaneous types cause common skin warts, plantar warts, flat warts, and thread-like (filiform) warts. These cutaneous warts are benign. Certain mucosal types (referred to as low risk) are associated with warts or papillomas of mucous membranes, including the upper respiratory tract and anogenital, oral, nasal, and conjunctival areas. Other mucosal types (referred to as high risk) can cause precancers and cancers, including cervical, anogenital, and oropharyngeal cancers.

Warts are common benign lesions, although they may be associated with significant clinical problems. Common **skin warts** are dome-shaped with conical projections that give the surface a rough appearance. Skin warts usually are painless and multiple, occurring commonly on the hands and around or under the nails. When small dermal vessels become thrombosed, black dots appear in the warts.

Plantar warts on the foot often are larger than warts at other sites and may not project through much of the skin surface. They can be painful when walking and are characterized by marked hyperkeratosis, sometimes with black dots.

Flat warts commonly are found on the face and extremities of children and adolescents. Flat warts usually are small, multiple, and flat topped, seldom exhibit papillomatosis, and rarely cause pain. **Filiform warts** occur on the face and neck.

Anogenital warts, also called **condylomata acuminata,** are skin-colored warts with a papular, flat, or cauliflower-like surface that range in size from a few millimeters to several centimeters. These warts often occur in groups, and may be found on the penis, urethra, scrotum, vulva, anal or perianal areas and, less commonly, in the vagina or on the cervix. Warts usually are painless, although they may cause itching, burning, local pain, or bleeding and may have significant psychological impact.

Invasive cancers attributable to HPV include those of the cervix, vagina, vulva, penis, anus, and oropharynx (back of throat, base of tongue, and tonsils). Cervical cancer is the most common HPV-attributable cancer in the female population.[1] Oropharyngeal cancer is the most common HPV-attributable cancer in the male population and the most common HPV-related cancer overall in the United States. Anogenital low-grade squamous intraepithelial lesions (LSILs) can result from infection with low-risk or high-risk HPV types, whereas high-grade squamous intraepithelial lesions (HSILs) result mostly from persistent infection with high-risk HPV types. In the cervix, HSILs include cervical intraepithelial neoplasia (CIN) grades 2 or 3, and adenocarcinoma in situ (AIS), which are precancerous lesions. LSIL and HSIL are lesions detected through routine screening with cytologic testing (Papanicolaou [Pap] test); tissue biopsy is required to make the diagnosis of CIN.

Recurrent respiratory papillomatosis (RRP) is a rare condition characterized by recurring papillomas in the larynx or other areas of the upper or lower respiratory tract. Onset can occur in childhood or adulthood. The disease is referred to as juvenile-onset RRP (JORRP) when it occurs before 12 years of age and as adult-onset RRP (AORRP) when it occurs at an older age. JORRP is believed to result most frequently from vertical transmission of HPV at the time of delivery. JORRP is diagnosed most commonly in children between 2 and 5 years of age, with manifestations of voice change (eg, hoarseness or abnormal cry), stridor, chronic cough, or respiratory distress.

---

[1] The terms female and male refer to sex assigned at birth.

Respiratory papillomas can cause respiratory tract obstruction in young children, and repeated surgeries often are needed. Most cases of JORRP are caused by HPV 6 or 11. AORRP most frequently occurs between 20 and 40 years of age, with causal HPV infections most likely acquired through sexual behavior. Most cases of JORRP and AORRP are caused by HPV 6 or 11. Prevalence of HPV type 6 in JORRP (50%–70%) and AORRP (~60%) is generally higher than that of HPV 11 (6%–29%).

Epidermodysplasia verruciformis is a rare, inherited disorder believed to be a consequence of a deficiency of cell-mediated immunity, resulting in an abnormal susceptibility to certain HPV types and manifesting as chronic cutaneous lesions and skin cancers. Lesions may resemble flat warts or pigmented plaques covering the torso and upper extremities. Most appear during the first decade of life, but malignant transformation, which occurs in 30% to 60% of affected people, usually is delayed until adulthood.

ETIOLOGY: HPVs are small, nonenveloped, double-stranded DNA viruses of the *Papillomaviridae* family, which are grouped into genera, species, and types based on DNA sequence variation. More than 200 types are recognized, but specific tissue tropism and disease associations are limited to date to less than 40 types. Types 6 and 11 cause anogenital warts (condylomata acuminata), recurrent respiratory papillomatosis, and conjunctival papillomas but rarely are found in cancer. High-risk HPV types (HPV 16, 18, 31, 33, 35, 39, 45, 51, 52, 56, 58, 59, 66, and 68) can be detected in almost all cervical precancers and invasive cervical cancers. Approximately 50% of cervical cancers worldwide are attributable to HPV type 16; 70% are attributable to either type 16 or 18. The majority of other HPV-related cancers—anogenital cancers (vulvar, vaginal, penile, anal) and oropharyngeal cancers—also are attributable to HPV type 16. Infection with a high-risk HPV type is considered necessary but not sufficient to cause cancer. The vast majority of people with an HPV infection will not develop cancer. Risk of developing cancer precursors or cancers is greater in people with certain immunocompromising conditions, such as human immunodeficiency virus (HIV) infection, cellular immune deficiencies, organ transplantation, and autoimmune diseases.

EPIDEMIOLOGY: Virtually all adults will be infected with some type of HPV during their lives. In the United States, it is estimated that 42 million people are infected with disease-associated HPV and 13 million people acquire a new anogenital HPV infection each year. Although HPV is common in the general population, specific risk factors include higher lifetime number of sex partners, earlier age at first sex, and immunocompromising conditions, including HIV infection. Groups that are disproportionately affected include transgender women and gay, bisexual, and other men who have sex with men.

Nongenital hand and foot warts occur commonly among school-aged children. Acquisition can occur through casual contact and is facilitated by minor skin trauma. Autoinoculation can result in spread of lesions. The intense and often widespread appearance of cutaneous warts in people with compromised cellular immunity (particularly those who have undergone transplantation or who have HIV infection) suggests that alterations in T-lymphocyte immunity may impair clearance of infection.

Genital HPV infections are transmitted by intimate contact through sexual intercourse or other close genital contact. In female individuals in the United States, the highest prevalence of infection is in 20- to 24-year-olds. Most infections are subclinical and clear spontaneously within 1 or 2 years. Cancer is an uncommon outcome of infection that generally requires decades of persistent infection with high-risk HPV types. There are more than 33 000 cases of HPV-attributable cancers annually in the United States. HPV-attributable cervical cancer accounts for approximately one third of new HPV-attributable cancer cases and 4000 deaths annually in the United States. HPV-attributable oropharyngeal cancer accounts for more than one third of new HPV-attributable cancer cases per year. HPV is the cause of at least 90% of all cervical cancers, 70% to 90% of oropharyngeal cancers, and most vulvar, vaginal, penile, and anal cancers.

Rarely, HPV infection is perinatally transmitted to a child during passage through an infected birth canal at delivery, or postnatally transmitted from nongenital sites. When anogenital warts are diagnosed in a child, the possibility of sexual abuse must be considered while noting the possibility of vertical transmission to neonates (see STI Evaluation After Sexual Assault of a Prepubertal Child, p 184, and Table 2.5, p 183).

The **incubation period** for symptoms of warts is estimated to range from 3 to 6 months. The period from infection to LSIL is likely similar. The period from infection to neoplastic changes is usually years to decades.

DIAGNOSTIC TESTS: Most cutaneous and anogenital warts can be diagnosed through clinical inspection. Serologic testing for HPV antibodies does not inform clinical decisions and is not commercially available. HPV-associated cervical lesions are detected through screening methods (described below). Anal, vulvar, vaginal, and penile lesions may be identified using visual inspection, sometimes using magnification; in some cases, cytologic screening is used and suspicious lesions are biopsied, but to date there is no routine screening recommended for cancers at these sites. Many dentists screen for oral cancer but there is no widely implemented screening program.

For all anogenital, oropharyngeal, and respiratory tract precancers and cancers, diagnosis is made histologically. Identifying the presence of HPV requires detection of viral nucleic acid (DNA or RNA) in a cellular sample from the lesion. Routine cervical cancer screening guidelines have been established by multiple professional societies (see Cervical Cancer Screening, p 508). Because high-risk HPV is a sensitive biomarker for cervical disease, primary screening with nucleic acid amplification tests (NAATs) for high-risk HPV types is increasingly favored for female individuals starting at age 25 years. The increased sensitivity of HPV testing allows longer screening intervals for people with negative test results. HPV tests may also be used in combination with cytologic testing in female individuals 30 years or older and for triage of equivocal cytology test abnormalities (atypical squamous cells of undetermined significance [ASCUS]) in those 21 years or older. Clinical HPV testing requires use of an assay approved by the US Food and Drug Administration (FDA) conducted in a CLIA-approved laboratory. There are differences in the appropriate clinical applications for each of these assays, including whether they can be used as an initial standalone test (ie, without cervical cytology) or in a primary screening algorithm; none is recommended for use in female individuals younger than 21 years or for male individuals. Criteria for abnormalities that require colposcopic evaluation and biopsy are included as part of professional societies' guidelines.

TREATMENT[1]: There is no FDA-approved treatment for HPV infection. Treatment may be directed toward lesions caused by HPV.

Regression of **nongenital and genital warts** occurs in approximately 30% of cases within 6 months and 90% within several years, even without treatment. Most methods of treatment of cutaneous warts use chemical or physical destruction of the infected epithelium, including cryotherapy with liquid nitrogen, laser or surgical removal of warts, application of salicylic acid products, or application of topical immune-modulating agents. Many agents used for treatment of warts have not been tested for safety and efficacy in children, and some are contraindicated in pregnancy.

Daily treatment with tretinoin has been useful for widespread flat warts in children. Systemic treatments, including cimetidine, have been used for refractory warts with variable success. Treatments for genital warts are characterized as patient-applied or provider administered. Interventions include ablational/excisional treatments, topical antiproliferative medications, or immune-modulating medications. Oral warts can be removed through cryotherapy, electrocautery, or surgical excision. Although most forms of therapy are successful for initial removal of warts, treatment may not eradicate HPV infection from the surrounding tissue and recurrences are common.

Cancer precursor lesions that are identified in the cervix (eg, AIS, CIN 2, CIN 3) or elsewhere in the genital tract may require excision or destruction. Treatment of cervical lesions can cause substantial economic, emotional, and reproductive adverse effects, including higher risk of preterm birth and perinatal mortality. Management of invasive cervical and other anogenital and oropharyngeal cancers requires a specialist and should be conducted according to current guidelines.

Respiratory papillomatosis is difficult to treat and is best managed by an experienced otolaryngologist. Local recurrence is common, and repeated surgical debulking procedures are often necessary to relieve airway obstruction, especially in young children because of their small airway diameter. Extension or dissemination of respiratory papillomas from the larynx into the trachea, bronchi, or lung parenchyma happens rarely but results in increased morbidity and mortality; malignant transformation occurs rarely. Intralesional interferon, oral indole-3-carbinole, systemic or intralesional bevacizumab, intralesional cidofovir, and HPV vaccination have been used as investigational treatments; however, efficacy with any of these is unproven.

INFECTION PREVENTION AND CONTROL MEASURES IN HEALTH CARE SETTINGS: Standard precautions are recommended.

CONTROL MEASURES AND CARE OF EXPOSED PEOPLE: Sexual abuse should be considered if anogenital warts are found in a child. When anogenital warts are found in a child who is prepubertal, the patient should be referred to a child abuse management pediatrician for an abuse evaluation (see STI Evaluation After Sexual Assault of a Prepubertal Child, p 184, and Table 2.5, p 183). Suspected child sexual abuse should be reported to the appropriate local agency.

Most cancer-causing HPV infections can be prevented by vaccination (see below). Delaying sexual debut and minimizing the lifetime number of sex partners are other modes of reducing risk of HPV infection. Consistent and correct use of latex condoms

---

[1] Centers for Disease Control and Prevention. Sexually transmitted infections treatment guidelines, 2021. *MMWR Recomm Rep*. 2021;70(RR-4):1-187. Available at: **www.cdc.gov/std/treatment-guidelines/hpv.htm**

may reduce the risk of anogenital HPV infection when infected areas are covered or protected by the condom. The degree and duration of contagiousness in patients with a history of genital HPV infection is unknown. People with genital warts should refrain from sex with new partners while warts are present and should inform their current sex partners, who also may benefit from a clinical evaluation for anogenital warts or other sexually transmitted infections.

Although JORRP is believed to be caused by perinatal transmission of HPV types 6 and 11 during passage through the birth canal, this condition has occurred in infants born by cesarean delivery. Because the preventive value of cesarean delivery is unknown, it should not be performed solely to prevent transmission of HPV to the newborn infant.

Cervical Cancer Screening. Female individuals who have received HPV vaccine should continue to have regular cervical cancer screening. HPV vaccines do not provide protection against all HPV types associated with development of cervical cancer and do not alter the course of infections existing before vaccination. Several professional organizations offer guidance on cervical cancer screening, including the American College of Obstetricians and Gynecologists (**www.acog.org**), the American Cancer Society (**www.cancer.org**), the American Society for Colposcopy and Cervical Pathology (**www.asccp.org**), and the US Preventive Services Task Force (**www. uspreventiveservicestaskforce.org**). These organizations, with one exception, all recommend that cervical cytologic testing begin at 21 years of age for all healthy female individuals, regardless of sexual history (the American Cancer Society recommends testing begin at 25 years of age). HIV-infected female adolescents who have initiated sexual intercourse should have cervical cytologic screening (liquid-based or Pap smear) performed twice at 6-month intervals during the first year after diagnosis of HIV infection, and if the results are normal, annually thereafter (**https:// clinicalinfo.hiv.gov/en/guidelines**). Sexually active female adolescents who have had an organ transplant or are receiving long-term corticosteroid therapy also should undergo similar cervical cytologic screening.

HPV Vaccines. Three HPV vaccines have been licensed by the FDA for use in the United States, but only one, Gardasil 9, a 9-valent vaccine (types 6, 11, 16, 18, 31, 33, 45, 52, and 58), licensed in 2014, is currently on the US market. A quadrivalent vaccine (4vHPV [types 6, 11, 16, and 18], Gardasil) was licensed in 2006, and a bivalent vaccine (2vHPV [types 16 and 18], Cervarix) was licensed in 2009.

Immunogenicity. More than 97% of healthy vaccine recipients develop antibodies to HPV vaccine types after vaccination. Antibody titers are higher in adolescents aged 9 through 15 years compared with those 16 through 26 years of age.

Antibody titers for all HPV vaccines decrease over time but plateau by 18 to 24 months after vaccination. Follow-up studies through 8 and 10 years after 4vHPV and 2vHPV vaccination, respectively, have shown no waning of protection. Studies of 9vHPV vaccine have found that antibody titers after 2 doses administered 6 to 12 months apart to 9- through 14-year-olds are similar to 3 doses administered to women 16 through 26 years of age, the age group in which efficacy was demonstrated in clinical trials.

Efficacy. 4vHPV and 2vHPV have been shown to be highly effective in preventing cervical precancers related to HPV types 16 and 18 in clinical trials among females

15 through 26 years of age. 4vHPV has been shown to be highly effective in preventing genital warts related to HPV types 6 and 11 in clinical trials among female and male individuals 16 through 26 years of age. 4vHPV also has been shown to be highly effective in preventing anal precancers in male individuals 16 through 26 years of age. 9vHPV has been shown in a clinical trial among female individuals 16 through 26 years of age to provide 97% protection against the additional 5 HPV types in the 9-valent product (31, 33, 45, 52, and 58) and to produce noninferior immunogenicity for the 4 HPV types in the quadrivalent product (6, 11, 16, and 18). Clinical trials of 2vHPV and 4vHPV have been conducted in female individuals older than 26 years; in those without evidence of prior HPV vaccine type infection, efficacy has been demonstrated for a combined endpoint of vaccine-type infection and cervical precancers. HPV vaccines have not been proven to have a therapeutic effect on existing HPV infection or disease and do not offer protection against progression of infection to disease from HPV acquired before immunization. Therefore, HPV vaccines are most effective when administered before exposure to any of the HPV types included in the vaccine.

Assessment of the full impact of HPV vaccination on anogenital and oropharyngeal cancers will take decades, given the natural history of HPV-driven oncogenesis. However, studies have already demonstrated significant reductions in HPV-related outcomes since the vaccines were introduced, including declines in vaccine-type HPV prevalence, anogenital warts, JORPP, cervical precancers, and cervical cancers. Long-term follow-up studies are being conducted to determine the duration of protection for all HPV vaccines.

Vaccine Recommendations.[1] The American Academy of Pediatrics (AAP) and the Advisory Committee on Immunization Practices (ACIP) of the Centers for Disease Control and Prevention recommend routine HPV vaccination for all adolescents. The AAP recommends starting the series between the ages of 9 and 12 years, at an age the pediatric health care professional deems optimal for acceptance and completion of the vaccination series. The ACIP recommends starting the series at age 11 or 12 years and states that vaccination can be administered starting at age 9 years. When HPV vaccination is initiated at 9 or 10 years of age, other adolescent vaccines (eg, MenACWY and Tdap) still are recommended to be administered at 11 to 12 years of age.

Pediatric health care professionals are encouraged to recommend HPV vaccination as they do other routine childhood and adolescent vaccines. Research has demonstrated that parents are influenced by effectively delivered recommendations and personal testimonials from their child's pediatrician. Opportunities to prevent cancers and deaths are being missed by clinicians who describe HPV vaccine as a sexually transmitted infection vaccine rather than a cancer prevention vaccine or who fail to inform patients and their parents or guardians that HPV vaccination is routinely recommended.

Catch-up HPV vaccination is recommended for all people through age 26 years who are not adequately vaccinated. Catch-up HPV vaccination is not recommended

---

[1] Meites E, Szilagyi PG, Chesson HW, Unger ER, Romero JR, Markowitz LE. Human papillomavirus vaccination for adults: updated recommendations of the Advisory Committee on Immunization Practices. *MMWR Morb Mortal Wkly Rep*. 2019;68(32):698–702. Available at: **www.cdc.gov/mmwr/volumes/68/wr/mm6832a3.htm**

for all adults 27 years or older. Instead, shared clinical decision-making regarding HPV vaccination is recommended for some adults 27 through 45 years of age who are not adequately vaccinated.

Dosage and Administration. HPV vaccine is administered in either 2 or 3 doses of 0.5 mL, intramuscularly, preferably in a deltoid muscle.

- For people initiating vaccination before their 15th birthday, the recommended schedule is 2 doses of HPV vaccine, with the second dose administered 6 to 12 months after the first dose (minimum interval 5 months).
- For people initiating vaccination on or after their 15th birthday, the recommended schedule is 3 doses of HPV vaccine. In a 3-dose schedule, the second dose should be administered at least 1 to 2 months after the first dose (minimum interval 4 weeks), and the third dose should be administered 6 months after the first dose (minimum interval 5 months after first dose, and 12 weeks after second dose).
- People considered adequately vaccinated are those:
  - Who initiated vaccination before their 15th birthday and received 2 doses of any HPV vaccine (9vHPV, 4vHPV, or 2vHPV) at the recommended dosing schedule (0, 6–12 months), or 3 doses of any HPV vaccine at the recommended dosing schedule (0, 1–2, 6 months).
  - Who initiated vaccination on or after their 15th birthday and received 3 doses of any HPV vaccine (9vHPV, 4vHPV, or 2vHPV) at the recommended dosing schedule (0, 1–2, 6 months). (Also see section on recommendations for special populations, below).
- If the vaccine schedule is interrupted, the vaccine series can be continued with the next recommended dose and does not need to be restarted.
- 9vHPV may be used to complete a series started with 4vHPV or 2vHPV.
- There is no recommendation regarding additional vaccination with 9vHPV for people who previously completed a 4vHPV or 2vHPV vaccination series.
- Evidence of past HPV exposure or current HPV infection or disease, such as abnormal cytologic test results, cervical lesions, anogenital warts, or a positive HPV DNA test result, are not contraindications to HPV immunization. People in the recommended age ranges still should receive HPV vaccine to protect against any HPV types not already acquired.
- HPV vaccines can be coadministered with any live or non-live vaccine indicated at the same visit.

Recommendations for Special Populations. HPV vaccines are not live vaccines. For people ages 9 through 26 years with immunocompromising conditions (including primary or secondary immunocompromising conditions that might reduce cell-mediated or humoral immunity, such as B-lymphocyte antibody deficiencies, T-lymphocyte complete or partial defects, HIV infection, malignant neoplasms, transplantation, autoimmune disease, or immunosuppressive therapy), a 3-dose schedule of HPV vaccine is recommended regardless of age at initiation. Immune response and vaccine efficacy in immunocompromised people might be less than that in immunocompetent people.

For children with a history of sexual abuse or assault, the HPV vaccination series should be started at 9 years of age, because they may be at higher risk of repeat abuse or assault.

Vaccine Adverse Events, Precautions, and Contraindications. Studies of more than 15 000 people in clinical trials for each of the HPV vaccines have shown no serious safety concerns. In addition, more than 135 million doses of HPV vaccines have been distributed in the United States without evidence for serious safety concerns. Injection site discomfort or pain, redness, and swelling are the most commonly reported local adverse events. Systemic symptoms after HPV vaccine include headache, fever, nausea, dizziness, and fatigue/malaise. Syncope (fainting) has been reported in adolescents after receipt of any vaccination, including HPV vaccine. Despite common misinformation disseminated mainly on the internet and through social media, HPV vaccine has not been associated with ovarian damage, infertility, or postural orthostatic tachycardia syndrome (POTS).

HPV vaccines can be administered to people with minor acute illnesses. Other considerations include:

- Immunization of people with moderate or severe acute illnesses should be deferred until after their condition improves.
- HPV vaccines are produced in yeast and are contraindicated in people with a history of immediate hypersensitivity to any vaccine component, including yeast.
- HPV vaccines are not recommended for use during pregnancy because of limited information about safety. The health care professional should inquire about pregnancy in patients who are known to be sexually active, but a pregnancy test is not required before starting the HPV vaccination series. If a vaccine recipient becomes pregnant, subsequent doses should be postponed until the person is no longer pregnant. If a dose has been administered inadvertently during pregnancy, no intervention is needed. Data to date show no evidence of adverse effect of any HPV vaccine on outcomes of pregnancy. Health care professionals can report inadvertent administrations of 9vHPV to pregnant people by calling the vaccine manufacturer at 1-877-888-4231.
- HPV vaccines can be administered to lactating people.
- Vaccine providers, particularly when vaccinating adolescents, should observe patients (with patients seated or lying down) for 15 minutes after vaccination to decrease the risk for injury should they faint and as is recommended for all vaccines. If syncope develops, patients should be observed until symptoms resolve.

Influenza

CLINICAL MANIFESTATIONS: Influenza illness typically begins with sudden onset of fever, often accompanied by nonproductive cough, chills or rigors, diffuse myalgia, headache, and malaise. Subsequently, respiratory tract symptoms including sore throat, nasal congestion, rhinitis, and cough become more prominent. Less commonly, abdominal pain, nausea, vomiting, and diarrhea are associated with influenza illness. In some children, influenza can appear as an upper respiratory tract illness or as a febrile illness with few respiratory tract symptoms. In infants, influenza can produce a nonspecific sepsis-like illness, and in infants and young children, influenza can cause otitis media, croup, pertussis like-illness, bronchiolitis, or pneumonia. Acute myositis secondary to influenza can present with calf tenderness and refusal to walk.

Although most children with influenza recover fully after 3 to 7 days of illness, complications may occur, even in previously healthy children. Neurologic complications associated with influenza range from febrile seizures to severe encephalopathy and encephalitis with status epilepticus, resulting in neurologic sequelae or death. Reye syndrome, now a very rare condition, has been associated with influenza infection and the use of aspirin therapy during the illness. Children with influenza or suspected influenza should not be given aspirin, and children with diseases that necessitate long-term aspirin therapy or salicylate-containing medication, including juvenile idiopathic arthritis or Kawasaki disease, should be recognized as being at increased risk for complications from influenza. Death from influenza-associated myocarditis has been reported. Invasive secondary infections or coinfections with *Staphylococcus aureus* (including methicillin-resistant *S aureus* [MRSA]), *Streptococcus pneumoniae,* group A streptococcus, or other bacterial pathogens can result in severe disease and death.

ETIOLOGY: Influenza viruses are orthomyxoviruses of 3 genera or types (A, B, and C). Annual epidemics are caused by influenza virus types A and B, and both influenza A and B virus antigens are included in seasonal influenza vaccines. Type C influenza viruses can cause sporadic mild influenza-like illness in children. Type C antigens are not included in influenza vaccines. Influenza A viruses are further classified into subtypes based on their surface antigens, hemagglutinin (HA) and neuraminidase (NA). Examples of these virus subtypes include H1N1 and H3N2 influenza A viruses. Specific antibodies to these antigens, especially to hemagglutinin, are important determinants of immunity.

A minor antigenic variation that leads to changes in the HA or NA surface proteins of influenza A or B viruses is termed *antigenic drift.* Antigenic drift occurs continuously and results in new strains of influenza A and B viruses, resulting in seasonal epidemics.

A major antigenic variation that leads to new subtypes containing a unique HA and/or NA is termed *antigenic shift.* If the new virus subtype infects humans and is transmitted efficiently from person to person in a sustained manner, a pandemic can occur because the human population has little or no preexisting immunity to the newly emerged influenza strain. Antigenic shift occurs only among influenza A viruses and has produced 4 influenza pandemics in the 20th and 21st centuries, the most recent in 2009. As with previous antigenic shifts, the 2009 pandemic influenza A (H1N1pdm09) viral strain subsequently replaced the previously circulating seasonal influenza A (H1N1) strain in the ensuing influenza seasons.

Humans of all ages may sporadically be infected with emerging influenza A viruses of swine or avian origin. Most notable among avian influenza viruses are A (H5N1), which emerged in 1997 in Hong Kong, and A (H7N9), first detected in 2013 in China, both of which have been associated with severe disease and high case fatality rates. Since 2017, the Asian (H7N9) subtype is considered the influenza virus with the highest potential pandemic risk.

EPIDEMIOLOGY: Influenza is highly contagious. The virus is spread person to person, primarily through large-particle respiratory droplet transmission (eg, coughing or sneezing), which requires close proximity between the person who is the source and the person who is the recipient because droplets generally only travel short distances. Another mode of transmission comes from contact with influenza virus from droplet-contaminated hands or surfaces, where it can remain viable for up to 24 hours, with transfer from hands to mucosal surfaces of the face. Airborne transmission via small-particle aerosols in the vicinity of the infectious individual also may occur. Patients may be infectious 24 hours before onset of symptoms. Viral shedding in nasal secretions usually peaks during the first 3 days of illness and ceases within 7 days but prolonged shedding (10 days or longer) can occur in young children and immunocompromised patients.

Influenza activity in the United States typically occurs anytime from October to May, commonly peaking between December and February. Seasonal epidemics can last 8 to 12 weeks or longer. Circulation of 2 or 3 influenza virus strains in a community may be associated with a prolonged influenza season and may produce bimodal peaks in activity.

Seasonal influenza epidemics are associated with an estimated 9.3 to 41 million illnesses, 140 000 to 710 000 hospitalizations, and 12 000 to 52 000 respiratory and circulatory deaths annually in the United States. The CDC estimates that on average, 8% (range, 3%–11%) of the US population develops symptomatic influenza illness during a typical season, depending on the circulating strains. During community outbreaks of influenza, the highest influenza incidence occurs among children, ranging from 10% to 40%, particularly school-aged children. Secondary spread to adults and other children within a family is common. Spread within schools can be a driver of more widespread transmission within the community.

Hospitalization rates are highest in those younger than 5 years and are similar to hospitalization rates among people 65 years and older. Although rates vary across studies (190–480 per 100 000 population) because of differences in methodology and severity of influenza seasons, children younger than 2 years consistently are at a substantially higher risk of hospitalization than are older children. Rates of hospitalization and morbidity attributable to complications, such as pneumonia, are greater in children with high-risk conditions, including chronic pulmonary diseases such as asthma, neurologic and neurodevelopmental disorders, hemodynamically significant cardiac disease, obesity, immunosuppression, metabolic diseases such as diabetes mellitus, and hemoglobinopathies such as sickle cell disease. However, 40% to 50% of all children hospitalized with influenza have no known underlying conditions, and almost half of children who die from influenza do not have an underlying high-risk condition. The total number of reported annual influenza-related deaths in the United States, including both chronically ill and previously healthy children, usually ranges from 35 to 199, with higher numbers reported in some seasons; actual numbers of deaths likely exceed the reported values.

Information about influenza surveillance is available through **www.cdc.gov/flu/weekly.**

The **incubation period** usually is 1 to 4 days, with a mean of 2 days.

DIAGNOSTIC TESTS: Influenza testing should be performed in children with signs and symptoms of influenza when test results are anticipated to impact clinical management (eg, to inform the decision to initiate antiviral or antibiotic therapy, pursue other diagnostic testing, or initiate infection prevention and control measures). The decision to test is related to the level of local influenza activity, clinical suspicion for influenza, and the sensitivity and specificity of commercially available influenza tests (Table 3.26). These include rapid molecular tests for influenza called nucleic acid amplification tests (NAATs) as part of single-plex or multiplex assays, immunofluorescence assays

Table 3.26. Summary of Influenza Diagnostic Tests

Influenza Diagnostic Test	Method	Availability	Typical Processing Time	Sensitivity	Types Detected
Rapid influenza diagnostic tests (RIDTs)[a]	Antigen detection	Wide	<15 min	Moderate	A and B
Rapid molecular assays[b]	Nucleic acid amplification	Wide	15–30 min	High	A and B
Molecular assays (including RT-PCR)[c]	Nucleic acid amplification	Limited	1–8 h	High	A and B
Direct and indirect Immunofluorescence antibody assays[c]	Antigen detection	Wide	1–4 h	Moderate	A and B
Rapid cell culture (shell vials and cell mixtures)[c]	Virus isolation	Limited	1–3 days	High	A and B
Tissue cell culture[c]	Virus isolation	Limited	3–10 days	High	A and B

RT-PCR indicates reverse transcriptase-polymerase chain reaction. May be single-plex or multiplex, real time, and other RNA-based assays.

[a] Most rapid influenza diagnostic tests are CLIA waived.
[b] Some rapid influenza molecular assays are CLIA waived, depending on the specimen.
[c] Not CLIA waived. Requires laboratory expertise.

Adapted from **www.cdc.gov/flu/professionals/diagnosis/overview-testing-methods.htm.**

(direct [DFA] or indirect [IFA] fluorescent antibody staining) for antigen detection, rapid influenza diagnostic tests (RIDTs) based on antigen detection, rapid cell culture (shell vial culture), and viral tissue cell culture (conventional) for virus isolation. The optimal choice of influenza test depends on the clinical setting.

The sensitivity and specificity of any influenza test varies by the type of test used (Table 3.26), the time from illness onset, specimen quality and source, and specimen handling and processing. To diagnose influenza in the outpatient or inpatient setting, testing should occur as soon after illness onset as possible, because the quantity of virus shed decreases rapidly as illness progresses. Nasopharyngeal swab specimens have the highest yield of upper respiratory tract specimens for detection of influenza viruses. Mid-turbinate nasal swab or wash specimens are also acceptable. Testing with combined nasal and throat swab specimens may increase the detection of influenza viruses over single specimens from either site (particularly over throat swab specimens alone). Using flocked swabs likely improves influenza virus detection over nonflocked swabs.

When influenza is circulating in the community, hospitalized patients with signs and symptoms of influenza should be tested with a molecular NAAT with high sensitivity and specificity. For patients with respiratory failure receiving mechanical ventilation, including patients with negative influenza testing results on upper respiratory tract specimens, endotracheal aspirate or bronchoalveolar lavage (BAL) fluid specimens should be obtained. Nonrespiratory specimens such as blood, plasma, serum, cerebrospinal fluid, urine, and stool should not be used for routine diagnosis of influenza.

At-home tests are available for children as young as 2 years. The use of at-home test results to inform treatment decisions should be informed by the sensitivity and specificity of the test, the prevalence of influenza in the community, and the presence and duration of compatible signs and symptoms.

Results of influenza testing should be properly interpreted in the context of clinical findings and local community influenza activity, because the prevalence of circulating influenza viruses influences the positive and negative predictive values of these influenza screening tests. False-positive results are more likely to occur during periods of low influenza activity; false-negative results are more likely to occur during periods of peak influenza activity.

TREATMENT: In the United States, 3 classes of antiviral medications with different mechanisms of action currently are approved for treatment or prophylaxis of influenza infections. Two of these classes are used in clinical management of influenza disease: 3 drugs in the neuraminidase inhibitor class (oral oseltamivir, inhaled zanamivir, and intravenous peramivir) and 1 drug in the cap-dependent endonuclease inhibitor class (oral baloxavir marboxil). Guidance for use of these antiviral agents is summarized in Table 3.27 and at **https://publications.aap.org/redbook/resources/15189** and **www.cdc.gov/flu/professionals/antivirals/index.htm.** Recommended dosages for drugs approved for treatment and prophylaxis of influenza are provided in Table 4.10 (p 1044).

Oseltamivir is the preferred antiviral medication for patients with influenza A and B. The US Food and Drug Administration (FDA) has approved oseltamivir for influenza treatment in children as young as 2 weeks of age. However, the available pharmacokinetic and safety data suggest that oseltamivir can be used to treat influenza in both term and preterm infants from birth, because benefits of therapy are likely to outweigh possible risks of treatment. Initiation of antiviral therapy should be based on signs and symptoms consistent with influenza infection and epidemiologic factors. Provision of antiviral therapy does not require a positive test result for influenza.

Inhaled zanamivir is an acceptable alternative for children 7 years and older. Intravenous peramivir is approved for use in people 6 months and older. Oral baloxavir is approved for people 5 years and older.

Resistance to oseltamivir and zanamivir has been documented in less than 1% of the tested influenza viral samples during the past seasons. Decreased susceptibility to baloxavir has been reported in Japan, where use has been more common; surveillance for resistance among circulating influenza viruses is ongoing in the United States but remains rare. Each year, options for treatment or chemoprophylaxis of influenza in the United States will depend on influenza strain resistance patterns.

Regardless of influenza vaccination status, antiviral treatment should be offered as early as possible to the following individuals:
• Any hospitalized child with suspected or confirmed influenza disease, regardless of the duration of symptoms;

Table 3.27. Antiviral Drugs for Influenza[a]

Drug (Trade Name)	Virus	Adminis- tration	Treatment Indications	Chemopro- phylaxis Indications	Adverse Effects
Oseltamivir (Tamiflu)	A and B	Oral twice daily for 5 days	Birth or older[b]	3 mo or older	Nausea, vomiting, headache; skin reactions; diarrhea (children <1 year)
Zanamivir (Relenza)	A and B	Inhalation twice daily for 5 days	7 y or older	5 y or older	Bronchospasm, skin reactions
Peramivir (Rapivab)	A and B[c]	Intravenous as a single dose	6 m or older	Not recommended	Diarrhea, skin reactions
Baloxavir marboxil (Xofluxa)[d]	A and B	Oral as a single dose	5 y or older	5 y or older	Nausea, vomiting, diarrhea

[a]Recommended dosages for drugs approved for treatment and prophylaxis of influenza are provided in Table 4.10 (p 1044). For current recommendations about treatment and chemoprophylaxis of influenza, including specific dosing information, see **https://publications.aap.org/redbook** and **www.cdc.gov/flu/professionals/antivirals/index.htm.** Antiviral susceptibilities of viral strains are reported weekly at **www.cdc.gov/flu/weekly/fluactivitysurv.htm.**

[b]Approved by the FDA for children as young as 2 weeks of age. Given available pharmacokinetic data and limited safety data, the AAP believes that oseltamivir can be used to treat influenza in both term and preterm infants from birth because benefits of therapy are likely to outweigh possible risks of treatment.

[c]Peramivir efficacy is based on clinical trials in which the predominant influenza virus type was influenza A; a limited number of subjects infected with influenza B virus were enrolled.

[d]Long-acting endonuclease inhibitor with different mechanism of action than neuraminidase inhibitors. Greater activity on influenza B reported compared with oseltamivir. No data on use in pregnancy or breastfeeding. Not recommended in severely immunocompromised patients.

- Any child, inpatient or outpatient, with severe, complicated, or progressive illness attributable to influenza, regardless of the duration of symptoms or presence of high-risk conditions; and
- Any child, inpatient or outpatient, with influenza virus infection of any severity who is at high risk of complications of influenza, regardless of the duration of symptoms.

Antiviral treatment may be considered for the following individuals in the outpatient setting:
- Any child with suspected or confirmed influenza disease who is not at high risk for influenza complications, if treatment can be initiated within 48 hours of illness onset; and
- Any child with suspected or confirmed influenza disease whose siblings or household contacts are either younger than 6 months or at high risk for influenza complications.

Children with severe influenza should be evaluated carefully for possible coinfection with bacterial pathogens (eg, *S aureus* or *S pneumoniae*) that might require antimicrobial therapy.

The most common adverse effects of oseltamivir are nausea and vomiting. Postmarketing reports, almost exclusively from Japan, have noted self-injury and delirium with use of oseltamivir among pediatric patients, but other data suggest that these occurrences may have been related to influenza disease itself rather than antiviral therapy. An FDA review of controlled clinical trial data and ongoing surveillance did not establish a link between oseltamivir (or any influenza antiviral medication) and neurologic or psychiatric events. Zanamivir use has been associated with bronchospasm in some people and is not recommended for use in patients with chronic respiratory diseases, such as asthma or chronic obstructive pulmonary disease, which increase the risk of bronchospasm. Zanamivir is contraindicated in patients with milk protein allergy. The most common adverse effects of baloxavir are nausea, vomiting, and diarrhea.

Control of fever with acetaminophen or another appropriate nonsalicylate-containing antipyretic agent may be important in some children, because fever and other symptoms of influenza could exacerbate underlying chronic conditions. Children and adolescents with influenza should not receive aspirin or any salicylate-containing products because of the potential risk of developing Reye syndrome.

INFECTION PREVENTION AND CONTROL MEASURES IN HEALTH CARE SETTINGS: In addition to standard precautions, droplet precautions are recommended for children hospitalized with influenza or an influenza-like illness for the duration of illness.

CONTROL MEASURES:

Influenza Vaccines.[1] All people 6 months and older should be vaccinated annually against influenza. Two types of influenza vaccines are available for children: inactivated (non-live) influenza vaccines (IIVs), which contain no live virus and are given via intramuscular (IM) injection; and the live attenuated influenza vaccine (LAIV), which is given as a nasal spray. All influenza vaccines are formulated to protect against the same viral strains. The influenza virus strains selected for inclusion in the seasonal vaccine may change yearly in anticipation of the predominant influenza strains expected to circulate in the northern hemisphere in the upcoming influenza season on the basis of influenza circulation in the southern hemisphere and/or in the northern hemisphere's prior season. All pediatric influenza vaccines available in the United States since the 2019–2020 season are quadrivalent, containing 2 influenza A strains and 2 influenza B strains. All licensed pediatric vaccines in the United States are manufactured using virus grown in eggs (egg-based), except for 1 non-live cell-based vaccine. One recombinant vaccine is licensed for individuals 18 years and older. The age indication and dose vary among licensed influenza vaccines for children (see Fig 3.12, p 518). FDA-approved formulations of licensed influenza vaccines are available for children 6 months and older (see Table 3.28, p 519). The American Academy of Pediatrics (AAP) has no preference for any type of vaccine (IIV or LAIV) or formulation over another.

An adjuvanted, cell-based vaccine designed to protect against H5N1 in the event of a pandemic has been approved for children 6 months or older. Recommendations for its use would be made in the event that such a pandemic develops.

Immunogenicity and Dosing in Children. Children 9 years and older require only 1 dose of influenza vaccine annually, regardless of their influenza immunization history.

---

[1] American Academy of Pediatrics, Committee on Infectious Diseases. Policy statement. Recommendations for prevention and control of influenza in children, 2023-2024. *Pediatrics.* 2023;152(4):e2023063722

FIG 3.12. AVAILABLE INFLUENZA VACCINES IN THE UNITED STATES, BY FDA-LICENSED AGE INDICATION

Vaccine Type	6 through 23 mo	2 through 3 y	4 through 17 y	18 through 49 y	50 through 64 y	≥65 y
IIV4s (egg-based)	Afluria Quadrivalent Fluarix Quadrivalent FluLaval Quadrivalent Fluzone Quadrivalent					
IIV4 (cell-based)	Flucelvax Quadrivalent					
RIV4 (recombinant)				Flublok Quadrivalent		
Adjuvanted IIV3 and IIV4 (egg-based)						Fluad
High-dose IIV3 (egg-based)						Fluzone High-dose
LAIV4 (egg-based)			FluMist Quadrivalent			

Children 6 months through 8 years of age who are receiving the influenza vaccine for the first time or who have received only 1 dose before the upcoming influenza season should receive 2 doses of influenza vaccine administered at least 4 weeks apart. For children requiring 2 doses, vaccination should not be delayed to obtain a specific product for either dose. Any available, age-appropriate vaccine can be used. The doses do not need to be the same brand, and a child may receive a combination of IIV and LAIV if appropriate for age and health status. Protection against disease is achieved 1 to 2 weeks after the second dose. For children 8 years of age who require 2 doses of influenza vaccine, both doses should be administered even if the child turns age 9 years between dose 1 and dose 2.

Coadministration With Other Vaccines. Influenza vaccines can be administered simultaneously with other live and non-live vaccines, including COVID-19 vaccines. Receipt of recommended childhood vaccines during a single visit has important benefits of protecting children against many infectious diseases and minimizing the number of visits that parents or caregivers and children must make.

Recommendations for Influenza Immunization.[1-3] All people 6 months and older should receive influenza vaccine annually. Influenza vaccine should be offered as soon as it

[1] Grohskopf LA, Blanton LH, Ferdinands JM, et al. Prevention and control of seasonal influenza with vaccines: recommendations of the Advisory Committee on Immunization Practices—United States, 2022–23 influenza season. *MMWR Recomm Rep.* 2022;71(RR-1):1–28. For updates, see **www.cdc.gov/flu**

[2] American Academy of Pediatrics, Committee on Infectious Diseases. Policy statement. Recommendations for prevention and control of influenza in children, 2023–2024. *Pediatrics.* 2023;152(4):2023063772

[3] American Academy of Pediatrics, Committee on Infectious Diseases. Technical report. Recommendations for Prevention and Control of Influenza in Children, 2023–2024. *Pediatrics.* 2023;152(4):2023063773

Table 3.28. Schedule for Influenza Vaccine Dosing by Age[a]

Age	Dose, mL[b]	No. of Doses	Route[c]
6 through 35 mo	0.25	1–2[d]	Intramuscular (Afluria, Fluzone)[e]
	0.5	1–2[d]	Intramuscular (Fluzone, Fluarix, FluLaval, Afluria, Flucelvax)
3 y through 8 y	0.5	1–2[d]	Intramuscular
9 y through 17 y	0.5	1	Intramuscular
18 y or older	0.5	1	Intramuscular
2 y through 49 years (healthy)	0.2	1–2[d]	Intranasal (Flumist)

[a]Manufacturers include Sanofi Pasteur (Fluzone Quadrivalent, split-virus vaccines licensed for people 6 months or older, Fluzone High-Dose, and Flublok Quadrivalent, recombinant vaccine licensed for people 18 years or older), Seqirus (Afluria Quadrivalent, split virus vaccine for people 6 months and older; Flucelvax Quadrivalent cell-based vaccine licensed for people 6 months and older, and Fluad adjuvanted trivalent vaccine for people 65 years and older), GlaxoSmithKline Biologicals (Fluarix Quadrivalent and FluLaval Quadrivalent split-virus vaccines licensed for people 6 months or older), and AstraZeneca (live attenuated influenza vaccine for otherwise healthy persons 2–49 years of age).

[b]From: Grohskopf LA, Blanton LH, Ferdinands JM, et al. Prevention and control of seasonal influenza with vaccines: recommendations of the Advisory Committee on Immunization Practices—United States, 2022–23 influenza season. *MMWR Recomm Rep.* 2022;71(RR-1):1–28. Available at: **www.cdc.gov/mmwr/volumes/71/rr/rr7101a1.htm.** Dosages are those recommended in recent years. Refer to the product circular each year to ensure that the appropriate dosage is given for each available formulation.

[c]For adults and older children, the recommended site of immunization is the deltoid muscle. For infants and young children, the preferred site is the anterolateral aspect of the thigh.

[d]Two doses administered at least 4 weeks apart are recommended for children 6 months through 8 years who are receiving influenza vaccine for the first time, who have received a single dose prior to the start of the current season or whose immunization history is unknown.

[e]The 0.25-mL prefilled syringes for Afluria are no longer available. For children aged 6 through 35 months, a 0.25-mL dose must be obtained from a multidose vial for Afluria, or from a single-dose or a multidose vial for Fluzone.

becomes available, especially to children who require 2 doses, with the recommended dose(s) ideally received by the end of October (**www.cdc.gov/flu/**). Providers should continue to offer vaccine until the vaccine expiration date (typically June 30, marking the end of the influenza season), because influenza circulation is unpredictable. Particular efforts should focus on vaccination of all children and adolescents with factors associated with an elevated risk of complications from influenza, including the following:

- Age <5 years, and especially <2 years, regardless of the presence of underlying medical conditions.
- Residence in a chronic care facility or nursing home.
- Chronic pulmonary disease (including asthma, cystic fibrosis, and compromised respiratory function, eg, tracheostomy or requiring mechanical ventilation), hemodynamically significant cardiovascular disease (except hypertension alone), or renal (including chronic kidney disease, end-stage kidney disease, and dialysis), hepatic (including chronic liver disease and cirrhosis), hematologic (including sickle cell disease and other hemoglobinopathies), or metabolic disorders (including diabetes mellitus).

- Immunosuppression attributable to any cause, including that caused by medications (see Special Considerations) or by human immunodeficiency virus (HIV) infection (see Human Immunodeficiency Virus Infection, p 489).
- Neurologic and neurodevelopment conditions (including disorders of the brain, spinal cord, peripheral nerve, and muscle such as cerebral palsy, epilepsy, stroke, intellectual disability, moderate-to-severe developmental delay, muscular dystrophy, or spinal cord injury).
- Being pregnant or in the postpartum period during the influenza season.
- Receipt of long-term aspirin therapy or salicylate containing medications (including those with Kawasaki disease and rheumatologic conditions) because of increased risk of Reye syndrome.
- Extreme obesity (not well defined in children but could consider body mass index ≥99th percentile for age).

Special Considerations. The optimal time to provide inactivated influenza vaccine to children with malignant neoplasms is not well defined, but generally vaccine should be administered ≥2 weeks before cytotoxic chemotherapy when clinically possible. In children receiving immunosuppressive chemotherapy, influenza immunization may result in a less robust response than in immunocompetent children. IIV should be deferred in children who have received anti-B lymphocyte therapies in the previous 6 months until there is evidence of B lymphocyte recovery. Children who have completed chemotherapy ≥3 months prior generally have adequate rates of seroconversion. Transplantation recipients should receive IIV vaccination starting 4 to 6 months after hematopoietic cell transplantation and 3 months after solid organ transplantation (SOT), although IIV may be considered ≥1 month after SOT during the influenza season.

Corticosteroids administered daily for brief periods or every other day seem to have a minimal effect on antibody response to influenza vaccine. Prolonged administration (eg, ≥14 days) of high doses of corticosteroids (ie, a dose of prednisone of either 2 mg/kg or greater or a total of 20 mg/day or greater for children who weigh 10 kg or more or an equivalent dose of other corticosteroids) may impair antibody response. Influenza immunization can be deferred during the time of receipt of high-dose corticosteroids, provided deferral does not compromise the likelihood of immunization before the start of influenza season (see Vaccine Administration, p 52).

Children with hemodynamically unstable cardiac disease are at high risk of complications of influenza. The immune response to and safety of IIV in these children are comparable to the immune response and safety in healthy children.

Breastfeeding. Breastfeeding is not a contraindication for influenza immunization. Special effort should be made to vaccinate all persons who are breastfeeding during the influenza season if they were not vaccinated during pregnancy.

Influenza Control in Peri- and Postpartum Settings. Strategies to decrease the likelihood of transmission from a birth parent to the newborn child during the birth hospitalization are provided at **www.cdc.gov/flu/professionals/infectioncontrol/peri-post-settings.htm.**

Close Contacts of High-Risk Patients. Immunization of everyone who is in close contact with children younger than 5 years or children with high-risk conditions (see Recommendations for Influenza Immunization, p 518) is an important strategy to ensure protection for these children who may not benefit from adequate protection from vaccination alone.

Health Care Personnel. The AAP supports mandatory annual immunization programs for health care personnel (HCP), because HCP frequently come into contact with patients at high risk of influenza illness in clinical settings.[1]

Reactions, Adverse Effects, and Contraindications. The most common reactions after IIV administration are local injection site pain and tenderness. Fever may occur within 24 hours after immunization in approximately 10% to 35% of children younger than 2 years but rarely in older children and adults. Mild systemic symptoms, such as nausea, lethargy, headache, muscle aches, and chills, may occur after administration of IIV. LAIV may result in nasal congestion, rhinorrhea, and sore throat, as well as wheezing, particularly in younger children and those with chronic respiratory diseases such as asthma.

Anaphylaxis after receipt of any influenza vaccine is a contraindication to influenza vaccination. Children who have had an allergic reaction after a previous dose of any influenza vaccine should be evaluated by an allergist to help determine the vaccine component responsible for the reaction and whether or not future receipt of an influenza vaccine is appropriate. Children who are allergic to gelatin (very rare) should receive IIV rather than LAIV.

Minor illnesses, with or without fever, are not contraindications to the use of influenza vaccines, including among children with mild upper respiratory infection symptoms or allergic rhinitis. In children with a moderate to severe febrile illness (eg, high fever, active infection, requiring hospitalization, etc), on the basis of the judgment of the clinician, vaccination should be deferred until resolution of the illness. Similarly, children with an amount of nasal congestion that would notably impede vaccine delivery into the nasopharyngeal mucosa should have LAIV vaccination deferred until resolution, or should receive IIV since nasal congestion would not impact its delivery. LAIV is contraindicated in immunocompromised hosts and pregnant individuals as well as in patients with asplenia or central nervous system anatomic barrier defects (eg, cochlear implant, congenital dysplasia of the inner ear, persistent cerebrospinal fluid communication with nasopharynx/oropharynx) (see Table 1.17, p 94). LAIV may be administered to healthy household and other close contacts of people with altered immunocompetence (see Household Members of Immunocompromised Patients, p 103).

Although most influenza vaccines are produced in eggs and contain measurable amounts of egg protein, they are well tolerated by recipients with egg allergy of any severity. Special precautions for recipients of IIV or LAIV with egg allergy are not warranted, as the rate of anaphylaxis after administration is no greater in recipients with egg allergy versus those without egg allergy or from other universally recommended vaccines.

History of Guillain-Barré syndrome (GBS) following influenza vaccine is considered a precaution for the administration of influenza vaccines. Data on the risk of GBS following vaccination with seasonal influenza vaccine are variable and have been inconsistent across seasons. GBS is rare, especially in children, and there is a lack of evidence on risk of GBS following influenza vaccine in children. The decision not to immunize should be thoughtfully balanced against the potential morbidity and mortality associated with influenza for that individual.

[1] Bernstein HH; Starke JR; and the American Academy of Pediatrics, Committee on Infectious Diseases. Policy statement: Influenza immunization for all health care personnel: keep it mandatory. *Pediatrics*. 2015;136(4):809-818 (Reaffirmed March 2020)

Chemoprophylaxis. Chemoprophylaxis with influenza antivirals should not be considered a substitute for immunization. If not contraindicated, influenza vaccine always should be offered, even after influenza virus has begun circulating in the community. Health care professionals should inform recipients of antiviral chemoprophylaxis that the risk of influenza is lowered but still remains while taking medication, and susceptibility to influenza returns when medication is discontinued.

Chemoprophylaxis is not a contraindication to immunization with IIV and does not interfere with the immune response to IIV. Chemoprophylaxis should not be administered in conjunction with LAIV immunization, because antivirals will interfere with LAIV replication. On the basis of drug half-lives, it is prudent to assume interference is possible during the following periods: (1) for oseltamivir and zanamivir, from 48 hours before to 2 weeks after LAIV; (2) for peramivir, from 5 days before to 2 weeks after LAIV; and (3) for baloxavir, from 17 days before to 2 weeks after LAIV. Chemoprophylaxis is not recommended for infants younger than 3 months, unless the situation is judged critical, because of limited safety and efficacy data in this age group.

Antiviral options for influenza chemoprophylaxis are listed in Table 3.27 (p 516), with dosing information provided in Table 4.10 (p 1044). For current recommendations about chemoprophylaxis against influenza, see **www.cdc.gov/flu/professionals/antivirals/index.htm** or **https://publications.aap.org/redbook/resources/15189.**

Public Health Reporting. All influenza-associated pediatric deaths as well as all infections with a novel influenza A virus are nationally notifiable and should be reported to the Centers for Disease Control and Prevention (CDC) through state health departments.

Kawasaki Disease

CLINICAL MANIFESTATIONS: Kawasaki disease is a vasculitis of medium-sized arteries. The diagnosis is made in patients with fever in addition to the presence of the following clinical criteria:
1. Bilateral injection of the bulbar conjunctivae with limbic sparing and without exudate;
2. Erythematous mouth and pharynx, strawberry tongue, and/or red, cracked lips;
3. A polymorphous, generalized, erythematous rash, often with accentuation in the groin, which can be morbilliform, maculopapular, scarlatiniform, or erythema multiforme-like;
4. Changes in the peripheral extremities consisting of erythema of the palms and soles and firm, sometimes painful, induration of the hands and feet, often followed by periungual desquamation;
5. Acute, nonsuppurative, usually unilateral, anterior cervical lymphadenopathy with at least 1 node ≥1.5 cm in diameter.

The diagnosis of classic (or complete) Kawasaki disease is based on the presence of ≥5 days of fever and ≥4 of the 5 principal features above. The diagnosis may be made with only 4 days of fever if ≥4 principal clinical findings are present without alternative explanation. Individual clinical manifestations may appear and self-resolve rather than all being present simultaneously. It is important to inquire about previous presence of relevant manifestations when evaluating for persistent fever.

The correct diagnosis may be delayed in patients who present with fever and unilateral neck swelling, which mistakenly is believed to be attributable to bacterial lymph node or para- or retropharyngeal infection. A distinguishing clinical and imaging feature in these cases is that suppuration is not observed in Kawasaki disease. Concurrent viral upper respiratory infection sometimes is present in patients with Kawasaki disease and, even if confirmed by virus detection, should not delay treatment of Kawasaki disease. (An exception is the patient with fever, exudative conjunctivitis, and exudative pharyngitis, in whom adenovirus is detected. In such cases, Kawasaki disease is considered unlikely.)

The following mucocutaneous or laboratory findings should prompt a search for an alternative diagnosis to Kawasaki disease: bullous, vesicular, or petechial rash; oral ulcers; pharyngeal or conjunctival exudates; generalized lymphadenopathy or splenomegaly; or leukopenia or relative lymphocyte predominance. Prior infection with SARS-CoV-2, the virus that causes COVID-19, increases the likelihood of multisystem inflammatory syndrome in children (MIS-C) as the cause in a child presenting with symptoms suggestive of Kawasaki disease (see Coronavirus Disease 2019 [COVID-19], p 234). Although features of MIS-C overlap with those of Kawasaki disease, MIS-C has a wider spectrum of manifestations and a more severe illness course, with more than half of the patients developing hypotension or shock requiring admission to an intensive care unit. Patients with MIS-C have a median age of 9 years (compared with 2 years in Kawasaki disease), are more commonly Black or Hispanic (compared with being more likely of Asian ancestry in Kawasaki disease), and show greater elevation of inflammatory markers. More than 80% of patients with MIS-C also present with cardiac injury with high concentrations of troponin and brain natriuretic peptide, and some develop arrhythmia or left ventricle dysfunction. Although evidence of recent SARS-CoV-2 infection is necessary to diagnose MIS-C, such evidence does not rule out a diagnosis of Kawasaki disease because of the widespread occurrence of SARS-CoV-2 infection.

The diagnosis of incomplete Kawasaki disease should be considered in children with unexplained fever who have only 2 or 3 principal clinical criteria. Supportive laboratory and echocardiography data should be obtained when considering the diagnosis of incomplete Kawasaki disease. In 2017, the American Heart Association (AHA) published updated guidelines for the diagnosis, treatment, and long-term management of Kawasaki disease,[1] which provides an algorithm for diagnosis and treatment of suspected incomplete Kawasaki disease (reproduced in Fig 3.13). A high index of suspicion for Kawasaki disease should be maintained for infants, particularly those younger than 6 months, because compared with older children, infants have heightened risk of incomplete manifestations, delayed diagnosis, and development of coronary artery abnormalities. Kawasaki disease should be considered in infants younger than 12 months with prolonged unexplained fever, with or without aseptic meningitis, with evidence of systemic inflammation, even with fewer than 2 of the principal clinical features of Kawasaki disease; the AHA recommends

---

[1] McCrindle BW, Rowley AH, Newburger JW, et al; American Heart Association Rheumatic Fever, Endocarditis, and Kawasaki Disease Committee of the Council on Cardiovascular Disease in the Young; Council on Cardiovascular and Stroke Nursing; Council on Cardiovascular Surgery and Anesthesia; and Council on Epidemiology and Prevention. Diagnosis, treatment, and long-term management of Kawasaki disease: a scientific statement for health professionals from the American Heart Association. *Circulation.* Published online March 29, 2017; **www.ahajournals.org/doi/full/10.1161/ CIR.0000000000000484**

FIG 3.13. EVALUATION OF SUSPECTED INCOMPLETE KAWASAKI DISEASE[a]

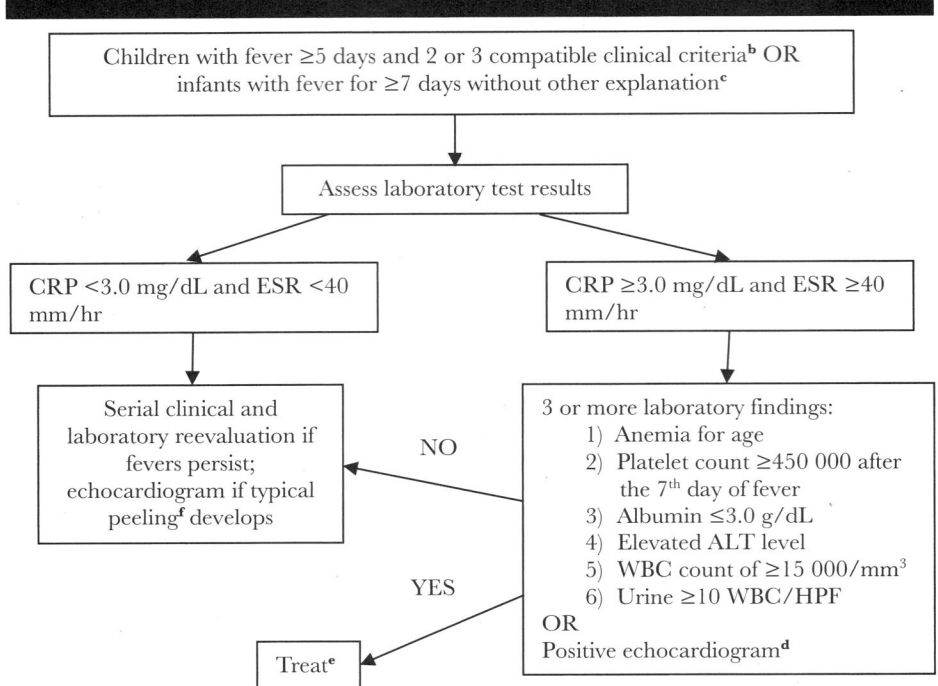

CRP indicates C-reactive protein; ESR, erythrocyte sedimentation rate; ALT, alanine aminotransferase; WBC, white blood cell; HPF, high-powered field.

[a] In the absence of a "gold standard" for diagnosis, this algorithm cannot be evidence based but rather represents the informed opinion of the expert committee. Consultation with an expert should be sought anytime assistance is needed.

[b] See text for clinical findings of Kawasaki disease.

[c] Infants ≤6 months of age are the most likely to develop prolonged fever without other clinical criteria for Kawasaki disease; these infants are at particularly high risk of developing coronary artery abnormalities.

[d] Echocardiography is considered positive for purposes of this algorithm if any of 3 conditions are met: z score of left anterior descending coronary artery or right coronary artery ≥2.5; coronary artery aneurysm is observed; or ≥3 other suggestive features exist, including decreased left ventricular function, mitral regurgitation, pericardial effusion, or z scores in left anterior descending coronary artery or right coronary artery of 2 to 2.5.

[e] Treatment should be given within 10 days of fever onset. See text for indications for treatment after the tenth day of fever.

[f] Typical peeling begins under the nail beds of fingers and toes.

Source: McCrindle BW, Rowley AH, Newburger JW, et al; American Heart Association Rheumatic Fever, Endocarditis, and Kawasaki Disease Committee of the Council on Cardiovascular Disease in the Young; Council on Cardiovascular and Stroke Nursing; Council on Cardiovascular Surgery and Anesthesia; and Council on Epidemiology and Prevention. Diagnosis, treatment, and long-term management of Kawasaki disease: a scientific statement for health professionals from the American Heart Association. *Circulation.* Published online March 29, 2017; **www.ahajournals.org/doi/full/10.1161/ CIR.0000000000000484**

echocardiography in all infants with 7 days of fever without another source. Other presentations of Kawasaki disease include infants and children with a shock-like syndrome in whom an inciting infection is not confirmed and those with presumed bacterial cervical lymphadenitis or para- or retropharyngeal phlegmon that fail to respond to appropriate antibiotic therapy.

If coronary artery aneurysm or dilatation is evident (z score ≥ 2.0 for the left anterior descending or right coronary arteries) in any patient evaluated for fever, a presumptive diagnosis of Kawasaki disease should be made. A normal early echocardiographic study is typical and does not exclude the diagnosis but may be useful in evaluation of patients with suspected incomplete Kawasaki disease. In one study, 80% of patients with Kawasaki disease who ultimately developed coronary artery disease had abnormalities (defined as a z score ≥ 2.5) on an echocardiogram obtained during the first 10 days of illness.

Other clinical features of Kawasaki disease include irritability, abdominal pain, diarrhea, and vomiting. Other examination and laboratory findings include urethritis with sterile pyuria (70% of cases), mild anterior uveitis, mild elevation of serum hepatobiliary enzyme concentrations (50%), arthralgia or arthritis (10%–20%), marked irritability with cerebrospinal fluid pleocytosis (40%), hydrops of the gallbladder (<10%), pericardial effusion of at least 1 mm (<5%), myocarditis manifesting as congestive heart failure (<5%), and cranial nerve palsy (<1%). Patients typically have multiple elevated acute phase reactants, such as C-reactive protein (CRP), erythrocyte sedimentation rate (ESR), platelets (after the first week of illness), and white blood cells (with left shift). They commonly have a normocytic, normochromic anemia. Persistent resting tachycardia and a hyperdynamic precordium are common findings, and an S3 gallop can be present. Fine desquamation in the groin area can occur in the acute phase of disease (Fink sign). Inflammation or ulceration may be observed at the inoculation scar of previous bacille Calmette-Guérin immunization. Rarely, Kawasaki disease can present with acute shock; these children often have significant thrombocytopenia attributable to consumption coagulopathy, which also causes a low ESR. Group A streptococcal or *Staphylococcus aureus* toxic shock syndrome should be excluded in such cases.

The average duration of fever in untreated Kawasaki disease is 10 days; however, fever can last 2 weeks or longer. After fever resolves, untreated patients can remain anorexic and/or irritable with decreased activity for 2 to 3 weeks. During this phase, periungual desquamation of the fingers and toes and fine peeling of the hands and feet may occur. Transverse lines across the nails (Beau lines) sometimes are noted month(s) later. Recurrent disease develops in approximately 1% to 2% of patients in the United States a median of 1.5 years after the index episode. The recurrence rate is 3.5% in Asian and Pacific Islander populations, and up to 9% in children of Filipino ancestry.

Coronary artery abnormalities are serious sequelae of Kawasaki disease, occurring in 20% to 25% of untreated children. Increased risk of developing coronary artery abnormalities is associated with male sex; age <12 months or >8 years; fever for more than 10 days; white blood cell count >15 000/mm^3; high relative neutrophil (>80%) and band count; low hemoglobin concentration (<10 g/dL); hypoalbuminemia, hyponatremia, or thrombocytopenia; and fever persisting or recurring >36 hours after completion of immune globulin intravenous (IGIV) administration.[1] Aneurysms of the coronary arteries most typically occur between 1 and 4 weeks after onset of illness; onset later than 6 weeks is extremely uncommon. Giant coronary artery aneurysms (internal diameter ≥ 8 mm or z score ≥ 10) are highly predictive of long-term complications. Aneurysms occurring in other medium-sized arteries (eg, iliac, femoral, renal, and axillary vessels) are uncommon and do not occur in the absence of significant

[1] The terms male and female refer to sex assigned at birth.

coronary abnormalities. In addition to coronary artery disease, carditis can involve the pericardium, myocardium, or endocardium, and mitral or aortic regurgitation or both can develop.

In children with only mild coronary artery dilation, coronary artery dimensions often return to baseline within 6 to 8 weeks after onset of disease. Approximately 50% of coronary aneurysms (but only a small proportion of giant aneurysms) regress by echocardiography to normal luminal size within 1 to 2 years, although this process can result in luminal stenosis or a poorly compliant, fibrotic vessel wall or both.

The current case fatality rate for acute Kawasaki disease in the United States and Japan is less than 0.2%. The principal cause of death is myocardial infarction resulting from coronary artery occlusion attributable to thrombosis or progressive stenosis. The relative risk of mortality is highest within 6 weeks of onset of acute symptoms, but myocardial infarction and sudden death can occur months to years after the acute episode. There is no current evidence that the vasculitis of Kawasaki disease predisposes to premature atherosclerotic coronary artery disease.

ETIOLOGY: The etiology is unknown. Epidemiologic and clinical features suggest an infectious and/or an environmental cause or trigger in genetically susceptible individuals. The disease was first described in 1967 by Dr. Tomisaku Kawasaki in a landmark paper titled "Acute Febrile Mucocutaneous Syndrome With Lymphoid Involvement With Specific Desquamation of the Fingers and Toes in Children" in the Japanese journal *Arerugi* ("Allergy"). This is now known universally as Kawasaki disease, although he did not use that term himself. Dr. Kawasaki died on June 5, 2020, at age 95.

EPIDEMIOLOGY: Peak age of occurrence in the United States is 6 to 24 months. Fifty percent of patients are younger than 2 years, and 80% are younger than 5 years; cases are uncommon in children older than 8 years, but rare cases have occurred even in young adults. The prevalence of coronary artery abnormalities is higher if treatment (IGIV) is delayed. The male-to-female ratio is approximately 1.5:1. In the United States, 4000 to 5500 cases are estimated to occur each year; the incidence is highest in children of Asian ancestry. More cases, including clusters, occur during winter and spring. Little evidence indicates person-to-person or common-source spread.

The **incubation period** is unknown.

DIAGNOSTIC TESTS: No specific diagnostic test is available. The diagnosis is made based on the presence of established clinical criteria (see Clinical Manifestations, p 522) after consideration of other possible illnesses, such as staphylococcal or streptococcal toxin-mediated disease; drug reactions (eg, Stevens-Johnson syndrome); MIS-C; measles, adenovirus, Epstein-Barr virus, parvovirus B19, or enterovirus infections; rickettsial disease; leptospirosis; rat bite fever; systemic-onset juvenile idiopathic arthritis; and reactive arthritis. The identification of a respiratory virus by molecular testing does not exclude the diagnosis of Kawasaki disease in infants and children who otherwise have met diagnostic criteria. A markedly increased ESR and/or serum C-reactive protein (CRP) concentration during the first 2 weeks of illness and an increased platelet count ($>450\,000/mm^3$) on days 10 to 21 of illness are almost universal laboratory features. ESR and platelet count usually are normal within 6 to 8 weeks; CRP concentration returns to normal much sooner.

TREATMENT: Management during the acute phase is directed at decreasing inflammation of the myocardium and coronary artery wall and providing supportive care. Therapy should be initiated as soon as the diagnosis is established or strongly suspected. Once the acute phase has subsided, therapy is directed at prevention of thrombosis for patients with coronary artery abnormalities.

Primary Treatment

Immune Globulin Intravenous. A single dose of IGIV, 2 g/kg, administered over 10 to 12 hours, results in rapid resolution of fever and other clinical and laboratory indicators of acute inflammation in approximately 85% of patients and has been proven to reduce the risk of coronary artery aneurysms from 17% to 4%. IGIV plus aspirin (see below) is the treatment of choice and should be initiated as soon as the diagnosis is established or strongly suspected and alternative diagnoses are unlikely, whether or not coronary artery abnormalities are detected. Despite prompt treatment with IGIV and aspirin, approximately 2% to 4% of patients develop coronary artery aneurysms even when treatment is initiated before the onset of coronary artery abnormalities.

Efficacy of therapy initiated later than the 10th day of illness or after detection of coronary artery aneurysms has not been evaluated fully. However, therapy with IGIV and aspirin should be provided for patients in whom the diagnosis is made more than 10 days after the onset of fever who have manifestations of continuing inflammation (ie, elevated ESR or CRP ≥3.0 mg/dL) plus either fever or coronary artery luminal dimension z score >2.5.

IGIV infusion reactions (chills and hypotension) are not uncommon. Occasionally, Coombs-positive hemolytic anemia can complicate IGIV therapy. The risk of hemolysis is increased in patients receiving high/repeated IGIV doses (usually ≥2 g/kg) and those with blood groups A, B, or AB, and usually occurs within 5 to 10 days of infusion. Aseptic meningitis can result from IGIV therapy and resolves quickly without neurologic sequelae. IGIV infusion results in elevation of the ESR; therefore, ESR is not a useful test to monitor disease activity after infusion; CRP is not affected by IGIV administration and can be used.

Aspirin. Aspirin is used for its anti-inflammatory (high-dose) and antithrombotic (low-dose) activity, although aspirin alone does not decrease the risk of coronary artery abnormalities. Guidelines vary with regard to dose. High-dose aspirin (ranging from 30–100 mg/kg per day, depending on country) therapy usually is given until the patient has been afebrile for 48 to 72 hours. This is followed by low-dose aspirin (3 to 5 mg/kg/day, in a single daily dose) until a follow-up echocardiogram 2 to 8 weeks after onset of illness is normal or is continued indefinitely for children in whom coronary artery abnormalities are present. In general, ibuprofen should be avoided in children with coronary aneurysms taking aspirin, because ibuprofen and other nonsteroidal anti-inflammatory drugs with known or potential effects on the cyclooxygenase pathway interfere with the antiplatelet effect of aspirin to prevent thrombosis. Because of the potential risk of Reye syndrome in patients with influenza or varicella receiving salicylates, parents of children receiving aspirin should be instructed to contact their child's physician promptly if the child develops symptoms of or is exposed to either of these diseases. The child and all household contacts older than 6 months should receive influenza vaccine according to seasonal recommendations. Inactivated (non-live) influenza vaccine (not live attenuated influenza vaccine) should be used in the child receiving aspirin. Family members can receive either IIV or live attenuated influenza vaccine.

Adjunctive Therapies for Primary Treatment. The following are 2017 consensus recommendations of the AHA[1]: (1) single-dose pulse methylprednisolone should not be administered with IGIV as routine primary therapy for patients with Kawasaki disease; and (2) patients believed to be at high risk for development of coronary artery aneurysms may benefit from primary adjunctive therapy. Risk factors for development of aneurysms includes baseline z score ≥ 2, age <12 months, Asian ancestry, and high inflammation at baseline. Additional anti-inflammatories to be considered in high-risk patients include administration of a longer course of corticosteroids (eg, prednisolone, 2 mg/kg/day IV, divided every 8 hours until afebrile, then an oral corticosteroid until CRP normalizes, with subsequent tapering over 2–3 weeks) or anticytokine biologics such as infliximab together with IGIV and aspirin. Any consideration of additional anti-inflammatory adjunctive therapy (eg, anticytokine biologics) in a patient believed to be at high risk should be discussed in consultation with an expert in Kawasaki disease.

Management of IGIV Resistance and Retreatment. Patients should be monitored daily for fever for a week after IGIV infusion. Approximately 30% of patients who receive IGIV, 2 g/kg, plus aspirin have fever within the first 36 hours after completing the IGIV infusion, which is not an indication of therapeutic failure. However, 10% to 20% of treated patients have recrudescent or persistent fever beyond 36 hours and less than 7 days after completion of their IGIV infusion and are termed IGIV resistant. In these situations, the diagnosis of Kawasaki disease should be reevaluated. If Kawasaki disease still is considered to be most likely, treatment for Kawasaki disease should be intensified as these children have an increased risk of developing coronary artery aneurysms as compared to children with Kawasaki disease who respond to the initial dose of IGIV. In such cases, retreatment with IGIV (2 g/kg) or infliximab (10 mg/kg) may be given and high-dose aspirin should be continued. As an alternative, corticosteroids may be given. In 1 large randomized, controlled study, infliximab as a single infusion was safer (less risk of hemolytic anemia) and more effective (reduced need for additional therapy and shorter hospitalization) when compared with a second infusion of IGIV. Evidence of alteration of coronary artery outcomes associated with different therapies is limited.

Management of patients with Kawasaki disease refractory to a second dose of IGIV, infliximab, or a course of corticosteroids has included use of cyclosporine, other immune modulating therapies, or plasma exchange but should be undertaken in consultation with an expert in Kawasaki disease.[1]

Cardiac Care.[1] Echocardiography should be performed at the time of suspected diagnosis and repeated at 2 weeks, and in most patients, 6 to 8 weeks after diagnosis in children with normal coronary arteries on initial evaluation. Coronary abnormalities

---

[1] For further information on the diagnosis and management of Kawasaki disease, see McCrindle BW, Rowley AH, Newburger JW, et al; American Heart Association Rheumatic Fever, Endocarditis, and Kawasaki Disease Committee of the Council on Cardiovascular Disease in the Young; Council on Cardiovascular and Stroke Nursing; Council on Cardiovascular Surgery and Anesthesia; and Council on Epidemiology and Prevention. Diagnosis, treatment, and long-term management of Kawasaki disease: a scientific statement for health professionals from the American Heart Association. *Circulation.* Published online March 29, 2017. Available at: **www.ahajournals.org/doi/full/10.1161/CIR.0000000000000484**

warrant closer follow-up with echocardiography. Children at higher risk—for example, children with persistent or recrudescent fever after initial IGIV, baseline coronary artery abnormalities, or very young patients—may require more frequent echocardiograms to guide the need for additional therapies. Children should be assessed during this time for conduction abnormalities, systolic and diastolic dysfunction, and valvular regurgitation. The care of patients with significant cardiac abnormalities should involve a pediatric cardiologist experienced in management of patients with Kawasaki disease and in assessing echocardiographic studies of coronary arteries in children.

Long-term management of Kawasaki disease should be based on the extent of coronary artery involvement. In patients with persistent moderately large coronary artery aneurysms that are not large enough to warrant anticoagulation, clopidogrel (0.2–1 mg/kg/day) to antagonize adenosine diphosphate-mediated platelet activation in combination with prolonged low-dose aspirin are recommended.

Development of giant coronary artery aneurysms (eg, luminal diameter $\geq$8 mm, z score $\geq$10) usually requires addition of anticoagulant therapy, such as warfarin or low-molecular weight heparin, to prevent thrombosis. The AHA has provided recommendations regarding criteria for systemic anticoagulation and frequency of echocardiography in those with coronary aneurysms.[1] The use of non-vitamin K oral anticoagulants (eg, apixaban) is under evaluation and being used in some centers.

Subsequent Immunization. Measles- and varicella-containing vaccines should be deferred until 11 months after receipt of IGIV, 2 g/kg, for treatment of Kawasaki disease because of possible interference with development of an adequate immune response (see Table 1.11, p 69). If the child's risk of exposure to measles or varicella within this period is high, the child should be immunized and then reimmunized at least 11 months after administration of IGIV. Live attenuated varicella-containing vaccines should be avoided during high-dose aspirin therapy because of a theoretical concern of Reye syndrome. The schedule for administration of non-live childhood vaccines should not be interrupted.

INFECTION PREVENTION AND CONTROL MEASURES IN HEALTH CARE SETTINGS: Standard precautions are indicated.

CONTROL MEASURES: None.

Kingella kingae Infections

CLINICAL MANIFESTATIONS: The most common infections attributable to *Kingella kingae* are pyogenic arthritis, osteomyelitis, and bacteremia. Other diseases caused by *K kingae* include spondylodiscitis, tenosynovitis, endocarditis (*K kingae* belongs to the HACEK group of organisms), meningitis, ocular infections, and pneumonia. *K kingae* infections typically occur in children between 6 and 48 months of age, with most cases

---

[1] Giglia TM, Massicotte MP, Tweddell JS, et al. Prevention and treatment of thrombosis in pediatric and congenital heart disease: a scientific statement from the American Heart Association. American Heart Association Congenital Heart Defects Committee of the Council on Cardiovascular Disease in the Young, Council on Cardiovascular and Stroke Nursing, Council on Epidemiology and Prevention, and Stroke Council. *Circulation.* 2013;128(24):2622-2703

occurring in children younger than 2 years, although infections can occur in other age groups. Children with invasive *K kingae* infections other than endocarditis usually present with low-grade fever and normal or only mildly elevated white blood cell counts and acute phase reactants; a high index of suspicion must be maintained for diagnosis. Affected children frequently have concurrent symptoms of respiratory or gastrointestinal tract disease.

K kingae is a primary cause of skeletal infections in the first 4 years of life. *K kingae* pyogenic arthritis generally is monoarticular and most commonly involves the knee, hip, or ankle. *K kingae* osteomyelitis most often involves the femur or tibia. The organism also shows an unusual predilection for the small joints and bones of the chest wall and of the hand and foot. Compared with the clinical manifestations of pyogenic arthritis and osteomyelitis in immunocompetent children caused by other pathogens, skeletal infections caused by *K kingae* can be milder and the clinical course can be more insidious, often resulting in a subacute presentation. Involvement of the apophysis or epiphysis is not unusual in *K kingae* osteomyelitis. Evolution to chronicity or long-term sequelae are rare; however, Brodie abscesses of bone attributable to *K kingae* have been reported.

K kingae bacteremia can occur in previously healthy young children and in children with preexisting chronic medical problems.

ETIOLOGY: *K kingae* is a gram-negative, encapsulated organism that belongs to the *Neisseriaceae* family. It is a fastidious, facultative anaerobic, β-hemolytic coccobacillus that appears as pairs or short chains with tapered ends. It often resists decolorization, sometimes resulting in misidentification as a gram-positive organism.

EPIDEMIOLOGY: The usual habitat of *K kingae* is the human posterior pharynx. The organism colonizes young children more frequently than older children or adults and can be transmitted among children in child care centers, occasionally causing clusters of cases. Infection may be associated with preceding or concomitant viral infections that cause hand, foot, and mouth disease, herpetic gingivostomatitis, or nonspecific upper respiratory tract infections.

The **incubation period** relative to acquisition of colonization is not well defined.

DIAGNOSTIC TESTS: *K kingae* can be isolated from blood, synovial fluid, bone, cerebrospinal fluid, respiratory tract secretions, and other fluid or tissues. Patients with pyogenic arthritis or osteomyelitis attributable to *K kingae* often have negative blood cultures. The organism grows best in aerobic conditions with enhanced carbon dioxide. *K kingae* is difficult to isolate on routinely used solid media. Therefore, synovial fluid and bone aspirates from patients with suspected *K kingae* infection should be inoculated on both solid media and into an aerobic blood culture vial and held for 5 to 7 days to maximize recovery. Once recovered in culture, standard biochemical tests readily identify the organism; alternatively, mass spectrometry of bacterial cellular components may be used for rapid identification.

When available, nucleic acid amplification tests (NAATs) markedly improve detection of *K kingae* in young children with culture-negative skeletal infections. Molecular tests that amplify the species-specific *rtx*A, *cpn*60, and *mdh* genes have higher sensitivity than those targeting the 16S rRNA gene. There currently are no NAATs cleared by the US Food and Drug Administration for *K kingae*, and such tests are available only in specialty laboratories.

TREATMENT: *K kingae* usually is highly susceptible to penicillins and cephalosporins, but in vitro susceptibility to oxacillin is relatively reduced. Nearly all isolates are susceptible to aminoglycosides, macrolides, tetracyclines, and fluoroquinolones. Isolates are resistant to clindamycin, glycopeptide antibiotics (eg, vancomycin), and trimethoprim (although most strains are susceptible to trimethoprim-sulfamethoxazole). Occasional isolates in parts of the United States and other countries have demonstrated beta-lactamase production resulting in low-level resistance to penicillin and ampicillin. The beta-lactamase producing strains are susceptible to beta-lactam/beta-lactamase inhibitor combinations and to cephalosporins.

Ampicillin-sulbactam or a first- or second-generation cephalosporin is recommended as initial therapy for children with osteoarticular infections suspected to be attributable to *K kingae* (definitive therapy can be determined after beta-lactamase production of the isolate is known). For more invasive or severe infections (eg, endocarditis), treatment with a third-generation cephalosporin or, if beta-lactamase production has been ruled out, ampicillin plus an aminoglycoside should be considered. Skeletal system infections usually require 2 to 4 days of intravenous antibiotic therapy, following which a change to an oral antibiotic may be made if the patient's fever has subsided, the clinical condition has improved, and the serum C-reactive protein level is declining. Generally, there is no need for surgical interventions other than a bone or synovial fluid diagnostic aspiration. A total of 2 to 3 weeks of antibiotics suffice for uncomplicated cases of *K kingae* septic arthritis and spondylodiscitis.[1] If an adjacent bone is involved, the antibiotic treatment should probably be extended to 3 to 4 weeks.[2] Patients with *K kingae* endocarditis are administered antibiotics for 4 to 7 weeks.

INFECTION PREVENTION AND CONTROL MEASURES IN HEALTH CARE SETTINGS: Standard precautions are recommended.

CONTROL MEASURES: None. Although small clusters of cases have been reported in child care facilities in multiple countries, antimicrobial prophylaxis in contacts of a case is not standard practice. Rifampin administration to close contacts at a dosage of 20 mg/kg/day in 2 divided doses for 2 days, alone or in combination with amoxicillin (80 mg/kg/per day) in 2 divided doses for 2 or 4 days, has been used in the setting of an outbreak. Although no further cases of the disease have been detected in the affected facilities following antibiotic administration, antimicrobial prophylaxis is not standard practice. Public health advice should be sought if more than a single case is identified in young children with close contact.

Legionella Infections

CLINICAL MANIFESTATIONS: Legionellosis is primarily associated with 2 clinically and epidemiologically distinct illnesses: **Legionnaires' disease** and **Pontiac fever**; extrapulmonary legionellosis occurs much less frequently. Legionnaires' disease presents as pneumonia characterized by fever, chills, cough with or without chest pain, and

---

[1] Woods CR, Bradley JS, Chatterjee A, et al. Clinical practice guideline by the Pediatric Infectious Diseases Society (PIDS) and the Infectious Diseases Society of America (IDSA): 2023 Guideline on diagnosis and management of acute bacterial arthritis in pediatrics. *J Pediatr Infect Dis Soc*. 2023;Nov 6:piad089

[2] Woods CR, Bradley JS, Chatterjee A, et al. Clinical practice guideline by the Pediatric Infectious Diseases Society and the Infectious Diseases Society of America: 2021 Guideline on diagnosis and management of acute hematogenous osteomyelitis in pediatrics. *J Pediatr Infect Dis Soc*. 2021;10(8):801-844

progressive respiratory distress. Legionnaires' disease can be associated with headache, myalgia, and gastrointestinal tract, central nervous system, and renal manifestations. Overall case fatality rate for Legionnaires' disease (including adults) is approximately 10%. Sites of extrapulmonary legionellosis in children can include liver, spleen, and brain. In addition, persistent cervical lymphadenitis caused by *Legionella* species has been reported. In adults, extrapulmonary legionellosis includes endocarditis, graft infections, joint infections, and cutaneous manifestations including wound infections. Pontiac fever is a milder, self-limited febrile illness without pneumonia that is characterized by an abrupt onset of an influenza-like illness (fever, myalgia, headache, weakness).

ETIOLOGY: *Legionella* species are fastidious, small, gram-negative, aerobic bacilli that grow on buffered charcoal yeast extract (BCYE) media. They constitute a single genus in the family *Legionellaceae*. At least 30 of the more than 60 known *Legionella* species have been implicated in human disease, but the most common species causing infections in the United States is *Legionella pneumophila*, with most isolates belonging to serogroup 1.

EPIDEMIOLOGY: Legionnaires' disease is usually acquired through inhalation of aerosolized water containing *Legionella* species. Rarely, transmission occurs via microaspiration of *Legionella*-containing water. *Legionella longbeachae*, common in some geographic areas such as Australia and New Zealand, is generally acquired through exposure to contaminated soil or compost. In general, Legionnaires' disease and Pontiac fever are not spread person to person. Outbreaks of Legionnaires' disease are commonly associated with buildings or structures that have complex water systems, such as hotels and resorts, long-term care facilities, hospitals, and cruise ships. Sources of infection include *Legionella*-containing water aerosolized from potable water systems (eg, through showerheads or faucets), cooling towers (parts of centralized air-conditioning systems for large buildings), hot tubs, decorative fountains, and other aerosolizing devices (eg, and humidifiers and respiratory therapy equipment). Multiplication of *Legionella* organisms in water sources occurs optimally in temperatures between 25°C (77°F) and 45°C (113°F), although *Legionella* organisms have been recovered from water outside this temperature range.

According to the Centers for Disease Control and Prevention's National Notifiable Disease Surveillance System data, Legionnaires' disease cases have increased by almost 9-fold since 2000; almost 10 000 cases were reported in 2018. Most cases of Legionnaires' disease are sporadic, although they may be associated with unidentified outbreaks or clusters. Health care-associated infections most commonly are related to contamination of the hot water supply. Legionnaires' disease should be considered in the differential diagnosis of patients who develop pneumonia during or after their hospitalization. Legionnaires' disease is more common among older individuals (>50 years), males, smokers, and people with weakened immune systems, malignancy, or chronic disease.[1] Infection in children is rare. Severe disease has occurred in children with malignancy, severe combined immunodeficiency, chronic granulomatous disease, organ transplantation, end-stage renal disease, underlying pulmonary disease, and those treated with systemic corticosteroids or other immunosuppressive agents. Health care-associated cases of *Legionella* infection in newborn infants, including severe

[1] The terms male and female refer to sex assigned at birth.

and sometimes fatal cases, have been associated with a *Legionella*-containing water source. Severe and fatal infections in neonates have occurred after birth in water (eg, use of a birthing pool or hot tub).[1]

The **incubation period** for Legionnaires' disease is generally 5 to 6 days but can range from 2 to 14 days. For Pontiac fever, the **incubation period** generally is 1 to 3 days but can be as short as 4 hours.

DIAGNOSTIC TESTS: When a patient is suspected of having Legionnaires' disease, testing should include both culture of a lower respiratory tract specimen and urine antigen testing. Detection of *Legionella* infection from clinical specimens using validated nucleic acid amplification tests (NAATs) is becoming more widely available.

Genus and species-specific NAAT-based assays, including multiplex assays, have been developed that detect *Legionella* DNA in lower respiratory tract specimens, isolates, and blood. NAATs can detect species and serogroups other than *L pneumophila* serogroup 1 and can be performed with quick turnaround. Additionally, the results are less likely to be affected by antibiotic use, because the assay detects genetic material as opposed to a viable organism.

Detection of *Legionella* lipopolysaccharide antigen in urine by commercially available immunoassays is highly specific. This test detects only *L pneumophila* serogroup 1, and thus other testing methods are needed to detect other *L pneumophila* serogroups and other *Legionella* species. Urinary antigen test sensitivity may be increased with increased disease severity.

Culture remains an important diagnostic tool, because it can detect all *Legionella* species and *L pneumophila* serogroups and can generate isolates for further investigation, including whole genome sequencing, which can be helpful in outbreak investigations. Recovery of *Legionella* organisms from lower respiratory tract secretions, lung tissue, pleural fluid, or other normally sterile fluid specimens using buffered charcoal yeast extract (BCYE) media provides definitive evidence of infection, but the sensitivity of culture is laboratory dependent. Specimens should be plated onto both nonselective BCYE and selective BCYE media containing appropriate antimicrobial agents and incubated at 35°C to 37°C for up to 14 days. Suspicious colonies are commonly identified by demonstrating growth dependence on L-cysteine followed by further confirmation and characterization by serologic or molecular tests.

Direct detection of the bacterium in lower respiratory tract specimens by direct immunofluorescent assay is rarely performed, because the specificity is technician dependent and the sensitivity is lower than that for culture or urine immunoassay.

Detection of serum immunoglobulin (Ig) M antibodies is not useful for diagnosis. The positive predictive value of a single elevated IgG titer is low and does not provide definitive evidence of acute infection. A fourfold increase in *L pneumophila*-specific IgG antibody titer, as measured by indirect immunofluorescent antibody (IFA), confirms a recent infection. However, this serologic result is not useful for treatment decisions, because convalescent titers take 3 to 4 weeks to increase (and may be delayed for 8 to 12 weeks). Antibodies to several gram-negative organisms, including *Pseudomonas* species, *Bacteroides fragilis*, and *Campylobacter jejuni*, can cause false-positive IFA test results.

---

[1] Nolt D, O'Leary ST, Aucott SW; American Academy of Pediatrics, Committee on Infectious Diseases, Committee on Fetus and Newborn. Risks of infectious diseases in newborns exposed to alternative perinatal practices. *Pediatrics*. 2022;149(2):e2021055554

TREATMENT: Patients with Legionnaires' disease should receive antimicrobial agents. Intravenously administered azithromycin or levofloxacin (or another fluoroquinolone for respiratory tract infection) is recommended. Once the patient is improved clinically, oral therapy can be substituted. Doxycycline is an alternative agent; however, *L longbeachae* often is resistant. Duration of therapy is generally 5 to 10 days with azithromycin and 7 to 14 days with other drugs, with the longer courses of therapy for patients who are immunocompromised or who have severe disease. Some patients who are immunocompromised or have complicated infections may require extended therapy.

Antimicrobial treatment for patients with Pontiac fever is not recommended, because the disease is self-limiting.

INFECTION PREVENTION AND CONTROL MEASURES IN HEALTH CARE SETTINGS: Standard precautions are recommended.

CONTROL MEASURES: The development and implementation of water management programs is the most effective strategy for prevention of Legionnaires' disease infections associated with buildings that have large or complex water systems or with high-risk devices such as cooling towers, hot tubs, decorative fountains, or other centrally installed aerosolizing devices. In 2017, the Centers for Medicare and Medicaid Services (CMS) released a survey and certification memo stating that health care facilities should develop and adhere to the American Society of Heating, Refrigerating and Air-Conditioning Engineers (ASHRAE)-compliant water management programs.[1] The Centers for Disease Control and Prevention Toolkit for Controlling *Legionella* in Common Sources of Exposure[2] and ASHRAE Guideline 12-2020[3] are resources that can help facilities develop water management programs to identify hazardous conditions and implement steps to minimize the risk associated with *Legionella* organisms and other waterborne pathogens in building water systems. Adequate levels of disinfectant should be maintained in all building water systems. Hospitals should maintain hot water at the highest temperature allowable by state regulations or codes, preferably stored at 60°C (140°F) or greater with a minimum return temperature of 49°C (120°F); precautions should be taken to avoid scalding. Facilities should store and circulate cold water at temperatures below the favorable range for *Legionella* (25–45°C, 77–113°F) to minimize waterborne *Legionella* growth. *Legionella* may grow at temperatures as low as 20°C (68°F). Some hospitals may choose to perform periodic testing of water samples from the hospital's potable water system to detect *Legionella* bacteria.

When 1 presumptive health care-associated case of *Legionella* infection is identified or when 2 or more possible health care-associated cases occur within 12 months, a

---

[1] Centers for Medicare and Medicaid Services. Requirement to Reduce *Legionella* Risk in Healthcare Facility Water Systems to Prevent Cases and Outbreaks of Legionnaires Disease (LD). Memo No. 17-30-Hospitals/CAHs/NHs. Centers for Medicare and Medicaid Services; 2018. Available at: **www.cms.gov/Medicare/Provider-Enrollment-and-Certification/SurveyCertificationGenInfo/Policy-and-Memos-to-States-and-Regions-Items/Survey-And-Cert-Letter-17-30-**

[2] Centers for Disease Control and Prevention. Toolkit for Controlling *Legionella* in Common Sources of Exposure. Available at: **www.cdc.gov/legionella/wmp/control-toolkit/index.html**

[3] American Society of Heating, Refrigerating and Air-Conditioning Engineers. Managing the Risk of Legionellosis Associated with Building Water Systems. ASHRAE Guideline 12-2020. ASHRAE; 2020. Available at: **www.techstreet.com/ashrae/standards/guideline-12-2020-managing-the-risk-of-legionellosis-associated-with-building-water-systems?product_id=2111422**

full epidemiologic and environmental investigation for the source of *Legionella* organisms in the health care facility is recommended. A presumptive health care-associated case is a patient with 10 or more days of continuous stay at a health care facility during the 14 days before onset of symptoms. A possible health care-associated case is a patient who spent a portion of the 14 days at a health care facility before onset of symptoms.

Hospitals with solid organ or hematopoietic cell transplantation programs should maintain a high index of suspicion for legionellosis, use sterile water for the filling and terminal rinsing of nebulization devices, and consider performing routine testing for *Legionella* species in the potable water supply of the transplant unit. For remedial disinfection, shock chlorination can be used. In addition, targeted application of point-of-use water filters and water restrictions can be immediately implemented and can prevent exposure while remediation is performed and its efficacy verified. Optional supplemental measures for long-term control of *Legionella* in potable water to prevent health care-associated infections include copper-silver ionization; addition of chlorine, monochloramine, or chlorine dioxide; and ultraviolet light when implemented as part of a comprehensive water management program.

Public Health Reporting. Infection with *Legionella* species is a nationally notifiable disease in the United States. Health care providers should promptly report legionellosis cases to the local or state health department.

Leishmaniasis

CLINICAL MANIFESTATIONS:

Cutaneous Leishmaniasis. After inoculation by the bite of an infected female phlebotomine sand fly (approximately 2–3 mm long), parasites proliferate locally in mononuclear phagocytes, leading to an erythematous papule that typically enlarges slowly to become a nodule and then an ulcerative lesion with raised, indurated borders. Ulcerative lesions may become dry and crusted or may develop a moist granulating base with overlying exudate. Lesions can persist as nodules, papules, or plaques and may be single or multiple. Lesions commonly appear on exposed areas of the body (eg, face and extremities) and may be accompanied by satellite lesions, sporotrichoid-like nodules, and regional adenopathy. Spontaneous resolution of lesions may take weeks to years, depending, in part, on the *Leishmania* species/strain, and usually results in a flat, atrophic scar.

Mucosal Leishmaniasis (Espundia). Mucosal leishmaniasis traditionally refers to a metastatic sequela of New World cutaneous infection resulting from dissemination of the parasite from the skin to the naso-oropharyngeal/laryngeal mucosa. This form of leishmaniasis typically is caused by species in the *Viannia* subgenus. Mucosal involvement attributable to local extension of cutaneous facial lesions has a different pathophysiology. Mucosal disease usually becomes evident clinically months to years after the original cutaneous lesions have healed, although mucosal and cutaneous lesions may be noted simultaneously, and some affected people have had subclinical cutaneous infection. Untreated mucosal leishmaniasis can progress to cause ulcerative destruction of the mucosa (eg, perforation of the nasal septum) and facial disfigurement.

Visceral Leishmaniasis (Kala-Azar). After cutaneous inoculation by an infected sand fly, the parasite spreads throughout the reticuloendothelial system (ie, within macrophages in spleen, liver, and bone marrow) leaving no or a minimal skin lesion at the bite site. Clinical manifestations include fever, weight loss, hepatosplenomegaly, pancytopenia (anemia, leukopenia, and thrombocytopenia), hypoalbuminemia, and hypergammaglobulinemia. Hemophagocytic lymphohistiocytosis has been reported as a complication of visceral leishmaniasis. Peripheral lymphadenopathy is common in East Africa (eg, South Sudan). Some patients in South Asia (the Indian subcontinent) develop grayish discoloration of their skin; this manifestation gave rise to the Hindi term kala-azar ("black sickness"). Untreated, advanced cases of visceral leishmaniasis almost always are fatal, either directly from the disease or from complications, such as secondary bacterial infections or hemorrhage. Visceral infection can, alternatively, be asymptomatic or have few symptoms. Latent visceral infection can reactivate years to decades after exposure in people who become immunocompromised (eg, because of coinfection with human immunodeficiency virus [HIV] or immunosuppressive/immunomodulatory therapy). Some patients develop post-kala-azar dermal leishmaniasis (PKDL) during or after treatment of visceral leishmaniasis.

Post-Kala-Azar Dermal Leishmaniasis. PKDL is a dermatosis that generally develops as a sequela after apparent successful cure from visceral leishmaniasis. In the Indian subcontinent variant, polymorphic lesions (coexistence of macules/patches along with papulonodules) are prevalent, whereas the Sudanese variant has papular or nodular lesions.

ETIOLOGY: In the human host, *Leishmania* species are obligate intracellular protozoan parasites of mononuclear phagocytes. Together with *Trypanosoma* species, they constitute the family *Trypanosomatidae*. Approximately 20 *Leishmania* species (in the *Leishmania* and *Viannia* subgenera) are known to infect humans. Cutaneous leishmaniasis typically is caused by Old World species *Leishmania tropica, Leishmania major,* and *Leishmania aethiopica* and by New World species *Leishmania mexicana, Leishmania amazonensis, Leishmania (Viannia) braziliensis, Leishmania (V) panamensis, Leishmania (V) guyanensis,* and *Leishmania (V) peruviana.* Mucosal leishmaniasis typically is caused by species in the *Viannia* subgenus, especially *L (V) braziliensis* but also *L (V) panamensis* and *L (V) guyanensis.* Most cases of visceral leishmaniasis are caused by *Leishmania donovani* or *Leishmania infantum (Leishmania chagasi* is synonymous). *L donovani* and *L infantum* also can cause cutaneous and mucosal leishmaniasis, although people with typical cutaneous leishmaniasis caused by these organisms rarely develop visceral leishmaniasis. Recently, emerging foci of both cutaneous and visceral infection with *Leishmania (Mundinia)* species have been reported from the Caribbean, Ghana, and Southeast Asia. PKDL has been reported to be caused primarily by *L donovani*, both in the Indian subcontinent and Sudan.

EPIDEMIOLOGY: Leishmaniasis is a zoonosis in most settings, with mammalian reservoir hosts, such as rodents or dogs. Some transmission cycles are anthroponotic: infected humans are the primary or only reservoir hosts of *L donovani* in South Asia (potentially also in East Africa) and of *L tropica*. Congenital and parenteral (ie, shared needles, blood transfusion) transmission also have been reported.

Leishmaniasis has been endemic in more than 90 countries in the tropics, subtropics, and southern Europe. Visceral leishmaniasis (50 000–90 000 new cases annually) is found in focal areas in the Old World; in parts of Asia (particularly South, Southeast,

Southwest, and Central Asia), Africa (East and Central Africa, including a recent outbreak in Chad), the Middle East, and southern Europe; and in the New World, particularly in Brazil. In 2020, most (>90%) of the world's reported cases of visceral leishmaniasis occurred in 10 countries: Brazil, China, Eritrea, Ethiopia, India, Kenya, Somalia, South Sudan, Sudan, and Yemen.

Cutaneous leishmaniasis is more common (0.6 to 1 million new cases annually). Approximately 90% of cutaneous leishmaniasis occurs in the Americas, the Mediterranean basin, parts of the Middle East, and Central Asia. Ten countries, Afghanistan, Algeria, Brazil, Colombia, Iraq, Libya, Pakistan, Peru, the Syrian Arab Republic, and Tunisia, accounted for over 85% of new cases of cutaneous leishmaniasis in 2020. In general, the geographic distribution of leishmaniasis cases identified in the United States reflects immigration from and travel patterns to regions with endemic disease. Autochthonous human cases of cutaneous leishmaniasis, mostly associated with *L mexicana*, have been reported in several southwest states including Texas, Oklahoma, and Arizona.

PKDL is confined mainly to 2 regions with endemic kala-azar: the Indian subcontinent (India, Nepal, Sri Lanka, and Bangladesh) and East Africa, mainly Sudan, although case reports have emanated from China, Iraq, and Iran. In the Indian subcontinent, transmission of visceral leishmaniasis is anthroponotic, whereas in Sudan it is zoonotic and anthroponotic; therefore, patients with PKDL are the proposed disease reservoir of visceral leishmaniasis in the Indian subcontinent. Young adults are affected more commonly in the Indian subcontinent and children are affected more commonly in Sudan.

Incubation periods for the various forms of leishmaniasis range from weeks to years. The primary skin lesions of cutaneous leishmaniasis typically appear within several weeks of exposure. The **incubation period** of visceral infection usually ranges from approximately 2 to 6 months. PKDL in Sudan develops within 6 months of treatment but in India can develop decades after cure of visceral leishmaniasis.

DIAGNOSTIC TESTS: Definitive diagnosis is made by detecting the parasite (amastigote stages) in infected tissue (eg, of aspirates, scrapings, touch preparations, or histologic sections) by light-microscopic examination of slides stained with Giemsa, hematoxylin and eosin, or other stains, by in vitro culture (available at reference laboratories), or increasingly by molecular methods (detection of parasite DNA by nucleic acid amplification tests [NAATs]). The latter are reported to be more sensitive than microscopy or culture. The SMART-Leish NAAT used by the US military leishmaniasis diagnostic laboratory is cleared by the US Food and Drug Administration (FDA). In cutaneous and mucosal disease, tissue can be obtained by a 3-mm punch biopsy, lesion scrapings, or needle aspiration of the raised nonnecrotic edge (biopsy) or the ulcer base of the lesion. In visceral leishmaniasis, although the sensitivity is highest (approximately 95%) for splenic aspiration, the procedure can be associated with life-threatening hemorrhage; bone marrow aspiration is safer and generally preferred. Other potential sources of specimens include liver, lymph node, and, in some patients (eg, those coinfected with HIV), whole blood or buffy coat. Identification of *Leishmania* species (eg, via isoenzyme analysis of cultured parasites or molecular approaches) may affect prognosis and influence treatment decisions. The Centers for Disease Control and Prevention (CDC) (**www.cdc.gov/parasites/leishmaniasis**) can assist in all aspects of diagnostic testing. Serologic testing usually is not helpful in the evaluation of potential cases of cutaneous leishmaniasis but can provide supportive evidence for diagnosis of visceral or mucosal leishmaniasis, particularly if the patient is immunocompetent. The rK39 immunochromatographic assay is FDA cleared for presumptive diagnosis of visceral leishmaniasis and is commercially available.

TREATMENT: Guidelines published in 2016 from the Infectious Diseases Society of America and the American Society of Tropical Medicine and Hygiene provide a detailed approach to diagnosis and treatment.[1] Systemic antileishmanial treatment always is indicated for patients with symptomatic visceral or mucosal leishmaniasis, whereas not all patients with cutaneous leishmaniasis need to be treated or require systemic therapy (see Drugs for Parasitic Infections, p 1068, for specific treatment recommendations). Consultation with infectious disease or tropical medicine specialists and with staff of the CDC Division of Parasitic Diseases and Malaria is recommended (telephone: 404-718-4745; e-mail: **parasites@cdc.gov**; CDC Emergency Operations Center [after business hours and on weekends]: 770-488-7100). The relative merits of various treatment approaches/regimens for an individual patient should be considered, taking into account that the therapeutic response may vary, not only for different *Leishmania* species but also for the same species in different geographic regions. Special considerations apply in the United States regarding availability of particular medications. For example, currently the pentavalent antimonial compounds (eg, sodium stibogluconate) are not available except under an investigator-initiated investigational new drug application.

Liposomal amphotericin B is approved by the FDA for treatment of visceral leishmaniasis. The oral agent miltefosine is approved for treatment of cutaneous, mucosal, and visceral leishmaniasis; the FDA-approved indications are limited to infections caused by particular *Leishmania* species and to patients who are at least 12 years of age, weigh at least 30 kg (66 lb), and are not pregnant or breastfeeding during and for 5 months after the treatment course.

INFECTION PREVENTION AND CONTROL MEASURES IN HEALTH CARE SETTINGS: Standard precautions are recommended.

CONTROL MEASURES: The best way for travelers to prevent leishmaniasis is by protecting themselves from sand fly bites. Vaccines and drugs for preventing infection are not available. To decrease the risk of being bitten, travelers should take the following measures:

• Stay in well-screened or air-conditioned areas when feasible. Avoid outdoor activities, especially from dusk to dawn, when sand flies generally are most active.
• When outside, wear long-sleeved shirts, long pants, and socks.
• Apply insect repellent on uncovered skin and under the ends of sleeves and pant legs. Follow instructions on the label of the repellent. The most effective repellents generally are those that contain the chemical N,N-diethyl-meta-toluamide (DEET) (see Prevention of Mosquito-borne and Tick-borne Infections, p 207).
• Spray clothing items with a pyrethroid-containing insecticide several days before travel, and allow them to dry. The insecticide should be reapplied after every 5 washings. Permethrin should never be applied to skin.

[1] Aronson N, Herwaldt BL, Libman M, et al. Diagnosis and treatment of leishmaniasis: clinical practice guidelines by the Infectious Diseases Society of America (IDSA) and the American Society of Tropical Medicine and Hygiene (ASTMH). *Clin Infect Dis.* 2016;63(12):e202-e264

- Spray living and sleeping areas with an insecticide.
- Use a bed net tucked under the mattress if not sleeping in an area that is well screened or air conditioned. If at all possible, a bed net that has been soaked in or sprayed with a pyrethroid-containing insecticide should be used; the insecticide will be effective for several months if the bed net is not washed. Because sand flies are much smaller than mosquitoes and can penetrate through smaller holes, fine-mesh netting, which may be uncomfortable in hot weather, is needed for an effective physical barrier against sand flies if the bed net is not impregnated.
- Purchase bed nets, repellents containing DEET, and permethrin before traveling.

Other considerations for prevention of leishmaniasis include early, effective treatment of infected persons, particularly those infected with anthroponotically transmitted parasites for which competent vectors exist; and treatment (to prevent potential congenital transmission) of pregnant people with visceral leishmaniasis. Leukoreduction filtering of blood products may decrease risk of acquiring visceral leishmaniasis through transfusion.

Leprosy

CLINICAL MANIFESTATIONS: Leprosy (Hansen's disease) is a curable infection primarily involving skin, peripheral nerves, and mucosa of the upper respiratory tract. The clinical forms of leprosy reflect the cellular immune response to *Mycobacterium leprae* and, in turn, the number, size, structure, and bacillary content of the lesions. The organism has unique tropism for peripheral nerves, and all forms of leprosy exhibit nerve involvement. Leprosy skin lesions are quite varied and may present as macular hypopigmented or erythematous anesthetic lesions, discolored patches, scaly plaques, sharply defined macules with central clearing, painless ulcers, or nodules. Leprosy lesions usually do not itch or hurt. They lack sensation to heat, touch, and pain but otherwise may be difficult to distinguish from other common maladies. There may be madarosis (loss of eyelashes or eyebrows). Although the nerve injury caused by leprosy is irreversible, early diagnosis and drug therapy can prevent sequelae.

Leprosy manifests over a broad clinical and histopathologic spectrum. In the United States, the Ridley-Jopling scale is used to classify patients according to the histopathologic features of their lesions and organization of the underlying granuloma. The scale is as follows: (1) tuberculoid; (2) borderline tuberculoid; (3) mid-borderline; (4) borderline lepromatous; and (5) lepromatous. A simplified scheme introduced by the World Health Organization for circumstances in which pathologic examination and diagnosis is unavailable is based purely on clinical skin examination. This scheme classifies leprosy by the number of skin patches as either paucibacillary (1–5 lesions, usually tuberculoid or borderline tuberculoid) or multibacillary (>5 lesions, usually mid-borderline, borderline lepromatous, or lepromatous). Patients in the tuberculoid spectrum have active cell-mediated immunity with low antibody responses to *M leprae* and few well-defined lesions containing few bacilli. Lepromatous spectrum cases have high antibody responses with little cell-mediated immunity to *M leprae* and several somewhat diffuse lesions usually containing numerous bacilli.

Serious consequences of leprosy occur from immune reactions and nerve involvement with resulting anesthesia, which can lead to repeated unrecognized trauma, ulcerations, fractures, and even bone resorption. Leprosy is a leading cause of permanent physical disability among communicable diseases worldwide. Eye involvement can occur, especially corneal scarring, and patients should be examined by an ophthalmologist. A diagnosis of leprosy should be considered in any patient with a hypoesthetic or anesthetic skin rash or skin patches who has a history of residence or travel in areas with endemic leprosy or exposure to armadillos.

Leprosy Reactions. Acute clinical exacerbations reflect abrupt changes in the immunologic balance. These reactions are especially common during initial years of treatment but can occur in the absence of therapy. Two major types of leprosy reactions (LRs) are observed. Type 1 (reversal reaction [LR-1]) is observed predominantly in borderline tuberculoid and borderline lepromatous leprosy and is the result of a sudden increase in effective cell-mediated immunity. Acute tenderness and swelling at the site of cutaneous and neural lesions with development of new lesions are major manifestations. Ulcerations can occur, but polymorphonuclear leukocytes are absent from the LR-1 lesion. Fever and systemic toxicity are uncommon. Type 2 (erythema nodosum leprosum [LR-2]) occurs in borderline and lepromatous forms as a systemic inflammatory response. Tender, red subcutaneous papules or nodules resembling erythema nodosum can occur along with high fever, migrating polyarthralgia, painful swelling of lymph nodes and spleen, iridocyclitis, and rarely, nephritis.

ETIOLOGY: Leprosy is caused by *M leprae* and *M lepromatosis*. The organisms can be differentiated only genetically. They manifest an identical spectrum of clinical symptoms and are equally susceptible to antibiotics typically used to treat leprosy. They are obligate intracellular, rod-shaped bacteria that can have variable findings on Gram stain and are weakly acid-fast on standard Ziehl-Neelsen staining. They are best visualized using the Fite stain. Leprosy bacilli have not been cultured successfully in vitro. They are the only bacteria known to infect Schwann cells of peripheral nerves, and demonstration of acid-fast bacilli in peripheral nerves is pathognomonic for leprosy.

EPIDEMIOLOGY: Leprosy is considered a neglected tropical disease and is most prevalent in tropical and subtropical zones. It is not highly infectious. Several human genes have been identified that are associated with susceptibility to *M leprae*, and a minority of people appear to be genetically susceptible to the infection. Accordingly, spouses of leprosy patients are not likely to develop leprosy, but biological parents, children, and siblings who are household contacts of untreated patients with leprosy are at higher risk.

Transmission is believed to be most effective through long-term close contact with an infected individual and likely occurs through respiratory shedding of organisms. The 9-banded armadillo (*Dasypus novemcinctus*) is a recognized nonhuman reservoir of *M leprae*, and zoonotic transmission has been reported in the southern United States. There are reports of *M leprae* infection among 9-banded armadillos as well as the 6-banded armadillo (*Euphractus sexcinctus*) in both Central and South America, mainly Argentina and Brazil. In addition, red squirrels (*Sciuris vulgarus*) in the British Isles may carry *M leprae* and *M lepromatosis*, and groups of chimpanzees in East Africa also have been found to carry *M leprae*. People living with human immunodeficiency virus (HIV) infection do not appear to be at increased risk of becoming infected with *M leprae*. However, concomitant HIV infection and leprosy can lead to worsening of leprosy symptoms during HIV treatment and resulting immune reconstitution inflammatory syndrome. Like many other chronic infectious diseases, onset of leprosy is associated increasingly with use of anti-inflammatory autoimmune therapies and immuno-logic senescence among elderly patients. Little is known about transmission during pregnancy and in the peripartum period. Further guidance on managing pregnant people and infants is available at **http://internationaltextbookofleprosy.org/chapter/pregnancy-and-children**.

More than 200 000 cases including 15 000 children are diagnosed with leprosy annually worldwide. More than 65% of the world's patients with leprosy reside in South and Southeast Asia, primarily India. Other areas of high endemicity include Angola, Brazil, the Central African Republic, Democratic Republic of Congo, Madagascar, Mozambique, the Republic of the Marshall Islands, South Sudan, the Federated States of Micronesia, and the United Republic of Tanzania. Approximately 6500 people with leprosy currently live in the United States, with approximately 150 to 200 new cases presenting each year. The majority of leprosy cases reported in the United States occur among residents of Arkansas, California, Florida, Hawaii, Louisiana, New York, and Texas or among immigrants and other people who lived or worked in countries with endemic leprosy.

The **incubation period** usually is 3 to 5 years but may range from 1 to 20 years. The average age at onset varies according to endemicity within a population. All age groups are susceptible.

DIAGNOSTIC TESTS: There are no diagnostic tests or methods to detect subclinical leprosy. Histopathologic examination of a skin biopsy by an experienced pathologist is the best method of establishing the diagnosis and establishing disease classification. Formalin fixed or paraffin embedded biopsies can be sent to the National Hansen's Disease (Leprosy) Program (NHDP [800-642-2477; **www.hrsa.gov/hansens-disease/diagnosis/biopsy.html**]). Acid-fast bacilli may be found in slit smears or biopsy specimens of skin lesions from patients with lepromatous (multibacillary) forms of the disease but rarely are visualized from patients with the paucibacillary tuberculoid and indeterminate (first lesion with slightly diminished sensation) forms of disease. A nucleic acid amplification test (NAAT) for *M leprae* and *M lepromatosis* is available at the NHDP, as are molecular tests for genetic mutations associated with drug resistance and strain typing based on single nucleotide polymorphisms and other genomic elements. Tuberculin skin tests and interferon-gamma release assays are not used to diagnose leprosy.

TREATMENT: Leprosy is curable. Therapy for patients with leprosy should be undertaken in consultation with an expert in leprosy. The NHDP (**www.hrsa.gov/hansens-disease**; 800-642-2477) provides consultation on clinical and pathologic issues and information about local Hansen's disease clinics and clinicians who have experience with the disease. The open access International Textbook of Leprosy (**http://internationaltextbookofleprosy.org/**) is another valuable resource. Prevention of permanent nerve damage and disability is an important goal of treatment and requires education of and self-awareness by the patient. Combination antimicrobial therapy can be obtained free of charge from the NHDP in the United States and from the World Health Organization in other countries (**www.hrsa.gov/hansensdisease/diagnosis/recommendedtreatment.html**).

It is important to treat infections with more than 1 antimicrobial agent to prevent development of antimicrobial-resistant organisms. Most patients are treated with dapsone and rifampin for 12 months (tuberculoid disease) or dapsone, rifampin, and clofazimine for 24 months (lepromatous disease). Regimens and doses for children are available and should be chosen with assistance from NHDP. Resistance to all 3 drugs has been documented but is extremely rare. Before beginning antimicrobial therapy, patients should be tested for glucose-6-phosphate dehydrogenase deficiency, have baseline complete blood cell counts and serum aminotransferase results documented, and be evaluated for any evidence of tuberculosis infection, especially if infected with HIV. This consideration is important to avoid monotherapy of active tuberculosis with rifampin while treating active leprosy. The infectivity of leprosy patients to others ceases within only a few days of initiating standard multidrug therapy.

Management of leprosy reactions is complex and expert guidance should be sought. Reactions should be treated aggressively to prevent peripheral nerve damage. Treatment with prednisone (1 mg/kg per day, orally) can be initiated for short-term management and rescue situations. Long-term use of prednisone should incorporate a sparing agent such as methotrexate. LR-2 may be treated with thalidomide (100–400 mg/day for 4 days). Thalidomide is available through Bristol-Meyers Squibb and is used under strict supervision (**www.celgeneriskmanagement.com** or 888-423-5436). Thalidomide is not approved for use in children younger than 12 years. Most patients can be treated on an outpatient basis. Rehabilitative measures, including surgery and physical therapy, may be necessary for some patients.

All patients with leprosy should be educated about signs and symptoms of neuritis and cautioned to report them immediately so that corticosteroid therapy can be instituted. Patients should receive counseling because of the social and psychological effects of this disease.

Relapse of disease after completing multidrug therapy is rare (0.01%–0.14%); the presentation of new skin patches usually is attributable to a late type 1 reaction (LR-1). When it does occur, relapse usually is attributable to reactivation of drug-susceptible organisms. People with relapses of disease require another course of multidrug therapy.

INFECTION PREVENTION AND CONTROL MEASURES IN HEALTH CARE SETTINGS: Standard precautions are indicated; isolation is not required.

CONTROL MEASURES: Leprosy is a reportable disease in the United States. Newly diagnosed cases should be reported to state public health authorities, the Centers for Disease Control and Prevention, and the NHDP. Household contacts should be examined initially, but long-term follow-up of asymptomatic contacts is not warranted. Chemoprophylaxis is not recommended.

There are no vaccines approved for use in the United States. A single bacille Calmette-Guérin (BCG) immunization is reported to be from 28% to 60% protective against leprosy, and BCG vaccine is used as an adjunct to drug therapy in Brazil. However, BCG vaccine administration also may precipitate leprosy among subclinically infected individuals. The effectiveness of combined drug and immunotherapy is unknown.

Leptospirosis

CLINICAL MANIFESTATIONS: Leptospirosis is an acute febrile disease with varied manifestations. The severity of disease ranges from asymptomatic or subclinical to a self-limited systemic febrile illness (approximately 90% of patients) to a life-threatening illness that can include jaundice, renal failure (oliguric or nonoliguric), myocarditis, hemorrhage (particularly pulmonary), aseptic meningitis, or refractory shock. Clinical presentation may be mono- or biphasic. Classically described biphasic leptospirosis has an acute septicemia phase usually lasting up to 1 week, when *Leptospira* organisms are present in blood, followed by a second immune-mediated phase that begins 1 to 3 days later and is less likely to respond to antimicrobial therapy. Regardless of its severity, the acute phase is characterized by nonspecific symptoms, including fever, chills, headache, myalgia, nausea, vomiting, or rash. Distinct clinical findings include notable conjunctival suffusion without purulent discharge (28%–99% of cases) and myalgia of the calf and lumbar regions (40%–97% of cases). Manifestations of the immune phase are more variable and milder than the initial illness. The hallmark of the immune phase is aseptic meningitis; uveitis typically is a late finding (4–8 months after the illness has begun) but can occur within 2 weeks. Supportive therapies are appropriate during this phase. Severe manifestations include jaundice and renal dysfunction (Weil syndrome), pulmonary hemorrhage, cardiac arrhythmias, and circulatory collapse. Abnormal potassium (high or low) and/or magnesium (low) levels may require aggressive management. The estimated case fatality rate is 5% to 15% with severe illness, although it can increase to >50% in patients with pulmonary hemorrhage syndrome.

ETIOLOGY: Leptospirosis is caused by pathogenic spirochetes of the genus *Leptospira*. Leptospires are classified by species and subdivided into more than 300 antigenically defined serovars and grouped into serogroups on the basis of antigenic relatedness. Currently, the molecular classification divides the genus into 2 clades: pathogens (consisting of 39 species that cause infection in humans and animals) and saprophytes (consisting of 28 noninfectious species found in the natural environment) as determined by average nucleotide identity (ANI). All leptospires are tightly coiled spirochetes, obligately aerobic, with an optimum growth temperature of 28°C to 30°C.

EPIDEMIOLOGY: Leptospirosis is among the most important zoonoses globally, affecting people in resource-abundant and resource-limited countries in both urban and rural contexts. It has been estimated that more than 1 million people worldwide are infected annually (95% confidence interval [CI], 434 000–1 750 000), with approximately 58 900 deaths (95% CI, 23 800–95 900) occurring each year. The reservoirs for *Leptospira* species include a wide range of wild and domestic animals, including rodents, dogs, livestock (cattle, pigs), and horses that may shed organisms asymptomatically for years. Leptospira organisms excreted in animal urine may remain viable in moist soil or water for weeks to months in warm climates. Humans usually become infected via entry of leptospires through contact of mucosal surfaces (especially conjunctivae) or abraded skin with urine-contaminated environmental sources such as soil and water. Infection also may be acquired through direct contact with infected animals or their tissues, urine, or other body fluids. Epidemics are associated with seasonal flooding and natural disasters, including hurricanes and monsoons. Populations in regions of high endemicity in the tropics and subtropics likely encounter *Leptospira* organisms during routine activities of daily living. People predisposed by occupation include abattoir and sewer workers, miners, veterinarians, farmers, and military personnel. Recreational exposures and clusters of disease have been associated with adventure travel, sporting events including triathlons, and wading, swimming, or boating in contaminated water, particularly during flooding or following heavy rainfall. Common history includes head submersion in or swallowing water during such activities. Person-to-person transmission is not described convincingly.

The **incubation period** usually is 5 to 14 days, and the range 2 is to 30 days.

DIAGNOSTIC TESTS: Clinical features and routine laboratory findings are not specific for leptospirosis; a high index of suspicion must be maintained for diagnosis. *Leptospira* organisms can be isolated from blood during the early septicemic phase (first week) of illness, from urine specimens starting approximately 1 week after symptom onset, and from cerebrospinal fluid when clinical signs of meningitis are present. Specialized culture media are required but are not available routinely in most clinical laboratories. *Leptospira* organisms can be subcultured to specific *Leptospira* semi-solid medium (ie, EMJH) from blood culture bottles used in automated systems within 1 week of inoculation. Isolation of the organism may be difficult, requiring incubation for up to 16 weeks, weekly darkfield microscopic examination, and avoidance of contamination. Sensitivity of culture for diagnosis is low. Isolated leptospires are identified either by serologic methods using agglutinating antisera or by molecular methods.

Serum specimens should be obtained to facilitate diagnosis, and paired acute and convalescent sera are recommended, ideally collected 10 to 14 days apart. Antibodies develop by 5 to 10 days after onset of illness, but increases in antibody concentration may not be detected until more than 10 days after onset, especially if antimicrobial therapy is initiated early. Antibodies can be measured by commercially available immunoassays, most of which are based on sonicates of the saprophyte *Leptospira biflexa*. These assays have variable sensitivity according to regional differences of the various *Leptospira* species and timing of patient presentation, as immunoassays are more sensitive in the convalescent phase of illness. In populations with high endemicity, background reactivity requires establishing both regionally relevant diagnostic criteria and diagnostic versus background titers. Antibody increases can be transient, delayed, or absent in some patients, which may be related to antibiotic use, bacterial virulence, immunogenetics of the individual, or other unknown factors. Microscopic agglutination, the reference standard serologic test, is performed only in select reference laboratories.

Immunohistochemical and immunofluorescent techniques can detect leptospiral antigens in infected tissues. Nucleic acid amplification tests (NAATs) for detection of *Leptospira* DNA in clinical specimens, such as polymerase chain reaction (PCR) assays, are available but are sensitive only in acute specimens and sometimes convalescent urine. *Leptospira* DNA can be detected in whole blood during the first 7 days of illness, with highest sensitivity between days 1 and 4; *Leptospira* DNA can be found after 7 days of illness in urine and may be detectable for weeks to months in the absence of antimicrobial treatment. *Leptospira* DNA also can be detected in cerebrospinal fluid from symptomatic patients with clinical signs of meningitis.

TREATMENT: Although most leptospirosis cases are mild and resolve without antibiotics, therapy should be initiated as soon as possible after clinical recognition to prevent disease progression and to reduce urine shedding of organisms. Intravenous penicillin is the drug of choice for patients with severe infection requiring hospitalization. Penicillin G, even when given as late as 7 days into the course of illness, has been shown to decrease the duration of fever, systemic symptoms, and persistence of associated laboratory abnormalities and may prevent development of leptospiruria.

A Jarisch-Herxheimer reaction (an acute febrile reaction accompanied by headache, myalgia, and a worsening of symptoms lasting less than 24 hours) can develop after initiation of penicillin therapy, as with other spirochetal infections. Parenteral cefotaxime, ceftriaxone, and doxycycline have demonstrated equal efficacy to penicillin G for treatment of severe leptospirosis in randomized clinical trials. For patients with mild disease, oral doxycycline has been shown to shorten the course of illness and decrease occurrence of leptospiruria. Doxycycline may be used regardless of patient age. Ampicillin or amoxicillin also can be used to treat mild disease. Azithromycin was reported to be as effective as doxycycline in a clinical trial. Severe cases require appropriate supportive care, including fluid and electrolyte replacement. Patients with oliguric renal insufficiency require prompt dialysis, and those with pulmonary hemorrhage may require mechanical ventilation to improve clinical outcome.

INFECTION PREVENTION AND CONTROL MEASURES IN HEALTH CARE SETTINGS: Standard precautions are recommended for patient care. Contact precautions are advised for potential exposure to urine.

CONTROL MEASURES:
- Immunization of livestock, horses, and dogs can prevent clinical disease attributable to infecting serovars contained within the vaccine. Immunization may not prevent the shedding of leptospires in urine of animals and, thus, contamination of environments with which humans may come in contact.
- Rodent-control programs may be useful in areas with endemic infection.
- Swimming, immersion, and swallowing water should be avoided in bodies of potentially contaminated fresh water.
- Appropriate protective clothing, boots, and gloves should be worn by people with exposure to urine or potentially contaminated water or mud, such as during floods.
- Doxycycline, 200 mg, administered orally once a week to adults, may provide effective prophylaxis against clinical disease and could be considered for high-risk groups with short-term exposure, but infection may not be prevented and adverse gastrointestinal tract events are common. Indications for prophylactic doxycycline use for children have not been established.

Listeria monocytogenes Infections
(Listeriosis)

CLINICAL MANIFESTATIONS: Listeriosis is an uncommon infection caused by *Listeria monocytogenes* that manifests as invasive disease or as self-limited gastroenteritis. Transmission predominantly is foodborne. Invasive disease can occur in previously well children but occurs most frequently among pregnant people and their fetuses or newborns, older adults, and people of all ages with impaired cell-mediated immunity. Infection during pregnancy can be asymptomatic or associated with a nonspecific febrile illness with myalgia, back pain, and occasionally gastrointestinal tract symptoms. Common adverse outcomes include spontaneous abortion, fetal death, preterm delivery, and neonatal infection or death. Fetal infection generally results from transplacental transmission following bacteremia in the pregnant person, although other mechanisms include inhalation of infected amniotic fluid and infection ascending from vaginal colonization of the birthing parent. When listeriosis is diagnosed in a neonate, a history of recent illness in the birthing parent compatible with *Listeria* infection is obtained in approximately 65% of cases. Amnionitis during labor, brown staining of amniotic fluid, or asymptomatic perinatal infection can occur.

Neonates can present with early- or late-onset disease. Preterm birth, pneumonia, and septicemia are common when infection occurs within the first week of life. An erythematous rash with small, pale papules characterized histologically by granulomas, termed "granulomatosis infantisepticum," can occur in severe newborn infection. Late-onset infections typically occur between 7 to 30 days of age and usually result in meningitis. Late-onset infection may result from acquisition of the organism during passage through the birth canal or, rarely, from environmental sources. Health care-associated nursery outbreaks have been reported.

Beyond the neonatal period, invasive listeriosis usually presents as bacteremia, meningitis with or without parenchymal brain involvement, and less commonly brain abscess or endocarditis. *L monocytogenes* also can cause rhombencephalitis (brain stem encephalitis) in otherwise healthy adolescents and young adults. Outbreaks of gastro-enteritis caused by food contaminated with a very large inoculum of *L monocytogenes* have been reported.

ETIOLOGY: *L monocytogenes* is a facultatively anaerobic, nonspore-forming, nonbranching, motile, gram-positive rod that multiplies intracellularly. It has been assigned to the family *Listeriaceae* along with 5 other traditional and several more recently named species. The organism grows readily on blood agar and produces β-hemolysis. *L monocytogenes* serotypes 1/2a, 4b, and 1/2b grow well at refrigerator temperatures (4°C–10°C).

EPIDEMIOLOGY: *L monocytogenes* causes approximately 1000 cases of invasive disease annually in the United States, and approximately 15% of cases are associated with pregnancy. Pregnant people have a 10 to 20 times higher risk of infection compared with other healthy adults. The mortality rate is highest among older adults and immunocompromised people, including neonates. The saprophytic organism is distributed widely in the environment and is an important cause of illness in ruminants. Foodborne transmission causes outbreaks and sporadic infections in humans. Common food sources include deli-style, ready-to-eat meats, particularly poultry; unpasteurized milk[1]; and soft cheeses, including Mexican-style cheese. Approximately 25% of global outbreaks are attributable to foods not traditionally associated as sources of *L monocytogenes*, such as ice cream and fresh and frozen fruits and vegetables. Listeriosis is a relatively rare foodborne illness (<1% of reported foodborne illness in the United States) but has the highest case fatality rate (20%) among all foodborne pathogens tracked by the Centers for Disease Control and Prevention (CDC **[www.cdc.gov/foodnet/ index.html]**). The incidence of listeriosis decreased substantially in the United States during the 1990s, when regulatory agencies began enforcing rigorous screening guidelines for *L monocytogenes* in processed foods and better detection methods became available to identify contaminated foods. The prevalence of stool carriage of *L monocytogenes* among healthy, asymptomatic adults is estimated to be 1% to 5%.

The **incubation period** for invasive disease is longer for pregnancy-associated cases (2–4 weeks or occasionally longer) than for nonpregnancy-associated cases (1 to

---

[1] American Academy of Pediatrics, Committee on Infectious Diseases, Committee on Nutrition. Consumption of raw or unpasteurized milk and milk products by pregnant women and children. *Pediatrics.* 2014;133(1):175-179 (Reaffirmed November 2019)

14 days). The **incubation period** for gastroenteritis following ingestion of a large inoculum is 24 hours; illness typically lasts 2 to 3 days.

DIAGNOSTIC TESTS: *L monocytogenes* can be recovered readily on blood agar from cultures of blood, cerebrospinal fluid (CSF), meconium, placental or fetal tissue specimens, amniotic fluid, and other infected tissue specimens, including joint, pleural, or peritoneal fluid. Attempts to recover the organism from clinical specimens from nonsterile body sites, including stool, should include the use of selective medium such as Oxford agar or PALCM, as well as enrichment in a *Listeria*-selective broth. Gram stain of meconium, placental tissue, biopsy specimens of the rash of early-onset infection, or CSF from an infected patient may demonstrate the organism. Although gram-positive rods, the organisms can be gram-variable and can resemble diphtheroids, cocci, or diplococci.

A multiplex polymerase chain reaction diagnostic panel designed to detect agents of meningitis and encephalitis in CSF is cleared by the US Food and Drug Administration and contains *L monocytogenes* as one of its target organisms; however, its clinical sensitivity is unknown, and parallel culture of CSF should be performed to allow for molecular characterization, especially for outbreak detection.

Another method for identification of *Listeria* isolates is matrix-assisted laser desorption/ionization–time-of-flight (MALDI-TOF) mass spectrometry.

TREATMENT: No controlled trials have established the drug(s) of choice or duration of therapy for invasive listeriosis. Combination therapy using ampicillin and a second agent (typically gentamicin) in doses appropriate for meningitis is recommended for severe infections. Use of an alternative second agent that is active intracellularly (eg, trimethoprim-sulfamethoxazole [contraindicated in infants younger than 2 months], fluoroquinolones, linezolid, or rifampin) is supported by case reports in adults. If these alternatives are used, susceptibility should be confirmed, because resistance to these agents has been reported. In the penicillin-allergic patient, options include penicillin desensitization or use of either trimethoprim-sulfamethoxazole or a fluoroquinolone, both of which have been used successfully as monotherapy for *Listeria* meningitis and in the setting of brain abscess. Treatment failures with vancomycin have been reported. Cephalosporins are not active against *L monocytogenes*.

For bacteremia without associated central nervous system infection, 10 to 14 days of treatment is recommended. For *L monocytogenes* meningitis, most experts recommend a minimum of 3 weeks of treatment. Longer courses are necessary for patients with endocarditis or parenchymal brain infection (cerebritis, rhombencephalitis, brain abscess). Iron may enhance the pathogenicity of *L monocytogenes*; iron supplements should be withheld until treatment for listeriosis is complete. Brain imaging near the end of the anticipated duration of therapy allows diagnosis of parenchymal involvement of the brain, which may require prolonged therapy.

INFECTION PREVENTION AND CONTROL MEASURES IN HEALTH CARE SETTINGS: Standard precautions are recommended.

CONTROL MEASURES:
- Antimicrobial therapy for *Listeria* infection diagnosed during pregnancy may prevent fetal or perinatal infection and its consequences.
- Neonatal listeriosis complicating successive pregnancies is virtually unknown, so intrapartum antimicrobial therapy is not recommended for people with a history of perinatal listeriosis.

- General and specific guidelines for preventing listeriosis from foodborne sources are provided in Table 3.29.
- Trimethoprim-sulfamethoxazole, given as pneumocystis prophylaxis for those with acquired immunodeficiency syndrome, transplant recipients, or others on long-term, high-dose corticosteroids, effectively prevents listeriosis.

Public Health Reporting. Listeriosis is a nationally notifiable disease in the United States. Cases should be reported promptly to the state or local health department to facilitate early recognition and control of common-source outbreaks. Clinical isolates should be forwarded to a public health laboratory for genetic sequencing.

Table 3.29. Recommendations for Preventing Foodborne Listeriosis (www.cdc.gov/listeria/prevention.html)

General recommendations:

Washing and handling food

- **Rinse** raw fruits and vegetables thoroughly under running tap water before eating, cutting, or cooking. Even if the produce will be peeled, it should still be washed first.
- **Scrub** firm produce, such as melons and cucumbers, with a clean produce brush.
- **Dry** the produce with a clean cloth or paper towel.
- **Separate** uncooked meats and poultry from vegetables, cooked foods, and ready-to-eat foods.

Keep your kitchen and environment cleaner and safer

- Wash hands, knives, countertops, and cutting boards after handling and preparing uncooked foods.
- Be aware that *Listeria monocytogenes* can grow in foods in the refrigerator. Use an appliance thermometer, such as a refrigerator thermometer, to check the temperature inside your refrigerator. The refrigerator temperature should be 40°F or colder and the freezer temperature should be 0°F or colder.
- Clean up all spills in your refrigerator right away, especially juices from hot dog and lunch meat packages, raw meat, and raw poultry.
- Clean the inside walls and shelves of your refrigerator with hot water and liquid soap, then rinse.

Cook meat and poultry thoroughly

- Thoroughly cook raw food from animal sources, such as beef, pork, or poultry to a safe internal temperature. For a list of recommended temperatures for meat and poultry, visit the safe minimum cooking temperatures chart at **FoodSafety.gov (www.foodsafety.gov/keep/charts/mintemp.html)**.

Safety tips for eating melons

- Consumers and food preparers should wash their hands with warm water and soap for at least 20 seconds *before* and *after* handling any whole melon such as cantaloupe, watermelon, or honeydew.
- Scrub the surface of melons, such as cantaloupes, with a clean produce brush under running water and dry them with a clean cloth or paper towel before cutting. Be sure that your scrub brush is sanitized after each use to avoid transferring bacteria between melons.
- Eat cut melon right away or refrigerate it.
- Keep cut melon refrigerated at 41°F or colder and for no more than 7 days.
- Throw away cut melons left at room temperature for more than 4 hours.

Store foods safely

- Use precooked or ready-to-eat food as soon as you can. Do not store the product in the refrigerator beyond the use-by date; follow USDA refrigerator storage time guidelines, especially for hot dogs and luncheon and deli meats.

Table 3.29. Recommendations for Preventing Foodborne Listeriosis (www.cdc.gov/listeria/prevention.html), continued

- Cover leftovers with airtight lids or enclose in plastic wrap or aluminum foil. Use leftovers within 3 to 4 days.

Choose safer foods

- Do not drink raw (unpasteurized) milk[a] (**www.cdc.gov/foodsafety/rawmilk/raw-milk-index.html** and **http://pediatrics.aappublications.org/content/pediatrics/early/2013/12/10/peds.2013-3502.full.pdf**) and do not eat foods that have unpasteurized milk in them.
- Find more specific information about this topic on the CDC Listeriosis Prevention website (**www.cdc.gov/listeria/prevention.html**).

Recommendations for people at higher risk, such as pregnant people, people with weakened immune systems, and older adults, in addition to the recommendations listed above:

Meats

- Avoid eating hot dogs, lunch meats, cold cuts, other deli meats (such as bologna), or fermented or dry sausages unless they are heated to an internal temperature of 165°F or until steaming hot just before serving.
- Pay attention to labels. Do not eat refrigerated pâté or meat spreads from a deli or meat counter or from the refrigerated section of a store.
- Do not eat soft cheese, such as feta, queso blanco, queso fresco, brie, Camembert, blue-veined, or panela (queso panela) unless it is labeled as "MADE WITH PASTEURIZED MILK."
- Be aware that Mexican-style cheeses made from pasteurized milk, such as queso fresco, have caused *Listeria* infections, most likely because they were contaminated during cheese-making.

Seafood

- Do not eat cold smoked fish unless it is canned or shelf-stable or it is in a cooked dish, such as a casserole.
- Do not eat refrigerated smoked fish, such as salmon, trout, whitefish, cod, tuna, and mackerel.

Raw sprouts

- Do not eat raw or lightly cooked sprouts of any kind (including alfalfa, clover, radish, and mung bean sprouts) (**www.cdc.gov/foodsafety/foods-linked-illness.html#sprouts**).

[a] American Academy of Pediatrics, Committee on Infectious Diseases, Committee on Nutrition. Consumption of raw or unpasteurized milk and milk products by pregnant women and children. *Pediatrics*. 2014;133(1):175-179 (Reaffirmed November 2019).

Lyme Disease[1]
(Lyme Borreliosis, *Borrelia burgdorferi* sensu lato Infection)

CLINICAL MANIFESTATIONS: Clinical manifestations of Lyme disease are divided into 3 stages: early localized, early disseminated, and late manifestations. Early localized disease, the most common manifestation of Lyme disease in children, is characterized by a distinctive lesion, erythema migrans (EM). An EM lesion appears at the site of the tick bite days to weeks later, beginning as a red macule or papule that usually expands to form a large (≥5 cm in diameter) annular, erythematous lesion, classically

[1] Lantos PM, Rumbaugh J, Bockenstedt LK, et al. Clinical practice guidelines by the Infectious Diseases Society of America (IDSA), American Academy of Neurology (AAN), and American College of Rheumatology (ACR): 2020 Guidelines for the prevention, diagnosis and treatment of Lyme disease. *Clin Infect Dis.* 2021;72(1):e1-e48. Available at: **www.idsociety.org/practice-guideline/lyme-disease/**

with central clearing creating a bull's-eye pattern. The lesion typically is painless and nonpruritic. EM lesions can vary greatly in size and shape and can be confused with other skin conditions (eg, cellulitis or ring worm). For images demonstrating the range of manifestations of EM rashes as well as rashes that can be confused with EM, see **www.cdc.gov/lyme/signs_symptoms/rashes.html.** Factors that distinguish erythema migrans from a local allergic reaction to a tick bite include larger size, gradual expansion, and lack of pruritis.

Early disseminated Lyme disease can present with multiple EM lesions, cranial neuritis (cranial nerve VII most common), meningitis, radiculitis, or carditis. Lyme meningitis can present with simultaneous cranial neuropathy or papilledema. Lyme carditis can present with syncope, palpations, or fatigue. First-degree atrioventricular block is the abnormality identified on electrocardiography (ECG) most commonly. Systemic symptoms, such as low-grade fever, arthralgia, myalgia, headache, and fatigue, may be present during the early localized or early disseminated stages. Ophthalmic manifestations (eg, conjunctivitis, optic neuritis, keratitis, and uveitis) are uncommon.

The most common manifestation of late Lyme disease in children is mono- or oligoarticular large joint arthritis, most frequently involving the knee. Children with Lyme arthritis have joint swelling out of proportion to pain or disability. If arthrocentesis is performed, synovial fluid white blood cells will be elevated. Children with Lyme arthritis have lower peripheral blood neutrophilia and inflammatory markers compared with children with pyogenic arthritis. Children with early Lyme disease treated with appropriate antimicrobial agents rarely develop late manifestations.

Lyme disease is not believed to produce a congenital infection syndrome. No causal relationship between Lyme disease in a pregnant person and abnormalities of pregnancy or congenital disease caused by *Borrelia burgdorferi* sensu lato complex has been documented. No evidence exists that Lyme disease can be transmitted via human milk.

ETIOLOGY: In the United States, Lyme disease is caused by the spirochete *Borrelia burgdorferi* sensu stricto and rarely, in the upper Midwest, by the recently discovered *Borrelia mayonii*. In Eurasia, *B burgdorferi*, *Borrelia afzelii*, and *Borrelia garinii* cause borreliosis.

EPIDEMIOLOGY: Almost 35 000 cases of confirmed and probable Lyme disease were reported in the United States in 2019, though the actual number of cases is likely at least 10-fold greater because of underreporting. Lyme disease occurs primarily in 2 distinct geographic regions of the United States, with more than 95% of cases occurring in the Northeast, Mid-Atlantic, and upper Midwestern states. Over the past 2 decades, Lyme disease has expanded considerably into states that border this region. Transmission also occurs at a low level on the West Coast, with some focal areas of endemicity in central and northern California. The occurrence of cases in the United States correlates with the distribution and frequency of infected tick vectors—*Ixodes scapularis* in eastern and Midwest states and *Ixodes pacificus* in western states. Climate change likely has contributed to the expansion of the range of these tick vectors (see **www.epa.gov/climate-indicators/climate-change-indicators-lyme-disease**). In Southern states, *Ixodes scapularis* ticks do not feed commonly on competent reservoir mammals and are less likely to bite humans because of different questing habits. Individuals with cases reported from states with low endemic transmission most often are exposed or infected during travel, although some cases may be misdiagnoses resulting from false-positive or misinterpreted test results. History of travel to areas with endemic transmission can guide clinical decision making.

Most cases of early localized and early disseminated Lyme disease occur between April and October, with a peak in June and July. People of all ages can be affected, but incidence in the United States is highest among children 5 through 9 years of age and adults 55 through 69 years of age. Lyme arthritis occurs throughout the year without a seasonal peak.

With lesion(s) similar to erythema migrans, "southern tick-associated rash illness" (STARI) has been reported mainly in south central and southeastern states without endemic *B burgdorferi* infection. The etiology is unknown. STARI results from the bite of the lone star tick, *Amblyomma americanum*, which is abundant in southern states and is biologically incapable of transmitting *B burgdorferi*. Patients with STARI may present with constitutional symptoms in addition to erythema migrans, but STARI has not been associated with any of the disseminated complications of Lyme disease. Appropriate treatment of STARI is unknown.

Lyme disease also is endemic in eastern Canada, Europe, states of the former Soviet Union, China, Mongolia, and Japan. The primary tick vector in Europe is *Ixodes ricinus*, and the primary tick vector in Asia is *Ixodes persulcatus*. Clinical manifestations vary somewhat from those seen in the United States. European Lyme disease can cause the skin lesions borrelial lymphocytoma and acrodermatitis chronica atrophicans and is more likely to produce neurologic disease, whereas arthritis is uncommon. These differences are attributable to the different genospecies of *Borrelia* responsible for European Lyme disease.

Patients with Lyme disease can be infected simultaneously with agents of babesiosis, anaplasmosis, and hard tick-borne relapsing fever (see Babesiosis, p 253; *Ehrlichia, Anaplasma,* and Related Infections, p 361; and *Borrelia* Infections Other Than Lyme Disease [Relapsing Fever], p 274). These diagnoses should be suspected in patients who manifest high fever, have hematologic abnormalities consistent with these infections, or do not respond as expected to therapy prescribed for Lyme disease, such as fever persisting for more than 1 day after starting treatment. Patients with Lyme disease may be coinfected with Powassan virus (deer tick virus) in the United States or with tick-borne encephalitis virus if infection was acquired in Europe.

The **incubation period** in the United States for Lyme disease from tick bite to appearance of single or multiple erythema migrans lesions ranges from 3 to 32 days, with a median time of 11 days. Late manifestations such as arthritis can occur months after the tick bite. Most children who develop Lyme disease do not recall a tick bite; absence of tick bite history should not be used to exclude disease.

DIAGNOSTIC TESTS: Diagnosis of Lyme disease rests first and foremost on the recognition of a consistent clinical illness in people who have had plausible geographic exposure. Information on areas of existing and emerging Lyme disease risk is available from the CDC (**www.cdc.gov/lyme/datasurveillance/lyme-disease-maps.html**). In patients with an EM lesion, Lyme disease is diagnosed based of the characteristic appearance of this skin lesion coupled with likely exposure in areas of known incidence. As the sensitivity of serologic testing is low during early infection (<50% with a solitary EM lesion), treatment should be initiated without serologic testing.

Diagnosis of extracutaneous Lyme disease, including late-stage disease, requires a typical clinical illness, plausible geographic exposure, and a positive serologic test result. The standard testing method for Lyme disease is a 2-tier serologic algorithm. Detailed serologic testing guidelines from the Association of Public Health Laboratories can be found at **www.aphl.org/aboutAPHL/publications/ Documents/ID-2021-Lyme-Disease-Serologic-Testing-Reporting.pdf.** The initial screening test identifies antibodies to a whole-cell sonicate, to peptide antigen, or to recombinant antigens of *B burgdorferi* using an enzyme-linked immunosorbent assay (ELISA or EIA) or immunofluorescent antibody (IFA) test.

If the first-tier EIA result is negative, the patient is considered seronegative and no further testing is indicated. If the result is equivocal or positive, then a second-tier test is required to confirm the result. There are 2 options for second tier testing: (1) a western immunoblot, which is part of the standard 2-tiered testing algorithm; or (2) an EIA test that has been cleared specifically by the US Food and Drug Administration (FDA) for use as a second-tier confirmatory test, which is part of the modified 2-tiered testing algorithm (**www.cdc.gov/mmwr/volumes/68/wr/mm6832a4. htm?s_cid=mm6832a4_w**).

Two-tier serologic testing is essential because of the characteristics of Lyme antibody tests. False-positive results on first-tier tests are common and can be explained partly by antigenic components of *B burgdorferi* that are not specific to this species. Cross-reactive antibodies may be produced in response to spirochetes in normal oral flora, other spirochetal infections (including syphilis), other acute infections, and certain autoimmune diseases. In areas with endemic infection, previous infection with seroconversion may have occurred, and a seropositive patient's current symptoms may be coincidental. Patients with active Lyme disease almost always have objective signs of infection (eg, an EM lesion, facial nerve palsy, arthritis). Nonspecific symptoms commonly accompany these specific signs but almost never are the only evidence of Lyme disease. Serologic testing for Lyme disease should not be performed for individuals without symptoms or signs suggestive of Lyme disease and plausible geographic exposure.

Second-tier testing with immunoglobulin (Ig) M and IgG immunoassays should be performed only as part of a validated 2-tier serologic testing algorithm. The Western immunoblot assay (performed as part of a standard 2-tier testing algorithm) tests for presence of antibodies to specific *B burgdorferi* antigens, including IgM antibodies to 3 spirochetal antigens (the 23/24, 39, and 41 kDa polypeptides) and IgG antibodies to 10 spirochetal antigens (the 18, 23/24, 28, 30, 39, 41, 45, 60, 66, and 93 kDa polypeptides). Many clinical laboratories report presence of antibody to each of 13 bands, describing each band as positive or negative. However, a positive immunoblot result is defined as presence of at least 2 IgM bands or 5 IgG bands. Physicians must be careful not to misinterpret a positive band as a positive test result or interpret a result as positive despite presence of 4 or fewer IgG bands. IgG antibodies to flagella protein, the p41 band, are present in 30% to 50% of healthy people.

A second-tier IgM result performed as part of standard or modified 2-tier testing can be falsely positive. IgM assays are useful only for patients in the first 4 weeks after symptom onset and should be disregarded in patients who have had symptoms for longer than 4 weeks. Most untreated patients with disseminated Lyme disease will have a positive IgG result by week 4 of symptoms.

Most patients with early disseminated disease and virtually all patients with late Lyme disease have antibodies against *B burgdorferi*. Some patients with early Lyme disease treated with antimicrobial agents never develop detectable antibodies against *B burgdorferi;* they are cured and are not at risk of late disease. Development of antibodies in patients treated for early Lyme disease does not indicate lack of cure or presence of persistent infection. Ongoing infection without development of antibodies ("seronegative Lyme") has not been demonstrated. Once antibodies develop, they may persist for many years. Tests for antibodies should not be repeated or used to assess success of treatment.

Current evidence indicates that patients with *B mayonii* infection develop a serologic response similar to that of patients infected with *B burgdorferi*. Standardized 2-tier testing can be expected to have positive results in patients with *B mayonii* infection. Some assays marketed in the United States have reduced sensitivity for European strains of *B burgdorferi*. For patients potentially infected in Europe, check with the test provider or laboratory director to select tests that have been validated for this purpose.

Nucleic acid amplification tests (NAATs) for *B burgdorferi* can be performed on synovial fluid or tissue, blood, or cerebrospinal fluid but currently are not cleared by the FDA. Sensitivity of Lyme NAATs of cerebrospinal fluid is very low; this test should not be obtained routinely for diagnosis of central nervous system infections. NAAT of joint fluid or synovial tissue may be considered in addition to serology in patients for whom the diagnosis of Lyme arthritis is being considered.

A number of tests for Lyme disease have been found to be invalid on the basis of independent testing or to be too nonspecific to exclude false-positive results. These include urine tests for *B burgdorferi*, CD57 assay, novel culture techniques, and antibody panels that differ from those recommended as part of standardized 2-tier testing. Although these tests are available from some clinical laboratories, they are not FDA cleared and are not appropriate diagnostic tests for Lyme disease.

TREATMENT: Consensus practice guidelines for assessment, treatment, and prevention of Lyme disease have been published jointly by the Infectious Diseases Society of America, American Academy of Neurology, and American College of Rheumatology and are available at **www.idsociety.org/practice-guideline/lyme-disease.** Care of children should follow recommendations in Table 3.30. Antimicrobial therapy for nonspecific symptoms or for asymptomatic seropositivity is not recommended. Antimicrobial agents administered for durations not specified in Table 3.30 are not recommended. Alternative diagnostic approaches or therapies without adequate validation and publication in peer-reviewed scientific literature are discouraged.

Early Localized Disease With Erythema Migrans (Single or Multiple). Doxycycline, amoxicillin, or cefuroxime axetil can be used to treat children of any age who present with EM lesions. Azithromycin is a second-line antimicrobial agent for EM, and its use should be limited to patients with EM in whom other antibiotic classes are contraindicated; it has not been studied sufficiently to warrant use in manifestations of Lyme disease other than EM. Selection of an oral antimicrobial agent for treatment of EM should be based on the following considerations: presence of neurologic disease (for which doxycycline is the drug of choice), drug allergy, adverse effects, frequency of administration (doxycycline and cefuroxime axetil are administered twice a day, amoxicillin is administered 3 times a day), ability to minimize sun exposure (photosensitivity may

Table 3.30. Recommended Treatment of Lyme Disease in Children

Disease Category	Drug(s) and Dose
Erythema migrans (single or multiple) (any age)	Doxycycline, 4.4 mg/kg per day, orally, divided into 2 doses (maximum 200 mg/day) for 10 days **OR** Amoxicillin, 50 mg/kg per day, orally, divided into 3 doses (maximum 1.5 g/day) for 14 days **OR** Cefuroxime axetil, 30 mg/kg per day, orally, in 2 divided doses (maximum 1 g/day) for 14 days **OR,** for a patient unable to take a beta-lactam or doxycycline, Azithromycin,[a] 10 mg/kg/day, orally, once daily for 7 days
Isolated facial palsy	Doxycycline, 4.4 mg/kg per day, orally, divided into 2 doses (maximum 200 mg/day), for 14–21 days[b]
Arthritis	An oral agent as for early localized disease, for 28 days
Persistent arthritis after first course of therapy	Retreat using an oral agent as for first-episode arthritis for an additional 28 days **OR** Ceftriaxone sodium, 50–75 mg/kg, IV, once a day (maximum 2 g/day) for 14–28 days
Atrioventricular heart block or carditis	An oral agent as for early localized disease, for 14 days (range 14–21 days) **OR** Ceftriaxone sodium, 50–75 mg/kg, IV, once a day (maximum 2 g/day) for 14 days (range 14–21 days for a hospitalized patient); oral therapy (using an agent as for early localized disease) can be substituted when the patient is stabilized or discharged, to complete the 14- to 21-day course
Meningitis	Doxycycline, 4.4 mg/kg per day, orally, divided into 1 or 2 doses (maximum 200 mg/day) for 14–21 days **OR** Ceftriaxone sodium, 50–75 mg/kg, IV, once a day (maximum 2 g/day) for 14–21 days

IV indicates intravenously.

[a] Because of concerns for lower efficacy, macrolide antibiotics including azithromycin are considered second line agents, and should be reserved for patients in whom other antibiotic classes are contraindicated. Azithromycin has not been sufficiently studied for manifestations of Lyme disease other than erythema migrans.

[b] There is insufficient evidence on whether corticosteroids are safe with Lyme facial palsy.

be associated with doxycycline use), likelihood of coinfection with *Anaplasma phagocytophilum* or *Ehrlichia muris*-like agent (neither is sensitive to beta-lactam antimicrobial agents), and when *Staphylococcus aureus* cellulitis cannot be distinguished easily from EM (doxycycline is effective against most strains of methicillin-sensitive and methicillin-resistant *S aureus*). EM should be treated orally for 10 days if doxycycline is used and for 14 days if amoxicillin or cefuroxime axetil is used. Treatment of EM results in resolution of the skin lesion within several days of initiating therapy and almost always prevents development of later stages of Lyme disease. Because STARI may be indistinguishable from early Lyme disease and questions remain about appropriate treatment, some physicians treat STARI with the same antimicrobial agents orally as for Lyme disease.

Early Disseminated Disease. Oral antimicrobial agents are appropriate and effective for most manifestations of disseminated Lyme disease. Doxycycline is preferred therapy for facial nerve palsy caused by *B burgdorferi* in children of any age, because amoxicillin is unlikely to reach therapeutic levels in the central nervous system. The risks and benefits of concurrent corticosteroid therapy for Lyme disease-associated facial nerve palsy are unknown.

A growing body of evidence suggests that oral doxycycline is effective for treatment of Lyme meningitis and may be used as an alternative to hospitalization and parenteral ceftriaxone or penicillin G therapy in children well enough to be treated as outpatients. Lumbar puncture is indicated for a child with a stiff neck and other symptoms of meningitis in whom the possibility of a bacterial (nonspirochetal) meningitis cannot be ruled out. Neurologic disease is treated for 14 to 21 days.

Late Disseminated Disease. Children with Lyme arthritis are treated with oral antimicrobial agents (eg, doxycycline, amoxicillin, or cefuroxime axetil) for 28 days. Children with no or minimal response to an initial course of oral antibiotics should be retreated with a second course of either parenteral or oral therapy; guidelines from multiple societies express a slight preference for parenteral therapy.[1] A second course of treatment may be considered for those with a partial response; specialty consultation may be helpful in these circumstances.

Approximately 10% to 15% of patients treated for Lyme arthritis will develop persistent synovitis that can last for months to years. Theories of pathophysiology include delayed resolution of inflammation because of slow clearance of nonviable bacteria following treatment versus an autoimmune mechanism. Misdiagnosis also should be considered (ie, Lyme antibodies in serum present from a previous infection or cross-reacting because of another disorder). Persisting synovitis following Lyme disease, termed "postantibiotic Lyme arthritis," is a strongly HLA-associated phenomenon. Patients with persistent synovitis despite repeat treatment should be managed initially with nonsteroidal anti-inflammatory drugs; referral to a rheumatologist may be appropriate for more severe cases. Arthroscopic synovectomy rarely is required for disabling or refractory cases.

Persistent Post-treatment Symptoms. Some patients have prolonged, persistent symptoms following standard treatment for Lyme disease. This phenomenon may not be unique to Lyme disease but rather a more general occurrence during convalescence from systemic illness. Patients with persistent symptoms following Lyme disease usually respond to symptomatic treatment and recover gradually.

Several double-blind, randomized, placebo-controlled trials have found that retreatment with additional antimicrobial agents for patients with residual post-treatment Lyme disease subjective symptoms may be associated with harm and does

---

[1] Lantos PM, Rumbaugh J, Bockenstedt LK, et al. Clinical practice guidelines by the Infectious Diseases Society of America (IDSA), American Academy of Neurology (AAN), and American College of Rheumatology (ACR): 2020 Guidelines for the prevention, diagnosis and treatment of Lyme disease. *Clin Infect Dis.* 2021;72(1):e1-e48. Available at: **www.idsociety.org/practice-guideline/lyme-disease/**

not offer benefit.[1–4] Administration of additional antimicrobial agents to a patient who has been given standard treatment for Lyme disease and continues to have symptoms is discouraged strongly. Retreatment is appropriate for subsequent acute infections caused by *B burgdorferi*.

Pregnancy. Tetracyclines are contraindicated in pregnancy. Doxycycline has not been studied adequately during pregnancy to make a recommendation regarding its use. Otherwise, therapy is the same as recommended for nonpregnant people.

INFECTION PREVENTION AND CONTROL MEASURES IN HEALTH CARE SETTINGS: Standard precautions are recommended.

CONTROL MEASURES:

Ticks. See Prevention of Mosquito-borne and Tick-borne Infections (p 207).

Chemoprophylaxis. Even in areas of high endemicity (the coastal northeast), where 30% to 50% of *I scapularis* ticks harbor *B burgdorferi*, risk of Lyme disease following a recognized tick bite is low, although it increases with duration of attachment. Testing of the tick for spirochete infection has poor predictive value and is not recommended.

Studies of doxycycline prophylaxis have been conducted in adults and older children (≥12 years). Benefits of prophylaxis may outweigh risks when the bite is high risk, defined as those that occur in areas of high endemicity; the bite was from an identified *Ixodes* species tick; the tick was attached for >36 hours; and prophylaxis can be started within 72 hours of tick removal. A single prophylactic 200-mg dose (or 4.4 mg/kg for children weighing less than 45 kg) of doxycycline can be used in children of any age to reduce risk of acquiring Lyme disease after a high-risk tick bite. Amoxicillin prophylaxis has not been studied sufficiently but likely would require a longer course than doxycycline because of its shorter half-life and is not recommended. There are no clinical data to support antibiotic prophylaxis for anaplasmosis, ehrlichiosis, babesiosis, or Rocky Mountain spotted fever.

Blood Donation. No documented cases of *B burgdorferi* transmission have occurred to date as a result of spirochete transmission via blood transfusion. Patients with active Lyme disease should not donate blood, because spirochetemia can occur in early disease. Patients who have been treated for Lyme disease can be considered for blood donation.

Vaccines. Multiple vaccine candidates are currently under development for both adults and children.

Public Health Reporting. Lyme disease is a nationally notifiable disease in the United States.

[1] Feder HM, Johnson BJ, O'Connell S, et al; Ad Hoc International Lyme Disease Group. A critical appraisal of "chronic Lyme disease." *N Engl J Med*. 2007;357(14):1422–1430

[2] Lantos PM, Rumbaugh J, Bockenstedt LK, et al. Clinical practice guidelines by the Infectious Diseases Society of America (IDSA), American Academy of Neurology (AAN), and American College of Rheumatology (ACR): 2020 Guidelines for the prevention, diagnosis and treatment of Lyme disease. *Clin Infect Dis*. Published online November 30, 2020. Available at: **www.idsociety.org/practice-guideline/lyme-disease/**

[3] Berende A, ter Hofstede HJ, Vos FJ, et al. Randomized trial of longer-term therapy for symptoms attributed to Lyme disease. *N Engl J Med*. 2016;374(13):1209–1220

[4] Marzec NS, Nelson C, Waldron PR, et al. Serious bacterial infections acquired during treatment of patients given a diagnosis of chronic Lyme disease—United States. *MMWR Morb Mortal Wkly Rep*. 2017;66(23):607–609

Lymphatic Filariasis
(Bancroftian, Malayan, and Timorian)

CLINICAL MANIFESTATIONS: Lymphatic filariasis is caused by infection with the filarial parasites *Wuchereria bancrofti*, *Brugia malayi*, or *Brugia timori*. Adult worms cause lymphatic dilatation and dysfunction, which result in abnormal lymph flow and eventually may lead to lymphedema in the legs, scrotal area (for *W bancrofti* only), and arms. Recurrent secondary bacterial infections hasten progression of lymphedema to the more severe form known as elephantiasis. Although the infection occurs commonly in young children living in areas with endemic lymphatic filariasis, chronic manifestations, such as hydrocele and lymphedema, occur infrequently in people younger than 20 years. Most filarial infections remain clinically asymptomatic, causing only subclinical lymphatic dilatation and dysfunction. Lymphadenopathy, most frequently of the inguinal, crural, and axillary lymph nodes, is the most common clinical sign of lymphatic filariasis in children. There can be an acute inflammatory response that progresses from the lymph node distally (retrograde) along the affected lymphatic vessel, usually in the limbs. Accompanying systemic symptoms, such as headache or fever, generally are mild. In postpubertal male individuals, adult *W bancrofti* organisms are found most commonly in the intrascrotal lymphatic vessels; thus, inflammation around dead or dying adult worms may present as funiculitis (inflammation of the spermatic cord), epididymitis, or orchitis.[1] A tender granulomatous nodule may be palpable at the site of dying or dead adult worms. Chyluria can occur as a manifestation of bancroftian filariasis. Tropical pulmonary eosinophilia, characterized by cough, fever, wheezing, marked eosinophilia, and high serum immunoglobulin (Ig) E concentrations, is a rare manifestation of lymphatic filariasis.

ETIOLOGY: Filariasis is caused by 3 filarial nematodes in the family *Filaridae*: *W bancrofti*, *B malayi*, and *B timori*.

EPIDEMIOLOGY: The parasite is transmitted by the bite of infected mosquitoes of various genera, including *Culex, Aedes, Anopheles,* and *Mansonia*. *W bancrofti*, the most prevalent cause of lymphatic filariasis, is found in Haiti, the Dominican Republic, Guyana, northeast Brazil, sub-Saharan and North Africa, and Asia, extending from India through the Indonesian archipelago to the western Pacific islands. Humans are the only definitive host for the parasite. *B malayi* is found mostly in China, Southeast Asia, parts of India, and some Pacific islands. *B timori* is restricted to certain islands at the eastern end of the Indonesian archipelago. Adult worms live for an average of 5 to 8 years, and reinfection is common. They release microfilariae into the bloodstream, which can infect mosquitoes and may be present in a patient's blood for decades, although individual microfilariae have a lifespan between 3 and 12 months. The adult worm is not transmissible from person to person or by blood transfusion; microfilariae can be transmitted by transfusion, but they do not develop into adult worms.

The **incubation period** is not well established; the period from acquisition to the appearance of microfilariae in blood can be 3 to 12 months, depending on the species of parasite.

---

[1] The term male refers to sex assigned at birth.

DIAGNOSTIC TESTS: Diagnosis requires epidemiologic risk and consistent laboratory findings (identification of microfilariae or antibody). Microfilariae generally can be detected microscopically on blood smears obtained at night (10 PM–4 AM), although variations in the periodicity of microfilaremia have been described depending on the parasite strain and the geographic location. Adult worms or microfilariae can be identified based on general morphology, size, and presence or absence of a sheath in Giemsa-stained fluid or tissue specimens obtained at biopsy. Serologic enzyme immunoassays are available, but interpretation of results is affected by cross-reactions of filarial antibodies with antibodies against other helminths. Antifilarial antibody tests are available through the Laboratory of Parasitic Diseases at the National Institutes of Health (301-496-5399), the Centers for Disease Control and Prevention (CDC [**www.cdc.gov/dpdx**; 404-718-4745; **parasites@cdc.gov**]), and commercial laboratories. Assays for circulating filarial antigen of *W bancrofti* are available commercially but are not cleared for use by the US Food and Drug Administration (FDA), nor are they available in the United States. Nucleic acid amplification tests (NAATs) can detect parasite-specific DNA in fluids and tissues with high sensitivity and specificity, but none are FDA cleared. Ultrasonography can be used to visualize adult worms. Patients with lymphedema may no longer have microfilariae or antifilarial antibody present.

TREATMENT: The main goal of treatment of an infected person is to kill the adult worm. Diethylcarbamazine citrate (DEC), which is both microfilaricidal and active against the adult worm, is the drug of choice for lymphatic filariasis (see Drugs for Parasitic Infections, p 1068). DEC can be obtained from the CDC (404-718-4745; **parasites@cdc.gov**; or **www.cdc.gov/parasites/lymphaticfilariasis**). DEC is contraindicated in patients who may also have onchocerciasis or loiasis because of the possibility of exacerbation of skin or eye involvement or severe adverse effects. Before DEC therapy for lymphatic filariasis or loiasis, onchocerciasis should be excluded in all patients with a consistent exposure history because of the possibility of severe exacerbations of skin and eye involvement (Mazzotti reaction). People coinfected with *Lao loa* and *Onchocerca volvulus* should not be treated with DEC until the onchocerciasis is treated. Treatment with DEC should be undertaken by a specialist with experience in treating lymphatic filariasis, because DEC therapy has been associated with life-threatening adverse events, including encephalopathy and renal failure in people with high levels of circulating *L loa* microfilariae. Ivermectin is effective against the microfilariae of *W bancrofti* and the 2 *Brugia* species but has no effect on the adult parasite and is, therefore, not recommended typically. Albendazole also has demonstrated macrofilaricidal activity. Two- or 3-drug combination therapies have been used in the Global Program for Elimination of Lymphatic Filariasis. Doxycycline, a drug that targets *Wolbachia* species, an intracellular rickettsial-like bacterial endosymbiont in adult worms, has been shown to be macrofilaricidal and has been used in combination with DEC.

Antifilarial chemotherapy has been shown to have limited efficacy for reversing or stabilizing lymphedema in its early forms. Doxycycline, in limited studies, has been shown to decrease the severity of lymphedema. Complex decongestive physiotherapy can be effective for treating lymphedema and requires strict attention to hygiene in the affected anatomic areas. Prompt identification and treatment of bacterial superinfections, particularly streptococcal and staphylococcal infections, and careful treatment of intertriginous and ungual fungal infections are important aspects of therapy for lymphedema. Surgery may be indicated for management of hydrocele. Chyluria originating in the bladder responds to fulguration; chyluria originating in the kidney is difficult to correct.

INFECTION PREVENTION AND CONTROL MEASURES IN HEALTH CARE SETTINGS: Standard precautions are recommended.

CONTROL MEASURES: Annual mass drug administration of DEC and albendazole; albendazole and ivermectin; or ivermectin, DEC, and albendazole, to decrease or possibly eliminate transmission, has been instituted in selected settings. The use of insecticide-treated bed nets also has been shown to decrease transmission. No vaccine is available for lymphatic filariasis.

Lymphocytic Choriomeningitis Virus

CLINICAL MANIFESTATIONS: Child and adult infections with lymphocytic choriomeningitis virus (LCMV) are asymptomatic in approximately one third of cases. Symptomatic infection may result in a mild to severe illness, which can include fever, malaise, myalgia, retro-orbital headache, photophobia, anorexia, and nausea and vomiting. Sore throat, cough, arthralgia or arthritis, and orchitis also may occur. Initial symptoms may last from a few days to 3 weeks. Leukopenia, lymphopenia, thrombocytopenia, and elevation of lactate dehydrogenase and aspartate aminotransferase occur frequently. A biphasic febrile course is common; after a few days without symptoms, the second phase may occur in up to half of symptomatic patients, consisting of neurologic manifestations that vary from aseptic meningitis to severe encephalitis. Transverse myelitis, eighth nerve deafness, Guillain-Barré syndrome, and hydrocephalus also have been reported. Extraneural disease has included reports of myocarditis and dermatitis. Rarely, LCMV has caused a disease resembling viral hemorrhagic syndrome. Transmission of LCMV through organ transplantation and infection in other immunocompromised populations can result in fatal disseminated infection with multiple organ failure.

Current prevalence and seasonality are not known, because diagnostic testing is not often performed. Recovery without sequelae is the usual outcome, but convalescence may take several weeks, with asthenia, poor cognitive function, headaches, and arthralgia. LCMV infection should be suspected in presence of: (1) aseptic meningitis or encephalitis, especially during periods of colder weather; (2) febrile illness, followed by brief remission, followed by onset of neurologic illness; and (3) cerebrospinal fluid (CSF) findings of lymphocytosis and hypoglycorrhachia.

Infection during pregnancy has been associated with spontaneous abortion. Congenital infection may cause severe CNS abnormalities, including hydrocephalus, chorioretinitis, intracranial calcifications, cortical malformations, cerebellar hypoplasia, microcephaly, and intellectual or developmental disabilities. Extracerebral abnormalities are rare but may include ascites, hepatosplenomegaly, cardiomegaly, myocardial hyperechogenicity, pleural or myocardial effusion, hydrops, skin abnormalities, and fetal growth restriction. Congenital LCMV infection should be included in the differential diagnosis whenever intrauterine infections with toxoplasma, rubella, cytomegalovirus, herpes simplex virus, enterovirus, parechovirus, Zika virus, *Treponema pallidum*, varicella-zoster virus, or parvovirus B19 are being considered.

ETIOLOGY: LCMV is a single-stranded RNA virus that belongs to the family *Arenaviridae*. Other members of this family included in the genus *Mammarenaviruses* are Lassa virus and the New World *Arenaviruses* Junin, Machupo, Guanarito, Sabiá, and Chapare.

EPIDEMIOLOGY: LCMV is a chronic infection of common house mice, which often are infected asymptomatically and chronically shed virus in urine and other excretions. Congenital murine infection is common and results in a normal-appearing litter with chronic viremia and particularly high virus excretion. In addition, hamsters, laboratory mice, and guinea pigs can have chronic infection and can be sources of human infection. Humans are infected mostly by inhalation of aerosol generated by rodents shedding virus from the urine, feces, blood, or nasopharyngeal secretions. Other less likely routes of entry of infected secretions include conjunctival and other mucous membranes, ingestion, and cuts in the skin. The disease is observed more frequently in young adults. Transmission has occurred transplacentally and through solid organ transplantation from an infected organ donor. Laboratory-acquired LCMV infections have occurred, both through infected laboratory animals and contaminated tissue-culture stocks.

The **incubation period** usually is 6 to 13 days and occasionally is as long as 3 weeks.

DIAGNOSTIC TESTS: Patients with central nervous system disease have a mononuclear pleocytosis with 30 to 8000 cells in CSF. Hypoglycorrhachia, as well as mild increase in protein, may occur. LCMV usually can be isolated from CSF obtained during the acute phase of illness and, in severe disseminated infections, also from blood, urine, and nasopharyngeal secretion specimens. Nucleic acid amplification tests (NAATs) available through reference or commercial laboratories can be used on serum during the acute stage and on CSF during the neurologic phase; however, none of these assays are cleared by the US Food and Drug Administration (FDA). Serum specimens from the acute and convalescent phases of illness can be tested for increases in antibody titers by enzyme immunoassays and neutralization tests. Demonstration of virus-specific immunoglobulin M antibodies in serum or CSF specimens is useful. In congenital infections, diagnosis usually is suspected when ocular or neurologic signs develop, and diagnosis usually is made by serologic testing. In immunosuppressed patients, seroconversion can take several weeks. Diagnosis can also be made by immunohistochemical assay of fixed tissues.

TREATMENT: Management is supportive. In vitro data suggest that ribavirin and favipiravir have activity against LCMV. However, favipiravir is not approved in the United States for any indication, and intravenous ribavirin is available only from the manufacturer through an emergency investigational new drug (eIND) application.

INFECTION PREVENTION AND CONTROL MEASURES IN HEALTH CARE SETTINGS: Standard precautions are recommended.

CONTROL MEASURES: Infection can be controlled by preventing rodent infestation in animal and food storage areas. Because the virus is excreted for long periods of time by rodent hosts, attempts should be made to monitor laboratory and commercial colonies of mice and hamsters for infection. Pet rodents or wild mice in a patient's home should be considered likely sources of infection. Guidelines for minimizing risk of human LCMV infection associated with rodents are available[1] (also see Appendix VII, Diseases Transmitted by Animals [Zoonoses], p 1157). Although the risk of LCMV infection from pet rodents is low, pregnant people should avoid exposure to wild or pet rodents and their aerosolized excreta. Pregnant people also should avoid working in the laboratory with LCMV.

Malaria

CLINICAL MANIFESTATIONS: The classic symptoms of malaria, which may be paroxysmal, are high fever with chills, rigor, sweats, and headache. Young children often present only with fever and nonspecific symptoms, which may include nausea, vomiting, diarrhea, cough, tachypnea, arthralgia, myalgia, and abdominal and back pain. Anemia and thrombocytopenia are common. Hepatosplenomegaly frequently is present in infected children in areas with endemic malaria and may be present in adults and in people previously not infected with malaria. Severe disease occurs more frequently in people without immunity acquired as a result of previous infection; young children; pregnant people, especially primigravidae; and those who are immunocompromised.

Infection with *Plasmodium falciparum*, one of the 5 *Plasmodium* species that naturally infect humans, manifests most commonly as a nonspecific febrile illness often without localizing signs. Severe disease may occur with any of the infecting species but is caused most commonly by *P falciparum*. Severe *P falciparum* malaria may manifest as one of the following clinical syndromes, many of which also may be seen with other malaria species, and all of which are medical emergencies and may be fatal unless treated promptly:

- **Impaired consciousness,** characterized by altered mental status, which may progress to **cerebral malaria,** defined by presence of coma (Blantyre coma scale ≤2) and often accompanied by multiple seizures; cerebral malaria has a mortality rate of 15% to 20%;
- **Multiple seizures** (2 or more in 24 hours), which, in the absence of coma, have a low mortality rate;
- **Severe anemia** (hemoglobin of ≤5 g/dL in children <12 years of age; hemoglobin ≤7 g/dL in children ≥12 years of age and adults) attributable to dyserythropoiesis, high parasitemia and hemolysis, sequestration of infected erythrocytes to capillaries and venules, coagulopathy, and hemolysis of infected erythrocytes associated with hypersplenism; late-onset hemolytic anemia has been described following treatment of severe disease with artemisinin derivatives;
- **Metabolic acidosis** (base deficit of >8 mEq/L, or, if not available, a bicarbonate of <15 mmol/L or a venous lactate of ≥5 mmol/L), usually attributed to lactic acidosis, hypovolemia, liver dysfunction, and impaired renal function, and clinically manifesting as respiratory distress (rapid, deep, labored breathing);
- **Hypoglycemia,** which can present with metabolic acidosis and hypotension associated with hyperparasitemia and is associated with increased mortality; it also can be a consequence of quinine or quinidine-induced hyperinsulinemia;

---

[1] Centers for Disease Control and Prevention. Update: interim guidance for minimizing risk for human lymphocytic choriomeningitis virus infection associated with pet rodents. *MMWR Morb Mortal Wkly Rep.* 2005;54(32):799–801

- **Acute kidney injury,** which likely is multifactorial, is common in severe malaria in children and associated with increased mortality; acute renal failure, caused by acute tubular necrosis, is more common in adults than children;
- **Pulmonary edema and acute respiratory distress syndrome,** which are more common in adults than children;
- **Prostration,** in which a child is unable to sit, stand, or walk without assistance;
- **Significant bleeding,** including recurrent or prolonged bleeding from the nose, gums, or venipuncture sites; hematemesis; or melena;
- **Vascular collapse and shock or impaired perfusion,** associated with concurrent bacteremia, hypothermia, or adrenal insufficiency;
- **Jaundice** (serum bilirubin >3 mg/dL), secondary to hemolysis of infected blood cells, coagulopathy, and/or hepatic dysfunction; or
- **Hyperparasitemia** (parasitemia >5%).

Syndromes primarily associated with *Plasmodium vivax* and *Plasmodium ovale* infection are as follows:
- **Anemia** attributable to acute parasitemia, leading to hemolysis;
- **Hypersplenism** with risk of splenic rupture;
- **Thrombocytopenia,** which may be severe with *P vivax*;
- **Pulmonary edema,** which may occur after initial treatment of *P ovale;* and
- **Relapse of infection,** for as long as 3 to 5 years after the primary infection, attributable to latent hepatic stages (hypnozoites).

Syndromes associated with *Plasmodium malariae* infection include:
- **Chronic asymptomatic parasitemia,** which persists at undetectable levels for as long as decades after the primary infection; and
- **Nephrotic syndrome** resulting from deposition of immune complexes in the kidney.

Plasmodium knowlesi is a nonhuman primate malaria parasite that also can infect humans and has been misdiagnosed as *P malariae* infection, which causes more benign infection. Disease can be characterized by very rapid replication of the parasite and hyperparasitemia resulting in severe disease. *P knowlesi* infection should be treated aggressively, because hepatorenal failure and subsequent death have been documented.

Congenital malaria resulting from perinatal transmission occurs infrequently, with increased risk among newborn children of primigravidae in areas with endemic infection. Most congenital cases have been caused by *P vivax* and *P falciparum; P malariae* and *P ovale* account for fewer than 20% of such cases. Manifestations can resemble those of neonatal sepsis, including fever and nonspecific symptoms of poor appetite, irritability, and lethargy.

ETIOLOGY: The genus *Plasmodium* includes species of intraerythrocytic parasites that infect a wide range of mammals, birds, and reptiles. The 5 species that infect humans are *P falciparum, P vivax, P ovale, P malariae,* and *P knowlesi.* Coinfection with multiple species has been documented.

EPIDEMIOLOGY: Malaria is endemic throughout tropical areas of the world and is acquired primarily from the bite of the female *Anopheles* genus of mosquito. Half of the world's population lives in areas where transmission occurs. Worldwide, 247 million cases and 619 000 deaths were reported in 2021 (**www.who.int/publications/i/item/9789240064898).** Approximately 10% of cases are severe malaria, which have a significantly higher chance of death. Most deaths occur in children younger than 5 years. Infection by the malaria parasite poses substantial risks to pregnant people and their fetuses, especially primigravidae in areas with endemic infection, and may result in spontaneous abortion and stillbirth. Malaria contributes to low birth weight in countries where *P falciparum* or *P vivax* is endemic.

Risk of malaria is highest, but variable, for residents of and travelers to sub-Saharan Africa, Papua New Guinea, and the Solomon Islands; risk is intermediate on the Indian subcontinent, and is low in most of Southeast Asia and Latin America. Potential for malaria reintroduction exists in areas where malaria has been eliminated, and local transmission has recently been detected in the United States (**https:// emergency.cdc.gov/han/2023/han00494.asp**). Climate change and interannual variation also affect the geographic range of malaria. Health care professionals can check the Centers for Disease Control and Prevention (CDC) website for the most current information (**www.cdc.gov/malaria**) to determine malaria endemicity when providing pretravel malaria advice or evaluating a febrile returned traveler.

Nearly all of the 1823 malaria cases reported in the United States in 2018 resulted from infection acquired outside the United States.[1] Locally acquired cases of malaria have been identified in Texas and Florida in 2023, the first such local transmission in 20 years (**https://emergency.cdc.gov/han/2023/han00494.asp**). Uncommon modes of malaria transmission are congenital, through transfusion or transplant, or through use of contaminated needles or syringes.

P falciparum and *P vivax* are the most prevalent species worldwide. *P falciparum* malaria is prevalent in Africa, Papua New Guinea, and on the island of Hispaniola (Haiti and the Dominican Republic). *P vivax* malaria is prevalent on the Indian subcontinent and in Central America. *P vivax* and *P falciparum* species are the most common malaria species in southern and Southeast Asia, Oceania, and South America. *P malariae*, although much less common, has a wide distribution. *P ovale* malaria occurs most frequently in West Africa but has been reported in other areas. Reported cases of human infections with *P knowlesi* have been from certain countries of Southeast Asia, specifically Borneo, Malaysia, Philippines, Thailand, Myanmar, Singapore, and Cambodia.

Relapses may occur in *P vivax* and *P ovale* infections because of a persistent hepatic (hypnozoite) stage of infection. Recrudescence of *P falciparum* and *P malariae* infection occurs when a persistent low-density parasitemia produces recurrence of symptoms of the disease, such as when incomplete treatment or drug resistance prevents elimination of the parasite. Asymptomatic parasitemia can occur in individuals with partial immunity.

Drug resistance in both *P falciparum* and *P vivax* has been evolving throughout areas with endemic malaria, generally proportional to the use of particular drugs in a population. The spread of chloroquine-resistant *P falciparum* strains throughout the world dates back to the 1960s. Chloroquine-resistant *P vivax* has been reported in Indonesia, Papua New Guinea, the Solomon Islands, Myanmar, India, and Guyana. *P falciparum* resistance to sulfadoxine-pyrimethamine is distributed throughout Africa and other endemic regions as well. Mefloquine resistance has been documented in Myanmar (Burma), Lao People's Democratic Republic (Laos), Thailand, Cambodia, and Vietnam. Resistance to artemisinin compounds has been reported across the same

[1] Centers for Disease Control and Prevention. Malaria surveillance—United States, 2018. *MMWR Surveill Summ.* 2022;71(8):1-29

region, and there are now reports of artemisinin resistance in Africa, although most such strains have, to date, still responded to artesunate or artemisinin combination treatment.

The **incubation period** (time to onset of malaria symptoms) in most cases ranges from as soon as 7 days after being bitten by an infected mosquito to about 30 days and is shortest for *P falciparum* and longest for *P malariae*. Antimalarial drugs discontinued before completing the recommended course of prophylaxis for *P falciparum* may delay symptoms for weeks to months. Relapses of *P vivax* and *P ovale* may occur months after initial infection.

DIAGNOSTIC TESTS: Definitive parasitologic diagnosis historically has been based on identification of *Plasmodium* parasites microscopically on stained blood films (Giemsa stain preferred). There is an increasing range of rapid diagnostic test methods available that detect specific malaria antigens in blood, one of which is approved by the US Food and Drug Administration (FDA) and is available for use by many hospitals and commercial laboratories. Rapid diagnostic testing is recommended to be conducted in parallel with routine microscopy to provide further information needed for patient treatment, such as the percentage of erythrocytes harboring parasites. Both positive and negative rapid diagnostic test results should be confirmed by microscopic examination, because low-level parasitemia may not be detected (ie, false-negative result), some *P falciparum* strains may not express the HRP-2 antigen targeted by many rapid test platforms, false-positive results occur, and mixed infections may not be detected accurately. Both thick and thin blood films should be examined. The thick film allows for concentration of the blood to find parasites that may be present at low density, whereas the thin film is most useful for species identification and determination of the density of red blood cells infected with parasites. If initial blood smears test negative for *Plasmodium* species but malaria remains a possibility, the smear should be repeated every 12 to 24 hours during a 72-hour period, ideally with at least 3 smears.

Confirmation and identification of the species of malaria parasites on the blood smear is essential in guiding therapy. Serologic testing generally is not helpful, except in epidemiologic surveys. A nucleic acid amplification test (NAAT) is available in reference laboratories and many state health departments, but same-day results may not be available to make treatment decisions. NAATs are most useful to confirm species of malaria and may be useful in cases in which there is a high clinical suspicion for malaria but blood smears are read as negative, as infections with *P ovale* and *P malariae* or infections in patients with treatment prior to obtaining blood smears may be present at very low levels of parasitemia that are difficult to detect with microscopy. Information about sensitivity of rapid diagnostic tests for the 3 less common species of malaria, *P ovale*, *P malariae*, and *P knowlesi*, is limited, but available data suggest low sensitivity. Additional information about rapid diagnostic testing for malaria is available on the CDC website. Species confirmation and antimalarial drug resistance marker testing is available at the CDC for all cases of malaria diagnosed in the United States (**www.cdc.gov/ malaria/diagnosis_treatment/index.html**).

TREATMENT: Choice of malaria treatment is based on the infecting species, possible drug resistance, and severity of disease. Assistance with management of malaria is available 24 hours a day through the CDC Emergency Operations Center (770-488-7100).

Treatment for malaria should not be delayed if malaria is suspected and rapid diagnosis is not available. Guidance on appropriate therapy for uncomplicated and severe malaria is presented in Table 4.11, Drugs for Parasitic Infections, beginning on p 1087. Patients with severe malaria require intensive care and parenteral treatment with intravenous (IV) artesunate. IV quinidine is no longer available in the United States. Use of artesunate without laboratory confirmation of malaria should be reserved for cases in which there is a strong clinical suspicion of severe malaria and prompt laboratory diagnosis is not available. Sequential blood smears to determine percentage of erythrocytes infected with parasites may be monitored to assess therapeutic efficacy. A review of available literature suggests exchange transfusion for severe disease is not efficacious in patients with end-organ involvement.

For patients with severe malaria in the United States or patients with malaria who are unable to tolerate an oral medication despite attempts, IV artesunate is the treatment of choice. CDC distribution of investigational IV artesunate was discontinued in September 2022, and IV artesunate now needs to be procured commercially and stocked by hospitals. Artesunate in the United States currently is very expensive, so every hospital should have a plan for stocking artesunate, obtaining artesunate if not stocked, or referring to a regional hospital that does stock artesunate. At hospitals where IV artesunate is not in stock, patients should receive an effective oral antimalarial in the interim while IV artesunate is obtained emergently from a commercial source, or should be referred to a regional hospital with artesunate available. If the patient is unable to tolerate oral medications, the medical team will need to consider alternative ways to administer oral medications while awaiting IV artesunate (eg, antiemetics before administering the antimalarial drug, or administering the drug via nasogastric tube). The preferred antimalarial for interim oral treatment is artemether-lumefantrine (Coartem) because of its fast onset of action. Other oral options include atovaquone-proguanil (Malarone), quinine, and mefloquine. Oral or intravenous clindamycin and tetracyclines, such as doxycycline, are not adequate for interim treatment. When IV artesunate arrives, the oral medication should be discontinued and parenteral treatment initiated.

Additional information on artesunate and guidelines for the treatment of malaria are available on the CDC website (**www.cdc.gov/malaria/diagnosis_treatment/artesunate.html** and **www.cdc.gov/malaria/resources/pdf/Malaria_Treatment_Table_202306.pdf**).

INFECTION PREVENTION AND CONTROL MEASURES IN HEALTH CARE SETTINGS: Standard precautions are recommended.

CONTROL MEASURES: Malaria is a nationally reportable disease in the United States. The RTS,S vaccine for malaria is used for malaria control in children living in endemic areas and is not available for travelers. Effective measures to reduce risk of acquiring malaria include control of *Anopheles* mosquito populations, protection against mosquito bites, treatment of infected people, and chemoprophylaxis (see Table 3.31). Measures to prevent contact with mosquitoes, especially from dusk to dawn (because of the nocturnal biting habits of most female *Anopheles* mosquitoes), include use of bed nets impregnated with insecticide, mosquito repellents (see Prevention of Mosquito-borne and Tick-borne Infections, p 207), and protective clothing. The most current information on country-specific malaria transmission, drug resistance, and

Table 3.31. Drugs to Consider for Use in Children for Malaria Prophylaxis[a]

Locale	Drug	Dosing	Timing	Adverse Effects and Contraindications	Other Considerations
Only chloroquine-sensitive areas	Chloroquine or hydroxy-chloroquine	Chloroquine dose: 5 mg/kg base (8.3 mg/kg salt), orally, once weekly, up to maximum adult dose 300 mg base Hydroxychloroquine dose: 5 mg/kg base (6.5 mg/kg salt), orally, once weekly, up to maximum 310 mg base	Begin 1–2 weeks before travel and take weekly throughout and for 4 weeks after leaving area	Most common adverse effects: gastrointestinal tract disturbance, headache, dizziness, blurred vision, pruritus, insomnia Can exacerbate psoriasis	Take with meals
Only mefloquine-sensitive areas	Mefloquine	≤9 kg: 4.6 mg/kg base (5 mg/kg salt), once weekly >9–19 kg: ¼ tablet, once weekly >19–30 kg: ½ tablet, once weekly >30–45 kg: ¾ tablet, once weekly >45 kg: 1 tablet, once weekly Each tablet contains 228 mg base (250 mg salt)	Begin ≥2 weeks before travel, then weekly on same day each week throughout and for 4 weeks after leaving area Initiating 2–3 weeks before travel can help assess tolerability	Most common adverse effects: gastrointestinal tract disturbance, headache, insomnia, vivid dreams, visual disturbance, anxiety, dizziness CONTRAINDICATED in travelers with a known hypersensitivity to the drug, and in those with active or recent history of depression, anxiety disorder, psychosis, schizophrenia, other major psychiatric disorder or seizures Do not use in those with cardiac conduction defects	Black box warning for neurologic (dizziness, vestibular problems, tinnitus) and psychiatric (anxiety, paranoia, depression, hallucinations) adverse effects that may occur at any time during drug use, and may last for months to years after the drug is stopped. Patients must be given copy of FDA medication guide May be given in all trimesters of pregnancy

Table 3.31. Drugs to Consider for Use in Children for Malaria Prophylaxis,[a] continued

Locale	Drug	Dosing	Timing	Adverse Effects and Contraindications	Other Considerations
All areas	Atovaquone-proguanil	Pediatric tablets, 62.5 mg atovaquone and 25 mg proguanil hydrochloride 5–8 kg: ½ tab >8–10 kg: ¾ tab >10–20 kg: 1 tab >20–30 kg: 2 tabs >30–40 kg: 3 tabs >40 kg: 1 adult tab (250 mg atovaquone/100 mg proguanil)	Start 1–2 days before travel, take daily throughout travel and for 7 days after leaving area	Most common adverse effects: abdominal pain, nausea, vomiting, headache Do not use in those with creatinine clearance <30 mL/min; not recommended for infants <5 kg, pregnant people, or people who are breastfeeding infants <5 kg	Take with meals Generally well tolerated Proguanil can increase warfarin effect; dosage adjustment may be needed
All areas	Doxycycline	2.2 mg/kg, up to maximum adult dose 100 mg/day	Start 1–2 days before travel, take daily throughout travel, and for 4 weeks after leaving area Licensed for use for 4 months but may be safely given up to 2 years	Most common adverse effects: photosensitivity, gastrointestinal disturbance Not recommended for pregnant people	Take with meals Also active against rickettsiae and leptospirae (hikers, campers, fresh water swimmers) Complete oral typhoid vaccine >72 hours before starting doxycycline

Table 3.31. Drugs to Consider for Use in Children for Malaria Prophylaxis,[a] continued

Locale	Drug	Dosing	Timing	Adverse Effects and Contraindications	Other Considerations
Short-duration travel (<6 months) to all areas	Primaquine	0.5 mg/kg base (0.8 mg/kg salt) up to adult dose of 30 mg base (52.6 mg salt) daily	Start 1–2 days before travel, take daily throughout travel, and for 7 days after leaving area	CONTRAINDICATED in those with G6PD deficiency and pregnant people Should not be given to lactating person unless infant has normal G6PD level	Test for G6PD deficiency before prescribing Also used for presumptive therapy (ie, terminal prophylaxis) to decrease risk of *P vivax* or *P ovale* relapse
Short-duration travel (<6 months) to all areas	Tafenoquine	In travelers 18 years and older: Loading dose: 200 mg once daily for 3 days before departure Maintenance regimen (while in malaria transmission area): 200 mg weekly Post-trip dose: 200 mg once, 7 days after the last weekly dose	Start 3 days before travel, weekly during the trip, and a single dose during the week after returning.	CONTRAINDICATED in those with G6PD deficiency and pregnant people Should not be given to lactating person unless infant has normal G6PD level	Test for G6PD deficiency using a quantitative test before prescribing Approved for 18 years and older for prophylaxis (and for antirelapse therapy in people ≥16 years) Also used for presumptive therapy (ie, terminal prophylaxis) to decrease risk of *P vivax* or *P ovale* relapse (different formulation and dosing schedule)

G6PD indicates glucose-6-phosphate dehydrogenase.

[a] No drug is 100% effective; always combine chemoprophylaxis with personal protection measures.

recommendations for travelers can be obtained by accessing the chapter on malaria in the *2024 CDC Yellow Book: Health Information for International Travel* (**wwwnc.cdc.gov/ travel/yellowbook/2024/infections-diseases/malaria**).

Chemoprophylaxis for Travelers to Areas With Endemic Malaria.[1] Drugs for prevention of malaria currently available in the United States include chloroquine, mefloquine, doxycycline, atovaquone-proguanil, primaquine, and tafenoquine (ages ≥18 years). Table 3.31 details use of these drugs for prophylaxis against malaria.

The appropriate chemoprophylactic regimen is determined by the traveler's risk of acquiring malaria at their destination(s) and by local prevalence of drug resistance. The travel itinerary should be reviewed in detail and compared with information on where malaria transmission occurs within a given country to determine whether the traveler will be traveling in a part of the country where malaria occurs and if antimalarial drug resistance has been reported in that location (see **wwwnc.cdc. gov/travel/yellowbook/2024/preparing/yellow-fever-vaccine-malaria- prevention-by-country**). Additional factors to consider are the patient's other medical conditions (including pregnancy), medications (to assess potential drug interactions), cost of the medicines, and potential adverse effects. Indications for prophylaxis for children are the same as those for adults. Pediatric dosages should be calculated based on the child's current weight, and children's dosages should never exceed adult dosages. Drugs used for malaria chemoprophylaxis generally are well tolerated, although adverse reactions can occur. Minor adverse reactions do not require stopping or adjusting drug dosage. Those who provide malaria chemoprophylaxis should provide travelers with information about management of mild adverse events, what to do in the event of serious adverse reactions, and what to do if doses are missed.

Medications for chemoprophylaxis of malaria should not be obtained at the destination, as quality of these products is unknown. Travelers also should avoid medications and combinations that are commonly prescribed abroad but not recommended in the United States. Chemoprophylaxis should begin before arrival in the area with endemic malaria.

Prophylaxis During Pregnancy and Lactation. Malaria during pregnancy carries significant risks for both the pregnant person and fetus. Malaria increases the risk of adverse outcomes in pregnancy, including abortion, preterm birth, and stillbirth. For these reasons and because no chemoprophylactic regimen is absolutely effective, people who are pregnant or likely to become pregnant should try to avoid travel to areas where they could contract malaria.

Pregnant people traveling to areas where chloroquine-resistant malaria has not been reported may take chloroquine prophylaxis. Harmful effects on the fetus have not been demonstrated when chloroquine is given in recommended doses for malaria prophylaxis. Pregnancy and lactation, therefore, are not contraindications for malaria prophylaxis with chloroquine.

Mefloquine chemoprophylaxis is recommended in all trimesters of pregnancy when exposure to chloroquine-resistant *P falciparum* is unavoidable. Lactating parents of infants may use mefloquine, or, when their infant weighs more than 5 kg, atovaquone-proguanil for prophylaxis when exposure to chloroquine-resistant

---

[1] For further information on prevention of malaria in travelers, see the biennial publication: *2024 CDC Yellow Book: Health Information for International Travel* (**wwwnc.cdc.gov/travel/yellowbook/2024/ infections-diseases/malaria**).

P falciparum is unavoidable. Primaquine and tafenoquine are contraindicated in pregnancy because of the unknown glucose-6-phosphate dehydrogenase (G6PD) status of the fetus.

Assessment for Malaria During Travel. Travelers to areas with endemic malaria should seek medical attention immediately if they develop fever. Malaria treatment is most effective if begun early in the course of disease, and delay of appropriate treatment can have serious or even fatal consequences. Travelers who develop malaria despite taking chemoprophylaxis should be treated with an appropriate antimalarial drug other than the one used for chemoprophylaxis. Although most cases of imported malaria are diagnosed ≤3 months from return to the United States, travelers should be advised that any fever or influenza-like illness that develops up to 1 year from departure from an area with endemic malaria requires medical evaluation, including appropriate blood testing to rule out malaria.

Prevention of Relapses. There is no test to determine the potential for relapses of *P vivax* or *P ovale* infection. Antirelapse therapy can be provided along with treatment of symptomatic infection or after leaving an endemic area following a prolonged stay. Presumptive antirelapse therapy, also known as terminal prophylaxis, uses a medication toward the end of the exposure period or immediately thereafter to prevent relapses or delayed onset clinical presentations of malaria caused by hypnozoites. Primaquine and tafenoquine (Krintafel, in patients 16 years and older, and only if coadministered with chloroquine or hydroxychloroquine) are approved for use to prevent relapses of *P vivax*. Both can be used to prevent *P ovale* relapse, but tafenoquine is not approved by the FDA for this use. Screening for G6PD deficiency using a quantitative test must be performed before using primaquine and tafenoquine, because both drugs can cause hemolysis in patients with G6PD deficiency.

Personal Protective Measures. All travelers to areas where malaria is endemic should be advised to use personal protective measures, including the following: (1) insecticide-impregnated mosquito nets while sleeping; (2) remaining in well-screened or air-conditioned areas at dusk and at night; (3) protective clothing, preferably permethrin treated; and (4) mosquito repellents (see Prevention of Mosquito-borne and Tick-borne Infections, p 207).

Measles

CLINICAL MANIFESTATIONS: Measles is an acute viral disease characterized by fever, cough, coryza, and conjunctivitis, followed by a maculopapular rash beginning on the face and spreading cephalocaudally and centrifugally. During the prodromal period, a pathognomonic enanthema (Koplik spots) may be present. Complications of measles, including otitis media, bronchopneumonia, laryngotracheobronchitis (croup), and diarrhea, occur commonly in young children and immunocompromised hosts. Acute encephalitis, which often results in neurologic deficits, occurs in approximately 1 of every 1000 cases. In the postelimination era in the United States, death, predominantly resulting from respiratory and neurologic complications, has occurred in 1 to 3 of every 1000 cases reported. Case fatality rates are increased in children younger than 5 years, pregnant people, and immunocompromised children, including children with leukemia, human immunodeficiency virus (HIV) infection, and severe malnutrition (including vitamin A deficiency). Sometimes the characteristic rash does not develop in immunocompromised patients.

Measles inclusion body encephalitis (MIBE) is a rare manifestation of measles infection in immunocompromised individuals usually presenting within 1 year of measles infection. Disease onset is subacute with progressive neurologic dysfunction occurring over weeks to months. Subacute sclerosing panencephalitis (SSPE) is a rare degenerative central nervous system disease characterized by behavioral and intellectual deterioration and seizures that generally occurs 7 to 11 years after wild-type measles virus infection. The highest rates occur in children infected before 2 years of age.

Several recent studies suggest that children who have had measles have blunted immune responses to other pathogens and increased mortality for several years after infection. This has been attributed to measles-induced suppression of cell-mediated immune function leading to immune amnesia and susceptibility to previously encountered antigens, including vaccine antigens. This effect is another reason why measles prevention is so important.

ETIOLOGY: Measles virus is an enveloped RNA virus with 1 serotype, classified as a member of the genus *Morbillivirus* in the *Paramyxoviridae* family.

EPIDEMIOLOGY: The only natural host of measles virus is humans. Measles virus is transmitted by direct contact with infectious droplets or by airborne spread. Measles is one of the most highly communicable of all infectious diseases; the attack rate in a susceptible individual exposed to measles is 90% in close-contact settings. Population immunity as high as 95% or greater is often needed to stop ongoing transmission. In temperate areas, the peak incidence of infection usually occurs during late winter and spring. In the prevaccine era, most cases of measles in the United States occurred in preschool- and young school-aged children, and few people remained susceptible by 20 years of age. Following implementation of routine childhood vaccination in the United States at 12 to 15 months of age, measles occurred more often in infants younger than 1 year and in older adolescents and adults who had not been adequately vaccinated. Infant susceptibility increases around the time when transplacentally acquired antibodies are no longer present. The childhood and adolescent immunization program in the United States began with licensure of the measles vaccine in 1963 and has resulted in a greater than 99% decrease in the reported incidence of measles, with declaration of measles elimination (ie, absence of endemic measles transmission for more than 1 year) in 2000.

From 1989 to 1991, the incidence of measles in the United States increased because of low immunization rates in preschool-aged children, especially in urban areas, and because of primary vaccine failures in children who had received 1 measles-containing vaccine dose. Following improved coverage in preschool-aged children and implementation of a routine second dose of measles, mumps, and rubella (MMR) vaccine for children, the incidence of measles has declined to extremely low levels (<1 case per 1 million population). Unfortunately, increasing numbers of cases and outbreaks of measles have occurred in many states in more recent years. The majority of these cases are linked to importation of measles by nonvaccinated international United States travelers from countries where measles is endemic, including countries in Western Europe, and subsequent internal spread among unimmunized subpopulations, including intentionally unimmunized children.

Progress continues toward global control and regional measles elimination, with a 94% drop in estimated measles deaths worldwide between 2000 and 2020.[1] By the end of 2021, 76 countries had been verified by independent regional commissions as having achieved or maintained measles elimination status. However, none of the World Health Organization (WHO) regions had achieved and sustained elimination, and no African Region country has yet been verified to have eliminated measles. WHO's Region of the Americas achieved verification of measles elimination in 2016; however, endemic measles transmission was reestablished in Venezuela (2016) and Brazil (2018).

Estimated coverage of first dose of measles-containing vaccine decreased from 86% in 2019 to 84% in 2020 and 81% in 2021 during the COVID-19 pandemic.[22] Worsening of suboptimal surveillance coupled with increased population susceptibility attributable to vaccine hesitancy and decreased routine vaccination during the COVID-19 pandemic remain major threats to global elimination of measles.

Lack of response to vaccine (ie, primary vaccine failure) occurs in as many as 7% of people who receive a single dose of measles-containing vaccine at 12 months or older. Most cases of measles in previously immunized children are attributable to primary vaccine failures, but waning immunity after immunization (ie, secondary vaccine failure) may be a factor in some cases. Primary vaccine failure was the main reason that in 1989 a 2-dose vaccine schedule was recommended routinely for children and high-risk adults.[3]

Patients infected with wild-type measles virus are contagious from 4 days before the rash through 4 days after appearance of the rash. Immunocompromised patients who may have prolonged excretion of the virus in respiratory tract secretions can be contagious for the duration of the illness. Patients with SSPE are not contagious.

The **incubation period** averages 11 to 12 days from exposure to onset of prodromal symptoms, and the average interval between exposure and appearance of rash is 14 days, with a range of 7 to 21 days. In SSPE, the mean **incubation period** of 84 cases reported between 1976 and 1983 was 10.8 years.

DIAGNOSTIC TESTS: Measles virus infection can be confirmed by: (1) detection of measles viral RNA by nucleic acid amplification test (NAAT); (2) detection of measles virus-specific immunoglobulin (Ig) M; (3) a fourfold increase in measles IgG antibody concentration in paired acute and convalescent serum specimens (collected at least 10 days apart); or (4) isolation of measles virus in cell culture. Detection of IgM in serum samples by enzyme immunoassay has been the preferred method for case confirmation; however, as the incidence of disease decreases, the positive predictive value of IgM detection decreases. For this reason, detection of viral RNA in throat, nasal, and posterior nasopharyngeal swab specimens; bronchial lavage samples; blood or urine samples (respiratory samples are preferred specimens, and sampling more than 1 site may increase sensitivity) is playing an increasing role in case confirmation. A serum sample as well as a throat swab specimen should be obtained from

[1] Centers for Disease Control and Prevention. Progress toward regional measles elimination—worldwide, 2000-2020. *MMWR Morb Mortal Wkly Rep.* 2021;70(45):1563-1569

[2] Minta AA, Ferrari M, Antoni S, et al. Progress toward regional measles elimination—worldwide, 2000-2021. *MMWR Morb Mortal Wkly Rep.* 2022;71(47):1489-1495

[3] Centers for Disease Control. Measles prevention. *MMWR Suppl.* 1989;38(9):1-18

any patient in whom measles is suspected. Many state public health laboratories, the Association of Public Health Laboratories Vaccine Preventable Disease Reference Centers (VPD-RCs), and the Measles Laboratory at the Centers for Disease Control and Prevention (CDC) can perform reverse transcriptase polymerase chain reaction (RT-PCR) assays to detect measles RNA. Isolation of measles virus in cell culture is not recommended for routine case confirmation, because isolation can take up to 2 weeks to complete.

The sensitivity of measles IgM assays varies by timing of specimen collection, immunization status of the patient, and the assay method itself. Up to 20% of assays for IgM may have a false-negative result in the first 72 hours after rash onset. If the measles IgM result is negative and the patient has a generalized rash lasting more than 72 hours, the measles IgM test should be repeated. Measles IgM is detectable for at least 1 month after rash onset in unimmunized people but might be absent or present only transiently in people immunized with 1 or 2 measles-containing vaccine doses. Therefore, a negative IgM test result should not be used to rule out the diagnosis in immunized people.

Detection of viral RNA by NAAT provides a rapid and sensitive method for case confirmation. It is important to collect samples for RNA detection as soon as possible after rash onset, because viral shedding declines with time after rash. Specimen timing and quality greatly influence the results of NAATs, so a negative result should not be the only criterion used to rule out a case of measles. Another advantage of collecting samples for molecular detection of the virus is that these samples can also be used to genotype the virus, which is important to determine patterns of importation and transmission.

In populations with high rates of measles-containing vaccine coverage, such as those in the United States, comprehensive serologic and virologic testing generally is not available locally and requires submitting specimens to state public health laboratories or the CDC. Individuals with a febrile rash illness who are seronegative for measles IgM and have negative NAAT results for measles should be tested for rubella using the same specimens.

TREATMENT: No specific antiviral therapy is available. Measles virus is susceptible in vitro to ribavirin, which has been administered by the intravenous and aerosol routes to treat severely affected and immunocompromised children with measles. However, no controlled trials have been conducted, and ribavirin is not licensed by the US Food and Drug Administration for treatment of measles. Intravenous ribavirin is available only from the manufacturer through an emergency investigational new drug (eIND) application.

Vitamin A. The WHO currently recommends vitamin A for all children with measles, regardless of their country of residence. Many US experts concur with administering vitamin A to all children in the United States with measles, regardless of hospitalization status. Vitamin A treatment of children with measles in resource-limited countries has been associated with decreased morbidity and mortality rates. Low serum concentrations of vitamin A also have been found in children in the United States, and children with more severe measles illness may have lower vitamin A concentrations. Vitamin A for treatment of measles is administered once daily for 2 days (ie, immediately on diagnosis and repeated the next day), at the following doses:

- 200 000 IU (60 000 μg retinol activity equivalent [RAE]) for children 12 months or older;
- 100 000 IU (30 000 μg RAE) for infants 6 through 11 months of age; and
- 50 000 IU (15 000 μg RAE) for infants younger than 6 months.
- An additional (ie, a third) age-specific dose of vitamin A should be given 2 through 6 weeks later to children with clinical signs and symptoms of vitamin A deficiency.

INFECTION PREVENTION AND CONTROL MEASURES IN HEALTH CARE SETTINGS: In addition to standard precautions, airborne transmission precautions are indicated for 4 days after the onset of rash in otherwise healthy children and for the duration of illness in immunocompromised patients. Exposed susceptible patients should be placed on airborne precautions for 21 days after last exposure (28 days if the patient received immune globulin as postexposure prophylaxis).[1]

CONTROL MEASURES:

Evidence of Immunity to Measles.[2] Evidence of immunity to measles includes any of the following:

1. Documentation of age-appropriate vaccination with a live measles-containing vaccine:
   - Preschool-aged children: 1 dose administered after the first birthday;
   - School-aged children (grades K–12): 2 doses; the first dose administered after the first birthday and the second dose administered at least 28 days after the first dose;
   - Adults not at high risk: 1 dose administered after the first birthday;
   - Adults at high risk (eg, students in postsecondary education institutions, health care workers, international travelers): 2 doses; the first dose administered after the first birthday and the second dose administered at least 28 days after the first dose;
2. Laboratory evidence of immunity;
3. Laboratory confirmation of disease; or
4. Born before 1957.

Care of Exposed People. Table 3.32 and Table 3.33 summarize the use of vaccine and immune globulin (IG) for postexposure prophylaxis in people who are not immuno-compromised or pregnant and people who are immunocompromised or pregnant, respectively.

Use of Vaccine. Available data suggest that measles vaccine, if administered within 72 hours of measles exposure to susceptible individuals, will provide protection or dis-ease modification in some cases. Measles-containing vaccine should be considered in all exposed individuals who are vaccine eligible and who have not been vaccinated or have received only 1 dose of vaccine (the second measles vaccine dose can be admin-istered ≥28 days after the first measles vaccine dose). If the exposure does not result in infection, the vaccine should induce protection against subsequent measles exposures. Immunization is the intervention of choice for control of measles outbreaks in schools and child care centers and for vaccine-eligible people 12 months and older and has been used starting at 6 months of age with good efficacy in previous measles epidemics in the United States.

---

[1] Centers for Disease Control and Prevention. Immunization of health-care personnel: recommendations of the Advisory Committee on Immunization Practices (ACIP). *MMWR Recomm Rep*. 2011;60(RR-7):1-45

[2] Centers for Disease Control and Prevention. Prevention of measles, rubella, congenital rubella syndrome, and mumps, 2013 summary: recommendations of the Advisory Committee on Immunization Practices (ACIP). *MMWR Recomm Rep*. 2013;62(RR-4):1-34

Table 3.32. Postexposure Prophylaxis (PEP) for People Exposed to Measles Who Are NOT Pregnant or Immunocompromised

Age Range	Measles Immune Status[a]	PEP Type Depending on Time After Initial Exposure		
		≤3 days (≤72 hours)	4–6 days	>6 days
All ages (≥6 mo)	Immune	PEP not indicated. Exposed person has documented immunity.		
<6 mo	Nonimmune (because of age[b])	• Administer immune globulin intramuscular (IGIM)[c] • Home quarantine[d]		• PEP not indicated (too late). • Home quarantine[d]
6–11 mo	Nonimmune	• Administer MMR vaccine (MMR vaccine preferred over immune globulin [IG]) • No quarantine needed.[e]	• Administer IGIM[c] • Home quarantine[d]	• PEP not indicated (too late). • Home quarantine[d]
≥12 mo	Nonimmune	• Administer MMR vaccine • No quarantine needed[e]	• IG PEP usually not administered[f] • Home quarantine,[d] then administer MMR vaccine to protect from future exposures	
≥12 mo	1 dose of MMR vaccine	• Administer 2nd MMR vaccine dose if ≥28 days from the first dose • No quarantine needed (person had 1 dose when exposed)		

Adapted from a table developed by New York City Department of Health: www1.nyc.gov/assets/doh/downloads/pdf/imm/pep-measles-providers.pdf. Additional source: Centers for Disease Control and Prevention. Prevention of measles, rubella, congenital rubella syndrome, and mumps, 2013. *MMWR Recomm Rep.* 2013;62(RR-4):1-34; and Gastanaduy P, Redd S, Clemmons N, et al. Chapter 7: Measles. In: Roush SW, Baldy LM, Kirkconnell Hall MA, eds. *Manual for the Surveillance of Vaccine-Preventable Diseases.* Centers for Disease Control and Prevention. Page last reviewed May 13, 2019. Available at: www.cdc.gov/vaccines/pubs/s0urv-manual/chpt07-measles.html

[a] Acceptable evidence of immunity includes written documentation of age-appropriate vaccination, laboratory evidence of immunity, laboratory confirmation of disease, or birth before 1957.

[b] MMR vaccine is not indicated in this age group.

[c] Dosing of IGIM is 0.5 mL/kg of body weight (max dose 15 mL).

[d] The quarantine period is 21 days after the last exposure; most health departments would extend the monitoring period to 28 days if IG is administered as PEP, because IG can prolong the incubation period. Decisions on whether exposed persons who received IG as PEP appropriately (ie, within 6-day window) should return to settings such as child care, school, or work (ie, not be quarantined) should include consideration of the immune status and intensity of contacts in the setting and presence of high-risk individuals. These persons should be excluded from health care settings.

[e] Quarantine is not needed for persons who received MMR as PEP appropriately (ie, within the 3-day window), although these persons should be excluded from health care settings for 21 days.

[f] IGIM is recommended for infants <12 months of age, and IG administered intravenously is recommended for nonimmune pregnant people and severely immunocompromised persons. IGIM can be given to other persons (eg, ≥12 months of age) who do not have evidence of measles immunity, but priority should be given to persons exposed in settings with intense, prolonged, close contact (eg, household, child care, classroom).

Table 3.33. Postexposure Prophylaxis (PEP) for People Exposed to Measles Who ARE Pregnant or Immunocompromised

Category	Measles Immune Status[a]	PEP Type Depending on Time After Initial Exposure		
		≤3 days (≤72 hours)	4–6 days	>6 days
Severely immunocompromised[b]	IG recommended regardless of measles immune status	• Administer immune globulin intravenous (IGIV)[c] • Home quarantine[d]		• PEP not indicated (too late) • Home quarantine[d]
Pregnant	Immune		• PEP not indicated	
	Nonimmune	• Administer IGIV[c] • Home quarantine[d]		• PEP not indicated (too late) • Home quarantine[d]

Adapted from a table developed by New York City Department of Health: **www1.nyc.gov/assets/doh/downloads/pdf/imm/pep-measles-providers.pdf**. Additional source: Centers for Disease Control and Prevention. Prevention of measles, rubella, congenital rubella syndrome, and mumps, 2013. *MMWR Recomm Rep*. 2013;62(RR-4):1-34; and Gastanaduy P, Redd S, Clemmons N, et al. Chapter 7: Measles. In: Roush SW, Baldy LM, Kirkconnell Hall MA, eds. *Manual for the Surveillance of Vaccine-Preventable Diseases*. Centers for Disease Control and Prevention. Page last reviewed May 13, 2019. Available at: **www.cdc.gov/vaccines/pubs/s0urv-manual/chpt07-measles.html**

[a] Acceptable evidence of immunity includes written documentation of age-appropriate vaccination, laboratory evidence of immunity, laboratory confirmation of disease, or birth before 1957.

[b] The degree of altered immunocompetence in a patient should be determined by a physician. Severely immunocompromised patients include patients with severe primary immunodeficiency; patients who have received a hematopoietic cell transplant until at least 12 months after finishing all immunosuppressive treatment, or longer in patients who have developed graft-versus-host disease; patients on treatment for acute lymphoblastic leukemia (ALL) within and until at least 6 months after completion of immunosuppressive chemotherapy; and patients with HIV with severe immunosuppression, which for children ≤5 years is defined as CD4+ T-lymphocyte percentage <15% and for children >5 years and adolescents is defined as a CD4+ T-lymphocyte percentage <15% or a CD4+ T-lymphocyte count <200 lymphocytes/mm³, and those who have not received MMR vaccine since receiving effective antiretroviral therapy. Additional severely immunocompromising conditions and medications are provided in Rubin LG, Levin MJ, Ljungman P, et al 2013 IDSA Clinical practice guideline for vaccination of the immunocompromised host. *Clin Infect Dis*. 2014;58(3):e44-e100:

[c] Dosing of IGIV is 400 mg/kg of body weight.

[d] The quarantine period is 21 days after the last exposure; most health departments would extend the monitoring period to 28 days if IG is administered as PEP because IG can prolong the incubation period. Decisions on whether exposed persons who received IG as PEP appropriately (ie, within 6-day window) should return to settings such as child care, school, or work (ie, not be quarantined) should include consideration of the immune status and intensity of contacts in the setting and presence of high-risk individuals. These persons should be excluded from health care settings.

Use of Immune Globulin. Either immune globulin intramuscular (IGIM) or immune globulin intravenous (IGIV) can be administered within 6 days of exposure to prevent or modify measles in people who do not have evidence of measles immunity. Concentrations of measles antibodies in IGIM or IGIV products produced internationally may be different from those of products available in the United States. The recommended dose of IGIM is 0.50 mL/kg (maximum 15 mL). IGIV is the recommended IG preparation for pregnant people without evidence of measles immunity and for severely immunocompromised hosts, regardless of immunologic or vaccination status, including patients with severe primary immunodeficiency; patients who have received a hematopoietic cell transplant, until at least 12 months after finishing all immunosuppressive treatment or longer in patients who have developed graft-versus-host disease; patients undergoing treatment for acute lymphoblastic leukemia, within and until at least 6 months after completion of immunosuppressive chemotherapy; people who have received a solid organ transplant; people with human immunodeficiency virus (HIV) infection who have severe immunosuppression (for people ≤5 years of age, defined as a CD4+ T-lymphocyte percentage <15%; for people >5 years of age, defined as a CD4+ T-lymphocyte percentage <15% **or** a CD4+ T-lymphocyte count <200 lymphocytes/mm^3); and patients younger than 12 months whose birthing parent received biologic response modifiers during pregnancy.[1,2] IGIV is recommended for these people because they may be at higher risk of severe measles and complications. IGIV also is recommended for people who weigh >30 kg, who would receive less than the recommended dose with IGIM preparations since the maximum volume administered is 15 mL. IGIV is administered at a dose of 400 mg/kg. For patients who already are receiving IGIV at regularly scheduled intervals, the usual dose of 400 mg/kg should be adequate for measles prophylaxis after exposures occurring within 3 weeks of receiving IGIV. For people routinely receiving immune globulin subcutaneous (IGSC) therapy, consult the prescribing information for specific dosing related to measles, because it may vary based on other product characteristics. IG is not indicated for household or other close contacts who have received 1 dose of vaccine at 12 months or older unless they are severely immunocompromised (as defined previously).

For children who receive IGIM for modification or prevention of measles after exposure, measles vaccine (if not contraindicated) should be administered 6 months after IGIM administration and 8 months after IGIV administration, provided the child is at least 12 months of age. Intervals vary between administration of other biologic products and measles-containing vaccines (see Table 1.11, p 69).

HIV Infection.[1] Children living with HIV who are exposed to measles require prophylaxis based on immune status and measles vaccine history. Children living with HIV with no to moderate immunosuppression who have evidence of immunity (eg, serologic evidence of immunity to measles or who received 2 doses of measles vaccine after initiation of ART) do not require any additional measures to prevent measles

---

[1] Centers for Disease Control and Prevention. Prevention of measles, rubella, congenital rubella syndrome, and mumps, 2013 summary: recommendations of the Advisory Committee on Immunization Practices (ACIP). *MMWR Recomm Rep.* 2013;62(RR-4):1-34

[2] Rubin LG, Levin MJ, Ljungman P, et al. 2013 IDSA Clinical practice guideline for vaccination of the immunocompromised host. *Clin Infect Dis.* 2014;58(3):e44-e100

following an exposure. Mildly or moderately immunocompromised people living with HIV without evidence of immunity to measles (eg, no serologic evidence of immunity to measles and who have not received 2 doses of measles vaccine after initiation of ART) should receive immune globulin intramuscular (IGIM) at a dose of 0.5 mL/ kg (maximum 15 mL). Severely immunocompromised hosts (for people ≤5 years of age, defined as a CD4+ T-lymphocyte percentage <15%; for people >5 years of age, defined as a CD4+ T-lymphocyte percentage <15% **or** a CD4+ T-lymphocyte count <200 lymphocytes/mm^3) who are exposed to measles should receive immune globulin intravenous (IGIV) prophylaxis, 400 mg/kg, after exposure to measles, regardless of prior vaccination status, because they may not be protected by the vaccine. Children living with HIV who have received IGIV within 3 weeks of exposure do not require additional passive immunization.

Health Care Personnel. To decrease health care-associated infection, immunization programs should be established to ensure that all people who work or volunteer in health care facilities (including students) have presumptive evidence of immunity to measles (see Immunization in Health Care Personnel, p 115).

Measles Vaccine Recommendations (see Table 3.34 for summary).

Use of MMR Vaccine. The only measles vaccines licensed in the United States are live attenuated strains. Measles-containing vaccines provided through the Expanded

Table 3.34. Recommendations for Measles Immunization[a]

Category	Recommendations
Unimmunized, no history of measles (12 through 15 mo of age)	MMR or MMRV vaccine is recommended at 12 through 15 mo of age; a second dose is recommended at least 28 days after the first dose (or 90 days for MMRV) and usually is administered at 4 through 6 y of age.
Children 6 through 11 mo of age in outbreak situations[b] or before international travel	Immunize with MMR vaccine, ideally at least 2 weeks prior to travel, but this dose is not considered valid, and 2 valid doses administered on or after the first birthday are required. MMRV should not be administered to children <12 mo of age.
Students in kindergarten, elementary, middle, and high school who have received 1 dose of measles vaccine at 12 mo of age or older	Administer the second dose.
Students in college and other postsecondary institutions who have received 1 dose of measles vaccine at 12 mo of age or older	Administer the second dose.
History of immunization before the first birthday	Dose not considered valid; immunize (2 doses).

Table 3.34. Recommendations for Measles Immunization,[a] continued

Category	Recommendations
History of receipt of inactivated measles vaccine or unknown type of vaccine, 1963–1967	Dose not considered valid; immunize (2 doses).
Further attenuated or unknown vaccine administered with IG	Dose not considered valid; immunize (2 doses).
Allergy to eggs	Immunize; no reactions likely (see text for details).
Neomycin allergy, nonanaphylactic	Immunize; no reactions likely (see text for details).
Severe hypersensitivity (anaphylaxis) to neomycin or gelatin	Avoid immunization.
Tuberculosis	Immunize (see Tuberculosis, p 888); if patient has untreated tuberculosis disease, start antituberculosis therapy before immunizing.
Measles exposure	Immunize or give IG, depending on circumstances (see Care of Exposed People, p 574, Table 3.32, and Table 3.33).
People with HIV	Immunize (2 doses) unless severely immunocompromised (see text, p 577); administration of IG if exposed to measles is based on degree of immunosuppression and measles vaccine history (see text, p 577).
Personal or family history of seizures	Immunize; advise parents of slightly increased risk of seizures.
IG or blood product recipient	Immunize at the appropriate interval (see Table 1.11, p 69).

HIV indicates human immunodeficiency virus; IG, immune globulin; MMR, measles, mumps, and rubella vaccine; MMRV, measles, mumps, rubella, and varicella vaccine.
[a] See text for details and recommendations for use of MMRV vaccine.
[b] See Outbreak Control (p 585).

Programme on Immunization in resource-limited countries meet the WHO standards and usually are comparable with the vaccines available in the United States. Measles vaccine is only available in the United States as combination formulations, which include MMR (M-M-R II, manufactured by Merck; and Priorix, manufactured by GSK) and measles, mumps, rubella, and varicella (MMRV [ProQuad], manufactured by Merck) vaccines; single-antigen measles vaccine no longer is available in the United States. Measles-containing vaccine in a dose of 0.5 mL can be administered subcutaneously or intramuscularly, depending on the specific vaccine formulation used; M-M-R II and MMRV can be given either subcutaneously or intramuscularly, while Priorix can be given only subcutaneously. Measles-containing vaccine can be administered simultaneously with other immunizations in a separate syringe at a separate site (see Simultaneous Administration of Multiple Vaccines, p 63).

Serum antimeasles antibodies develop in approximately 95% of children immunized at 12 months of age and 98% of children immunized at 15 months of age. Protection conferred by a single dose is durable in most people. A small proportion (5% or less) of immunized people may lose protection after several years. For measles elimination, 2 doses of measles-containing vaccine are required. More than 99% of people who receive 2 doses (separated by at least 28 days, and the first dose administered on or after the first birthday) develop serologic evidence of measles immunity. The second dose provides protection to those failing to respond to their primary measles immunization and, therefore, is not a booster dose. Immunization is not deleterious for people who already are immune. Immunized people do not transmit measles vaccine virus.

Improperly stored vaccine may fail to protect against measles. Since 1979, an improved stabilizer has been added to the vaccine that makes it more resistant to heat inactivation. For recommended storage of MMR and MMRV vaccines, see the manufacturers' package labels. MMRV vaccine must be stored frozen between −58°F and +5°F.

Age of Routine Immunization. The first dose of MMR vaccine should be administered at 12 through 15 months of age. Delays in administering the first dose contributed to large outbreaks in the United States from 1989 to 1991. The second dose is recommended routinely at school entry (ie, 4 through 6 years of age) but can be administered at an earlier age (eg, during an outbreak or before international travel) provided the interval between the first and second MMR doses is at least 28 days. Catch-up second-dose immunization should occur for all school-aged children (elementary, middle, high school) who have received only 1 dose, including at the adolescent visit at 11 through 12 years of age and older. If a child receives a dose of measles vaccine before 12 months of age, this dose is not counted toward the required number of doses; the universally recommended 2 doses are still required in the United States beginning at 12 through 15 months of age and separated by at least 28 days.

Use of MMRV Vaccine.[1]

- MMRV vaccine is indicated for simultaneous immunization against measles, mumps, rubella, and varicella among children 12 months through 12 years of age; MMRV vaccine is not indicated for people outside this age group. See Varicella-Zoster Infections, p 938, for recommendations for use of MMRV vaccine for the first dose.
- Children with HIV infection should not receive MMRV vaccine because of lack of safety data of the quadrivalent vaccine in children infected with HIV.
- MMRV vaccine may be administered with other vaccines recommended at 12 through 15 months of age or at 4 through 6 years of age (**https://redbook. solutions.aap.org/SS/Immunization_Schedules.aspx**).
- At least 28 days should elapse between a dose of measles-containing vaccine, such as MMR vaccine, and a dose of MMRV vaccine. However, the recommended minimal interval between 2 separate MMRV vaccine doses is 90 days.

Colleges and Other Institutions for Education Beyond High School. Colleges and other post-secondary educational institutions should require that all entering students have documentation of evidence of measles immunity (see Evidence of Immunity to Measles, p 574). Students without documentation of measles immunity should receive MMR vaccine on entry, followed by a second dose 28 days later, if not contraindicated.

---

[1] Centers for Disease Control and Prevention. Use of combination measles, mumps, rubella, and varicella vaccine: recommendations of the Advisory Committee on Immunization Practices (ACIP). *MMWR Recomm Rep.* 2010;59(RR−3):1−12

Immunization During an Outbreak. During an outbreak, MMR vaccine should be offered to all vaccine-eligible people exposed or in the outbreak setting who lack evidence of measles immunity. During a community-wide outbreak that affects infants, MMR vaccine has been shown to be efficacious and may be recommended for infants 6 through 11 months of age (see Outbreak Control, p 585). Doses received prior to the first birthday do not count toward the recommended 2-dose series.

International Travel. People traveling internationally (any country outside of the United States) should be immune to measles prior to travel. Infants 6 through 11 months of age should receive 1 dose of MMR vaccine at least 2 weeks before departure if possible, and then should receive a second dose of measles-containing vaccine at 12 through 15 months of age (at least 28 days after the initial measles immunization) and a third dose at 4 through 6 years of age. Children 12 months or older as well as adults who have received 1 dose and are traveling to areas where measles is endemic or epidemic should receive their second dose before departure, provided the interval between doses is 28 days or more.

International Adoptees. The US Department of State requires that internationally adopted children 10 years and older receive MMR vaccine before entry into the United States. Internationally adopted children who are younger than 10 years are exempt from Immigration and Nationality Act regulations pertaining to immunization of immigrants before arrival in the United States (see Children Who Received Immunizations Outside the United States or Whose Immunization Status is Unknown or Uncertain, p 119); adoptive parents are required to sign a waiver indicating their intention to comply with US immunization recommendations after their child's arrival in the United States.

Health Care Personnel.[1] Adequate presumptive evidence of immunity to measles for people who work in health care facilities is: (1) documented administration of 2 doses of live-virus measles vaccine with the first dose administered at ≥ 12 months of age and the second dose at least 28 days after the first; (2) laboratory evidence of immunity or laboratory confirmation of disease; or (3) birth before 1957. Birth before 1957 is not a guarantee of measles immunity, and therefore, facilities should consider vaccinating unimmunized personnel born before 1957 who lack laboratory evidence of immunity with 2 doses of MMR vaccine at the appropriate interval (see Immunization in Health Care Personnel, p 115). For recommendations during an outbreak, see Outbreak Control (p 585).

Adverse Events. A body temperature of 39.4°C (103°F) or higher develops in approximately 5% to 15% of vaccine recipients, usually between 5 and 12 days after receipt of MMR vaccine; fever generally lasts 1 to 2 days but may last as long as 5 days. Most people with fever do not have other symptoms. Transient rashes have been reported in approximately 5% of vaccine recipients. Although recipients who develop fever and/or rash are not considered contagious and are not at risk for long-term sequelae of measles, suspicion for wild-type measles may be high, especially if vaccine was administered as part of an outbreak response. Therefore, rapid differentiation of vaccine reactions from infections with wild-type virus is critical for guiding the public health response to outbreaks. Vaccine reactions can be laboratory confirmed by detecting

---

[1] Centers for Disease Control and Prevention. Immunization of health-care personnel: recommendations of the Advisory Committee on Immunization Practices (ACIP). *MMWR Recomm Rep.* 2011;60(RR–07):1–45

measles vaccine virus in respiratory secretions or urine followed by sequencing to determine genotype or by use of a NAAT for specific detection of measles vaccine strains (MeVa) that is available at the CDC and through state health departments.

Febrile seizures 5 to 12 days after immunization occur in 1 in 3000 to 4000 people immunized with MMR vaccine. Transient thrombocytopenia occurs in 1 in 22 000 to 40 000 people after administration of measles-containing vaccines, specifically MMR (see Thrombocytopenia, p 583). There is no evidence that reimmunization increases the risk of adverse events in people already immune to these diseases. Data indicate that only people who are not immune to the viruses in MMR tend to have adverse effects. Thus, events following a second dose of MMR vaccine would be expected to be substantially lower than after a first dose because most people who received a first dose would be immune.

Rates of most local and systemic adverse events for children immunized with MMRV vaccine are comparable with rates for children immunized with MMR and varicella vaccines administered concomitantly. However, recipients of a first dose of MMRV vaccine have a greater rate of fever 102°F (38.9°C) or higher than do recipients of MMR and varicella vaccine administered concomitantly (22% vs 15%, respectively). Febrile seizures occur in 1 in 1100 to 1400 children immunized with a first dose of MMRV vaccine at 12 through 23 months of age and in 1 in 2500 to 3000 children immunized with a first dose of MMR and varicella vaccines administered separately at the same visit. The period of risk for febrile seizures is from 5 to 12 days following receipt of the vaccine. The benefit of using MMRV instead of MMR and monovalent varicella vaccines separately is that the quadrivalent product results in 1 fewer injection. Either MMRV or separate MMR and varicella vaccines are an acceptable option for dose 1 at 12 through 15 months of age and pediatricians should discuss risks and benefits of the vaccine choices with the parents or caregivers. For the first dose of measles, mumps, rubella, and varicella vaccines at ages 48 months and older and for dose 2 at any age (15 months through 12 years), use of MMRV vaccine generally is preferred over separate injections of MMR and varicella vaccines to minimize the number of injections.

The reported frequency of central nervous system conditions, such as encephalitis and encephalopathy, after measles immunization is less than 1 per million doses administered in the United States. Because the incidence of encephalitis or encephalopathy after measles immunization in the United States is lower than the observed incidence of encephalitis of unknown cause, some or most of the rare reported severe neurologic disorders may be related temporally, rather than causally, to measles immunization. Multiple studies, as well as the National Academy of Medicine Vaccine Safety Review, refute a causal relationship between autism and MMR vaccine or between inflammatory bowel disease and MMR vaccine.

Precautions and Contraindications.

Febrile Illnesses. Children with minor illnesses, such as upper respiratory tract infections, may be immunized. Fever is not a contraindication to immunization. However, if other manifestations suggest a more serious illness, immunization should be deferred until the illness has resolved.

Allergic Reactions. Hypersensitivity reactions occur rarely and usually are minor, consisting of wheal-and-flare reactions or urticaria at the injection site. Reactions have been attributed to trace amounts of neomycin or gelatin or some other component in the vaccine formulation. Anaphylaxis is rare. Measles vaccine is produced in chicken embryo cell culture and does not contain significant amounts of egg white (ovalbumin) cross-reacting proteins. Children with egg allergy are at low risk of anaphylactic reactions to measles-containing vaccine (including MMR and MMRV). Skin testing of children for egg allergy is not predictive of reactions to MMR vaccine and is not recommended before administering MMR or other measles-containing vaccine. People with allergies to chickens or feathers are not at increased risk of reaction to the vaccine.

Measles-containing vaccine should not be administered to people who have had a severe allergic reaction to a previous dose of measles-containing vaccine or to a vaccine component.

Thrombocytopenia. Rarely, MMR vaccine can be associated with mild thrombocytopenia within 2 months of immunization, with a temporal clustering 2 to 3 weeks after immunization. Most cases of thrombocytopenia resolve within 1 week. Based on case reports, the risk of vaccine-associated thrombocytopenia may be higher for people who previously experienced thrombocytopenia, especially if it occurred in temporal association with earlier MMR immunization. The decision to immunize these children should be based on assessment of immunity after the first dose and the benefits of protection against measles, mumps, and rubella in comparison with the risks of recurrence of thrombocytopenia after immunization. The risk of thrombocytopenia is higher after the first dose of vaccine than after the second dose. There have been no reported cases of thrombocytopenia associated with receipt of MMR vaccine that have resulted in hemorrhagic complications or death in otherwise healthy people.

Recent Administration of IG or Other Blood Products. IG preparations interfere with the serologic response to measles vaccine for variable periods, depending on the dose of IG administered. Suggested intervals between IG or blood-product administration and measles immunization are provided in Table 1.11 (p 69). If vaccine is administered at intervals shorter than those indicated, as may be warranted if the risk of exposure to measles is imminent, the child should be reimmunized at or after the appropriate interval for immunization (and at least 28 days after the earlier immunization).

MMR vaccine should be administered at least 2 weeks before planned administration of IG, blood transfusion, or other blood products because of the theoretical possibility that antibody in those products could neutralize vaccine virus and interfere with successful immunization. If IG must be administered within 14 days after administration of MMR or MMRV, these vaccines should be administered again after the interval specified in Table 1.11 (p 69).

Tuberculosis. Tuberculin skin testing or interferon gamma release assay (IGRA) testing is not a prerequisite for MMR immunization. Antituberculosis therapy should be initiated before administering MMR vaccine to people with untreated tuberculosis infection or disease. Tuberculin skin or IGRA testing, if otherwise indicated, can be performed on the day of immunization with MMR vaccine. Otherwise, tuberculin skin or IGRA testing should be postponed for 4 to 6 weeks, because measles immunization temporarily may suppress tuberculin skin test reactivity and possibly affect IGRA testing.

Altered Immunity. Immunocompromised patients with disorders associated with increased severity of viral infections should not receive live-virus measles vaccine (the exception is people with HIV infection, unless they have evidence of severe immuno-suppression; see Immunization and Other Considerations in Immunocompromised Children, p 93, and HIV Infection, below). The risk of exposure to measles for immunocompromised patients can be decreased by immunizing their close susceptible contacts. Immunized people do not shed or transmit infectious measles vaccine virus. Management of immunodeficient and immunosuppressed patients exposed to measles can be facilitated by previous knowledge of their immune status. If possible, children should receive measles vaccine before initiating treatment with biologic response modifiers, such as tumor necrosis factor antagonists, and before transplantation, ideally with 2 doses. Severely immunocompromised patients should receive IG after measles exposure regardless of immunologic or vaccination status (see Care of Exposed People, p 574, Table 3.32, and Table 3.33).

Corticosteroids. For patients who have received high doses of corticosteroids ($\geq$2 mg/kg of body weight or $\geq$20 mg/day of prednisone or its equivalent for people who weigh $\geq$10 kg) for 14 days or more and who otherwise are not immunocompromised, the recommended interval between stopping the corticosteroids and immunization is at least 4 weeks (see Immunization and Other Considerations in Immunocompromised Children, p 93). In general, inhaled steroids do not cause immunosuppression and are not a contraindication to measles immunization.

HIV Infection.[1] Measles immunization (administered as MMR vaccine) is recommended for all people $\geq$12 months of age with HIV who do not have evidence of measles immunity and who do not have evidence of severe immunosuppression, because measles can be severe and sometimes is fatal in patients with HIV (see Human Immunodeficiency Virus Infection, p 489). For vaccination purposes, severe immuno-suppression for people $\leq$5 years of age is defined as a CD4+ T-lymphocyte percentage <15%, and for people >5 years of age is defined as a CD4+ T-lymphocyte percentage <15% **or** a CD4+ T-lymphocyte count <200 lymphocytes/mm^3. Severely immuno-compromised HIV-infected infants, children, adolescents, and young adults should not receive measles virus-containing vaccine. MMRV vaccine should not be administered to any infant or child with HIV, regardless of degree of immunosuppression, because of lack of safety data in this population. Children, adolescents, and adults with newly diagnosed HIV and without evidence of measles immunity should complete a 2-dose schedule with MMR vaccine as soon as possible after diagnosis, unless they have evidence of severe immunosuppression. People with perinatally acquired HIV who were vaccinated against measles prior to the establishment of effective ART should be considered unvaccinated and should be revaccinated with 2 doses of MMR vaccine once effective ART has been administered, unless they have other acceptable current evidence of measles immunity or unless they are severely immunocompromised. All members of the household of an HIV-infected person who lack evidence of measles immunity should receive 2 doses of MMR.

Personal or Family History of Seizures. Children with a personal or family history of seizures should be immunized after parents or guardians are advised that the risk of seizures after measles immunization is increased slightly. Children receiving anticonvulsants should continue such therapy after measles immunization.

---

[1] Rubin LG, Levin MJ, Ljungman P, et al. 2013 IDSA clinical practice guideline for vaccination of the immunocompromised host. *Clin Infect Dis.* 2014;58(3):309-318

Pregnancy. Measles-containing vaccine should not be administered to people known to be pregnant. People who receive MMR vaccine should not become pregnant for at least 28 days. This precaution is based on the theoretical risk of fetal infection, which applies to administration of any live-virus vaccine to people who might be pregnant or who might become pregnant shortly after immunization. No data from people who were inadvertently vaccinated while pregnant substantiate this theoretical risk. When immunizing adolescents and young adults against measles, recommended precautions include asking if they are pregnant, excluding people who are pregnant, and explaining the theoretical risks to others who may become pregnant. Pregnancy testing prior to immunization is not required.

Outbreak Control. Every suspected measles case should be reported immediately to the local health department, and every effort must be made to obtain laboratory evidence that would confirm that the illness is measles, especially if the illness may be the first case in the community. Subsequent prevention of spread of measles depends on prompt immunization of people at risk of exposure or people already exposed. People who have not been immunized, including those who have been exempted from measles immunization for medical reasons, should be excluded from school, child care, and health care settings until at least 21 days after the onset of rash in the last case of measles involved in the outbreak.

Schools and Child Care Facilities. During measles outbreaks in child care facilities, schools, and colleges and other institutions of higher education, all students, their siblings, and personnel born in 1957 or after who cannot provide evidence of measles immunity should be immunized. People receiving their second dose, as well as unimmunized people receiving their first dose as part of the outbreak-control program, may be readmitted immediately to the school or child care facility.

Health Care Facilities. If an outbreak occurs in an area served by a hospital or within a hospital, all employees and volunteers who cannot provide evidence of immunity to measles should receive 2 doses of MMR vaccine. Because some health care personnel born before 1957 have acquired measles in health care facilities, immunization with 2 doses of MMR vaccine is recommended for health care personnel without serologic evidence of immunity in this age category during outbreaks. Serologic testing before immunization is not recommended during an outbreak because rapid immunization is required to halt disease transmission. Health care personnel without evidence of immunity who have been exposed should be relieved of direct patient contact from the fifth day after the first exposure to the 21st day after the last exposure, regardless of whether they received vaccine or IG after the exposure. Health care personnel who become ill should be relieved of patient contact until 4 days after rash develops.

Meningococcal Infections

CLINICAL MANIFESTATIONS: Invasive meningococcal infection usually results in septicemia (35%–40% of cases), meningitis (~50% of cases), or both. Bacteremic pneumonia is less common (10% of cases). Rarely, *Neisseria meningitidis* is identified as a cause of occult bacteremia. The onset of invasive infections can be insidious and nonspecific, but the onset of septicemia (meningococcemia) typically is abrupt, with fever, chills, malaise, myalgia, limb pain, prostration, and a rash that initially can be macular or maculopapular but typically becomes petechial or purpuric within hours.

A similar rash can occur with viral infections or with severe sepsis attributable to other bacterial pathogens. In fulminant cases, purpura, limb ischemia, coagulopathy, pulmonary edema, shock, coma, and death can ensue within hours despite appropriate management. Signs and symptoms of meningococcal meningitis are indistinguishable from those associated with pneumococcal meningitis. In severe and fatal cases of meningococcal meningitis, increased intracranial pressure is a predominant presenting feature. Invasive infections can be complicated by arthritis, myocarditis, pericarditis, and endophthalmitis. Noninvasive meningococcal infections, such as conjunctivitis and urethritis, also occur. Chronic meningococcemia is a rare syndrome, mostly seen in young adults, that is characterized by a more prolonged course (>7 days) with intermittent fever, migratory arthralgia, and cutaneous lesions (erythematous macules, papules, nodules, petechiae, or purpura).

The overall case fatality rate for invasive meningococcal disease is 15% and is somewhat higher in older adults. Clinical predictors of mortality include coma, hypotension, leukopenia, and thrombocytopenia. A self-limiting postinfectious inflammatory syndrome occurs in fewer than 10% of cases, begins a minimum 4 days after onset of meningococcal infection, and most commonly presents as fever and arthritis or vasculitis with less common manifestations including iritis, scleritis, conjunctivitis, pericarditis, and polyserositis.

Sequelae associated with meningococcal disease occur in up to 20% of survivors and include hearing loss, neurologic disability, digit or limb amputations, and skin scarring. In addition, patients may experience subtle long-term neurologic deficits, such as impaired school performance, behavioral problems, and attention-deficit/hyperactivity disorder.

ETIOLOGY: *Neisseria meningitidis* is a gram-negative diplococcus with 12 confirmed serogroups based on capsular type.

EPIDEMIOLOGY: *N meningitidis* disease rates are highest in infants <1 year of age, followed by children 1 to 4 years of age, the very elderly (≥85 years), and adolescents and young adults 16 to 23 years of age. Household contacts of cases have 500 to 800 times the rate of disease of the general population. A predominance of US cases is observed in the winter, often noted 2 to 3 weeks following onset of influenza outbreaks, with a peak of cases in January, February, and March. Patients with persistent complement-component deficiencies (eg, C3, C5–C9, properdin, or factor D or factor H deficiencies), with anatomic or functional asplenia or human immunodeficiency virus infection (HIV), or treated with eculizumab or similar complement inhibitors are at increased risk of invasive and recurrent meningococcal disease. Asymptomatic colonization of the upper respiratory tract is most common in older adolescents and young adults and is the reservoir from which the organism is spread. Transmission occurs from person to person through droplets from the respiratory tract and requires close contact. Patients should be considered capable of transmitting the organism for up to 24 hours after initiation of effective antimicrobial treatment.

Distribution of meningococcal serogroups in the United States has shifted in the past 2 decades. Serogroups B accounts for most cases currently, followed by serogroups C, W, and Y and nongroupable (nonencapsulated) meningococci. Serogroup distribution varies by age, location, and time. In infants and children younger than 60 months, approximately two thirds of cases are caused by serogroup B. More than 75% of cases among adolescents and young adults are caused by serogroups B, C, Y, or W and, therefore, potentially are preventable with available vaccines.

Since the early 2000s, annual incidence rates for invasive meningococcal disease have decreased, and during 2019 approximately 375 cases occurred (incidence of 0.11 per 100 000 population) in the United States. The decrease in cases in the United States started before the 2005 introduction of ACWY meningococcal conjugate vaccine into the routine immunization schedule at age 11 through 12 years and the 2010 recommendation for a booster vaccine at age 16 years. Reasons for this decrease in incidence are postulated to be related to the increased use of influenza vaccine, reduction in the carriage rates, the use of meningococcal conjugate vaccines in preadolescents and adolescents, and changes in behavioral risk factors (eg, decreases in smoking and exposure to secondhand smoke among adolescents and young adults).

Strains belonging to groups A, B, C, W, X, and Y are implicated most commonly in invasive disease worldwide. Serogroup A has historically been associated with epidemics outside the United States, primarily in sub-Saharan Africa. A serogroup A meningococcal conjugate vaccine was introduced in the "meningitis belt" of sub-Saharan Africa starting in December 2010, and its widespread use has been associated with a marked reduction in serogroup A disease rates; recent outbreaks in the meningitis belt have been associated with serogroups C, W, and X. In Europe, Australia, and South America, the incidence of meningococcal disease ranged from 0.3 to 2 cases per 100 000 population in recent years. Serogroups B, C, W, and Y are most commonly reported in these regions. Rates of meningococcal disease declined globally (~70%) in 2020 during the COVID-19 pandemic; these declines may have been the result of masking, social distancing, and other measures controlling respiratory droplet spread.

Most cases of meningococcal disease are sporadic, with fewer than 10% associated with outbreaks. Outbreaks occur in communities and institutions, including child care centers, schools, colleges, and military recruit camps. Multiple outbreaks of serogroup B meningococcal disease have occurred on college campuses, and outbreaks of serogroup C meningococcal disease have been reported among men who have sex with men and among people lacking housing.

The **incubation period** for invasive disease is 1 to 10 days, usually less than 4 days.

DIAGNOSTIC TESTS: Cultures of blood and cerebrospinal fluid (CSF) are indicated for patients with suspected invasive meningococcal disease. Cultures of a petechial or purpuric lesion scraping, synovial fluid, and other usually sterile body fluid specimens sometimes are positive. Specimens for culture should be plated onto both sheep blood and chocolate agar and incubated at 35°C to 37°C with 5% carbon dioxide in a moist atmosphere. The organism is readily identified with standard biochemical tests as well as by the newer method of mass spectrometry of bacterial cell components. Antimicrobial susceptibility testing of invasive isolates is useful because of the occurrence of beta-lactamase producing strains and fluoroquinolone-resistant strains (ciprofloxacin is one of the agents used for prophylaxis of close contacts; antimicrobial testing should not delay administration of prophylaxis). A Gram stain of a petechial or purpuric scraping, CSF, or buffy coat smear of blood may reveal gram negative diplococci. Because *N meningitidis* can be a component of the nasopharyngeal flora, isolation of *N meningitidis* from this site is not helpful diagnostically. A serogroup-specific nucleic acid amplification test (NAAT) to detect *N meningitidis* from clinical specimens from

Table 3.35. Surveillance Case Definitions for Invasive Meningococcal Disease[a]

Confirmed case
- Detection of *Neisseria meningitidis*-specific nucleic acid in a specimen obtained from a normally sterile body site (eg, blood or cerebrospinal fluid [CSF]) using a validated polymerase chain reaction assay; or
- Isolation of *N meningitidis*
  - From a normally sterile body site (eg, blood or CSF, or less commonly, synovial, pleural, or pericardial fluid); or
  - From purpuric lesions

Probable case
- Detection of *N meningitidis* antigen
  - In formalin-fixed tissue by immunohistochemistry; or
  - In CSF by latex agglutination

Suspect case
- Clinical purpura fulminans in the absence of a positive blood culture; or
- Gram-negative diplococci, not yet identified, isolated from a normally sterile body site (eg, blood or CSF)

[a]https://ndc.services.cdc.gov/case-definitions/meningococcal-disease-2015/

usually sterile sites (eg, CSF) is useful particularly in patients who receive antimicrobial therapy before cultures are obtained. In the United States, commercially available multiplex polymerase chain reaction (PCR) assays have excellent sensitivity and specificity for detection of serogroups A, B, C, W, X, and Y. Antigen detection tests, primarily by latex agglutination, to detect select meningococcal polysaccharide types in CSF were developed more than 3 decades ago. These assays no longer are commonly used in the United States because of concerns about test sensitivity and specificity.

Surveillance case definitions for invasive meningococcal disease are provided in Table 3.35. Serologic typing and other characterization such as whole genome sequencing and genomic typing can be useful epidemiologic tools during a suspected outbreak to detect concordance among invasive strains.

TREATMENT: The priority in management of meningococcal disease is treatment of shock in meningococcemia and of raised intracranial pressure in severe meningitis. Empirical therapy for suspected meningococcal disease should include cefotaxime or ceftriaxone. Once the microbiologic diagnosis is established, treatment options include cefotaxime, ceftriaxone, penicillin G, or ampicillin. A course of 5 to 7 days of antimicrobial therapy is adequate. Because of recent detections of β-lactamase-producing *N meningitidis* in the United States, meningococcal isolate susceptibility to penicillin should be determined before switching to penicillin or ampicillin.[1] Ceftriaxone clears nasopharyngeal carriage effectively after 1 dose. For patients with a life-threatening penicillin allergy characterized by anaphylaxis, meropenem can be used with caution as the rate of cross-reactivity in penicillin-allergic adults is very low. In meningococcemia, early and rapid fluid resuscitation and early use of inotropic and ventilatory

[1] McNamara LA, Potts C, Blain AE, et al. Detection of ciprofloxacin-resistant, β-lactamase–producing *Neisseria meningitidis* serogroup Y isolates—United States, 2019–2020. *MMWR Morb Mortal Wkly Rep.* 2020;69(24):735–739

support may reduce mortality. The postinfectious inflammatory syndromes associated with meningococcal disease often respond to nonsteroidal anti-inflammatory drugs. Treating physicians should consider evaluating for conditions that increase risk of disease, such as underlying complement component deficiencies. In some studies, underlying complement deficiency has been identified in up to 10% to 50% of patients with meningococcal disease, although no recent data are available on complement deficiency prevalence among US patients with meningococcal disease.

INFECTION PREVENTION AND CONTROL MEASURES IN HEALTH CARE SETTINGS: In addition to standard precautions, droplet precautions are recommended until 24 hours after initiation of effective antimicrobial therapy.

CONTROL MEASURES:

Care of Exposed People.

Postexposure Chemoprophylaxis. Regardless of immunization status, close contacts including household contacts of all people with invasive meningococcal disease (see Table 3.36), whether endemic or in an outbreak situation, are at high risk of infection and should promptly receive chemoprophylaxis. Chemoprophylaxis should be provided even if the close contact has received a meningococcal vaccine. The decision to administer chemoprophylaxis to other contacts is based on risk of contracting invasive disease related to specific exposure to the secretions from the infected patient. Throat and nasopharyngeal cultures are not recommended, because these cultures are of no value in deciding who should receive chemoprophylaxis.

Table 3.36. Disease Risk for Contacts of People With Invasive Meningococcal Disease

High risk: chemoprophylaxis recommended (close contacts)
- Household contact
- Child care or preschool contact at any time during 7 days before onset of illness
- Direct exposure to index patient's secretions through kissing or through sharing toothbrushes or eating utensils, markers of close social contact, at any time during 7 days before onset of illness
- Mouth-to-mouth resuscitation, unprotected contact during endotracheal intubation at any time from 7 days before onset of illness to 24 h after initiation of effective antimicrobial therapy
- Frequently slept in same dwelling as index patient during 7 days before onset of illness
- Passengers seated directly next to the index case during airline flights lasting more than 8 hours (gate to gate), or passengers seated within one seat in any direction from an index case on a flight of any duration if the index case was coughing or vomiting during the flight

Low risk: chemoprophylaxis not recommended
- Casual contact: no history of direct exposure to index patient's oral secretions (eg, school or work)
- Indirect contact: only contact is with a high-risk contact, no direct contact with the index patient
- Health care personnel without direct exposure to patient's oral secretions

In outbreak or cluster
- Chemoprophylaxis for people other than people at high risk (close contacts) should be administered only after consultation with local public health authorities

Table 3.35 provides the surveillance case definition for invasive meningococcal disease. Table 3.36 provides prophylaxis recommendations for contacts of a person with invasive meningococcal disease, and Table 3.37 provides recommended prophylaxis regimens. Routine prophylaxis is not recommended for health care personnel unless they have had intimate exposure to respiratory tract secretions, such as occurs with unprotected mouth-to-mouth resuscitation, intubation, or suctioning before or

Table 3.37. Recommended Chemoprophylaxis Regimens for High-Risk Contacts and People With Invasive Meningococcal Disease

Age of Infants, Children, and Adults	Dose	Duration	Efficacy, %	Cautions
Rifampin[a]				
<1 mo	5 mg/kg per dose, orally, every 12 h	2 days		Discussion with an expert for infants <1 mo
≥1 mo	10 mg/kg per dose (maximum 600 mg), orally, every 12 h	2 days	90–95	Can interfere with efficacy of oral contraceptives and some seizure and anticoagulant medications; can stain soft contact lenses
Ceftriaxone				
<15 y	125 mg, intramuscularly	Single dose	90–95	To decrease pain at injection site, dilute with 1% lidocaine
≥15 y	250 mg, intramuscularly	Single dose	90–95	To decrease pain at injection site, dilute with 1% lidocaine
Ciprofloxacin[a,b]				
≥1 mo	20 mg/kg (maximum 500 mg), orally	Single dose	90–95	
Azithromycin	10 mg/kg (maximum 500 mg)	Single dose	90	Not recommended routinely; equivalent to rifampin for eradication of Neisseria meningitidis from nasopharynx in one study of young adults

[a] Not recommended for use in pregnant people.
[b] If fluoroquinolone-resistant strains of N meningitidis have been identified in a community, refer to Table 3.38.

Table 3.38. Recommended Approach to Chemoprophylaxis When Ciprofloxacin-Resistant Invasive Isolates Have Been Detected[a]

- Consult local or state public health officials on whether ciprofloxacin-resistant isolates have been detected and discuss approach (which may be refined depending on local epidemiology)
- Discontinue use of ciprofloxacin for prophylaxis of close contacts when both of the following threshold criteria have been met in the catchment area during a rolling 12-month period:
  - Two or more invasive meningococcal disease cases caused by ciprofloxacin-resistant strains have been reported, and
  - Cases caused by ciprofloxacin-resistant strains make up at least 20% of all reported invasive meningococcal disease cases
- Prescribe rifampin, ceftriaxone, or azithromycin instead of ciprofloxacin as prophylaxis when the threshold criteria have been reached
- Implement updated prophylaxis guidance in all counties within the catchment area (or other geographic area as determined by local or state public health officials)
- Maintain updated prophylaxis guidance until a full 24 months have passed without any invasive meningococcal disease cases caused by ciprofloxacin-resistant strains having been reported in the catchment area

[a]Adapted from **www.cdc.gov/meningococcal/outbreaks/changing-prophylaxis-antibiotics.html**.

less than 24 hours after antimicrobial therapy was initiated. Chemoprophylaxis ideally should be initiated within 24 hours after the index patient is identified; prophylaxis is not indicated if more than 2 weeks have passed since the last exposure. If antimicrobial agents other than ceftriaxone or cefotaxime (each of which will eradicate nasopharyngeal carriage) are used for treatment of invasive meningococcal disease, the index patient should receive chemoprophylaxis before hospital discharge to eradicate nasopharyngeal carriage of *N meningitidis*.

Ciprofloxacin-resistant strains of *N meningitidis* have been detected over the past 17 years.[1,2] Prophylaxis failures and antimicrobial resistance among meningococcal isolates should be monitored and reported to the local or state public health department to inform meningococcal prophylaxis recommendations. The Centers for Disease Control and Prevention (CDC) has provided guidance on meningococcal disease prophylaxis in areas with ciprofloxacin resistance (see Table 3.38 and **www.cdc.gov/meningococcal/outbreaks/changing-prophylaxis-antibiotics.html**).

Meningococcal Vaccines. In the United States, 3 meningococcal vaccines are licensed and available for use in children and adults against serogroups A, C, W, and Y (MenACWY), and 2 vaccines are licensed for people 10 through 25 years of age against serogroup B (MenB). All 3 MenACWY vaccines are protein-polysaccharide conjugate vaccines, while the 2 MenB vaccines are protein-based vaccines using 2 different technologies. In addition, the US Food and Drug Administration licensed a MenABCWY pentavalent meningococcal vaccine on October 20, 2023, for persons 10 through

[1] Centers for Disease Control and Prevention. Emergence of fluoroquinolone-resistant *Neisseria meningitidis*—Minnesota and North Dakota, 2007–2008. *MMWR Morb Mortal Wkly Rep.* 2008;57(7):173-175

[2] McNamara LA, Potts C, Blain AE, et al. Detection of ciprofloxacin-resistant, β-lactamase–producing *Neisseria meningitidis* serogroup Y isolates—United States, 2019–2020. *MMWR Morb Mortal Wkly Rep.* 2020;69(24):735–739

Table 3.39. Recommended Meningococcal Vaccines for Immunocompetent Children and Adults[a]

Age	Vaccine	Status
Meningococcal ACWY Vaccines		
2 mo through 10 y	MenACWY-D[b] (Menactra) or MenACWY-CRM[c] (Menveo) or MenACWY-TT[d] (MenQuadfi)	**Not routinely recommended;** see Table 3.40 (p 594) for recommendations for people at increased risk
11 through 21 y	MenACWY-D or MenACWY-CRM or MenACWY-TT	• 11 through 18 y of age, with first dose at age 11–12 y and booster dose at age 16 y (give booster only if first dose administered prior to 16th birthday) • 19 through 21 y of age, not routinely recommended but may be administered as catch-up immunization for those who have not received a dose after their 16th birthday or who become at increased risk for meningococcal disease
Meningococcal B Vaccines		
10 y through 15 y	MenB-FHbp[e] (Trumenba) or MenB-4C[f] (Bexsero)	**Not routinely recommended** see Table 3.40 (p 594) for recommendations for people at increased risk
16 y through 23 y	MenB-FHbp or MenB-4C	• Administer based on shared clinical decision-making with preferred age of 16 y through 18 y and 2-dose series recommended • For MenB-4C (Bexsero), dose 1 administered initially, then followed by dose 2 administered ≥1 month later • For MenB-FHbp (Trumenba), dose 1 administered initially, then followed by dose 2 administered 6 months later; in setting of serogroup B meningococcal outbreak, a 3-dose vaccine series administered at 0, 1–2, and 6 months See Table 3.40 (p 594) for recommendations for people at increased risk

Table 3.39. Recommended Meningococcal Vaccines for Immunocompetent Children and Adults,[a] continued

Age	Vaccine	Status
Meningococcal ABCWY Vaccine		
10 through 25 y	MenABCWY[g]	May be used when both MenACWY and MenB are indicated at the same visit[h]

[a] Please see full recommendations on Meningococcal Vaccination: Recommendations of the Advisory Committee on Immunization Practices, United States, 2020 at **www.cdc.gov/mmwr/volumes/69/rr/rr6909a1.htm**

[b] Licensed for people 9 months through 55 years of age but should not be used before 2 y of age in patients with asplenia or HIV to avoid interference with the immune response to the pneumococcal conjugate vaccine. In all patients (not just those with asplenia or HIV infection), administration of MenACWY-D 30 days after diphtheria and tetanus toxoids and acellular pertussis (DTaP) vaccine interferes with the immune response for all four meningococcal serogroups; therefore, MenACWY-D should be administered either before or at the same time as DTaP, or alternatively one of two other MenACWY vaccines could be used.

[c] Licensed for people 2 months through 55 years of age.

[d] Licensed for people 2 years of age and older.

[e] Licensed for people 10 years through 25 years of age.

[f] Licensed for people 10 years through 25 years of age.

[g] Composed of MenACWY-TT (Nimenrix) and MenB-FHbp (Trumenba).

[h] 1) Healthy individuals aged 16–23 years of age (routine schedule) when shared clinical decision making favors administration of MenB vaccination; or 2) individuals aged 10 years and older at increased risk of meningococcal disease (eg, because of persistent complement deficiencies, complement inhibitor use, or functional or anatomic asplenia) for whom both vaccines are due.

25 years of age; it is composed of Pfizer's Trumenba (serogroup B) and Nimenrix (serogroups ACWY) vaccines. Tables 3.39 and 3.40 provide recommendations on meningococcal vaccines.

Serogroup A, C, W, and Y Vaccines. Meningococcal groups A, C, W, and Y polysaccharide diphtheria toxoid conjugate vaccine (MenACWY-D [Menactra]) is licensed for use in people 9 months through 55 years of age. Meningococcal groups A, C, W, and Y oligosaccharide diphtheria CRM_{197} conjugate vaccine (MenACWY-CRM [Menveo]) is licensed for use in people 2 months through 55 years of age. Meningococcal groups A, C, W, and Y polysaccharide tetanus toxoid conjugate vaccine (MenACWY-TT [MenQuadfi]) is licensed for use in people 2 years and older. Each is administered intramuscularly as a 0.5-mL dose. Dosing during the primary series varies by product, age, and underlying risk for disease.

Recommendations for use of MenACWY vaccine are as follows[1] (Tables 3.39 and 3.40):

- Adolescents should be immunized routinely with 1 dose at the 11- through 12-year health care visit (see **https://redbook.solutions.aap.org/SS/Immunization_Schedules.aspx**), when immunization status and other preventive health services can be addressed. A booster dose at 16 years of age is recommended for adolescents immunized at 11 through 12 years of age.
- Adolescents who receive their first dose at age 13 to 15 years should receive a booster dose at age 16 to 18 years; the booster dose can be administered at any time, as long as a minimum interval of 8 weeks between doses is maintained.
- Adolescents who receive a first dose after their 16th birthday do not need a booster dose unless they become at increased risk for meningococcal disease.

[1] Mbaeyi SA, Bozio CH, Duffy J, et al. Meningococcal vaccination: recommendations of the Advisory Committee on Immunization Practices, United States, 2020. *MMWR Recomm Rep.* 2020;69(RR-9):1–41

Table 3.40. Recommended Immunization Schedule and Intervals for People at Increased Risk of Invasive Meningococcal Disease[a,b,c]

Age	Subgroup	Primary Immunization	Booster Dose
Meningococcal ACWY Vaccines			
2 through 23 mo of age	Children who: • have persistent complement deficiencies (including complement inhibitor use) • have functional or anatomic asplenia • have human immunodeficiency virus (HIV) infection • travel to or are residents of countries where meningococcal disease is hyperendemic or epidemic • are at risk during a community outbreak attributable to an A,C,W,Y vaccine serogroup	**MenACWY-CRM (Menveo):** 4 doses at 2, 4, 6, and 12 mo In children initiating vaccination at 7 through 23 mo of age, MenACWY-CRM is to be administered as a 2-dose series, with the second dose administered in the second year of life and at least 3 mo after the first dose **MenACWY-D (Menactra):** MenACWY-D SHOULD NOT BE USED before 2 y of age in children with asplenia or HIV to avoid interference with the immune response to the pneumococcal conjugate vaccine (PCV) series For children aged ≥9 mo who are at increased risk because of complement deficiency, travel or an outbreak, MenACWY-D can be administered as a 2-dose series at 9 and 12 months (3 months apart; may be administered ≥8 weeks apart in travelers) **MenACWY-TT (MenQuadfi):** SHOULD NOT BE USED before 2 y of age because not approved in this age group	Person remains at increased risk and first dose received at age: • **2 mo through 6 y of age:** Should receive additional dose of MenACWY 3 y after primary immunization. Boosters should be repeated every 5 y.[d]

Table 3.40. Recommended Immunization Schedule and Intervals for People at Increased Risk of Invasive Meningococcal Disease,[a,b,c] continued

Age	Subgroup	Primary Immunization	Booster Dose
≥2 y[f]	People who: • have persistent complement deficiencies • have functional or anatomic asplenia • have HIV infection	2 doses of either **MenACWY-CRM** or **MenACWY-D**[e] or **MenACWY-TT**, 8–12 wk apart **MenACWY-D** (Menactra) may be used if at least 4 wk after completion of PCV doses	• **2 y through 6 y of age:** Should receive additional dose of MenACWY 3 y after primary immunization. Boosters should be repeated every 5 y.[d] • **≥7 y of age:** should receive an additional dose of MenACWY 5 y after primary immunization. Boosters should be repeated every 5 y.[d]
≥2 y[f]	People who: • are at risk during a community outbreak attributable to an A,C,W,Y vaccine serogroup • travel to or are residents of countries where meningococcal disease is hyperendemic or epidemic • college freshmen living in residence halls and military recruits • are laboratory workers routinely exposed to isolates of *Neisseria meningitidis*	1 dose of **MenACWY-CRM** or **MenACWY-D**[e] or **MenACWY-TT**	
Meningococcal B Vaccines			
≥10 y[g]	People who: • have persistent complement deficiencies (including complement inhibitor use) • have functional or anatomic asplenia	2-dose series of **MenB-4C**, ≥1 mo apart OR 3-dose series of **MenB-FHbp,** with 2nd and 3rd doses administered 1–2 and 6 mo after initial doses	**For subgroup at increased risk:** • Other than outbreak: booster[g] 1 year following completion of a MenB primary series followed by MenB booster every 2–3 years thereafter.[d]

Table 3.40. Recommended Immunization Schedule and Intervals for People at Increased Risk of Invasive Meningococcal Disease,[a,b,c] continued

Age	Subgroup	Primary Immunization	Booster Dose
	• are laboratory workers routinely exposed to isolates of *N meningitidis* • are at increased risk, as determined by public health officials, because of a serogroup B meningococcal disease outbreak		• For outbreak: booster[h] if it has been ≥1 year since completion of a MenB primary series (≥6 months interval might also be considered by public health officials).

[a] Please see full recommendations on Meningococcal Vaccination: Recommendations of the Advisory Committee on Immunization Practices, United States, 2020 at **www.cdc.gov/mmwr/volumes/69/rr/rr6909a1.htm**

[b] Includes children who have persistent complement deficiencies (eg, C3, C5-C9, properdin, or factor D or factor H or receiving eculizumab or ravulizumab) or anatomic or functional asplenia; travelers to or residents of countries in which meningococcal disease is hyperendemic or epidemic; and children who are part of a community outbreak of a vaccine-preventable serogroup.

[c] The pentavalent MenABCWY vaccine may be used when both MenACWY and MenB are indicated at the same visit: 1) healthy individuals aged 16–23 years of age (routine schedule) when shared clinical decision making favors administration of MenB vaccination; or 2) individuals aged 10 years and older at increased risk of meningococcal disease (eg, because of persistent complement deficiencies, complement inhibitor use, or functional or anatomic asplenia) for whom both vaccines are due.

[d] If person remains at increased risk of meningococcal disease.

[e] When MenACWY-D and DTaP are being administered to children 4 through 6 years of age, preference should be given to simultaneous administration of the 2 vaccines or administration of MenACWY-D before administration of DTaP, because administration of MenACWY-D 1 month after Daptacel has been shown to reduce meningococcal antibody response to MenACWY-D. Alternatively, one of two other MenACWY vaccines could be used.

[f] Meningococcal polysaccharide vaccine is no longer available in the United States.

[g] According to the Advisory Committee on Immunization Practices, people >25 years who are at increased risk for meningococcal B disease can receive MenB vaccine (no preference for MenB vaccine, but the same vaccine should be used for full series).

[h] The same MenB vaccine should be used for boosters as was used in the primary series.

• People 19 to 21 years of age who have not received a dose after their 16th birthday can receive a single MenACWY dose as part of catch-up vaccination.

• Routine childhood immunization with meningococcal conjugate vaccines is not recommended for children 2 months through 10 years of age because of the low proportion of infections that are preventable with MenACWY vaccine.

• People at increased risk of invasive meningococcal disease (defined, by age, in the subgroup column of Table 3.40) should be immunized with a meningococcal conjugate vaccine beginning at 2 months of age. Table 3.40 also details dosing recommendations for each of the 3 MenACWY vaccines in these increased-risk populations.

• Because of their high risk for invasive pneumococcal disease, children with functional or anatomic asplenia or HIV infection should not be vaccinated with MenACWY-D (Menactra) before age 2 years to avoid interference with the immune response to pneumococcal conjugate vaccine; only MenACWY-CRM (Menveo) should be used in this group. MenACWY-TT (MenQuadfi) should not be used in this situation because it is only approved in children ≥2 years of age.

- When MenACWY-D (Menactra) is administered 30 days after diphtheria and tetanus toxoids and acellular pertussis vaccine (DTaP), it interferes with the immune response to all four meningococcal serogroups. Therefore, MenACWY-D (Menactra) should be administered either before or at the same time as DTaP. Alternatively, Menveo or MenQuadfi (if ≥2 years of age) may be administered instead of Menactra.

Serogroup B Meningococcal Vaccines. MenB-FHbp (Trumenba) is based on a surface-exposed lipoprotein named factor H binding protein (FHbp). MenB-FHbp can be administered as either a 2- or 3-dose series (0 and 6 months; or 0, 1–2, and 6 months), depending on risk factors for disease and on outbreak conditions (see Tables 3.39 and 3.40).

MenB-4C (Bexsero, GSK) contains 4 antigenic components: 1 FHbp fusion protein, NadA, NHBA fusion protein, and outer membrane vesicles. It is administered as a 2-dose series (0, ≥1 month [see Tables 3.39 and 3.40]).

Data on effectiveness against clinical disease endpoints and duration of protection for either vaccine in the age groups for which they are licensed in the United States are limited. Recommendations for use of a MenB vaccine are as follows[1] (Tables 3.39 and 3.40):

- People 10 years and older at increased risk for meningococcal disease should receive a MenB vaccine, using the same vaccine product for all doses in the vaccination series. Vaccination may further activate complement, and as a result, patients with complement-mediated diseases may experience increased symptoms of their underlying disease, such as hemolysis, following vaccination.
- A MenB vaccine series may be considered for people 16 through 23 years of age on the basis of shared clinical decision making (decided in the context of the provider-patient relationship and joint decision making), with a preferred age at vaccination of 16 through 18 years. If MenB vaccine is elected to be administered, the same vaccine product should be used for all doses. MenB vaccine may be administered with other vaccines at the same visit but at a different injection site.

Serogroup A, B, C, W, and Y Meningococcal Vaccine. A pentavalent meningococcal vaccine composed of Pfizer's Trumenba (serogroup B) and Nimenrix (serogroups ACWY) vaccines was licensed by the FDA on October 20, 2023, for persons 10 through 25 years of age. It may be used when both MenACWY and MenB are indicated at the same visit for: 1) healthy individuals aged 16 through 23 years of age (routine schedule) when shared clinical decision making favors administration of MenB vaccination; or 2) individuals aged 10 years and older at increased risk of meningococcal disease (eg, because of persistent complement deficiencies, complement inhibitor use, or functional or anatomic asplenia) for whom both vaccines are due. The licensed B component vaccines are not interchangeable by manufacturer. Administration of a B component vaccine (MenB or MenABCWY) requires that subsequent B component vaccine doses be from the same manufacturer. The minimum interval for Pfizer's MenABCWY vaccine is 6 months. Individuals at increased risk of meningococcal disease who are recommended to receive additional doses of MenACWY and MenB less than 6 months after a dose of pentavalent meningococcal vaccine should instead receive separate MenACWY and MenB-FHbp vaccines.

Immunization During Eculizumab Therapy.[1] Use of complement inhibitors (eg, eculizumab [Soliris] and its long-acting derivative ravulizumab [Ultomiris]; monoclonal antibody therapies that block C5) is associated with a substantially increased risk for

---

[1] Mbaeyi SA, Bozio CH, Duffy J, et al. Meningococcal vaccination: recommendations of the Advisory Committee on Immunization Practices, United States, 2020. *MMWR Recomm Rep.* 2020;69(RR-9):1–41

meningococcal disease. Eculizumab use is associated with an approximately 2000-fold increased incidence of meningococcal disease. Eculizumab and ravulizumab recipients should receive both MenACWY and MenB vaccines. Because these monoclonal antibodies inhibit terminal complement activation and opsonophagocytic killing of meningococci, patients receiving them are still at risk for invasive meningococcal disease even if they develop antibodies following vaccination. Providers, therefore, should also consider antimicrobial prophylaxis (usually penicillin prophylaxis) for the duration of eculizumab or ravulizumab treatment and until immunocompetence is restored once the monoclonal antibody therapy is stopped, to potentially reduce the risk for meningococcal disease.

Reimmunization/Booster Doses. Children previously immunized with a meningococcal conjugate vaccine (ACWY or B) who are at ongoing increased risk for meningococcal disease should receive booster immunizations (see Table 3.40). If a child was vaccinated with MenACWY vaccine because of an outbreak or travel at <10 years of age, the adolescent doses are still needed. For MenB vaccine, the same vaccine product used in the primary series should be used for booster doses.

Immunization During Outbreaks. During an outbreak, additional cases can occur several weeks or more after onset of disease in the index case; therefore, meningococcal vaccine is recommended when an outbreak is caused by a serogroup prevented by a meningococcal vaccine.

Adverse Events. Common adverse events after quadrivalent meningococcal conjugate vaccines include pain, erythema, and swelling at the injection site; headache; fatigue; and irritability. Similar adverse effects are observed after MenB vaccines, although effects are more common and may be more severe, and often include myalgia. Syncope can occur after any vaccination and is most common among adolescents and young adults. Adolescents should be seated or lying down during vaccination and ideally remain that way for at least 15 minutes after immunization to avert syncopal episodes and secondary injuries. If syncope develops, patients should be observed until symptoms resolve.[1] Syncope following receipt of a vaccine is not a contraindication to subsequent doses.

Pregnant People.[2] Pregnant and lactating people should receive MenACWY vaccine if indicated. Because limited data are available for MenB vaccination during pregnancy, vaccination with MenB should be deferred unless the person is at increased risk and, after consultation with their health care provider, the benefits of vaccination are considered to outweigh the potential risks.

Counseling and Public Education. When a case of invasive meningococcal disease is detected, the physician should provide accurate and timely information about meningococcal disease and the risk of transmission to families and contacts of the infected person and provide or arrange for chemoprophylaxis (which may be accomplished together with the public health department). Some experts recommend that all patients with invasive meningococcal disease be evaluated for a complement component deficiency; screening can be accomplished with inexpensive CH50 and AH50 testing. If a specific complement component deficiency is detected, patients should receive a MenACWY vaccine series if 2 months or older and a MenB series if 10 years or older. Patients and parents should be counseled about the risk of recurrent invasive

---

[1] Centers for Disease Control and Prevention. Syncope after vaccination—United States, January 2005–July 2007. *MMWR Morb Mortal Wkly Rep.* 2008;57(17):457–460

[2] Mbaeyi SA, Bozio CH, Duffy J, et al. Meningococcal vaccination: recommendations of the Advisory Committee on Immunization Practices, United States, 2020. *MMWR Recomm Rep.* 2020;69(No. RR-9):1–41

meningococcal disease and the need for immediate medical evaluation when fever develops. Patients on eculizumab or ravulizumab or with other complement deficiencies should be counseled about the risk of invasive infection. Public health questions, such as whether a mass immunization program or an expanded chemoprophylaxis program is needed, should be referred to the local or state public health department. In appropriate situations, early provision of information in collaboration with the health department to schools or affected groups, and to the media may help minimize public anxiety and unrealistic or inappropriate demands for intervention.

Public Health Reporting. All confirmed, suspected, and probable cases of invasive meningococcal disease (see Table 3.35) must be immediately reported to the appropriate public health department. Meningococcal disease is a nationally notifiable condition. Timely reporting can facilitate early administration of chemoprophylaxis to close contacts, recognition and containment of outbreaks, and characterization of isolates so that appropriate prevention recommendations can be implemented rapidly.

Human Metapneumovirus

CLINICAL MANIFESTATIONS: Human metapneumovirus (hMPV) causes acute respiratory tract illness in people of all ages but is most common in children, especially those younger than 5 years. In infants, hMPV is a common cause of bronchiolitis. In children, hMPV also causes asthma exacerbations, croup, pneumonia, upper respiratory tract infections, and acute otitis media; these may be accompanied by fever. Healthy, young children generally have mild or moderate symptoms when infected with hMPV, but some can develop severe disease requiring hospitalization. Encephalitis has been reported rarely. As with other respiratory viral infections, secondary bacterial pneumonia can occur. Children with underlying cardiopulmonary disease and those born preterm, especially at a gestational age <32 weeks, are at higher risk for hospitalization, suffer more severe disease, and require longer stays and supplementary oxygen administration. hMPV infection in immunocompromised patients can result in severe disease, and fatalities have been reported in hematopoietic cell or lung transplant recipients. Among adults, hMPV is associated with acute exacerbations of chronic obstructive pulmonary disease (COPD) and pneumonia. Recurrent infections can occur throughout life and, in people without medical conditions, are usually mild or asymptomatic.

ETIOLOGY: hMPV is an enveloped single-stranded nonsegmented negative-sense RNA virus in the genus *Metapneumovirus* of the family *Pneumoviridae*. Phylogenetic analyses, based on sequence differences in the fusion (F) and attachment (G) surface glycoproteins, have identified 2 major hMPV antigenic lineages further subdivided into 2 clades within each lineage for a total of 5 genotypes (designated A1, A2a, A2b, B1, and B2). Viruses from these different clades cocirculate each year in varying proportions.

EPIDEMIOLOGY: Humans are the only host. Transmission occurs by direct or close contact with contaminated secretions via large particle aerosols, droplets, or fomites. Health care-associated infections have been reported.

In temperate climates, hMPV circulation usually occurs during late winter and early spring, overlapping with the latter part of the respiratory syncytial virus (RSV) season, but typically peaks 1 to 2 months later than RSV. Sporadic infections may occur throughout the year, and summer outbreaks have occasionally been described in closed settings. In otherwise healthy infants, the duration of viral shedding is 1 to 2 weeks. Prolonged shedding (weeks to months) has been reported in severely immunocompromised individuals.

Serologic studies suggest that nearly all children are infected at least once by 5 years of age. The incidence of hospitalizations attributed to hMPV is lower than that attributed to RSV but comparable to influenza and parainfluenza 3 in children younger than 5 years. Large studies have shown that hMPV is detected among 5% to 15% of children with medically attended lower respiratory tract illnesses. Worldwide, models have estimated >14 million annual cases of lower respiratory tract infections secondary to hMPV in children younger than 5 years. Overall annual rates of hospitalization associated with hMPV infection are highest in the first year of life but occur throughout childhood. In infants, the peak age of hospitalization is 6 to 12 months (compared with 2 to 3 months for RSV). Coinfection with other respiratory viruses occurs.

The **incubation period** is 3 to 9 days.

DIAGNOSTIC TESTS: Nucleic acid amplification tests (NAATs) are the diagnostic method of choice for hMPV. Several NAATs for hMPV are available commercially and have been approved for use by the US Food and Drug Administration. These include reverse transcriptase polymerase chain reaction (RT-PCR) tests for hMPV alone or in multiplex RT-PCR respiratory pathogen panels. hMPV is difficult to isolate in cell culture. Direct fluorescent antibody (DFA) testing for hMPV detection in respiratory specimens is available in some reference laboratories, with reported sensitivity of 85%. Serologic testing is only used in research settings.

TREATMENT: Treatment is supportive. In vitro studies and animal models have shown that ribavirin and some preparations of immune globulin intravenous have activity against hMPV. There are anecdotal reports using these therapies in humans, but there are no controlled clinical data available to assess whether these have therapeutic benefit, and their use is not routinely recommended. Antimicrobial agents are not indicated in the treatment of infants hospitalized with uncomplicated hMPV bronchiolitis or pneumonia unless evidence exists for the presence of a concurrent bacterial infection. Additional management recommendations for infants with bronchiolitis can be found in the bronchiolitis guidelines from the American Academy of Pediatrics.[1]

INFECTION PREVENTION AND CONTROL MEASURES IN HEALTH CARE SETTINGS: In addition to standard precautions, contact and droplet precautions are recommended for the duration of hMPV-associated illness. In immunocompromised patients, the duration of precautions should be extended because of possible prolonged shedding.

CONTROL MEASURES: Appropriate respiratory and hand hygiene and cough etiquette should be followed. Control of health care-associated hMPV infection depends on adherence to contact and droplet precautions, and routine cleaning and sanitizing of potentially contaminated surfaces. Exposure to hMPV-infected people, including other patients, staff, and family members, may not be recognized because illness may be mild.

Preventive measures outside the health care setting include emphasizing hand and respiratory hygiene in all settings. Commonly used surfaces should be cleaned and sanitized routinely.

---

[1] American Academy of Pediatrics, Subcommittee on Diagnosis and Management of Bronchiolitis. Clinical practice guideline: the diagnosis, management, and prevention of bronchiolitis. *Pediatrics.* 2014;134(5):e1474-e1502

Microsporidia Infections
(Microsporidiosis)

CLINICAL MANIFESTATIONS: Clinical presentations of microsporidia infections are diverse and vary according to the causal species and route of infection. They can be grouped broadly into intestinal, ocular, and disseminated infections. Infection may also be asymptomatic. Patients with symptomatic intestinal infection have watery, non-bloody diarrhea; nausea; and diffuse abdominal pain. Abdominal cramping can occur. Symptomatic intestinal infection, often manifested by protracted diarrhea, is most common in immunocompromised people, especially in organ transplant recipients and people with human immunodeficiency virus (HIV) infection with low CD4+ T-lymphocyte counts (<100 cells/μL). Complications include malnutrition, progressive weight loss, and failure to thrive. Ocular infections most often affect the cornea, and disseminated infections can lead to biliary tract, cerebral, respiratory, muscle, and genitourinary involvement (see Table 3.41). Chronic infection in immunocompetent people is rare.

ETIOLOGY: Microsporidia are obligate intracellular, spore-forming organisms historically classified as parasites but closely related to fungi; their taxonomic position continues to

Table 3.41. Clinical Manifestations of Microsporidia Infections

Microsporidia	Clinical Manifestation
Anncaliia algerae	Myositis, ocular infection, cellulitis, myositis, disseminated disease
Anncaliia connori	Disseminated disease, ocular infection
Anncaliia vesicularum	Myositis
Encephalitozoon cuniculi	Encephalitis, hepatitis, peritonitis, ocular infection, sinusitis, osteomyelitis, pulmonary disease, disseminated disease
Encephalitozoon hellem	Ocular infection, disseminated disease, sinusitis, pneumonitis, nephritis, urethritis, cystitis
Encephalitozoon intestinalis	Diarrhea, cholangitis, disseminated infection, skin infection, ocular infection
Enterocytozoon bieneusi	Diarrhea, acalculous cholecystitis, pulmonary disease
Microsporidium africanum	Ocular infection
Microsporidium ceylonensis	Ocular infection
Nosema ocularum	Ocular infection
Pleistophora species	Myositis, disseminated disease, sinusitis
Trachipleistophora anthropophthera	Disseminated infection, encephalitis, ocular infection
Trachipleistophora hominis	Myositis, sinusitis, encephalitis, ocular infection, disseminated disease
Tubulinosema acridophagus	Disseminated infection, myositis
Vittaforma corneae	Ocular infection, urinary tract infection, diarrhea

Adapted from: Han B, Weiss LM. Microsporidia: obligate intracellular pathogens within the fungal kingdom. *Microbiol Spectr.* 2017;5(2).

See also: **www.cdc.gov/dpdx/microsporidiosis/**

be debated. More than 1400 species belonging to about 200 genera have been identified with at least 15 reported in human infection (Table 3.41). *Enterocytozoon bieneusi* and *Encephalitozoon intestinalis* are the pathogens reported most commonly in humans and are associated most often with chronic diarrhea in people with HIV infection.

EPIDEMIOLOGY: Most microsporidia infections are transmitted by oral ingestion of spores. Microsporidia spores commonly are found in surface water, and strains responsible for human infection have been identified in municipal water supplies and ground water. Spores can survive for extended periods in the environment. Several studies indicate that waterborne transmission occurs. Donor-derived infections in organ transplant recipients have been documented. Person-to-person spread by the fecal-oral route also occurs. Spores also have been detected in other body fluids, but their role in transmission is unknown. Data suggest the possibility of zoonotic and vector-borne transmission.

The **incubation period** is unknown.

DIAGNOSTIC TESTS: Infection with gastrointestinal tract microsporidia can be documented by microscopic identification of spores in stool or biopsy specimens. The laboratory should be alerted and specific stains for microsporidia requested, because routine ova and parasite examination usually does not detect microsporidia spores. Microsporidia spores can be detected in formalin-fixed or unfixed stool, other fluid, or tissue specimens stained with a chromotrope-based stain (a modification of the trichrome stain) and examined by an experienced microscopist. Fluorescent techniques including calcofluor or Fungi-Fluor also can be used to detect organisms in stool or tissue sections. Identification and diagnostic confirmation of species requires transmission electron microscopy or molecular methods (nucleic acid amplification test [NAAT]), which are available for *E bieneusi*, *E intestinalis*, *Encephalitozoon hellem*, and *Encephalitozoon cuniculi*. The value of serologic testing, when available, has not been substantiated.

TREATMENT: Restoration of immune function is critical for control of microsporidia infection in immunocompromised individuals. Effective antiretroviral therapy is the primary initial treatment for these infections in people with HIV infection and can result in resolution of symptoms even without specific therapy against microsporidia. Albendazole is the drug of choice for systemic infections caused by microsporidia other than *E bieneusi* infection, which may respond to fumagillin (see Table 4.11, Drugs for Parasitic Infections, p 1068). Fumagillin for systemic use is not available in the United States; it is associated with bone marrow toxicity, and recurrence of diarrhea is common after therapy is discontinued. Limited data suggest that nitazoxanide may be effective for treatment of *E bieneusi* gastroenteritis in patients with acquired immunodeficiency syndrome (AIDS). Topical fumagillin is used to treat ocular microsporidial infection. Topical voriconazole (1%) and topical fluoroquinolones have been reported effective for treatment of microsporidial ocular infection, but more study is needed. Supportive care for malnutrition and dehydration may be necessary. Antimotility agents may be useful to control chronic diarrhea.

INFECTION PREVENTION AND CONTROL MEASURES IN HEALTH CARE SETTINGS: In addition to standard precautions, contact precautions are recommended for diapered and incontinent children for the duration of illness.

CONTROL MEASURES: In patients with HIV infection and other immunocompromised people, attention to hand hygiene, drinking bottled or boiled water, and avoiding unpeeled fruits and vegetables may decrease exposure. No chemoprophylactic regimens are known to be effective in preventing microsporidiosis, although continuation of treatment regimens is recommended as secondary prophylaxis in individuals with HIV infection until immune reconstitution.

Molluscum Contagiosum

CLINICAL MANIFESTATIONS: Molluscum contagiosum is a benign viral infection of the skin with no systemic manifestations. It usually is characterized by 1 to 20 discrete, 2- to 5-mm-diameter, flesh-colored to translucent, dome-shaped papules, some with central umbilication. Lesions commonly occur on the trunk, face, and extremities but rarely are generalized. Molluscum contagiosum is a self-limited epidermal infection with individual lesions often spontaneously resolving in 6 to 12 months but some taking as long as 3 to 4 years to disappear completely. An eczematous reaction (molluscum dermatitis) encircling the lesions is common. People with atopic dermatitis and immunocompromising conditions, including human immunodeficiency virus infection and patients with congenital DOCK8 deficiency or CARD11 mutations, tend to have more widespread and prolonged eruptions, which often are recalcitrant to therapy.

ETIOLOGY: Molluscum contagiosum virus is the sole member of the genus *Molluscipoxvirus*, family *Poxviridae*. DNA subtypes of molluscum contagiosum virus can be differentiated, but the specific subtype probably is insignificant in pathogenesis. Other poxviruses include the agents of smallpox, mpox, vaccinia, and cowpox.

EPIDEMIOLOGY: Humans are the only known source of the virus, which is spread by direct contact with lesions, including scratching, shaving, sexual contact, or fomites. Vertical transmission has been linked with neonatal molluscum contagiosum infection. Lesions can be disseminated by autoinoculation. Infectivity generally is low, but occasional outbreaks may occur in facilities such as child care centers. The period of communicability is unknown.

The **incubation period** is generally between 2 and 7 weeks but may be as long as 6 months.

DIAGNOSTIC TESTS: The diagnosis usually can be made clinically from the characteristic appearance of umbilicated papules. Side lighting of the individual lesions may enhance the visibility of the umbilication. Handheld dermoscopy can be useful in identifying orifices (umbilications) along with white amorphous structures with a surrounding crown of vessels. Wright or Giemsa staining of cells expressed from the central core of a lesion reveals characteristic intracytoplasmic inclusions. Electron microscopic examination of these cells identifies typical poxvirus particles. The virus does not grow readily in culture. Serologic testing is not available routinely for clinical practice. If uncertainty persists in the differential diagnosis (eg, warts, trichoepithelioma, tuberous sclerosis), nucleic acid amplification tests (NAATs) are available at certain reference centers. Adolescents and young adults with genital molluscum contagiosum should prompt a screening for other sexually transmitted infections.

TREATMENT: There is no consensus on management of molluscum contagiosum in children and adolescents. Genital lesions in sexually active patients should be treated to prevent spread to sexual contacts. Nongenital lesions in healthy people are typically self-limited, so treatment may be unnecessary. However, therapy may be warranted to (1) alleviate discomfort, including itching; (2) reduce autoinoculation; (3) limit transmission of the virus to close contacts; (4) reduce cosmetic concerns; and (5) prevent secondary infection.

Physical destruction of the lesions is the most rapid and effective means of curing molluscum contagiosum. Modalities available include curettage, cryodestruction with liquid nitrogen, electrodesiccation, and chemical agents designed to initiate a local inflammatory response (podophyllin, tretinoin, cantharidin, 25%–50% trichloroacetic acid, liquefied phenol, silver nitrate, tincture of iodine, or potassium hydroxide). Although randomized controlled trials have been conducted for the use of cantharidin, the evidence for most of these other modalities remains anecdotal. Cantharidin was approved by the US Food and Drug Administration (FDA) on July 21, 2023, for treatment of molluscum. In addition, berdazimer gel was approved by the FDA for treatment of molluscum on January 5, 2024. When treatment is desired, the most support exists for cryotherapy, curettage, or cantharidin. These treatments require an experienced health care professional, as they can result in postprocedural pain, irritation, dyspigmentation, and scarring. Because physical destruction of the lesions is painful, appropriate local anesthesia may be required, particularly in young children.

Cidofovir is a cytosine nucleotide analogue with in vitro activity against molluscum contagiosum; successful intravenous treatment of immunocompromised adults with severe involvement has been reported. However, use of cidofovir should be reserved for extreme cases because of potential carcinogenicity and known toxicities (neutropenia and potentially permanent nephrotoxicity) associated with systemic administration of cidofovir. Successful treatment using compounded formulations of topical cidofovir has been reported in both adult and pediatric cases, most of whom were immunocompromised. Solitary genital lesions in children usually are not acquired by sexual transmission and do not necessarily denote sexual abuse, as other modes of direct contact with the virus, including autoinoculation, may result in genital infection.

INFECTION PREVENTION AND CONTROL MEASURES IN HEALTH CARE SETTINGS: Standard precautions are recommended.

CONTROL MEASURES: No control measures are known for isolated cases. For outbreaks, which are common in the tropics, restricting direct person-to-person contact and sharing of potentially contaminated fomites, such as towels and bedding, may decrease spread. Molluscum contagiosum should not prevent a child from attending child care or school or from swimming in public pools. Covering lesions is not necessary for child care, but when possible, localized lesions not covered by clothing may be covered with a gas-permeable dressing followed by under wrap and tape when participating in sports activities.[1] When children will be entering swimming pools, a watertight bandage can be placed on visible lesions. Bandages should be changed daily or when soiled.

Moraxella catarrhalis Infections

CLINICAL MANIFESTATIONS: *Moraxella catarrhalis* is commonly implicated in acute otitis media (AOM), otitis media with effusion, and sinusitis. AOM caused by *M catarrhalis* occurs predominantly in younger infants and frequently is recovered from middle ear and sinuses as part of mixed infections. Since introduction of the conjugate pneumococcal vaccine, *M catarrhalis* appears to be recovered in a greater proportion of children

---

[1] Davies HH, Jackson MA, Rice SG; American Academy of Pediatrics, Committee on Infectious Diseases. Infectious diseases associated with organized sports and outbreak control. *Pediatrics*. 2017;140(4):e20172477

undergoing tympanocentesis. *M catarrhalis* was recovered from 15% of children with AOM undergoing tympanocentesis between 2015 and 2019; however, it is unclear whether this represents an increase in cases attributable to *M catarrhalis* or a decrease in pneumococcal disease. *M catarrhalis* can cause pneumonia with or without bacteremia in immunocompetent infants and has been recovered from children with aspirated foreign body complicated by secondary infection. It is more commonly recovered from children with chronic lung disease or impaired host defenses, such as leukemia with neutropenia or congenital immunodeficiency. In immunocompromised children, often no focus of infection is identified. Other clinical manifestations include hypotension with or without a rash that is indistinguishable from that observed in meningococcemia; neonatal meningitis; and focal infections, such as preseptal cellulitis, bacterial tracheitis, urethritis, osteomyelitis, or septic arthritis. Rare manifestations include endocarditis, peritonitis, shunt-associated ventriculitis, meningitis, and mastoiditis. Health care-acquired *M catarrhalis* bacteremia has been reported in hospitalized children with transnasal devices (nasogastric tube, elemental diet tube, or nasotracheal tube); foci of infection in these cases have included pneumonia or bronchitis. Other health care-associated outbreaks of *M catarrhalis* have been described.

ETIOLOGY: *M catarrhalis* is a gram-negative aerobic diplococcus.

EPIDEMIOLOGY: *M catarrhalis* is part of the normal microbiota of the upper respiratory tract of humans. At least two thirds of children are colonized within the first year of life. The mode of transmission is presumed to be direct contact with contaminated respiratory tract secretions or droplet spread. Infection is most common in infants and young children but also occurs in immunocompromised people of all ages. The duration of carriage by children with infection or colonization and the period of communicability are unknown. Recent studies suggest early colonization with *M catarrhalis* is associated with a stable microbiome and low risk for recurrent respiratory tract infection.

DIAGNOSTIC TESTS: The organism can be isolated on blood or chocolate agar culture media after incubation in air or with increased carbon dioxide. On Gram stain, *Moraxella* species are short and plump gram-negative cocci, usually occurring in pairs or short chains and are mostly catalase and cytochrome oxidase positive. Nucleic acid amplification tests (NAATs) for *M catarrhalis* have been developed but currently are used for research purposes only. The significance of *M catarrhalis* detection from clinical specimens requires clinical correlation; isolation of *M catarrhalis* from respiratory cultures may often represent colonization rather than infection.

TREATMENT: Almost all strains of *Moraxella* species produce beta-lactamase and are resistant to amoxicillin, unlike other common pathogens causing acute otitis media. *M catarrhalis* are typically susceptible to ampicillin-sulbactam (and amoxicillin-clavulanate), second- or third-generation cephalosporins, trimethoprim sulfamethoxazole, macrolides, and fluoroquinolones. Empiric and definitive therapy will depend on the severity of illness and type of infection, immunocompetence of the patient, and susceptibility of the isolate. The organism is resistant to clindamycin, vancomycin, and oxacillin. Macrolide-resistant isolates have been reported from Asia, but resistant strains only rarely have been identified in the United States or Western Europe.

INFECTION PREVENTION AND CONTROL MEASURES IN HEALTH CARE SETTINGS: Standard precautions are recommended.

CONTROL MEASURES: None.

Mpox

CLINICAL MANIFESTATIONS: The presentation of mpox (formerly known as monkey-pox) is similar to but milder than that of smallpox, prior to its eradication.

Clinical Presentation Associated With Classic Mpox Infections. Classic mpox infection generally involves a prodromal illness that may last several days and is characterized by fever, lymphadenopathy, malaise, sore throat, and headache, followed by the development of a characteristic diffuse rash. The rash typically involves many lesions, begins on the face, and spreads to other parts of the body including the extremities (often with involvement of palms and soles) and trunk. Generally, there are more lesions on the face and extremities than the trunk (centrifugal distribution). Classically, lesions begin as macules that progress to papules, firm vesicles, and deep-seated pustules, which can develop central umbilication and be painful until the healing phase begins. The lesions are typically in the same stage of evolution in a particular area on the body. Crusting and resolution occur over a period of 2 to 4 weeks. Lymphadenopathy in the submandibular, cervical, axillary, or inguinal regions usually occurs during the prodromal period or, rarely, with rash onset. An enanthem characterized by oral lesions on the tongue and other areas of the mouth may develop shortly before the appearance of cutaneous lesions. Ocular involvement can lead to keratitis, corneal scarring, and blindness. Other complications can include vomiting and diarrhea leading to severe dehydration, pneumonia, encephalitis, sepsis, hemorrhagic lesions, bacterial skin infection, pregnancy loss, congenital infection, and preterm delivery. Deaths have occurred. Coinfections, including with varicella zoster virus, have been reported.

Clinical Presentation Associated With 2022 Global Mpox Outbreak. In May 2022, a global outbreak of mpox began, primarily infecting men who have sex with men. Most people infected with mpox virus in this outbreak had mild or absent prodromal symptoms. Occasionally, one or more prodromal symptoms (eg, fever, lymphadenopathy, malaise, sore throat, headache) developed concurrently with the onset of skin lesions. Lesions varied in size, and for some patients were much smaller than those associated with classic mpox and were fewer in number (ie, a single lesion or a few scattered lesions). In many cases, the rash was prominent in the anogenital region and associated with proctitis and rectal complaints (eg, severe rectal pain, tenesmus). Lesions in differing stages of rash progression occurred side-by-side. Fulminant and fatal infection occurred in persons with severe immunocompromise, including uncontrolled human immunodeficiency virus (HIV) infection.

Mpox is typically self-limited and resolves over 2 to 4 weeks. It can be confused with other illnesses, particularly varicella. Generally, varicella in children is not associated with a febrile prodrome or prominent lymphadenopathy, both of which can occur with mpox, particularly the classic clinical presentation of mpox. Mpox lesions develop into firm pustules, and historically (although not always) are in the same stage in the same area of the body, whereas varicella is in multiple stages of rash in the same area. Classic mpox lesions are typically more prominent on the face and extremities, versus varicella, which typically has a higher number of lesions on the trunk. Other common pediatric conditions that can be confused with mpox include hand, foot, and mouth disease; molluscum contagiosum; scabies; insect bites; allergic reactions; and drug eruptions. Genital or perianal lesions can look similar to a variety of sexually transmitted infections (STIs) (eg, syphilis, herpes simplex virus, lymphogranuloma venereum), and people have been coinfected with mpox virus and other STIs.

ETIOLOGY: Monkeypox virus, which causes mpox disease, is a member of the *Poxviridae* family (genus *Orthopoxvirus*). Other members of this genus that can infect humans include cowpox virus, vaccinia virus, and smallpox (variola).

EPIDEMIOLOGY: Mpox virus has 2 clades. Clade I (previously called the Congo Basin clade of mpox virus) is associated with a 11% case fatality rate in Africa in individuals without prior smallpox vaccination. Clade II (previously called the West African clade of mpox virus) is associated with a 1% case fatality rate in Africa. Clade IIb was associated with the 2022 global mpox outbreak. Disease severity, regardless of clade, is believed to be increased in pregnant people, young children, people who have atopic dermatitis and other exfoliative skin conditions, and people who are immunocompromised. The classic presentation of mpox has occurred after exposures to either clade in central and west African countries where mpox virus is endemic.

Mpox virus is spread most commonly by direct contact with lesion material, body fluids, or indirectly via fomites, such as contaminated clothing and bedding. It can also be spread by respiratory secretions, occurring when there is exposure to saliva and possibly prolonged face to face contact. A person is considered infectious from prodromal illness onset until all skin lesion crusts have fallen off and a new layer of skin has formed. The animal reservoir for classic mpox has not yet been determined, although small mammals, including rodents, are suspected; humans and other nonhuman primates can be infected and present with disease. Mpox can be acquired by the scratch or bite of an infected animal, through exposure to contaminated animal products, or through fomites (eg, shared towels and bedding).

During the 2022 global mpox outbreak, cases in adolescents were reported resulting from sexual contact; nonsexual transmission also occurred. Cases in children younger than 12 years occurred in the setting of skin-to-skin contact with a household member with mpox during routine caregiving activities (an instance of fomite transmission through shared towels was also reported). No anogenital lesions were reported among the 28 children younger than 12 years of age.[1]

The **incubation period** for mpox is 3 to 17 days (average, 5–13 days).

DIAGNOSTIC TESTS: Mpox virus can be detected in a swab of a lesion or a lesion crust or exudate (unroofing or aspirating a lesion is not recommended) by *Orthopoxvirus* or mpox-specific nucleic acid amplification tests (NAATs). Diagnostic testing is available through the US Laboratory Response Network (LRN), through consultation with state or local public health departments, and through some commercial laboratories. A positive NAAT result for *Orthopoxvirus* in the epidemiologic setting of a known mpox outbreak may be treated as a presumptive case, if collected from a patient with a compatible clinical presentation and epidemiologic risk factors. Specimens can also be sent to the Centers for Disease Control and Prevention (CDC) for mpox virus-specific characterization, including a NAAT assay specific for mpox virus, immunohistochemistry in tissue for *Orthopoxvirus*, serology for *Orthopoxvirus*, and genetic sequencing. Anti-*Orthopoxvirus* immunoglobulin M may be useful to diagnose mpox in a patient 4 to

---

[1] Hennessee I, Shelus V, McArdle CE, et al. Epidemiologic and clinical features of children and adolescents aged <18 years with monkeypox—United States, May 17–September 24, 2022. *MMWR Morb Mortal Wkly Rep.* 2022;71(44);1407–1411

56 days after rash onset who has not been vaccinated with a smallpox or mpox vaccine within the past 60 days.

Testing for other STIs and HIV should be performed for patients with anogenital lesions as coinfections occur.

TREATMENT: Most patients with mpox have self-limited disease. Patients should be counseled not to touch their eyes. Patients with ocular or periorbital lesions should be treated promptly because of the risk of developing keratitis and potentially permanent visual problems; these patients should have a consultation with an ophthalmologist regarding management and discussion of ocular therapy, such as topical trifluridine. Patients with severe disease (eg, hemorrhagic disease, confluent lesions, secondary bacterial infections, sepsis, encephalitis, lesions on the penile foreskin or strictures involving the urethral meatus, or severe involvement of other anatomic areas including anorectal lesions interfering with bowel movements, oral lesions associated with severe dysphagia, or other complicated or severe conditions, including conditions requiring hospitalization) and those at risk for severe disease (eg, patients with immunocompromising conditions, patients who are pregnant or breastfeeding, children younger than 1 year, patients with a condition affecting skin integrity) should also be considered for antiviral treatment. Management of patients with severe or complicated disease or those at risk for severe disease should be discussed with an expert in infectious diseases.

Pain can be severe, particularly when there are genital, rectal, or anal lesions. A variety of over-the-counter treatment modalities, including sitz baths, can be helpful. Information on pain management in mpox infections is described at **www.cdc.gov/poxvirus/mpox/clinicians/pain-management.html.**

Antiviral Agents. Guidance is available from the CDC (**www.cdc.gov/poxvirus/mpox/clinicians/treatment.html** and **www.cdc.gov/poxvirus/monkeypox/clinicians/people-with-HIV.html**). Tecovirimat (TPOXX or ST-246) was approved by the US Food and Drug Administration (FDA) for the treatment of smallpox and has been shown to be active against mpox virus in animal models; it is the preferred treatment for mpox patients who would benefit from antivirals. As of August 2023, tecovirimat is available through an expanded access investigational new drug (EA-IND) protocol for intravenous treatment of mpox for those who weigh at least 3 kg and for oral administration for those who weigh at least 13 kg (see **www.accessdata.fda.gov/drugsatfda_docs/label/2022/214518s000lbl.pdf; www.cdc.gov/poxvirus/monkeypox/clinicians/treatment.html#anchor_1655488137245;** and Table 4.10, p 1044). At least weekly monitoring of renal function is indicated in children and adolescents receiving intravenous tecovirimat.

Vaccinia immune globulin intravenous (VIGIV) is licensed for the treatment of complications of vaccinia vaccination; effectiveness for mpox is unknown. The CDC has an EA-IND for use in mpox (**www.fda.gov/media/78174/download).** To discuss use of VIGIV, the CDC clinical consultation team can be accessed by email (**eocevent482@cdc.gov**) or if urgent, through the CDC Emergency Operations Center (770-488-7100).

Brincidofovir (a lipophilic derivative of cidofovir that can be given orally and does not appear to have renal toxicity) has been approved for smallpox treatment. There is an FDA-authorized single patient emergency use IND for brincidofovir for mpox (**www.cdc.gov/poxvirus/monkeypox/clinicians/treatment.html#anchor_1655488353796** and **www.accessdata.fda.gov/**

drugsatfda_docs/label/2021/214460s000,214461s000lbl.pdf). It can be used in patients who have significant progression on tecovirimat, develop recrudescence of disease after initial improvement on tecovirimat, or have a contraindication for tecovirimat (see Table 4.10, p 1044).

Cidofovir is licensed for treatment of cytomegalovirus retinitis in patients with AIDS, is commercially available, and has activity against orthopoxviruses in studies, but the effectiveness for treating people with severe mpox is unknown. It has dose-dependent nephrotoxicity (**www.accessdata.fda.gov/drugsatfda_docs/label/1999/020638s003lbl.pdf**).

INFECTION PREVENTION AND CONTROL MEASURES IN HEALTH CARE SETTINGS:
A patient suspected of having mpox should be placed in a private room, and a health care professional should use a National Institute for Occupational Safety and Health-approved particulate respirator equipped with an N95 or higher respirator, gown, gloves, and eye protection. If an aerosol-generating procedure is performed, the patient should be placed in a private room equipped with negative-pressure ventilation with high-efficiency particulate air filtration. Good hand hygiene should be practiced, and extreme care should be taken with materials that may have been contaminated by the patient's lesions, crusts, or body fluids, so as not to create aerosols or contaminate additional items. Hospital infection control personnel and the state (and/or local) health department should be notified about the patient.

Mpox patients who do not require hospitalization can be isolated at home. General guidance on isolation and mpox is available on the CDC website (**www.cdc.gov/poxvirus/mpox/clinicians/infection-control-home.html** and **www.cdc.gov/poxvirus/mpox/clinicians/isolation-procedures.html**). During the infectious period, an infected patient should avoid contact with others when possible, and with pets. Ideally, one person should provide care to an infected child. The caregiver should wear a respirator or well-fitting mask when caring for the patient, cover areas of broken skin with bandages and clothing to the extent possible, and avoid direct skin-to-skin contact with the rash. The caregiver should wear gloves when changing bandages or when skin contact may occur. Gloves should be disposed of after each use, followed by handwashing. If any clothing (whether on the caregiver or the child) comes into contact with the rash, it should be laundered. Patients 2 years and older should wear a well-fitting mask, and lesions should be covered when interacting with the caregiver (or other in the household). Skin lesions should be covered when possible. Additional information, including information on laundering and cleaning is available on the CDC website (**www.cdc.gov/poxvirus/mpox/clinicians/pediatric.html** and **www.cdc.gov/poxvirus/mpox/if-sick/cleaning-disinfecting.html**).

CONTROL MEASURES:

Preexposure Immunization. Laboratory workers handling mpox specimens or a member of a high-risk group, as identified by public health, may be eligible for vaccination and for booster doses. Recommendations from the CDC Advisory Committee on Immunization Practices (ACIP) are available.[1]

---

[1] Rao AK, Petersen BW, Whitehill F, et al. Use of JYNNEOS (smallpox and monkeypox vaccine, live, non-replicating) for preexposure vaccination of persons at risk for occupational exposure to orthopoxviruses: recommendations of the Advisory Committee on Immunization Practices—United States, 2022. *MMWR Morb Mortal Wkly Rep.* 2022;71(22):734–742

JYNNEOS is a live, **nonreplicating** vaccinia vaccine that was approved by the FDA in 2019 for the prevention of mpox and smallpox in persons 18 years or older who are at high risk for mpox. It is given as a 2-dose series, separated by 28 days. It has an emergency use authorization (EUA) for use in children younger than 18 years (**www.fda.gov/media/160774/download**). There is also an EUA for intradermal dosing and administration in patients 18 years or older. In October 2023, the ACIP voted to recommend vaccination with the 2-dose JYNNEOS vaccine series for persons aged 18 years and older at risk for mpox, defined as: 1) gay, bisexual, and other men who have sex with men, transgender, or nonbinary people who in the past 6 months have had a new diagnosis of ≥1 sexually transmitted infection, more than one sex partner, sex at a commercial sex venue, or sex in association with a large public event in a geographic area where mpox transmission is occurring; 2) sexual partners of persons with the risks described in above; or 3) persons who anticipate experiencing any of the above.

ACAM2000 is a licensed live, **replicating** vaccinia virus vaccine to prevent smallpox and may be used to protect against mpox under FDA's EA-IND mechanism. It is a lyophilized, single-dose vaccine (for primary administration) that requires a bifurcated needle for administration. Inadvertent transmission of the vaccine virus from ACAM2000 may occur from vaccine recipients to their household contacts. Children who are immunocompromised or have atopic skin disease are at increased risk of serious complications following contact transmission, including progressive vaccinia and eczema vaccinatum. Information on these vaccines can be found on the CDC website (**www.cdc.gov/poxvirus/monkeypox/clinicians/smallpox-vaccine.html**). Detailed information about contraindications to preexposure smallpox immunization and adverse reactions to vaccination can be found in the ACAM2000 package insert and medication guide (**www.fda.gov/BiologicsBloodVaccines/Vaccines/ApprovedProducts/ucm180810.htm**). VIGIV, available through the CDC, is licensed for certain complications of ACAM2000 vaccination (**www.cdc.gov/smallpox/clinicians/vaccine-medical-management6.html**). CDC medical staff can be reached through the CDC emergency operations center at 770-488-7100.

Care of Exposed People. Cases of febrile rash illness for which mpox is considered should be reported to state or local health departments, who will investigate potential contacts and provide recommendations that may include symptom monitoring for 21 days and postexposure prophylaxis. Asymptomatic exposed persons do not need to quarantine but should monitor for symptoms.

Use of Vaccine. Postexposure immunization within 4 days of exposure with JYNNEOS or ACAM2000 vaccines may prevent mpox. If unable to vaccinate within that time, vaccinating up 14 days after exposure may still provide protection against severe disease. State and local health officials should be consulted on the use of vaccine for exposed individuals.

Care of Exposed Neonates. Infants born to people with suspected or confirmed mpox should undergo early bathing and postexposure prophylaxis. Although the optimal strategy for postexposure prophylaxis of newborn infants born to infected persons has not been defined, VIGIV should be considered, and consultation with an expert in pediatric infectious diseases is recommended. Infants should stay in a separate room and not have direct contact with parent(s) or caregivers infected with mpox virus. Breastfeeding should be delayed during the isolation period of the breastfeeding parent, and human milk should be pumped and discarded. Neonates should be monitored closely for signs of mpox (eg, fever, lymphadenopathy, rash, symptoms of illness) for 21 days following birth/contact with the infected person. Monitoring should include daily temperature checks and full skin examinations. This monitoring can be performed by a health care professional or the person taking care of the neonate. Additional recommendations are available at **www.cdc.gov/poxvirus/mpox/clinicians/pediatric.html.**

Public Health Reporting. Mpox is a nationally notifiable disease and should be reported immediately to the state or local health department.

Mumps

CLINICAL MANIFESTATIONS: Mumps is a systemic disease typically characterized by pain and swelling of one or more of the salivary glands, usually the parotid glands. Nonspecific symptoms may precede parotitis, including fever, myalgia, anorexia, malaise, and headache. Approximately one fifth of infections in unvaccinated people may be asymptomatic. The frequency of asymptomatic infection in vaccinated persons is unknown, but mumps symptoms are usually milder and complications less common among vaccinated people. Parotitis occurs in 95% of symptomatic individuals and may be unilateral initially with involvement of the contralateral parotid gland in 70% of cases. Emergence of contralateral parotitis within weeks to months after apparent recovery has been described. Orchitis is the most frequently reported postpubertal complication and occurs in approximately 30% of those who are unvaccinated and 6% of those who are vaccinated. Unilateral testicular involvement is common. Approximately half of patients with mumps orchitis develop testicular atrophy of affected testicles. More than 50% of people with mumps have cerebrospinal fluid pleocytosis, but fewer than 1% have symptoms of viral meningitis. Uncommon complications include oophoritis, pancreatitis, encephalitis, hearing loss (either transient or permanent), arthritis, thyroiditis, mastitis, glomerulonephritis, myocarditis, endocardial fibroelastosis, thrombocytopenia, cerebellar ataxia, and transverse myelitis. In the absence of an immunization program, mumps typically occurs during childhood. Infection in adults is more likely to result in complications. Although mumps virus can cross the placenta, no evidence exists that this transmission results in congenital malformation.

ETIOLOGY: Mumps is an enveloped RNA virus with 12 genotypes in the genus *Rubulavirus* in the family *Paramyxoviridae*. The genus also includes human parainfluenza virus types 2 and 4. Other common infectious causes of parotitis include Epstein-Barr virus, adenovirus, human herpes virus 6, parainfluenza virus types 1 and 3, influenza A virus, enteroviruses, human immunodeficiency virus (HIV), nontuberculous mycobacterium, and gram-positive (eg, *Staphylococcus aureus*) and gram-negative bacteria.

EPIDEMIOLOGY: Mumps occurs worldwide, and humans are the only known natural hosts. The virus is spread by contact with infectious respiratory tract secretions and saliva. Mumps virus is the only known cause of epidemic parotitis. Historically, the peak incidence of mumps was between January and May and among children younger than 10 years. Mumps vaccine was licensed in the United States in 1967 and recommended for routine childhood immunization in 1977. After implementation of the

2-dose measles, mumps, and rubella vaccine (MMR) recommendation in 1989 for measles control in the United States, mumps declined by 99%. From 2000 to 2005, there were fewer than 300 reported cases per year. However, there has been an increase in the number of reported mumps cases with peak years in 2006, 2016-2017 (more than 6000 cases each year), and 2019 (more than 3500 cases). Most cases during these peak years occurred in high-density, close-contact settings (eg, university campuses, military barracks) among young adults and persons who previously received 2 doses of MMR. Complications (eg, orchitis) have occurred following mumps outbreaks in college populations. Transmission of mumps has been reported to occur from asymptomatic, fully vaccinated individuals in close-contact social settings, leading to widespread outbreaks. Although secondary vaccine failure attributable to waning vaccine-derived immunity is believed to be an important contributing factor for mumps outbreaks among vaccinated individuals, antigenic differences between currently circulating wild-type strains and the vaccine strain, or lower incidence of subclinical immunologic boosting because of lack of exposure to wild-type virus may also play a role.

The **incubation period** usually is 16 to 18 days, but cases may occur from 12 to 25 days after exposure. The period of maximum communicability begins 2 days before parotitis onset. The recommended isolation period is 5 days after onset of parotid swelling. However, virus has been detected in patients' saliva as early as 7 days before and until 9 days after onset of swelling. Mumps virus has been isolated from urine and seminal fluids up to 14 days after onset of parotitis.

DIAGNOSTIC TESTS: Unvaccinated and vaccinated people with parotitis, orchitis, or oophoritis without other apparent cause should undergo diagnostic testing for mumps virus. Mumps can be confirmed by detection of mumps virus nucleic acid by nucleic acid amplification tests (NAATs) in buccal swab specimens (Stenson duct exudates), throat or oral swab specimens, urine, or cerebrospinal fluid. The parotid gland should be massaged for 30 seconds prior to buccal swab specimen collection. The mumps NAAT, developed by the Centers for Disease Control and Prevention (CDC) and available at the CDC, many state public health departments, and the Vaccine Preventable Disease Reference Centers (VPD-RC), is highly sensitive and specific. Other NAATs for mumps may be available at clinical or commercial laboratories, but the performance measures of these tests are not well characterized. Mumps virus may be isolated in cell culture using a variety of cell types, using either standard or rapid isolation and identification techniques. However, molecular detection of viral RNA by NAAT is the preferred test for confirmation of mumps infection.

Samples for mumps virus detection should be obtained soon after clinical diagnosis of mumps, preferably within 1 to 3 days after symptom onset. Vaccinated individuals may shed virus for a shorter period (less than 1 week) and may shed smaller amounts of virus. Failure to detect mumps virus RNA by NAAT in samples from a person with clinically compatible mumps symptoms does not rule out mumps as a diagnosis.

Testing for mumps-specific immunoglobulin (Ig) M antibody, IgG seroconversion, or a significant increase between acute and convalescent IgG antibody titer can also aid in the diagnosis of mumps, but these serologic assays do not confirm a diagnosis of mumps. In previously vaccinated patients who acquire mumps, IgM response may be transient, delayed, or not detected. Collection of serum 3 to 10 days after parotitis onset improves the ability to detect IgM. A negative IgM in a person with clinically compatible mumps symptoms does not rule out mumps as a diagnosis. In vaccinated patients, collection of acute and convalescent phase serum samples to demonstrate a fourfold increase in IgG titer is not recommended, because by the time of onset of symptoms, IgG titers may already be elevated such that detection of a fourfold increase in titer is not possible.

To distinguish wild-type mumps virus from vaccine virus in a person with clinically compatible mumps symptoms who was recently vaccinated, it is necessary to obtain a buccal/oral swab specimen for genotyping. Serologic tests cannot differentiate between an exposure to vaccine and an exposure to wild-type mumps virus.

TREATMENT: Management is supportive.

INFECTION PREVENTION AND CONTROL MEASURES IN HEALTH CARE SETTINGS: In addition to standard precautions, droplet precautions are recommended until 5 days after onset of parotid swelling.

CONTROL MEASURES:

Evidence of Immunity to Mumps. Presumptive evidence of immunity to mumps includes any of the following:

1. Documentation of age-appropriate vaccination with a live mumps virus-containing vaccine:
   - Preschool-aged children: 1 dose after their first birthday;
   - School-aged children (grades K–12) and adults at high risk (ie, health care personnel, international travelers, and students at postsecondary educational institutions): 2 doses after their first birthday, with the second dose administered at least 28 days after the first dose;
   - Adults not at high risk: 1 dose;
2. Laboratory evidence of immunity (Note: although the presence of mumps-specific IgG is considered evidence of prior exposure to mumps vaccine or mumps virus and is considered evidence of immunity for most situations [eg, employment], it does not necessarily predict protection against mumps disease, and equivocal tests should be considered negative);
3. Laboratory confirmation of disease; or
4. Born before 1957 (note: health care workers of any age are not considered immune unless they have had 2 immunizations separated by at least 28 days or have serologic evidence of immunity).

School and Child Care. Children and young adults should be excluded for 5 days from onset of parotid gland swelling. When determining means to control outbreaks, exclusion of students without evidence of immunity from affected schools and schools judged by local public health authorities to be at risk of transmission should be considered. If implemented, unimmunized students should be excluded until at least 26 days after onset of parotitis in the last person with mumps. Excluded students can be readmitted after receipt of a dose of MMR vaccine at the discretion of local or state health department.

Care of Exposed People. Mumps vaccine has not been demonstrated to be effective in preventing infection or decreasing the severity of infection if administered after exposure.

However, people without evidence of immunity who are exposed to mumps still should receive MMR vaccine (or measles, mumps, rubella, and varicella vaccine

[MMRV]), because immunization will provide protection against subsequent exposures. Immunization during the incubation period presents no increased risk of adverse events. Immune globulin (IG) preparations are not effective as postexposure prophylaxis for mumps.

During an outbreak, all people should be brought up-to-date on age-appropriate vaccinations (1 dose or 2 doses, depending on age; see below).

Mumps Vaccine. The only mumps vaccines licensed in the United States are live attenuated strains. Mumps vaccine is only available in the United States as combination formulations, which include MMR (M-M-R II, manufactured by Merck; and Priorix, manufactured by GSK) and MMRV vaccines. Vaccine is administered by subcutaneous injection of 0.5 mL of MMR vaccine (licensed for people 12 months or older) or MMRV vaccine (licensed for children 12 months through 12 years of age). Monovalent mumps vaccine is no longer is available in the United States.

Vaccine Recommendations.
- The first dose of MMR or MMRV (see MMRV-specific recommendations in Varicella-Zoster Infections, p 938) should be administered routinely to children at 12 through 15 months of age, with a second dose of MMR or MMRV administered at 4 through 6 years of age. The second dose of MMR or MMRV may be administered before 4 years of age, provided at least 28 days have elapsed since the first dose. MMR or MMRV is not harmful if administered to a person already immune to one or more of the viruses from previous infection or immunization.
- People should be immunized unless they have evidence of mumps immunity (p 613). Adequate immunization is 2 doses of mumps-containing vaccine (≥28 days apart) for school-aged children and adults at high risk (ie, health care personnel, students at postsecondary educational institutions, and international travelers). Because mumps is endemic throughout most of the world, unless they have evidence of immunity, people 12 months or older should be offered 2 doses of MMR before beginning travel. Children younger than 12 months need not receive mumps vaccine before travel, but they may receive it as MMR starting at 6 months of age if measles immunization is indicated. If a child receives a dose of mumps vaccine before 12 months of age, this dose is not counted toward the recommended number of doses, and 2 additional doses are recommended beginning at 12 through 15 months of age and separated by at least 28 days.
- During a mumps outbreak, people previously vaccinated with 2 doses who are identified by public health authorities as being part of a group or population at increased risk for acquiring mumps should receive a third dose of MMR (or MMRV if age appropriate). Active and passive surveillance have not identified any new or unexpected short-term safety concerns following receipt of a third dose of mumps-containing vaccine. People who have evidence of presumptive immunity for mumps other than receipt of 2 doses also should receive a dose of MMR (or MMRV if age appropriate) if they are part of the group at increased risk. No additional dose is recommended for people who already received 3 or more doses before the outbreak.
- Health care personnel born before 1957 should receive 2 doses of MMR unless they have laboratory evidence of immunity or disease.
- A mumps-containing vaccine may be administered with other vaccines at different injection sites and with separate syringes (see Simultaneous Administration of Multiple Vaccines, p 63).

- Vaccine documentation is required in multiple states for attendance in lower and higher educational institutions and is an effective public health tool to maximize immunization rates.

   Adverse Reactions. Adverse reactions associated with the mumps component of US-licensed MMR or MMRV vaccines are rare. Orchitis, parotitis, and low-grade fever may occur. Causality has not been established for nerve deafness, aseptic meningitis, encephalitis, rash, pruritus, and purpura. Allergic reactions also are rare. Other reactions that occur after immunization with MMR or MMRV may be attributable to other components of the vaccines (see Adverse Event sections in Measles, p 581, Rubella, p 740, and Varicella-Zoster Infections, p 948).

   A second dose of MMR or MMRV is not associated with an increased incidence of reactions relative to the first dose.

Precautions and Contraindications. See Measles, p 582, Rubella, p 740, and, if MMRV is used, Varicella-Zoster Infections, p 949.

   Febrile Illness. Children with minor illnesses, such as upper respiratory tract infections, should be immunized. Fever is not a contraindication to immunization. However, if other manifestations suggest a more serious illness, the child should not be immunized until recovered.

   Allergies. Hypersensitivity reactions occur rarely and usually are minor, consisting of wheal-and-flare reactions or urticaria at the injection site. Reactions have been attributed to trace amounts of neomycin or gelatin or some other component in the vaccine formulation.

   Anaphylaxis is rare. MMR and MMRV are produced in chicken embryo cell culture and do not contain significant amounts of egg white (ovalbumin) cross-reacting proteins, so children with egg allergy are at low risk of anaphylactic reactions. Skin testing of children for egg allergy is not predictive of reactions to MMR or MMRV and, therefore, is not required before administering vaccine. People with allergies to chickens or feathers are not at increased risk of reaction to the vaccine. People who have experienced anaphylactic reactions to gelatin or topically or systemically administered neomycin should receive mumps vaccine only in settings where such reactions could be managed and after consultation with an allergist or immunologist. Most often, however, neomycin allergy manifests as contact dermatitis, which is not a contraindication to receiving mumps vaccine (see Measles, p 570).

   Recent Administration of IG. Administration of MMR or MMRV should be delayed from 3 to 11 months following receipt of specific blood products or IG (see Table 1.11, p 69). When possible, MMR should be administered at least 2 weeks before planned administration of IG, blood transfusion, or other blood products because of the theoretical possibility that antibody will neutralize vaccine virus and interfere with successful immunization. If IG must be administered within 14 days after administration of MMR or MMRV, these vaccines should be readministered after the interval specified in Table 1.11 (p 69).

   Altered Immunity. Patients with immunodeficiency diseases and those receiving immunosuppressive therapy or expected to receive such therapy within 4 weeks, including high doses of systemically administered corticosteroids, alkylating agents, antimetabolites, or radiation, or people who are otherwise immunocompromised should not receive live attenuated vaccines including MMR or MMRV (see Immunization and Other Considerations in Immunocompromised Children, p 93).

Exceptions are patients with human immunodeficiency virus (HIV) infection who are not severely immunocompromised. MMR vaccine is recommended for all people ≥12 months of age with HIV who do not have evidence of severe immunosuppression (see Human Immunodeficiency Virus Infection, p 489). For vaccination purposes, severe immunosuppression for people ≤5 years of age is defined as a CD4+ T-lymphocyte percentage <15%, and for people >5 years of age is defined as a CD4+ T-lymphocyte percentage <15% **or** a CD4+ T-lymphocyte count <200 lymphocytes/mm^3. Severely immunocompromised HIV-infected infants, children, adolescents, and young adults should not receive MMR. MMRV vaccine should not be administered to any infant or child with HIV, regardless of degree of immunosuppression, because of lack of safety data in this population.

The risk of mumps exposure for patients with altered immunity can be decreased by immunizing their close susceptible (ie, household) contacts. Vaccine recipients cannot transmit mumps vaccine virus.

After cessation of immunosuppressive therapy, MMR immunization should be deferred for at least 3 months (except for corticosteroid recipients [see next paragraph]). This interval is based on the assumptions that immunologic responsiveness will have been restored in 3 months and the underlying disease for which immunosuppressive therapy was given is in remission or under control. However, because the interval can vary with the intensity and type of immunosuppressive therapy, radiation therapy, underlying disease, and other factors, a definitive recommendation for an interval after cessation of immunosuppressive therapy when mumps vaccine (as MMR) can be administered safely and effectively often is not possible.

Corticosteroids. Children receiving ≥2 mg/kg per day of prednisone or its equivalent, or ≥20 mg/day if they weigh 10 kg or more, for 14 days or more and who otherwise are not immunocompromised should not receive live-virus vaccines until 4 weeks after discontinuation (see Immunization and Other Considerations in Immunocompromised Children, p 93).

Pregnancy. Conception should be avoided for 4 weeks after mumps immunization because of the theoretical risk associated with live-virus vaccine. Susceptible postpubertal people should not be immunized if they are known to be pregnant. However, mumps immunization during pregnancy has not been associated with congenital malformations (see Immunization in Pregnancy, p 89).

Tuberculosis. Tuberculin skin testing or interferon gamma release assay (IGRA) testing is not a prerequisite for MMR immunization. Antituberculosis therapy should be initiated before administering MMR vaccine to people with untreated tuberculosis infection or disease. Tuberculin skin or IGRA testing, if otherwise indicated, can be performed on the day of immunization with MMR vaccine. Otherwise, tuberculin skin or IGRA testing should be postponed for 4 to 6 weeks, because measles immunization temporarily may suppress tuberculin skin test reactivity and possibly affect IGRA testing.

Public Health Reporting. Mumps is a nationally notifiable disease in the United States.

Mycoplasma pneumoniae and Other *Mycoplasma* Species Infections

CLINICAL MANIFESTATIONS: *Mycoplasma pneumoniae* is a frequent cause of upper and lower respiratory tract infections in children, including pharyngitis, acute bronchitis, and pneumonia. Acute otitis media is uncommon. Bullous myringitis, once considered pathognomonic for mycoplasma, now is known to occur with other pathogens as well. Sinusitis and croup are rare. Symptoms are variable and include cough, malaise, fever, and occasionally headache. Acute bronchitis and upper respiratory tract illness caused by *M pneumoniae* generally are mild and self-limited. Approximately 25% of infected school-aged children will develop pneumonia with cough and rales on physical examination within days after onset of constitutional symptoms. Cough, initially nonproductive, can become productive, persist for 3 to 4 weeks, and be accompanied by wheezing. Approximately 10% of children with *M pneumoniae* infection will exhibit a rash, which most often is maculopapular. Radiographic abnormalities are variable; bilateral diffuse infiltrates or focal abnormalities, such as consolidation, pleural effusion, or hilar adenopathy, can occur.

Unusual manifestations include nervous system disease (eg, aseptic meningitis, encephalitis, acute disseminated encephalomyelitis, cerebellar ataxia, transverse myelitis, and peripheral neuropathy) as well as myocarditis, pericarditis, arthritis (particularly in immunocompromised hosts), erythema nodosum, polymorphous mucocutaneous eruptions (eg, Stevens-Johnson syndrome or reactive infection mucocutaneous eruption [RIME], formerly referred to as *Mycoplasma*-induced rash and mucositis [MIRM] syndrome), hemolytic anemia, thrombocytopenic purpura, hemophagocytic syndromes, and postinfectious glomerulonephritis. Severe pneumonia with pleural effusion can occur, particularly in patients with sickle cell disease, Down syndrome, immunodeficiencies, and chronic cardiorespiratory disease. Acute chest syndrome and pneumonia have been associated with *M pneumoniae* in patients with sickle cell disease. Infection also has been associated with exacerbations of asthma.

Several other *Mycoplasma* species colonize mucosal surfaces of humans and can produce disease in children. *Mycoplasma hominis* infection has been reported in neonates and children (both immunocompetent and immunocompromised). Intra-abdominal abscess, septic arthritis, endocarditis, pneumonia, meningoencephalitis, brain abscess, and surgical wound infection have been attributed to *M hominis*. *Mycoplasma genitalium* causes urethritis among male individuals and is the etiology of approximately 15% to 20% of nongonococcal urethritis (NGU), 20% to 25% of nonchlamydial NGU, and 40% of persistent or recurrent urethritis.[1] Among female individuals, *M genitalium* has been associated with cervicitis, pelvic inflammatory disease, preterm delivery, spontaneous abortion, and infertility, with an approximately twofold increase in the risk for these outcomes among women with *M genitalium*. Female individuals with *M genitalium* are also frequently asymptomatic, and the consequences associated with asymptomatic *M genitalium* infection are unknown.

ETIOLOGY: Mycoplasmas are pleomorphic bacteria that lack a cell wall. They are classified in the family *Mycoplasmataceae*, which includes the *Mycoplasma* and *Ureaplasma* genera.

EPIDEMIOLOGY: Mycoplasmas are ubiquitous in animals and plants, but *M pneumoniae* causes disease only in humans. *M pneumoniae* is transmissible by respiratory droplets during close contact. Outbreaks have been described in hospitals, military bases, colleges, and summer camps. Occasionally, *M pneumoniae* causes ventilator-associated pneumonia. *M pneumoniae* is a leading cause of pneumonia in school-aged children and young adults but is an infrequent cause of community-acquired pneumonia (CAP) in

---

[1] The terms male, female, men, and women refer to sex assigned at birth.

children younger than 5 years. In the United States, an estimated 2 million infections are caused by *M pneumoniae* each year. Overall, approximately 10% to 20% of cases of CAP in hospitalized patients are believed to be caused by *M pneumoniae*. Infections occur throughout the world, in any season, and in all geographic settings. In family studies, approximately 30% of household contacts develop pneumonia. Asymptomatic carriage after infection may occur for weeks to months. Immunity after infection is not long lasting.

The **incubation period** usually is 2 to 3 weeks (range, 1–4 weeks), which can contribute to lengthy outbreaks.

DIAGNOSTIC TESTS: Nucleic acid amplification tests (NAATs) for *M pneumoniae* are available commercially and increasingly are replacing other tests, because NAATs performed on respiratory tract specimens (nasal wash, nasopharyngeal swab, oropharyngeal swab, sputum, and bronchoalveolar lavage fluid) are rapid, have sensitivity and specificity between 80% and 100%, and yield positive results earlier in the course of illness. Several assays are cleared by the US Food and Drug Administration (FDA) for diagnostic use, including an assay targeting *M pneumoniae* alone and multiplex assays that simultaneously target other respiratory pathogens as well. Identification of *M pneumoniae* by NAAT or culture in a patient with compatible clinical manifestations suggests causation. However, attributing a nonclassic clinical disorder to *M pneumoniae* is problematic, because the organism can colonize the respiratory tract for several weeks after acute infection (even after appropriate antimicrobial therapy) and has been detected by NAAT in 17% to 25% of asymptomatic children 3 months to 16 years of age. NAAT of body fluids for *M hominis* is available at reference laboratories and may be helpful diagnostically.

Serologic tests using immunofluorescence and enzyme immunoassays that detect *M pneumoniae*-specific immunoglobulin (Ig) M, IgA, and IgG antibodies are available commercially. IgM antibodies generally are not detectable within the first 7 days after onset of symptoms. Although the presence of IgM antibodies may indicate recent *M pneumoniae* infection, false-positive test results occur, and antibodies may persist in serum for several months or even years and, thus, may not indicate acute infection. IgM antibodies may not be elevated in older children and adults who have had recurrent *M pneumoniae* infection. Serologic diagnosis is best accomplished by demonstrating a fourfold or greater increase in IgG antibody titer between acute and convalescent serum specimens. Complement-fixation assay results should be interpreted cautiously, because the assay is both less sensitive and less specific than is immunofluorescent assay or enzyme immunoassay. Measurement of serum cold hemagglutinin titer has limited value, because titers of ≥1:64 are present in only 50% to 75% of patients with pneumonia caused by *M pneumoniae*, and lower titers are nonspecifically present during respiratory viral infections.

Mycoplasma organisms lack cell walls and so are not visible by cell-wall specific stains (eg, Gram stain) using light microscopy. *M pneumoniae* and *M hominis* can be grown in special enriched broth and agar media such as SP4 or on commercially available mixed liquid broth/agar slant media. However, most clinical laboratories lack the capacity to perform culture isolation and culture and identification may take longer than 21 days. *M genitalium* culture can take up to several months, and technical laboratory capacity is limited to research settings. A NAAT for *M genitalium* is FDA cleared for use with urine and urethral, penile meatal, endocervical, and vaginal swab samples.

Molecular tests for macrolide (ie, azithromycin) or quinolone (ie, moxifloxacin) resistance markers are limited in the United States. However, molecular assays that incorporate detection of mutations associated with macrolide resistance are under evaluation.

The diagnosis of mycoplasma-associated central nervous system disease is challenging, both because disease may not be the result of direct invasion and because there is no reliable single test for cerebrospinal fluid to establish a diagnosis.

TREATMENT: Evidence of benefit of antimicrobial therapy for nonhospitalized children with lower respiratory tract disease attributable to *M pneumoniae* is limited. Most children with CAP attributable to *M pneumoniae* have a relatively mild, self-limited illness, but effective antibiotic therapy may be more important with more severe infections. The usual course of antimicrobial therapy for pneumonia is 7 to 10 days, except for azithromycin, for which it usually is 5 days.

Antimicrobial therapy is not routinely recommended for preschool-aged children with CAP, because viral pathogens are responsible for the great majority of cases.[1] There is no evidence that treatment of other possible manifestations of *M pneumoniae* infection (eg, upper respiratory tract infection) with antimicrobial agents alters the course of illness. However, despite limited data, it is reasonable to treat severe extra-pulmonary infections such as central nervous system disease or septic arthritis in an immunocompromised patient with an expectation that it may shorten the duration and severity of illness.

Because mycoplasmas lack a cell wall, they inherently are resistant to beta-lactam agents. Macrolides, including azithromycin, clarithromycin, and erythromycin, are the preferred antimicrobial agents for treatment of *Mycoplasma* pneumonia in school-aged children who have moderate to severe infection and those with underlying conditions, such as sickle cell disease.[1] Fluoroquinolones, tetracyclines (doxycycline), and pleuromutilins (the latter only approved in people 18 years and older) are 3 other classes of antibiotics to which *M pneumoniae* is susceptible.

Although macrolide-resistant strains of *M pneumoniae* have been identified, the majority of strains are susceptible, and the clinical implications of resistance are unclear. Treatment of hospitalized children with CAP attributable to a macrolide-resistant *M pneumoniae* using a fluoroquinolone has been shown in some studies to shorten the duration of fever and the length of hospitalization, but other studies have found no difference. *M hominis* usually is resistant to erythromycin and azithromycin but is variably susceptible to clindamycin, tetracyclines, and fluoroquinolones.

M genitalium is susceptible in vitro to macrolides, tetracyclines, and fluoroquinolones; however, resistance to macrolides has been rapidly increasing and has been confirmed in multiple studies. Prevalence of molecular markers for macrolide resistance, which highly correlates with treatment failure, range from 44% to 90% in the United States, Canada, Western Europe, and Australia. Although the majority of *M genitalium* strains are sensitive to moxifloxacin, resistance has been reported. Resistance-guided therapy has demonstrated cure rates of >90% and should be used whenever possible. As part of this approach, doxycycline is provided as initial empiric therapy,

[1] Bradley JS, Byington CL, Shah SS, et al. The management of community-acquired pneumonia in infants and children older than 3 months of age: clinical practice guidelines by the Pediatric Infectious Diseases Society and the Infectious Diseases Society of America. *Clin Infect Dis.* 2011;53(1):e25-e76

which reduces the organism load and facilitates organism clearance, followed by either azithromycin for macrolide-sensitive strains or moxifloxacin for macrolide-resistant strains. If resistance testing is not available, doxycycline 100 mg twice daily for 7 days is provided followed by moxifloxacin 400 mg once daily for 7 days. Data are limited regarding use of minocycline in instances of treatment failure.

INFECTION PREVENTION AND CONTROL MEASURES IN HEALTH CARE SETTINGS: In addition to standard precautions, droplet precautions are recommended for the duration of symptomatic illness with *M pneumoniae*.

CONTROL MEASURES FOR *M PNEUMONIAE* INFECTIONS: Hand hygiene decreases household transmission of respiratory pathogens and should be encouraged.

Tetracycline or azithromycin prophylaxis for close contacts has been shown to limit transmission in family and institutional outbreaks. However, antimicrobial prophylaxis for asymptomatic exposed contacts is not recommended routinely, because most secondary illnesses are generally mild and self-limited. Prophylaxis with a macrolide or a tetracycline (doxycycline) can be considered for people at increased risk of severe illness with *M pneumoniae*, such as children with sickle cell disease who are close contacts of a person who is acutely ill with *M pneumoniae* infection.

Nocardiosis

CLINICAL MANIFESTATIONS: Immunocompetent children typically develop cutaneous or lymphocutaneous disease with pustular or ulcerative lesions following soil contamination of a skin injury. Deep-seated tissue infection may follow traumatic soil-contaminated wounds. Immunocompromised people may develop invasive disease (pulmonary disease, which may disseminate, in particular to the central nervous system). At-risk people include those with chronic granulomatous disease, chronic obstructive pulmonary disease (COPD), impaired cell-mediated immunity including human immunodeficiency virus (HIV) infection, diseases requiring long-term systemic corticosteroid/immunosuppressive therapy, and autoimmune disease; people having received tumor necrosis factor inhibitors; and solid organ or hematopoietic cell transplant recipients, especially if calcineurin inhibitor levels are high. Pulmonary disease commonly manifests as rounded nodular infiltrates that can undergo cavitation; the infection may be acute, subacute, or chronic suppurative. The most common clinical symptoms include fever, cough, pleuritic chest pain, chills, and headache. Nocardia has a propensity to spread hematogenously to the brain (single or multiple abscesses) from the lungs. The organism also may spread to the skin (pustules, pyoderma, abscesses, mycetoma), or occasionally to other organs. *Nocardia* organisms can be recovered from respiratory specimens of patients with cystic fibrosis, but the clinical significance of this pathogen in these patients is unclear.

ETIOLOGY: *Nocardia* are gram-positive, aerobic, intracellular, nonmotile, filamentous bacteria in the order *Actinomycetales*. Cell walls of *Nocardia* organisms contain mycolic acid and thus may be described as "acid fast" or "partially acid fast" using the modified Kinyoun or Fite Faraco acid-fast staining and light microscopy.

EPIDEMIOLOGY: *Nocardia* species are ubiquitous environmental saprophytes, living in soil, organic matter, and fresh or sea water. Infections caused by *Nocardia* species typically are the result of environmental exposure through inhalation of soil or dust particles or through traumatic inoculation with a soil-contaminated object. The most prevalent species reported from human clinical sources in the United States are *Nocardia nova* complex, *Nocardia farcinica*, *Nocardia cyriacigeorgica*, and *Nocardia abscessus* complex; there is geographic variation by infecting species. Primary cutaneous infection and mycetoma most often are associated with *Nocardia brasiliensis*. Other less common pathogenic species include *Nocardia brevicatena* complex, *Nocardia otitidiscaviarum* complex, *Nocardia pseudobrasiliensis*, and *Nocardia transvalensis* complex.

Health care-associated or person-to-person transmission has been reported rarely. Animal-to-human transmission is not known to occur.

The **incubation period** is unknown.

DIAGNOSTIC TESTS: Isolation of *Nocardia* species from clinical specimens can require extended incubation periods, often 2 to 3 weeks. Specimens from sterile sites can be inoculated directly onto enriched solid media such as trypticase soy agar supplemented with 5% sheep blood, chocolate, brain-heart infusion, Sabouraud dextrose agars, and buffered charcoal yeast extract (BCYE) agar. Colonies look like white snowballs because of aerial hyphae. Specimens from nonsterile or contaminated sites, such as tissue or sputum, should be inoculated onto selective media, such as Thayer Martin or BCYE supplemented with vancomycin, with a minimum incubation of 3 weeks. Recovery of *Nocardia* species from tissue can be improved if the laboratory is requested to observe cultures for up to 4 weeks in an appropriate liquid medium at optimal growth temperature (between 25°C and 35°C for most species). Stained smears of sputum, body fluids, or pus demonstrating beaded, branching rods that stain weakly gram positive and partially acid-fast by the modified Kinyoun method suggest the diagnosis. The Brown-Brenn tissue Gram stain method and Grocott-Gomori methenamine silver stains are recommended to demonstrate microorganisms in tissue specimens.

Accurate identification of *Nocardia* isolates paired with antimicrobial susceptibility testing greatly enhances selection of appropriate antimicrobial therapy. Because of variability of phenotypic traits and difficulty growing organisms on commercial biochemical testing media, accurate identification is accomplished through molecular methods. Matrix-assisted laser desorption/ionization–time-of-flight (MALDI-TOF) mass spectrometry is often the first method used to identify the *Nocardia* isolate down to the species level, with other complementary methods used as necessary, such as 16S rRNA gene sequence analysis of full length or nearly full-length (~1440 bp) sequences, or whole genome analysis. Serologic tests for *Nocardia* species are not useful except for an enzyme-linked immunosorbent assay used to determine the presence of antibodies to *N brasiliensis* mycetoma.

Most experts recommend neuroimaging with or without cerebrospinal fluid examination in patients with pulmonary disease, even with a nonfocal neurologic examination, given the propensity of these organisms to infect the central nervous system.

TREATMENT: Rapid and accurate identification of *Nocardia* isolates and antimicrobial susceptibility testing are essential tools for successful treatment of nocardiosis. *Nocardia* species possess intrinsic resistance to multiple drugs. Antimicrobial susceptibility testing recommended by the Clinical and Laboratory Standards Institute (CLSI) is complex and generally requires a specialty or reference laboratory. Such testing should guide therapy and is recommended for all strains from patients with invasive disease, when patients are unable to tolerate a sulfonamide, or for patients in whom sulfonamide therapy fails.

Trimethoprim-sulfamethoxazole (TMP/SMX) is the drug of choice for mild infections. Certain *Nocardia* species including *N farcinica*, *N nova*, and *N otitidiscaviarum* may demonstrate intrinsic resistance to TMP/SMX. If infection does not respond to TMP/SMX, a fluoroquinolone or a carbapenem may be considered, although most *Nocardia* species are resistant to ertapenem. Linezolid has excellent activity against all *Nocardia* species but is not recommended for long-term administration because of hematologic and possible neurologic toxicity. Other agents with specific *Nocardia* coverage include clarithromycin *(N nova)* and amoxicillin-clavulanate (*N brasiliensis* and *N abscessus* complex). Pediatric data are lacking for many of these agents in the treatment of nocardiosis. Immunocompetent patients with lymphocutaneous disease usually respond after 6 to 12 weeks of monotherapy.

Combination drug therapy is recommended for patients with serious disease (pulmonary infection, disseminated disease, central nervous system involvement) and for infection in immunocompromised hosts. Initial combination treatment should include TMP/SMX, amikacin, and either linezolid, imipenem, or meropenem (resistance noted for some strains of *N brasiliensis*) until susceptibilities are available. Ceftriaxone is an alternative agent, but resistance is noted for many strains of *N farcinica*, *N transvalensis* complex, and *N otitidiscaviarum* complex. Immunocompromised patients and patients with serious disease should be treated for 6 to 12 months and for at least 3 months after apparent cure because of the propensity for relapse. Patients living with HIV may need even longer therapy, and suppressive therapy should be considered for life in the absence of immune reconstitution. Patients with central nervous system disease should be monitored with serial neuroimaging studies.

Drainage of abscesses is beneficial, and removal of infected foreign bodies (eg, central venous catheters) is recommended.

INFECTION PREVENTION AND CONTROL MEASURES IN HEALTH CARE SETTINGS: Standard precautions are recommended.

CONTROL MEASURES: People with weakened immune systems should be advised to cover their skin when working with soil. TMP/SMX administered 3 times per week for prophylaxis against *Pneumocystis jirovecii* generally is ineffective in preventing nocardiosis.

Norovirus and Sapovirus Infections

CLINICAL MANIFESTATIONS: Abrupt onset of vomiting and/or watery diarrhea, accompanied by abdominal cramps and nausea, are characteristic of norovirus and sapovirus gastroenteritis. Symptoms typically last from 24 to 72 hours. However, more prolonged courses of illness can occur, particularly among elderly people, young children, and hospitalized patients. Norovirus illness is recognized as a cause of chronic gastroenteritis in immunocompromised patients. Systemic manifestations, including fever, myalgia, malaise, anorexia, and headache, may accompany gastrointestinal tract symptoms.

ETIOLOGY: *Norovirus* and *Sapovirus* are genera in the family *Caliciviridae* and are 23- to 40-nm, nonenveloped, single-stranded RNA viruses. Noroviruses are genetically diverse and are classified into 10 genogroups of which viruses from genogroups (G) I and GII cause most of the infections in humans. Globally, GII genotype 4 viruses have caused the majority of outbreaks in recent decades (although some other genotypes have dominated in parts of Asia). Sapovirus genogroups I, II, IV, and V cause acute gastroenteritis with symptoms indistinguishable to norovirus in humans. At least 19 different sapovirus genogroups have been recognized.

EPIDEMIOLOGY: Norovirus causes illness in an estimated 1 in 15 Americans each year, resulting in 109 000 hospitalizations and 900 deaths annually. Nearly 1 million children (particularly those younger than 5 years) seek medical care because of norovirus. Deaths occur primarily among the elderly. As a result of the success of rotavirus vaccines, noroviruses have become the predominant cause of medically attended acute gastroenteritis in the United States, causing both sporadic cases and outbreaks. Outbreaks of sapovirus infection are relatively rare, with a prevalence in children younger than 5 years ranging from 3% to 17%.

Outbreaks with high attack rates tend to occur in semi-closed communities, such as long-term care facilities, schools, child care centers, and cruise ships. Transmission occurs via the fecal-oral or vomitus-oral routes, either directly person to person or indirectly by ingesting contaminated food or water or by touching surfaces contaminated with the virus and then touching the mouth. Common-source outbreaks have been described after ingestion of ice, shellfish, and a variety of ready-to-eat foods, including salads, berries, and bakery products, usually contaminated by infected food handlers. Transmission via vomitus has been documented, and exposure to contaminated surfaces and aerosolized vomitus has been implicated in some outbreaks. Asymptomatic shedding of norovirus is common across all age groups, with the highest prevalence in children.

Most norovirus strains bind to histo-blood group antigens, which are expressed on intestinal epithelial cells and are genetically regulated by the fucosyltransferase 2 (FUT2) gene. Individuals with a functional FUT2 gene are referred to as "secretors" whereas nonsecretors have a single point mutation in FUT2 making them nonsusceptible to most norovirus infections.

The **incubation period** for both norovirus and sapovirus is 12 to 48 hours. Viral shedding may start before onset of symptoms, peaks several days after exposure, and in some cases, may persist for ≥4 weeks. Prolonged shedding (>6 months) has been reported in immunocompromised hosts. Infection occurs year-round but is more common during the colder months of the year.

DIAGNOSTIC TESTS: Molecular diagnostic methods, such as nucleic acid amplification tests (NAATs) of stool samples, are the most sensitive means to detect norovirus and sapovirus. Several multiplex NAATs for the detection of gastrointestinal tract pathogens are cleared by the US Food and Drug Administration, with the majority including norovirus testing and some also including sapovirus testing. In children, interpretation of multipathogen test results may be complicated by coinfection with other enteric pathogens.

State and local public health laboratories use reverse transcriptase quantitative polymerase chain reaction (RT-qPCR) or multipathogen platforms for detection of norovirus and sapovirus RNA in clinical specimens. Both norovirus and sapovirus can be genotyped by amplification and sequencing of small regions of the capsid regions. Laboratory and epidemiologic support for investigation of suspected viral gastroenteritis outbreaks in the United States is available through local and state health departments.

TREATMENT: Supportive therapy includes oral or intravenous rehydration solutions to replace and maintain fluid and electrolyte balance. In transplant recipients with chronic diarrhea, some experts consider reduction in immunosuppressive medications, if feasible, and/or use of nitazoxanide.[1]

INFECTION PREVENTION AND CONTROL MEASURES IN HEALTH CARE SETTINGS: In addition to standard precautions, contact precautions are recommended for suspected cases of acute gastroenteritis attributable to norovirus infection until 48 hours after symptom resolution.

CONTROL MEASURES: Appropriate hand hygiene is the most important method to prevent norovirus and sapovirus infections and control transmission. This hand hygiene is best accomplished by thorough handwashing with running water and plain or antiseptic soap. Washing hands with soap and water after contact with a patient with norovirus or sapovirus infection is more effective than using alcohol-based hand sanitizers for reducing transmission.

Several factors favor transmission of noroviruses, including low infectious dose, large numbers of virus particles excreted, prolonged shedding, and persistence of the virus in the environment. The risk of infection can be decreased by standard measures for control of vomiting and diarrhea, such as educating child care providers and food handlers about infection control, maintaining cleanliness of surfaces and food preparation areas, using appropriate disinfectants (principally sodium hypochlorite [chlorine bleach]), excluding caregivers or food handlers who are ill and for at least 2 days after symptoms stop, and exercising appropriate hand hygiene, as discussed previously. If a source of transmission can be identified (eg, contaminated food or water) during an outbreak, then specific interventions to interrupt transmission can be effective.

Infants and children should be excluded from child care centers until stools are contained in the diaper or when toilet-trained children no longer have accidents using the toilet and when stool frequency becomes no more than 2 stools above that child's normal frequency for the time the child is in the program, even if the stools remain loose.

Public Health Reporting. Sporadic cases are not nationally notifiable, but outbreaks should be reported to local and state public health authorities as required and to the Centers for Disease Control and Prevention via the National Outbreak Reporting System (NORS) (**www.cdc.gov/nors**)**,** and laboratory test data including genotype information should be submitted to CaliciNet (**www.cdc.gov/norovirus/reporting/calicinet/index.html**).

Onchocerciasis
(River Blindness, Filariasis)

CLINICAL MANIFESTATIONS: Onchocerciasis primarily affects skin, subcutaneous tissues, and eyes. Subcutaneous, nontender nodules containing male and female adult worms can be up to several centimeters in diameter and are more common over bony prominences. Nodules tend to be found on the lower torso, pelvis, and lower extremities in patients infected in Africa, whereas in patients infected in South America,

---

[1] Angarone M, Snydman D; American Society of Transplantation Infectious Diseases Community of Practice. Diagnosis and management of diarrhea in solid-organ transplant recipients: Guidelines from the American Society of Transplantation Infectious Diseases Community of Practice. *Clin Transplant.* 2019;33(9):e13550

nodules are located more often on the upper body (the head and trunk). After the worms mature, fertilized female worms produce prelarval stages called microfilariae that migrate to the dermis and may cause a papular dermatitis. Pruritus often is intense, resulting in patient-inflicted excoriations over the affected areas. After years, skin can become lichenified and hypo- or hyperpigmented. Microfilariae may invade ocular structures, leading to inflammation of the cornea, iris, ciliary body, retina, choroid, and optic nerve. Loss of visual acuity and blindness can result over time if the disease is left untreated. Infection has also been associated with development of epilepsy.

ETIOLOGY: *Onchocerca volvulus* is a filarial nematode.

EPIDEMIOLOGY: *O volvulus* has no significant animal or environmental reservoir. Humans are infected when infectious larvae are transmitted through the bites of *Simulium* species flies (black flies). Black flies breed in fast-flowing streams and rivers (hence, the colloquial name for the disease, "river blindness"). Transmission of the parasite occurs primarily in equatorial Africa, but small foci are found in Venezuela, Brazil, and Yemen. Prevalence is greatest among people who live near vector breeding sites. The infection is not transmissible by person-to-person contact, blood transfusion, or breastfeeding; congenital transmission does not occur. Infection in travelers to areas with endemic infection who stay less than 6 to 12 months is uncommon.

The **incubation period** from infective bite to adult worm nodules is 6 to 12 months, and to microfilariae in the skin usually is 12 to 18 months but can be as long as 3 years.

DIAGNOSTIC TESTS: Direct microscopic examination of a 1- to 2-mm biopsy specimen of the epidermis and upper dermis (taken from the posterior iliac crest or other areas with highest suspicion for local microfilariae), incubated in saline, can reveal emerging microfilariae. Multiple skin snips may be needed to make a diagnosis, and in children in whom clinical suspicion of onchocerciasis is high, use of a nucleic acid amplification test (NAAT) may increase diagnostic yield if microscopic examination is negative. Microfilariae are not found in blood. Adult worms may be demonstrated in excised nodules that have been sectioned and stained. A slit-lamp examination of an involved eye may reveal motile microfilariae in the anterior chamber or "snowflake" corneal lesions. Eosinophilia is common. Specific serologic tests and detection of microfilariae in skin by NAAT are available in the United States in research and public health laboratories, including those of the National Institutes of Health and Centers for Disease Control and Prevention. Ultrasonography of nodules may visualize adult worms.

TREATMENT: Ivermectin and moxidectin are approved in the United States for treatment of onchocerciasis, although moxidectin is not yet available commercially (see Drugs for Parasitic Infections, p 1068). Patients from areas with endemic *Loa loa* infection should be screened for *L loa* and should referred to an expert if coinfected with *O volvulus* and *L loa*, as treatment of patients with high levels of circulating *L loa* microfilaremia with ivermectin rarely can result in fatal encephalopathy. Ivermectin can be used in younger children weighing more than 15 kg. Treatment decreases pruritus and dermatitis as well as the risk of developing severe ocular disease but does not kill the adult worms (which can live for more than a decade) and, thus, is not curative. Treatment with ivermectin is administered every 6 months until asymptomatic. Moxidectin, as a single oral dose for patients 12 years and older, has superior and more durable efficacy in reducing microfilariae in skin compared with a single dose of ivermectin. Safety and efficacy of repeated doses of moxidectin have not been studied, but on the basis of the duration of microfilarial suppression observed in the available studies, yearly dosing of moxidectin until asymptomatic is reasonable. Adverse reactions to treatment are caused by death of microfilariae and can include rash, edema, fever, myalgia, and rarely, asthma exacerbation and hypotension. Such reactions are more common in people with higher skin loads of microfilariae and decrease with repeated treatment in the absence of reexposure. Precautions to ivermectin/moxidectin treatment include pregnancy (class C drug), central nervous system disorders, and coinfection with *L loa* (see Lymphatic Filariasis, p 557). Ivermectin usually is compatible with breastfeeding, but because low levels of drug are found in human milk after treatment of the lactating person, most experts recommend delaying treatment of a breastfeeding person until the infant is >7 days of age.

A 6-week course of doxycycline can be used in addition to ivermectin or moxidectin to kill adult worms through depletion of their endosymbiotic rickettsia-like bacteria *Wolbachia*, which appear to be required for survival of *O volvulus*. Doxycycline may be used regardless of age in nonpregnant patients to obviate the need for years of ivermectin treatment. Doxycycline treatment may be initiated 1 week after treatment with ivermectin/moxidectin; for patients without symptoms, a 4- to 6-week course of doxycycline may be given, followed by a dose of ivermectin/moxidectin. There are no studies of the safety of simultaneous treatment.

The microfilaricide diethylcarbamazine (DEC) is contraindicated for the treatment of onchocerciasis, because it may cause adverse ocular reactions. Nodules can be removed surgically, but medical treatment still should be offered, because not all nodules may be detectable clinically or accessible surgically.

INFECTION PREVENTION AND CONTROL MEASURES IN HEALTH CARE SETTINGS: Standard precautions are recommended.

CONTROL MEASURES: Repellents and protective clothing (long sleeves and pants) can decrease exposure to bites from black flies, which bite by day. Treatment of vector breeding sites with larvicides is effective for controlling black fly populations. Vector control, however, largely has been supplanted by community-wide mass ivermectin administration programs. A highly successful global initiative being led by the World Health Organization has distributed hundreds of millions of ivermectin treatments (donated by the drug manufacturer for this purpose) in communities with endemic onchocerciasis. As a result of these programs, morbidity and transmission largely have been eliminated from the Americas (where most mass treatment programs now have halted) and markedly curtailed throughout Africa.

Paracoccidioidomycosis
(Formerly Known as South American Blastomycosis)

CLINICAL MANIFESTATIONS: Most disease occurs in adults (90%–95% of cases). The site of initial infection is the lungs. Clinical patterns include subclinical infection or progressive disease that can be either acute-subacute (juvenile type) or chronic (adult type). Constitutional symptoms, such as fever, malaise, anorexia, and weight loss, are common in both adult and juvenile forms.

In the juvenile form, the initial pulmonary infection usually is asymptomatic, and manifestations are related to dissemination of infection to the reticuloendothelial system, resulting in enlarged lymph nodes and involvement of liver, spleen, and bone marrow. Skin lesions are observed regularly and are located typically on the face, neck, and trunk. Involvement of bones, joints, and mucous membranes is less common. Enlarged lymph nodes occasionally coalesce and form abscesses or fistulas. The chronic form of the illness can be localized to the lungs or can disseminate. Oral mucosal lesions are observed in half of the cases, and skin involvement is common but occurs in a smaller proportion than in patients with the acute-subacute form. Infection can be latent for years before causing illness.

ETIOLOGY: *Paracoccidioides brasiliensis* is a thermally dimorphic fungus with yeast and mycelia (mold) phases. *P brasiliensis* complex contains 5 different phylogenetic lineages (S1a, S1b, PS2, PS3, and PS4). *Paracoccidioides lutzii* also causes paracoccidioidomycosis.

EPIDEMIOLOGY: The infection occurs in Latin America, from Mexico to Argentina, with 80% of cases in Brazil. The natural reservoir is unknown although soil is suspected; most disease is associated with agricultural work. The mode of transmission is unknown but most likely occurs via inhalation of contaminated soil or dust; person-to-person transmission does not occur. The armadillo is a known reservoir of *P brasiliensis*.

The **incubation period** is highly variable, ranging from 1 month to decades. Cases have been diagnosed outside endemic regions, so prior residence in Latin America is an important determinant in raising suspicion of the infection.

DIAGNOSTIC TESTS: Diagnosis is confirmed by visualization of fungal elements. Round, multiple-budding yeast cells with a distinguishing pilot's wheel appearance can be seen in preparations of sputum, bronchoalveolar lavage specimens, scrapings from ulcers, and material from lesions or in tissue biopsy specimens. Specimens can be prepared with several procedures, including wet or KOH wet preparations, or histologic staining with hematoxylin and eosin, silver, or periodic-acid Schiff. The mycelia form of *P brasiliensis* can be cultured on most enriched media, including Mycosel or Sabouraud dextrose agar, at 25°C to 30°C. Cultures should be held at least 8 weeks. The appearance of the mycelia form is not distinctive, and identification requires conversion to the yeast phase or DNA sequence determination. Complement fixation and immunodiffusion serologic tests are available for antibody detection. Semiquantitative immunodiffusion is the preferred test, with sensitivity around 80% and specificity >95%, and is the most widely available test in endemic regions.

TREATMENT[1]: Oral therapy with itraconazole is the treatment of choice for less severe or localized infection. Serum trough concentrations of itraconazole should be 1 to 2 µg/mL. A trough level should be checked 10 days or later following initiation to ensure adequate drug exposure. When measured by high-pressure liquid chromatography, both itraconazole and its bioactive hydroxyitraconazole metabolite are reported, the sum of which should be considered in assessing the trough concentration. The itraconazole oral solution formulation is preferred over the capsule formulation because of improved absorption, and should be taken on an empty stomach.

[1] Thompson GR III, Le T, Chindamporn A, et al. Global guideline for the diagnosis and management of the endemic mycoses: an initiative of the European Confederation of Medical Mycology in cooperation with the International Society for Human and Animal Mycology [Erratum in: *Lancet Infect Dis.* 2021;21(11):e341]. *Lancet Infect Dis.* 2021;21(12):e364-e374

However, a super bioavailable (SUBA) itraconazole is now approved by the Food and Drug Administration for the treatment of pulmonary and extrapulmonary blastomycosis in individuals 18 years or older, with pharmacokinetic studies of this formulation demonstrating less variable absorption than conventional itraconazole capsules and a similar side effect profile; data in children are lacking.

Voriconazole may be as effective as itraconazole, including when there is central nervous system involvement, but has not been studied as extensively. Close monitoring of voriconazole serum trough concentrations is critical for both efficacy and safety. Most experts agree that voriconazole trough concentrations should be measured on day 3 or later after initiating treatment and for children, therapeutic trough concentrations are 2 to 6 µg/mL. It is important to individualize dosing in patients following initiation of voriconazole therapy, because there is high interpatient variability in metabolism.

Isavuconazole has been efficacious in adults, but there are limited pediatric data for paracoccidioidomycosis.

Optimal duration of therapy is unknown, but prolonged therapy for 9 to 18 months is necessary to minimize the relapse rate, and children with severe disease can require a longer course. See Table 4.8 (p 1026) for dosing.

Trimethoprim-sulfamethoxazole orally is an inferior alternative to itraconazole, and treatment must be continued for 18 months or longer to lessen risk of relapse, which occurs in 10% to 15% of optimally treated patients. Amphotericin B generally is given only for initial treatment of severe paracoccidioidomycosis for 2 to 4 weeks. Intravenous trimethoprim-sulfamethoxazole is another option. Children treated initially by the intravenous route can transition to orally administered therapy after clinical improvement has been observed, usually after 3 to 6 weeks.

Serial serologic testing by complement fixation or semiquantitative immunodiffusion is useful for monitoring the response to therapy. The expected response is a progressive decline in titers after 1 to 3 months of treatment with stabilization at a low titer for years or even for life.

INFECTION PREVENTION AND CONTROL MEASURES IN HEALTH CARE SETTINGS: Standard precautions are recommended.

CONTROL MEASURES: None.

Paragonimiasis

CLINICAL MANIFESTATIONS: There are 2 major forms of paragonimiasis: 1) primary pulmonary disease with or without extrapulmonary manifestations caused by adult flukes and their eggs, and 2) extrapulmonary disease caused by aberrant migrating immature flukes, sometimes resulting in a visceral larva migrans syndrome.

Pulmonary infections mostly are asymptomatic or result in mild symptoms but may be associated with chronic cough, chest pain, and dyspnea, often of insidious onset and often misdiagnosed as pulmonary tuberculosis, malignancy, or chronic obstructive pulmonary disease. During worm migration in the lungs, migratory infiltrates may be noted on serial imaging. Heavy infestations cause paroxysms of coughing, which often produce blood-tinged, foul-smelling sputum that is brown because of the presence of the pigmented *Paragonimus* eggs and hemosiderin. Hemoptysis can be severe. Eosinophilic pleural effusion, pneumothorax, bronchiectasis, and pulmonary fibrosis with clubbing can develop.

Extrapulmonary manifestations may involve the liver, spleen, abdominal cavity, intestinal wall, intra-abdominal lymph nodes, skin, pericardium, or central nervous system, with meningoencephalitis, seizures, and space-occupying tumors attributable to invasion of the brain by adult flukes. Cerebral paragonimiasis is the most common extrapulmonary manifestation, is more common in children, and typically presents with seizure, headache, visual disturbance, or motor or sensory dysfunction. Extrapulmonary paragonimiasis also is associated with migratory subcutaneous nodules, which contain juvenile worms. Symptoms tend to subside after approximately 5 years but can persist for as many as 20 years.

ETIOLOGY: Paragonimiasis is caused by the lung fluke (trematode, flat worm) *Paragonimus*. In Asia, pulmonary paragonimiasis with or without extrapulmonary manifestations is caused by adult flukes and eggs of *Paragonimus westermani* and *Paragonimus heterotremus*. In Africa, the adult flukes and eggs of *Paragonimus africanus* and *Paragonimus uterobilateralis* produce the disease. *Paragonimus kellicotti* is the endemic species in North America.

Adult flukes of *P westermani* are up to 12 mm long and 7 mm wide and occur throughout Asia. A triploid parthenogenetic form of *P westermani*, which is larger, produces more eggs, and elicits greater disease, has been described in Japan, Korea, Taiwan, and parts of eastern China. *P heterotremus* occurs in Southeast Asia, adjacent parts of China, and India. *P africanus* and *P uterobilateralis* are found in the rainforests of West and Central Africa.

Extrapulmonary paragonimiasis (ie, visceral larva migrans syndrome) can be caused by larval stages of *Paragonimus skrjabini* and *Paragonimus miyazakii*. The worms rarely mature in infected human tissues. *P skrjabini* occurs in China, whereas *P miyazakii* occurs in Japan. *Paragonimus mexicanus* and *Paragonimus ecuadoriensis* occur in Mexico, Costa Rica, Ecuador, and Peru.

EPIDEMIOLOGY: Transmission occurs when raw or undercooked freshwater crabs or crayfish, including pickled and soy sauce-marinated products, containing larvae (metacercariae) are ingested. Numerous cases of *P kellicotti* infection have occurred when people have ingested uncooked or undercooked crayfish while canoeing or camping in the Midwestern United States. In North America, disease also has been caused by *P westermani* present in imported crab. A less common mode of transmission that also may occur is human infection through ingestion of meat from a paratenic host, most commonly ingestion of raw pork, usually from wild pigs, containing the juvenile stages of *Paragonimus* species (described as occurring in Japan). Humans are accidental ("dead-end") hosts for *P skrjabini* and *P miyazakii* in visceral larva migrans. These flukes cannot mature in humans and do not produce eggs. *Paragonimus* species also infect a variety of other mammals, such as canids, mustelids, felids, and rodents, which serve as animal reservoir hosts.

The **incubation period** is variable. Egg production begins approximately 9 to 13 weeks after ingestion of *P westermani* metacercariae.

DIAGNOSIS: Paragonimiasis should be considered in patients with unexplained fever, cough, eosinophilia, and pleural effusion or other chest radiographic abnormalities who have eaten raw or undercooked crab or crayfish. Microscopic examination of stool, sputum, pleural fluid, cerebrospinal fluid, and other tissue specimens may reveal operculate eggs. A Western blot serologic antibody test based on *P westermani* antigen, available at the Centers for Disease Control and Prevention (CDC), is sensitive and specific; antibody concentrations detected by immunoblot decrease slowly after the infection is cured by treatment. Charcot-Leyden crystals and eosinophils in sputum are useful diagnostic elements. Peripheral blood eosinophilia also is characteristic. Chest radiographs may appear normal or may resemble radiographs from patients with tuberculosis or malignancy.

TREATMENT: Praziquantel is the treatment of choice (see Drugs for Parasitic Infections, p 1068) and typically is associated with high cure rates, as demonstrated by cessation of egg production and resolution of radiographic lesions in the lungs. The drug also is effective for some extrapulmonary manifestations. An alternative drug for patients unable to take praziquantel (eg, because of previous allergic reaction) is triclabendazole. Triclabendazole is a narrow-spectrum anthelmintic with activity against *Fasciola* and *Paragonimus;* it is approved by the US Food and Drug Administration (FDA) only for fascioliasis. In patients with central nervous system paragonimiasis, a short course of steroids may be beneficial, in addition to praziquantel, to reduce the inflammatory response associated with dying flukes. Other supportive care, including anti-epileptics and shunt placement, may be needed.

INFECTION PREVENTION AND CONTROL MEASURES IN HEALTH CARE SETTINGS: Standard precautions are recommended. There is no person-to-person transmission.

CONTROL MEASURES: Crabs and crayfish should be cooked for several minutes to at least 145°F [63°C]. Meat from wild pigs should be cooked to an internal temperature of at least 160°F [71°C] before eating. Control of animal reservoirs is not possible.

Parainfluenza Viral Infections

CLINICAL MANIFESTATIONS: Human parainfluenza viruses (hPIVs) are the major cause of laryngotracheobronchitis (croup) and also cause bronchiolitis and pneumonia as well as upper respiratory tract infection.[1] hPIV type 1 (hPIV1) and, to a lesser extent, hPIV type 2 (hPIV2) are the most common pathogens associated with croup. hPIV type 3 (hPIV3) most commonly is associated with bronchiolitis and pneumonia in infants and young children. Infections with hPIV type 4 (hPIV4) are less well characterized but have been associated with both upper and lower respiratory tract infections. Longitudinal studies have demonstrated that upper respiratory infections caused by viruses, including hPIVs, can be associated with acute otitis media, which is frequently a mixed viral-bacterial infection. Rarely, hPIVs have been isolated from patients with parotitis, myopericarditis, aseptic meningitis, encephalitis, febrile seizures, and Guillain-Barré syndrome. hPIV infections can exacerbate symptoms of chronic lung disease and asthma in children and adults. In children with immunodeficiency and recipients of hematopoietic cell transplants, hPIVs, most commonly hPIV3, can cause refractory infections with persistent shedding, severe pneumonia with extrapulmonary dissemination, and even fatal disease. hPIV infections do not confer complete protective immunity; therefore, reinfections can occur with all serotypes and at any age, but reinfections usually are mild and limited to the upper respiratory tract.

---

[1] American Academy of Pediatrics, Subcommittee on Diagnosis and Management of Bronchiolitis. Clinical practice guideline: the diagnosis, management, and prevention of bronchiolitis. *Pediatrics.* 2014;134(5):e1474-e1502

ETIOLOGY: hPIVs are enveloped single-stranded negative-sense RNA viruses classified in the family *Paramyxoviridae*. Four antigenically distinct types—1, 2, 3, and 4 (with 2 subtypes, 4A and 4B)—that infect humans have been identified. hPIV1 and hPIV3 are in the genus *Respirovirus*, and hPIV2 and hPIV4 are classified in the genus *Rubulavirus*.

EPIDEMIOLOGY: hPIVs are transmitted from person to person by direct contact with contaminated nasopharyngeal secretions through large respiratory tract droplets and fomites. hPIV infections can be sporadic or associated with outbreaks of acute respiratory tract disease. Seasonal patterns of infection are distinct, predictable, and cyclic in temperate regions. Different serotypes have distinct epidemiologic patterns. hPIV1 tends to produce outbreaks of respiratory tract illness, usually croup, in the autumn of every other year. A major increase in the number of cases of croup in the autumn usually indicates a hPIV1 outbreak. hPIV2 also can cause outbreaks of respiratory tract illness in the autumn, but hPIV2 outbreaks tend to be less severe, irregular, and less common. hPIV3 is endemic and usually is prominent during spring and summer in temperate climates but often continues into autumn, especially in years when autumn outbreaks of hPIV1 or hPIV2 are absent. hPIV4 seasonal patterns are not as well characterized, but studies have shown that infections with hPIV4 had year-round prevalence with peaks during the fall and winter.

The age of primary infection varies with serotype. Primary infection with all types usually occurs by 5 years of age. Infection with hPIV3 more often occurs in infants and is a frequent cause of bronchiolitis and pneumonia in this age group. By 12 months of age, 50% of infants have acquired hPIV3 infection. Infections with hPIV1 and, to a lesser extent, hPIV2 are more likely to occur between 1 and 5 years of age. Acquisition of hPIV4 also occurs more often during preschool years.

Immunocompetent children with primary hPIV infection may shed virus for up to 1 week before onset of clinical symptoms and for 1 to 3 weeks after symptoms have disappeared, depending on serotype. Severe lower respiratory tract disease with prolonged shedding of the virus can occur in immunocompromised individuals. In these patients, infection may disseminate, with reports of extrapulmonary dissemination to brain, myocardium, and pericardium.

The **incubation period** ranges from 2 to 6 days. Symptoms can develop from 2 to 10 days after exposure and typically last up to 7 to 10 days, although viral shedding can persist for several weeks.

DIAGNOSTIC TESTS: Nucleic acid amplification tests (NAATs) are the preferred diagnostic method for detection and differentiation of hPIVs and have become the standard method in clinical practice. hPIVs are included in many multiplex polymerase chain reaction (PCR)-based respiratory pathogen panels, although hPIV4 is less commonly included. hPIVs may be isolated from nasopharyngeal secretions in cell culture, usually within 4 to 7 days of culture inoculation. Serologic diagnosis, made by a significant increase in antibody titer between acute and convalescent serum specimens, is less useful, because results are delayed and infection may not always be accompanied by a significant homotypic antibody response.

TREATMENT: Specific antiviral therapy is not available. Pharmacologic therapy focuses on decreasing airway edema via corticosteroids and nebulized epinephrine, which are mainstays of treatment. Patients with mild croup can often be managed with supportive care at home, although data have shown benefit for outpatients with mild croup who receive steroids. Oral, intramuscular, and nebulized corticosteroids (ie, budesonide) have been demonstrated to decrease the severity and duration of symptoms and hospitalization in patients with moderate to severe laryngotracheobronchitis. Nebulized epinephrine is typically used in conjunction with corticosteroids for moderate to severe croup, and repeated doses may be needed for patients with severe croup. Antimicrobial agents should be reserved for documented secondary bacterial infections. Use of ribavirin (usually inhaled), with or without concomitant administration of immune globulin intravenous (IGIV), has been reported anecdotally in immunocompromised patients with severe pneumonia; however, controlled studies are lacking and this use is not routinely recommended.

INFECTION PREVENTION AND CONTROL MEASURES IN HEALTH CARE SETTINGS: In addition to standard precautions, contact and droplet precautions are recommended for the duration of hPIV-associated illness. In immunocompromised patients, the duration of precautions should be extended because of possible prolonged shedding.

CONTROL MEASURES: Appropriate respiratory hygiene and cough etiquette should be followed. Exposure to hPIV-infected people, including other patients, staff, and family members, may not be recognized, both because illness may be mild and because infected people may shed virus for up to 1 week before onset of clinical symptoms. Additional infection control measures should be considered in certain settings (eg, child care centers, nursing homes) when respiratory infections have been identified.

Parasitic Diseases

Parasites are among the most common causes of morbidity and mortality in children worldwide. Outside the tropics and subtropics, parasitic diseases occur among travelers and immigrants. Toxocariasis occurs in the United States, most commonly in the South. Malaria infections in the United States occur among people who have traveled to regions with ongoing malaria transmission, and the diagnosis should be considered when evaluating fever in a returned traveler. Local transmission of malaria has recently been detected as well in the United States (**https://emergency.cdc.gov/han/2023/han00494.asp**). Certain parasitic infections have long latency periods, and the diseases they cause, such as Chagas disease, neurocysticercosis, schistosomiasis, and strongyloidiasis, are encountered in immigrants from or travelers to regions with endemic infection. Clinicians need to be aware of where these infections may be acquired, their clinical presentations, methods of diagnosis, and how to prevent infection. A number of human parasitic infections are discussed in individual chapters in Section 3; diseases are arranged alphabetically. Table 3.42 provides details on some infrequently encountered parasitic diseases not discussed elsewhere.

Consultation and assistance in diagnosis and management of parasitic diseases are available from the Centers for Disease Control and Prevention (CDC), state health departments, and university departments or hospitals that have divisions of travel medicine, tropical medicine, infectious diseases, international or global health, and public health.

Drugs for Parasitic Infections can be found beginning on p 1068; information in the table is compiled from recommendations from the CDC and other sources. Treatment recommendations may vary based on expert opinion, and because some commonly used drugs do not have approved indications for a specific parasitic

Table 3.42. Selected Parasitic Diseases Not Covered Elsewhere[a]

Disease and/or Agent	Where Infection May Be Acquired	Definitive Host	Intermediate Host	Modes of Human Infection	Diagnostic Laboratory Tests in Humans	Parasitic Form Causing Human Disease	Common Manifestations in Humans
Angiostrongylus cantonensis (neurotropic disease)	Widespread in the tropics, particularly Pacific Islands and Southeast Asia; also in Central and South America, the Caribbean, Africa, and the United States	Rats	Snails and slugs	Eating raw or improperly cooked infected mollusks, including inadvertent ingestion on raw produce; possibly other modes	Eosinophils in CSF; rarely, identification of larvae in CSF; serologic testing and CSF NAAT not commercially available	Larval worms	Eosinophilic meningitis with severe headache, neck stiffness, nausea, vomiting, paresthesias or hyperesthesias, peripheral eosinophilia
Angiostrongylus costaricensis (gastrointestinal tract disease)	Central and South America, the Caribbean	Rodents	Snails and slugs	Eating raw or improperly cooked infected mollusks, including inadvertent ingestion on raw produce; possibly other modes	Identification of larvae and eggs in tissue (not stool); NAAT and serologic testing not commercially available	Larval worms	Eosinophilic enterocolitis with abdominal pain, fever, nausea, vomiting, diarrhea (may mimic appendicitis), peripheral eosinophilia

Table 3.42. Selected Parasitic Diseases Not Covered Elsewhere,[a] continued

Disease and/or Agent	Where Infection May Be Acquired	Definitive Host	Intermediate Host	Modes of Human Infection	Diagnostic Laboratory Tests in Humans	Parasitic Form Causing Human Disease	Common Manifestations in Humans
Anisakiasis (*Anisakis* and *Pseudoterranova* species)	Cosmopolitan, most common where eating raw fish is practiced	Marine mammals	Certain saltwater fish, squid, and octopus	Eating raw, pickled, or undercooked infected marine fish or squid or octopus	Identification of recovered larvae on endoscopy or within tissue biopsies; serologic testing and NAAT not available in the United States	Larval worms	Abdominal pain, nausea, vomiting, diarrhea, allergic reactions
Capillariasis-intestinal disease (*Capillaria philippinensis*)	Philippines, Thailand	Humans, fish-eating birds	Freshwater fish	Ingestion of raw or undercooked infected fish	Eggs and parasite in feces or biopsies of small intestine	Larvae and mature worms	Abdominal pain, diarrhea, vomiting, weight loss
Clonorchis sinensis, *Opisthorchis viverrini*, *Opisthorchis felineus* (liver flukes)	East Asia, Southeast Asia, Central and Eastern Europe, Russian Federation	Humans, cats, dogs, other mammals	Certain freshwater snails	Eating raw or undercooked infected freshwater fish, crabs, crayfish	Eggs in stool, bile, or duodenal fluid Serologic testing, antigen tests, and NAAT not commercially available	Larvae and mature flukes	Abdominal pain; nausea, vomiting, diarrhea, hepatobiliary disease; cholangiocarcinoma

Table 3.42. Selected Parasitic Diseases Not Covered Elsewhere,[a] continued

Disease and/or Agent	Where Infection May and/or Be Acquired	Definitive Host	Intermediate Host	Modes of Human Infection	Diagnostic Laboratory Tests in Humans	Parasitic Form Causing Human Disease	Common Manifestations in Humans
Dracunculiasis (*Dracunculus medinensis*) (Guinea worm)	Foci in Africa; global eradication nearly achieved, 13 human cases worldwide in 2022; 2 during the first half of 2023[b]	Humans, dogs	Crustacea (copepods)	Drinking water infested with infected copepods	Identification of emerging or adult worm in subcutaneous tissues; serology available but not necessary	Adult female worms	Emerging roundworm; inflammatory response; systemic and local blister or ulcer in skin
Fascioliasis (liver flukes; *Fasciola hepatica*)	Worldwide; predominantly in the tropics	Sheep and cattle most important; other ruminants	Certain freshwater snails	Eating raw freshwater plants (eg, watercress) or drinking water contaminated with larvae	Identifying eggs in stool, duodenal fluid, or bile; serologic testing; examination of surgical specimens	Larvae and mature flukes	Abdominal pain nausea, vomiting; hepatobiliary disease

Table 3.42. Selected Parasitic Diseases Not Covered Elsewhere,[a] continued

Disease and/or Agent	Where Infection May Be Acquired	Definitive Host	Intermediate Host	Modes of Human Infection	Diagnostic Laboratory Tests in Humans	Parasitic Form Causing Human Disease	Common Manifestations in Humans
Fasciolopsiasis (intestinal flukes; *Fasciolopsis buski*)	East Asia, Southeast Asia	Humans, pigs, dogs	Certain freshwater snails	Eating raw plants (eg, bamboo shoots, watercress, water chestnuts) contaminated with larvae	Eggs or worm in feces or duodenal fluid; serologic testing not commercially available	Larvae and mature flukes	Diarrhea, constipation, vomiting, anorexia, edema of face and legs, ascites

CSF indicates cerebrospinal fluid; NAAT, nucleic acid amplification test.

[a] For recommended drug treatment, see Drugs for Parasitic Infections (p 1068).

[b] For progress toward global eradication (which will be the second human disease eradicated, after smallpox), see **www.cartercenter.org/health/guinea_worm/index.html**.

infection or a particular age group. Specific expertise or multiple sources should be consulted especially when there is a lack of familiarity with the parasite or the drugs recommended for treatment. The CDC distributes several drugs that are not available commercially in the United States for treatment of parasitic diseases. To request these drugs, a physician must contact the CDC Parasitic Diseases Inquiries office (see Appendix I, Directory of Resources, p 1134; Monday-Friday 8 am–4 pm: 404-718-4745, and outside these hours 24/7: 770-488-7100; email: **parasites@cdc.gov**). Consultation with a medical officer from the CDC is required before a drug is released for a patient. For drugs and consultation regarding malaria, a separate CDC hotline is available Monday-Friday 9 am–5 pm (770-488-7788) and outside these hours 24/7 (770-488-7100).

Parechovirus Infections

CLINICAL MANIFESTATIONS: Parechoviruses (PeVs) primarily cause disease in young infants and present in a similar manner to enteroviruses, with febrile illness, exanthems (maculopapular, erythroderma, and/or palmar and plantar erythema), sepsis-like syndrome (frequently with leukopenia), and/or central nervous system disease. The latter includes meningitis (typically with little or no pleocytosis), encephalitis (typically white-matter predominant), seizures, and apnea; long-term neurodevelopmental sequelae may occur. Infections (particularly with HPeV-3) in neonates or very young infants may be severe, with manifestations that include sepsis, hepatitis and coagulopathy, myocarditis, pneumonia, and/or meningoencephalitis; long-term sequelae or death may occur. PeV infections in older infants and toddlers have been associated with generally mild upper and lower respiratory tract disease and gastroenteritis (although causation has not been established consistently) and a variety of other less common manifestations, including acute flaccid paralysis, acute disseminated encephalomyelitis, myalgia and myositis, herpangina, hand-foot-and-mouth disease, sudden infant death syndrome, and hemophagocytic lymphohistiocytosis.

ETIOLOGY: PeVs are small, nonenveloped, single-stranded, positive-sense RNA viruses in the family *Picornaviridae*. The *Parechovirus* genus consists of 6 species, *Parechovirus* A through F. *Parechovirus* A (formerly named human *Parechovirus*) includes at least 19 PeV types (designated HPeV1–19) and is the only species known to cause human disease. HPeV-1 and HPeV-2 previously were classified as echoviruses 22 and 23, respectively. HPeV-1 and HPeV-3 have been implicated in disease most frequently.

EPIDEMIOLOGY: Humans are the primary reservoir for PeV-A, although infection in primates has been demonstrated. PeV-A infections have been reported worldwide. Seroepidemiologic studies suggest that PeV-A infections occur commonly during early childhood. In some studies, most school-aged children have serologic evidence of prior infection, but seroprevalence appears to vary by geographic region and specific PeV-A type. PeV infections frequently are asymptomatic. Symptomatic infection is most frequent in children younger than 2 years, with the most severe disease occurring in infants (especially younger than 6 months of age infected with HPeV-6).

Transmission appears to occur via the fecal-oral and respiratory routes, from symptomatic or asymptomatic individuals. On the basis of reports of very early onset neonatal disease, in utero and perinatal transmission also may occur. Certain PeV-A types may circulate throughout the year, while infections by other types (eg, HPeV-3) occur more commonly during summer and fall months in temperate climates. Multiple PeV-A types may circulate in a community during the same time period. Community outbreaks and health care-associated transmission in neonatal and pediatric hospital units have been observed. Virus is shed from the upper respiratory tract for 1 to 3 weeks and in stool for less than 2 weeks to as long as 6 months. Shedding may occur in the absence of illness or continue after symptoms resolve.

The **incubation period** for PeV infections has not been defined.

DIAGNOSTIC TESTS: Parechovirus-specific molecular tests such as nucleic acid amplification tests (NAATs) represent the best available diagnostic method. Some assays may not detect all PeV-A types. Enterovirus NAATs will not detect PeVs (and vice versa). PeVs can be detected by molecular assays in stool, rectal and throat swab specimens, nasopharyngeal aspirates, tracheal secretions, blood, and cerebrospinal fluid. Certain multiplex NAATs designed to detect multiple bacterial and viral agents of meningitis and encephalitis, including PeVs, in cerebrospinal fluid are available. The PeV type can be identified by partial or complete sequencing of the viral protein 1 region, typically through reverse transcriptase-polymerase chain reaction (RT-PCR) amplification. Serologic assays have been developed for research but are not available commercially for diagnostic purposes.

TREATMENT: No specific therapy is available for PeV infections. Immune globulin intravenous (IGIV) has been used in some published case reports of neonates with severe PeV infections.

INFECTION PREVENTION AND CONTROL MEASURES IN HEALTH CARE SETTINGS: In addition to standard precautions, contact precautions are appropriate for infants and young children for the duration of PeV illness. Cohorting of infected neonates may be effective in controlling hospital nursery outbreaks.

CONTROL MEASURES: Hand hygiene and environmental cleaning are important in decreasing spread of PeVs within families and institution.

Parvovirus B19
(Erythema Infectiosum, Fifth Disease)

CLINICAL MANIFESTATIONS: Infection with parvovirus B19 is clinically recognized most often as erythema infectiosum (EI), or fifth disease, which is characterized by a distinctive rash that may be preceded by mild systemic symptoms, including fever in 15% to 30% of patients. Fifth disease is so named because it was fifth in a list of historical classifications of common skin rash illnesses in children. The facial rash can be intensely red with a "slapped cheek" appearance that often is accompanied by circumoral pallor. A symmetric, macular, lace-like, and often pruritic rash occurs on the trunk, moving peripherally to involve the arms, buttocks, and thighs. The rash can fluctuate in intensity and can recur with environmental changes, such as temperature and exposure to sunlight, for weeks to months. A brief, mild, nonspecific illness consisting of fever, malaise, myalgia, and headache often precedes the characteristic exanthem by approximately 7 to 10 days. Arthralgia and arthritis occur in fewer than 10% of infected children but commonly occur among adults, especially women. Knees are involved most commonly in children, but a symmetric polyarthropathy of knees, fingers, and other joints is common in adults.

Table 3.43. Clinical Manifestations of Parvovirus B19 Infection

Conditions	Usual Hosts
Erythema infectiosum (EI, fifth disease)	Immunocompetent children
Polyarthropathy syndrome	Immunocompetent adults (more common in women)
Chronic anemia/pure red cell aplasia	Immunocompromised hosts
Transient aplastic crisis	People with hemolytic anemia (ie, sickle cell disease)
Hydrops fetalis/congenital anemia	Fetus (first 20 weeks of pregnancy)
Petechial, papular-purpuric gloves-and-socks syndrome (PPGSS)	Immunocompetent children and young adults

Parvovirus B19 can cause asymptomatic or subclinical infections. Other manifestations (Table 3.43) include a mild respiratory tract illness with no rash, a rash atypical for EI that may be rubelliform or petechial, papular-purpuric gloves-and-socks syndrome (PPGSS; painful and pruritic papules, petechiae, and purpura of hands and feet, often with fever and an enanthem), polyarthropathy syndrome (arthralgia and arthritis in adults in the absence of other manifestations of EI), chronic erythroid hypoplasia with severe anemia in immunodeficient patients, and transient aplastic crisis lasting 7 to 10 days in patients with hemolytic anemias (eg, sickle cell disease and autoimmune hemolytic anemia). Patients with transient aplastic crisis may have a prodromal illness with fever, malaise, and myalgia, but rash usually is absent. In addition, parvovirus B19 infection sometimes has been associated with decreases in numbers of platelets, lymphocytes, and neutrophils. In rare cases, parvovirus B19 infection has been associated with acute hepatitis, myocarditis, encephalopathies, hemophagocytic lymphohistiocytosis, and nephrotic syndrome in children and young adults. Parvovirus B19 infection occurring during pregnancy can cause fetal hydrops, intrauterine growth restriction, isolated pleural and pericardial effusions, and fetal death, but the virus is not a proven cause of congenital anomalies. The risk of fetal death is between 2% and 6% when infection occurs during pregnancy. The greatest risk appears to occur during the first half of pregnancy.

ETIOLOGY: Parvovirus B19 is a small, nonenveloped, single-stranded DNA virus in the family *Parvoviridae*, genus *Erythroparvovirus*. Three distinct genotypes of the virus have been described that appear to have variable geographic distribution, but there is no evidence of differences of virologic or disease characteristics among the genotypes. Parvovirus B19 replicates in human erythrocyte precursors, which accounts for some of the clinical manifestations following infection. Parvovirus B19-associated red blood cell aplasia is related to cell death of erythrocyte precursors. Other findings are believed to be associated with the immunologic response.

EPIDEMIOLOGY: Parvovirus B19 is distributed worldwide; humans are the only known hosts. Modes of transmission include contact with respiratory tract secretions, percutaneous exposure to blood or blood products, and vertical transmission. The virus is quite resistant and can survive in the environment at least for days (or longer). Parvovirus B19 infections are ubiquitous, and cases of EI can occur sporadically or in outbreaks in schools, particularly during late winter and early spring. Secondary spread among susceptible household members is common, with infection occurring in approximately 50% of susceptible contacts in some studies. The transmission rate in schools is lower, but infection can be an occupational risk for school and child care personnel, with approximately 20% of susceptible contacts becoming infected. In young children, antibody seroprevalence generally is 5% to 10%. In most communities, approximately 50% of young adults and often more than 90% of elderly people are seropositive.

The **incubation period** from acquisition of parvovirus B19 to onset of initial symptoms (fever, runny nose, fatigue, myalgia) is between 4 and 14 days but can be as long as 21 days. Rash and arthralgias tend to occur at least a few days after initial viral symptoms. Timing of the presence of high levels of parvovirus B19 DNA in serum and respiratory tract secretions indicates that people with EI are likely infectious before rash onset and are unlikely to be infectious after onset of the rash and/or joint symptoms. In contrast, patients with aplastic crises are contagious from before the onset of symptoms through at least the week after onset. Symptoms of PPGSS can occur in association with viremia and before development of antibody response, and affected patients should be considered infectious.

DIAGNOSTIC TESTS: In an immunocompetent host, detection of serum parvovirus B19-specific immunoglobulin (Ig) M antibodies is the preferred diagnostic test for an acute or recent parvovirus B19-associated rash illness. A positive IgM test result indicates that infection probably occurred within the previous 2 to 3 months. IgM antibodies can be detected in 90% or more of patients at the time of the EI rash and by the third day of illness in patients with transient aplastic crisis. Serum IgG antibodies appear by approximately day 2 of EI and persist for life; therefore, presence of parvovirus B19 IgG is not necessarily indicative of acute infection. These assays are available through commercial laboratories and some state public health department laboratories.

Serum IgM and IgG assays are not reliable in immunocompromised patients. The optimal method for detecting transient aplastic crisis or chronic infection in the immunocompromised patient is demonstration of high titer of viral DNA by a quantitative nucleic acid amplification test (NAAT). Such patients generally have $>10^6$ parvovirus B19 DNA copies/mL of plasma. Currently, there are no NAATs cleared by the US Food and Drug Administration for the qualitative or quantitative detection of parvovirus B19 DNA, but such assays are available through select commercial and reference laboratories and sometimes in larger hospital-based laboratories. With the availability of a World Health Organization (WHO) nucleic acid standard for parvovirus B19 DNA, assay results can be reported in international units per mL (IU/mL) to allow for comparison across assays. False-negative results can occur with NAATs that do not detect all 3 genotypes. Because parvovirus B19 DNA can be detected at low levels by NAAT in serum for months and even years after the acute viremic phase when infectious virus no longer appears to be present, detection of low levels of DNA does not necessarily indicate acute infection. Low levels of parvovirus B19 DNA also can be detected by NAAT in tissues (skin, heart, liver, bone marrow), independent of active disease. A qualitative NAAT may be used on amniotic fluid as an aid to diagnosis of hydrops fetalis. Parvovirus B19 cannot be propagated in standard cell culture.

TREATMENT: For most patients, only supportive care is indicated. Patients with aplastic crisis may require transfusions of blood products. Immune globulin intravenous (IGIV) therapy often is effective and should be used for the treatment of parvovirus B19 infection-induced anemia in immunodeficient patients. The optimal dosing regimen and duration of treatment have not been established. Reduction of immune suppression also should be attempted, if possible. There are no approved specific antivirals for the treatment of parvovirus B19. Some cases of parvovirus B19 infection in pregnancy concurrent with hydrops fetalis have been treated successfully with intrauterine blood transfusions of the fetus.

INFECTION PREVENTION AND CONTROL MEASURES IN HEALTH CARE SETTINGS: In addition to standard precautions, droplet precautions are recommended for hospitalized children with aplastic crises, children with PPGSS or immunosuppressed patients with chronic infection and anemia for the duration of hospitalization. For patients with transient aplastic or erythrocyte crisis, these precautions should be maintained for 7 days or until the reticulocyte count has recovered from suppression to at least 2%. Neonates who had hydrops attributable to parvovirus B19 in utero do not require isolation if the hydrops is resolved at the time of birth. Pregnant health care workers should be informed of the potential risks to their fetus from parvovirus B19 infections and about preventive measures that may decrease these risks (eg, attention to strict infection control procedures).

CONTROL MEASURES:
- Pregnant people who are exposed to children at home or at work (eg, teachers or child care providers) are at increased risk of infection with parvovirus B19. However, in view of the high prevalence of parvovirus B19 infection, the low incidence of adverse effects on the fetus, and the fact that avoidance of child care or classroom teaching can decrease but not eliminate the risk of exposure, routine exclusion of pregnant people from the workplace where EI is occurring is not required. People capable of becoming pregnant who are concerned can undergo serologic testing for IgG antibody to parvovirus B19 to determine their susceptibility to infection.
- Pregnant people who discover that they have been in contact with children who were in the incubation period of EI or with children who were in aplastic crisis should have the relatively low potential risk of infection explained to them. The American College of Obstetricians and Gynecologists recommends that pregnant people exposed to parvovirus B19 should have serologic testing performed to determine susceptibility and possible evidence of acute parvovirus B19 infection.[1] Pregnant people with evidence of acute parvovirus B19 infection should be monitored closely (eg, serial ultrasonographic examinations) by their obstetric provider. In pregnant people with suspected or proven intrauterine parvovirus B19 infection, amniotic fluid and fetal tissues should be considered infectious, and contact precautions should be used in addition to standard precautions if exposure is likely.
- Children with EI may attend child care or school, because they no longer are contagious once the rash appears.
- Transmission of parvovirus B19 is decreased through use of routine infection control practices, including hand hygiene.

---

[1] American College of Obstetricians and Gynecologists. Cytomegalovirus, parvovirus B19, varicella zoster, and toxoplasmosis in pregnancy. Practice Bulletin No. 151. *Obstet Gynecol.* 2015;125(6):1510–1525

- Viral DNA may persist in blood and high levels may indicate the presence of infectious virus. The US Food and Drug Administration has issued guidance for use of nucleic acid amplification tests to reduce the possible risk of parvovirus B19 transmission by plasma-derived products (**www.fda.gov/ucm/groups/fdagov-public/@fdagov-bio-gen/documents/document/ucm078510.pdf**). The goal is to identify and prevent the use of plasma-derived products containing high levels of virus. Parvovirus B19 viral loads in manufacturing pools should not exceed 10^4 IU/mL.

Pasteurella Infections

CLINICAL MANIFESTATIONS: The most common manifestation is cellulitis at the site of a bite or scratch of a cat, dog, or other domestic or wild animal. Cellulitis typically develops within 12 to 24 hours of the injury and includes warmth, swelling, erythema, tenderness, and serosanguinous to purulent drainage at the wound site. Regional lymphadenopathy, chills, and fever can also occur. The most frequent local complications related to deep penetration of the teeth or claws of the biting animal are abscesses and tenosynovitis, but septic arthritis and osteomyelitis also occur. Other less common manifestations include septicemia, central nervous system infections (meningitis is the most common, although brain abscess and subdural empyema have been observed), ocular infections (eg, conjunctivitis, corneal ulcer, endophthalmitis), endocarditis, respiratory tract infections (eg, pneumonia, pulmonary abscesses, pleural empyema, epiglottitis), appendicitis, hepatic abscess, granulomatous hepatitis, peritonitis, ventriculoperitoneal shunt infection, and urinary tract infection. Infection in the neonate is rare but may present as early onset fulminant sepsis with or without meningitis from vertical transmission or later with sepsis and/or meningitis or focal infections after animal exposures (sometimes without known bites, scratches, or licks). People with liver disease, solid organ transplant, or underlying host defense abnormalities are predisposed to bacteremia with *Pasteurella multocida*. Those with chronic pulmonary or renal conditions may be predisposed to lung or kidney infections, respectively.

ETIOLOGY: The genus *Pasteurella* is one of 5 genera of human pathogens classified in the family *Pasteurellaceae;* the other genera are *Actinobacillus, Aggregatibacter, Haemophilus,* and *Mannheimia.* Members of the genus *Pasteurella* are nonmotile, facultatively anaerobic, mostly catalase and oxidase positive, nitrate reducing, gram-negative coccobacilli that are primarily respiratory tract colonizers and pathogens in animals. The most common human pathogen is *P multocida.* Most human infections are caused by the following species or subspecies: *P multocida* subspecies *multocida* (causing more than 50% of infections), followed by *Pasteurella canis, P multocida* subspecies *septica, Pasteurella stomatis,* and *Pasteurella dagmatis.*

EPIDEMIOLOGY: *Pasteurella* species have a worldwide distribution. They colonize the upper respiratory tract of 70% to 90% of cats, 25% to 50% of dogs, and many other wild and domestic animals including large cats, lions, tigers, panthers, swine, rats, opossums, rabbits, and fowl. Transmission most frequently occurs from the bite, scratch, or lick of a previous wound by a cat or dog. Infected cat bite wounds contain *Pasteurella* species more often than do dog bite wounds. Rarely, respiratory tract spread occurs from animals to humans, and in 5% to 15% of all cases, no animal exposure can be identified. The highest rates of infection occur in children younger than 5 years and in adults older than 55 years of age. Human-to-human transmission has been documented vertically, horizontally from colonized people, and through contaminated blood products.

The **incubation period** usually is less than 24 hours.

DIAGNOSTIC TESTS: The isolation of *Pasteurella* species from a normally sterile body site (eg, blood, joint fluid, bone, cerebrospinal fluid, pleural fluid, peritoneal fluid, or suppurative lymph nodes) establishes the diagnosis of systemic infection. Recovery of the organism from a superficial site, such as drainage from a skin lesion subsequent to an animal bite, must be interpreted in the context of other potential pathogens isolated, as mixed infection may occur. *Pasteurella* species are somewhat fastidious but may be cultured on several media generally used in clinical laboratories, including tryptic soybean digest agar with 5% sheep blood and chocolate agars, at 35°C to 37°C without increased carbon dioxide concentration. Although they resemble several other organisms morphologically, laboratory identification to the genus level generally is not difficult, although species and subspecies differentiation is more challenging. Newer laboratory methods, including polymerase chain reaction (PCR) amplification of the 16S rRNA gene followed by sequencing and identification of cellular components by matrix-assisted laser desorption/ionization–time-of-flight (MALDI-TOF) mass spectroscopy, have significantly improved species identification.

TREATMENT: The drug of choice is penicillin. Penicillin resistance is rare, but beta-lactamase–producing strains have been recovered. Other oral agents that usually are effective include ampicillin, amoxicillin, amoxicillin-clavulanate, cefuroxime axetil, cefixime, cefpodoxime, cefdinir, trimethoprim-sulfamethoxazole, azithromycin, doxycycline, and fluoroquinolones. Parenteral third-generation cephalosporins, including ceftriaxone and cefotaxime, demonstrate excellent in vitro activity. Oral and parenteral antistaphylococcal penicillins and first-generation cephalosporins including cephalexin are not as active and therefore not recommended for treatment. *Pasteurella* species usually are resistant to vancomycin, clindamycin, and erythromycin. For patients who are allergic to beta-lactam agents, trimethoprim-sulfamethoxazole, azithromycin, and the fluoroquinolones are alternative choices, but clinical experience with these agents is limited. For suspected polymicrobial infected bite wounds, oral amoxicillin-clavulanate or, for severe infection, intravenous ampicillin-sulbactam or piperacillin-tazobactam can be given. The duration of therapy usually is 7 to 10 days for local infections and 10 to 14 days for more severe infections. Duration of antimicrobial therapy for optimal outcomes for bone and joint infections is unknown but likely 3 to 6 weeks depending on clinical course. Endocarditis may require 4 to 6 weeks. Wound drainage or débridement may be necessary.

INFECTION PREVENTION AND CONTROL MEASURES IN HEALTH CARE SETTINGS: Standard precautions are recommended.

CONTROL MEASURES: Limiting contact with wild animals and education about appropriate contact with domestic animals can help to prevent *Pasteurella* infections (see Bite Wounds, p 202). Parents should not allow pets to lick infants and children on the face or on pre-existing skin injuries. Wounds from animal bites and scratches should be irrigated, cleansed, and débrided promptly. Following a bite wound, antimicrobial prophylaxis for selected children, depending on host factors and the type of animal bite wound, should be initiated according to the recommendations in Table 2.9, p 203, and the risk of rabies exposure and tetanus immunization status should be assessed.

Pediculosis Capitis[1]
(Head Lice)

CLINICAL MANIFESTATIONS: Itching is the most common symptom of head lice infestation, but many children are asymptomatic. Adult lice (2–3 mm long, tan to grayish-white, with claws on all 6 legs) or eggs (match hair color) and nits (empty egg casings, white) are found on the hair and are most readily apparent behind the ears and near the nape of the neck. Excoriations and crusting caused by secondary bacterial infection may occur and often are associated with regional lymphadenopathy. Head lice usually deposit their eggs on a hair shaft 1 to 2 mm from the scalp. Because hair grows at a rate of approximately 1 cm per month, duration of infestation can be estimated by the distance of the nit from the scalp.

ETIOLOGY: *Pediculus humanus capitis* is the head louse. Both nymphs and adult lice feed on human blood.

EPIDEMIOLOGY: Head lice infestation in the United States is most common in children attending child care, preschool, and elementary school. It is not a sign of poor hygiene, and all socioeconomic groups are affected. Head lice infestation is not influenced by hair length, hair texture, or frequency of shampooing or brushing. Head lice are not a health hazard and are not responsible for spread of any disease. Transmission occurs mainly by direct head-to-head contact with hair of infested people. Transmission by contact with personal belongings, such as combs, hair brushes, sporting gear, and hats, is uncommon. Head lice survive <1 day at room temperature away from the scalp, and their eggs cannot hatch at a lower ambient temperature than that near the scalp.

The **incubation period** from the laying of eggs to hatching of the first nymph usually is about 8 to 9 days (range 7 to 12 days). Lice mature to the adult stage approximately 7 days later.

DIAGNOSTIC TESTS: Identification of eggs, nymphs, and adult lice with the naked eye is possible; diagnosis can be confirmed by using a hand lens, dermatoscope (epiluminescence microscope), or traditional microscope. Nymphal and adult lice shun light and move rapidly to conceal themselves. Wetting the hair with water, oil, or a conditioner to "slow down" the movement of the lice and using a fine-tooth comb may improve ability to diagnose infestation and shorten inspection time. It is important to differentiate nits from dandruff, hair casts (a layer of follicular cells that slide easily off the hair shaft), plugs of desquamated cells, external hair debris, and fungal infections of the scalp. Finding nits attached firmly within ¼ inch of the base of the hair shaft suggests that a person has had infestation, but because nits remain affixed firmly to hair even after hatching or when dead, their mere presence (particularly >1 cm from the scalp) is not a conclusive sign of an active infestation.

TREATMENT: Treatment should be initiated only if there is a diagnosis of active head lice infestation. A number of effective pediculicidal agents are available to treat head lice infestation (see Drugs for Parasitic Infections, p 1068, and Table 3.44). Costs and recommended age ranges vary by product. Safety is a major concern with pediculicides, because head lice infestation, itself, presents minimal risk to the host. Instructions

[1] Nolt D, Moore S, Yan AC, Melnick L; American Academy of Pediatrics, Committee on Infectious Diseases, Committee on Practice and Ambulatory Medicine, Section on Dermatology. Head Lice. *Pediatrics*. 2022;150(4):e2022059282

Table 3.44. Pediculicides for the Treatment of Head Lice

Product	Brand Name	Recommended Age Range	Retreatment Interval (If Needed)	Availability
Permethrin 1% lotion	Multiple products	≥2 mo	9–10 days	Over the counter
Pyrethrins + piperonyl butoxide shampoo	Example: Rid	≥24 mo	9–10 days	Over the counter
Ivermectin 0.5% lotion	Sklice	≥6 mo	Single use	Over the counter
Malathion 0.5%	Ovide	≥6 y (safety not established for ages <6 y)	7–9 days if live lice are seen after initial dose	Prescription
Spinosad 0.9% suspension	Natroba	≥6 mo (safety not established for ages <4 y)	7 days if live lice are seen after initial dose	Prescription
Ivermectin (oral)	Stromectol	Any age, if weight ≥15 kg	7–10 days	Prescription

on proper use of any product should be explained carefully. Extra amounts should not be used, and multiple products should not be used concurrently. If medication gets into a child's eyes, it should be flushed out immediately with water. Skin exposure to pediculicide should be limited. Hair should be rinsed over a sink rather than during a shower or bath after topical pediculicide application, and warm rather than hot water should be used to minimize skin absorption attributable to vasodilation. Hair should not be shampooed as part of the rinse process nor for 24 to 48 hours after product is washed out.

Therapy can be initiated with over-the-counter 1% permethrin lotion or with pyrethrin combined with piperonyl butoxide, both of which have good safety profiles. Prevalence of clinical resistance to these products is highly variable from community to community and country to country. Information about these agents and others are listed below and in Table 3.44 and in Drugs for Parasitic Infections (p 1068). Drugs vary in their residual activity and no treatment is 100% ovicidal. Retreatment may be needed after eggs present at the time of initial treatment have hatched but before new eggs are produced; retreatment intervals vary by product.

- **Permethrin (1%) lotion.** Permethrin is available without a prescription in a 1% lotion and is approved for infants 2 months or older. Infested hair and scalp are washed first with a nonconditioning shampoo and towel-dried. Permethrin then is applied to the scalp and entire length of wet hair, left for 10 minutes, and then rinsed off with water. Permethrin has a low potential for toxic effects and can be highly effective. Although residual permethrin is designed to kill emerging nymphs, many experts advise a second treatment 9 to 10 days after the first treatment if live lice are seen in the interim. An alternate treatment schedule on days 0, 7, and 13-15 has been proposed based on the longest possible life cycle of head lice.

- **Pyrethrin-based shampoo products.** Pyrethrins formulated with piperonyl butoxide are available without a prescription as shampoos or mousse preparations for children 24 months or older. The product is applied to dry hair in sufficient amounts to saturate the scalp and entire length of the hair, left for 10 minutes, and then rinsed off with water. Repeat application 9 to 10 days after the first application is necessary to kill newly hatched lice.

- **Ivermectin (0.5%) lotion.** Ivermectin, a widely used anthelmintic agent, appears to prevent newly hatched lice (nymphs) from surviving. The lotion is applied to dry hair in sufficient amounts to saturate the scalp and entire length of the hair, left for 10 minutes, and then rinsed off with water. It is effective in most patients when given as a single application on dry hair and may be used in children 6 months and older.

- **Oral ivermectin.** Oral ivermectin is not approved by the US Food and Drug Administration (FDA) for treatment of head lice in pediatrics but is FDA approved for treatment of head lice in adults and has pediatric indications for other parasitic infections. It has been administered as a single oral dose of 200 µg/kg or 400 µg/kg, with a second dose given after 7 to 10 days. The 400-µg/kg dose has been shown to be comparable or more effective than 0.5% malathion lotion. Ivermectin should not be used for this indication in children weighing less than 15 kg, because it blocks essential neural transmission if it crosses the blood-brain barrier and young children may be at higher risk of this adverse drug reaction.
  - ◆ Oral and topical forms of ivermectin for veterinary use are available without a prescription. The dose of active ingredients, presence of inactive ingredients, and different production standards render these products inappropriate for treatment of head lice in humans.

- **Malathion (0.5%) lotion.** This organophosphate pesticide is available only by prescription as a lotion. Malathion lotion is applied to dry hair in sufficient amounts to saturate the scalp and entire length of the hair, left to dry naturally, and then washed off after 8 to 12 hours by washing and rinsing the hair. The product should be reapplied 7 to 9 days later if live lice are seen in the interim. The high alcohol content of the lotion makes it highly flammable; during treatment the lotion or lotion-coated hair should not be exposed to lighted cigarettes (no smoking around the individual during hair treatment), open flames, or electric heat sources such as hair dryers or curling irons. Malathion should not be used in children younger than 6 years, because safety and effectiveness have not been assessed by the FDA for those children.

- **Spinosad (0.9%) suspension.** Spinosad has a broad spectrum of activity against insects, including lice. The suspension is applied to dry hair in sufficient amounts to saturate the scalp and entire length of the hair, left for 10 minutes, and then rinsed off with water. A second treatment is applied 7 days later if live lice are seen in the interim. This product contains benzyl alcohol and should not be used in infants younger than 6 months, because systemic absorption may lead to benzyl alcohol toxicity.

- **Abametapir (0.74%) lotion** (not available in the United States). Abametapir inhibits metalloproteinases, which have a role in physiological processes critical to egg development and survival of lice. Abametapir lotion is applied to dry hair in sufficient amounts to coat the hair and scalp thoroughly, left on for 10 minutes, and then rinsed off. Treatment involves a single application. This product contains benzyl alcohol and should not be used in infants younger than 6 months, because systemic absorption may lead to benzyl alcohol toxicity. For 2 weeks after abametapir application, the treated individual should avoid taking drugs that are substrates of CYP3A4, CYP2B6, or CYP1A2.

- Lindane (marketed as Kwell), although FDA approved for treatment of head lice, no longer is recommended by the American Academy of Pediatrics because of toxicity.

Detection of living lice on scalp inspection 24 hours or more after treatment suggests incorrect use of pediculicide, hatching of lice after treatment, reinfestation, or resistance to therapy, because pediculicides kill lice shortly after application. After excluding incorrect use, retreatment with a different pediculicide followed by a second application (with the exception of single-use topical ivermectin) at the intervals specified above and in Drugs for Parasitic Infections (p 1068) is recommended in such situations. See Fig 3.14 for a treatment algorithm.

Data are lacking to determine whether heat therapy or suffocation of lice by application of occlusive agents, such as petroleum jelly, olive oil, butter, fat-containing mayonnaise, or desiccating methods are effective methods of treatment. Vinegar-based products claim to loosen the "glue" that attaches the nits to the hair, although clinical benefit has not been demonstrated.

Itching or mild burning of the scalp caused by inflammation of the skin in response to topical therapeutic agents can persist for many days after lice are killed; this is not a reason for retreatment. Topical corticosteroid and oral antihistamine agents may be beneficial for relieving these signs and symptoms.

Manual removal of nits after successful treatment with a pediculicide is helpful to decrease diagnostic confusion and to decrease the small risk of self-reinfestation and social stigmatization. Fine-toothed nit combs designed for this purpose are available, although the type of comb is less important than the actual action of combing.

INFECTION PREVENTION AND CONTROL MEASURES IN HEALTH CARE SETTINGS: Standard precautions plus contact precautions are recommended until the patient has been treated with an appropriate pediculicide.

CONTROL MEASURES: Household and other close contacts should be examined and treated if infested. Bedmates of infested people should be treated prophylactically at the same time as the infested household members and contacts, even if bedmates do not have identifiable live lice. Children should not be excluded or sent home early from school or child care because of head lice, because head lice have a low contagion in these settings (see Table 2.3, p 149). Parents of children with infestation (ie, at least 1 live, crawling louse) should be notified and informed that their child should be treated. The presence of nits alone does not justify treatment.

"No-nit" policies requiring that children be free of nits before they return to a child care facility or school should be discouraged. Nits farther from the scalp are easier to discover but are of no consequence. Routine classroom or schoolwide screening for lice is discouraged, because it is not an accurate or cost-effective way of lowering the incidence of head lice in the school setting. Parents who are educated on the diagnosis of lice infestation may screen their own children's heads for lice regularly (perhaps monthly) and if the child is symptomatic.

FIG 3.14. TREATMENT ALGORITHM FOR HEAD LICE[a,b]

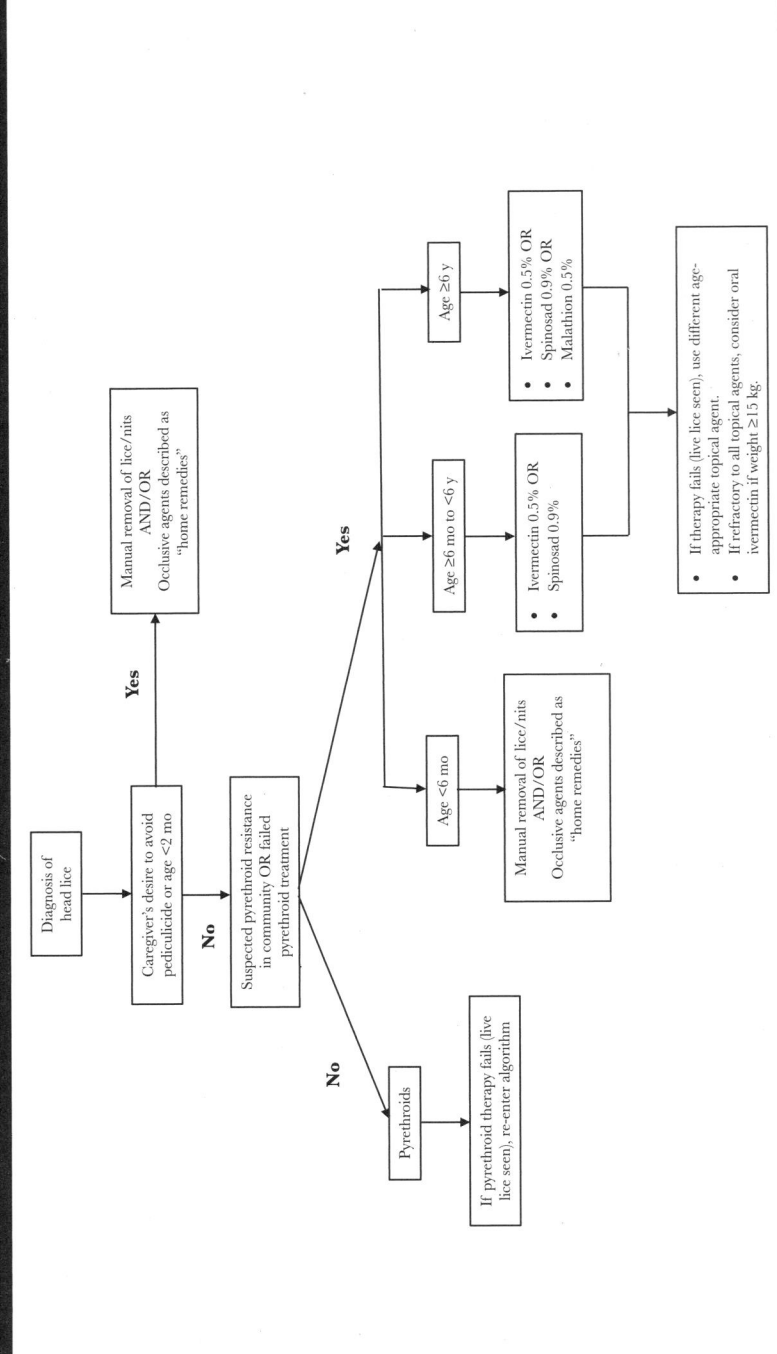

[a]Cost and insurance formulary coverage for individual patients should be considered by the prescriber.

[b]Modified from Nolt D, Moore S, Yan AC, Melnick L; American Academy of Pediatrics, Committee on Infectious Diseases, Committee on Practice and Ambulatory Medicine, Section on Dermatology. Head Lice. *Pediatrics.* 2022;150(4):e2022059282

Supplemental measures generally are not required to eliminate an infestation. Head lice rarely are transferred via fomites from shared headgear, clothing, combs, or bedding. Special handling of such items, therefore, is not likely to be useful; protective headgear should not be refused because of fear of head lice. If desired, hats, bedding, clothing, and towels worn or used by the infested person in the 2-day period just before treatment is started can be machine-washed and dried using the hot water and hot air cycles, respectively, because lice and eggs are killed by exposure for 5 minutes to temperatures greater than 130°F. Clothing and items that are not washable can be dry cleaned or sealed in a plastic bag and stored for 2 weeks. Brushes and combs can be soaked in hot water (at least 130°F) for 5 to 10 minutes. Vacuuming furniture and floors can remove an infested person's hairs that might have viable eggs attached. Pediculicide spray is not necessary and should not be used. Treatment of dogs, cats, or other pets is not indicated, because they do not play a role in transmission of human head lice.

Pediculosis Corporis
(Body Lice)

CLINICAL MANIFESTATIONS: Patients affected with pediculosis corporis characteristically seek medical attention because of intense itching, particularly at night. The pruritus is an allergic reaction to bites, which manifest as small erythematous macules, papules, and excoriations, primarily on the trunk. In heavily bitten areas of the body, typically around the mid-section (waist, groin, upper thighs), the skin can become thickened and darkened. Secondary bacterial infection of the skin (pyoderma) caused by scratching is common.

ETIOLOGY: *Pediculus humanus corporis* (or *humanus*) is the body louse. Both nymphs and adult lice feed on human blood.

EPIDEMIOLOGY: Body lice live in clothes or bedding used by infested people, lay their eggs on or near the seams of clothing, and only move to the skin to feed before retreating. Body lice cannot survive away from a blood source for longer than 5 to 7 days at room temperature. Body lice generally are restricted to people living in crowded conditions without access to regular bathing (at least weekly) or changes of clean clothing (refugees, victims of war or natural disasters, people lacking housing). Under these conditions, body lice can spread rapidly through direct contact with others or indirect contact with contaminated clothing or bedding. In contrast with head and pubic lice, body lice are well-recognized vectors of disease (eg, epidemic typhus, trench fever, epidemic relapsing fever, and bacillary angiomatosis).

The **incubation period** from laying eggs to hatching of the first nymph is approximately 1 to 2 weeks, depending on ambient temperature. Lice mature and can reproduce 9 to 19 days after hatching.

DIAGNOSTIC TESTS: Seams of clothing should be examined for eggs (nits), nymphs, and adult lice (2–4 mm) if body louse infestation is suspected. Nits and lice may be seen with the naked eye; diagnosis can be confirmed by using a hand lens, dermatoscope (epiluminescence microscope), or traditional microscope. Adult and nymphal body lice seldom are seen on the body because they generally are sequestered in clothing.

TREATMENT: Treatment consists of improving hygiene, including bathing and regular (at least weekly) changes to clean clothes and bedding. Infested materials can be discarded or decontaminated by machine-washing and drying using the hot water and hot air cycles, respectively; by dry cleaning; by sealing in a plastic bag and storing for 2 weeks; or by pressing with a hot iron. Temperatures exceeding 130°F for 5 minutes are lethal to lice and eggs. Pediculicides for patients usually are not necessary if materials are laundered at sufficiently hot temperatures at least weekly. People with abundant body hair may require full-body treatment with a pediculicide, because lice and eggs occasionally may adhere to body hair. Guidance for the choice and application of pediculicide (if desired for treatment) is the same as for head lice (see Pediculosis Capitis, p 644; and Drugs for Parasitic Infections, p 1068).

INFECTION PREVENTION AND CONTROL MEASURES IN HEALTH CARE SETTINGS: In addition to standard precautions, contact precautions are recommended and should continue until the patient's clothing and bedding have been cleaned effectively.

CONTROL MEASURES: The most important factor in the control of body lice infestation is the ability to change and wash clothing. Close contacts should be examined and treated appropriately. Clothing, beds, bedding, and towels from infested persons should not be shared until articles are treated. Fumigation or dusting with chemical insecticides sometimes is necessary to control and prevent certain diseases (epidemic typhus) that are spread by body lice.

Pediculosis Pubis
(Pubic Lice, Crab Lice)

CLINICAL MANIFESTATIONS: Pruritus of the anogenital area is a common symptom in pubic lice infestations ("crabs" or "phthiriasis"). Adult lice (1–2 mm long and flattened, tan to grayish-white with 4 of its 6 legs terminating in crab-like claws) or eggs (match hair color) and nits (empty egg casings, white) are found on hair, particularly near the hair-skin junction. The parasite most frequently is found in the pubic region, but infestation can involve other coarse body hair, including the eyelashes, eyebrows, beard, axilla, legs, perianal area, and rarely, the scalp. A characteristic sign of heavy pubic lice infestation is the presence of bluish or slate-colored macules (maculae ceruleae) on the chest, abdomen, or thighs.

ETIOLOGY: *Pthirus pubis* is the pubic or crab louse. Both nymphs and adult lice feed on human blood. Pubic lice are not a health hazard and are not responsible for the spread of any disease.

EPIDEMIOLOGY: Pubic lice infestations are more prevalent in teenagers and young adults and usually are spread through sexual contact. Transmission by contact with contaminated items, such as bed linens, towels, or shared clothing, can occur. Pubic lice on the eyelashes or eyebrows of prepubertal children (likely the only areas of coarse hair) may be evidence of sexual abuse, although rarely it may instead be a manifestation of shared sleeping arrangements with infested individuals or fomites. Animals do not get or spread pubic lice.

The **incubation period** from the laying of eggs to the hatching of the first nymph is 6 to 10 days. Adult lice become capable of reproducing 2 to 3 weeks after hatching. Adult pubic lice can survive away from a host for up to 48 hours, and their eggs can remain viable for up to 10 days under suitable environmental conditions.

DIAGNOSTIC TESTS: Identification of eggs (nits), nymphs, and lice with the naked eye is possible, although it can be difficult to detect lice unless they have had a recent blood meal. The diagnosis can be confirmed by using a hand lens, traditional microscope, or dermatoscope (epiluminescence microscope) to examine hair shafts. Pubic lice may be difficult to find because of low numbers, and they do not crawl as quickly as head and body lice. If crawling lice are not seen, finding nits in the pubic area strongly suggests infestation and should lead to treatment.

TREATMENT[1]: All areas of the body with coarse hair should be examined for evidence of pubic lice infestation. Lice and their eggs can be removed manually (hand-picking or wet-combing with a lice comb), or the hairs can be shaved to eliminate infestation immediately; topical pediculicides should still be used even when the affected area is shaved. Caution should be used when inspecting, removing, or treating lice on or near the eyelashes. No high-quality data exist for treatment of pubic lice, and thus treatment is extrapolated from head lice. Recommended therapies include either permethrin 1% cream rinse (applied to affected areas and washed off after 10 minutes) or pyrethrins with piperonyl butoxide (applied to the affected areas and washed off after 10 minutes). Both treatments should be repeated in 9 to 10 days. Reported clinical resistance of head lice to permethrin and pyrethrins has been increasing and may be extrapolated to pubic lice, although data are lacking. Reevaluation is recommended after 1 week if symptoms persist. Retreatment might be necessary if lice are found or if eggs are observed at the hair-skin junction. If no clinical response is achieved to one of the recommended regimens, treatment with malathion (0.5% lotion applied to affected areas and washed off after 8–12 hours) or oral ivermectin (250 µg/kg orally, repeated in 7–14 days) is recommended.

Infested people should be examined for other sexually transmitted infections (see Sexually Transmitted Infections in Adolescents and Children, p 179). Pubic lice on the eyelashes or eyebrows of prepubertal children should prompt evaluation for sexual abuse (see Sexual Assault and Abuse in Children and Adolescents/Young Adults, p 182).

INFECTION PREVENTION AND CONTROL MEASURES IN HEALTH CARE SETTINGS: In addition to standard precautions, contact precautions are recommended until the patient has been treated with an appropriate pediculicide.

CONTROL MEASURES: Pubic lice are highly contagious; thus, all sexual contacts within the previous month should be treated. Patients should be advised to avoid sexual contact until they and their sex partners have been treated successfully, bedding and clothing have been decontaminated, and reevaluation has been performed to rule out persistent infestation if persons are still symptomatic. Bedding, towels, and clothing used in the preceding 3 days should be decontaminated by machine washing and drying using the hot water and hot air cycles, respectively, because lice and eggs are killed by exposure for 5 minutes at temperatures greater than 130°F. Clothing and items that are not washable can be dry cleaned or sealed in a plastic bag and stored for 2 weeks.

---

[1] Centers for Disease Control and Prevention. Sexually transmitted infections treatment guidelines, 2021. *MMWR Recomm Rep.* 2021;70(RR-4):1-187. Available at: **www.cdc.gov/std/treatment-guidelines/**

Pelvic Inflammatory Disease

CLINICAL MANIFESTATIONS: Pelvic inflammatory disease (PID) comprises a spectrum of inflammatory disorders of the female upper genital tract, including any combination of endometritis, parametritis, salpingitis, oophoritis, tubo-ovarian abscess, and pelvic peritonitis.[1] Acute PID is difficult to diagnose because of the wide variation in symptoms and signs. Symptoms of acute PID include unilateral or bilateral lower abdominal or pelvic pain, fever, vomiting, abnormal vaginal discharge, irregular vaginal bleeding, and pain with intercourse. The severity of symptoms varies widely and may range from indolent to severe. Patients occasionally present with right upper quadrant abdominal pain resulting from peritoneal adhesions related to perihepatitis (Fitz-Hugh-Curtis syndrome). Many episodes of PID go undiagnosed and untreated because the patient and/or health care professional fails to recognize the implications of mild or nonspecific symptoms and signs. Subclinical PID is defined as inflammation of the upper reproductive tract in the absence of signs and symptoms of acute PID, and there is a growing body of evidence that this represents a large proportion of all PID cases. In both clinically apparent and subclinical PID, inflammation occurs within the reproductive tract, which scars or damages the fallopian tubes or surrounding structures. Clinicians should maintain a high degree of suspicion for PID when female patients of reproductive age present with mild or nonspecific findings.

Examination findings vary but may include oral temperature >101°F (>38.3°C), lower abdominal tenderness with or without peritoneal signs, abnormal cervical or vaginal discharge, tenderness with lateral motion of the cervix, cervical friability, uterine tenderness, unilateral or bilateral adnexal tenderness, and adnexal fullness. Pyuria (presence of white blood cells [WBCs] on urine microscopy), abundant WBCs on saline microscopy of vaginal fluid, an elevated erythrocyte sedimentation rate, elevated C-reactive protein, and/or an adnexal mass demonstrated by abdominal or transvaginal ultrasonography are findings that support a diagnosis of PID.

Complications of PID include perihepatitis (Fitz-Hugh-Curtis syndrome) and tubo-ovarian abscess/complex formation. Long-term sequelae include tubal scarring that can cause infertility in an estimated 10% to 20% of affected individuals, ectopic pregnancy in an estimated 9%, and chronic pelvic pain in an estimated 18%. Factors that may increase the likelihood of infertility are delay in diagnosis or in initiation of antimicrobial therapy, younger age at time of infection, chlamydial infection, recurrent PID, and PID determined to be severe by laparoscopic examination.

Any prepubertal child with PID needs to be assessed for sexual abuse (see Sexual Assault and Abuse in Children and Adolescents/Young Adults, p 182). Mandatory reporters should follow their state's regulations for reporting.

ETIOLOGY: *Neisseria gonorrhoeae* and *Chlamydia trachomatis* are the pathogens most commonly associated with PID, although only approximately half of PID cases have evidence of these bacterial pathogens. A number of organisms other than *N gonorrhoeae* and *C trachomatis* that are present in the vaginal flora have been isolated from upper genital tract cultures of people with PID, including anaerobes (such as *Prevotella* species), *Gardnerella vaginalis*, *Haemophilus influenzae*, *Streptococcus agalactiae*, and enteric gram-negative rods. Additionally, cytomegalovirus, *Mycoplasma hominis*, and *Ureaplasma*

---

[1] The terms female, woman/women, and male refer to sex assigned at birth.

urealyticum might be associated with some instances of PID. Therefore, PID is managed as a polymicrobial infection. In more than half of cases, however, no organism is identified from routine lower genital tract swab specimens (ie, endocervical or vaginal swab specimens). *Mycoplasma genitalium* also has been implicated in the etiology of PID in some studies, although the natural history of *M genitalium* in females remains unclear. PID may also be secondary to other causes of peritonitis, such as ruptured appendicitis.

EPIDEMIOLOGY: Although many of the issues pertaining to high-risk sexual behavior and acquisition of sexually transmitted infections (STIs) are common to both adolescents and adults, they often are intensified among adolescents because of both behavioral and biological predispositions. Female adolescents and young adults can be at higher risk of STIs and PID because of behavioral factors such as inconsistent barrier contraceptive use, douching, greater number of concurrent sex partners, and use of alcohol and other substances that may impair judgment while engaging in sexual activity. Use of condoms may reduce the risk of PID. Female adolescents and young adults also have an increased biologic susceptibility to STIs. Cervical ectopy increases risk of chlamydia and gonorrhea infection by exposing columnar epithelium to a potential infectious inoculum.

An **incubation period** for PID is undefined.

DIAGNOSTIC TESTS[1]: Centers for Disease Control and Prevention (CDC) criteria for clinical diagnosis and presumptive treatment of PID are presented in Table 3.45. Many individuals with PID have subtle or nonspecific symptoms or are asymptomatic, and a diagnosis of PID usually is based on imprecise clinical findings. A clinical diagnosis of symptomatic PID has a positive predictive value for salpingitis of 65% to 90% compared with laparoscopy. No single historical, physical, or laboratory finding is both sensitive and specific for the diagnosis of acute PID. Because of the difficulty of diagnosis and the potential for damage to reproductive health, providers should maintain a low threshold for the clinical diagnosis of PID.

A cervical or vaginal swab specimen should be obtained from individuals with suspected PID to perform a nucleic acid amplification test (NAAT) for *C trachomatis* and *N gonorrhoeae*. A swab specimen for culture of *N gonorrhoeae* may be collected from the cervix or vagina to allow susceptibility testing to be performed. The most specific criteria for diagnosing PID include endometrial biopsy with histopathologic evidence of endometritis; transvaginal ultrasonography or magnetic resonance imaging techniques showing thickened, fluid-filled tubes with or without free pelvic fluid or tubo-ovarian complex or Doppler ultrasonography suggesting pelvic infection (eg, tubal hyperemia); or laparoscopic findings consistent with PID. A diagnostic evaluation that includes some of these more extensive procedures might be warranted in some cases. Endometrial biopsy is warranted in patients undergoing laparoscopy who do not have visual evidence of salpingitis, because endometritis may be the only sign of PID.

In addition to determining whether WBCs are present in cervicovaginal secretions, a wet mount or NAAT of vaginal fluid will assist in the identification of trichomoniasis or bacterial vaginosis. Serologic testing for HIV and syphilis also should be performed.

---

[1] Centers for Disease Control and Prevention. Sexually transmitted infections treatment guidelines, 2021. *MMWR Recomm Rep.* 2021;70(RR-4):1-187. Available at: **www.cdc.gov/std/treatment-guidelines/pid.htm**

Table 3.45. Criteria for Clinical Diagnosis and Presumptive Treatment of Pelvic Inflammatory Disease (PID)[a]

Minimum Criteria

Presumptive treatment for PID should be initiated in sexually active female adolescents and young adults at risk for STIs if they are experiencing pelvic or lower abdominal pain, if no cause for the illness other than PID can be identified, or if one or more of the following **minimum clinical criteria** are present on pelvic examination:

- Cervical motion tenderness

or

- Uterine tenderness

or

- Adnexal tenderness

One or more of the following **additional criteria** can be used to enhance the specificity of the minimum clinical criteria and support a diagnosis of PID:

- Oral temperature >101°F (>38.3°C);
- Abnormal cervical mucopurulent discharge or cervical friability;
- Presence of abundant numbers of WBC on saline microscopy of vaginal fluid;
- Elevated erythrocyte sedimentation rate;
- Elevated C-reactive protein; and
- Laboratory documentation of cervical infection with *Neisseria gonorrhoeae* or *Chlamydia trachomatis*.

Most people with PID have either mucopurulent cervical discharge or evidence of WBCs on a microscopic evaluation of a saline preparation of vaginal fluid (ie, wet prep). If the cervical discharge appears normal and no WBCs are observed on the wet prep of vaginal fluid, the diagnosis of PID is unlikely, and alternative causes of pain should be considered. A wet prep of vaginal fluid also can detect the presence of concomitant infections (eg, bacterial vaginosis and trichomoniasis).

[a] Adapted from Centers for Disease Control and Prevention. Sexually transmitted infections treatment guidelines, 2021. *MMWR Recomm Rep*. 2021;70(RR-4):1-187. Available at: **www.cdc.gov/std/treatment-guidelines/pid.htm.**

The possibility of coexisting early pregnancy must always be assessed in patients who are being evaluated for PID.

TREATMENT[1]: A sexually active female adolescent or young adult with lower abdominal pain who exhibits uterine, adnexal, or cervical motion tenderness on bimanual examination should be treated for PID if no other cause is identified. To minimize risks of progressive infection and subsequent infertility, treatment should be initiated at the time of clinical diagnosis, and therapy should be completed, regardless of the STI test results.

Among patients with mild to moderate PID, there is no difference in clinical course, recurrent PID, chronic pelvic pain, or infertility rates between those hospitalized and those treated on an outpatient basis for PID. The decision to hospitalize adolescent or young adult patients with acute PID should be based on

[1] Centers for Disease Control and Prevention. Sexually transmitted infections treatment guidelines, 2021. *MMWR Recomm Rep*. 2021;70(RR-4):1-187. Available at: **www.cdc.gov/std/treatment-guidelines/pid.htm**

the provider's judgment and whether any of the following suggested criteria are relevant:

- Surgical emergencies (eg, appendicitis) cannot be excluded;
- The patient has tubo-ovarian abscess;
- The patient is pregnant;
- The patient has severe illness, nausea and vomiting, or high fever;
- The patient is unable to follow or tolerate an outpatient oral regimen; or
- There is no clinical response to oral antimicrobial therapy.

Whether treated on an inpatient or outpatient basis, the antimicrobial regimen chosen should provide empiric, broad-spectrum coverage directed against the most common causative agents, including *N gonorrhoeae* and *C trachomatis*, and anaerobic organisms, even if these pathogens are not identified in lower genital tract specimens. If a *N gonorrhoeae* culture is positive, antimicrobial susceptibility testing should guide subsequent therapy. Addition of metronidazole to the PID regimen can effectively eradicate anaerobic organisms from the upper genital tract.

Table 4.4 (p 1007) lists the parenteral regimens recommended by the CDC for treatment of hospitalized patients and the intramuscular/oral regimens recommended for the treatment of patients in the outpatient setting. For management of females hospitalized and managed initially with the parenteral therapy options listed in Table 4.4, clinical experience should guide decisions regarding transition to oral therapy, which usually can be initiated within 24 to 48 hours of clinical improvement. In patients with tubo-ovarian abscesses, at least 24 hours of inpatient observation is recommended. Because of the pain associated with intravenous (IV) infusion, doxycycline should be administered orally when possible. Oral and IV administration of doxycycline and metronidazole provide similar bioavailability. Intramuscular/oral therapy (Table 4.4, p 1007) can be considered for individuals with mild-to-moderately severe acute PID who can be managed in the outpatient setting from the outset, because the clinical outcomes among patients treated with these regimens are similar to those treated with intravenous therapy. Patients who do not respond to intramuscular/oral therapy within 72 hours should be reevaluated to confirm the diagnosis and be administered intravenous therapy. Patients should demonstrate clinical improvement (eg, defervescence; reduction in direct or rebound abdominal tenderness; and reduction in uterine, adnexal, cervical motion tenderness) within 3 days after initiation of therapy. If no clinical improvement has occurred within 72 hours after outpatient intramuscular/oral therapy, hospitalization, assessment of the antimicrobial regimen, and additional diagnostics (including consideration of diagnostic laparoscopy for alternative diagnoses) are recommended.

If a person with an intrauterine device (IUD) receives a diagnosis of PID, the IUD does not need to be removed. However, the patient should have close clinical follow-up, and if there is no clinical improvement 48 to 72 hours after treatment initiation, removal of the IUD may be considered.

Pregnancy. Pregnant people with suspected PID are at high risk for morbidity and pre-term delivery. These patients should be hospitalized and treated with IV antimicrobials in consultation with an infectious disease specialist.

INFECTION PREVENTION AND CONTROL MEASURES IN HEALTH CARE SETTINGS: Standard precautions are recommended.

CONTROL MEASURES:
- All individuals who have received a diagnosis of chlamydial or gonococcal PID should be retested 3 months after treatment, regardless of whether their sex partners were treated. If retesting at 3 months is not possible, retest whenever the patient next presents for medical care in the 12 months following treatment.
- Male sexual partners of a person with PID during the 60 days preceding the onset of symptoms should be evaluated, tested, and presumptively treated for chlamydia and gonorrhea, regardless of the etiology of PID or pathogens isolated from the patient with PID. If the last sexual intercourse was >60 days before onset of symptoms or diagnosis, the most recent sex partner should be treated.
- To minimize disease transmission, patients should be instructed to abstain from sexual intercourse until therapy is completed, symptoms have resolved, and sex partners have been adequately treated.
- The patient and sexual partner(s) should be encouraged to use condoms consistently and correctly.
- The patient should be screened for other STIs, including human immunodeficiency virus, gonorrhea, chlamydia, and syphilis.
- Unimmunized or incompletely immunized patients should complete the immunization series for human papillomavirus and hepatitis B (**https://redbook. solutions.aap.org/SS/Immunization_Schedules.aspx**).
- The diagnosis of PID provides an opportunity to educate the adolescent about STI prevention, including abstinence, consistent use of barrier methods of protection, immunization, and the importance of receiving periodic STI screening.

Pertussis (Whooping Cough)

CLINICAL MANIFESTATIONS: Pertussis begins with mild upper respiratory tract symptoms similar to the common cold (catarrhal stage) and progresses to cough, usually paroxysms of cough (paroxysmal stage), characterized by inspiratory whoop (gasping) after repeated cough on the same breath, which commonly is followed by post-tussive emesis. Fever is absent or minimal. Symptoms wane gradually over weeks to months (convalescent stage). Cough illness in immunized children and adults can range from typical to very mild. The duration of classic pertussis is 6 to 10 weeks. Complications among adolescents and adults include syncope, weight loss, sleep disturbance, incontinence, rib fractures, and pneumonia; among adults, complications may increase with age. Pertussis is most severe when it occurs during the first 6 months of life, particularly in preterm and unimmunized infants. Disease in infants younger than 6 months can be atypical with a short catarrhal stage, followed by gagging, gasping, bradycardia, or apnea as prominent early manifestations; absence of whoop; and prolonged convalescence. Complications among infants include pneumonia, pulmonary hypertension, and severe coughing spells with associated conjunctival hemorrhage, hernia, and hypoxia. Seizures (0.9%), encephalopathy (less than 0.5%), apnea, acute respiratory distress syndrome, and death can occur in infants with pertussis. Approximately a third of infants with pertussis in the United States are hospitalized. Case fatality rates are approximately 1.1% in infants younger than 2 months and 0.1 in infants 2 through 11 months of age. Immunization with tetanus and diphtheria toxoids and acellular pertussis vaccine (Tdap) during each pregnancy and an infant's receipt of at least some doses of pertussis vaccine reduce morbidity and mortality in young infants.

ETIOLOGY: Pertussis is caused by a fastidious, gram-negative, pleomorphic bacillus, *Bordetella pertussis.* Other *Bordetella* species can cause sporadic prolonged cough illness in people, including *Bordetella parapertussis, Bordetella bronchiseptica* (the cause of canine kennel cough), and *Bordetella holmesii.*

EPIDEMIOLOGY: Humans are the only known hosts of *B pertussis.* Transmission occurs by close contact with infected individuals via large respiratory droplets generated by coughing or sneezing. Cases occur year-round, typically with a late summer-autumn peak. Neither infection nor immunization provides lifelong immunity. Waning immunity is predominantly responsible for increased cases reported in school-aged children, adolescents, and adults. Additionally, waning immunity in pregnant people who have not received Tdap vaccine during that pregnancy results in low concentrations of transplacentally transmitted antibody and an increased risk of pertussis in very young infants. Reported incidence is cyclic and had been increasing since the early 1990s until the start of the COVID-19 pandemic in 2020. Pertussis is highly contagious. As many as 80% of susceptible household contacts of symptomatic infant cases are infected with *B pertussis,* with symptoms in these contacts varying from mild to classic pertussis. Siblings and adults with cough illness are important sources of pertussis infection for young infants. Infected people are most contagious during the catarrhal stage through the third week after onset of paroxysms or until 5 days after the start of effective antimicrobial treatment. Factors affecting the length of communicability include age, immunization status or previous infection, and receipt of appropriate antimicrobial therapy.

The **incubation period** is 7 to 10 days, with a range of 5 to 21 days.

DIAGNOSTIC TESTS: Culture previously was considered the "gold standard" for laboratory diagnosis of pertussis but is not optimally sensitive and has largely been replaced by nucleic acid amplification tests (NAATs). Culture requires collection of an appropriate nasopharyngeal swab specimen, obtained either by aspiration or with polyester or flocked rayon swabs. Specimens must not be allowed to dry during prompt transport to the laboratory. Culture results can be negative if obtained from a previously immunized person, if antimicrobial therapy has been started, if more than 2 weeks has elapsed since cough onset, or if the specimen is not collected or handled appropriately. Testing nasopharyngeal swab specimens by rolling on slides and staining with direct fluorescent antibodies (DFA) is not recommended because of nonspecific cross-reactions.

NAATs cleared by the US Food and Drug Administration (FDA), including polymerase chain reaction (PCR) assays, are commercially available as standalone tests or as multiplex assays and are the most commonly used laboratory method for detection of *B pertussis* because of greater sensitivity and more rapid turnaround time. The PCR test requires collection of an adequate nasopharyngeal specimen using a polyester or flocked swab or nasopharyngeal wash or aspirate. Calcium alginate swabs can be inhibitory to PCR and should not be used. The PCR test has optimal sensitivity during the first 3 weeks of cough and is unlikely to be useful if a patient has been receiving antimicrobial therapy for more than 5 days. The Centers for Disease Control and Prevention (CDC) has released a "best practices" document to guide pertussis PCR assays (**www.cdc.gov/pertussis/clinical/diagnostic-testing/diagnosis-pcr-bestpractices.html**) as well as a video demonstrating optimal specimen collection.

Most PCR assays target a multicopy insertion gene sequence (IS481) found in *B pertussis* as well as the less commonly encountered *B holmesii* and some strains of *B bronchiseptica*. Several multiplex PCR assays test for both *B pertussis* and *B parapertussis* utilizing differing DNA targets for each pathogen. Multiple DNA target sequences are required to distinguish among clinically relevant *Bordetella* species.

Serologic tests for pertussis infection may be helpful for diagnosis, especially late in illness, but are not commonly used. The CDC and FDA have developed a pertussis serologic test that has been used by state public health laboratories during outbreaks; however, no commercial kit is cleared by the FDA for diagnostic use. In the absence of recent immunization, an elevated serum immunoglobulin (Ig) G antibody to pertussis toxin (PT) present 2 to 8 weeks after onset of cough is suggestive of recent *B pertussis* infection. For single serum specimens, an IgG anti-PT value of approximately 100 IU/mL or greater (using an assay calibrated to standard reference sera) has been recommended. IgA and IgM assays lack adequate sensitivity and specificity and should not be used for the diagnosis of pertussis.

An increased white blood cell count attributable to absolute lymphocytosis is suggestive of pertussis in infants and young children but often is absent in older people with pertussis and may be only mildly abnormal in some infants. A markedly elevated white blood cell count is associated with a poor prognosis in young infants.

TREATMENT: Antimicrobial therapy administered during the catarrhal stage may ameliorate the disease. Antimicrobial therapy is indicated before test results are received if the clinical history is strongly suggestive of pertussis or the patient is at high risk of severe or complicated disease (eg, an infant). A 5-day course of azithromycin is the appropriate first-line choice for treatment and for postexposure prophylaxis (PEP [see Table 3.46]). After the paroxysmal cough is established, antimicrobial agents have no discernible effect on the course of illness but are recommended to limit spread of organisms to others. Resistance of *B pertussis* to macrolide antimicrobial agents has been reported but rarely in the United States. Penicillins and cephalosporins are not effective against *B pertussis.* Trimethoprim-sulfamethoxazole is an alternative for patients older than 2 months who cannot tolerate macrolides or who are infected with a macrolide-resistant strain, but studies evaluating trimethoprim-sulfamethoxazole as treatment for pertussis are limited. When administered in the first 6 weeks of life, oral erythromycin and, to a lesser degree azithromycin, are associated with increased risk of infantile hypertrophic pyloric stenosis (IHPS), but azithromycin remains the drug of choice for treatment or prophylaxis of pertussis in very young infants.

Young infants are at increased risk of respiratory failure attributable to apnea or secondary bacterial pneumonia and are at risk of cardiopulmonary failure and death from severe pulmonary hypertension. Hospitalization is most common in infants younger than 6 months. Characteristics that would suggest the need for hospitalization of infants with pertussis include young age, respiratory distress, inability to feed, cyanosis or apnea, and seizures. Hospitalized young infants with pertussis should be managed in a setting/facility where these complications can be recognized and managed urgently. Exchange transfusions or leukopheresis have been reported to be life-saving in infants with progressive pulmonary hypertension and markedly elevated lymphocyte counts.

Because data on the clinical effectiveness of antibiotic treatment on *B parapertussis* are limited, treatment decisions should be based on clinical judgment, with particular attention to special populations that may be at increased risk for severe *B parapertussis*

Table 3.46. Recommended Antimicrobial Therapy and Postexposure Prophylaxis for Pertussis in Infants, Children, Adolescents, and Adults[a]

| Age | Recommended Drugs | | | Alternative |
	Azithromycin	Erythromycin	Clarithromycin	TMP-SMX
Younger than 1 mo	10 mg/kg/day as a single dose daily for 5 days[b,c]	40 mg/kg/day in 4 divided doses for 14 days	Not recommended	Contraindicated at younger than 2 mo
1 through 5 mo	10 mg/kg/day as a single dose daily for 5 days[b]	40 mg/kg/day in 4 divided doses for 14 days	15 mg/kg/day in 2 divided doses for 7 days	2 mo or older: TMP, 8 mg/kg/day; SMX, 40 mg/kg/day in 2 doses for 14 days
6 mo or older and children	10 mg/kg as a single dose on day 1 (maximum 500 mg), then 5 mg/kg/day as a single dose on days 2 through 5 (maximum 250 mg/day)[b,d]	40 mg/kg/day in 4 divided doses for 7–14 days (maximum 2 g/day)	15 mg/kg/day in 2 divided doses for 7 days (maximum 1 g/day)	2 mo or older: TMP, 8 mg/kg/day; SMX, 40 mg/kg/day in 2 doses for 14 days
Adolescents and adults	500 mg as a single dose on day 1, then 250 mg as a single dose on days 2 through 5[b,d]	2 g/day in 4 divided doses for 7–14 days	1 g/day in 2 divided doses for 7 days	TMP, 320 mg/day; SMX, 1600 mg/day in 2 divided doses for 14 days

SMX indicates sulfamethoxazole; TMP, trimethoprim.

[a]Centers for Disease Control and Prevention. Recommended antimicrobial agents for the treatment and postexposure prophylaxis of pertussis: 2005 CDC guidelines. *MMWR Recomm Rep.* 2005;54(RR-14):1–16

[b]Azithromycin should be used with caution in people with prolonged QT interval and certain proarrhythmic conditions.

[c]Preferred macrolide for this age because of risk of idiopathic hypertrophic pyloric stenosis associated with erythromycin.

[d]A 3-day course of azithromycin for PEP or treatment has not been validated and is not recommended.

disease, including infants, elderly people, and immunocompromised people. Limited available data suggest that *B parapertussis* is less susceptible to antimicrobial agents than *B pertussis,* although some studies indicate that macrolides, trimethoprim-sulfamethoxazole, and ciprofloxacin generally have activity against *B parapertussis. B bronchiseptica* has intrinsic resistance to macrolide antibiotics.

INFECTION PREVENTION AND CONTROL MEASURES IN HEALTH CARE SETTINGS:
In addition to standard precautions, droplet precautions are recommended for 21 days

from onset of cough if appropriate antimicrobial therapy is not administered or for 5 days after initiation of effective therapy.

CONTROL MEASURES:

Care of Exposed People. Individuals, regardless of immunization status and in all settings, who have been in close contact with a person infected with pertussis should be monitored closely for respiratory tract symptoms for 21 days after last contact with the infected person. Close contacts with cough should be evaluated. People in child care settings (both workers and children), schools (both teachers and students), and health care settings with confirmed pertussis should be excluded from child care, school, or work until completion of 5 days of the recommended course of antimicrobial therapy. Untreated individuals should be excluded until 21 days have elapsed from cough onset.

Household and Other Close Contacts. PEP is recommended for all household contacts of the index case and other close contacts, including children in child care, regardless of immunization status. (**www.cdc.gov/pertussis/pep.html**). When considering a nonhousehold contact with an uncertain amount of exposure, PEP should be administered if the contact personally is at high risk or will have close contact with a person at high risk of severe pertussis (eg, young infant, pregnant person, person who has contact with infants). If 21 days have elapsed since onset of cough in the index case, PEP has limited value but may be considered for households or in situations with high-risk contacts. The agents, doses, and duration of PEP are the same as for treatment of pertussis (see Table 3.46). Prophylaxis for people exposed to *B parapertussis* is not recommended.

Close contacts who are unimmunized or underimmunized should have pertussis immunization initiated or continued as soon as possible using age-appropriate products according to the recommended schedule; this includes off-label use of tetanus toxoid, reduced-content diphtheria toxoid, and acellular pertussis vaccine (Tdap) in children 7 through 9 years of age who did not complete the diphtheria and tetanus toxoids and acellular pertussis vaccine (DTaP) series (see Table 3.47). Because pertussis-containing vaccines are non-live, they can be administered concomitantly with PEP.

Child Care. Pertussis vaccine and PEP should be administered as recommended for household and other close contacts. In the setting of known pertussis exposure, children and child care providers who are symptomatic should be excluded from the child care setting, pending evaluation by a physician.

Schools. Use of PEP for large groups of students usually is not recommended, especially in the setting of widespread community transmission, but exceptions for specific individuals can be considered. This occurs when close contact simulates household exposure or when pertussis in the exposed person may result in severe medical consequences. Public health officials should be consulted for recommendations to control pertussis transmission in schools. The immunization status of close contacts should be reviewed, and appropriate vaccines administered when indicated. Parents and teachers should be notified about possible exposures to pertussis. Exclusion of exposed people with cough illness within 21 days of last exposure should be considered pending evaluation by a physician.

Health Care Settings.[1] Health care facilities should maximize efforts to immunize all health care personnel (HCP) with Tdap. All HCP should observe droplet

---

[1] Centers for Disease Control and Prevention. Immunization of health-care personnel. Recommendations of the Advisory Committee on Immunization Practices (ACIP). *MMWR Recomm Rep.* 2011;60(RR-07):1–45

Table 3.47. Composition and Recommended Use of Vaccines With Tetanus Toxoid, Diphtheria Toxoid, and Acellular Pertussis Components Licensed and Available in the United States[a]

Pharmaceutical	Manufacturer	Recommended Use
DTaP (Infanrix)	GlaxoSmithKline Biologicals	**All 5 doses,** children 6 wk through 6 y of age.
DTaP (Daptacel)	Sanofi Pasteur	**All 5 doses,** children 6 wk through 6 y of age.
DTaP-hepatitis B-IPV (Pediarix)	GlaxoSmithKline Biologicals	**First 3 doses, children 6 wk through 6 y of age; usual use** at 2, 4, and 6 months of age; then 2 doses of DTaP are needed to complete the 5-dose series before 7 y of age.
DTaP-IPV/Hib (Pentacel)	Sanofi Pasteur	**First 4 doses, children 6 wk through 4 y of age; usual use** at 2, 4, 6, and 15 through 18 mo of age; then 1 dose of DTaP is needed to complete the 5-dose series before 7 y of age.
DTaP-IPV-hepatitis B-Hib (Vaxelis)	Merck/Sanofi Pasteur	**First 3 doses, children 6 wk through 4 y of age: usual use** at 2, 4, and 6 months of age; then 2 doses of DTaP are needed to complete the 5-dose series before 7 y of age.
DTaP-IPV (Kinrix)	GlaxoSmithKline Biologicals	**Booster dose** for **fifth dose** of DTaP and **fourth dose** of IPV at 4 through 6 y of age.
DTaP-IPV (Quadracel)	Sanofi Pasteur	**Booster dose** for **fifth dose** of DTaP and **fourth dose** of IPV at 4 through 6 y of age.
Tdap (Boostrix)	GlaxoSmithKline Biologicals	**Single dose** at 11 y or older. Can be used in place of Td. One dose recommended during EACH pregnancy, optimally between 27 and 36 weeks' gestation.
Tdap (Adacel)	Sanofi Pasteur	**Single dose** at 11 y or older. Can be used in place of Td. One dose recommended during EACH pregnancy, optimally between 27 and 36 weeks' gestation.

DTaP indicates pediatric formulation of diphtheria and tetanus toxoids and acellular pertussis vaccines; FHA, filamentous hemagglutinin; Hib, *Haemophilus influenzae* type b vaccine; IPV, inactivated (non-live) poliovirus; PT, pertussis toxoid; Td, tetanus and reduced diphtheria toxoids (for children 7 years of age or older and adults); Tdap, adolescent/adult formulation of tetanus toxoid, reduced diphtheria toxoid, and acellular pertussis vaccine.

[a] DTaP recommended schedule is 2, 4, 6, and 15 through 18 months and 4 through 6 years of age. The fourth dose can be administered as early as 12 months of age, provided 6 months have elapsed since the third dose was administered. The fifth dose is not necessary if the fourth dose was administered on or after the fourth birthday. Refer to manufacturers' product information for comprehensive product information regarding indications and use of the vaccines listed.

precautions when examining a patient with pertussis (see Infection Prevention and Control in Health Care Settings). People exposed to a patient with pertussis should be evaluated by infection control personnel for postexposure management and follow-up.

Recommendations of the CDC are as follows:

- PEP is recommended for all HCP (even if immunized with Tdap) who have been exposed to pertussis and are likely to expose patients at risk of severe pertussis (eg, hospitalized neonates and pregnant women). Other exposed HCP either should receive PEP or should be monitored daily for 21 days after exposure and treated at the onset of signs and symptoms of pertussis.
- Other people (patients, caregivers) defined as close contacts or high-risk contacts of a patient or HCP with pertussis should receive PEP (and immunization when indicated), as recommended for household contacts (see Table 3.46, p 659).
- HCP with symptoms of pertussis (or HCP with any respiratory illness within 21 days of exposure to pertussis who did not receive PEP) should be excluded from work for at least the first 5 days of the recommended antimicrobial therapy. HCP with symptoms of pertussis who do not accept antimicrobial therapy should be excluded from work for 21 days from onset of cough.

Immunization.

Vaccine Products. Acellular-component pertussis vaccines (DTaP) replaced previously used diphtheria, tetanus, and whole-cell pertussis vaccine (DTwP or DTP) exclusively in 1997; see Table 3.47 for products. All pertussis vaccines in the United States are combined with diphtheria and tetanus toxoids; none contains thimerosal as a preservative. DTaP products may be formulated as combination vaccines that contain other vaccine components. Adolescent and adult formulations, known as Tdap vaccines, contain reduced quantities of diphtheria toxoid and some pertussis antigens compared with DTaP.

Dose and Route. Each 0.5-mL dose of DTaP or Tdap is administered intramuscularly. Use of a decreased volume of individual doses of pertussis vaccines or multiple doses of decreased-volume (fractional) doses is not recommended.

Interchangeability of Acellular Pertussis Vaccines. Insufficient data exist on the safety, immunogenicity, and efficacy of DTaP vaccines from different manufacturers when administered interchangeably for the primary series in infants. In circumstances in which the type of DTaP product(s) received previously is unknown or the previously administered product(s) is not readily available, any DTaP vaccine licensed for use in the primary series may be used. There is no need to match Tdap vaccine manufacturer with DTaP vaccine manufacturer used for earlier doses.

Recommendations for Routine Childhood Immunization With DTaP. Five doses of pertussis-containing vaccine are recommended prior to entering school. The first dose of DTaP may be administered as early as 6 weeks of age, followed by 2 additional doses at intervals of approximately 2 months. The fourth dose of DTaP is recommended at 15 through 18 months of age, and the fifth dose of DTaP is administered at 4 through 6 years of age. The fourth dose can be administered as early as 12 months of age, provided 6 months have elapsed since the third dose was administered. If the fourth dose of pertussis vaccine is delayed until after the fourth birthday, the fifth dose is not recommended.

Other recommendations are as follows:

- Simultaneous administration of DTaP and all other recommended vaccines is acceptable. Vaccines should not be mixed in the same syringe unless the specific combination is licensed by the FDA (see Simultaneous Administration of Multiple Vaccines, p 63, and *Haemophilus influenzae* Infections, p 400).

- Inadvertent administration of Tdap instead of DTaP to a child younger than 7 years as either dose 1, 2, or 3 of the DTaP series does not count as a valid dose; DTaP should be administered as soon as is feasible.
- Inadvertent administration of Tdap instead of DTaP to a child younger than 7 years of age as either dose 4 or 5 can be counted as valid for DTaP dose 4 or 5.
- During a pertussis outbreak in the community, public health authorities may recommend starting DTaP immunization as early as 6 weeks of age, with doses 2 and 3 in the primary series administered at intervals as short as 4 weeks.
- Children younger than 7 years who have begun but not completed their primary immunization schedule with DTwP outside the United States should receive DTaP to complete the pertussis immunization schedule.
- DTaP is not licensed or recommended for people 7 years or older.

Combined Vaccines. Several pertussis-containing combination vaccines are licensed for use (see Table 3.47, p 661) and may be used when feasible and when any components are indicated and none is contraindicated.

Recommendations for Scheduling Pertussis Immunization for Children Younger Than 7 Years in Special Circumstances.

- For children who have received fewer than the recommended number of doses of pertussis vaccine but who have received the recommended number of diphtheria and tetanus toxoid vaccine doses for their age, DTaP should be administered to complete the recommended pertussis immunization schedule.
- The total number of doses of diphtheria and tetanus toxoids (as DTaP or DTwP) should not exceed 6 before the seventh birthday.
- Although *B pertussis* infection confers protection against recurrent infection, the duration of protection is unknown. Age-appropriate DTaP dose(s) or a Tdap dose should be administered to complete the standard or catch-up immunization series on schedule in people who have had pertussis infection. No minimum interval between disease and immunization is needed.

Adverse Events After DTaP Immunization in Children Younger Than 7 Years.

- **Local and febrile reactions.** Reactions to DTaP can occur within several hours of immunization and subside spontaneously within 48 hours without sequelae. Most commonly, these include redness, swelling, induration, and tenderness at the injection site as well as drowsiness and irritability. Less common reactions include anorexia, vomiting, crying, and slight to moderate fever.
- **Limb swelling** involving the entire thigh or upper arm has been reported in 2% to 3% of vaccine recipients after administration of the fourth and fifth doses of DTaP in that extremity. Although thigh swelling may interfere with walking, most children have no limitation of activity; the condition resolves spontaneously and has no sequelae. Entire limb swelling is not a contraindication to further DTaP, Tdap, or Td immunization.
- A review by the National Academy of Medicine (NAM) based on case-series reports found evidence of a rare yet likely causal relationship between receipt of tetanus toxoid-containing vaccines and **brachial neuritis.** However, the frequency of this event has not been determined.
- **Seizures.** In contrast to DTwP, no increased risk of seizures has been observed after DTaP administration. A small increased risk for febrile seizures after DTaP when administered simultaneously with inactivated (non-live) influenza vaccine was observed in a study by the CDC Vaccine Safety Datalink project. However, neither

the CDC Advisory Committee on Immunization Practices (ACIP) nor the American Academy of Pediatrics recommends administering vaccines on separate days.

- **Hypotonic-hyporesponsive episode.** Hypotonic-hyporesponsive episodes (HHEs) (also termed "collapse" or "shock-like state") occur significantly less often after immunization with DTaP than previously shown with DTwP and are not a contraindication to subsequent dose(s).

- **Other reactions.** Severe anaphylactic reactions are rare after pertussis immunization. Transient urticarial rashes that occur occasionally after pertussis immunization, unless appearing immediately (ie, within minutes), are unlikely to be anaphylactic (IgE- mediated) in origin.

Contraindications and Precautions to DTaP Immunization.

Contraindications to DTaP and Tdap occur only very rarely, and in questioning about them, providers should probe whether a true contraindication actually exists. DTaP and Tdap contraindications are limited to **only** the following:

- **Severe allergic reaction (eg, anaphylaxis)** to a dose of DTaP or Tdap or to a vaccine component (Td) is a contraindication to DTaP, Tdap, or Td. Because of the importance of tetanus vaccination, people who experience anaphylactic reactions should be referred to an allergist to determine whether they have a specific allergy to tetanus toxoid and can be desensitized to tetanus toxoid.

- **Encephalopathy (eg, coma, decreased level of consciousness, or prolonged seizures) not attributable to another identifiable cause** within 7 days after administration of a previous dose of diphtheria and tetanus toxoids and pertussis vaccine (DTwP, DTaP, or Tdap) is a contraindication to the pertussis component.

Precautions to DTaP and Tdap:

- **Guillain-Barré syndrome** within 6 weeks after a previous dose of tetanus toxoid-containing vaccine is a **precaution** to further doses of DTaP, Tdap, or Td.

- Moderate or severe acute illness with or without a fever is a reason to defer administration of any vaccine until the person has recovered.

- **Evolving neurologic disorder** generally is a reason to defer DTaP or Tdap immunization temporarily to reduce confusion about reason(s) for a change in the clinical course. Note that as of 2023 DT is no longer available in the United States (**www.cdc.gov/vaccines/vpd/dtap-tdap-td/hcp/recommendations. html** and **www.cdc.gov/vaccines/vpd/dtap-tdap-td/hcp/td-offlabel. html**) (see Diphtheria, p 357, and Tetanus, p 848). For young children with a contraindication to pertussis-containing vaccines, vaccine providers may administer Td for all recommended remaining doses in place of DTaP. Td contains a lower dose (approximately 1/12th the amount) of diphtheria toxoid compared with DT. The impact of this lower dose on the protection provided against diphtheria in young children is uncertain. Available evidence suggests young children who receive Td in place of DTaP may have suboptimal protection against diphtheria.

Recommendations for Routine Adolescent Immunization With Tdap.[1,2] Adolescents 11 years and older should receive a single dose of Tdap instead of Td for booster immunization

[1] Centers for Disease Control and Prevention. Prevention of pertussis, tetanus, and diphtheria with vaccines in the United States: recommendations of the Advisory Committee on Immunization Practices, 2018. *MMWR Morb Mortal Wkly Rep.* 2018;67(2):1-44

[2] Havers FP, Moro PL, Hunter P, Hariri S, Bernstein H. Use of tetanus toxoid, reduced diphtheria toxoid, and acellular pertussis vaccines: updated recommendations of the Advisory Committee on Immunization Practices—United States, 2019. *MMWR Morb Mortal Wkly Rep.* 2020;69(3):77–83

against tetanus, diphtheria, and pertussis. The preferred age for Tdap immunizations is 11 through 12 years of age.

- Adolescents who received Td but not Tdap should receive a single dose of Tdap to provide protection against pertussis regardless of time since receipt of Td.
- Simultaneous administration of Tdap and all other recommended vaccines is recommended when feasible.
- Inadvertent administration of DTaP instead of Tdap in people 7 years and older is counted as a valid dose of Tdap.

Recommendations for Scheduling Tdap in Children 7 Years and Older Who Did Not Complete Recommended DTaP Doses Before 7 Years of Age.[1]

- Children 7 through 10 years of age who have not completed their immunization schedule with DTaP before 7 years of age or who have an unknown vaccine history should receive at least 1 dose of Tdap. If further dose(s) of tetanus and diphtheria toxoids are needed in a catch-up schedule, either Td or Tdap can be used. The preferred schedule is Tdap followed by Td or Tdap at 2 months and 6 to 12 months (if needed).
- Children 7 through 9 years of age who receive Tdap or DTaP for any reason should receive the adolescent Tdap booster at 11 through 12 years of age.
- A Tdap or DTaP dose received by a 10 year-old for any reason can count as the adolescent Tdap booster dose.

Recommendations for Adolescent and Adult Immunization With Tdap in Special Situations.[1]

Despite the burden of pertussis in the community, a decision analysis conducted by the CDC concluded that a routine second dose would have a limited effect on overall disease rates. However, repeat doses of Tdap are generally well tolerated, and either Td or a Tdap can be used regardless of prior receipt of Tdap for catchup immunization of individuals 7 years and older, for the routine decennial tetanus-diphtheria booster, and for wound prophylaxis when indicated. Special situations for use of Tdap, or repeated use of Tdap off label, are provided in the following sections.

Use of Tdap in Pregnancy.[2] Tdap is approved for use by the US Food and Drug Administration (FDA) for use in the third trimester of pregnancy to prevent pertussis in infants younger than 2 months of age. In order to protect infants, who have a high risk for severe or fatal pertussis, the ACIP recommends that a dose of Tdap be administered during **each** pregnancy, irrespective of the pregnant individual's prior history of receiving Tdap or having had pertussis. Immunization during pregnancy leads to transplacental transfer of antibody that has been shown to provide protection to the infant. Tdap may be administered at any time during pregnancy, but current evidence suggests that immunization early in the interval between 27 and 36 weeks of gestation will maximize passive antibody transfer to the infant. For people not previously vaccinated with Tdap and in whom Tdap was not administered during pregnancy for some reason, Tdap should be administered immediately postpartum. Postpartum Tdap is

[1] Havers FP, Moro PL, Hunter P, Hariri S, Bernstein H. Use of tetanus toxoid, reduced diphtheria toxoid, and acellular pertussis vaccines: updated recommendations of the Advisory Committee on Immunization Practices—United States, 2019. *MMWR Morb Mortal Wkly Rep.* 2020;69(3):77–83

[2] Centers for Disease Control and Prevention. Prevention of pertussis, tetanus, and diphtheria with vaccines in the United States: recommendations of the Advisory Committee on Immunization Practices, 2018. *MMWR Morb Mortal Wkly Rep.* 2018;67(2):1-44

not recommended for people who have received a previous Tdap dose unless they are due for their decennial tetanus booster.

Protection of Young Infants: The Cocoon Strategy. Tdap vaccination during each pregnancy is the preferred strategy for protecting young infants from pertussis in the early months of life. In addition, the American Academy of Pediatrics, CDC, American College of Obstetricians and Gynecologists, American Academy of Family Physicians, American College of Nurse-Midwives, American Academy of Physician Associates, and National Association of Pediatric Nurse Practitioners recommend the "cocoon" strategy to help protect infants from pertussis by immunizing those around them. This strategy may offer indirect protection by decreasing their likelihood of acquisition and subsequent development of clinical pertussis. Immunizing parents or other adult family contacts in the pediatric office setting could increase immunization coverage for this population.[1]

- Underimmunized children younger than 7 years should receive DTaP, and underimmunized children 7 years and older should receive Tdap (see previous discussion).
- All adolescents and adults should have received a single dose of Tdap, ideally at least 2 weeks before beginning close contact with the infant. There is no minimum interval required between Tdap and prior Td.
- Cough illness in contacts of neonates should be investigated and managed promptly, with consideration given for azithromycin prophylaxis for the neonate if pertussis contact is likely (see Control Measures).

Special Situations.

- **Wound management.**[2] A tetanus toxoid–containing vaccine is indicated for wound management when >5 years have passed since the last tetanus toxoid–containing vaccine dose. If a tetanus toxoid–containing vaccine is indicated for persons aged ≥11 years, Tdap is preferred for persons who have not previously received Tdap or whose Tdap history is unknown. If a tetanus toxoid–containing vaccine is indicated for a pregnant person, Tdap should be used. For nonpregnant persons with documentation of previous Tdap vaccination, either Td or Tdap may be used if a tetanus toxoid–containing vaccine is indicated.
- **Pregnant people for whom tetanus booster is due.** If Td booster immunization is indicated during pregnancy (ie, 10 years or more since previous Td), Tdap should be administered, preferably early in the interval between weeks 27 and 36 of gestation.
- **Pregnant people with unknown or incomplete tetanus vaccination.** To ensure protection against maternal and neonatal tetanus, pregnant people who never have been immunized against tetanus should receive 3 doses of Td-containing vaccines during pregnancy. The recommended schedule is 0, 4 weeks, and 6 to 12 months, and at least 1 Tdap dose should be used in this series, preferably early in the interval between 27 and 36 weeks of gestation; either Td or Tdap can be used to complete the series.

[1] Lessin HR; Edwards KM; American Academy of Pediatrics, Committee on Practice and Ambulatory Medicine, Committee on Infectious Diseases. Immunizing parents and other close family contacts in the pediatric office setting. *Pediatrics.* 2012;129(2):e247-e253

[2] Havers FP, Moro PL, Hunter P, Hariri S, Bernstein H. Use of tetanus toxoid, reduced diphtheria toxoid, and acellular pertussis vaccines: updated recommendations of the Advisory Committee on Immunization Practices—United States, 2019. *MMWR Morb Mortal Wkly Rep.* 2020;69(3):77–83

Health Care Professionals. The CDC recommends a single dose of Tdap as soon as is feasible for HCP of any age who previously have not received Tdap. There is no minimum interval suggested or required between Tdap and prior Td.

In certain cases (eg, documented transmission in the health care setting), revaccination of HCP with Tdap may be considered (**www.cdc.gov/vaccines/vpd/ pertussis/tdap-revac-hcp.html**). In such a case, Tdap is not a substitute for infection prevention and control measures, including PEP for exposed HCP. If implemented, HCP who work with infants or pregnant people should be prioritized for revaccination.

Hospitals and ambulatory care facilities should provide Tdap for HCP and maximize immunization rates (eg, education about the benefits of immunization or mandatory requirement, convenient access, and provision of Tdap at no charge).

Recommendations for Adult Immunization With Tdap. The CDC recommends administration of a single dose of Tdap universally for adults of any age who previously have not received Tdap, with no minimum interval required between Tdap and prior dose of Td.

Adverse Events After Administration of Tdap. Local adverse events after administration of Tdap in adolescents and adults are common but usually are mild. Systemic adverse events also are common but usually are mild (eg, any fever, 3%–14%; any headache, 40%–44%; tiredness, 27%–37%). Postmarketing data suggest that these events occur at approximately the same rate and severity as following receipt of Td.

Contraindications, Precautions, and Deferral of Use of Tdap in Adolescents and Adults. Anaphylaxis that occurred after any component of the vaccine is a **contraindication** to Tdap (see Tetanus, p 848, for additional recommendations regarding tetanus immunization). In individuals with **latex allergy,** package inserts should be consulted regarding latex content.

History of **Guillain-Barré syndrome** within 6 weeks of a dose of a tetanus toxoid vaccine is a **precaution** to Tdap immunization. If the decision is made to continue tetanus toxoid immunization, Tdap is preferred if indicated. A history of severe **Arthus hypersensitivity reaction** after a previous dose of a tetanus or diphtheria toxoid-containing vaccine administered less than 10 years previously should lead to **deferral** of Tdap or Td immunization for 10 years after administration of the tetanus or diphtheria toxoid-containing vaccine.

Public Health Reporting. Pertussis is a nationally notifiable disease in the United States.

Pinworm Infection
(Enterobius vermicularis)

CLINICAL MANIFESTATIONS: Pinworm infection (enterobiasis) commonly is asymptomatic but may cause pruritus ani and, rarely, pruritus vulvae. Pruritus ani can be severe enough to cause sleep disturbance. Bacterial superinfections can result from scratching and excoriation of the irritated area. Pinworms have been found in the lumen of the appendix, and in some cases, these intraluminal parasites have been associated with signs of acute appendicitis, but they have also been observed in histologically normal appendices removed for incidental reasons. Urethritis, vaginitis, salpingitis, or pelvic peritonitis uncommonly may occur from aberrant migration of an adult worm from the perineum. Eosinophilic enterocolitis has been reported, although peripheral eosinophilia generally is not seen in any form of enterobiasis. No proof of a causal relationship has been established for pinworms causing nonspecific clinical findings such as grinding of teeth at night, weight loss, or enuresis.

ETIOLOGY: *Enterobius vermicularis* is a nematode helminth (roundworm).

EPIDEMIOLOGY: Enterobiasis occurs worldwide and commonly clusters within families. Prevalence rates are higher in preschool- and school-aged children, in primary caregivers of infected children, and in institutionalized people. An estimated 40 million people in the United States have been infected with pinworms, with a prevalence as high as 20% to 30% in some age groups and communities.

Initial infection occurs by ingestion of contaminated food, or contact with hands, clothing, bedding, or other items contaminated with eggs. Infection may also occur by person-to-person transmission, including during sexual activity or via fecal-oral or oral-genital contact. Eggs hatch and release larvae in the small intestine, and adult worms then locate themselves usually in the cecum, appendix, and ascending colon. Adult male worms die soon after copulating. Gravid female worms migrate, usually at night while the host is resting, to the perianal area to deposit eggs containing larvae, which mature in 6 to 8 hours. Female worms begin to oviposit after 30 days and have an overall lifespan of up to 100 days. Adult female worms and eggs may induce intense perianal pruritus, leading to an autoinfection cycle during which the area is scratched and then eggs are lodged on the hands and under the fingernails and ingested when hands are put in the mouth. Retroinfection, in which newly hatched larvae migrate back into the rectum, has been hypothesized, but its role in transmission of infection is uncertain. A person remains infectious as long as female pinworms are discharging eggs on perianal skin. Eggs may remain infective in an indoor environment for up to 2 weeks. Humans are the only known natural hosts. Pets are not reservoirs of infection.

The **incubation period** from ingestion of an egg until an adult gravid female worm migrates to the perianal region is 2 to 6 weeks or longer.

DIAGNOSTIC TESTS: Diagnosis is established via the classic cellulose tape test ("Scotch tape test") or with a commercially available pinworm paddle test, which is a clear plastic paddle coated with an adhesive surface on one side that is pressed on both sides of the perianal region during the night or at the time of waking and before bathing. The tape or paddle is then pressed on a slide and eggs can be visualized by microscopy. Eggs are 50 to 60 microns by 20 to 30 microns and flattened on one side, giving them a "bean-shaped" appearance. Testing on 3 different days will increase the sensitivity from around 65% for a single test to approximately 90%. Adult female worms, which are white and measure 8 to 13 mm, also can be seen in the perineal region. Stool examination is not helpful, because worms or eggs are found infrequently (only in about 10% or less) in the stool. Neither peripheral eosinophilia nor elevated immunoglobulin E concentrations are typical because of low pinworm invasiveness and, if present, should not be attributed to pinworm infection.

TREATMENT: Several drugs will treat pinworms (see Drugs for Parasitic Infections, p 1068), including pyrantel pamoate, mebendazole, and albendazole. Pyrantel pamoate, available as an over-the-counter drug in the United States, is significantly less expensive than the prescription benzimidazole medications mebendazole and albendazole. Albendazole currently is not approved by the US Food and Drug Administration for treatment of pinworms. Each medication has high potency against adult pinworms, but overall effectiveness of therapy depends on existing larval and egg burden in the child and reinfection from close contacts. Each medication (pyrantel pamoate or a benzimidazole) is recommended to be given in a single dose and repeated in 2 weeks, in order to treat nematodes developed from eggs or larvae during that period. For children younger than 2 years, in whom experience with these 3 drugs is limited and use is off-label, risks and benefits should be considered before drug administration. Ivermectin has been evaluated and is partially effective, but should not be used in children weighing less than 15 kg, because it blocks essential neural transmission if it crosses the blood-brain barrier and young children may be at higher risk of this adverse drug reaction. Because reinfection is common even when effective therapy is given, treatment of the entire household as a group should be considered. Repeated infections should be treated by the same method as the first infection. Vaginitis is self-limited and does not require separate treatment. "Pulse" treatment with a single dose of mebendazole every 14 days for a period of 16 weeks has been used in refractory cases with multiple recurrences. Alternative diagnoses in cases being attributed to recurrent pinworm infections can include *Dipylidium caninum*, which is characterized by proglottid segments being visible in the stool, and is definitively diagnosed by stool ova and parasite analysis and treated with praziquantel (see Other Tapeworm Infections [Including Hydatid Disease], p 845, and Table 4.11, p 1068), as well as, uncommonly, delusional parasitosis.

INFECTION PREVENTION AND CONTROL MEASURES IN HEALTH CARE SETTINGS: Standard precautions are indicated.

CONTROL MEASURES: Control is difficult in child care centers and schools, because the rate of reinfection is high. In institutions, mass and simultaneous treatment, repeated in 2 weeks, can be successful. Hygienic measures, such as bathing in the morning to remove eggs, frequent hand hygiene, and clipping of fingernails, all are helpful for decreasing the risk of autoinfection and continued transmission. Bed linens and underclothing of infected children should be handled carefully, should not be shaken (to avoid scattering eggs), and should be laundered promptly.

Pityriasis Versicolor
(Formerly Tinea Versicolor)

CLINICAL MANIFESTATIONS: Pityriasis versicolor (formerly tinea versicolor) is a common and benign superficial infection of the skin, classically manifesting on the seborrheic (sebum-rich) areas of the upper trunk (chest, shoulders, upper arms) and neck. Most patients are asymptomatic, although some may complain of pruritus. In infants and children, the infection is likely to involve the face, particularly the temples. Infection can include other areas, including the scalp, genital area, and thighs. Symmetrical involvement with ovoid discrete or coalescent lesions of varying size is typical; these macules or patches vary in color, even in the same person. White, pink, tan, or brown coloration is often surmounted by faint dusty scales. Lesions fail to tan during the summer and are relatively darker than the surrounding skin during the winter, hence the term versicolor. The differential diagnosis includes pityriasis alba, vitiligo, seborrheic dermatitis, pityriasis rosea, pityriasis lichenoides, progressive macular hypopigmentation, and dyschromatosis universalis hereditaria. Coexisting pityrosporum folliculitis also can occur, particularly in immunocompromised patients. More exuberant cases of pityriasis versicolor have been documented in the context of therapy with immunosuppressive systemic agents, including ixekizumab and immune checkpoint inhibitors for melanoma. Invasive infections can occur in neonates, particularly those receiving total parenteral nutrition with lipids.

ETIOLOGY: Pityriasis versicolor is caused by several species of the *Malassezia furfur* complex, a group of lipid-dependent yeasts that exist on healthy skin in yeast phase and causes clinical lesions only when substantial growth of hyphae occurs. Moisture, heat, and the presence of lipid-containing sebaceous secretions encourage rapid overgrowth of hyphae.

EPIDEMIOLOGY: Pityriasis versicolor can occur in any climate or age group but tends to favor adolescents and young adults. Living in hot and humid climates, sweating excessively, or a weakened immune system allows the fungus to flourish. Pityriasis versicolor is not contagious.

The **incubation period** is unknown.

DIAGNOSTIC TESTS: The presence of symmetrically distributed faintly scaling macules and patches of varying color concentrated on the upper back and chest is close to diagnostic. The "evoked scale" sign is when the clinician uses thumb and forefinger to stretch the skin, eliciting a visible white patch of scale overlying the affected area, which is still visible when the affected area is released. Another technique to evoke scales is scraping the involved skin with a scalpel blade or glass microscope slide, again yielding a pale and fuzzy scale that is confined to the lesion. Involved areas fluoresce yellow-green under Wood lamp evaluation. Potassium hydroxide wet mount prep of scraped scales reveals the classic "spaghetti and meatballs" short hyphae and clusters of yeast forms. Because this yeast is a common inhabitant of the skin, fungal culture from the skin surface is nondiagnostic. To grow the fungus in the laboratory, samples from pustules (if folliculitis is present) or sterile sites should be placed in media enriched with olive oil or another long-chain fatty acid.

TREATMENT: Multiple topical and systemic agents are efficacious, and recommendations vary substantially depending on expert opinion. For uncomplicated cases, most experts recommend initiating therapy with topical agents. The most cost-effective treatments are selenium sulfide shampoo/lotion and clotrimazole cream. Selenium sulfide shampoo is used for 3 to 7 days; application is once daily for 5 to 10 minutes, followed by rinsing. Topical azole therapy (eg, clotrimazole cream) is applied twice daily for 2 to 3 weeks. Adherence with these agents may be low because of unpleasant adverse effects (the shampoo has a sulfur-like odor) or duration and anatomic extent of required therapy. Other effective topical agents include ketoconazole and off-label bifonazole, miconazole, econazole, oxiconazole, terbinafine, and ciclopirox, as well as zinc pyrithione shampoo. Shampoos are easier to disperse, particularly on wet skin, than topical creams, and may increase compliance. One randomized controlled trial demonstrated that topical retinoids such as adapalene gel can produce clinical benefit either as monotherapy or in conjunction with topical ketoconazole cream when used twice daily for 4 weeks.

Treatment response is measured by resolution of scale and/or disappearance of "spaghetti and meatball" microscopic findings. Restoration of normal pigmentation may take months after successful treatment.

Recurrence following discontinuation of therapy may approach 60% to 80%, and preventive treatments sometimes are used to decrease recurrences. Off-label regimens to decrease recurrence include use of the aforementioned shampoos/lotions on a weekly or monthly basis.

Systemic therapy is reserved for resistant infection or extensive involvement. Medications, including fluconazole, itraconazole, and pramiconazole, are not approved by the US Food and Drug Administration (FDA) for pityriasis versicolor. Fluconazole (preferred) can be administered at 300 mg weekly for 2 to 4 weeks or itraconazole 200 mg daily for 1 week. Although oral agents may be easier to use than topical agents, they are not necessarily more effective and have possible serious adverse effects. Drug interactions can occur when using oral drugs, and monitoring for liver toxicity must be considered in patients receiving systemic therapy, particularly if they receive multiple courses. Although ketoconazole can treat pityriasis versicolor effectively, the FDA reaffirmed in 2016 that it strongly discourages use of systemic ketoconazole for uncomplicated skin and nail infections because of significant risks of liver toxicity, adrenal insufficiency, and interactions with multiple medications, which have resulted in at least 1 fatality. In several studies, topical therapy has appeared to be equivalent or superior to systemic therapy.

INFECTION PREVENTION AND CONTROL MEASURES IN HEALTH CARE SETTINGS: Standard precautions are recommended.

CONTROL MEASURES: The organism that causes pityriasis versicolor is commensal and resides on normal skin.

Plague

CLINICAL MANIFESTATIONS: Naturally acquired plague most commonly presents in the primary **bubonic form,** with fever and a painful swollen regional lymph node (bubo). Buboes develop most commonly in the inguinal region but also occur in axillary or cervical areas. Less commonly, plague manifests in the primary **septicemic form** without localizing signs (fever, hypotension, purpuric skin lesions, intravascular coagulopathy, organ failure) or as primary **pneumonic plague** (cough, fever, dyspnea, and hemoptysis) and rarely as **meningitic**, **pharyngeal**, **cutaneous, ocular**, or **gastrointestinal plague.** Occasionally, patients present with mild lymphadenitis or prominent gastrointestinal tract symptoms, which may obscure the correct diagnosis. Secondary pneumonic or other forms of plague can occur via hematogenous dissemination of bacteria. Untreated, plague often progresses to overwhelming sepsis and death. Plague was known as the Black Death in 14th century Europe because of the tissue necrosis that it induces.

ETIOLOGY: Plague is caused by *Yersinia pestis,* a pleomorphic, bipolar-staining (with Giemsa, Wright, and Wayson stains), facultative intracellular gram-negative coccobacillus. *Y pestis* is a member of the *Enterobacterales* order, along with more common *Yersinia* species and other enteric bacteria.

EPIDEMIOLOGY: Plague is a zoonotic infection primarily maintained in rodents and their fleas. Humans are incidental hosts who develop bubonic or primary septicemic manifestations, typically through the bite of infected rodent fleas or through direct contact with tissues of infected animals. Primary pneumonic plague is acquired by inhalation of respiratory tract droplets from a human or animal with pneumonic plague. Only the pneumonic form has been shown to be transmitted from person to person. Plague enzootic foci are found in parts of Asia, Africa, and the Americas. Most human plague cases are reported from rural, underdeveloped areas and mainly occur as isolated cases or in small, focal clusters. In the United States, plague is endemic in western states, with most cases reported from New Mexico, Colorado, Arizona, and California.[1] Cases of plague in states without endemic plague have been identified in travelers returning from these states.

Y pestis has also been identified as a potential bioterrorism agent, particularly through widespread dispersal of an aerosolized form. Such an event would have potential for a large number of pneumonic plague cases. Contamination of food and water with *Y pestis* would be expected to result in cases of pharyngeal or gastrointestinal plague, and release of infected fleas would be expected to produce a range of illness similar to naturally occurring plague, but with a higher number of cases.

The **incubation period** is 2 to 8 days for bubonic plague and 1 to 6 days for primary pneumonic plague.

DIAGNOSTIC TESTS: Diagnosis of plague usually is confirmed by culture of *Y pestis* from blood, bubo aspirate, sputum, or another clinical specimen. The organism is slow growing but not fastidious and can be isolated on sheep blood agar with typical "fried-egg" colonies appearing after 48 to 72 hours of incubation. *Y pestis* has a bipolar (safety-pin) appearance when stained with Wright-Giemsa or Wayson stains. Neither automated, commercially available biochemical identification systems nor matrix-assisted laser desorption/ionization–time-of-flight (MALDI-TOF) mass spectrometry are reliable for identification of *Y pestis*, as they may misidentify the organism. Identification of suspected isolates of *Y pestis* should be based on guidelines recommended for "sentinel level" clinical microbiology laboratories using preliminary characterization tests, followed by definitive identification performed at the state or federal public health laboratory. Nucleic acid amplification tests (NAATs) and immunohistochemical (IHC) staining for rapid diagnosis of *Y pestis* are available in some reference and public health laboratories.

Presumptive laboratory evidence of plague includes detection of *Y pestis* by NAAT or IHC from a clinical specimen or a positive serum antibody titer from a single specimen. Confirmatory laboratory evidence of plague includes isolation of the organism in culture with positive identification by *Y pestis* bacteriophage lysis or seroconversion, defined as a fourfold or greater increase in serum antibody to the F1 antigen between paired specimens obtained 4 to 6 weeks apart.

Laboratory-acquired cases, including fatal cases, have been reported. Biosafety level 3 practices, containment equipment, and facilities are recommended for all manipulation of suspect cultures. Isolates suspected as *Y pestis* should be reported immediately to the state health department.

TREATMENT: After obtaining diagnostic specimens, appropriate antibiotic therapy should be started immediately for any patient suspected of having plague. Pediatric treatment recommendations[2] are as follows (see also Table 3.48):

---

[1] Kwit N, Nelson C, Kugeler K, et al. Human plague—United States, 2015. *MMWR Morb Mortal Wkly Rep.* 2015;64(33):918-919

[2] Nelson CA, Meaney-Delman D, Fleck-Derderian S, Cooley KM, Yu PA, Mead PS. Antimicrobial treatment and prophylaxis of plague: recommendations for naturally acquired infections and bioterrorism response. *MMWR Morb Mortal Wkly Rep.* 2021;70(3):1-27

Table 3.48. Antimicrobial Dosing for Treatment of Plague in Children and Neonates[a]

Drug	Dosage per kg per Day
Ciprofloxacin[b]	20–30 mg/kg, divided in 2 or 3 doses IV (maximum 400 mg/dose IV) 30–45 mg/kg, divided in 2 or 3 doses PO (maximum 500 mg/dose TID or 750 mg/dose BID) Neonates 20–30 mg/kg, divided in 2 or 3 doses IV
Levofloxacin[b]	<50 kg: 16 mg/kg, divided in 2 doses IV/PO (maximum 250 mg/dose) ≥50 kg: 500–750 mg once daily IV/PO Neonates 20 mg/kg, divided in 2 doses IV
Gentamicin[c]	4.5-7.5 mg/kg once daily IV/IM Neonates ≤7 days: 4 mg/kg once daily IV/IM 8–28 days: 5 mg/kg once daily IV/IM
Streptomycin[d]	30 mg/kg, divided in 2 doses IV/IM (maximum dose 1 g/dose) Neonates 30 mg/kg, divided in 2 doses IV/IM
Doxycycline[b]	<45 kg: 4.4 mg/kg load, then 4.4 mg/kg, divided in 2 doses IV/PO ≥45 kg: 200 mg load, then 200 mg divided in 2 doses IV/PO Neonates 4.4 mg/kg load, then 4.4 mg/kg, divided in 2 doses IV
Chloramphenicol[c,e]	50–100 mg/kg, divided in 4 doses IV (maximum 1 g/dose) Meningitis ≥29 days to ≥17 years: 100 mg/kg, divided in 4 doses IV (maximum 1 g/dose) Neonates: Meningitis 8–28 days: 50 mg/kg, divided in 2 doses IV ≤7 days: 25 mg/kg once daily IV All other forms ≤14 days: 25 mg/kg, divided in 4 doses IV/IM 15–28 days: 50 mg/kg, divided into 4 doses IV/IM
Moxifloxacin[b]	≥3 months to ≤23 months: 12 mg/kg, divided in 2 doses IV/PO 2 to 5 years: 10 mg/kg, divided in 2 doses IV/PO 6 to 11 years: 8 mg/kg, divided in 2 doses IV/PO 12 to ≤17 years, <45 kg: 8 mg/kg, divided in 2 doses IV/PO (maximum 200 mg/dose) 12 to ≤17 years, ≥45 kg: 400 mg once daily IV/PO

BID indicates twice per day; IM, intramuscular; IV, intravenous; PO, oral; TID, three times per day.

All dosages are applicable for all forms of disease, except for chloramphenicol, which is dosed as above.

[a] Adapted from Nelson CA, Meaney-Delman D, Fleck-Derderian S, Cooley KM, Yu PA, Mead PS. Antimicrobial treatment and prophylaxis of plague: recommendations for naturally acquired infections and bioterrorism response. *MMWR Morb Mortal Wkly Rep*. 2021;70(3):1-27.

[b] Data on use in neonates are extremely limited.

[c] Not currently approved by the Food and Drug Administration (FDA) for the treatment of plague.

[d] The intramuscular formulation of streptomycin has been given intravenously in an off label use (the intravenous formulation is not approved by FDA).

[e] Chloramphenicol is generally contraindicated for infants aged <6 months because of the risk for serious blood dyscrasias or circulatory collapse (gray baby syndrome), because of the severity of meningitis, it is still a treatment option. Levofloxacin can be used for treatment of plague meningitis in neonates and older children and moxifloxacin for plague meningitis for infants ≥3 months of age. After clinical improvement, chloramphenicol can be reduced to a lower dose of 12.5 mg/kg every 6 hours in adults and administered orally. Serum concentration monitoring should be performed when available, especially in children. Chloramphenicol is not considered a first-line drug for nonmeningitis forms of plague; rather, it is considered an alternative drug.

- Monotherapy with gentamicin, streptomycin, ciprofloxacin, or levofloxacin is recommended for naturally acquired primary bubonic or pharyngeal plague without signs of sepsis or secondary pneumonic plague and for early/mild primary pneumonic or septicemic plague.
- Doxycycline is a first-line option for treatment of naturally acquired bubonic or pharyngeal plague but is an alternative antibiotic for naturally acquired pneumonic plague.
- Dual therapy with 2 distinct antibiotic classes is recommended for initial treatment of patients with naturally acquired severe septicemic or pneumonic plague, or for infection following intentional release of *Y pestis* (eg, acts of bioterrorism). Dual therapy can be considered for patients with naturally acquired primary bubonic disease with large buboes. The recommended drugs are those listed in the first bullet.
- Alternative antibiotics for pneumonic, septicemic, bubonic, or pharyngeal plague are listed in the Centers for Disease Control and Prevention (CDC) plague guidance.
- Dual therapy with 2 distinct antibiotic classes is recommended for initial treatment of patients who present with signs of meningitis or who are later found to have meningitis. The recommended antibiotics are chloramphenicol in combination with moxifloxacin or levofloxacin. If chloramphenicol is unavailable, a first-line or alternative nonfluoroquinolone antibiotic for the treatment of primary pneumonic or septicemic plague should be substituted as part of a dual class regimen that includes moxifloxacin or levofloxacin.
- Because of the potential for engineered antimicrobial resistance, if bioterrorism is suspected, dual therapy with 2 distinct classes of antibiotics should be used for all patients until susceptibility patterns are known.

A neonate born to a person infected with plague at or around the time of delivery should be treated if the infant is symptomatic, using the antibiotic regimens described (levofloxacin may be considered rather than chloramphenicol in the case of meningitis because of the toxicity of chloramphenicol in neonates; consultation with an expert in pediatric infectious diseases is recommended). An asymptomatic neonate born to a person infected with *Y pestis* within 7 days of delivery should receive antimicrobial prophylaxis (see Care of Exposed People) if the birthing person is untreated or has only recently begun treatment (<48 hours before delivery). If the neonate is asymptomatic and the birthing person has been sufficiently treated and is improving, observation of the infant is acceptable.

The duration of antibiotic treatment for all forms of plague, including meningitis, is 10 to 14 days; treatment duration can be extended for patients with ongoing fever or other concerning signs or symptoms. Drainage of abscessed buboes may be necessary; drainage material is considered infectious.

INFECTION PREVENTION AND CONTROL MEASURES IN HEALTH CARE SETTINGS:
For patients with bubonic or septicemic plague, standard precautions are recommended. If aspiration of a bubo or another procedure that may generate sprays or splashes is performed, contact and droplet precautions should be used; health care personnel should wear appropriate personal protective equipment including a mask, eye protection (such as googles or face shield), gown, and gloves. For patients with suspected pneumonic plague, respiratory droplet precautions in addition to standard precautions should be initiated immediately and continued for 48 hours after initiation of effective antibiotic treatment and until clinical improvement with decreased sputum production is documented.

CONTROL MEASURES:

Care of Exposed People. All people with exposure to a known or suspected source of plague, such as *Y pestis*-infected fleas or infectious tissues, in the previous 6 days, should be offered antibiotic prophylaxis or be cautioned to report fever greater than 38.3°C (101.0°F) or other illness to their physician. Postexposure prophylaxis is recommended for people with close and sustained exposure (less than 2 meters) to a patient with pneumonic plague, who were not wearing adequate personal protective equipment (per standard and droplet precautions). Pneumonic transmission typically occurs in the later stages of disease in patients with hemoptysis, thereby placing caregivers and health care professionals at higher risk. Isolation of exposed, asymptomatic people is not recommended. For children, including those younger than 8 years, doxycycline, levofloxacin, or ciprofloxacin is recommended. The benefits of prophylactic therapy should be weighed against the risks. Prophylaxis is administered for 7 days (see Table 3.49). In the case of an intentional release of *Y pestis*, postexposure prophylaxis should be started rapidly for exposed persons; specific recommendations regarding appropriate antibiotics will be issued by the public health authority. Recommendations will be guided by what is known about the strain. For further discussion, including alternative agents, see **www.cdc.gov/mmwr/volumes/70/rr/rr7003a1.htm.**

Breastfeeding. There are no reports of suspected *Y pestis* transmission from human milk, and the risk is believed to be low. Breastfeeding parents with bubonic or septicemic plague and those taking antibiotic prophylaxis after exposure to *Y pestis* can continue to breastfeed their infants. A breastfeeding parent with pneumonic plague may continue to breastfeed if receiving antibiotic treatment and the infant is receiving antibiotic treatment or postexposure prophylaxis for *Y pestis*. Because of the risk of person-to-person transmission of pneumonic plague, a parent with primary or secondary pneumonic plague whose infant is not receiving antibiotic treatment or prophylaxis should avoid direct breastfeeding until the parent has received antibiotic treatment for ≥48 hours and demonstrated clinical improvement. The parent's expressed milk may be fed to the infant. The CDC has guidance about breastfeeding and drugs or metabolites

Table 3.49. Antimicrobial Dosing for Postexposure Prophylaxis for Plague in Neonates and Children[a]

Drug	Dosage per kg per Day
Ciprofloxacin[b]	30 mg/kg, divided in 2 doses PO (maximum 750 mg/dose) Neonates 30 mg/kg, divided in 2 doses PO
Levofloxacin[b]	<50 kg: 16 mg/kg, divided in 2 doses PO (maximum 250 mg/dose) ≥50 kg: 500–750 mg once daily PO Neonates 20 mg/kg, divided in 2 doses PO
Doxycycline[b]	<45 kg: 4.4 mg/kg, divided in 2 doses PO ≥45 kg: 200 mg divided in 2 doses PO Neonates 4.4 mg/kg, divided in 2 doses PO

PO indicates oral.

[a] Adapted from Nelson CA, Meaney-Delman D, Fleck-Derderian S, Cooley KM, Yu PA, Mead PS. Antimicrobial treatment and prophylaxis of plague: recommendations for naturally acquired infections and bioterrorism response. *MMWR Morb Mortal Wkly Rep.* 2021;70(3):1-27.

[b] Data on use in neonates are extremely limited.

present in human milk, potential consequences to infants, and specific recommendations regarding antibiotics.[1]

Other Measures. People living in areas with endemic plague should be informed about the importance of eliminating sources of rodent food and harborage near residences, the role of dogs and cats in bringing plague-infected rodent fleas into peridomestic environments, the need for flea control and confinement of pets, and the importance of avoiding contact with sick and dead animals. Other preventive measures include surveillance of rodent populations and use of rodent control measures and insecticides by health authorities when surveillance indicates the occurrence of plague epizootics. For additional information on laboratory safety, see the CDC *Biosafety in Microbiological and Biomedical Laboratories* manual (**www.cdc.gov/labs/pdf/SF__19_308133-A_BMBL6_00-BOOK-WEB-final-3.pdf**).

Vaccine. There is no vaccine currently licensed for use in the United States. New vaccines based on recombinant capsular subunit protein F1 and the low-calcium response V antigen (LcrV) are under evaluation.

Public Health Reporting. Infection with *Y pestis* is nationally reportable. In the United States, *Y pestis* is classified as a select agent, and the possession and transport of the organism requires adherence to strict federal guidelines. State public health authorities should be notified immediately of any suspected cases of human plague.

Pneumocystis jirovecii Infections

CLINICAL MANIFESTATIONS: Symptomatic infection with *Pneumocystis jirovecii* is extremely rare in healthy people. However, in immunocompromised infants and children, *P jirovecii* can cause a respiratory illness characterized by dyspnea, tachypnea, significant hypoxemia, nonproductive cough, chills, fatigue, and fever. The intensity of these signs and symptoms may vary, and in some immunocompromised children and adults, the onset may be acute and fulminant. Most children with *Pneumocystis* pneumonia are significantly hypoxic. Chest radiographs often show bilateral diffuse interstitial or alveolar disease but may appear normal in early disease. Atypical radiographic findings may include lobar, miliary, cavitary, and nodular lesions. The mortality rate in immunocompromised patients ranges from 5% to 40% in treated patients and approaches 100% without therapy.

Extrapulmonary *Pneumocystis* organisms, often associated with a localized inflammatory reaction, are found in <2.5% of adults and children living with human immunodeficiency virus (HIV). This can occur without concurrent *Pneumocystis* pneumonia and can be located at multiple noncontiguous sites. Involved sites have included the ear, eye, thyroid, spleen, gastrointestinal tract, peritoneum, stomach, duodenum, small intestine, transverse colon, liver, and pancreas. Less frequently involved sites include the adrenal glands, muscle, bone marrow, heart, kidney, ureter, lymph nodes, meninges, and cerebral cortex.

ETIOLOGY: Nomenclature for *Pneumocystis* species has evolved. Human *Pneumocystis* is called *Pneumocystis jirovecii*, although the familiar acronym PCP (originally *Pneumocystis*

---

[1] Nelson CA, Meaney-Delman D, Fleck-Derderian S, Cooley KM, Yu PA, Mead PS. Antimicrobial treatment and prophylaxis of plague: recommendations for naturally acquired infections and bioterrorism response. *MMWR Morb Mortal Wkly Rep.* 2021;70(3):1-27

carinii pneumonia) still is used commonly among clinicians. *P jirovecii* is an atypical fungus (based on DNA sequence analysis) with several morphologic and biologic similarities to protozoa, including susceptibility to a number of antiprotozoal agents but resistance to most antifungal agents. In addition, the organism exists as 2 distinct morphologic forms: the 5- to 7-μm-diameter cysts, which contain up to 8 intracystic bodies or sporozoites, and the smaller, 1- to 5-μm-diameter trophozoite or trophic form.

EPIDEMIOLOGY: *Pneumocystis* species are ubiquitous in mammals worldwide and have a tropism for respiratory tract epithelium. Asymptomatic or mild human infection occurs early in life, with more than 85% of healthy children showing seropositivity by 20 months of age. Animal models and studies of patients with acquired immunodeficiency syndrome (AIDS) do not support the existence of latency and suggest that disease after the second year of life is likely reinfection.

The single most important factor in susceptibility to PCP is the status of cell-mediated immunity of the host, reflected by a marked decrease in percentage and numbers of CD4+ T-lymphocytes or a decrease in CD4+ T-lymphocyte function. In resource-limited countries and in times of famine, *Pneumocystis* pneumonia can occur in epidemics, primarily affecting malnourished infants and children. In industrialized countries, PCP occurs almost entirely in immunocompromised people with deficient cell-mediated immunity, particularly people with HIV infection, recipients of immunosuppressive therapy after solid organ and hematopoietic cell transplantation, people undergoing treatment for hematologic malignancy, and children with primary immunodeficiency syndromes. Although onset of disease can occur at any age, PCP most commonly occurs in children living with HIV in the first year of life, with peak incidence at 3 through 6 months of age. In patients with cancer, the disease can occur during remission or relapse of the malignancy.

The incidence of PCP has dramatically decreased in the United States as a result of antiretroviral therapy for people living with HIV and the general adoption of recommendations for prophylaxis. Despite this decrease, it is still one of the leading opportunistic infections among people living with HIV, particularly those not aware of their infection or not receiving antiretroviral therapy or who are not adherent with their indicated PCP prophylaxis.

Animal studies have demonstrated animal-to-animal transmission by the airborne route; human-to-human transmission has been suggested by molecular epidemiology and global clustering of PCP cases in several studies. Outbreaks in hospitals have been reported. Vertical transmission has been postulated but never proven. The period of communicability is unknown.

The **incubation period** is unknown, but outbreaks of PCP in transplant recipients have demonstrated a median of 53 days from exposure to clinically apparent infection.

DIAGNOSTIC TESTS: A definitive diagnosis of PCP is made by microscopic visualization of organisms (*Pneumocystis* cysts) in lung tissue or respiratory tract secretion specimens. Bronchoscopy with bronchoalveolar lavage (BAL) is the diagnostic procedure of choice for most infants and children. Methenamine silver stain, toluidine blue stain, and fluorescently conjugated monoclonal antibody are useful tools for identifying the thick-walled cysts of *P jirovecii*. Sporozoites (within cysts) and trophozoites are identified with Giemsa or modified Wright-Giemsa stain. A cyst wall, trophozoite, and immunofluorescent antibody stain is recommended for each specimen studied. The sensitivity of all microscopy-based methods depends on the skill of the laboratory technician and the quality of the specimen.

Nucleic acid amplification tests (NAATs) to diagnose PCP are becoming more widely available. They are highly sensitive with a variety of specimen types from the respiratory tract, including nasopharyngeal aspirates. However, there are currently no US Food and Drug Administration (FDA)-cleared NAATs for *P jirovecii*. Because highly sensitive NAATs may detect colonization with these organisms, results from such assays must be interpreted in the context of clinical presentation.

Limited data suggest that serum 1,3-β-D-glucan (BG) assay, which is available as an FDA-cleared test in the United States for invasive fungal infections, may be a potential marker for *Pneumocystis* infection. This compound is a component of the cell wall of the cyst stage of the organism and may be found in high concentrations in serum of patients infected with *P jirovecii*; however, most other fungi also secrete the compound during infection, so correlation with clinical presentation is imperative.

TREATMENT[1]**:** The drug of choice is trimethoprim-sulfamethoxazole (TMP-SMX), usually administered intravenously. Oral therapy should be reserved for patients with mild disease who do not have malabsorption or diarrhea and for patients with a favorable clinical response to initial intravenous therapy. See Table 4.3 (p 993) for dosages. Duration of therapy is 21 days. The rate of adverse reactions to TMP-SMX (eg, rash, neutropenia, anemia, thrombocytopenia, renal toxicity, hepatitis, nausea, vomiting, and diarrhea) is higher in children living with HIV than in patients without HIV. It is not necessary to discontinue therapy for mild adverse reactions (eg, vomiting). At least half of patients with more severe reactions that include rash require interruption of therapy. Desensitization to TMP-SMX may be considered after the acute reaction has abated.

Pentamidine, administered intravenously, is an alternative drug for treatment of *Pneumocystis* infection in children and adults who cannot tolerate TMP-SMX or who have severe disease and have not responded to TMP-SMX after 5 to 7 days of therapy. The therapeutic efficacy of intravenous pentamidine in adults with PCP is similar to that of TMP-SMX. Pentamidine is associated with a high incidence of adverse reactions, including renal toxicity, pancreatitis, diabetes mellitus, electrolyte abnormalities, hypoglycemia, hyperglycemia, hypotension, cardiac arrhythmias, fever, and neutropenia. Aerosolized pentamidine should not be used for treatment, because its efficacy is limited.

Atovaquone is approved for oral treatment of mild to moderate PCP in adults who are intolerant of TMP-SMX. Experience with use of atovaquone in children is limited, although a study comparing the efficacy of bacterial prophylaxis of atovaquone-azithromycin versus TMP-SMX noted that prevention of PCP was equivalent between the 2 drug regimens. Adverse reactions to atovaquone are limited to rash, nausea, and diarrhea.

Other potentially useful drugs for mild to moderate PCP in adults include clindamycin with primaquine (adverse reactions are rash, nausea, and diarrhea), dapsone with trimethoprim (associated with neutropenia, anemia, thrombocytopenia,

---

[1] Panel on Opportunistic Infections in Children with and Exposed to HIV. Guidelines for the Prevention and Treatment of Opportunistic Infections in Children with and Exposed to HIV. Department of Health and Human Services. Available at: **https://clinicalinfo.hiv.gov/en/guidelines/pediatric-opportunistic-infection**

Table 3.50. Dosing of Oral Prednisone in the Treatment of *Pneumocystis* pneumonia[a,b]

Age	Days 1–5	Days 6–10	Days 11–21
<13 y	1 mg/kg/dose, twice daily	0.5 mg/kg/dose, twice daily	0.5 mg/kg/dose daily
≥13 y	40 mg, twice daily	40 mg daily	20 mg daily

[a] The maximum doses should not exceed the dose for children older than 13 years.
[b] For those unable to take oral therapy, intravenous methylprednisolone can be administered as follows: 1 mg/kg/dose every 6 hours on days 1 through 7; 1 mg/kg/dose twice daily on days 8 through 9; 0.5 mg/kg/dose twice daily on days 10 and 11; and 1 mg/kg/dose once daily on days 12–16.

methemoglobinemia, rash, and aminotransferase elevation), and trimetrexate with leucovorin. Experience with the use of these combinations in children is limited.

On the basis of studies in both adults and children, a course of corticosteroids is recommended in patients with moderate to severe PCP (as defined by an arterial oxygen pressure [PaO_2] of less than 70 mm Hg in room air or an arterial-alveolar gradient ≥35 mm Hg), starting within 72 hours of diagnosis. The recommended scheduled dosing of oral prednisone during treatment is presented in Table 3.50.

Coinfection with other organisms, such as cytomegalovirus, histoplasmosis, or *Streptococcus pneumoniae*, has been reported in children living with HIV. Children with dual infections may have more severe disease.

Chemoprophylaxis. Chemoprophylaxis is highly effective in preventing PCP among high-risk groups. Prophylaxis against a first episode of PCP is indicated for many patients with significant immunosuppression, including people living with HIV (see Table 3.51 and Human Immunodeficiency Virus Infection, p 489) and people with primary or acquired cell-mediated immunodeficiency.

The recommended drug regimen for PCP prophylaxis for all immunocompromised patients is TMP-SMX. Acceptable dosing intervals and schedules are presented in Table 3.52. For patients who cannot tolerate TMP-SMX, alternative oral choices include atovaquone or dapsone. Atovaquone is effective and safe but expensive. Dapsone is effective and inexpensive but associated with more serious adverse effects than atovaquone. Aerosolized pentamidine is recommended for children who cannot tolerate TMP-SMX, atovaquone, or dapsone and are old enough to use a Respirgard II nebulizer. Intravenous pentamidine has been used but is not recommended for prophylaxis unless no other options are available. Another drug combinations with potential for prophylaxis is pyrimethamine-sulfadoxine, although experience in children for this indication is limited.

In children living with HIV, risk of PCP is associated with age-specific CD4+ T-lymphocyte cell counts and percentages that define severe immunosuppression (Immune Category 3). Because CD4+ T-lymphocyte counts and percentages can decline rapidly in infants with HIV, prophylaxis for PCP is recommended for all infants born to a person living with HIV in resource-limited settings beginning at 4 to 6 weeks of age and continuing until 12 months of age unless a diagnosis of HIV has been excluded presumptively or definitively, in which case prophylaxis should be discontinued (see Table 3.52). Children who are HIV infected or whose HIV status is indeterminate should continue prophylaxis throughout the first year of life. In the United

Table 3.51. Recommendations for *Pneumocystis jirovecii* Pneumonia (PCP) Prophylaxis for Human Immunodeficiency Virus (HIV)-Exposed Infants and Children, by Age and HIV Infection Status[a]

Age and HIV Infection Status	Initiation of PCP prophylaxis[b]	Discontinuation of PCP prophylaxis[b]
Birth through 4 to 6 wk of age, HIV exposed or HIV infected	No prophylaxis	Not applicable
4 to 6 wk through 12 mo of age		
HIV infected or indeterminate	Prophylaxis	Administer throughout first year of life
HIV infection presumptively or definitively excluded[c]	No prophylaxis	Not applicable
1 through 5 y of age, HIV infected	Prophylaxis if: CD4+ T-lymphocyte count is less than 500 cells/μL or percentage is less than 15%[d]	Discontinue if antiretroviral therapy (ART) administered for >6 months, and the following have been sustained for >3 consecutive months: CD4+ T-lymphocyte count 500 cells/μL or greater or percentage is 15% or greater
6 y of age or older, HIV infected	Prophylaxis if: CD4+ T-lymphocyte count is less than 200 cells/μL or percentage is less than 15%[d]	Discontinue if ART administered for >6 months, and the following have been sustained for >3 consecutive months: CD4+ T-lymphocyte count 200 cells/μL or greater or percentage is 15% or greater

[a] Panel on Opportunistic Infections in Children with and Exposed to HIV. Guidelines for the Prevention and Treatment of Opportunistic Infections in Children with and Exposed to HIV. Department of Health and Human Services. Available at: **https://clinicalinfo.hiv.gov/en/guidelines/pediatric-opportunistic-infection**

[b] Children who have had PCP should receive lifelong ("secondary") PCP prophylaxis unless/until they have been on ART for at least 6 months and their CD4+ T-lymphocyte cell counts and percentages achieve and maintain designated age-specific values greater than those indicative of severe immunosuppression (Immune Category 3) for at least 3 months (see Human Immunodeficiency Virus Infection, p 489).

[c] See Human Immunodeficiency Virus Infection, p 489.

[d] Prophylaxis should be considered on a case-by-case basis for children who might otherwise be at risk of PCP, such as children with rapidly declining CD4+ T-lymphocyte counts or percentages.

Table 3.52. Drug Regimens for *Pneumocystis jirovecii* Pneumonia Prophylaxis for Children 4 Weeks and Older[a]

Recommended daily dose:

Trimethoprim-sulfamethoxazole (trimethoprim, 5–10 mg/kg per day; and sulfamethoxazole, 25–50 mg/kg per day, orally). The total daily dose should not exceed 320 mg TMP and 1600 mg SMX.

Acceptable dosing intervals and schedules:
- In divided doses twice daily, given 3 days per week on consecutive days or on alternate days
- In divided doses twice daily, given 2 days per week on consecutive days or on alternate days
- Total dose once daily, given 7 days per week

Alternative regimens if trimethoprim-sulfamethoxazole is not tolerated:
- **Atovaquone**
  - **children 1 through 3 mo of age and older than 24 mo through 12 y of age:** 30 mg/kg (maximum 1500 mg), orally, once a day
  - **children 4 through 24 mo of age:** 45 mg/kg (maximum 1500 mg), orally, once a day
  - **children older than 12 y:** 1500 mg, orally, once a day
- **Dapsone (children 1 mo or older)**
  2 mg/kg (maximum 100 mg), orally, once a day or 4 mg/kg (maximum 200 mg), orally, every week
- **Aerosolized pentamidine (children 5 y or older)**
  300 mg, inhaled monthly via Respirgard II nebulizer

[a]Panel on Opportunistic Infections in Children with and Exposed to HIV. Guidelines for the Prevention and Treatment of Opportunistic Infections in Children with and Exposed to HIV. Department of Health and Human Services. Available at: **https://clinicalinfo.hiv.gov/en/guidelines/pediatric-opportunistic-infection**

States, in HIV-exposed infants who are deemed low risk for HIV seroconversion, PCP prophylaxis is not indicated unless there is evidence of HIV transmission in the infant.

For children with HIV ages 12 months or older, initiation and discontinuation of PCP prophylaxis is detailed in Table 3.51. In patients with AIDS who had PCP, prophylaxis should be initiated at the end of therapy for acute infection. In most cases, secondary prophylaxis can be discontinued using the same criteria as for primary prophylaxis (see Table 3.51). Prophylaxis should be continued at least through 12 months of life for infants with HIV, or lifelong if CD4+ T-lymphocyte counts or percentages do not exceed the thresholds shown in Table 3.51 in response to antiretroviral therapy.

Prophylaxis for PCP is recommended for children who have received hematopoietic cell transplants (HCTs)[1] or solid organ transplants; children with hematologic malignancies (eg, leukemia or lymphoma) and some nonhematologic malignancies; children with severe cell-mediated immunodeficiency, including children who received adrenocorticotropic hormone for treatment of infantile spasms; and children who otherwise are immunocompromised and who have had a previous episode of PCP. For this diverse group of immunocompromised hosts, the risk of PCP varies with duration and

[1] Center for International Blood and Marrow Research; National Marrow Donor program; European Blood and Marrow Transplant Group; American Society of Blood and Marrow Transplantation; Canadian Blood and Marrow Transplant Group; Infectious Diseases Society of America; Society for Healthcare Epidemiology of America; Association of Medical Microbiology and Infectious Disease Canada; Centers for Disease Control and Prevention. Guidelines for preventing infectious complications among hematopoietic cell transplant recipients: a global perspective. *Biol Blood Marrow Transplant.* 2009;15(10):1143-1238

intensity of chemotherapy, with other immunosuppressive therapies, with coinfection with immunosuppressive viruses (eg, cytomegalovirus), and local epidemiologic rates of PCP. Guidelines for allogeneic HCT recipients recommend that PCP prophylaxis be initiated at engraftment (or before engraftment, if engraftment is delayed) and administered for at least 6 months in autologous HCT recipients and for at least 1 year in allogeneic transplant recipients, especially matched unrelated or haploidentical transplants who may receive in vivo T-lymphocyte depletion with antithymocyte globulin (ATG) or with Campath (alemtuzumab). Prophylaxis should be continued in all children receiving ongoing or intensified immunosuppressive therapy (eg, prednisone or cyclosporine) or in children with chronic graft-versus-host disease. Guidelines for PCP prophylaxis for solid organ transplant recipients are less definitive. In general, PCP prophylaxis is recommended for all solid organ transplant recipients for at least 6 to 12 months posttransplant, although longer durations should be considered. For lung and small bowel transplant recipients, as well as any transplant patient with a history of prior PCP infection or chronic cytomegalovirus disease, lifelong prophylaxis may be indicated.

INFECTION PREVENTION AND CONTROL MEASURES IN HEALTH CARE SETTINGS: Standard precautions are recommended. Some experts recommend that because of the theoretical risk for airborne transmission, patients with PCP should not share a room with other immunocompromised patients, especially patients who are not receiving PCP prophylaxis. Data are insufficient to support this recommendation as standard practice.

CONTROL MEASURES: Appropriate therapy for infected patients and prophylaxis in immunocompromised patients are the only available means of control. Detailed guidelines for children, adolescents, and adults with HIV have been issued by the Department of Health and Human Services.[1,2]

Poliovirus Infections

CLINICAL MANIFESTATIONS: Approximately 70% of poliovirus infections in susceptible children are asymptomatic. Nonspecific illness with low-grade fever and sore throat (minor illness) occurs in approximately 25% of infected people, and viral meningitis (nonparalytic polio), sometimes accompanied by paresthesias, occurs in 1% to 5% of patients a few days after the minor illness has resolved. Rapid onset of asymmetric acute flaccid paralysis with areflexia of the involved limb (paralytic poliomyelitis) occurs in fewer than 1% of infections, with residual paresis in approximately two thirds of patients. Classical paralytic polio begins with a minor illness characterized by fever, sore throat, headache, nausea, constipation, and/or malaise for several days, followed by a symptom-free period of 1 to 3 days. Rapid onset of paralysis then follows.

---

[1] Panel on Opportunistic Infections in Children with and Exposed to HIV. Guidelines for the Prevention and Treatment of Opportunistic Infections in Children with and Exposed to HIV. Department of Health and Human Services. Available at: **https://clinicalinfo.hiv.gov/en/guidelines/pediatric-opportunistic-infection**

[2] Panel on Guidelines for the Prevention and Treatment of Opportunistic Infections in Adults and Adolescents with HIV. Guidelines for the Prevention and Treatment of Opportunistic Infections in Adults and Adolescents with HIV. National Institutes of Health, Centers for Disease Control and Prevention, HIV Medicine Association, and Infectious Diseases Society of America. Available at: **https://clinicalinfo.hiv.gov/en/guidelines/adult-andadolescent-opportunistic-infection**

Typically, paralysis is asymmetric and affects the proximal muscles more than the distal muscles. Cranial nerve involvement (bulbar poliomyelitis) and paralysis of the diaphragm and intercostal muscles may lead to impaired respiration requiring assisted ventilation. Sensation usually is intact. The cerebrospinal fluid (CSF) profile is characteristic of viral meningitis, with mild pleocytosis and lymphocytic predominance.

Adults who contracted paralytic poliomyelitis during childhood may develop the noninfectious post-polio syndrome 15 to 40 years later, characterized by slow and irreversible exacerbation of weakness in the muscle groups affected during the original infection. Muscle and joint pain also are common manifestations. The estimated incidence of post-polio syndrome in poliomyelitis survivors is 25% to 40%.

ETIOLOGY: Polioviruses are classified as members of the family *Picornaviridae*, genus *Enterovirus*, in the species enterovirus C, and include 3 serotypes. They are nonenveloped, positive-sense, single-stranded RNA viruses that are stable in moderate environmental conditions. Acute paralytic disease may be caused by naturally occurring (wild) polioviruses (WPVs) or by circulating vaccine-derived polioviruses (cVDPVs) that have acquired virulence properties that are indistinguishable from WPVs as a result of sustained person-to-person transmission in the absence of adequate population immunity. Rarely, oral poliovirus vaccine (OPV) viruses may cause vaccine-associated paralytic poliomyelitis (VAPP) in vaccine recipients or their close contacts. People with primary (but not acquired) B-lymphocyte immunodeficiencies are at increased risk both of VAPP and of persistent infection (immunodeficiency-associated vaccine-derived polioviruses, or iVDPVs) from vaccine virus.

EPIDEMIOLOGY: Humans are the only natural reservoir for poliovirus. Spread is by contact with feces and/or respiratory secretions. Infection is more common in infants and young children and occurs at an earlier age among children living in poor hygienic conditions. In temperate climates, poliovirus infections are most common during summer and autumn; in the tropics, the seasonal pattern is less pronounced. With continuing progress toward global polio eradication, more cases of paralytic disease are now caused by cVDPVs than by wild polioviruses.

The last cases of poliomyelitis attributable to indigenously acquired WPVs in the United States were reported in 1979. Subsequently, there have been rare, imported cases and rare cases of VAPP (6–8 people annually) prior to the shift in US immunization policy in 1997 from use of OPV to a sequential inactivated (non-live) poliovirus (IPV) vaccine/OPV schedule. Implementation of an all-IPV vaccine schedule in 2000 halted the occurrence of VAPP cases in the United States. In 2011, a case of iVDPV serotype 2 (iVDPV2) was reported in a patient with common variable immunodeficiency who was chronically infected for about 12 years. In 2022, a case of poliomyelitis attributable to cVDPV serotype 2 (cVDPV2) occurred in an unvaccinated young adult who was part of an undervaccinated community.[1] Strong efforts to increase vaccination in undervaccinated communities are essential to prevent cases of poliomyelitis, even in the United States.

WPV serotype 2 (WPV2) and WPV serotype 3 (WPV3) were declared eradicated by the World Health Organization (WHO) in 2015 and 2019, respectively; the last

---

[1] Link-Gelles R, Lutterloh E, Schnabel Ruppert P, et al. Public health response to a case of paralytic poliomyelitis in an unvaccinated person and detection of poliovirus in wastewater—New York, June–August 2022. *MMWR Morb Mortal Wkly Rep.* 2022;71(33):1065-1068

WPV2 poliomyelitis case was detected in 1999 in India, and the last WPV3 poliomyelitis case occurred in Nigeria in 2012. WPV serotype 1 (WPV1) now accounts for all cases attributable to wild poliovirus. WPV1 remains endemic in Afghanistan and Pakistan, and in 2022, there was importation of WPV1 into Malawi and Mozambique.

Because the only source of disease from serotype 2 poliovirus was related to vaccine use, there was a global switch from trivalent OPV (tOPV) to bivalent OPV (bOPV) in April 2016, thus ending all routine immunization with live serotype 2 poliovirus-containing oral vaccines. Concurrent recommendations were made for all countries to provide at least 1 dose of IPV to all vaccinees. Following this vaccine change, the remaining risk of serotype 2 infection comes from continued transmission of serotype 2 OPV viruses administered before the switch, ongoing cVDPV outbreaks, long-term iVDPV2 excreters, and breach of containment at facilities maintaining serotype 2 polioviruses. Containment of infectious and potentially infectious materials containing polioviruses by destroying the materials or transferring material to accredited polio essential facilities is an important part of the strategy for global polio eradication. The National Authority for the Containment of Polio at the Centers for Disease Control and Prevention (CDC) is responsible for containment activities in the United States **(www.cdc.gov/orr/poliaviruscontainment/index.htm).**

Communicability of poliovirus is greatest shortly before and after onset of clinical illness, when the virus is present in the throat and excreted in high concentrations in feces. Virus persists in the throat for approximately 1 to 2 weeks after onset of illness and is excreted in feces for an average of 3 to 6 weeks. In recipients of OPV, virus also persists in the throat for 1 to 2 weeks and is excreted in feces for several weeks, although in rare cases, excretion for more than 2 months can occur. Immunocompromised patients with significant primary B-lymphocyte immune deficiencies have excreted iVDPV for periods of more than 30 years.

The **incubation period of nonparalytic polio** is 3 to 6 days. For the onset of poliomyelitis, the **incubation period to paralysis** usually is 7 to 21 days (range, 3–35 days).

DIAGNOSTIC TESTS: Poliovirus can be detected in specimens from the pharynx and feces, less commonly from urine, and rarely from CSF by isolation in cell culture or a nucleic acid amplification test (NAAT). The relatively low sensitivity of isolation in cell culture from CSF is likely attributable to low viral load. Fecal material and pharyngeal swab specimens are most likely to yield virus in cell culture.

The diagnostic test of choice for confirming polio is viral culture of stool specimens and throat swab specimens obtained as early in the course of illness as possible. There currently are nucleic acid amplification tests for enteroviruses from CSF and at least several multiplexed assays that detect enteroviruses, in addition to other bacterial and viral agents. Such commonly used molecular tests for enteroviruses will detect poliovirus but will not differentiate poliovirus from other enteroviruses and, therefore, are insufficient to demonstrate that poliovirus is the etiology of disease. In these situations, additional testing of the virus will be necessary to confirm the diagnosis of poliovirus-related disease.

NAATs generally have sensitivity that is comparable to or better than cell culture and may be more likely to identify poliovirus in CSF. Two or more stool and throat swab specimens for enterovirus isolation or detection by NAAT should be obtained at least 24 hours apart from patients with suspected paralytic poliomyelitis as early in the course of illness as possible, ideally within 14 days of onset of symptoms. Poliovirus may be excreted intermittently, and a single negative test result does not rule out infection.

Molecular methods have replaced neutralization for identification and typing to differentiate wild type from vaccine derived virus strains.

Because OPV no longer is available in the United States, the chance of exposure to OPV viruses has become remote. Therefore, if a poliovirus is isolated in the United States, the isolate should be reported immediately to the state health department and sent to the CDC through the state health department for further testing.

TREATMENT: Management is supportive. There are no antiviral agents approved by the US Food and Drug Administration for the treatment of poliovirus infections. Several poliovirus antivirals are in early stage development, however, including pocapavir (a capsid inhibitor), which is being evaluated in combination with V-7404 (a protease inhibitor). However, safety and dosing information for these products is limited, especially in children.

INFECTION PREVENTION AND CONTROL MEASURES IN HEALTH CARE SETTINGS: In addition to standard precautions, contact precautions are indicated for infants and young children for the duration of hospitalization.

CONTROL MEASURES:

Immunization of Infants and Children.

Vaccines. Only IPV is available in the United States. IPV contains the 3 serotypes, which are grown in Vero cells or human diploid cells and inactivated with formaldehyde. IPV also is available in combination with other childhood vaccines (see Table 1.10, p 65). In 2016, bivalent live attenuated oral poliovirus vaccine (bOPV), which contains types 1 and 3 poliovirus serotypes, became the primary vaccine used in low- and middle-income countries that rely on OPV for routine infant immunization. bOPV is produced in monkey kidney cells or human diploid cells.

Immunogenicity and Efficacy. Both IPV and OPV, in their recommended schedules, are highly immunogenic and effective in preventing poliomyelitis. Administration of IPV results in seroconversion in 95% or more of vaccine recipients to each of the 3 serotypes after 2 doses and results in seroconversion in 99% to 100% of recipients after 3 doses. Immunity probably is lifelong. Following exposure to live poliovirus, most IPV-immunized children will excrete virus from stool but not from the oropharynx. Stool excretion quantities and duration are modestly reduced compared with shedding from unimmunized people. Immunization with 3 or more doses of OPV induces excellent serum antibody responses and substantial intestinal immunity against poliovirus reinfection. A 3-dose series of OPV, as formerly used in the United States, results in sustained, probably lifelong immunity. After 3 doses of OPV, seroconversion rates are lower in some low-income countries, likely because of chronic enteropathy and interference by other enteric pathogens with the replication of the OPV vaccine strains.

Administration With Other Vaccines. Either IPV or OPV may be administered concurrently with other routinely recommended childhood vaccines (see Simultaneous Administration of Multiple Vaccines, p 63). For administration of combination vaccines containing IPV (see Table 1.10, p 65) with other vaccines and interchangeability of the combined vaccine with other vaccine products, see Pertussis (p 656), Hepatitis B (p 437), *Haemophilus influenzae* Infections (p 400), and *Streptococcus pneumoniae* [Pneumococcal] Infections (p 810).

Adverse Reactions. Most adverse reactions to IPV are mild and self-limited (eg, injection site pain and fever). Serious reactions to IPV are rare. Because IPV may contain trace amounts of streptomycin, neomycin, and polymyxin B, allergic reactions are possible in recipients with hypersensitivity to one or more of these antimicrobial agents. Allergic reactions to other ingredients or components of IPV are also possible.

OPV can cause VAPP. Before exclusive use of IPV in the United States beginning in 2000, the overall risk of VAPP associated with OPV was approximately 1 case per 2.4 million doses of OPV distributed. The rate of VAPP following the first dose, including vaccine recipient and contact cases, was approximately 1 case per 750 000 doses.

Schedule.[1] Four doses of IPV are recommended for routine immunization of all infants and children in the United States.

Refugee and Immigrant Children. Refugee and immigrant children should meet recommendations of the Advisory Committee on Immunization Practices of the CDC for poliovirus vaccination, which include protection against all 3 poliovirus serotypes by age-appropriate vaccination with IPV or trivalent OPV (tOPV). Only written documentation or receipt of IPV or tOPV constitutes proof of vaccination according to US polio vaccination recommendations. If OPV was administered prior to April 1, 2016, OPV can be counted as tOPV. If OPV was administered after April 1, 2016, it may not be counted as tOPV unless the written documentation denotes that it is tOPV. For children incompletely immunized with tOPV, the series should be completed with IPV according to the catch-up schedule outlined below. In the absence of adequate written vaccination records, vaccination or revaccination in accordance with the age appropriate IPV schedule for the United States is recommended. Serologic testing to assess immunity no longer is available.[2]

- The first 2 doses of the 4-dose IPV series should be administered at 2-month intervals beginning at 2 months of age (minimum age, 6 weeks), and a third dose is recommended at 6 through 18 months of age. Doses may be administered at 4-week intervals when accelerated protection is indicated.
- Administration of the third dose at 6 months of age has the potential advantage of enhancing the likelihood of completion of the primary series and does not compromise seroconversion.
- A fourth and final dose in the series should be administered at 4 years or older and at a minimum interval of 6 months from the third dose.
- The final dose in the IPV series at 4 years or older should be administered regardless of the number of previous doses; a fourth dose is not necessary if the third dose was administered at 4 years or older and a minimum of 6 months after the second dose.
- When IPV is administered in combination with other vaccines at 2, 4, 6, and 12 through 15 months of age, it is necessary to administer a fifth and final dose of IPV at 4 years or older. The minimum interval from dose 4 to dose 5 should be at least 6 months.

---

[1] Centers for Disease Control and Prevention. Updated recommendations of the Advisory Committee on Immunization Practices (ACIP) regarding routine poliovirus vaccination. *MMWR Morb Mortal Wkly Rep.* 2009;58(30):829-830

[2] Marin M, Patel M, Oberste S, Pallansch MA. Guidance for assessment of poliovirus vaccination status and vaccination of children who have received poliovirus vaccine outside the United States. *MMWR Morb Mortal Wkly Rep.* 2017;66(1):23-25

- If a child misses an IPV dose at 4 through 6 years of age, the child should receive a booster dose as soon as feasible. More information on the polio vaccine schedule can be found at: **www.cdc.gov/vaccines/schedules/hcp/imz/child-adolescent.html.**

   OPV remains the vaccine of choice for global eradication, although the Strategic Advisory Group of Experts on Immunization (SAGE) of the WHO has recommended that all countries currently using bOPV now include 2 doses of IPV into their routine immunization schedules to mitigate the risk of VDPV serotype 2 poliomyelitis.[1] A novel OPV serotype 2 vaccine (nOPV2), which provides comparable protection but is more genetically stable than serotype 2 monovalent OPV, is available to countries through the WHO Emergency Use Listing procedures for deployment in responding to cVDPV2 outbreaks **(https://polioeradication.org/nopv2/).**

   Children Incompletely Immunized. Children who have not received the recommended doses of poliovirus vaccines on schedule should receive sufficient doses of IPV to complete the immunization series for their age **(http://aapredbook.aappublications.org/site/resources/izschedules.xhtml).**

Vaccine Recommendations for Adults. Most adults residing in the United States are presumed to be immune to poliovirus from previous immunization and have only a small risk of exposure to wild poliovirus in the United States. For those traveling to areas where poliovirus infection occurs, immunization or booster should be provided as per CDC guidance **(wwwnc.cdc.gov/travel/yellowbook/2024/infections-diseases/poliomyelitis).** Countries are considered to have active poliovirus circulation if they have ongoing endemic circulation, active outbreaks, or environmental evidence of active circulation with either WPV or VDPVs.

   For unimmunized adults, primary immunization with IPV is recommended. Adults without documentation of vaccination history should be considered unimmunized. Two doses of IPV should be administered at intervals of 1 to 2 months (4–8 weeks); a third dose is administered 6 to 12 months after the second dose. If time does not allow 3 doses of IPV to be administered according to the recommended schedule before protection is required, the following alternatives are recommended:

- If protection is not needed until 8 weeks or more, 3 doses of IPV should be administered at least 4 weeks apart (eg, at weeks 0, 4, and 8).
- If protection is not needed for 4 to 8 weeks, 2 doses of IPV should be administered at least 4 weeks apart (eg, at weeks 0 and 4).
- If protection is needed in fewer than 4 weeks, a single dose of IPV should be administered.

   The remaining doses of IPV to complete the primary immunization schedule should be administered subsequently at the recommended intervals if the person remains at an increased risk.

   Recommendations in other circumstances are as follows:

- **Incompletely immunized adults.** Adults who previously received less than a full primary series of OPV or IPV should receive the remaining required doses of IPV, a minimum of 4 weeks since the last dose.

---

[1] World Health Organization. Weekly Epidemiological Record. 2020;95:596-598. Available at: **https://apps.who.int/iris/bitstream/handle/10665/337100/WER9548-eng-fre.pdf**

- **Adults who are at an increased risk of exposure to WPV or cVDPV and who previously completed primary immunization with OPV or IPV.** These adults can receive a single dose of IPV. Available data do not indicate the need for more than a single lifetime booster dose with IPV.

  Travelers also may be affected by WHO and CDC polio vaccination recommendations for people residing for 4 or more consecutive weeks in countries with ongoing poliovirus transmission and who are traveling to polio-free countries.[1]

- All residents and long-term visitors (defined as a duration of more than 4 weeks) should receive an additional dose of IPV between 4 weeks and 12 months before international travel and have the dose documented.

- Residents and long-term visitors who currently are in those countries who must travel with fewer than 4 weeks' notice and have not been vaccinated with OPV or IPV within the previous 4 weeks to 12 months should receive a dose at least by the time of departure.

The list of countries affected by this recommendation can be found online (**http://polioeradication.org/polio-today/polio-now/public-health-emergency-status/**).

Precautions and Contraindications to Immunization.

Immunocompromised People. Immunocompromised patients, including people with human immunodeficiency virus (HIV) infection; combined immunodeficiency; abnormalities of immunoglobulin synthesis (ie, antibody deficiency syndromes); leukemia, lymphoma, or generalized malignant neoplasm; or people receiving immunosuppressive therapy with pharmacologic agents (see Immunization and Other Considerations in Immunocompromised Children, p 93) or radiation therapy should receive IPV. OPV should not be used. The immune response to IPV in immunocompromised patients may vary depending on their level of immunosuppression.

Household Contacts of Immunocompromised People or People With Altered Immune States or Immunosuppression Attributable to Therapy for Other Disease. IPV is recommended for these people, and OPV should not be used. If OPV inadvertently is introduced into a household of an immunocompromised person, close contact between the patient and the OPV recipient should be minimized for approximately 4 to 6 weeks after immunization. Household members should be counseled on practices that will minimize exposure of the immunocompromised to excreted poliovirus vaccine. These practices include exercising hand hygiene after contact with the child by all and avoiding diaper changing by the immunosuppressed person.

Pregnancy. If a pregnant person is at increased risk of exposure and protection against polioviruses is needed, IPV is recommended. There is no evidence that IPV is unsafe in pregnant people or their developing fetuses.

Hypersensitivity or Anaphylactic Reactions to IPV Vaccine or Antimicrobial Agents Contained in IPV. IPV is contraindicated for people who have experienced an anaphylactic reaction after a previous dose of IPV attributable to any component of the vaccine.

Breastfeeding. Breastfeeding is not a contraindication to IPV or OPV administration.

Reporting of Adverse Events After Immunization. Any case of VAPP should be reported to the Vaccine Adverse Event Reporting System (VAERS). This and other reporting

---

[1] Centers for Disease Control and Prevention. Interim CDC guidance for polio vaccination for travel to and from countries affected by wild poliovirus. *MMWR Morb Mortal Wkly Rep.* 2014;63(27):591-594

requirements for adverse events following IPV and OPV are listed in the VAERS Table of Reportable Events (**https://vaers.hhs.gov/docs/VAERS_Table_of_Reportable_Events_Following_Vaccination.pdf**). In addition, reporting is encouraged for any clinically significant adverse event following a vaccination, even if uncertainty exists as to whether a vaccine caused the event (see Understanding Vaccine Evaluation and Safety as an Approach to Addressing Parental Concerns, p 27).

Public Health Reporting. A suspected case of poliomyelitis or a nonparalytic poliovirus infection, regardless of whether the virus is suspected to be WPV or VDPV, should be considered a **public health emergency** and **reported immediately** to the state health department; this results in an immediate epidemiologic investigation. Poliomyelitis should be considered in the differential diagnosis of all cases of acute flaccid paralysis, including Guillain-Barré syndrome, transverse myelitis, and acute flaccid myelitis (acute neurologic illness associated with limb weakness in children, which is associated with enterovirus D68 and less commonly with enterovirus A71, or other nonpolio enteroviruses; see Enterovirus [Nonpoliovirus], p 369).[1] If the course is compatible clinically with poliomyelitis, specimens should be obtained for virologic studies (see Diagnostic Tests, p 684). If evidence implicates wild poliovirus or a VDPV infection, an intensive investigation will be conducted, and a public health decision will be made about the need for supplementary immunizations, choice of vaccine, and other actions. Because most people who transmit poliovirus either are clinically asymptomatic or have a minor illness, the source person who transmitted virus to the patient with paralytic polio may be difficult to identify (eg, there may be no known contact with someone who traveled to an area with endemic or epidemic polio). Therefore, pediatricians should be guided by the clinical presentation in deciding whether a child with acute paralysis might have polio and warrant reporting the suspected case to public health authorities.

Polyomaviruses (BK, JC, and Other Polyomaviruses)

CLINICAL MANIFESTATIONS: BK virus (BKV) infection and JC virus (JCV) infection in humans usually occur in childhood and seemingly result in lifelong persistence. More than 80% of adults are seropositive for BKV. Primary infection with BKV in immunocompetent children generally is asymptomatic, although it may result in mild upper respiratory tract symptoms. BKV is more likely to cause disease in immunocompromised people, including hemorrhagic cystitis in hematopoietic cell transplant recipients and interstitial nephritis and ureteral stenosis in renal transplant recipients. BKV-associated nephropathy occurs in 3% to 8% of renal transplant recipients and less frequently in other solid organ transplant recipients. The primary symptom of BKV-associated hemorrhagic cystitis among immunocompromised children is painful hematuria; blood clots in the urine and secondary obstructive nephropathy also can occur. Often, however, BKV nephropathy is asymptomatic, and therefore should be suspected in any renal transplant recipient with allograft dysfunction. More than half of renal allograft patients with BKV-associated nephropathy may experience allograft loss.

---

[1] Centers for Disease Control and Prevention. Acute neurologic illness of unknown etiology in children—Colorado, August–September 2014. *MMWR Morb Mortal Wkly.* 2014;63(40):901-902

JCV is the cause of progressive multifocal leukoencephalopathy (PML), a demyelinating disease of the central nervous system that occurs in severely immunocompromised patients, including patients with acquired immunodeficiency syndrome (AIDS), patients receiving intensive chemotherapy, hematopoietic cell or solid organ transplant recipients, and patients receiving various monoclonal antibody therapies for treatment of autoimmune, oncologic, and neurologic diseases. PML, the only known disease caused by JCV, occurs in approximately 3% to 5% of untreated adults with acquired immunodeficiency syndrome (AIDS) but is rare in children with AIDS. Symptoms include cognitive disturbance, hemiparesis, ataxia, cranial nerve dysfunction, and aphasia. Lytic infection of oligodendrocytes by JCV is the primary mechanism of pathogenesis for PML. In the absence of restored T-lymphocyte function, PML almost always is fatal. PML is an AIDS-defining illness in people with human immunodeficiency virus (HIV) infection.[1] Approximately 50% to 60% of adults are infected by JCV, with infections being acquired during adolescence and early adulthood.

Of the polyomaviruses catalogued to date, 14 have been detected in humans, but only a few have been associated with disease, including BK and JC viruses. The Merkel cell polyomavirus (MCPyV) has been detected in >80% of Merkel cell carcinomas, which are rare neuroendocrine tumors of the skin. The trichodysplasia spinulosa-associated polyomavirus (TSPyV) has been identified in tissue from patients with trichodysplasia spinulosa, a rare follicular disease of immunocompromised patients that primarily affects the face. The KI polyomavirus (KIPyV) and WU polyomavirus (WUPyV) have been identified in respiratory tract secretions, primarily in association with known pathogenic viruses of the respiratory tract. Human polyomaviruses 6 and 7 (HPyV6 and HPyV7) have been detected as asymptomatic inhabitants of human skin. Human polyomavirus 9 (HPyV9) has been detected in the serum of some renal transplant recipients. The natural history, prevalence, and pathogenic potential of these recently discovered human polyomaviruses have not been established.

ETIOLOGY: Polyomaviruses are members of the family *Polyomaviridae*. BKV, JCV, WUPyV, and KIPyV are members of the genus *Betapolyomavirus;* MCPyV, TSPyV, HPyV9, HPyV12, and New Jersey polyomavirus are members of the genus *Alphapolyomavirus*; HPyV6, HPyV7, Malawi polyomavirus, and St. Louis polyomavirus are members of the genus *Deltapolyomavirus*. They are nonenveloped viruses with a circular double-stranded DNA genome with icosahedral symmetry of the capsid ranging 40 to 50 nm in diameter. One of the biological characteristics of the polyomaviruses is the maintenance of a chronic viral infection in their host with few or no symptoms. Symptomatic disease caused by human polyomavirus infections occurs almost exclusively in immunosuppressed people. Four genotypes of BKV have been identified; genotype 1 BKV accounts for the majority of cases of BKV nephropathy.

EPIDEMIOLOGY: Humans are the only known natural hosts for BKV and JCV. The mode of transmission of BKV and JCV is uncertain, but the respiratory route and the oral route by water or food have been postulated. BKV and JCV are ubiquitous in the human population, with BKV infection occurring in early childhood and JCV

---

[1] Panel on Opportunistic Infections in Children with and Exposed to HIV. Guidelines for the Prevention and Treatment of Opportunistic Infections in Children with and Exposed to HIV. Department of Health and Human Services. Available at: **https://clinicalinfo.hiv.gov/en/guidelines/pediatric-opportunistic-infection**

infection occurring primarily in adolescence and adulthood. BKV persists in the renal epithelial and urothelial cells and gastrointestinal tract of healthy subjects, with urinary excretion occurring in 3% to 5% of healthy adults. JCV persists in the kidney, gastrointestinal tract, and brain of healthy people. The prevalence of urinary excretion of JCV increases with age.

DIAGNOSTIC TESTS: Detection of BKV T-antigen by immunohistochemical analysis of renal biopsy material with characteristic cytopathic changes is the gold standard for diagnosis of BKV-associated nephropathy, but nucleic acid amplification tests (NAATs) are the most sensitive tools for rapid viral screening for polyomaviruses and quantification of viral load. Prospective monitoring of BK viral DNA load in plasma using NAATs is common after renal transplantation to monitor for BKV-associated nephropathy. Detection of BKV nucleic acid in plasma by NAAT is associated with an increased risk of BKV-associated nephropathy, especially when BKV viral loads exceed 10 000 genomes/mL, but detection of BKV in urine of renal transplant recipients is common and does not predict BKV disease after renal transplantation. Both BKV and JCV can be propagated in cell culture, but culture plays no role in the laboratory diagnosis of infection attributable to these agents. Antibody assays are used commonly to detect presence of specific antibodies against individual viruses, but their use in clinical practice is limited.

Diagnosis of BKV-associated hemorrhagic cystitis is made clinically when other causes of urinary tract bleeding are excluded. Among hematopoietic cell transplant recipients, detection of BKV by NAAT in urine is common (more than 50%), but BKV-associated hemorrhagic cystitis is much less common (10%–15%). Prolonged urinary shedding of BKV and detection of BKV in plasma after hematopoietic cell transplantation has been associated with increased risk of developing BKV-associated hemorrhagic cystitis. Urine cytologic testing may suggest urinary shedding of BKV on the basis of presence of decoy cells, which resemble renal carcinoma cells, but decoy cells do not have high sensitivity or specificity for BKV disease.

A confirmed diagnosis of PML attributable to JCV requires a compatible clinical syndrome and magnetic resonance imaging or computed tomographic findings showing lesions in the brain white matter coupled with brain biopsy findings. JCV can be demonstrated by in situ hybridization, electron microscopy, or immunohistochemistry of brain biopsy or autopsy material. There are no FDA-cleared NAATs for detection of JCV. Diagnosis of PML can be facilitated when JCV DNA is detected in cerebrospinal fluid by a NAAT, which may obviate the need for a brain biopsy. Early in the course of PML, false-negative NAAT results have been reported, so repeat testing is warranted when clinical suspicion of PML is high. Measurement of JCV DNA concentrations in cerebrospinal fluid samples may be a useful marker for managing PML in patients with AIDS who are receiving antiretroviral therapy.

TREATMENT: Multiple studies evaluating treatment options for polyomavirus diseases are ongoing (**www.clinicaltrials.gov**). At this time there is no proven antiviral therapy for BKV nephropathy. Closely monitored reduction of immunosuppression remains the mainstay of treatment. Efficacy of other agents used as adjunctive therapy (immune globulin intravenous [IGIV], leflunomide, cidofovir) has not been established. Fluoroquinolones are not recommended for prophylaxis or treatment of BKV-associated nephropathy based on results of prospective, controlled studies.

Most patients with BKV-hemorrhagic cystitis after hematopoietic cell transplantation require only supportive care because restoration of immune function by cell engraftment ultimately will control BKV replication. In severe cases, surgical intervention may be required to stop bladder hemorrhage. Parenteral and/or intravesicular cidofovir have been used for treatment, but data from prospective, controlled studies on its efficacy and safety are lacking. Use of systemic cidofovir must be balanced against its high risk of nephrotoxicity. Adoptive transfer of BKV-specific T lymphocytes has been used with varying success at some transplant centers.

Restoration of immune function (eg, antiretroviral therapy for patients with AIDS) is necessary for survival of patients with PML. Cidofovir has not been shown to be effective for treatment of PML. For patients with monoclonal antibody-associated PML (eg, natalizumab), plasmapheresis and/or immune stimulatory agents (eg, granulocyte colony-stimulating factor) may be useful to improve outcomes. Infusion of allogeneic BKV-specific T-lymphocytes, IL-7 homologues, and the use of monoclonal antibodies to inhibit programmed cell death protein 1 (PD-1) have shown encouraging results for patients with PML but remain experimental at this time.

INFECTION PREVENTION AND CONTROL MEASURES IN HEALTH CARE SETTINGS: Standard precautions are recommended.

CONTROL MEASURES: None.

Prion Diseases: Transmissible Spongiform Encephalopathies

CLINICAL MANIFESTATIONS: Prion diseases, or transmissible spongiform encephalopathies (TSEs), constitute a group of rare, rapidly progressive, universally fatal, transmissible neurodegenerative diseases of humans and animals characterized by neuronal degeneration, reactive gliosis, and most often, spongiform degeneration in the cerebral cortical, subcortical, and cerebellar gray matter,. These findings are accompanied by accumulation of an abnormal misfolded, partially protease-resistant "prion" (proteinaceous infectious) protein. The normal protease-sensitive isomer of the protein is called "cellular" prion protein or PrP^C. The protease-resistant pathogenic form of the prion protein is variably called PrP^{res}, scrapie prion protein (PrP^{sc}, named for the first known prion disease affecting sheep), or as suggested by the World Health Organization, TSE-associated PrP (PrP^{TSE}). PrP^{TSE} distributes widely, albeit unevenly, throughout the central nervous system, sometimes forming plaques of varying morphologies.

Human prion diseases include several sporadic, genetic, and acquired diseases: Creutzfeldt-Jakob disease (CJD), variably protease-sensitive prionopathy (VPSPr), Gerstmann-Sträussler-Scheinker disease, fatal familial insomnia and sporadic fatal insomnia, kuru, and variant CJD (vCJD, caused by the agent of bovine spongiform encephalopathy [BSE], commonly called "mad cow" disease). CJD can be sporadic (approximately 85% of cases), genetic (approximately 10%–15% of cases), or iatrogenic (fewer than 1% of cases). Sporadic CJD most commonly is a disease of older adults (median age of death in the United States, 68 years) but also has been described in adolescents and young adults. Iatrogenic CJD has been acquired through intramuscular injection of contaminated cadaveric pituitary hormones (growth hormone and human gonadotropin), dura mater allografts, corneal transplantation, use of contaminated instruments in neurosurgery, and electroencephalographic probe electrodes.

In 1996, an outbreak of a new variant of CJD (vCJD) was linked to consumption of beef from BSE-infected cattle in the United Kingdom and France, with index cases occurring in teenagers. Since the end of 2003, 4 presumptive cases of transfusion-transmitted vCJD have been reported: 3 clinical cases as well as 1 asymptomatic case in which PrP^{TSE} was detected in the spleen and lymph nodes but not brain tissues. A fifth possible iatrogenic vCJD infection was reported in the United Kingdom, affecting a patient with hemophilia, also asymptomatic, who had PrP^{TSE} in the spleen; preclinical vCJD was attributed to treatment with plasma-derived coagulation factor fractionated in the United Kingdom; the plasma product implicated in transmitting vCJD was never marketed in the United States.

The best-known prion diseases affecting animals include scrapie of sheep and goats, BSE of cattle, and a chronic wasting disease (CWD) of North American deer, elk, and moose (**www.cdc.gov/prions/index.html**). CWD recently was detected in reindeer and moose (European elk) in Norway, Sweden, and Finland. Except for vCJD, no human prion disease has been attributed convincingly to infection with an agent of animal origin.

CJD manifests most typically as a rapidly progressive neurologic disease with escalating defects in memory, personality, and other higher cortical functions. Approximately one third of patients have cerebellar dysfunction at presentation, including ataxia, incoordination, and dysarthria. Iatrogenic CJD also may manifest as dementia with cerebellar signs. Myoclonus develops in at least 80% of affected patients at some point in the course of disease. Death usually occurs in weeks to months (median, 4–5 months); only 10% to 20% of patients with sporadic CJD survive for more than 1 year.

vCJD is distinguished from classic CJD by younger age at onset (median age at death around 28 years), early "psychiatric" manifestations, and other features such as painful sensations in the limbs, delayed onset of overt neurologic signs, relative absence of diagnostic electroencephalographic changes, and a more prolonged duration of illness (median, 13–14 months). A high proportion of people with vCJD, but not classic CJD, exhibit high signal abnormalities on T2-weighted brain magnetic resonance imaging in the pulvinar region of the posterior thalamus (known as the "pulvinar sign"). Neuropathologic examination in vCJD reveals highly reproducible pathology with spongiform vacuolation and numerous "florid" plaques (compact flower-like amyloid plaques surrounded by vacuoles) and exceptionally striking punctate deposition of PrP^{TSE} in the basal ganglia. PrP^{TSE} is detectable by immunohistochemistry in the tonsils, appendix, spleen, and lymph nodes of patients with vCJD.

ETIOLOGY: The proteinaceous infectious particle (or prion) widely believed to cause human and animal prion diseases consists of PrP^{TSE}, the misfolded form of PrP^{C}, a ubiquitous normal sialoglycoprotein of unknown function found on the surfaces of neurons and many other cells of humans and animals. It has been postulated by some authorities that sporadic CJD and atypical forms of BSE may result from a spontaneous structural change of host-encoded PrP^{C} into the self-replicating pathogenic PrP^{TSE} form. Prion propagation is proposed to occur by a "recruitment" reaction in which abnormal PrP^{TSE} serves as a template to convert PrP^{C} molecules into misfolded PrP^{TSE} molecules that precipitate in saline-detergent solutions, resist digestion with some proteolytic enzymes, and have a high potential to aggregate. Experimental efforts to confirm this hypothesis have yielded inconsistent results.

EPIDEMIOLOGY: Sporadic CJD is rare, occurring in the United States at a rate of approximately 1 to 1.5 cases per million people annually. Lifetime risk of CJD in the United States is approximately 1 in 6 239 people. Onset of disease peaks in the 60- through 74-year age group. Case-control studies of sporadic CJD have identified no consistent environmental risk factor. No increase in cases of sporadic CJD has been observed in people previously transfused with blood or blood components or injected with human plasma derivatives. The rate of sporadic CJD is not increased in patients with several diseases treated by repeated blood transfusions (eg, thalassemia and sickle cell disease) or in patients with hemophilia treated with human plasma derivatives. The American Red Cross traced a number of recipients of blood transfusions from donors later diagnosed with sporadic CJD; no cases of CJD were identified in recipients, some of whom survived for many years. Taken together, this information suggests that any risk of transfusion-transmitted sporadic CJD must be very low and appropriately regarded as theoretical. Except in families with genetic forms of the disease, CJD has not been reported in progeny of mothers who died with CJD. Genetic forms of prion diseases are expressed as autosomal dominant disorders with variable penetrance associated with a variety of mutations of the PrP-encoding gene (*PRNP*) located on chromosome 20. On average, genetic CJD begins approximately 10 years earlier than does sporadic CJD, but age at onset varies widely, even for members of the same family harboring identical mutations.

As of April 2021 (**www.eurocjd.ed.ac.uk/data_tables**), the total number of vCJD cases reported was 178 patients in the United Kingdom, 28 in France, 5 in Spain, 4 in Ireland, 4 in the United States, 3 in the Netherlands, 3 in Italy, 2 in Portugal, 2 in Canada, and 1 each in Taiwan, Japan, and Saudi Arabia. Two of the 4 patients in the United States, 2 of the 4 in Ireland, and 1 each of the patients in France, Canada, and Taiwan are believed to have acquired vCJD during residence in the United Kingdom. A study using statistical analysis of probability density of exposure to BSE concluded that 2 vCJD patients in the United States and another in Canada probably were infected during childhood residence in the Kingdom of Saudi Arabia. On the basis of animal inoculation studies, comparative PrP immunoblotting, and epidemiologic investigations, almost all cases of vCJD are believed to have resulted from exposure to tissues from cattle infected with BSE. Authorities suspect that the Japanese patient was infected during a short visit of 24 days to the United Kingdom in 1990, 12 years before onset of vCJD. Most patients with vCJD were younger than 30 years at onset, and several were adolescents. Median age at death of the 175 primary UK vCJD cases was 27 years. The ages at death of the 3 iatrogenic vCJD transfusion-transmitted cases were 32, 69, and 75 years; they developed typical vCJD 6.3 to 8.5 years after transfusions with nonleukoreduced red blood cells from apparently healthy individuals who donated the blood 1.4 to 3.5 years before onset of vCJD, demonstrating that blood contained the infectious agent during a substantial part of the asymptomatic incubation period. One patient with hemophilia, also showing no clinical signs of prion disease, probably was infected through injections of human plasma-derived clotting factors.

The **incubation periods** for iatrogenic classic CJD vary by route of exposure and range from about 14 months to at least 42 years. No transfusion-transmitted cases of nonvariant forms of CJD have been recognized.

DIAGNOSTIC TESTS: The diagnosis of human prion diseases can be made with certainty only by neuropathologic examination of affected brain tissue, usually obtained at autopsy. Immunodetection methods for PrP such as immunohistochemistry with sections and Western blot with saline-detergent extracts can be used to test brain tissues. Electroencephalography (EEG), magnetic resonance imaging (MRI), and cerebrospinal fluid (CSF) testing can be used to diagnose prion disease in living patients. In most patients with classic CJD, characteristic 1-cycle to 2-cycles per second triphasic sharp-wave discharges on EEG tracing indicate CJD. The likelihood of finding this abnormality is enhanced by serial EEG recordings.

Validated assays that detect 2 protein markers, 14-3-3 and tau, in CSF showed 83% to 90% sensitivity and 78% specificity. These proteins, sometimes detected in other neurologic diseases, are surrogate nonspecific markers found in CSF, probably as a result of the death of neurons.

Brain MRI is a highly sensitive and specific diagnostic tool for CJD, demonstrating hyperintensity in the basal ganglia and/or at least 2 cortical areas (excluding the frontal lobe) on diffusion-weighted imaging (DWI) or fluid attenuated inversion recovery (FLAIR) sequences.

No validated blood test is available. Recent promising developments exploit the in vivo prion replication process to amplify and detect even minute amounts of prions in biological samples. One such technique, real-time quaking-induced conversion (RT-QuIC), has been applied successfully in the clinical diagnosis of CJD in CSF samples with high specificity and sensitivity.[1] RT-QuIC also has been applied to diagnose CJD in olfactory epithelium brushings and, with additional validation, may be used in clinical settings.[2] RT-QuIC has not been applied successfully to blood samples. Some success has been reported with blood samples tested using another PrP^{TSE} amplification technique called protein misfolding cyclic amplification (PMCA).[3] These are currently "research-use-only" tests not marketed for human diagnosis.

Any person bearing a pathogenic mutation of the *PRNP* gene (not a normal polymorphism) with progressive neurologic signs suggestive of a TSE can be presumed to have a prion disease. Because no unique nucleic acid has been detected in prions causing TSEs, nucleic acid amplification tests (NAATs) are not possible. Brain biopsies for patients with possible CJD should be considered only when other potentially treatable diseases remain in the differential diagnosis. Complete postmortem examination of the brain is encouraged to confirm the clinical diagnosis of prion disease, to detect emerging forms of CJD, such as vCJD, and to survey for potential zoonotic transmission of CWD. State-of-the-art diagnostic testing, including assays of 14-3-3 and tau and RT-QuIC in CSF, *PRNP* gene sequencing, histopathology and Western blot analysis of brain to identify and characterize PrP^{TSE}, as well as expert neuropathologic consultation, are offered by the National Prion Disease Pathology Surveillance Center (telephone, 216-368-0587; **www.cjdsurveillance.com**). Clinical specimens that may

---

[1] Zerr I. Laboratory diagnosis of Creutzfeld-Jakob disease. *N Engl J Med*. 2022;386(14):1345-1350

[2] Orrú CD, Bongianni M, Tonoli G, et al. A test for Creutzfeldt-Jakob disease using nasal brushings. *N Engl J Med*. 2014;371(6):519-529

[3] Kramm C, Pritzkow S, Lyon A, Nichols T, Morales R, Soto C. Detection of prions in blood of cervids at the asymptomatic stage of chronic wasting disease. *Sci Rep*. 2017;7(1):17241

contain prions, particularly specimens with substantial amounts of infectivity, including brain, spinal cord, and CSF, should be handled with extreme caution. Amounts of infectivity can be significantly but not completely inactivated by physical or chemical means commonly used in the laboratory. Potentially contaminated laboratory waste should be steam autoclaved, when possible, at 134°C, and then sent to incineration as medical-pathological waste.

TREATMENT: No treatment has stopped or slowed the progressive neurodegeneration in prion diseases. Experimental treatments are being studied. Supportive therapy aids in managing dementia, spasticity, rigidity, and seizures occurring during the course of illness. Compassionate counseling and emotional support should be offered to families of affected people. Skilled genetic counseling is indicated for genetic disease, taking into account that penetrance has been variable in some kindreds in which people with a *PRNP* mutation survived to an advanced age without developing neurodegenerative disease. A family support and patient advocacy group, the CJD Foundation (telephone 800-659-1991; **www.cjdfoundation.org**), offers helpful information and advice together with information for professionals.

INFECTION PREVENTION AND CONTROL MEASURES IN HEALTH CARE SETTINGS: Standard precautions are recommended. Available evidence indicates that even prolonged intimate contact with CJD patients has not transmitted disease. Tissues with high levels of infectivity (eg, brain, eyes, spinal cord) and instruments in contact with those tissues are considered biohazards; incineration, prolonged autoclaving at high temperature and pressure after thorough cleaning, and, especially, exposure to a solution of 1 N or greater sodium hydroxide for 1 hour has been reported to decrease markedly or eliminate infectivity of contaminated surgical instruments. Work surfaces can be decontaminated effectively by exposure to 5.25% or stronger sodium hypochlorite (NaOCl, undiluted household chlorine bleach), but many surgical instruments corrode when exposed to NaOCl. The Centers for Disease Control and Prevention (CDC) offers advice for dealing with CJD patients (**www.cdc.gov/prions/index.html**) and recommendations for CJD infection control. Information on distribution of infectivity in various tissues and specific decontamination protocols are available online (**www.cdc.gov/prions/cjd/infection-control.html** and **apps.who.int/iris/bitstream/handle/10665/66707/WHO_CDS_CSR_APH_2000.3.pdf**). Person-to-person transmission of sporadic CJD by blood, milk, saliva, urine, or feces has not been reported. Body fluids should be handled using standard infection control procedures. Universal blood precautions, recommended for all patients, should be sufficient to prevent bloodborne transmission of TSEs.

CONTROL MEASURES: Immunization against prion diseases is not available, and no protective immune response to infection has been demonstrated. Iatrogenic transmission of CJD through cadaveric pituitary hormones has been obviated by use of recombinant products. Recognition that CJD had been spread by transplantation of infected dura mater allografts and corneal transplantation led to improved sourcing of those materials. After reports of transfusion-transmitted vCJD in the United Kingdom, blood establishments implemented more stringent blood and plasma donor selection criteria and improved collection protocols. Health care professionals should follow their state's prion disease reporting requirements and indicate CJD or other prion disease diagnoses appropriately on death certificates; the CDC uses mortality data from the United

States to help monitor prion diseases. In addition, any suspected or confirmed diagnosis of a prion disease of special public health concern (eg, any suspected iatrogenic TSE, vCJD, or human TSE with onset before age of 55 years) should be reported promptly to the appropriate state or local health departments and to the CDC (telephone, 404-639-3091 or 404-639-4435; **www.cdc.gov/prions/cjd/index.html**). Current precautionary policies of the US Food and Drug Administration to reduce the risk of transmitting CJD by human blood or blood products are available online (**www.fda.gov/regulatory-information/search-fda-guidance-documents/recommendations-reduce-possible-risk-transmission-creutzfeldt-jakob-disease-and-variant-creutzfeldt**). General information about BSE and CWD is available from the US Food and Drug Administration (**www.fda.gov/AnimalVeterinary/ResourcesforYou/AnimalHealthLiteracy/ucm136222.htm**), from the US Department of Agriculture (**www.usda.gov/topics/animals/bse-surveillance-information-center**), from the CDC (**www.cdc.gov/prions/bse/index.html**), and from the World Organization for Animal Health (**www.oie.int/en/animal-health-in-the-world/bse-portal/**).

Pseudomonas aeruginosa Infections

CLINICAL MANIFESTATIONS: *Pseudomonas aeruginosa* causes a variety of localized and systemic infections including otitis externa, mastoiditis, folliculitis, cellulitis, ecthyma gangrenosum, wound infection, ocular infection, pneumonia, osteomyelitis, bacteremia, endocarditis, meningitis, peritonitis, and urinary tract infection. It is a common cause of health care-associated infections (particularly in the presence of invasive devices), infections in immunocompromised children, pulmonary infections in children with cystic fibrosis, and infections in children with burns. *Pseudomonas* ophthalmia occurs predominantly in preterm infants and presents with eyelid edema and erythema, purulent discharge, and pannus formation. It can progress to corneal perforation, endophthalmitis, sepsis, and meningitis.

ETIOLOGY: *P aeruginosa* is an aerobic, gram-negative, nonfermenting bacillus that is commonly found in the environment. It is a member of the *Pseudomonas* genus and the *Pseudomonadaceae* family. The organism has multiple virulence factors, including the ability to form biofilms. *P aeruginosa* can convert to a mucoid phenotype, particularly in the setting of prolonged colonization, such as in individuals with cystic fibrosis.

EPIDEMIOLOGY: *P aeruginosa* is an opportunistic pathogen, causing infections in immunocompromised hosts (particularly those with neutropenia or poor granulocyte function), those with indwelling devices, burns, or cystic fibrosis. Children with cystic fibrosis commonly develop chronic endobronchial colonization with *P aeruginosa*, which is often associated with a more rapid decline in pulmonary function. Children with cystic fibrosis can share epidemic strains of *P aeruginosa*. Hospital-acquired *P aeruginosa* infections include ventilator-associated pneumonia, catheter-associated urinary tract infections, surgical site infections, and peritonitis associated with peritoneal dialysis. Community-associated infections include "hot tub" folliculitis, otitis externa after swimming in fresh water, osteomyelitis after a puncture wound (particularly through a sneaker), and endocarditis in people who inject drugs. It is a common cause of "contact lens" keratitis. Auricular chondritis has occurred after upper ear piercing. Outbreaks of infection have occurred from contaminated bronchoscopes.

P aeruginosa has intrinsic resistance to a variety of antibiotics and circulating strains are often multidrug resistant. Resistance may emerge during therapy. Production of beta-lactamases, loss of outer membrane proteins, and multidrug efflux pumps are common. Carbapenemase-producing strains (most commonly IMP and VIM) also occur.

The **incubation period** is variable depending on the host and site of colonization/infection. Incubation period for folliculitis following immersion in a whirlpool is a few hours to several days after exposure.

DIAGNOSTIC TESTS: Diagnosis is established by growth of *P aeruginosa* from culture of clinical specimens. Isolates may be identified by traditional biochemical tests, by a variety of commercially available biochemical test systems, by matrix-assisted laser desorption/ionization–time-of-flight (MALDI-TOF) mass spectrometry of bacterial cell components, or by molecular methods.

TREATMENT:

- Empiric combination therapy from different antimicrobial classes (eg, adding a fluoroquinolone or an aminoglycoside to an antipseudomonal β-lactam) may be indicated in severe sepsis, in patients with neutropenia, in patients who recently received broad-spectrum β-lactams, or in settings where antibiotic resistance is high to increase the probability of covering the infecting organism prior to knowing its identification and susceptibility.
- Cultures and susceptibilities should be sent prior to initiation of empiric therapy and therapy adjusted as per susceptibility data. In most patients, therapy can be simplified to a single active agent; there are no data to support continuation of combination therapy for an isolate susceptible to an appropriate antipseudomonal drug (see below). When the clinical course is complicated or when there is multidrug resistance to commonly used anti-pseudomonal agents (eg, antipseudomonal beta-lactam agents), it is recommended that an expert in infectious diseases assist in the management, particularly in the setting of carbapenem resistance.
- An important component of treatment is timely source control (ie, removal of catheters and devices, drainage of abscesses).
- Antimicrobial agents that have activity against *P aeruginosa* include piperacillin-tazobactam, ceftazidime, cefepime, aztreonam, ciprofloxacin, levofloxacin, meropenem, and imipenem/cilastatin (see Tables of Antibacterial Drugs, p 987); however, susceptibility patterns vary regionally, and local epidemiology and individual patient antibiotic exposure history should inform empiric therapy. Aminoglycosides are often used as adjunctive therapy (but not as monotherapy beyond urinary tract infections). Polymyxins (ie, colistin and polymyxin B) can be considered in the setting of highly resistant organisms but should not be used as first-line treatments if newer agents (eg, imipenem/cilastatin-relebactam, ceftazidime-avibactam, ceftolozane-tazobactam, or cefiderocol [experience for this agent is limited in children]) are available because of the general lower efficacy and higher adverse event rates of polymyxins compared with these newer agents.
- Management of children with cystic fibrosis should occur in conjunction with an expert in cystic fibrosis. Treatment for pulmonary exacerbation often includes 2 antipseudomonal agents in patients known to be chronically colonized with *P aeruginosa*. The Cystic Fibrosis Foundation recommends early eradication of *P aeruginosa*

with inhaled tobramycin (300 mg twice daily for 28 days). Once *P aeruginosa* becomes established, it can persist for years. Chronic suppressive treatment with inhaled antibiotics can decrease the bacterial burden. Inhaled antibiotics are generally not indicated for pulmonary exacerbations.

- Management of *Pseudomonas* neonatal ophthalmia urgently requires a combination of systemic and topical therapy, because systemic antibiotics alone have poor penetration in the anterior chamber of the eye. The diagnosis should be suspected when Gram-stained specimens of exudate contain gram-negative bacilli and should be confirmed by culture. Ophthalmology consultation is recommended.
- Duration of therapy is based on clinical and bacteriologic response of the patient and the site(s) of infection. Most bloodstream infections, ventilator-associated pneumonias, and urinary tract infections in immunocompetent people beyond the neonatal period can be treated with 7 days of antibiotic therapy if source control is achieved. In immunocompromised hosts (eg, those with neutropenia) and neonates, the duration of antibiotic therapy is usually 10 to 14 days.

INFECTION PREVENTION AND CONTROL MEASURES IN HEALTH CARE SETTINGS: Standard precautions for routine patients are recommended. For carbapenemase-producing organisms, contact precautions are indicated.[1] The Cystic Fibrosis Foundation recommends implementation of contact precautions in addition to standard precautions for care of all patients with cystic fibrosis in inpatient or ambulatory care settings, regardless of respiratory tract cultures.

CONTROL MEASURES: The Cystic Fibrosis Foundation recommends that all cystic fibrosis care centers limit contact between patients. This includes inpatient, outpatient, and social settings. When in a health care setting, patients with cystic fibrosis should wear a mask while outside of a clinic examination room or a hospital room. Education of patients and families about hand hygiene and appropriate personal hygiene is recommended.

Q Fever (*Coxiella burnetii* Infection)

CLINICAL MANIFESTATIONS: Approximately half of acute Q fever infections result in symptoms. Acute and chronic forms of the disease exist, and both can present as fever of unknown origin. Q fever is rare in children. Acute Q fever is typically characterized by abrupt onset of fever and is often accompanied by chills, headache, weakness, cough, and other nonspecific systemic symptoms. Illness typically is self-limited, although a relapsing febrile illness lasting for several months has been documented in children. Gastrointestinal tract symptoms, such as diarrhea, vomiting, abdominal pain, and anorexia, are reported in 50% to 80% of children. Rash has been observed in some patients. Q fever pneumonia usually manifests with a mild cough and shortness of breath but can progress to respiratory distress. Chest radiographic patterns are variable. In immunocompromised patients, a nodular pattern accompanied by a halo of ground-glass opacification and vessel connection, or findings suggestive of a necrotizing process, may be seen. More severe manifestations of acute Q fever include

---

[1] Centers for Disease Control and Prevention. Facility Guidance for Control of Carbapenem Resistant Enterobacteriaceae (CRE) November 2015 Update. Available at: **www.cdc.gov/hai/pdfs/cre/CRE-guidance-508.pdf**

hepatitis, hemolytic-uremic syndrome, myocarditis, pericarditis, encephalitis, meningitis, hemophagocytosis, lymphadenitis, cholecystitis, and rhabdomyolysis. The presence of anticardiolipin antibodies during acute Q fever has been associated with severe complications in adults. People who are infected during pregnancy may be at risk for miscarriage or preterm delivery. Chronic (persistent, localized) Q fever can present as blood culture-negative endocarditis, vascular infection, chronic relapsing or multifocal osteomyelitis, chronic hepatitis, or infection of the reproductive organs. Osteomyelitis is a common presentation of chronic Q fever in children. Children who are immunocompromised or have underlying valvular heart disease may be at higher risk of chronic Q fever.

ETIOLOGY: *Coxiella burnetii,* the cause of Q fever, previously was considered to be a rickettsial organism but is a gram-negative intracellular bacterium that belongs to the order *Legionellales,* family *Coxiellaceae.* It shares many features, including relatedness of several virulence genes, with *Legionella pneumophila.* The infectious form of *C burnetii* is highly resistant to heat, desiccation, and disinfectant chemicals and can persist for long periods of time in the environment. *C burnetii* is classified as a category B bioterrorism agent by the Centers for Disease Control and Prevention (CDC).

EPIDEMIOLOGY: Q fever is a zoonotic infection that has been reported worldwide, including in every state in the United States. The "Q" comes from "query" fever, the name of the disease until its etiologic agent was identified in the 1930s. *C burnetii* infection usually is asymptomatic in animals, but can cause abortions when introduced into naïve herds, particularly in goats. Many different species can be infected, although cattle, sheep, and goats are the primary reservoirs for human infection. Tick vectors may be important for maintaining animal and bird reservoirs but are not believed to be important in transmission to humans. Humans most often acquire infection by inhalation of fine-particle aerosols of *C burnetii* generated from birthing fluids or other excreta of infected animals or through inhalation of dust contaminated by these materials. Infection can occur by exposure to contaminated materials, such as wool, straw, bedding, or laundry. Windborne particles containing infectious organisms can travel long distances, contributing to sporadic cases for which no apparent animal contact can be demonstrated. Unpasteurized dairy products also can contain the organism.[1] Seasonal trends occur in farming areas with predictable frequency, and the disease often coincides with the livestock birthing season in spring.

The **incubation period** is 14 to 22 days, with a range from 9 to 39 days, depending on the inoculum size. Chronic Q fever can develop months to years after initial infection.

DIAGNOSTIC TESTS: Serologic evidence of a fourfold increase in phase II immunoglobulin (Ig) G via immunofluorescent assays (IFAs) between paired sera obtained 3 to 6 weeks apart is the most commonly used method to diagnose acute Q fever. A single high serum phase II IgG titer (≥1:128) by IFA in the convalescent stage may be considered as evidence of probable infection. Confirmation of persistent (chronic) Q fever is based on an increasing phase I IgG titer (typically ≥1:1024) **and** an identifiable nidus of infection (eg, endocarditis, vascular infection, osteomyelitis, chronic hepatitis). Use

---

[1] American Academy of Pediatrics, Committee on Infectious Diseases, Committee on Nutrition. Consumption of raw or unpasteurized milk and milk products by pregnant women and children. *Pediatrics.* 2014;133(1):175-179 (Reaffirmed November 2019)

of a nucleic acid amplification test (NAAT) on whole blood or serum may be useful in the first 2 weeks of symptom onset and before antimicrobial administration. Although a positive NAAT result can confirm the diagnosis, a negative NAAT result does not rule out Q fever. NAATs and serologic testing for *C burnetii* are available through state public health laboratories and from some commercial diagnostic laboratories. Detection of *C burnetii* in tissues (eg, heart valve) by immunohistochemistry or NAAT can also confirm a diagnosis of chronic Q fever. However, NAAT results may be negative in up to 66% of patients with endocarditis attributable to Q fever. Isolation of *C burnetii* from blood or tissue using tissue culture, embryonated eggs, or animal inoculation can be performed only in special laboratories with biosafety level 3 facilities because of the potential hazard to laboratory workers.

TREATMENT: Acute Q fever generally is a self-limited illness, and many patients recover without antimicrobial therapy. However, early treatment is effective in shortening illness duration and symptom severity and should be initiated in all symptomatic patients. For symptomatic patients with suspected Q fever, immediate empiric therapy should be given because laboratory results are often negative early in the illness onset before the production of quantifiable antibody. Doxycycline administered for 14 days is the drug of choice for patients with severe infections and can be used for acute Q fever regardless of patient age. Pregnant people and patients allergic to doxycycline can be treated with trimethoprim-sulfamethoxazole.

Chronic Q fever is much more difficult to treat, and relapses can occur despite appropriate therapy, necessitating repeated courses of therapy. For Q fever endocarditis in adults, the recommended therapy is a combination of doxycycline and hydroxychloroquine for a minimum of 18 months. There are limited data available on effective treatment of chronic Q fever in children, and in some cases, surgical replacement of infected tissue and/or surgical débridement may be required. In the few cases of pediatric chronic Q fever in the published literature, the combination of doxycycline plus hydroxychloroquine has been the most commonly used treatment.

INFECTION PREVENTION AND CONTROL MEASURES IN HEALTH CARE SETTINGS: Standard precautions are recommended for routine care. Airborne precautions should be used for patients who are undergoing procedures that could cause aerosolization or for pregnant people with Q fever who are delivering.

CONTROL MEASURES: Strict adherence to proper hygiene when handling infected parturient animals or their excreta can help decrease the risk of infection in the farm setting, as can ensuring that people do not consume unpasteurized milk and milk products.[1] Improved prescreening of animal herds used by research facilities may decrease the risk of infection. Biosafety level 2 practices and facilities are recommended for nonpropagative laboratory procedures involving *C burnetii* and biosafety level 3 practices for all propagative procedures and necropsy of infected animals. Special safety practices are recommended during high-risk worker exposures in biomedical facilities that house sheep and goats. Vaccines for domestic animals and people working in high-risk occupations have been developed but are not licensed in the United States. A small number of high-risk children in Australia have safely received the vaccine.

---

[1] American Academy of Pediatrics, Committee on Infectious Diseases, Committee on Nutrition. Consumption of raw or unpasteurized milk and milk products by pregnant women and children. *Pediatrics.* 2014;133(1):175-179 (Reaffirmed November 2019)

Additional information about Q fever, is available on the CDC website (**www. cdc.gov/qfever/index.html**).

Public Health Reporting. Q fever is a nationally notifiable disease, and all human cases should be reported to the state or local health department.

Rabies

CLINICAL MANIFESTATIONS: Infection with rabies virus and other lyssaviruses characteristically produces nonspecific prodromal symptoms (eg, low grade fever, myalgias) followed by an acute illness with rapidly progressive central nervous system manifestations that may include anxiety, radicular pain, dysesthesia or pruritus, hydrophobia, unconsciousness, and dysautonomia. Some patients may have paralysis. Illness almost invariably progresses to death. The differential diagnosis of acute encephalitic illnesses of unknown cause or with features of Guillain-Barré syndrome should include rabies.

ETIOLOGY: Rabies virus is a single-stranded RNA virus classified in the *Rhabdoviridae* family, *Lyssavirus* genus. The genus *Lyssavirus* currently contains 17 species and 1 related unclassified virus species divided into 3 phylogroups.

EPIDEMIOLOGY: Understanding the epidemiology of rabies has been aided by viral variant identification using monoclonal antibodies and nucleotide sequencing. In the United States, human cases have decreased steadily since the 1950s, reflecting widespread immunization of dogs and the availability of effective human prophylaxis after exposure to a rabid animal. From 2009 through 2021, 21 of 30 cases of human rabies reported in the United States were acquired indigenously. Among the indigenously acquired cases, all but 5 were associated with bats. Despite the large focus of rabies in raccoons in the eastern United States, only 3 cases during this time period were found to have the raccoon rabies virus variant. Historically, 2 cases of human rabies were attributable to probable aerosol exposure in laboratories, and 2 unusual cases have been attributed to possible airborne exposures in caves inhabited by millions of bats, although alternative infection routes cannot be discounted. Transmission also has occurred by transplantation of organs, corneas, and other tissues from patients dying of undiagnosed rabies.

Rabies virus variants from bats perpetuate throughout the United States except Hawaii, which remains "rabies free." Wildlife, including bats, raccoons, skunks, foxes, and mongoose, are the most important potential sources of infection for humans and domestic animals in the United States and its territories, but the prevalence of each of these differs geographically (see **www.cdc.gov/rabies/location/usa/ surveillance/wild_animals.html** for a map of rabies variants by reservoir hosts). The virus is present in saliva and is transmitted by bites or, rarely, by contamination of mucosa or skin lesions by saliva or other potentially infectious material (eg, neural tissue). Worldwide, most rabies cases in humans result from dog bites in areas where canine rabies is enzootic. The largest burden of disease is in rural, low-income populations because of inadequate implementation of control measures and lack of access to postexposure prophylaxis. Half of the 59 000 estimated yearly global deaths occur in children. The World Health Organization (WHO) has developed a plan in collaboration with partner organizations to eliminate canine rabies by 2030 (**www.who.int/ publications/i/item/WHO-UCN-NTD-VVE-2021.1**). Most rabid dogs, cats, and ferrets shed virus for a few days before there are obvious signs of illness. No case of human rabies in the United States has been attributed to a dog, cat, or ferret that has remained healthy throughout the standard 10-day period of confinement after an exposure.

The **incubation period** in humans averages 1 to 3 months but ranges from days to years.

DIAGNOSTIC TESTS: Infection in animals can be diagnosed by demonstration of the presence of rabies virus antigen in brain tissue using a direct fluorescent antibody (DFA) test, direct rapid immunohistochemical test (dRIT), or a pan-lyssavirus real-time polymerase chain reaction (PCR) assay. Suspected rabid animals should be euthanized in a manner that preserves brain tissue for appropriate laboratory diagnosis. Diagnosis in suspected human cases can be made postmortem by either immunofluorescent or immunohistochemical examination of brain tissue or by detection of viral nucleotide sequences. Antemortem diagnosis can be made by DFA testing on skin biopsy specimens from the nape of the neck, by isolation of the virus from saliva or other clinical specimens, by detection of antibody in serum (neutralization or indirect fluorescent antibody methods generally are used) in people without a history of immunization and in cerebrospinal fluid (CSF) regardless of immunization history, or by detection of viral nucleotide sequences in saliva, skin, or other tissues. In order for rabies to be ruled out in a patient, specimens from saliva, serum, CSF and skin biopsy must all be tested. No single test is sufficiently sensitive because of the unique nature of rabies pathobiology. State or local health departments should be consulted before submission of specimens to the Centers for Disease Control and Prevention (CDC). Consultation with public health authorities facilitates cases inconsistent with rabies to be identified before specimens are collected and enables appropriate collection and transport of materials to be arranged when rabies testing is indicated. Step-by-step instructions can be found at **www.cdc.gov/rabies/resources/specimen-submission-guidelines.html.**

TREATMENT: There is no specific treatment. Once symptoms have developed, neither rabies vaccine nor rabies immune globulin (RIG) improves the prognosis. Experimental therapies have been tried but are often not successful (for additional information, see **www.cdc.gov/rabies/specific_groups/hcp/human_rabies. html** and **www.mcw.edu/rabies**). Reasons for the rare instances of patient survival after clinical presentation of rabies are poorly understood.

INFECTION PREVENTION AND CONTROL MEASURES IN HEALTH CARE SETTINGS: Standard precautions are recommended, including face mask, eye protection, gown, and gloves for procedures and patient care activities that could generate splashes or sprays or when contact with potentially infectious fluids is anticipated. If the patient has bitten another person or potentially infectious material from the patient has contaminated an open wound or mucous membrane, the involved area should be washed thoroughly with soap and water, and risk assessment should be completed to determine whether postexposure prophylaxis should be administered (see Care of Exposed People, p 706).

CONTROL MEASURES: In the United States, animal rabies is common. Education of children to avoid contact with bats and stray or wild animals is of primary importance. Inadvertent contact of family members and pets with potentially rabid animals, such as raccoons, foxes, and skunks, may be decreased by securing garbage and pet food outdoors to decrease attraction of domestic and wild animals. Chimneys and other potential entrances for wildlife, including bats, should be identified and covered. Bats should be excluded from human living quarters (although some restrictions on exclusion may apply based on the conservation status of the bat species and local regulations). International travelers to areas with enzootic canine rabies should be warned to avoid exposure to stray dogs, and if traveling to an area with enzootic infection where immediate access to medical care or availability of biologic agents is limited, preexposure prophylaxis is indicated in addition to postexposure prophylaxis if an exposure occurs.

Exposure Risk and Decisions to Administer Prophylaxis. Exposure to rabies results from a break in the skin caused by the teeth of a rabid animal or by contamination of scratches, abrasions, or mucous membranes with saliva or other potentially infectious material, such as neural tissue, from a rabid animal. The decision to immunize a potentially exposed person should be made in consultation with the state or local health department, which can provide information on risk of rabies in a particular area for each species of animal and in accordance with the guidance in Table 3.53. Consultation with experts at the CDC may be helpful to guide decisions on prophylaxis (**www.cdc.gov/rabies/resources/contacts.html**).

In the United States and Puerto Rico, all mammals are believed to be susceptible, but bats, raccoons, skunks, foxes, and mongooses are reservoir species more likely to

Table 3.53. Rabies Postexposure Prophylaxis Guide

Animal Type	Evaluation and Disposition of Animal	Postexposure Prophylaxis Recommendations
Dogs, cats, and ferrets	Healthy and available for 10 days of observation Rabid or suspected of being rabid[a] Unknown (escaped)	Prophylaxis only if animal develops signs of rabies[b] Immediate immunization and RIG[c] Consult public health officials for advice
Bats, skunks, raccoons, foxes, mongooses,[c] and most other carnivores; groundhogs	Regarded as rabid unless geographic area is known to be free of rabies or until animal proven negative by laboratory tests[a]	Immediate immunization and RIG[c]
Livestock, rodents, and lagomorphs (rabbits, hares, and pikas)	Consider individually	Consult public health officials; bites of squirrels, hamsters, guinea pigs, gerbils, chipmunks, rats, mice and other rodents, rabbits, hares, and pikas almost never require rabies postexposure prophylaxis

RIG indicates rabies immune globulin.

[a] The animal should be euthanized and tested as soon as possible. Holding for observation is not recommended. Immunization is discontinued if immunofluorescent test result for the animal is negative.

[b] During the 10-day observation period, at the first sign of rabies in the biting dog, cat, or ferret, prophylaxis of the exposed person with RIG (human) and vaccine should be initiated. The animal should be euthanized immediately and tested.

[c] See text.

be infected than are other animals.[1] Postexposure prophylaxis typically should be initiated as soon as possible following a high-risk exposure; however, if the animal is available for observation (ie, dogs, cats, ferrets) or can be euthanized and tested (eg, bats and other wildlife), public health authorities may recommend delaying postexposure prophylaxis pending these results. Alternatively, if postexposure prophylaxis has been initiated and subsequent testing shows that the exposing animal was not rabid, postexposure prophylaxis can be discontinued. In many cases, persons who discontinue postexposure prophylaxis after 3 doses can be considered previously immunized. Cattle, horses, and other large mammals occasionally are infected. Bites of small rodents (such as squirrels, hamsters, guinea pigs, gerbils, chipmunks, mice, and rats) and lagomorphs (rabbits, hares, and pikas) rarely require prophylaxis, because these animals almost never are found to be infected with rabies and have not been known to transmit rabies to humans. Rabies in larger rodents, such as groundhogs, is more prevalent and presents a higher risk compared to small rodents. Additional factors must be considered when deciding whether postexposure prophylaxis is indicated. An unprovoked attack may be more suggestive of a rabid animal than a bite that occurs during attempts to feed or handle an animal. Properly immunized dogs, cats, and ferrets have only a minimal chance of developing rabies. However, in rare instances, rabies has developed in properly immunized animals.

Postexposure prophylaxis for rabies is recommended for all people bitten by animals that are suspected to be rabid unless laboratory tests prove that the animal does not have rabies. The CDC Advisory Committee on Immunization Practices (ACIP) recommends dogs, cats, and ferrets be observed for 10 days after exposure, if healthy and available to observe.[2] If the animal shows clinical signs of rabies, the exposed person should begin prophylaxis. Postexposure prophylaxis also is recommended for people who report an open wound, scratch, or mucous membrane that has been contaminated with saliva or other potentially infectious material (eg, brain tissue) from an animal suspected to be rabid. The injury inflicted by a bat bite or scratch may be small and not readily evident, so any direct contact with a bat should prompt consideration of postexposure prophylaxis regardless of the visible presence of a bite or scratch. The circumstances of contact with a bat may preclude accurate recall (eg, a bat in the room of a deeply sleeping or medicated person or a previously unattended child, especially an infant or toddler who cannot reliably communicate about a potential bite). Hence, postexposure prophylaxis may be indicated, following proper risk assessment, for situations in which a bat physically is present in the same room if a bite or mucous membrane exposure cannot reliably be excluded, unless prompt testing of the bat has excluded rabies virus infection. In the wild, approximately 1% of bats are infected with rabies. Among bats that have contact with humans (and therefore are being tested for rabies), approximately 6% to 12% are infected with rabies. Prophylaxis should be initiated as soon as possible after bites by known or suspected rabid animals.

---

[1] Centers for Disease Control and Prevention. Human rabies—Puerto Rico, 2015. *MMWR Morb Mortal Wkly Rep*. 2017;65(52):1474-1476

[2] Centers for Disease Control and Prevention. Human rabies prevention: United States, 2008. Recommendations of the Advisory Committee on Immunization Practices. *MMWR Recomm Rep*. 2008;57(RR-3):1-28

Risk Assessments for Contacts of Humans With Rabies. Risk assessment for the administration of postexposure prophylaxis is recommended for people who report a possibly infectious exposure (eg, bite, scratch, or open wound or mucous membrane contaminated with saliva or other infectious material, such as tears, CSF, or brain tissue) to a human with rabies. Rabies virus transmission after exposure to a human with rabies has not been documented convincingly in the United States, except after tissue or organ transplantation from donors who died of unsuspected rabies encephalitis. Casual contact with an infected person (eg, by touching a patient) or contact with noninfectious fluids or tissues (eg, blood or feces) alone does not constitute an exposure and is not an indication for prophylaxis. Administration of postexposure prophylaxis to hospital contacts of patients with rabies is required only in situations in which potentially infectious material (such as saliva, CSF, or brain tissue) comes into direct contact with broken skin or mucous membranes. In cases in which people are using the protective equipment appropriate for the given interaction with the patient, there likely will be no risk of exposure.

Handling of Animals Suspected of Having Rabies. An animal that is suspected of having rabies and has bitten a human should be humanely captured, confined, euthanized, and tested. Alternatively, as noted earlier, if the dog, cat, or ferret appears healthy, it can be observed by a veterinarian for 10 days by order of public health authorities. If signs of rabies develop, the animal should be humanely euthanized in a manner to allow its head to be removed and shipped to a qualified laboratory for examination. Instructions for packing can be found at **www.cdc.gov/rabies/resources/ specimen-submission-guidelines.html;** freshly frozen and shipped with dry ice is preferred to refrigerated specimens.

Other biting animals that may have exposed a person to rabies virus should be reported immediately to the state, local health department, animal control or police. Management of animals depends on the species, the circumstances of the bite, and the epidemiology of rabies in the area. Previous immunization of an animal may not preclude the necessity for euthanasia and testing. Because clinical manifestations of rabies in a wild animal cannot be interpreted reliably, a wild mammal suspected of having rabies should be euthanized at once, and its brain should be examined for evidence of rabies virus infection. The exposed person need not receive prophylaxis if the result of rapid examination of the brain by a qualified test is negative for rabies virus infection.

Care of Exposed People.

Local Wound Care. The immediate objective of postexposure prophylaxis is to prevent virus from entering neural tissue. Prompt and thorough local treatment of all lesions is essential, because virus may remain localized to the area of the bite for a variable time. All wounds should be flushed thoroughly and cleaned with soap and water. Quaternary ammonium compounds (such as benzalkonium chloride) no longer are considered superior to soap. The need for tetanus prophylaxis and measures to control bacterial infection should be considered. The wound can be loosely sutured but only after RIG is infiltrated around the wound. For severe facial wounds, which often also are infected with bacteria, better cosmesis results from single sutures, widely placed, several hours after local instillation of RIG, followed by plastic surgery days later.

Prophylaxis (see Table 3.53, p 704). After wound care is completed, concurrent use of passive (RIG) and active (rabies vaccine) immunization is optimal, with the exceptions of people who previously have received complete vaccination regimens (preexposure [see **www.cdc.gov/mmwr/volumes/71/wr/mm7118a2.htm**] or postexposure) with a cell culture vaccine or people who have been vaccinated with other types of rabies vaccines and have previously had a documented rabies virus-neutralizing antibody titer; these people should receive only vaccine. Prophylaxis should begin as soon as possible after exposure is confirmed, ideally within 24 hours. Although not ideal, a delay of several days or more may not compromise effectiveness, and prophylaxis should be initiated if reasonably indicated, regardless of the interval between exposure and initiation of therapy. Physicians can obtain expert counsel from their state or local health departments when uncertain about administering these products.

Active Immunization (Postexposure). Human diploid cell vaccine (HDCV) and purified chicken embryo cell vaccine (PCECV) are licensed in the United States (see Table 3.54). A 1.0-mL dose of vaccine is injected intramuscularly in the deltoid area or other nongluteal muscle mass (virus-neutralizing antibody responses in adults who received vaccine in the gluteal area sometimes have been inferior to those who received vaccine in the deltoid muscle). In infants and young children, the anterolateral aspect of the thigh is used for intramuscular injection of vaccine. For a previously unvaccinated immunocompetent person, vaccine is administered on the first day of postexposure prophylaxis (day 0), and repeated doses are administered on days 3, 7, and 14

Table 3.54. US Food and Drug Administration-Licensed Rabies Vaccines[a] and Rabies Immune Globulin Products

Category	Product	Manufacturer	Dose and Route of Administration
Human rabies vaccine	Human diploid cell vaccine (HDCV) (Imovax Rabies)	Sanofi Pasteur	1 mL, IM
	Purified chicken embryo cell vaccine (PCECV) (RabAvert)	Novartis Vaccines and Diagnostics	1 mL, IM
Rabies immune globulin	Imogam Rabies-HT	Sanofi Pasteur	20 IU/kg, infiltrate around wound[b]
	HyperRab	Grifols USA	20 IU/kg, infiltrate around wound[b]
	Kedrab	Kedrion Biopharma	20 IU/kg, infiltrate around wound[b]

IM indicates intramuscular.
[a] Rabies vaccine adsorbed (RVA) is licensed in the United States but no longer is distributed in the United States.
[b] Any remaining volume should be administered intramuscularly.

after the first dose, for a total of 4 doses,[1] with 1 dose of RIG (based on body weight) administered on day 0. Rabies vaccine and RIG should never be administered in the same muscle.

For a person with altered immunocompetence, postexposure prophylaxis is the same vaccination regimen, however, an antibody titer of the recipient's serum should be evaluated to ensure the minimum antibody titer cut-off (0.5 IU/mL) has been reached or exceeded. The serum specimen can ideally be obtained with the fourth dose of rabies vaccine (ie, day 14) or up to 2 weeks after completion of the series. Serologic testing to document seroconversion after administration of a rabies vaccine series given for postexposure prophylaxis is only advised for recipients who may be immunocompromised, for people with deviations from the recommended vaccination schedule, or for those who initiated vaccination outside of the United States with a product of questionable quality. Ideally, a vaccination series should be initiated and completed with 1 vaccine product unless serious adverse reactions occur. Clinical studies evaluating efficacy or frequency of adverse reactions when the series is completed with a second product have not been conducted.

Care should be taken to ensure that the vaccine is administered intramuscularly. Vaccines licensed in the United States are not approved or packaged for intradermal administration in the postexposure setting, although the World Health Organization (WHO) has recommended postexposure intradermal regimens as an alternative to intramuscular administration for reasons of cost and availability, and these are used in some countries (**apps.who.int/iris/handle/10665/272364**).

ADVERSE REACTIONS AND PRECAUTIONS WITH HDCV AND PCECV. Reactions are uncommon in children. In adults, mild local reactions, such as pain, erythema, and swelling or itching at the injection site, are reported in 15% to 25%, and mild systemic reactions, such as headache, nausea, abdominal pain, muscle aches, and dizziness, are reported in 10% to 20% of recipients. Immune complex-like reactions in people receiving booster doses of HDCV have been observed, possibly because of interaction between propiolactone contained in the vaccine and human albumin. The reaction, characterized by onset 2 to 21 days after inoculation, begins with generalized urticaria and can include arthralgia, arthritis, angioedema, nausea, vomiting, fever, and malaise. The reaction is not life threatening, occurs in as many as 6% of adults receiving booster doses as part of a preexposure immunization regimen, and is rare in people receiving primary immunization with HDCV. Similar reactions with primary or booster doses have been reported with PCECV. If the patient has a serious allergic reaction to HDCV, PCECV may be administered according to the same schedule as HDCV, and vice-versa. If reactions following vaccine are mild, pretreatment with antihistamines just before the next vaccination can be considered. All suspected serious, systemic, paralytic, or anaphylactic reactions to rabies vaccine should be reported immediately to the Vaccine Adverse Event Reporting System (VAERS).

Rabies vaccines have been safely administered to pregnant people. Pregnancy is not a contraindication to use of vaccine or RIG after exposure.

Passive Immunization (Postexposure). RIG should be used concomitantly with the first dose of vaccine for postexposure prophylaxis to bridge the time between possible

[1] Centers for Disease Control and Prevention. Use of a reduced (4-dose) vaccine schedule for postexposure prophylaxis to prevent human rabies: recommendations of the Advisory Committee on Immunization Practices. *MMWR Recomm Rep.* 2010;59(RR–02):1–9

infection and antibody production induced by the vaccine (see Table 3.54). If vaccine is not available immediately, RIG should be administered alone, and vaccination should be started as soon as possible. If RIG is not available immediately, vaccine should be administered, and RIG should be administered subsequently if obtained within 7 days after initiating vaccination. If administration of both vaccine and RIG is delayed, both should be used regardless of the interval between exposure and treatment.

Only human RIG is available in the United States; the recommended dose is 20 IU/kg. RIG should never be administered in the same syringe as vaccine. As much of the RIG dose as is safely possible should be used to infiltrate the wound(s) if present. The remainder is administered intramuscularly into muscle that is not the same one where rabies vaccine was administered. In cases of multiple severe wounds in which RIG is insufficient for infiltration, dilution in saline solution to an adequate volume (twofold or threefold) has been recommended to ensure that all wound areas receive infiltrate. For children with small muscle mass, it may be necessary to administer RIG at multiple sites. Since 2018, a concentrated RIG product, HyperRab, has been licensed for use in the United States; this product requires 5% dextrose in water to be used as the diluent (rather than normal saline) and may be preferable for infiltrating small wounds (eg, those from a bat). Passive antibody can, in some cases, slightly reduce the level of neutralizing antibodies in the response to rabies vaccines. Therefore, the recommended dose should ideally not be exceeded; however, up to 2 times the recommended RIG dose is typically not clinically significant. Hypersensitivity reactions to human RIG are rare.

Purified equine RIG containing rabies antibodies may be available outside the United States and generally is accompanied by a low rate of serum sickness (less than 1%). Equine RIG is administered at a dose of 40 IU/kg.

Management of Postexposure Prophylaxis In Previously Immunized People. Administration of RIG is not recommended for people who are considered "previously vaccinated." A previously vaccinated person is defined as someone who has received one of the recommended pre- or postexposure regimens of HDCV, PCECV, or rabies vaccine adsorbed (the latter is a vaccine no longer available in the United States). Also acceptable is receipt of another vaccine along with a documented rabies virus neutralizing titer. Such individuals should receive two 1.0-mL booster doses of HDCV or PCECV; the first dose ideally is administered as soon as possible after exposure, and the second dose is administered 3 days later.

Preexposure Control Measures, Including Vaccination. The relatively low frequency of reactions to HDCV and PCECV has made provision of preexposure vaccination practical for people in high-risk groups, including veterinarians, animal handlers, certain laboratory workers, and people moving or traveling to areas where canine rabies is common. Others, such as spelunkers (cavers) or animal rehabilitators, who may have frequent exposures to bats and other wildlife, also should be considered for preexposure prophylaxis. Please refer to Table 3.55 and the 2022 ACIP guidance for detailed recommendations (**www.cdc.gov/mmwr/volumes/71/wr/mm7118a2.htm**)[1]; note the

---

[1] Centers for Disease Control and Prevention. Use of a modified preexposure prophylaxis vaccination schedule to prevent human rabies: recommendations of the Advisory Committee on Immunization Practices. *MMWR Morb Mortal Wkly Rep.* 2022;71(18):619-627

Table 3.55. Rabies Preexposure Prophylaxis (PrEP) Recommendations in Immunocompetent and Immunocompromised Individuals[a]

Risk Category	Examples of Typical Population	PrEP Rabies Vaccine Recommendation	Assessment of Long-Term Immunogenicity[b]
Elevated risk for unrecognized and recognized exposures, including unusual or high-risk exposures	Individuals working with live rabies virus (research or vaccine production facilities or performing rabies testing)	IM rabies vaccine on days 0 and 7	Check rabies titers **every 6 months;** booster if titer <0.5 IU/mL
Elevated risk for unrecognized and recognized exposures	Individuals who frequently handle bats, have contact with bats, enter high-density bat environments, perform animal necropsies	IM rabies vaccine on days 0 and 7	Check rabies titers **every 2 years;** booster if titer <0.5 IU/mL
Elevated risk for recognized exposures, sustained risk	Individuals who interact with animals that could be rabid; occupational or recreational activities that involve contact with animals (veterinarians, technicians, animal control officers, persons who handle wildlife reservoir species, spelunkers)	IM rabies vaccine on days 0 and 7	• Check **one-time titer during years 1–3** after 2-dose primary series; booster if titer <0.5 IU/mL OR • **Provide IM rabies vaccine booster** no sooner than day 21 to no later than year 3 after completing the 2-dose primary series
Elevated risk for recognized exposures, risk not sustained	Similar population for risk category 3, but risk duration is ≤3 y	IM rabies vaccine on days 0 and 7	None
Low risk for exposure	Typical person living in the United States	None	None

Adapted from Rao AK, Briggs D, Moore SM, et al. Use of a modified preexposure prophylaxis vaccination schedule to prevent human rabies: recommendations of the Advisory Committee on Immunization Practices—United States, 2022. *MMWR Morb Mortal Wkly Rep*. 2022;71(18):619-627.
[a] If PrEP is provided to an immunocompromised individual, an antibody titer should be checked 2 to 4 weeks after completion of the 2-dose PrEP primary series and all booster doses; administer booster dose if titer <0.5 IU/mL. If 2 booster doses fail to elicit a titer ≥0.5 IU/mL, contact local or state public health authorities to provide case-specific guidance.
[b] Immunogenicity defined as rabies titer ≥0.5 IU/mL, obtained 2 to 4 weeks after completing the recommended primary vaccination schedule.

risk categories and recommendations, including those regarding serologic testing. In children, the most common reason for preexposure prophylaxis is travel.

HDCV and PCECV are licensed in the United States for intramuscular administration. The preexposure prophylaxis schedule is two 1-mL intramuscular injections each, administered on days 0 and 7. This series of immunizations has resulted in development of rabies virus-neutralizing antibodies in immunocompetent people properly immunized.

For immunocompromised persons, serum should be collected no sooner than 1 week after the second PrEP dose, but ideally 2 to 4 weeks after. Up to 2 additional doses should be administered before public health authorities are consulted for guidance for persons who have not reached or exceeded the minimum acceptable antibody titer cut-off of 0.5 IU/mL.

Persons who have received preexposure immunization and are exposed to rabies should receive booster doses of vaccine at days 0 and 3 as postexposure prophylaxis (see "Management of Postexposure Prophylaxis in Previously Immunized People," above).

Public Health. A variety of approved public health measures, including vaccination of dogs, cats, and ferrets and management of the stray dog population and selected wildlife, are used to control rabies in animals.[1] In regions where oral vaccination of wildlife with recombinant rabies vaccine is undertaken, the prevalence of rabies among foxes, coyotes, and raccoons may be decreased. Unvaccinated dogs, cats, ferrets, or other pets bitten by a known rabid animal should be euthanized immediately. If the owner is unwilling to allow the animal to be euthanized, the animal should be placed in strict isolation for 6 months and immunized, at the latest, 1 month before release. The isolation should be instituted under the supervision of the appropriate public health authority. If the exposed animal has been immunized within 1 to 3 years, depending on the vaccine administered and local regulations, the animal should be revaccinated and observed for 45 days.

Public Health Reporting. A confirmatory diagnosis of rabies in humans or animals is reportable to the state health department and notifiable to the CDC. All suspected human cases of rabies should be reported promptly to state or local health departments.

Rat-Bite Fever

CLINICAL MANIFESTATIONS: Rat-bite fever is typically caused by infection with either *Streptobacillus moniliformis* or *Spirillum minus*. *S moniliformis* infection (streptobacillary fever or Haverhill fever) is characterized by relapsing fever, rash, and migratory polyarthritis, although variable presentations outside this classic triad increasingly are reported. There is an abrupt onset of fever, chills, muscle pain, vomiting, headache, and rarely (unlike *S minus*) lymphadenopathy. A maculopapular, purpuric, or petechial rash develops, predominantly on the peripheral extremities including the palms and soles, typically within a few days of fever onset. The skin lesions may become purpuric or confluent and may desquamate. The bite site usually heals promptly and exhibits no or minimal inflammation. Nonsuppurative migratory polyarthritis or arthralgia follows

---

[1] National Association of State Public Health Veterinarians Inc. Compendium of animal rabies prevention and control, 2011. *MMWR Recomm Rep.* 2011;60(RR-6):1-15

in approximately 50% of patients and especially affects the knees, followed by wrists, ankles, and occasionally hips. Symptoms of untreated infection may resolve within 2 weeks, but fever occasionally can relapse for weeks or months, and infection can lead to serious complications including soft tissue and solid-organ abscesses (brain, myocardium), septic arthritis, pneumonia, endocarditis, myocarditis, pericarditis, sepsis, and meningitis. The case fatality rate is 7% to 13% in untreated patients, and fatal cases have been reported in children.

With *S minus* infection ("sodoku"), a period of initial apparent healing at the site of the bite usually is followed by fever and ulceration, discoloration, swelling, and pain at the site (about 1 to 4 weeks later), regional lymphangitis and lymphadenopathy, and a distinctive rash of red or purple plaques. Arthritis is rare.

ETIOLOGY: The major causes of rat-bite fever are *S moniliformis*, a microaerophilic, facultatively anaerobic, gram-negative, pleomorphic bacillus, and *S minus*, a small, gramnegative, spiral-shaped bacterium with bipolar flagellar tufts. Other members of the *Streptobacillus* genus, including *Streptobacillus notomytis*, are rare causes of disease.

EPIDEMIOLOGY: Rat-bite fever is a zoonotic illness. The natural habitat of *S moniliformis* and *S minus* is the oropharynx and nasopharynx of rodents. *S moniliformis* is transmitted by bites, scratches, or exposure to oral secretions (eg, via kissing pet rodents) of infected rats, other rodents (eg, mice, gerbils, squirrels, weasels), or rodent-eating animals, including cats and dogs. Infection via contact with contaminated fomites (eg, rat cages or bedding) has been reported rarely. Haverhill fever refers to infection after ingestion of unpasteurized milk, water, or food contaminated with urine containing *S moniliformis* and may be associated with an outbreak of disease. *S minus* is transmitted by bites of rats and mice. *S moniliformis* infection accounts for almost all cases of ratbite fever in the United States; *S minus* infections occur primarily in Asia.

The **incubation period** for *S moniliformis* usually is less than 7 days but can range from 3 days to 3 weeks; for *S minus*, the **incubation period** is 7 to 21 days.

DIAGNOSTIC TESTS: *S moniliformis* is a fastidious, slow-growing organism isolated from blood, synovial fluid, abscesses, or aspirates from the bite lesion. Growth is best in bacteriologic media enriched with blood (15% rabbit blood seems optimal), serum, and ascitic fluid; cultures should be kept in 5% to 10% carbon dioxide atmosphere at 37°C. Sodium polyanethol sulfonate (SPS), a common anticoagulant in blood culture media, inhibits growth. The laboratory should be alerted that *S moniliformis* is suspected and asked to hold the culture for at least 1 week. Nucleic acid amplification tests (NAATs) are increasingly available in hospital and commercial laboratories. The use of 16S ribosomal RNA gene sequencing and matrix-assisted laser desorption/ionization-time of flight (MALDI-TOF) mass spectrometry improve the diagnostic sensitivity and specificity of culture-based practices.

S minus has not been recovered on artificial media but can be visualized by darkfield microscopy in wet mounts of blood, exudate of a lesion, and lymph nodes or by Giemsa or Wright stain of blood specimens.

TREATMENT: Penicillin G procaine administered intramuscularly or penicillin G administered intravenously for 7 to 10 days is the treatment for rat-bite fever caused by either agent; currently in the United States and other countries, intravenous administration is the more acceptable route. Conversion to oral penicillin after a minimum of 5 days of intravenous therapy can be considered in uncomplicated cases, to complete a full 10-day course. There is limited experience using ampicillin, cefuroxime, ceftriaxone, and cefotaxime for treatment. Doxycycline or streptomycin can be substituted when a patient has a serious allergy to penicillin or while awaiting laboratory results when rickettsial infections (eg, Rocky Mountain spotted fever) are also among the differential diagnoses. Patients with endocarditis should receive intravenous high-dose penicillin G for at least 4 weeks. The addition of streptomycin or gentamicin for initial therapy may be useful in severe infections including endocarditis.

INFECTION PREVENTION AND CONTROL MEASURES IN HEALTH CARE SETTINGS: Standard precautions are recommended.

CONTROL MEASURES: Exposed people should be observed for symptoms. Rat control is important in the control of disease. Rodents and other small pets are not recommended for children younger than 5 years or people with weakened immune systems, because they are at a greater risk for serious illness from pathogens that pets can carry. Adults should supervise the touching, feeding, or caring for pets by young children and hand washing for young children. People with frequent rodent exposure should wear gloves and avoid hand-to-mouth contact during animal handling. Regular hand hygiene should be practiced, and surfaces that the rodent contacted should be disinfected.

Respiratory Syncytial Virus

CLINICAL MANIFESTATIONS: Respiratory syncytial virus (RSV) causes acute respiratory tract infections in people of all ages and is one of the most common diseases of early childhood. Most infants infected with RSV experience upper respiratory tract symptoms, and 20% to 30% develop lower respiratory tract disease (eg, bronchiolitis and/or pneumonia) with the first infection. Signs and symptoms of bronchiolitis typically begin with rhinitis and cough, which may progress to increased respiratory effort with tachypnea, wheezing, rales, intercostal and/or subcostal retractions, grunting, and nasal flaring. Fever may, but does not always, occur. Infection with RSV during the first few weeks of life, particularly among preterm infants, may present with more general symptoms such as lethargy, irritability, and poor feeding, accompanied by minimal respiratory tract symptoms; these infants are at risk of developing apnea, even in the absence of other respiratory symptoms.

Most previously healthy infants who develop RSV bronchiolitis do not require hospitalization, and most who are hospitalized improve with supportive care and are discharged after 2 or 3 days. However, approximately 1% to 3% of all children in the first 12 months of life will be hospitalized because of severe RSV lower respiratory tract disease, with the highest rate of RSV hospitalizations occurring in the first 6 months of life. Factors that increase the risk of severe RSV lower respiratory tract illness include preterm birth, especially birth before 29 weeks of gestation; chronic lung disease of prematurity (CLD [formerly called bronchopulmonary dysplasia]); certain types of hemodynamically significant congenital heart disease (CHD), especially conditions associated with pulmonary hypertension; certain immunodeficiency states; and neurologic and neuromuscular conditions. Other risk factors with a more limited correlation with disease severity include low birth weight, maternal smoking during pregnancy, exposure to secondhand smoke in the household, family history of atopy, lack of breastfeeding, and household crowding. Mortality is rare when supportive care is available.

Children hospitalized for RSV bronchiolitis in infancy are at increased risk of recurrent wheezing in early childhood. The association between RSV infection early in life and subsequent asthma, however, remains incompletely understood. Infants who experience severe lower respiratory tract disease (eg, bronchiolitis or pneumonia) from RSV have an increased risk of developing asthma later in life. This association is also seen with other respiratory viral infections, particularly those caused by rhinoviruses. The unresolved question is whether the association between severe infection and reactive airway disease is causal and attributable to direct damage caused by viral replication and the host's response. Alternatively, the association may reflect a common genotype, indicating the same anatomic or immunologic abnormalities that predispose to asthma also predispose to severe viral lower respiratory tract disease. Results from 2 randomized, placebo-controlled trials demonstrated that providing RSV immunoprophylaxis with palivizumab to term and preterm infants had no measurable effect on medically attended wheezing, physician-diagnosed asthma, or lung function at 3 to 6 years of age.

Almost all children are infected by RSV at least once by 24 months of age, and reinfection throughout life is common. Particularly among otherwise healthy older children and adults, recurrent RSV infection manifests as mild upper respiratory tract illness and seldom involves the lower respiratory tract. However, serious disease involving the lower respiratory tract may develop in older children and adults, especially in immunocompromised people and elderly people, particularly those with cardiopulmonary comorbidities. Each year in the United States, the burden of RSV disease in adults ≥65 years of age includes approximately 2 200 000 symptomatic illnesses, approximately 177 000 hospitalizations, and approximately 14 000 deaths. This is comparable to influenza disease burden in this older age group.

ETIOLOGY: RSV is an enveloped, nonsegmented, negative-strand RNA virus of the genus *Orthopneumovirus* of the family *Pneumoviridae*. Human RSV exists as 2 antigenic subgroups, A and B, and often these cocirculate during the same RSV season. A consistent correlation between RSV subgroup and disease severity is unclear. The RSV envelope contains 3 surface glycoproteins: glycoprotein G, fusion protein F, and a small hydrophobic protein (SH). Antibodies directed against F and G are neutralizing and protective. G protein is involved in viral attachment to the cell and assists in the ability of the virus to evade host immunity. F protein enables viral penetration of the epithelial cell once viral attachment occurs. In contrast to G protein, F protein is relatively conserved, making it an attractive target for vaccine and monoclonal antibody development.

EPIDEMIOLOGY: Humans are the only source of infection. RSV usually is transmitted by direct or close contact with contaminated secretions, which may occur from exposure to large-particle droplets at short distances (typically <6 feet) or by self-inoculation after touching contaminated surfaces or fomites. Viable RSV can persist on environmental surfaces for several hours and for 30 minutes or more on hands.

RSV typically occurs in annual epidemics beginning in fall and continuing through early spring in temperate climates, although RSV seasonality was unusual during the COVID-19 pandemic and included significant circulation during the summer.[1] Spread among households and people in child care facilities, including adults, is common. Spread also can occur in the health care setting. The relationship between the presence of infectious virus and the duration of positive molecular testing is unclear. Most infections occur within 7 days of household exposure. The usual period of viral detection by molecular testing is 11 to 14 days, but it may be longer, especially in young infants, who may have positive test results for 3 to 4 weeks, and in immunosuppressed children, who may have positive test results for several months or longer.

The **incubation period** ranges from 2 to 8 days; 4 to 6 days is most common.

DIAGNOSTIC TESTS: Molecular diagnostic tests using reverse transcriptase-polymerase chain reaction (RT-PCR) assays have largely replaced viral isolation and antigen detection assays. Some commercially available assays are designed as multiplex assays to facilitate testing for multiple respiratory viruses from a single nasopharyngeal specimen. Some complex multiplex tests can distinguish between RSV A and B subgroups. Using RT-PCR assays, as many as 30% of symptomatic children will demonstrate the presence of a viral coinfection with 2 or more respiratory viruses. Whether symptomatic children who are coinfected with more than one virus experience more severe or even less severe disease is not clear.

Testing for seroconversion with acute and convalescent serum specimens is rarely performed for the purposes of diagnosing RSV infection and may not be reliable in infants because the immune response to RSV infection may be limited.

Rapid diagnostic assays, including direct fluorescent antibody (DFA) assays and enzyme or chromatographic immunoassays, are available for detection of viral antigen in nasopharyngeal specimens and are reliable in infants and young children. The sensitivity of these tests is lower than for the molecular diagnostics. As with all antigen detection assays, the predictive value is high during the peak season, but false-positive test results are more likely to occur when the incidence of disease is low, such as in the summer in temperate areas.

In most outpatient settings for children with bronchiolitis, routine specific respiratory viral testing has little effect on management and is not recommended.[2] Among hospitalized children with bronchiolitis, testing for viral etiology is not routinely recommended, although it can aid in limiting unnecessary antibiotics. Additionally, if patient cohorting is necessary, identification of the specific viral etiology of a respiratory infection will aid hospital infection prevention efforts.

TREATMENT[2]: No available treatment shortens the course of bronchiolitis or hastens the resolution of symptoms. Management of young children hospitalized with bronchiolitis is supportive and should include hydration, and careful assessment of respiratory status. Supplemental oxygen is recommended only when oxyhemoglobin saturation persistently decreases below 90% in a previously healthy infant. Data

[1] Hamid S, Winn A, Parikh R, et al. Seasonality of respiratory syncytial virus—United States, 2017-2023. *MMWR Morb Mortal Wkly Rep.* 2023;72(14):355-361

[2] Ralston SL, Lieberthal AS, Meissner HC, et al. Clinical practice guideline: the diagnosis, management, and prevention of bronchiolitis. *Pediatrics.* 2014;134(5):e1474-e1502

support the use of heated humidified high-flow nasal cannula treatment as rescue therapy in infants who have continued hypoxemia despite standard oxygen therapy. Nasal continuous positive airway pressure and heliox have been used for respiratory support in hospitalized infants with bronchiolitis who are at risk for progression to respiratory failure. Only limited data are available on the effectiveness of these therapies in bronchiolitis specifically caused by RSV. Because these therapies, as well as intubation and ventilation, typically are used in severely or critically ill infants with bronchiolitis, they should be used only in consultation with a critical care or pulmonary specialist.

Early studies with aerosolized ribavirin therapy demonstrated a small increase in oxygen saturation in small clinical trials; however, a decrease in the need for mechanical ventilation or a decrease in the length of stay was not shown. Because of limited evidence for a clinically relevant benefit, potential toxic effects, and high cost, routine use of aerosolized ribavirin is not recommended.

Alpha- and Beta-Adrenergic Agents. Beta-adrenergic agents are not recommended for care of wheezing associated with RSV bronchiolitis, and a trial of albuterol no longer is included as a recommended option in the management of RSV bronchiolitis.[1] Evidence does not support the use of nebulized epinephrine in children hospitalized with bronchiolitis.

Glucocorticoid Therapy. Controlled clinical trials among children with bronchiolitis have demonstrated that corticosteroids do not reduce hospital admissions and do not reduce length of stay for inpatients. Corticosteroid treatment should not be used for infants and children with RSV bronchiolitis.

Antimicrobial Therapy. Antimicrobial therapy is not indicated for infants with RSV bronchiolitis or pneumonia unless there is evidence of concurrent bacterial infection. A young child with a distinct viral lower respiratory tract infection (bronchiolitis) has a low risk (<1%) of bacterial meningitis. Bacterial lung infections and bacteremia are uncommon in this setting. Acute otitis media (AOM) caused by RSV or bacterial superinfection may occur in infants with RSV bronchiolitis. Oral antimicrobial therapy for treatment of otitis media may be considered if bulging of the tympanic membrane is present.[2]

INFECTION PREVENTION AND CONTROL MEASURES IN HEALTH CARE SETTINGS: In addition to standard precautions, contact and droplet precautions are recommended for the duration of RSV-associated illness. In immunocompromised patients, the duration of precautions should be extended because of possible prolonged shedding. In addition, a variety of measures have been demonstrated to reduce the risk of health care-associated transmission, including: (1) placing in single rooms or cohorting of symptomatic patients with dedicated staff; (2) emphasizing hand hygiene before and after direct contact with patients, after contact with inanimate objects in the direct vicinity of patients because of the likelihood of skin contamination from contact with respiratory secretions (alcohol-based gels and antibacterial hand soaps rapidly

---

[1] Ralston SL, Lieberthal AL, Meissner HC, et al. Clinical practice guideline: the diagnosis, management, and prevention of bronchiolitis. *Pediatrics.* 2014;134(5):e1474-e1502

[2] Lieberthal AS, Carroll AE, Chonmaitree T, et al. Clinical practice guideline: the diagnosis and management of acute otitis media. *Pediatrics. 2013*;131(3):e964-e999

inactivate RSV), and after glove removal; (3) excluding visitors with current or recent respiratory tract infections from health care settings; and (4) limiting young children visiting during the RSV season.

PREVENTION OF RSV INFECTIONS:

Active Immunization. Two RSV vaccines have been approved by the US Food and Drug Administration (FDA) for use in adults ≥60 years of age.[1] Both are recombinant stabilized prefusion F protein (preF) vaccines. One of these products is also approved for use during pregnancy to prevent lower respiratory tract disease (LRTD) and severe LRTD caused by RSV in infants from birth through 6 months of age. The vaccine is administered to the pregnant person as a single intramuscular injection at 32 through 36 weeks' gestation. In clinical trials, vaccine efficacy (VE) for prevention of severe RSV-associated LRTD within 90 days after birth was 81.8% (99.5% confidence interval [CI]: 40.6, 96.3), and within 180 days after birth was 69.4% (97.6% CI: 44.3%, 84.1%). Safety assessments for both the pregnant and infant populations were similar for vaccine and placebo recipients. A slightly higher percentage of premature births occurred in the vaccine recipients compared with placebo recipients (5.6% [95% CI: 4.9%, 6.4%] versus 4.7% [95% CI: 4.1%, 5.5%]), but this did not reach statistical significance and was seen 30 days or more following vaccine administration. The vaccine is recommended for use in all pregnant people at 32 through 36 weeks' gestation, using seasonal administration, to prevent RSV lower respiratory tract infection in infants.

Passive Immunization. Two monoclonal antibodies against RSV have been licensed by the FDA, palivizumab and nirsevimab. Nirsevimab's long half-life allows for administration of a single dose that provides protection across the entire RSV season, while palivizumab requires monthly administration. Nirsevimab is recommended for universal use in all infants under 8 months of age to prevent RSV-associated LRTD (see Nirsevimab Recommendations for First RSV Season, below). It also is recommended for high-risk infants 8 through 19 months of age to prevent RSV LRTD during their second RSV season. Infants in certain risk categories are recommended to receive palivizumab if nirsevimab is not available (see Nirsevimab Recommendations for Second RSV Season, below).

In clinical trials, nirsevimab's pooled efficacy in preventing medically attended RSV-associated LRTD was 79.0% (95% CI: 68.5%, 86.1%), efficacy in preventing RSV-associated LRTD with hospitalization was 80.6% (95% CI: 62.3%, 90.1%), and efficacy in preventing RSV-associated LRTD with ICU admission was 90.0% (95% CI: 16.4%, 98.8%).

Nirsevimab Recommendations for First RSV Season. Recommendations for use of nirsevimab for the infant's first RSV season are dependent on whether the infant's birthing parent received the RSV vaccine during pregnancy and the timing of administration of that vaccine (if given) relative to birth. If the birthing parent: (1) either did not receive RSV vaccine during pregnancy ≥14 days prior to birth or maternal RSV vaccine status is unknown; AND (2) the time of year is during

[1] Melgar M, Britton A, Roper LE, et al. Use of respiratory syncytial virus vaccines in older adults: recommendations of the Advisory Committee on Immunization Practices—United States, 2023. *MMWR Morb Mortal Wkly Rep.* 2023;72(34):793–801

October through March (see Timing of Nirsevimab Administration, below); AND (3) the infant is <8 months of age, then the infant is recommended to receive 1 dose of nirsevimab for protection during the first RSV season. The nirsevimab dose is 50 mg for infants weighing <5 kg and 100 mg for infants weighing ≥5 kg. If nirsevimab is administered, palivizumab should not be administered later that season. An algorithm that details which infants under 8 months of age should receive nirsevimab is provided in Fig 3.15.

Nirsevimab Recommendations for Second RSV Season. In addition, 1 dose of nirsevimab is recommended for infants and children 8 months through 19 months of age who are at increased risk for severe RSV disease and are entering their second RSV season (see Timing of Nirsevimab Administration, below). The dose for these older infants is 200 mg, administered as two 100-mg injections given at the same time at different injection sites. Nirsevimab is recommended for use during the second RSV season for patients in the following risk categories:

- Children with chronic lung disease of prematurity who required medical support (chronic corticosteroid therapy, diuretic therapy, or supplemental oxygen) anytime during the 6-month period before the start of the second RSV season
- Children with severe immunocompromise
- Children with cystic fibrosis who have either:
  - Manifestations of severe lung disease (previous hospitalization for pulmonary exacerbation in the first year of life or abnormalities on chest imaging that persist when stable), or
  - Weight-for-length <10th percentile
- American Indian or Alaska Native children

An algorithm that details which infants 8 months through 19 months of age should receive nirsevimab is provided in Fig 3.15.

Timing of Nirsevimab Administration.[1] Nirsevimab should be administered to eligible infants and children beginning shortly before the start of the RSV season, which in most of the continental United States is from October through the end of March. Infants born shortly before or during the RSV season should receive nirsevimab within 1 week of birth. Nirsevimab administration can occur during the birth hospitalization or in the outpatient setting. Optimal timing for nirsevimab administration is shortly before the RSV season begins; however, nirsevimab may be administered to age-eligible infants and children who have not yet received a dose at any time during the season. Only a single dose of nirsevimab is recommended for an RSV season.

Infants with prolonged birth hospitalizations related to prematurity or other causes should receive nirsevimab shortly before or promptly after hospital discharge. No evidence is available to support use of nirsevimab for prevention of hospital-acquired RSV infection, and nirsevimab is not recommended for this indication.

Because the timing of the onset, peak, and decline of RSV activity might vary geographically, administration schedules can be adjusted based on local epidemiology. RSV seasonality in tropical climates (including southern Florida, Guam, Hawaii,

---

[1] Jones JM, Fleming-Dutra KE, Prill MM, et al. Use of nirsevimab for the prevention of respiratory syncytial virus disease among infants and young children: recommendations of the Advisory Committee on Immunization Practices—United States, 2023. *MMWR Morb Mortal Wkly Rep.* 2023;72(34):920–925

FIG 3.15. RESPIRATORY SYNCYTIAL VIRUS (RSV) MONOCLONAL ANTIBODY PROPHYLAXIS DECISION ALGORITHM FOR INFANTS <8 MONTHS AND 8 THROUGH 19 MONTHS OF AGE

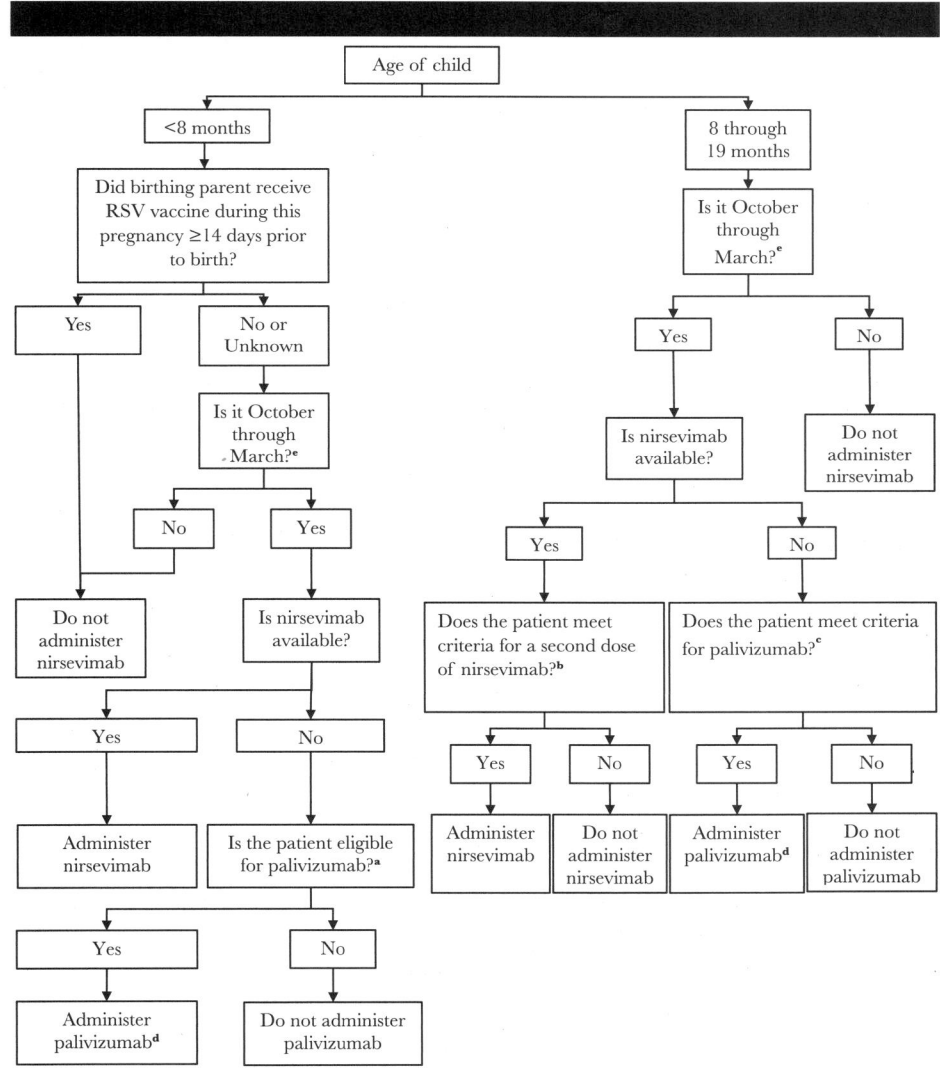

[a] Preterm infants with chronic lung disease of prematurity (CLD); infants with hemodynamically significant congenital heart disease (CHD); preterm infants without CLD or CHD but born before 29 weeks, 0 days gestation who are younger than 12 months at the start of the RSV season; children with anatomic pulmonary abnormalities or neuromuscular disorder; immunocompromised children; children with cystic fibrosis.

[b] Children with CLD who required medical support (chronic corticosteroid therapy, diuretic therapy, or supplemental oxygen) any time during the 6-month period before the start of the second RSV season; severe immunocompromise; cystic fibrosis who have either (1) manifestations of severe lung disease (previous hospitalization for pulmonary exacerbation in the first year of life or abnormalities on chest imaging that persist when stable), or (2) weight-for-length <10th percentile; American Indian or Alaska Native children.

FIG 3.15. RESPIRATORY SYNCYTIAL VIRUS (RSV) MONOCLONAL ANTIBODY PROPHYLAXIS DECISION ALGORITHM FOR INFANTS <8 MONTHS AND 8 THROUGH 19 MONTHS OF AGE, CONTINUED

[c] Preterm infants with CLD requiring require medical support (chronic corticosteroid therapy, diuretic therapy, or supplemental oxygen) during the 6-month period before the start of the second RSV season; immunocompromised children; children with cystic fibrosis with manifestations of severe lung disease (previous hospitalization for pulmonary exacerbation in the first year or abnormalities on chest radiography or chest computed tomography that persist when stable) or weight-for-length less than the 10th percentile.

[d] For recommendations on use of palivizumab, see Ralston SL, Lieberthal AL, Meissner HC, et al. Clinical practice guideline: the diagnosis, management, and prevention of bronchiolitis. *Pediatrics.* 2014;134(5):e1474-e1502; and Caserta MT, O'Leary ST, Munoz FM, Ralston SL; American Academy of Pediatrics, Committee on Infectious Diseases. Technical report. Palivizumab prophylaxis in infants and young children at increased risk of hospitalization for respiratory syncytial virus infection. *Pediatrics.* 2023;152(1):e20230618.

[e] In jurisdictions with seasonality that differs from most of the continental United States (eg, Alaska, jurisdictions with tropical climates), providers should follow state, local, or territorial guidance on timing of administration.

Puerto Rico, US-affiliated Pacific Islands, and US Virgin Islands) might differ from that of most of the continental United States or be unpredictable. In Alaska, RSV seasonality is less predictable, and the duration of RSV activity is often longer than the national average duration. Providers in these jurisdictions should consult state, local, or territorial guidance on timing of nirsevimab administration.

Coadministration With Other Vaccines. Nirsevimab is not expected to interfere with the immune response to other routine childhood immunizations, and simultaneous administration of nirsevimab with age-appropriate vaccines is recommended.

Palivizumab. If nirsevimab is not available, palivizumab may be used in high risk patients in their first or second RSV seasons (see Fig 3.15 for definitions of who qualifies). If nirsevimab becomes available during the course of the season and before the fifth dose of palivizumab, a single dose should be administered and no additional palivizumab doses should be given.

Use of Nirsevimab in Children Who Already Have Had RSV in That Season. Nirsevimab should be administered for the first (or if high risk patients, the second) RSV season regardless of whether the infant has already had an RSV infection at any time previously, including during the current season. Reinfection with RSV, even during the same season, can occur. If there is a shortage of nirsevimab, this recommendation for its use regardless of prior RSV infection may need to be modified until the shortage is resolved. Children who are moderately or severely ill with or without fever including those who have known current RSV infection should defer nirsevimab until recovery from the acute illness.

Cardiopulmonary Bypass. Children undergoing cardiac surgery with cardiopulmonary bypass should receive an additional dose of nirsevimab after surgery during RSV season if age-eligible.

For the first RSV season, if cardiac surgery with cardiopulmonary bypass is performed within 90 days after receiving nirsevimab, an additional dose should be administered based on body weight at the time of the additional dose (50 mg if less than 5 kg and 100 mg if ≥5 kg). If cardiac surgery with cardiopulmonary bypass is performed more than 90 days after receiving nirsevimab, an additional dose of 50 mg, regardless of body weight, should be administered.

For the second RSV season, if cardiac surgery with cardiopulmonary bypass is performed within 90 days after receiving nirsevimab, an additional dose of 200 mg, regardless of body weight, should be administered. If cardiac surgery with cardiopulmonary bypass is performed more than 90 days after receiving nirsevimab, an additional dose of 100 mg, regardless of body weight, should be administered.

Contraindications and Adverse Event Reporting.[1] Nirsevimab is contraindicated in persons with a history of severe allergic reaction (eg, anaphylaxis) after a previous dose or to a product component. Adverse reactions might occur after administration of nirsevimab alone, and should be reported to MedWatch online (**www.fda.gov/medwatch**), by fax, by mail, or by contacting FDA at 1-800-FDA-1088. Adverse reactions also might occur after the coadministration of nirsevimab with a vaccine, and these reactions should be reported to the Vaccine Adverse Event Reporting System (VAERS), with reports specifying that the patient received nirsevimab on the VAERS form (**https://vaers.hhs.gov**; 1-800-822-7967). When adverse reactions that occur after the coadministration of nirsevimab with a vaccine are reported to VAERS, additional reporting of the same adverse reactions to MedWatch is not necessary.

CONTROL MEASURES: A critical aspect of RSV prevention among high-risk infants is education of parents and other caregivers about the importance of decreasing exposure to and transmission of RSV. Preventive measures include limiting, where feasible, exposure to contagious settings (eg, child care centers); emphasis on hand hygiene in all settings, including the home, especially during periods when contacts of high-risk children have respiratory tract infections; and limiting exposure to secondhand smoke.

Rhinovirus Infections

CLINICAL MANIFESTATIONS: Rhinoviruses are the most frequent cause of the common cold, or rhinosinusitis. Typical clinical manifestations include sore throat, nasal congestion, and nasal discharge that initially is watery and clear but often becomes mucopurulent and viscous after a few days. Malaise, headache, myalgia, low-grade fever, cough, and sneezing may occur. Symptoms typically peak in severity after 2 to 3 days and have a median duration of 7 days but may persist for more than 10 days in approximately 25% of illnesses. Rhinoviruses also cause otitis media and lower respiratory tract infections (eg, bronchiolitis, pneumonia), particularly in infants, and are associated with approximately 60% to 70% of acute exacerbations of asthma in school-aged children.

ETIOLOGY: Rhinoviruses (RVs) are small, nonenveloped, single, positive-stranded RNA viruses classified into 3 species (RV-A, RV-B, and RV-C) in the family *Picornaviridae*, genus *Enterovirus*. Nearly 170 rhinovirus types have been identified by immunologic and molecular methods. Infection confers type-specific immunity, but protection is temporary.

---

[1] Jones JM, Fleming-Dutra KE, Prill MM, et al. Use of nirsevimab for the prevention of respiratory syncytial virus disease among infants and young children: recommendations of the Advisory Committee on Immunization Practices—United States, 2023. *MMWR Morb Mortal Wkly Rep*. 2023;72(34):920–925

EPIDEMIOLOGY: Rhinovirus infection is ubiquitous in human populations. It is most frequent in infancy and early childhood; more than 20% of infants experience their first rhinovirus infection before 6 months of age. Children typically experience 2 to 4 rhinovirus infections each year, and 93% of adults experience at least 1 rhinovirus infection annually. Rhinoviruses may cause up to two thirds of cases of the common cold. They can cause sinusitis and otitis media, either as the sole pathogen or with secondary bacterial infections. Rhinovirus infections are a major viral cause of exacerbations of asthma, cystic fibrosis, and chronic obstructive pulmonary disease and have been detected in the lower respiratory tract in patients of all ages hospitalized with wheezing or pneumonia. Rhinovirus infection is associated with increased mortality in hematopoietic cell transplant recipients.

Person-to-person transmission occurs by self-inoculation of contaminated secretions on hands or by large-particle aerosol spread. Infections occur throughout the year, but peak activity occurs during fall and spring. Multiple types circulate simultaneously, and the prevalent types circulating in a given population change from season to season. Viral shedding in nasopharyngeal secretions is most abundant during the first 2 to 3 days of infection and usually ceases by 7 to 10 days. Viral RNA may be detectable in nasal secretions by molecular testing for as long as 30 days, although low amounts of virus detected by nucleic acid amplification tests (NAATs) in an asymptomatic person are unlikely to result in transmission. Young age and child care attendance are associated with more frequent rhinovirus infections. Those at increased risk for severe illness include those born preterm with or without chronic lung disease, respiratory syncytial virus coinfection, congenital heart disease, underlying pulmonary disease, immunocompromise, and history of atopy in the birthing parent.

The **incubation period** usually is 2 to 3 days.

DIAGNOSTIC TESTS: Rhinovirus infection is diagnosed by detection of virus in respiratory secretions, although a specific viral diagnosis may not be useful clinically in terms of patient management. Because of the lack of common group antigens among the various types, antigen detection is not practical for clinical diagnosis. If a viral diagnosis is necessary, NAATs are the preferred method to identify rhinovirus infections, with several commercial assays cleared by the US Food and Drug Administration. Most of these assays are designed as multiplexed tests that detect a wide variety of viral and, in some cases, bacterial respiratory pathogens. In general, these assays cannot clearly distinguish rhinoviruses from enteroviruses because of the genetic similarity of the 2 groups. Given the prevalence of rhinovirus infection and the occurrence of shedding following infection, rhinovirus detection, even in symptomatic patients, may not be causal. Serologic diagnosis of rhinovirus infection is impractical because of the large number of antigenic types and the absence of a common antigen.

TREATMENT: Treatment is supportive. Over-the-counter cough and cold medications are not recommended for use in children younger than 2 years. No specific antiviral therapy is currently available for treatment of rhinovirus infections. Antimicrobial agents should not be used for prevention of secondary bacterial infection, because their use may promote the emergence of resistant bacteria and subsequently complicate treatment for a bacterial infection, and because of the risk of antibiotic-associated adverse effects (eg, *Clostridioides difficile* disease; see Antimicrobial Resistance and Antimicrobial Stewardship: Appropriate and Judicious Use of Antimicrobial Agents, p 978).

INFECTION PREVENTION AND CONTROL MEASURES IN HEALTH CARE SETTINGS: In addition to standard precautions, droplet precautions are recommended for symptomatic hospitalized infants and children for the duration of illness. Contact precautions should be added if copious moist secretions and close contact are likely to occur (eg, young infants). In symptomatic immunocompromised patients, the duration of contact precautions should be extended because of possible prolonged shedding.

CONTROL MEASURES: Appropriate respiratory hygiene and cough etiquette should be followed. Routine hand washing and alcohol-based hand sanitizers are effective for removal of rhinovirus from the hands.

Rickettsial Diseases

Rickettsial diseases comprise infections caused by bacterial species within the genera *Rickettsia* (endemic and epidemic typhus and spotted fever group rickettsioses), *Orientia* (scrub typhus), *Ehrlichia* (ehrlichiosis), *Anaplasma* (anaplasmosis), *Neoehrlichia,* and *Neorickettsia*. The genus *Rickettsia* is further divided into 4 groups based on serologic and genomic analyses, comprising the typhus group, spotted fever group, ancestral group, and transitional group.

CLINICAL MANIFESTATIONS: Early signs and symptoms can be nonspecific and often mimic viral illness. Rickettsial infections have many features in common. Fever, rash (especially in spotted fever and typhus group rickettsiae), headache, and myalgia are prominent features. The classic rash of Rocky Mountain spotted fever (RMSF) may not appear until 3 to 5 days after onset of symptoms, and approximately 10% of patients do not develop an identifiable rash. One or more inoculation eschars occur with many rickettsial diseases, especially most spotted fever group rickettsioses (but not RMSF), rickettsialpox, and scrub typhus. Systemic endothelial damage of small blood vessels resulting in increased vascular permeability is the hallmark pathologic feature of most severe spotted fever and typhus group rickettsial infections. Some rickettsial diseases, particularly RMSF, Mediterranean spotted fever, epidemic typhus, and scrub typhus, can rapidly become life threatening. Risk factors for severe disease include glucose-6-phosphate dehydrogenase deficiency, being male, and antecedent exposure to sulfonamides.[1]

Anecdotal information suggests that prior infection confers some short-term immunity. Documented reinfections with *Rickettsia* and *Ehrlichia* species have been described only rarely.

ETIOLOGY: Rickettsiae are small, coccobacillary gram-negative bacteria that are obligate intracellular pathogens and cannot be grown in cell-free media such as routine blood agar. *Orientia* and *Rickettsia* organisms reside free within the cytosol whereas

---

[1] The term male refers to sex assigned at birth.

Anaplasmataceae organisms reside in phagosomes. Currently recognized rickettsial pathogens of humans include more than 20 species of *Rickettsia*, 5 species of *Ehrlichia*, at least 2 species each of *Orientia* and *Anaplasma*, and *Neorickettsia sennetsu*. Tick-borne neoehrlichiosis caused by *Candidatus Neoehrlichia mikurensis* is an emerging, increasingly recognized disease in Asia and Europe.

EPIDEMIOLOGY: Rickettsial diseases have various hematophagous (blood-feeding) arthropod vectors that include ticks, fleas, mites, and lice. Except for *Rickettsia prowazekii*, the cause of epidemic typhus, humans are incidental hosts for rickettsial pathogens. Rickettsial life cycles typically involve one or more arthropod species as well as various mammalian reservoirs or amplifying hosts, and transmission to humans occurs during environmental or occupational exposures to infected arthropods. Geographic and seasonal occurrences of each rickettsial disease are related directly to distributions and life cycles of the specific vector.

    Incubation periods vary according to organism (see disease-specific chapters in Section 3).

Other Global Rickettsial Spotted Fever Infections. Other, epidemiologically distinct, flea-borne and tick-borne spotted fever rickettsioses have been recognized (also see **www.cdc.gov/otherspottedfever/**). These diseases can affect people living in, traveling to, or returning from areas where these pathogens are endemic. These infections have clinical and pathologic features that vary widely in severity. Most tick-borne rickettsioses present with an eschar at the site of the tick bite, and some present without rash or a sparse rash. Information about spotted fevers occurring outside the United States can be found at **www.cdc.gov/otherspottedfever/imported/index.html.** Causative agents of spotted fevers in the United States other than *R rickettsii* and of other rickettsial diseases most important for travelers include the following:

- *Rickettsia africae*, the causative agent of African tick bite fever that is endemic in sub-Saharan Africa, Oceania, and some Caribbean islands.

- *Rickettsia akari*, the causative agent of rickettsialpox, which occurs sporadically throughout the United States but is often reported from metropolitan centers in the eastern United States, particularly New York City (see Rickettsialpox, p 726).

- *Rickettsia conorii* and subspecies, the causative agents of Mediterranean spotted fever, Indian tick typhus, Israeli tick typhus, and Astrakhan spotted fever, that are endemic in southern Europe, Africa, the Middle East, and the Indian subcontinent.

- *Rickettsia parkeri*, a causative agent of eschar-associated infections in the Americas.

- *Rickettsia* 364D, the causative agent of Pacific Coast tick fever, an eschar-associated rickettsiosis in California.

DIAGNOSTIC TESTS: Group-specific antibodies are detectable in the serum of most patients by 7 to 10 days after onset of illness, but slower antibody responses can occur, particularly in some diseases of lesser severity, such as African tick bite fever. The utility of serologic testing during the acute illness generally is of limited value, and a negative serologic test result during the initial stage of the illness should never be used to exclude a diagnosis of rickettsial disease. Serologic assays provide an excellent method of retrospective confirmation when paired serum samples collected during the illness and 2 to 4 weeks later are tested in tandem and demonstrate a fourfold or greater increase in antibody titer. The indirect immunofluorescence antibody assay is recommended in most circumstances but cannot determine the causative agent to the species level. Treatment early in the course of illness can blunt or delay serologic responses. Once present, antibodies can persist for months or longer, and in some areas of the United States, 10% of people may have antibodies against *Rickettsia* or related organisms. Nucleic acid amplification tests (NAATs) can detect rickettsiae in whole blood or tissues collected during the acute stage of illness and before administration of antimicrobial agents; availability of these tests often is limited to reference and research laboratories. Immunohistochemical staining and NAATs of skin biopsy specimens from patients with rash or eschar lesions can help to diagnose rickettsial infections early in the course of disease. NAATs and sequencing of DNA collected during acute infection provide more accurate identification of the etiologic agent than serologic testing.

TREATMENT: Prompt initiation of treatment is indicated for all patients in all age groups with presumptive evidence of any rickettsial disease and is of paramount importance when there is clinical suspicion of a potentially life-threatening infection such as RMSF, ehrlichiosis, epidemic typhus, murine typhus, or scrub typhus. Treatment decisions should be made on the basis of clinical findings and epidemiologic data and never should be delayed until test results are known, because confirmatory laboratory tests are rarely available early in the course of illness. Therapy is less effective in preventing complications when disease remains untreated into the second week of illness. For all ages, the drug of choice for all rickettsioses, including RMSF and ehrlichiosis, is doxycycline. Treatment should be continued for at least 3 days after fever subsides and there is evidence of clinical improvement, with a typical minimum duration of therapy of 5 to 7 days. For patients with anaplasmosis, therapy should be extended for 10 days to provide appropriate length of therapy for possible coinfection with *Borrelia burgdorferi*. Antibiotic prophylaxis after a tick bite is not recommended to prevent any rickettsial infection.

CONTROL MEASURES: Limiting exposures to ticks, mites, chiggers, and their associated bites is the primary means of prevention (see Prevention of Mosquito-borne and Tick-borne Infections, p 207).

For more details, the following chapters in Section 3 on rickettsial diseases should be consulted:

- *Ehrlichia, Anaplasma,* and Related Infections, p 361 (or **www.cdc.gov/ ehrlichiosis/**).
- Rickettsialpox, p 726.
- Rocky Mountain Spotted Fever, p 727 (or **www.cdc.gov/rmsf/**).
- Louse-borne Typhus (Epidemic or Sylvatic Typhus), p 932.
- Murine Typhus (Endemic or Flea-borne Typhus), p 934.

Public Health Reporting. Several rickettsial diseases, including spotted fevers, ehrlichiosis, and anaplasmosis, are nationally notifiable diseases and should be reported to state and local health departments.

Rickettsialpox

CLINICAL MANIFESTATIONS: Rickettsialpox is a febrile, eschar-associated illness characterized by generalized, relatively sparse, erythematous, papulovesicular eruptions on the trunk, face, extremities (less often on palms and soles), and occasionally involving the oral mucous membranes. The rash may resemble chickenpox and develops 1 to 4 days after onset of fever and 3 to 10 days after appearance of an eschar at the site of the bite of an infected house mouse mite. Eschars are generally 0.5 to 2.5 cm, are most frequently found on the extremities and torso, and may be nontender or mildly tender. Regional lymph nodes proximal to the inoculation eschar often become enlarged and tender. Without specific antimicrobial therapy, systemic disease lasts approximately 7 to 14 days; manifestations include fever, headache, malaise, and myalgia. Less frequent manifestations include anorexia, vomiting, conjunctivitis, hepatitis, nuchal rigidity, and photophobia. The disease is mild compared with Rocky Mountain spotted fever, and although no rickettsialpox-associated deaths have been described, disease occasionally is severe enough to warrant hospitalization.

ETIOLOGY: Rickettsialpox is caused by *Rickettsia akari*, a gram-negative intracellular bacillus now classified with *Rickettsia felis* and *Rickettsia australis* within the transitional group of the genus *Rickettsia*, so named because they have features of both the spotted fever and typhus groups.

EPIDEMIOLOGY: The natural host for *R akari* in the United States is *Mus musculus*, the common house mouse. The organism is transmitted by the bite of the house mouse mite, *Liponyssoides sanguineus*. Disease risk is heightened in areas infested with house mice. The disease can occur wherever the hosts, pathogens, and humans coexist but most frequently is reported in large urban settings. In the United States, rickettsialpox has been described predominantly in metropolitan centers, especially in New York City, as well as Boston, Baltimore, and other large cities along the Atlantic coast. It has been confirmed in many other countries, including the Netherlands, Croatia, Ukraine, Turkey, Russia, South Korea, South Africa, and Mexico. All age groups can be affected. No seasonal pattern of disease occurs. The disease is not communicable but occurs occasionally among families or people cohabiting a house mouse mite-infested dwelling.

The **incubation period** is 6 to 15 days.

DIAGNOSTIC TESTS: Serologic tests for antibodies reactive with spotted fever group rickettsial antigens are the most frequently used diagnostic assays. Immunoglobulin (Ig) M and IgG are generally detected 7 to 15 days after illness onset. *R akari* can be isolated in cell culture from blood and eschar biopsy specimens during the acute stage of disease, but culture is not attempted routinely. Because antigens of *R akari* have extensive cross-reactivity with antigens of *Rickettsia rickettsii* (the cause of Rocky Mountain spotted fever) and other spotted fever-group rickettsiae, an indirect immunofluorescence antibody assay for *R rickettsii* can be used to demonstrate a fourfold or greater change in antibody titers between acute and convalescent serum specimens obtained 2 to 6 weeks apart. Use of *R akari* antigen is recommended for a more accurate diagnosis but may be available only in specialized research laboratories. Immunohistochemical testing of formalin-fixed, paraffin-embedded eschars or papulovesicle biopsy specimens at specialized reference laboratories can also detect rickettsiae in the samples and are useful diagnostic techniques, but because of antigenic cross-reactivity these assays are not able to confirm the etiologic agent. A polymerase chain reaction assay for detection of rickettsial DNA with subsequent sequence identification can confirm *R akari* infection but currently is not cleared by the US Food and Drug Administration for use in the United States.

TREATMENT: Doxycycline is the drug of choice in all age groups. The minimum course of therapy is 5 days. Treatment is continued for at least 3 days after resolution of fever and until there is clinical improvement. Doxycycline shortens the course of disease, and symptoms typically resolve within 12 to 48 hours after initiation of therapy. Chloramphenicol is an alternative drug but carries a risk of serious adverse events and is not available as an oral formulation in the United States. Use of chloramphenicol should be considered only in rare cases, such as for patients with an absolute contraindication to receiving doxycycline, because rickettsialpox usually is mild and self-limited. Untreated rickettsialpox usually resolves within 2 weeks.

INFECTION PREVENTION AND CONTROL MEASURES IN HEALTH CARE SETTINGS: Person-to-person spread of rickettsialpox has not been reported. Standard precautions are recommended.

CONTROL MEASURES: Application of residual acaricides can be used in heavily mite-infested environments to eliminate the vector. Rodent-control measures are important in limiting or eliminating spread of rickettsialpox but they should be conducted only in conjunction with acaricide application to ensure vector control. No specific management of exposed people is necessary.

Rocky Mountain Spotted Fever

CLINICAL MANIFESTATIONS: Rocky Mountain spotted fever (RMSF) is a systemic, predominantly small-vessel vasculitis that often involves a characteristic rash. Unlike many other spotted fever rickettsioses, eschars at sites of tick bites do not develop with RMSF. High fever, myalgia, headache (less commonly reported in young children), nausea, vomiting, and malaise are typical presenting symptoms. Abdominal pain and diarrhea can be present and may obscure the diagnosis. Children may also experience peripheral and/or periorbital edema. The rash usually appears 2 to 4 days following the onset of fever; a faint maculopapular rash first appears on the wrists, forearms, or ankles and spreads centripetally to involve the limbs and trunk. The rash associated with RMSF can also involve the palms and soles. Although development of a rash is a useful diagnostic sign, fewer than 50% of patients have a rash during the first 3 days of illness, the early rash may be faint, and rash can be absent altogether in up to 10% of patients. As the disease progresses, the rash can become petechial, which is indicative of worsening small-vessel vasculitis and regional extravasation of red cells. A petechial rash is also indicative of progressive injury to small blood vessels of other organs and tissues. Delayed onset or atypical appearance of the rash is a risk factor for misdiagnosis and poor outcome. Meningismus, altered mental status, cerebral edema leading to life-threatening increases in intracranial pressure, and/or coma can occur with the progression of disease. Thrombocytopenia, elevated liver aminotransferases, and hyponatremia are the laboratory abnormalities seen most frequently and worsen as disease progresses. White blood cell count is often normal until later stages of disease, but leukopenia and anemia can occur. When appropriate antibiotic therapy is initiated during the first few days of infection, patients typically recover completely, and fever resolves in the first 48 hours of treatment. If appropriate antimicrobial treatment is not initiated or is delayed past the fifth day of symptoms, the illness can be severe or life-threatening and can include prominent central nervous system, cardiac, pulmonary, gastrointestinal tract, and renal involvement; disseminated intravascular coagulation; necrosis of digits and gangrene; and shock leading to death. RMSF can progress rapidly, even in previously healthy people. Case fatality rates of untreated RMSF range from 20% to 80%, with a median time to death of 8 days. Significant long-term sequelae can occur in patients with severe RMSF, even if treated with appropriate antibiotics; these include neurologic (paraparesis; hearing loss; peripheral neuropathy; bladder and bowel incontinence; developmental and language delays; and cerebellar, vestibular, and motor dysfunction) and nonneurologic (disability from limb or digit amputation) sequelae.

ETIOLOGY: *Rickettsia rickettsii*, an obligate, intracellular, gram-negative bacillus and a member of the spotted fever group of rickettsiae, is the causative agent of RMSF. The primary targets of infection in mammalian hosts are endothelial cells lining the small blood vessels of all major tissues and organs. Diffuse small vessel vasculitis and vascular injury leads to increased permeability and tissue edema.

EPIDEMIOLOGY: The pathogen is transmitted to humans by the bites of several genera of hard ticks of the family *Ixodidae*. The principal recognized vectors of *R rickettsii* are *Dermacentor variabilis* (the American dog tick) in the eastern and central United States and *Dermacentor andersoni* (the Rocky Mountain wood tick) in the northern and western United States. *Rhipicephalus sanguineus* (the brown dog tick) has been confirmed as a vector of *R rickettsii* in Arizona and Mexico and may play a role in other regions. Ticks and their small mammal hosts serve as reservoirs of the pathogen in nature. Other wild animals and dogs have been found with antibodies to *R rickettsii*, but their role as natural reservoirs is not clear. Dogs can experience clinical symptoms similar to those described in humans. People with occupational or recreational exposure to the tick vector (eg, pet owners, animal handlers, and people who spend more time outdoors) are at increased risk of exposure to the organism. People of all ages can be infected. The period of highest incidence in the United States is from April to September, although RMSF can occur year-round in certain areas with endemic disease. The geographic ranges of many ticks, including those that transmit *R rickettsii* are expanding because of climate change. Laboratory-acquired infection is rare. Transmission has occurred on rare occasions by blood transfusion. There have been no documented cases of RMSF transmitted via organ transplantation, although it is theoretically possible.

RMSF is the most severe and frequently fatal rickettsial illness in the United States. Patients at higher risk for severe illness include those in whom treatment was delayed, children younger than 10 years, and patients with glucose-6-phosphate dehydrogenase (G6PD) deficiency. Children younger than 10 years are 5 times more likely than adults to die of RMSF.

Current national surveillance collects data on spotted fever rickettsioses, including RMSF. They are widespread in the United States, with most cases reported in the south Atlantic, southeastern, and south-central states. The incidence of spotted fever rickettsioses has increased in the past 2 decades; the reported cases in the southwestern United States are largely believed to be secondary to RMSF.

The **incubation period** is approximately 1 week (typical range, 3–12 days).

DIAGNOSTIC TESTS[1]**:** The diagnosis of RMSF must be made using clinical signs and symptoms and can be confirmed later using diagnostic tests. Treatment should never be delayed while awaiting laboratory confirmation or because of lack of history of tick bite; approximately half of RMSF cases occur in people who do not report a tick bite. The indirect immunofluorescence antibody (IFA) assay using *R rickettsii* antigen is considered the reference standard serologic assay. Both immunoglobulin (Ig) G and IgM antibodies begin to increase approximately 7 to 10 days after onset of symptoms; IgM is less specific, and IgG is the preferred test. Confirmation requires a fourfold or greater increase in antigen-specific IgG between serum specimens collected during the acute (first 1–2 weeks of illness) and convalescent stage (2–6 weeks following resolution of symptoms). An elevated acute titer may represent prior exposure to RMSF or another spotted fever group rickettsiae rather than acute infection, and a negative serologic test in the acute phase does not rule out diagnosis of RMSF. Low-level elevated antibody titers can be an incidental finding in a significant proportion of the general population in some regions. Cross-reactivity can be observed with antigens of other spotted fever group rickettsiae, including *Rickettsia parkeri* and *Rickettsia africae*. Enzyme-linked immunosorbent assays also can be used for assessing antibody presence in acute and convalescent sera but are less useful for quantifying changes in titer values.

RMSF can be diagnosed by detection of *R rickettsii* DNA in acute whole blood, tissue, and serum specimens by nucleic acid amplification tests (NAATs). *R rickettsii* typically does not circulate in large numbers in whole blood until advanced stages of disease; assays relying on detection of DNA can lack sensitivity, and a negative result does not rule out RMSF. Specimens used for NAATs should be obtained before doxycycline administration when possible, but initiation of treatment should not be delayed. Diagnosis can also be confirmed by detection of rickettsial DNA in biopsy or autopsy specimens by NAATs or immunohistochemical (IHC) visualization of rickettsiae in tissues, although these assays have limited availability.

R rickettsii also can be isolated from acute blood specimens or from infected tissues, but culture requires specialized cell culture techniques and a laboratory with a minimum biosafety level 3 designation. Cell culture cultivation of the organism must be confirmed by molecular methods.

TREATMENT[1]**:** Doxycycline is the drug of choice for treatment of RMSF in patients of any age and should be started as soon as RMSF is suspected. Physicians should treat empirically if RMSF is being considered and should not postpone treatment while awaiting laboratory confirmation. Treatment is most effective if initiated in the first 5 days of symptoms, and treatment started after that time is less likely to prevent death or other adverse outcomes. Antimicrobial treatment should be continued until

[1] Biggs HM, Behravesh CB, Bradley KK, et al. Diagnosis and management of tickborne rickettsial diseases: Rocky Mountain spotted fever and other spotted fever group rickettsioses, ehrlichioses, and anaplasmosis—United States. A practical guide for health care and public health professionals. *MMWR Recomm Rep.* 2016;65(RR-2):1–44

the patient has been afebrile for at least 3 days and has demonstrated clinical improvement; the usual minimum duration of therapy is 5 to 7 days but can be longer in severe cases. Resistance to doxycycline or relapses in symptoms after the completion of the recommended course has not been documented. Use of antimicrobial agents other than doxycycline increases risk of mortality. Chloramphenicol can be found in some references as an alternative treatment; however, its use is associated with a higher risk of fatal outcome. Chloramphenicol carries a risk of serious adverse events and is not available as an oral formulation in the United States. Sulfa-containing drugs are associated with clinical worsening and increase the likelihood of death from RMSF. Other antibiotics are not effective. In the case of severe doxycycline allergy, a specialist should be consulted to discuss risks, benefits, and alternatives. Doxycycline desensitization has been described. Experts at the Centers for Disease Control and Prevention (CDC) are available by telephone for consultation with health care providers at 1-800-CDC-INFO (1-800-232-4636).

INFECTION PREVENTION AND CONTROL MEASURES IN HEALTH CARE SETTINGS: Standard precautions are recommended.

CONTROL MEASURES: Limiting exposures to ticks and tick bites is the primary means of prevention (see Prevention of Mosquito-borne and Tick-borne Infections, p 207). Prophylactic use of antimicrobial agents to prevent RMSF is not recommended, even in children with a documented tick bite who are asymptomatic. People who were bitten by a tick in an area with endemic disease should be advised to see a health care provider should they develop signs or symptoms of RMSF. No licensed *R rickettsii* vaccine is available in the United States. Additional information is available on the Centers for Disease Control and Prevention's Web site (**www.cdc.gov/rmsf/**).

Rotavirus Infections

CLINICAL MANIFESTATIONS: The clinical manifestations of rotavirus vary and depend on whether it is the first infection or a reinfection. After 3 months of age, the first infection generally is the most severe. Infection begins with acute onset of vomiting followed 24 to 48 hours later by watery diarrhea; up to one third of patients will have high fevers. Symptoms usually last for 3 to 7 days but improve over time. In moderate to severe cases or with prolonged diarrhea, additional sequelae including dehydration, electrolyte abnormalities, and acidosis may occur. More severe cases are seen primarily among unvaccinated children 3 through 35 months of age. In certain immunocompromised children, including children with congenital cellular immunodeficiencies or severe combined immunodeficiency (SCID) and children who are hematopoietic cell or solid organ transplant recipients, severe, prolonged, and sometimes fatal rotavirus diarrhea can occur. Rotavirus RNA in cerebrospinal fluid (CSF) has been detected in children with rotavirus-associated seizures.

ETIOLOGY: Rotaviruses are segmented, nonenveloped, double-stranded RNA viruses belonging to the family *Reoviridae*, with at least 10 distinct groups (A through J). Group A viruses are the major causes of human disease, although rotaviruses of groups B and C have also been associated with acute gastroenteritis. An 11-gene typing system is used for rotavirus where the notations Gx-P[x]-Ix-Rx-Cx-Mx-Ax-Nx-Tx-Ex-Hx indicate the genotypes of the 6 structural viral proteins (VP7, VP4, VP6, VP1, VP2, VP3) and the 6 nonstructural proteins (NSP1, NSP2, NSP3, NSP4, NSP5/6), respectively.

The most prevalent genotypes circulating in the United States are: G1P[8], G2P[4], G3P[8], G4P[8], G9P[8], and G12P[8].

EPIDEMIOLOGY: Rotavirus is present in high titer in stools of infected patients several days before and may continue for at least 10 days after onset of clinical disease. Only a small inoculum (<100 viral particles/g of stool) is needed for transmission or to cause infection in a susceptible person, which occurs via the fecal-oral route. Rotavirus can remain viable for weeks to months on contaminated environmental surfaces and fomites (such as toys), which can also lead to transmission. Airborne droplet transmission has not been proven but may play a minor role in disease transmission. Spread within families and institutions is common. Rarely, common-source outbreaks from contaminated water or food have been reported.

The epidemiology and burden of rotavirus disease in the United States has changed dramatically following the introduction of rotavirus vaccines in 2006 and 2008. Before widespread use of these vaccines, rotavirus was the most common cause of community acquired gastroenteritis and health care-associated diarrhea in young children. Since the introduction of rotavirus vaccines in the United States, a biennial pattern has emerged, with small, short seasons (median 9 weeks) beginning in late winter/early spring in some years, alternating with years with extremely low circulation. Beginning in 2008, annual hospitalizations for rotavirus disease among US children younger than 5 years declined by approximately 75%, with an estimated 40 000 to 50 000 fewer rotavirus hospitalizations nationally each year. In case-control evaluations in the United States, the rotavirus vaccines have been found to be approximately 80% to 90% effective against rotavirus disease resulting in hospitalization. The vaccines also are highly effective in reducing emergency department visits for rotavirus disease. During a 4-year period after vaccine introduction, an estimated 177 000 hospitalizations, 242 000 emergency department visits, and 1.1 million outpatient visits for diarrhea were averted among US children younger than 5 years. A 20% reduction in seizure risk has also been associated with rotavirus vaccination.

The **incubation period** for rotavirus is short, usually less than 48 hours.

DIAGNOSTIC TESTS: It is not possible to diagnose rotavirus infection by clinical presentation or nonspecific laboratory tests. Diagnosis of rotavirus infection depends on direct viral detection from fecal specimens. Diagnostic enzyme immunoassays (EIAs) and rapid chromatographic immunoassays for group A rotavirus antigen detection in stool are available commercially. Given the marked reduction in rotavirus disease prevalence because of vaccine use, the positive predictive value of the immunoassays can be expected to be lower, and the negative predictive value can be expected to be higher, compared with the prevaccine period. Polymerase chain reaction (PCR)-based multipathogen detection systems that test stool for a panel of viral, bacterial, and parasitic gastrointestinal tract pathogens, including rotavirus, are being used more frequently. Although the advantages of such PCR-based systems are high throughput, increased sensitivity, and the ability to test for multiple pathogens in a single sample, the probability of coincidental detection of rotaviruses or other potential pathogens that may not be causing current symptoms complicates test interpretation. The virus from rotavirus vaccines can be detected in stool for at least 10 days after immunization.

Research and reference laboratories may have additional diagnostic assays including electron microscopy, polyacrylamide gel electrophoresis (PAGE) of viral RNA with silver staining, and viral culture. Genotyping and nucleotide sequencing can be used for surveillance purposes to identify circulating rotavirus G and P genotypes. These tests generally are not used for clinical diagnosis of rotavirus disease.

TREATMENT: No specific antiviral therapy is available. Oral or parenteral fluids and electrolytes are given to prevent or correct dehydration. Breastfeeding should continue through the diarrheal illness. Orally administered human immune globulin, administered as an investigational therapy in immunocompromised patients with prolonged infection, has decreased viral shedding and shortened the duration of diarrhea.

INFECTION PREVENTION AND CONTROL MEASURES IN HEALTH CARE SETTINGS: In addition to standard precautions, contact precautions are indicated for diapered or incontinent children for the duration of illness.

CONTROL MEASURES: Breastfeeding is associated with milder rotavirus disease and should be encouraged (see Breastfeeding and Human Milk, p 135).

Child Care. General measures for interrupting enteric transmission in child care centers are available (see Children in Group Child Care and Schools, p 145). Hand washing and cleaning surfaces with soap and water followed by disinfection is recommended. Bleach solutions or other products with confirmed virucidal activity against rotavirus can be used to inactivate rotavirus and may help prevent disease transmission resulting from contact with environmental surfaces (**www.cdc.gov/infectioncontrol/ guidelines/disinfection/disinfection-methods/chemical.html**). Infants and children with rotavirus diarrhea should be excluded from child care centers until stools are contained in the diaper or when toilet-trained children no longer have accidents using the toilet and when stool frequency becomes no more than 2 stools above that child's normal frequency, even if the stools remain loose.

Vaccines. Two rotavirus vaccines are licensed for use among infants in the United States: a live, oral human-bovine reassortant pentavalent rotavirus (RV5 [RotaTeq, Merck & Co Inc]) vaccine, administered as a 3-dose series; and a live, oral human attenuated monovalent rotavirus (RV1 [Rotarix, GlaxoSmithKline]) vaccine, administered as a 2-dose series. The products differ in composition and schedule of administration. The American Academy of Pediatrics and the Centers for Disease Control and Prevention do not express a preference for either vaccine.

The following are recommendations for use of rotavirus vaccines currently licensed in the United States[1] (see Table 3.56):

- Infants in the United States should be immunized routinely with a licensed rotavirus vaccine.
- Breastfeeding infants should be immunized according to the same schedule as non-breastfed infants.
- Immunization should not be initiated for infants 15 weeks, 0 days of age or older. For infants to whom the first dose of rotavirus vaccine is administered inadvertently at 15 weeks, 0 days of age or older, the remainder of the rotavirus immunization series should be completed according to the schedule.
- The maximum age for the last dose of rotavirus vaccine is 8 months, 0 days.
- The rotavirus vaccine series should be completed with the same product whenever possible. However, immunization should not be deferred if the product used for

---

[1] Centers for Disease Control and Prevention. Prevention of rotavirus gastroenteritis among infants and children. Recommendations of the Advisory Committee on Immunization Practices (ACIP). *MMWR Recomm Rep.* 2009;58(RR-2):1–25

Table 3.56. Recommended Schedule for Administration of Rotavirus Vaccine

Recommendation	RV5 (RotaTeq)	RV1 (Rotarix)
Number of doses in series	3	2
Recommended ages for doses	2, 4, and 6 months of age	2 and 4 months of age
Minimum age for first dose	6 weeks of age	6 weeks of age
Maximum age for first dose	14 weeks, 6 days of age	14 weeks, 6 days of age
Minimum interval between doses	4 weeks	4 weeks
Maximum age for last dose	8 months, 0 days of age	8 months, 0 days of age

previous doses is not available or is unknown. In this situation, the health care professional should continue or complete the series with the product available.
- If any dose in the series was RV5 vaccine or the product is unknown for any dose in the series, a total of 3 doses of rotavirus vaccine should be administered.
- Rotavirus vaccine can be administered concurrently with other childhood vaccines.
- Rotavirus vaccine may be administered at any time before, concurrent with, or after administration of any blood product, including antibody-containing blood products.
- If an infant regurgitates, spits out, or vomits during or after vaccine administration, the vaccine dose should not be repeated.
- If a recently immunized infant is hospitalized, standard precautions should be followed.

Considerations in special populations:
- Infants with transient, mild illness, with or without low-grade fever, may receive rotavirus vaccine.
- Infants who have had rotavirus gastroenteritis before receiving the full series of rotavirus immunization should begin or complete the schedule following the standard age and interval recommendations.
- Preterm infants may be immunized if the infant is at least 6 weeks of postnatal age and is clinically stable. Preterm infants should be immunized on the same schedule and with the same precautions as recommended for full-term infants. Rotavirus vaccine virus is shed by some infants in the weeks after vaccination. There are limited published studies examining the transmission of vaccine virus in hospital settings, including neonatal intensive care units, but health care-associated transmission has not been documented. Individual institutions may consider administering rotavirus vaccine at the recommended chronologic age to otherwise eligible infants during hospitalization, including in the neonatal intensive care unit. If not administered earlier, the first dose of vaccine should be administered at the time of discharge to eligible infants.
- Rotavirus vaccine should be administered to human immunodeficiency virus (HIV)-exposed and HIV-infected infants, irrespective of CD4+ T-lymphocyte percentage or count, according to the schedule for uninfected infants (see Human Immunodeficiency Virus Infection, p 489). Rotavirus vaccine may be indicated for infants with other acquired immunocompromising conditions if the potential benefit of protection outweighs the risk of adverse reaction.

- Infants living in households with immunocompromised people can be immunized. Highly immunocompromised patients should avoid handling diapers of infants who have been vaccinated with rotavirus vaccine for 4 weeks after vaccination.
- Infants living in households with pregnant people should be immunized.

Contraindications and precautions:
- Rotavirus vaccine should not be administered to infants who have a history of a severe allergic reaction (eg, anaphylaxis) after a previous dose of rotavirus vaccine or to a vaccine component.
- Known SCID or history of intussusception are contraindications for use of both rotavirus vaccines. Gastroenteritis, including severe diarrhea and prolonged shedding of vaccine virus, has been reported in infants who received live, oral rotavirus vaccines and later identified as having SCID.
- Consultation with experts should be sought prior to administering rotavirus vaccine in infants with altered immunocompetence other than SCID (eg, condition that affects the immune system, including cancer or treatment with drugs such as steroids, chemotherapy, or radiation) or with moderate to severe illness, including gastroenteritis and preexisting chronic intestinal tract disease.
- Infants exposed in utero to biologic response modifiers (BRMs) given to the pregnant person can have detectable drug concentrations for many months following delivery, resulting in concern for immunosuppression among infants in the 12 months after the last dose during pregnancy. Data are sparse on the safety of rotavirus vaccines in infants who were exposed to in utero to BRMs administered to the pregnant person. Considering that rotavirus disease is rarely life threatening in the United States, rotavirus vaccines should be avoided in infants for the first 12 months after the last in utero exposure to most BRMs. Exceptions include certolizumab, which is not transferred across the placenta because of its structure as a pegylated Fab fragment, and likely infliximab, although the data are more sparse for it; rotavirus vaccination of infants can be considered when treatment with either of these BRMs was administered to the pregnant person (see Biologic Response-Modifying Drugs Used to Decrease Inflammation, p 104). As more data become available for the other BRMs, recommendations are likely to change and consultation with an expert in pediatric infectious diseases is recommended.
- The tip caps of the prefilled oral applicators of the RV1 vaccine may contain natural rubber latex, so infants with a severe (anaphylactic) allergy to latex (eg, some patients with spina bifida or bladder extrophy) should preferentially receive RV5 vaccine, because dosing tubes of RV5 do not contain natural rubber latex.

Adverse Events. Postmarketing surveillance data from the United States, Australia, Mexico, Canada, and Brazil indicate that there is a small risk of intussusception from the currently licensed rotavirus vaccines. In the United States, the available data suggest the attributable risk is between approximately 1 and 5 excess intussusception cases per 100 000 vaccinated infants. The risk appears to be primarily during the first week following the first or second dose; data from Australia suggest some risk may extend up to 21 days following the first dose. In the United States as well as other parts of the world, the benefits of rotavirus vaccination in preventing severe rotavirus disease outweigh the risk of intussusception. Parents should be informed of the risk, the early signs and symptoms of intussusception, and the need for prompt care if these develop.

Postmarketing strain surveillance in the United States and other countries has revealed that RV5 vaccine reassortant strains have been detected occasionally in stool samples of children with diarrhea. In some of the reports, the reassortant virus seemed to cause diarrheal illness. An RV1 vaccine wild-type reassortant strain has also been reported outside the United States.

In 2010, porcine circovirus or porcine circovirus DNA was detected in both rotavirus vaccines. There is no evidence that this virus is a safety risk or causes illness in humans.

Rubella

CLINICAL MANIFESTATIONS:

Postnatal Rubella. Many cases of postnatal rubella are subclinical, with 25% to 50% of adults being asymptomatic. Clinical disease usually is mild and characterized by a generalized erythematous maculopapular rash, lymphadenopathy, and slight fever. The rash starts on the face, becomes generalized in 24 hours, and lasts a median of 3 days. Lymphadenopathy, which may precede rash, often involves posterior auricular or suboccipital lymph nodes, can be generalized, and lasts between 5 and 8 days. In addition, conjunctivitis, cough, headache, coryza, and palatal enanthema may occur 1 to 5 days prior to the rash. Transient polyarthralgia and polyarthritis rarely occur in children but are common in adolescents and adults, especially among females. Encephalitis (1 in 6000 cases) and thrombocytopenia (1 in 3000 cases) are complications.

Congenital Rubella Syndrome. Maternal rubella during pregnancy can result in miscarriage, fetal death, or a constellation of congenital anomalies (congenital rubella syndrome [CRS]). The most commonly described anomalies/manifestations associated with CRS are ophthalmologic (cataracts, pigmentary retinopathy, microphthalmos, congenital glaucoma), cardiac (patent ductus arteriosus, peripheral pulmonary artery stenosis), auditory (sensorineural hearing impairment), or neurologic (behavioral disorders, meningoencephalitis, microcephaly, developmental disabilities). Neonatal manifestations of CRS include growth restriction, interstitial pneumonitis, radiolucent bone disease, hepatosplenomegaly, thrombocytopenia, and dermal erythropoiesis (so-called "blueberry muffin" lesions). Mild forms of the disease can be associated with few or no obvious clinical manifestations at birth. Congenital defects primarily occur in the infants of people infected during the first trimester of pregnancy. CRS is one of the few known causes of autism.

ETIOLOGY: Rubella virus is an enveloped, positive-stranded RNA virus classified as a *Rubivirus* in the *Matonaviridae* family.

EPIDEMIOLOGY: Humans are the only natural host. Postnatal rubella is transmitted primarily through direct or droplet contact from nasopharyngeal secretions. The peak incidence of infection is during late winter and early spring. Immunity from wild-type or vaccine virus usually is lifelong, but reinfection on rare occasions has been demonstrated and rarely has resulted in CRS.

Rubella virus has been recovered from lens aspirates in children with congenital cataracts for several years, and a small proportion of infants with congenital rubella continue to shed virus in nasopharyngeal secretions and urine for 1 year or more, with transmission to susceptible contacts being possible (see Infection Prevention and Control Measures in Health Care Settings and Control Measures).

Persistent infection of rubella virus has been associated with Fuchs' uveitis, encephalitis, and granulomas, sometimes decades after the initial infection and/or vaccination. Both wild-type and vaccine viruses can persist for decades subclinically before disease emerges. Most cases occur among patients with various primary immunodeficiencies.

Before widespread use of rubella vaccine, rubella was an epidemic disease, occurring in 6- to 9-year cycles, with most cases occurring in children. In the postvaccine era, most cases in the mid-1970s and 1980s occurred in young unimmunized adults in outbreaks on college campuses and in occupational settings. More recent outbreaks have occurred in people born outside the United States or among unimmunized populations. The incidence of rubella in the United States has decreased by more than 99% from the prevaccine era (see Table 1.1, p 20).

Rubella was declared eliminated from the United States in 2004, and since 2012 all rubella cases reported in the United States had evidence that the patients contracted virus outside the United States. In addition, mothers of most children with CRS reported since 1998 were born outside the United States. A national serologic survey from 2009–2010 indicated that among children and adolescents 6 through 19 years of age, rubella seroprevalence was >97%. In 2003, the Pan American Health Organization (PAHO) adopted a resolution calling for elimination of rubella and CRS in the Americas by the year 2010. The strategy consisted of achieving high levels of measles-rubella vaccination coverage in the routine immunization program and in the supplemental vaccination campaigns, including adults, to rapidly reduce the number of people in the country susceptible to acute infection. This goal was accomplished while simultaneously strengthening epidemiologic surveillance to monitor impact. The last confirmed endemic rubella case in the Americas was diagnosed in Argentina in February 2009, and the last confirmed endemic CRS case was reported in Brazil in August 2009. In April 2015, the PAHO International Expert Committee for Verification of Measles and Rubella Elimination verified that the region of the Americas had achieved the rubella and CRS elimination goals.

The average **incubation period** of rubella virus is 17 days, with a range of 12 to 23 days. People infected with rubella are most contagious a week before and after the appearance of rash.

DIAGNOSTIC TESTS: Rubella infection can be confirmed by: (1) detection of rubella viral RNA by reverse transcriptase-polymerase chain reaction (RT-PCR); (2) detection of rubella virus-specific immunoglobulin (Ig) M; (3) a fourfold increase in rubella IgG antibody titer in paired acute and convalescent serum specimens (collected at least 10 days apart); or (4) isolation of rubella virus in cell culture. Neonates in whom there is concern for CRS should have both virologic and serologic testing performed.

Currently, the most reliable method of rubella diagnosis is detection of rubella virus RNA by RT-PCR. In most postnatal cases, viral RNA is detectable by RT-PCR within 3 days of rash onset, and in most congenital cases, viral detection is possible at birth and in some cases for up to 12 months. Nasopharyngeal and throat swab specimens are the preferred specimens for detecting rubella RNA in both suspected CRS and postnatal cases. Viral RNA also may be detectable in blood, urine, and cataract specimens, particularly in infants with congenital infection. Collection of 2 or more specimen types, for example nasopharyngeal swab and urine samples, can increase the likelihood of diagnosis. Genotyping, typically only available in public health laboratories, is critical for tracking the source of infection.

Detection of rubella-specific IgM antibody usually indicates primary infection. Most postnatal rubella cases are IgM-positive by 5 days after symptom onset. A second sample collected 10 days following the first is necessary to confirm or rule out rubella if the day 5 serum specimen is negative. For diagnosis of postnatally acquired rubella, a fourfold or greater increase in antibody titer between acute and convalescent periods or seroconversion between acute and convalescent IgG serum titers also indicate infection. Acute serum must be collected as close to rash onset as possible, preferably in the first 3 days after symptom onset. CRS can be confirmed by detection of rubella-specific IgM antibody usually within the first 6 months of life. Congenital infection also can be confirmed by stable or increasing serum concentrations of rubella-specific IgG over the first 7 to 11 months of life. Diagnosis of congenital rubella infection in children older than 1 year is difficult because of routine vaccination with measles, mumps, and rubella (MMR) vaccine.

Rubella virus can be isolated most consistently from throat or nasal swab specimens (and less consistently from urine) by inoculation of appropriate cell culture. Virus isolation is usually conducted to confirm virus shedding from patients. Laboratory personnel should be notified immediately that rubella is suspected, because specialized cell culture methods are required to isolate and identify the virus. Blood, urine, and cataract specimens also may yield virus, particularly in infants with congenital infection.

TREATMENT: Management is supportive.

INFECTION PREVENTION AND CONTROL MEASURES IN HEALTH CARE SETTINGS: In addition to standard precautions, for postnatal rubella droplet precautions are recommended for 7 days after onset of the rash. Contact isolation is indicated for children with proven or suspected congenital rubella until they are at least 1 year of age, unless rubella RT-PCR testing of 2 sets of clinical specimens (eg, throat/nasal swab and urine specimen) obtained 1 month apart after 3 months of age do not detect rubella virus RNA. In addition, droplet precautions can be considered if the infant has a respiratory illness or an aerosol-generating procedure is being performed. Infection control precautions should be considered in children with CRS up to 3 years of age who are hospitalized for congenital cataract extraction.

CONTROL MEASURES:

School and Child Care. Children with postnatal rubella should be excluded from school or child care for 7 days after onset of the rash. During an outbreak, children without evidence of immunity should be immunized or excluded for 21 days after onset of rash of the last case in the outbreak. Children with CRS should be considered contagious as indicated in the section above on Infection Prevention and Control Measures in Health Care Settings. When infants with CRS who are still potentially contagious are considered for placement in a group child care setting, public health authorities should be contacted for guidance. Caregivers of these infants should be made aware of the potential hazard of the infants to susceptible pregnant contacts. Rubella is an enveloped virus; alcohol-based hand rubs are generally effective against enveloped viruses. Surfaces and items contaminated with potentially infectious material should be disinfected. A 1% bleach solution or 70% ethanol are effective at inactivating rubella virus.

Care of Exposed People. Evidence of rubella immunity consists of documented receipt of at least 1 dose of rubella-containing vaccine on or after the first birthday or serologic evidence of immunity. People born prior to 1957 can be considered immune. Documented evidence of rubella immunity is especially important for people who could become pregnant. Prenatal IgG serologic screening for rubella immunity should be performed for all pregnant people. The cutoff value for rubella immunity is set at 10 IU/mL. People whose levels of rubella-specific IgG antibody are ≥10 IU/mL can be considered to have adequate evidence of rubella immunity. Those with rubella-specific IgG titer less than 10 IU/mL should receive rubella vaccine during the immediate postpartum period before discharge from the hospital. Vaccinated people capable of becoming pregnant who have received 1 or 2 doses of rubella-containing vaccine with rubella serum IgG titers less than 10 IU/mL should receive 1 additional dose of MMR vaccine (maximum of 3 doses) and do not need to be retested thereafter for serologic evidence of rubella immunity. When a pregnant person with unknown rubella immunity is exposed to rubella, a blood specimen should be obtained as soon as possible and tested for rubella antibody (IgG and IgM). An aliquot of frozen serum should be stored for possible repeated testing at a later time. The presence of rubella-specific IgG antibody at the time of exposure indicates that the person most likely is immune. If antibody is not detectable, a second blood specimen should be obtained 2 to 3 weeks later and tested concurrently with the frozen first specimen. If the second test result is negative, another blood specimen should be obtained 6 weeks after the exposure and also tested concurrently with the frozen first specimen; a negative test result in both the second and third specimens indicates that infection has not occurred, and a positive test result in the second or third specimen but not the first (seroconversion) indicates recent infection.

Immune Globulin. Administration of immune globulin (IG) to susceptible people experimentally exposed to rubella virus can prevent clinical rubella. However, there have also been many reports of the failure of IG to prevent the anomalies of congenital rubella. For this reason, the routine use of immune globulin intramuscular for the prevention of rubella in an exposed pregnant person is not recommended.

Vaccine. Rubella vaccine administered after exposure has not been demonstrated to prevent illness. Immunization of exposed nonpregnant people may be indicated, because if the exposure did not result in infection, then immunization will protect these people in the future. Immunization of a person who is incubating natural rubella or who already is immune is not associated with an increased risk of adverse reactions.

Rubella Vaccine.[1,2] The only rubella vaccines licensed in the United States are live attenuated strains. Rubella vaccine is only available in the United States as combination formulations, which include MMR (M-M-R II manufactured by Merck, and Priorix manufactured by GSK) and measles, mumps, rubella, and varicella (MMRV) vaccines. Both vaccines contain the rubella RA 27/3 strain. Vaccine can be administered simultaneously with other vaccines (see Simultaneous Administration of Multiple Vaccines, p 63, and Table 1.9, p 60). Serum antibody to rubella is induced in more than 95% of recipients after a single dose at 12 months or older. Clinical efficacy and challenge studies have demonstrated that 1 dose confers long-term immunity against clinical and

[1] Centers for Disease Control and Prevention. Prevention of measles, rubella, congenital rubella syndrome, and mumps, 2013 summary: recommendations of the Advisory Committee on Immunization Practices (ACIP). *MMWR Recomm Rep.* 2013;62(RR-4):1-34

[2] Krow-Lucal E, Marin M, Shepersky L, Bahta L, Loehr J, Dooling K. Measles, mumps, rubella vaccine (PRIORIX): recommendations of the Advisory Committee on Immunization Practices—United States, 2022. *MMWR Morb Mortal Wkly Rep.* 2022;71(46):1465–1470

asymptomatic infection in more than 90% of immunized people. However, both symptomatic (rare) and asymptomatic reinfection have occurred in immunized people.

Because of the 2-dose recommendations for measles- and mumps-containing vaccine (as MMR) and varicella vaccine (as MMRV), 2 doses of rubella vaccine are administered routinely. The 2-dose series provides an added safeguard against primary vaccine failures.

Vaccine Recommendations. At least 1 dose of live attenuated rubella-containing vaccine is recommended for people 12 months or older. The first dose is usually given at 12 through 15 months of age, with a second dose of MMR or MMRV at school entry at 4 through 6 years of age or sooner. People who have not received the dose at school entry should receive their second dose as soon as possible but optimally no later than 11 through 12 years of age (see Measles, p 570).

Special emphasis must continue to be placed on the immunization of at-risk postpubertal individuals, especially college students, military recruits, recent immigrants, health care professionals, teachers, and child care providers. People who were born in 1957 or after and who have not received at least 1 dose of vaccine or who have no serologic evidence of immunity to rubella are considered susceptible and should be immunized with MMR vaccine. Clinical diagnosis of infection is unreliable and should not be accepted as evidence of immunity.

Specific recommendations are as follows:

- People capable of becoming pregnant who lack documentation of presumptive evidence of rubella immunity should be immunized unless they are pregnant. Rubella-containing vaccine recipients should be advised not to become pregnant for 28 days after vaccination (see Precautions and Contraindications, p 740, for further discussion). Routine serologic testing before immunization of people who are capable of becoming pregnant is unnecessary and is a potential impediment to protection against rubella, because it requires 2 visits.
- During annual health care examinations, family planning visits, and visits to sexually transmitted infection clinics, people capable of becoming pregnant should be assessed for rubella susceptibility and, if deemed susceptible, should be immunized with MMR vaccine.
- Routine prenatal IgG screening for rubella immunity should be performed. If a pregnant person is found to be susceptible, rubella vaccine should be administered during the immediate postpartum period before discharge from the hospital.
- People who have rubella-specific IgG titers of ≥ 10 IU/mL can be considered to have adequate evidence of rubella immunity. Except for people capable of becoming pregnant, people who have an equivocal serologic test result should be considered susceptible to rubella unless they have documented receipt of 1 dose of rubella-containing vaccine or subsequent serologic test results indicate rubella immunity.
- Vaccinated people capable of becoming pregnant who have rubella serum IgG less than 10 IU/mL should receive 1 additional dose of MMR vaccine (maximum of 3 doses) and do not need to be retested thereafter for serologic evidence of rubella immunity.
- Breastfeeding is not a contraindication to postpartum immunization of the birthing parent (for additional information, see Breastfeeding and Human Milk, p 135).
- All susceptible health care personnel who may be exposed to patients with rubella or who provide care for pregnant patients, as well as people who work in educational

institutions or provide child care, should be immunized to prevent infection for themselves and to prevent transmission of rubella to pregnant people.[1]

Adverse Reactions.

- Of susceptible children who receive MMR or MMRV vaccines, fever develops in 5% to 15% from 6 to 12 days after immunization. Rash occurs in approximately 5% of immunized people. Mild lymphadenopathy occurs commonly. Febrile seizures occur slightly more frequently among children 12 through 23 months of age after administration of MMRV vaccine compared with MMR and varicella administered as separate injections during the same visit (see Measles, p 570).
- Joint pain, usually in small peripheral joints, has been reported in approximately 0.5% of young children following vaccination with a rubella-containing vaccine. Arthralgia and transient arthritis tend to be more common in susceptible postmenarcheal vaccine recipients, occurring in approximately 25% and 10%, respectively. Joint involvement usually begins 7 to 21 days after immunization and generally is transient. The incidence of joint manifestations after immunization is lower than after wild-type virus infection at the corresponding age.
- Transient paresthesia and pain in the arms and legs have rarely been reported.
- Central nervous system manifestations have been reported, but no causal relationship with rubella vaccine has been established.
- Other reactions that occur after immunization with MMR or MMRV are associated with the measles, mumps, and varicella components of the vaccine (see Measles, p 570, Mumps, p 611, and Varicella-Zoster Infections, p 938).

Precautions and Contraindications.

- **Pregnancy.** Rubella vaccine should not be administered to pregnant people. If vaccine is administered to an unknowingly pregnant person or the pregnancy occurs within 28 days of immunization, the patient should be counseled on the theoretical risks to the fetus. The theoretical maximum risk for CRS after vaccine administration is 0.2%, which is considerably lower than the risk with wild rubella virus or risk of non–CRS-induced congenital defects in pregnancy. Of the 2931 people immunized while pregnant who have been followed globally, 3.3% of offspring had subclinical infection, none had congenital defects, and 96.7% were not infected. In view of these observations, receipt of rubella vaccine during pregnancy is not an indication for termination of pregnancy.
- **Children of pregnant people.** Immunizing susceptible children who have a parent or other household contact who is pregnant does not pose a risk. Most immunized people intermittently shed small amounts of virus from the pharynx 7 to 28 days after immunization, but no evidence of transmission of the vaccine virus from immunized children has been found.
- **Febrile illness.** Children with minor illnesses, such as upper respiratory tract infection, may be immunized (see Understanding Vaccine Evaluation and Safety as an Approach to Addressing Parental Concerns, p 27). Fever is not a contraindication to immunization. However, if other manifestations suggest a more serious illness, the child should not be immunized until recovery has occurred.
- **Recent administration of IG.** IG preparations interfere with immune response to measles vaccine and theoretically may interfere with the serologic response to

---

[1] Centers for Disease Control and Prevention. Immunization of health-care personnel: recommendations of the Advisory Committee on Immunization Practices (ACIP). *MMWR Recomm Rep.* 2011;60(RR-7):1-45

rubella vaccine (see Table 1.11, p 69). If rubella vaccine is indicated postpartum for a person who has received anti-Rho (D) IG or blood products, suggested intervals are the same as used between IG administration and measles immunization (see Table 1.11, p 69).

- **Altered immunity.** Immunocompromised patients with disorders associated with increased severity of viral infections should not receive live-virus rubella vaccine (see Immunization and Other Considerations in Immunocompromised Children, p 93). Exceptions are patients with human immunodeficiency virus (HIV) infection who are not severely immunocompromised. MMR vaccine is recommended for all people ≥12 months of age with HIV who do not have evidence of severe immunosuppression (see Human Immunodeficiency Virus Infection, p 489). For vaccination purposes, severe immunosuppression for people ≤5 years of age is defined as a CD4+ T-lymphocyte percentage <15%, and for people > 5 years of age is defined as a CD4+ T-lymphocyte percentage <15% **or** a CD4+ T-lymphocyte count <200 lymphocytes/mm^3. Severely immunocompromised HIV-infected infants, children, adolescents, and young adults should not receive MMR. MMRV vaccine should not be administered to any infant or child with HIV, regardless of degree of immunosuppression, because of lack of safety data in this population. If possible, children receiving biologic response modifiers, such as anti-tumor necrosis factor-alpha (see Biologic Response-Modifying Drugs Used to Decrease Inflammation, p 104), should be immunized before initiating treatment.

- **Household contacts of immunocompromised people.** The risk of rubella exposure for patients with altered immunity is decreased by immunizing susceptible contacts. Although small amounts of vaccine virus may be isolated from the pharynx, no evidence of transmission of rubella vaccine virus from immunized children to immunocompromised contacts has been found. Precautions and contraindications appropriate for the measles, mumps, and varicella components of MMR or MMRV vaccines also should be reviewed before administration (see Measles, p 570, Mumps, p 611, and Varicella-Zoster Infections, p 938).

- **Corticosteroids.** For patients who have received high doses of corticosteroids (2 mg/kg or greater or more than 20 mg/day) for 14 days or more and who otherwise are not immunocompromised, the recommended interval between stopping the steroids and immunization is at least 4 weeks (see Immunization and Other Considerations in Immunocompromised Children, p 93) after steroids have been discontinued.

Tuberculosis. Tuberculin skin testing or interferon gamma release assay (IGRA) testing is not a prerequisite for MMR immunization. Antituberculosis therapy should be initiated before administering MMR vaccine to people with untreated tuberculosis infection or disease. Tuberculin skin or IGRA testing, if otherwise indicated, can be performed on the day of immunization with MMR vaccine. Otherwise, tuberculin skin or IGRA testing should be postponed for 4 to 6 weeks, because measles immunization temporarily may suppress tuberculin skin test reactivity and possibly affect IGRA testing.

Public Health Reporting. Accurate diagnosis and reporting of CRS are extremely important in assessing control of rubella. All birth defects in which rubella infection is suspected etiologically should be investigated thoroughly and reported to the CDC through local or state health departments.

Salmonella Infections

CLINICAL MANIFESTATIONS:

Nontyphoidal* Salmonella *Infection. Nontyphoidal *Salmonella* (NTS) infection is associated with a spectrum of illness ranging from asymptomatic gastrointestinal tract carriage to gastroenteritis, urinary tract infection, bacteremia, and focal infections, including meningitis, brain abscess, and osteomyelitis (to which people with sickle cell anemia are predisposed). The most common illness associated with NTS infection is gastroenteritis, with manifestations of diarrhea, abdominal cramps, and fever. The site of infection usually is the distal small intestine and colon. Sustained or intermittent bacteremia can occur, and focal infections are recognized in up to 10% of patients with NTS bacteremia. In the United States, the incidence of invasive NTS is highest among infants. Certain NTS serovars (eg, Dublin, Choleraesuis), although rare, are more likely to result in invasive infection than gastroenteritis. Invasive NTS disease in infants and toddlers, manifesting as severe clinical illness and accompanied by high case fatality rates, is prevalent in many parts of sub-Saharan Africa. *Salmonella* Typhimurium, *Salmonella* Enteritidis, and *Salmonella* I:4,[5],12:i:- (and, to a lesser extent, *Salmonella* Dublin) are the most frequent NTS serovars isolated from blood and cerebrospinal fluid. Severe anemia, malaria, human immunodeficiency virus (HIV), and malnutrition are known risk factors that contribute to the high case fatality rate (10%–30%). However, whole genome sequencing has revealed that most of the *Salmonella* Typhimurium and *Salmonella* I:4,[5],12:i:- isolates from infants and toddlers with invasive NTS disease in sub-Saharan Africa exhibit genomic degradation that renders them distinct from NTS associated with gastroenteritis in North America and Europe.

Enteric Fever. *Salmonella enterica* serovars Typhi, Paratyphi A, Paratyphi B, and Paratyphi C (which occurs rarely) can cause a protracted bacteremic illness referred to collectively as enteric fever (and as typhoid fever and paratyphoid fever). In older children, the onset of enteric fever typically is gradual, with manifestations such as fever, constitutional symptoms (eg, headache, malaise, anorexia, cough, and lethargy), abdominal pain, hepatomegaly, splenomegaly, dactylitis, and rose spots (visible in approximately 30% of patients). Change in mental status and shock may ensue. Myocarditis or endocarditis occur rarely. In infants and toddlers, invasive infection with enteric fever serovars can manifest as a mild, nondescript febrile illness accompanied by self-limited bacteremia or as an invasive infection in association with more severe clinical symptoms and signs, sustained bacteremia, and meningitis. Diarrhea (resembling pea soup) or constipation can be early features. Intestinal perforations or hemorrhage occurs in up to 10% of hospitalized adults and children with enteric fever. Prolonged untreated typhoid increases the risk for intestinal perforations. Relative bradycardia (pulse rate slower than would be expected for a given body temperature) has been considered a common feature of typhoid fever in adults but in children is neither a discriminating feature in the assessment of a febrile child from an area where enteric fever is endemic, nor a feature of the disease per se. Chronic carriage of *S* Typhi (excretion longer than 1 year) following acute typhoid infection is associated with cholelithiasis, increased age, and female sex.[1] Chronic carriage in children is uncommon.

---

[1] The term female refers to sex assigned at birth.

ETIOLOGY: *Salmonella* bacteria are gram-negative bacilli in the *Enterobacterales* order. Current taxonomy recognizes 3 *Salmonella* species: *S enterica* with 6 subspecies, *Salmonella bongori*, and *Salmonella subterranea*. *S enterica* subspecies *enterica* (also called subspecies I) is responsible for most infections in humans and other warm-blooded animals; the other *S enterica* subspecies and *S bongori* are usually isolated from cold-blooded animals. More than 2600 *Salmonella* serovars have been described. During 2017-2021, the most commonly reported human clinical isolates in the United States were *Salmonella* serovars Enteritidis, Newport, Typhimurium, and Javiana; these serovars accounted for approximately 45% of all human clinical *Salmonella* isolates in the United States during this period (**www.cdc.gov/ncezid/dfwed/BEAM-dashboard.html**). *S* Typhi belongs to O serogroup 9, along with many other common serovars including Enteritidis and Dublin. The relative prevalence of serovars varies by country, state, and county.

EPIDEMIOLOGY:

Nontyphoidal* Salmonella *Infection. Every year, NTS organisms are among the most common causes of laboratory-confirmed cases of enteric disease reported to the US Foodborne Diseases Active Surveillance Network (**wwwn.cdc.gov/foodnetfast**). The incidence of NTS infection is highest in children younger than 4 years. In the United States, rates of invasive infections and mortality are higher in infants, elderly people, and people with hemoglobinopathies (including sickle cell disease) and immunocompromising conditions (eg, malignant neoplasms, HIV infection). Most reported cases are sporadic, but widespread outbreaks, including health care-associated and institutional outbreaks, have been reported.

The incidence of foodborne cases of NTS gastroenteritis ranged from 16.6 to 19.6 per 100 000 in the period of 2015-2019, but fell to 13.3 per 100 000 in 2020. The incidence of diarrheal infections attributable to *Campylobacter* species, Shiga toxin-producing *Escherichia coli*, and *Shigella* species also decreased notably in 2020, likely as a result of the COVID-19 pandemic (**wwwn.cdc.gov/foodnetfast** and **www.cdc. gov/foodnet/reports/prelim-data-intro-2018.html**).

The principal reservoirs for NTS organisms include birds, mammals, reptiles, and amphibians. The major food vehicles of transmission to humans in industrialized countries include seeded vegetables and other produce as well as food of animal origin (such as poultry, beef, pork, eggs, and dairy products). Multiple other food vehicles (eg, peanut butter, frozen pot pies, powdered infant formula, cereal, and bakery products) have also been implicated in outbreaks in the United States and Europe. Other modes of transmission include ingestion of contaminated water or close contact with infected animals, mainly poultry (eg, chicks, chickens, ducks), reptiles or amphibians (eg, pet turtles, iguanas, geckos, bearded dragons, lizards, snakes, frogs, toads, newts, salamanders), and rodents (eg, hamsters, mice, guinea pigs) or other mammals (eg, hedgehogs). Reptiles and amphibians that live in tanks or aquariums can contaminate the water with bacteria, which can spread to people. Small turtles with a shell length of less than 4 inches are a well-known source of *Salmonella* infections. Because of this risk, the US Food and Drug Administration (FDA) has banned the interstate sale and distribution of these turtles since 1975. Animal-derived pet foods and treats have been linked to *Salmonella* infections as well, especially in young children.

A risk of transmission to others persists for as long as an infected person sheds NTS organisms. Twelve weeks after infection with the most common NTS serovars, approximately 45% of children younger than 5 years shed organisms, compared with 5% of older children and adults; antimicrobial therapy can prolong shedding. Approximately 1% of adults continue to shed NTS organisms for more than 1 year.

Enteric Fever. Although typhoid fever (approximately 300–400 cases annually) and paratyphoid fever (approximately 100 cases annually) are uncommon in the United States, these infections are highly endemic in many resource-limited countries, particularly in Asia. Consequently, most typhoid fever infections in US residents are acquired during international travel. Unlike NTS serovars, the enteric fever serovars (S Typhi, S Paratyphi A, S Paratyphi B, and S Paratyphi C) are restricted to human hosts, in whom they cause both clinical and subclinical infections. Chronic human S Typhi carriers (mostly involving chronic infection of the gall bladder in persons with cholelithiasis but occasionally involving infection of the urinary tract) constitute the long-term reservoir of typhoidal *Salmonella* in areas with endemic disease. Infection with enteric fever serovars implies ingestion of a food or water vehicle contaminated by a chronic carrier or a person with acute clinical or subclinical typhoidal *Salmonella* infection.

The **incubation period** for NTS gastroenteritis usually is 6 to 48 hours, but incubation periods of a week or more have been reported. For enteric fever, the **incubation period** usually is 7 to 14 days (range 3–60 days).

DIAGNOSTIC TESTS: Isolation of *Salmonella* from cultures of stool, blood, urine, bile (including duodenal fluid containing bile), and material from foci of infection is diagnostic. NTS gastroenteritis is diagnosed by stool culture or molecular testing; stool cultures should be obtained in all children with bloody diarrhea, or unexplained persistent or severe diarrhea. To evaluate for enteric fever, blood cultures (positive in 60% of patients with enteric fever) and stool cultures (positive in up to 30%) should be obtained for all children who present with unexplained fever after travel to resource-limited countries or contact with someone who has traveled internationally. In addition, blood cultures should be considered for patients at risk of severe illness (eg, age <3 months, those who are immunocompromised or have hemolytic anemia) and in patients with evidence of disseminated infection, bacteremia, or septicemia. Optimal recovery of *Salmonella* from stool is achieved with the use of enrichment broth and multiple selective agar plate media. Definitive identification requires confirmation by phenotypic methods (biochemical profiling and preliminary agglutination with high-quality typing sera, if available, in the hospital or state laboratory), molecular methods (such as polymerase chain reaction [PCR]-based assays), or mass spectrometry of cellular components and O serogroup determination. Serovar determination using validated antisera to identify O group and phase 1 and 2 flagella (H) antigens and Vi polysaccharide capsule or serotyping by whole genome sequencing are helpful for epidemiologic purposes and usually performed at public health laboratories.

Diagnostic tests to detect *Salmonella* antigens by enzyme immunoassay, latex agglutination, and monoclonal antibodies have been developed, as have commercial immunoassays that detect antibodies to antigens of enteric fever serovars. These tests are especially important in areas of the world where typhoid fever is endemic.

Several multiplex PCR platforms for detection of multiple viral, parasitic, and bacterial pathogens, including *Salmonella* organisms, directly in stool have been approved for diagnostic use by the FDA and are commercially available. Nevertheless, clinical microbiology laboratories should maintain culture capabilities for *Salmonella* species because antimicrobial susceptibility testing requires an isolate. In addition, isolates are useful for state public health laboratories to conduct genomic characterization of strains for outbreak detection and epidemiologic investigation.

If enteric fever is suspected, multiple cultures may be needed to isolate the pathogen. Blood, bone marrow, and bile (or duodenal fluid containing bile) comprise the highest-yield clinical specimens for culture. Bone marrow cultures are considered the gold standard and may be positive even when blood cultures are negative. *S* Typhi and *S* Paratyphi are often not recovered from stool culture. The sensitivity of blood culture and bone marrow culture in children with enteric fever is approximately 60% and 90%, respectively. The sensitivity of a single blood culture plus culture of bile (collected from a bile-stained duodenal string) is 90% for detecting *S* Typhi infection in children with clinical enteric fever. Collection of large but age-appropriate blood volumes is needed to optimize recovery of organisms from blood cultures.

The Centers for Disease Control and Prevention does not recommend using serologic tests, such as the Widal test, to diagnose acute typhoid, because these tests are difficult to interpret in populations in whom previous *Salmonella* infection or vaccination may result in a false-positive result. Isolate recovery remains important for guiding antimicrobial therapy for enteric fever, given that cases are increasingly caused by multidrug-resistant strains. Serologic testing may be helpful for identification of chronic carriers, who often have very elevated IgG Vi titers. However, Vi serologic testing is not useful if the individual has received a Vi polysaccharide vaccine within the previous year.

TREATMENT:

Nontyphoidal Salmonella *Infection.*

- Antimicrobial therapy usually is not indicated for patients with either asymptomatic infection or uncomplicated gastroenteritis caused by NTS serovars, because therapy does not shorten the duration of diarrheal disease, can prolong duration of fecal shedding, and increases symptomatic relapse rate.
- Antimicrobial therapy is recommended for gastroenteritis caused by NTS serovars in people at increased risk for invasive disease, including infants younger than 3 months and people with chronic gastrointestinal tract disease, neoplasms, hemoglobinopathies, HIV infection, or other immunocompromising conditions. It should also be considered for those experiencing severe symptoms, such as severe diarrhea or prolonged or high fever.
- If antimicrobial therapy is initiated in patients in the United States with presumed or proven NTS gastroenteritis, a blood and a stool culture should be obtained prior to antibiotic administration and an initial dose of ceftriaxone should be given. The patient who does not appear ill or have evidence of disseminated infection can be discharged on oral azithromycin pending blood culture results. Once susceptibilities are available, ampicillin/amoxicillin or trimethoprim-sulfamethoxazole may be considered for susceptible strains. A fluoroquinolone is an alternative option. For those who appear ill or have evidence of disseminated infection, hospitalization is required.

- For patients with bacteremia caused by NTS, evaluation for disseminated disease (meningitis, osteoarticular infection, endocarditis) should be considered. Blood cultures should be repeated until negative. Initial therapy with ceftriaxone should be administered. Transition from intravenous ceftriaxone to oral azithromycin or a fluoroquinolone to complete a 7- to 10-day course of therapy may be considered after the blood culture has cleared and focal disease has been excluded. Specific antimicrobial, route of administration, and duration of therapy will depend on antimicrobial susceptibilities, patient age and other host factors, clinical response, and geographic region and availability of antibiotics. Aminoglycosides have reduced efficacy and are not recommended for the treatment of any invasive *Salmonella* infections (including those attributable to *S* Typhi) despite in vitro sensitivity of strains.
- Treatment durations should be extended to 4 weeks for meningitis and 4 to 6 weeks for osteomyelitis or other focal metastatic infections. Evaluation for underlying immunodeficiency (eg, asplenia, HIV) should be considered for patients with invasive infection.
- Antibiotic-resistant nontyphoidal *Salmonella* strains are increasing. Ciprofloxacin-nonsusceptible strains increased from 2% in 2009 to 9% in 2020 (**www.cdc.gov/drugresistance/pdf/threats-report/2019-ar-threats-report-508.pdf** and **wwwn.cdc.gov/narmsnow/**).

Enteric Fever.
- Travel history and regional antibiotic resistance patterns should be carefully considered when choosing empiric antibiotic therapy for enteric fever. Most typhoid fever infections diagnosed in the United States are fluoroquinolone nonsusceptible; therefore, clinicians should not use fluoroquinolones as empiric therapy.
- Since 2016, Pakistan has had an ongoing large epidemic of extensively drug-resistant (XDR) *S* Typhi disease with resistance to ceftriaxone, ampicillin, ciprofloxacin, and trimethoprim-sulfamethoxazole (TMP-SMX); isolates are susceptible only to azithromycin and carbapenems.[1] XDR *S* Typhi has spread to many regions of Pakistan, and many confirmed cases of XDR typhoid have been documented in travelers returning from Pakistan to the United States, Canada, European countries, Taiwan, and Australia. More recently, XDR *S* Typhi has also been reported in US residents who did not travel internationally. Although the original Hyderabad, Pakistan XDR strain was sensitive to azithromycin, some areas of South Asia have since reported *S* Typhi with diminished sensitivity to azithromycin. Mass vaccination with World Health Organization prequalified Vi conjugate vaccine (Typbar-TCV, Bharat Biotech International, India) was conducted in Hyderabad, Pakistan, after which the incidence of XDR cases dropped markedly in the vaccinated population.
- For enteric fever caused by *S* Typhi that is known or suspected to be multidrug resistant (but not XDR), empiric therapy with a parenteral third-generation cephalosporin or azithromycin should be initiated. Azithromycin or a carbapenem antibiotic should be considered if the patient has traveled to Pakistan or Iraq in the 30 days before symptom onset because of ceftriaxone-resistant strains in those countries. Drugs of choice, route of administration, and duration of therapy are based on

---

[1] François Watkins LK, Winstead A, Appiah GD, et al. Update on extensively drug-resistant *Salmonella* serotype Typhi infections among travelers to or from Pakistan and report of ceftriaxone-resistant *Salmonella* serotype Typhi infections among travelers to Iraq—United States, 2018–2019. *MMWR Morb Mortal Wkly Rep.* 2020;69(20):618–622

susceptibility of the organism (or inferred susceptibility if this is not available), severity and site of infection, host characteristics, and clinical response. The optimal duration of therapy is unclear and depends on the antibiotic used. Most experts would treat for at least 7 to 10 days for uncomplicated disease, although in 1 trial of children with uncomplicated typhoid fever, a 5-day course of azithromycin was effective. If amoxicillin, TMP-SMX, or a fluoroquinolone are used on the basis of susceptibility testing, a 10- to 14-day course of therapy should be considered. Consultation with an expert in infectious diseases is recommended for management of severe and complicated cases.

- Relapse of typhoidal *Salmonella* infection can occur in up to 17% of patients within 4 weeks and is a particular risk for immunocompromised patients, who may require longer duration of treatment as well as retreatment. Relapse rates appear to be lower in those treated with oral ciprofloxacin or azithromycin compared with patients treated with oral TMP-SMX, amoxicillin, or parenteral ceftriaxone.

- The chronic typhoidal serovar carrier state may be eradicated by 4 weeks of oral therapy with ciprofloxacin in approximately 80% of people. High-dose parenteral ampicillin can be used if 4 weeks of oral fluoroquinolone therapy is not tolerated and if the strain is susceptible. Cholecystectomy followed by another course of antimicrobial agents may be indicated in some adults if antimicrobial therapy alone fails.

- Corticosteroids may be beneficial in children with severe enteric fever, which is characterized by delirium, obtundation, stupor, coma, or shock. These drugs should be reserved for critically ill patients in whom relief of manifestations of toxemia may be lifesaving. The usual regimen is high-dose dexamethasone, administered intravenously at an initial dose of 3 mg/kg, followed by 1 mg/kg, every 6 hours, for a total course of 48 hours.

- For enteric fever caused by *S* Typhi acquired from overseas travel, a stool culture should be performed on all contacts who traveled with the index case(s). If results are positive, treatment of contacts should be initiated with azithromycin until susceptibilities are known (due to high likelihood of fluroquinolone nonsusceptibility) and the contact should be monitored for development of any symptoms. Asymptomatic people in the United States who had contact with the index case(s) but did not travel overseas with them, should be evaluated on a case by case basis to determine necessity for culture of stool samples.

INFECTION PREVENTION AND CONTROL MEASURES IN HEALTH CARE SETTINGS: In addition to standard precautions, contact precautions should be used for diapered and incontinent children for the duration of illness. In children with enteric fever, precautions should be continued until culture results are negative for 3 consecutive stool specimens obtained at least 48 hours after cessation of antimicrobial therapy. For XDR typhoid, contact precautions should be used throughout the hospital stay.

CONTROL MEASURES: Important measures include proper food hygiene practices; treated water supplies; proper hand hygiene; adequate sanitation to dispose of human fecal waste; exclusion of infected people from handling food or providing health care; education on the risk of *Salmonella* infections from animal contact; prohibiting the sale of pet turtles; limiting exposure of children younger than 5 years and immunocompromised children to reptiles, amphibians, live poultry, and rodents at home, at school, and in child care and public settings (see Diseases Transmitted by Animals [Zoonoses], p 1157); reporting cases to appropriate health authorities; and investigating outbreaks. Eggs and other foods of animal origin should be cooked thoroughly. People should not eat raw eggs or foods containing raw eggs or consume unpasteurized milk or raw milk products.[1]

Child Care. Outbreaks of *Salmonella* illness in child care centers are rare but do occur. Specific strategies for controlling infection in out-of-home child care involve adherence to hygiene practices, including meticulous hand hygiene, and limiting exposure to certain animals. Animals at higher risk of causing salmonellosis, including reptiles, amphibians, and poultry, are not recommended in schools, child care settings, hospitals, or nursing homes (see Children in Group Child Care and Schools, p 145).

When NTS serovars are identified in a symptomatic child care attendee or staff member with enterocolitis, older children and staff members do not need to be excluded unless they are symptomatic. Stool cultures are not required for asymptomatic contacts. Likewise, children or staff members with NTS enterocolitis do not require negative culture results from stool samples; children can return to child care facilities if stools are contained in the diaper or when toilet-trained children are continent and when stool frequency becomes no more than 2 stools above that child's normal frequency for the time the child is in the program, even if the stools remain loose (see Children in Group Child Care and Schools, p 145).

When *S* Typhi infection is identified in a child care staff member, local or state health departments should be consulted regarding regulations for length of exclusion and testing, which may vary by jurisdiction. A directory of state and territorial, city and county, and tribal health departments can be found at **www.cdc.gov/publichealthgateway/healthdirectories/index.html.** Because typhoid and paratyphoid infections can be severe (with 77% of US pediatric cases resulting in hospitalization), exclusion of an infected child is warranted at least until negative results for 3 stool samples obtained at least 48 hours after cessation of antimicrobial therapy for *S* Typhi *or S* Paratyphi (see Children in Group Child Care and Schools, p 145).

Typhoid Vaccine. Two typhoid vaccines are licensed by the FDA for use in the United States: live, attenuated oral vaccine Ty21a for people 6 years or older, and the intramuscular Vi capsular polysaccharide vaccine (ViCPS) for people 2 years or older (see Table 3.57). The efficacy of these 2 vaccines ranges from 50% to 80%, but the duration of protection differs notably between the vaccines. Vaccine is selected on the basis of age of the child, need for booster doses, and possible contraindications (see Precautions and Contraindications, p 750) and reactions (see Adverse Events, p 750).

Recommended Use. In the United States, immunization is recommended only for the following people:

- **Travelers to areas where risk of exposure to *S* Typhi is recognized.** Risk is greatest for travelers to the Indian subcontinent, South and Southeast Asia, Latin America, the Caribbean, the Middle East, Africa, and parts of Oceania (eg, Samoa, Fiji) who may have prolonged exposure to contaminated food and drink. Travelers need to be cautioned that typhoid vaccine is not a substitute for careful selection of food and drink (see **www.cdc.gov/travel**).

---

[1] American Academy of Pediatrics, Committee on Infectious Diseases and Committee on Nutrition. Consumption of raw or unpasteurized milk and milk products by pregnant women and children. *Pediatrics*. 2014;133(1):175-179 (Reaffirmed November 2019)

Table 3.57. Commercially Available Typhoid Vaccines in the United States

Typhoid Vaccine	Type	Route	Minimum Age of Receipt	No. of Doses[a]	Booster Frequency, y
Ty21a	Live attenuated	Oral	6 years	4	5
ViCPS	Polysaccharide	Intramuscular	2 years	1	2

ViCPS: Vi capsular polysaccharide vaccine.
[a]Primary immunization. For further information on dosage, schedules, and adverse events, see text.

- **People with intimate exposure to a documented chronic *S* Typhi carrier,** as occurs with continued household contact.
- **Laboratory workers with frequent or potential contact with *S* Typhi.**
    Dosages. For primary immunization, the following dosage is recommended for each vaccine:
- **Typhoid vaccine live oral Ty21a (Vivotif).** Children (6 years and older) and adults should take 1 Ty21a enteric-coated capsule every other day for a total of 4 capsules. Each capsule of Ty21a should be swallowed whole (not chewed) with liquid, no warmer than 37°C (98°F), approximately 1 hour before a meal. Ty21a should be kept refrigerated, and all 4 doses must be taken to achieve maximal efficacy. Immunization should be completed at least 1 week before possible exposure.
- **Typhoid Vi polysaccharide vaccine (Typhim Vi).** Primary immunization of people 2 years and older with unconjugated Vi capsular polysaccharide vaccine (ViCPS) consists of one 0.5-mL (25-μg) dose administered intramuscularly. ViCPS should be administered at least 2 weeks before possible exposure.
- **Vi conjugate vaccine (not currently licensed or available in the United States).** This is a typhoid conjugate vaccine that consists of the Vi capsular polysaccharide of *S* Typhi linked to tetanus toxoid protein that is manufactured and licensed in India (Typbar-TCV). It is the first Vi conjugate to be prequalified by the World Health Organization (WHO). Typbar-TCV has been recommended by the WHO Scientific Advisory Group of Experts for use in infants as young as 6 months of age on the basis of results of clinical trials establishing its tolerability and immunogenicity in children 6 through 23 months of age, as well as in older children and adults. The vaccine is administered as a single intramuscular dose and provides greater protection against typhoid fever than the other available vaccines. Serum IgG Vi antibody appears to endure for several years among children living in areas with endemic infection. Mass vaccination of children in Hyderabad, Pakistan, demonstrated safety and effectiveness of Typbar-TCV in preventing typhoid attributable to the XDR *S* Typhi strain. Typbar-TCV is not licensed in the United States. However, if families with children younger than 2 years of age (and, hence, not able to receive the Typhim Vi vaccine) but older than 6 months are traveling to live in areas of South Asia where XDR *S* Typhi is circulating, parents of infants and toddlers can be advised to contact local pediatricians to have their young children vaccinated with this vaccine.
- **Protection against *S* Paratyphi A and *S* Paratyphi B.** No currently available vaccine provides protection against *S* Paratyphi A. Results of 2 field trials suggest that Ty21a may provide partial cross-protection against *S* Paratyphi B.

Booster Doses. In circumstances of continued or repeated exposure to *S* Typhi, periodic reimmunization is recommended to maintain immunity.

Continued efficacy for 7 years after immunization with Ty21a vaccine has been demonstrated; however, the manufacturer of Ty21a vaccine recommends reimmunization (completing the entire 4-dose series) every 5 years if continued or renewed exposure to *S* Typhi is expected.

ViCPS elicits a T-lymphocyte independent antigen response that does not create immunologic memory to allow boosting of serum Vi antibody titers following an initial immunization. The manufacturer of ViCPS recommends reimmunization every 2 years if continued or renewed exposure is expected.

Ty21a (which does not express Vi antigen) and ViCPS (which protects by stimulating serum IgG Vi antibody) mediate protection by distinct mechanisms. No data have been reported concerning use of one vaccine administered after primary immunization with the other.

Adverse Events. Ty21a vaccine is very well tolerated, but mild adverse reactions may occur; these include abdominal pain, nausea, diarrhea, vomiting, fever, headache, and rash or urticaria. Reported adverse reactions to ViCPS also are minimal and include fever, headache, malaise, myalgia, and local reaction of tenderness and pain, erythema, or induration of 1 cm or greater.

Precautions and Contraindications. A contraindication to administration of ViCPS vaccine is a history of hypersensitivity to any component of the vaccine. No safety data have been reported for typhoid vaccines in pregnant people. Ty21a vaccine is a live attenuated vaccine and should not be administered to immunocompromised people, including people known to be infected with HIV, pregnant people, or people with a phagocytic cell defect or chronic granulomatous disease.[1] The intramuscular ViCPS may be an alternative, although the expected immune response may not be achieved in some hosts. Ty21a should not be administered during acute febrile illness or gastrointestinal tract illness. Antimalarial drugs mefloquine and chloroquine and the combination antimalarials atovaquone/proguanil and pyrimethamine/sulfadoxine, at doses used for prophylaxis, can be administered with Ty21a. The manufacturer advises that other antimalarial agents be administered at least 3 days after the last dose of Ty21a.[2] Antimicrobial agents should be avoided from 3 days before the first dose through 3 days after the last dose of Ty21a.

Public Health Reporting. Notification of public health authorities, sending isolates (or specimens), and determination of serovar are of primary importance in detection and investigation of outbreaks.

Scabies

CLINICAL MANIFESTATIONS: Scabies is characterized by an intensely pruritic, erythematous eruption that may include papules, nodules, vesicles, or bullae caused by burrowing of adult female mites in upper layers of the epidermis, creating serpiginous

---

[1] Rubin LG, Levin MJ, Ljungman P, et al. 2013 IDSA clinical practice guideline for vaccination of the immunocompromised host. *Clin Infect Dis.* 2014;58(3):e44-e100

[2] Jackson BR, Iqbal S, Mahon B. Updated recommendations for the use of typhoid vaccine—Advisory Committee on Immunization Practices, United States, 2015. *MMWR Morb Mortal Wkly Rep.* 2015;64(11):305-308

burrows. Itching is most intense at night. Sites of predilection in older children and adults are the interdigital folds, flexor aspects of wrists, extensor surfaces of elbows, anterior axillary folds, waistline, thighs, navel, genitalia, areolae, abdomen, intergluteal cleft, and buttocks. In children younger than 2 years, the eruption more often is vesicular and often occurs in areas usually spared in older children and adults, such as the scalp, face, neck, palms, and soles. The eruption is caused by a hypersensitivity reaction to the parasite's proteins and products.

Characteristic scabietic burrows appear as thin, gray or white, serpiginous, thread-like lines. Excoriations are common, and most burrows are obliterated by scratching before a patient seeks medical attention. Occasionally, 2- to 5-mm red-brown nodules are present, particularly on covered parts of the body, such as the genitalia, groin, and axilla. These scabies nodules are a granulomatous response to dead mite antigens and feces; the nodules can persist for weeks and even months after effective treatment. Cutaneous secondary bacterial infection is a frequent complication and usually is caused by *Streptococcus pyogenes* or *Staphylococcus aureus*. Studies have demonstrated a rare correlation between scabies and development of poststreptococcal glomerulonephritis.

Crusted (formerly called Norwegian) scabies is an uncommon clinical syndrome characterized by a large number of mites and widespread, crusted, hyperkeratotic lesions. Crusted scabies usually occurs in people with debilitating conditions, people with developmental disabilities, or people who are immunocompromised, including patients receiving biologic response modifiers. Crusted scabies also can occur in otherwise healthy children after long-term use of topical corticosteroid therapy.

Postscabietic pustulosis is a reactive phenomenon that may follow successful treatment of primary infestation with scabies. Affected infants and young children manifest episodic crops of sterile, pruritic papules and pustules predominantly in an acral distribution, but lesions may extend to a lesser degree onto the torso.

ETIOLOGY: The mite *Sarcoptes scabiei* subspecies *hominis* is the cause of scabies. The adult female burrows in the stratum corneum of the skin and lays eggs. Larvae emerge from the eggs in 2 to 4 days and molt to nymphs and then to adults, which mate and produce new eggs. The entire cycle takes approximately 10 to 17 days. *S scabiei* subspecies *canis*, acquired from dogs with clinical mange, can cause a self-limited and mild infestation in humans, usually involving the area in direct contact with the infested animal.

EPIDEMIOLOGY: Humans are the source of infestation. Transmission usually occurs through prolonged close, personal contact. Even minimal contact with patients with crusted scabies or their immediate environment can result in transmission because of the large number of mites in exfoliating scales. Infestation acquired from dogs and other animals is uncommon, and these mites do not replicate in humans. Scabies of human origin can be transmitted as long as the patient remains infested and untreated, including during the interval before symptoms develop. Scabies is endemic in many countries and occurs worldwide sporadically and in epidemics, which may be cyclical in some settings. Scabies affects people from all socioeconomic levels without regard to age, gender, or standards of personal hygiene. Scabies in adults may be acquired sexually.[1]

---

[1] Centers for Disease Control and Prevention. Sexually transmitted infections treatment guidelines, 2021. *MMWR Recomm Rep.* 2021;70(RR-4):1-187

The **incubation period** in people without previous exposure usually is 4 to 6 weeks. People who previously were infested are sensitized and develop symptoms 1 to 4 days after repeated infestation with the mite; reinfestations usually are milder than the original episode.

DIAGNOSTIC TESTS: Diagnosis of scabies typically is made by clinical examination.[1] Diagnosis can be confirmed by identification of the mite, mite eggs, or scybala (feces) from scrapings of papules or intact burrows, preferably from the terminal portion where the mite generally is found. Mineral oil, microscope immersion oil, or water applied to skin facilitates collection of scrapings. A broad-blade scalpel is used to scrape the burrow. Scrapings and oil can be placed on a slide under a glass coverslip and examined microscopically under low power. Adult female mites average 330 to 450 μm in length. Skin scrapings provide definitive evidence of infestation but have low sensitivity. Handheld dermoscopy (epiluminescence microscopy) has been used to identify in vivo the pigmented mite parts or air bubbles corresponding to infesting mites within the stratum corneum. Reflectance in vivo microscopy and polymerase chain reaction assays on swabbed skin material are promising techniques with improved sensitivity and specificity.

TREATMENT: Topical permethrin 5% cream or off-label use of oral ivermectin both are effective agents for treatment of scabies (see Drugs for Parasitic Infections, p 1068). Most experts recommend starting with topical 5% permethrin cream as the drug of choice, particularly for infants (not approved for infants younger than 2 months), young children, and pregnant or nursing people. Permethrin kills the scabies mite and eggs. For children and adults, lotion or cream containing this scabicide should be applied over the entire body below the head and removed by bathing after 8 to 14 hours. Because scabies can affect the face, scalp, and neck in infants and young children, treatment of the entire head, neck, and body in this age group is required. Special attention should be given to trimming fingernails and ensuring application of medication to these areas. Two (or more) applications, each about a week apart, may be necessary to eliminate all mites.

A Cochrane review found that oral ivermectin is as effective as topical permethrin for treating scabies. Because ivermectin is not ovicidal, it is given as 2 doses, 7 to 14 days apart. Ivermectin is not approved for treatment of scabies by the US Food and Drug Administration (FDA). Oral ivermectin should be considered for patients who have failed treatment or who cannot tolerate topical permethrin.

Alternative drugs include 10% crotamiton cream or lotion (not FDA approved for children), 5% to 10% precipitated sulfur compounded into petrolatum, or Spinosad 0.9% suspension (approved by FDA in 2021 for adults and children 4 years and older). Lindane lotion (currently not available in the United States) generally should not be used for treatment of scabies because of safety concerns and availability of other treatments but may be used if all other medications cannot be tolerated or have failed.

Because scabietic lesions are the result of a hypersensitivity reaction to the mite, itching may not subside for several weeks despite successful treatment. Use of oral antihistamines and topical corticosteroids can help relieve itching. Topical or systemic antimicrobial therapy is indicated for secondary bacterial infections of excoriated lesions.

---

[1] Engelman D, Yoshizumi J, Hay RJ, et al. The 2020 International Alliance for the Control of Scabies consensus criteria for the diagnosis of scabies. *Br J Dermatol*. 2020;183(5):808-820

Treatment of crusted scabies can be difficult and typically requires multiple doses of both topical and oral therapy. The most commonly recommended medications are 5% topical permethrin cream and oral ivermectin. Duration of therapy depends on severity of the disease (**www.cdc.gov/parasites/scabies/ health_professionals/meds.html**).

INFECTION PREVENTION AND CONTROL MEASURES IN HEALTH CARE SETTINGS: In addition to standard precautions, contact precautions are recommended until the patient has been treated with an appropriate scabicide.

CONTROL MEASURES:

- Most experts recommend prophylactic therapy for household members, particularly those who have had prolonged direct skin-to-skin contact. Manifestations of scabies infestation can appear as late as 2 months after exposure, during which time the mite can be transmitted. Household members should be treated at the same time to prevent reinfestation. Bedding and clothing worn next to the skin during the 3 days before initiation of therapy should be laundered in a washer with hot water and dried using a hot cycle. Mites do not survive more than 3 days without skin contact. Clothing that cannot be laundered should be removed from the patient and stored for several days to a week to avoid reinfestation.
- Children should not be excluded or sent home early from school because of scabies (see Table 2.3, p 149). They can be treated at the end of the day and allowed to return to child care or school after the first course of treatment has been completed.
- Epidemics and localized outbreaks may require stringent and consistent measures to treat contacts. Health care workers and other caregivers who have had prolonged skin-to-skin contact with patients with infestation may benefit from prophylactic treatment.
- Environmental disinfestation is unnecessary and unwarranted in noncrusted scabies. Thorough vacuuming of environmental surfaces is recommended after use of a room by a patient with noncrusted scabies.
- People with crusted scabies and their close contacts must be treated promptly and aggressively to prevent outbreaks. Information about environmental disinfection for crusted scabies is available from the Centers for Disease Control and Prevention (**www.cdc.gov/parasites/scabies/health_professionals/crusted.html**).

Schistosomiasis

CLINICAL MANIFESTATIONS: Schistosomiasis (bilharziasis) is acquired by skin penetration of infecting larvae (cercariae, shed by freshwater snails). Initial infections often are asymptomatic. Skin manifestations include pruritus at the penetration site a few hours after water exposure, followed in 5 to 14 days by an intermittent pruritic, sometimes papular, eruption. More intense papular eruptions may occur more quickly and last for 7 to 10 days after exposure in people sensitized previously. Cercarial dermatitis (swimmer's itch) also can be caused by larvae of schistosome parasites of birds or other wildlife. These larvae can penetrate human skin but eventually die in the dermis and do not cause systemic disease.

Parasites capable of causing intestinal and urogenital schistosomiasis enter the bloodstream after penetration of the skin, migrate through the lungs, and eventually mature into adult worms that reside in the venous plexus that drains the intestines or, in the case of *Schistosoma haematobium*, the urogenital tract. Four to 8 weeks after exposure, worms develop into adults and females begin egg deposition, which can lead to an acute serum sickness-like illness (Katayama syndrome) that manifests as fever, malaise, cough, rash, abdominal pain, hepatosplenomegaly, diarrhea, nausea, lymphadenopathy, and/or eosinophilia. This syndrome is most common among non-immune hosts, such as travelers. Severity of symptoms associated with chronic infection is partially related to worm burden. People with low to moderate worm burdens may have only subclinical disease or relatively mild manifestations, such as growth stunting or anemia. Higher worm burdens are associated with a range of symptoms primarily caused by inflammation and local fibrosis triggered by the immune response to eggs produced by adult worms. Severe forms of chronic intestinal schistosomiasis (*Schistosoma mansoni* and *Schistosoma japonicum* infections) can result in hepatosplenomegaly, abdominal pain, bloody diarrhea, periportal fibrosis, portal hypertension, ascites, esophageal varices, and hematemesis. Urogenital schistosomiasis (*S haematobium* infections) can result in the bladder becoming inflamed and fibrotic. Urinary tract symptoms and signs include dysuria, urgency, microscopic and gross hematuria, secondary urinary tract infections, hydronephrosis, and nonspecific pelvic pain. *S haematobium* is associated with lesions of the lower genital tract (vulva, vagina, and cervix) in women, prostatitis and hematospermia in men, and certain forms of bladder cancer.[1] Other organ systems can be involved—for example, eggs can embolize to the lungs, causing pulmonary hypertension. Less commonly, eggs can lodge in the central nervous system, causing severe neurologic complications.

ETIOLOGY: The trematodes (flukes) *S mansoni*, *S japonicum*, *Schistosoma mekongi*, *Schistosoma guineensis*, and *Schistosoma intercalatum* cause intestinal schistosomiasis, and *S haematobium* causes urogenital disease. All species have similar life cycles.

EPIDEMIOLOGY: Persistence of schistosomiasis in a population depends on the local presence of an appropriate snail as an intermediate host. Eggs excreted in stool (*S mansoni*, *S japonicum*, *S mekongi*, *S intercalatum*, and *S guineensis*) or urine *(S haematobium)* into fresh water hatch into motile miracidia, which infect snails. After development and asexual replication in snails, cercariae emerge and penetrate the skin of humans in contact with water. In areas with endemic schistosomiasis, children are infected first when they accompany their parents to lakes, ponds, and other open fresh water sources. School-aged children typically are the most heavily infected people in the community because of prolonged wading and swimming in infected waters. Children have greater susceptibility to infection than older people because of a lack of high preexisting immunity to these parasites and are important in maintaining transmission through behaviors such as uncontrolled defecation and urination. Animals play an important zoonotic role (as a source of eggs) in maintaining the life cycle of *S japonicum*. Animal reservoirs may also play a role in areas of West Africa, where *S haematobium* has hybridized with the cattle parasite *Schistosoma bovis*. Infection is not transmissible by person-to-person contact or blood transfusion.

Distribution of schistosomiasis is focal and limited by presence of appropriate snail intermediate hosts, infected human reservoirs, and fresh water sources. *S mansoni* occurs throughout tropical Africa, in parts of several Caribbean islands, and in areas of Venezuela, Brazil, Suriname, and the Arabian Peninsula. *S japonicum* is found in

[1] The terms women and men refer to sex assigned at birth.

China, the Philippines, and Indonesia. *S haematobium* occurs in Africa and the Middle East; in 2014, local transmission of *S haematobium/S bovis* hybrids was reported in Corsica. *S mekongi* is found in Cambodia and Laos. *S intercalatum* is found in Central Africa, and *S guineensis* is found in West Africa. Adult worms of *S mansoni* usually survive for 5 to 7 years but can live as long as 30 years in the human host. Schistosomiasis can be diagnosed in patients many years after they have left an area with endemic transmission. (See Medical Evaluation for Infectious Diseases for Internationally Adopted, Refugee, and Other Immigrant Children, p 189.) Immunity is incomplete, and reinfection occurs commonly. Swimmer's itch can occur in all regions of the world after exposure to fresh water, brackish water, or salt water.

The **incubation period** is variable but is approximately 4 to 6 weeks for *S japonicum*, 6 to 8 weeks for *S mansoni*, and 10 to 12 weeks for *S haematobium*.

DIAGNOSTIC TESTS: Eosinophilia is common and may be intense in Katayama syndrome (acute schistosomiasis). Infection with *S mansoni* and other intestinal species is diagnosed by microscopic examination of stool specimens to detect characteristic eggs containing fully differentiated larvae, but results may be negative if performed too early in the course of infection. In light infections, several stool specimens examined by a concentration technique may be needed before eggs are found, or eggs may be seen in a biopsy of the rectal mucosa. *S haematobium* is diagnosed by examining urine for eggs; filtration or centrifugation and examination of the urinary sediment is required for optimum sensitivity. Egg excretion in urine often peaks between noon and 3 pm. Biopsy of the bladder or vaginal/cervical mucosa may be used to diagnose *S haematobium* infection. Urine reagent dipsticks commonly will be positive for blood. Serologic tests, available through the Centers for Disease Control and Prevention and some commercial laboratories, may be helpful for detecting light infections; results of these antibody-based tests remain positive for many years and are not useful in differentiating ongoing infection from past infection or reinfection. Serologic test results are negative during acute infection, turn positive 6 to 12 weeks or more after infection, and may be positive before eggs are detectable. Polymerase chain reaction and antigen tests for detection of schistosomes have been developed but are considered to be research tools at present.

Swimmer's itch, which is caused by the cercariae of certain schistosome species whose normal hosts are birds and nonhuman mammals, can be difficult to differentiate from other causes of dermatitis. A skin biopsy may demonstrate larvae, but their absence does not exclude the diagnosis. A history of exposure to water used by waterfowl may be helpful in making the diagnosis.

TREATMENT: The drug of choice for schistosomiasis caused by any species is praziquantel (see Drugs for Parasitic Infections, p 1068). Praziquantel does not kill developing worms, so treatment administered early (eg, 4 to 8 weeks after exposure) should be repeated 2 to 4 weeks later to improve parasitologic cure. Initial management of acute schistosomiasis and neuroschistosomiasis includes reduction of inflammation with steroids, although optimal dose and duration are uncertain. Initial treatment with praziquantel may exacerbate symptoms. The optimal timing of adding praziquantel is unknown; treating with this drug when inflammation has subsided generally is favored. Swimmer's itch is a self-limited disease that may require symptomatic treatment of the rash. More intense reactions may require a course of oral corticosteroids.

INFECTION PREVENTION AND CONTROL MEASURES IN HEALTH CARE SETTINGS: Standard precautions are recommended. Schistosomiasis cannot be transmitted from person to person or by the fecal-oral route.

CONTROL MEASURES: Elimination of the intermediate snail host is difficult to achieve in most areas. Mass or selective treatment of infected populations, sanitary disposal of human waste, water sanitation programs, and education about the source of infection are key elements of current control measures. Travelers to areas with endemic schistosomiasis should be advised to avoid any contact with freshwater streams, rivers, ponds, or lakes. Swimming and wading should occur only in chlorinated pools. Human schistosomiasis is not transmitted in sea water.

Shigella Infections

CLINICAL MANIFESTATIONS: *Shigella* species primarily infect the large intestine, resulting in clinical manifestations that range from watery or loose stools with minimal or no constitutional symptoms to more severe symptoms, including high fever or hypothermia, abdominal cramps or tenderness, tenesmus, lethargy, and mucoid stools with or without blood. Infection with *Shigella dysenteriae* serotype 1 often results in a more severe illness than infection with other *Shigella* species, with a higher risk of complications, including septicemia, pseudomembranous colitis, toxic megacolon, intestinal perforation, hemolysis, and hemolytic-uremic syndrome (HUS). Infections attributable to *S dysenteriae* serotype 1 have become less common but continue to be an important etiology of illness in low-resource settings. Generalized seizures have been reported among young children with shigellosis attributable to any serotype, although the pathophysiology and incidence are poorly understood. Seizures associated with shigellosis are self-limited and usually are associated with high fever or electrolyte abnormalities. Septicemia is rare during illness and is caused either by *Shigella* organisms or by translocation of gastrointestinal flora into the bloodstream through compromised intestinal mucosa. Septicemia occurs most often in neonates, malnourished children, and immunocompromised people with *S dysenteriae* serotype 1 infection but may occur in healthy children with non-*S dysenteriae* shigellosis. Septicemia presents a higher risk of death in those ill with shigellosis. Reactive arthritis with extraarticular manifestations is a rare complication that can develop weeks to months after shigellosis, especially in people expressing HLA-B27. Postinfectious irritable bowel syndrome can occur and may last for weeks to months.

ETIOLOGY: *Shigella* species are facultative anaerobic, gram-negative bacilli in the order *Enterobacterales*. Four species (with more than 40 serotypes) have been identified, with *Shigella sonnei* being the most common in the United States. The other species are *Shigella flexneri*, *S dysenteriae*, and *Shigella boydii*. In resource-limited settings, especially in Africa and Asia, *S flexneri* predominates, and *S dysenteriae* serotype 1 is associated with outbreaks. Shiga toxin, a potent cytotoxin produced by *S dysenteriae* serotype 1, enhances the virulence of this serotype at the colonic mucosa resulting in small blood vessel and renal damage, leading to HUS in some individuals. The Shiga toxin genes are phage-encoded and have been found in a small number of strains belonging to other *Shigella* species and serotypes, including *S flexneri* serotype 2a, *S dysenteriae* serotype 4, and *Shigella sonnei*. HUS has been associated with an infection attributable to *S sonnei* in an adult, although the non-*S dysenteriae* species are not commonly associated with HUS.

EPIDEMIOLOGY: Humans are the primary reservoir of *Shigella* species, although non-human primates are also able to be infected. The primary mode of transmission is the fecal-oral route, and transmission can occur via contact with a contaminated inanimate object, ingestion of contaminated food or water, or sexual contact. Houseflies and cockroaches also may be vectors facilitating physical transport of feces with *Shigella*. It is very easy to transmit *Shigella* infection, because ingestion of very few organisms is sufficient for infection to occur. Prolonged organism survival in water (up to 6 months) and food (up to 30 days) can occur. Children 5 years or younger attending child care settings and their caregivers, as well as people living in crowded conditions, are at increased risk of infection. Men who have sex with men are also at increased risk of shigellosis and are particularly at risk for multidrug-resistant strains. Infections attributable to *S flexneri*, *S boydii*, and *S dysenteriae* are slightly more common among adults than among children. Travel to resource-limited settings with inadequate sanitation can place travelers at risk of infection. Even without antimicrobial therapy, the carrier state usually ceases within 1 to 4 weeks after onset of illness; long-term carriage is uncommon and does not correlate with underlying intestinal dysfunction.

Antibiotic resistance is increasing among *Shigella* isolates, especially among international travelers, men who have sex with men, people who lack housing, and people who are immunocompromised. During 2020, a year impacted by the COVID-19 pandemic, preliminary data suggest that 38% of *Shigella* isolates tested in the United States were resistant to ampicillin, 63% were resistant to trimethoprim-sulfamethoxazole, 13% were resistant to azithromycin, 50% were resistant to ciprofloxacin, and 13% were resistant to ceftriaxone.[1] The Centers for Disease Control and Prevention (CDC) has been monitoring *Shigella* isolates that harbor 1 or more quinolone resistance mechanisms (ie, those with a minimum inhibitory concentration [MIC] of ≥ 0.12 µg/mL for ciprofloxacin) but that have in vitro susceptibility to fluoroquinolones **(https://emergency.cdc.gov/han/han00411.asp).** Additional data are needed to determine whether fluoroquinolone treatment outcomes and risk of illness transmission are impacted in patients with such isolates. Data from the National Antimicrobial Resistance Monitoring System (NARMS) indicate that many *Shigella* isolates with a quinolone resistance mechanism are nonsusceptible or resistant to many other commonly used first-line treatment agents. Since 2015, an increase in extensively drug-resistant (XDR) *Shigella* infections, defined as isolates resistant to azithromycin, ciprofloxacin, ceftriaxone, trimethoprim-sulfamethoxazole, and ampicillin, has been reported through national surveillance systems. In 2022, about 5% of *Shigella* infections reported to CDC were caused by XDR strains, compared with 0% in 2015 **(https://emergency.cdc.gov/han/2023/han00486.asp).**

The **incubation period** varies from 1 to 7 days but typically is 1 to 3 days.

DIAGNOSTIC TESTS: Isolation of *Shigella* organisms from feces or rectal swab specimens containing feces is diagnostic; sensitivity is improved by testing stool as soon as possible after it is passed, along with the use of enrichment broth media and selective agar plate media. If specimens cannot be transported to the testing laboratory within 2 hours, they should be transferred to appropriate transport media (eg, Cary-Blair or

[1] Centers for Disease Control and Prevention. National Antimicrobial Resistance Monitoring System (NARMS) Now: Human Data. Centers for Disease Control and Prevention; November 2021. Available at: **www.cdc.gov/narmsnow**

similar media) and kept and transported at 4°C. Definitive identification of the organism requires both biochemical profiling and serogrouping to differentiate *Shigella* from *Escherichia*. Identification by mass spectrometry of cellular components should not be used, because this method cannot distinguish between the 2 genera. The presence of fecal lactoferrin demonstrated on a methylene-blue stained stool smear is sensitive for the diagnosis of colitis but is not specific for shigellosis. Although bacteremia is rare, children who are severely ill, immunocompromised, or malnourished should have a blood culture obtained. Multiplex polymerase chain reaction (PCR) platforms for detection of multiple bacterial (including *Shigella*), viral, and parasitic pathogens have high sensitivity but will not distinguish between viable and nonviable organisms nor provide antimicrobial susceptibility results. To guide treatment, if needed, and to enable surveillance and outbreak detection, stool cultures are recommended if shigellosis is diagnosed using multiplex PCR platforms or other nonculture-based diagnostic tests. Other tests for bacterial detection, including qualitative and quantitative PCR assays, are available in research laboratories and some clinical laboratories. Isolates of *Shigella* species (or clinical specimens from positive nonculture diagnostic tests if reflex culturing is not possible) should be submitted as required to local or state public health laboratories.

TREATMENT:
- Although severe dehydration is rare with shigellosis, correction of fluid and electrolyte losses, preferably by oral rehydration solutions, is the mainstay of treatment.
- Most infections with *S sonnei* are self-limited (48 to 72 hours) and mild episodes do not require antimicrobial therapy.
- Antimicrobial treatment is recommended for patients with severe disease or with underlying immunosuppressive conditions; in these patients, empiric therapy should be given while awaiting culture and susceptibility results. Treatment is also indicated for symptomatic patients with culture-proven *Shigella* who require hospitalization, attend daycare, live in institutions or are involved in food handling. Available evidence suggests that antimicrobial therapy is somewhat effective in shortening duration of diarrhea and hastening eradication of organisms from feces; however, whether antimicrobial treatment reduces transmission is unclear.
- Antimicrobial susceptibility testing of clinical isolates is indicated to guide therapy because resistance to antimicrobial agents is common and increasing. Increasing antimicrobial resistance to azithromycin, ciprofloxacin, and ceftriaxone have been reported in the United States. For situations in which antibiotic treatment is indicated, oral administration is recommended, except for seriously ill patients, those with underlying immunodeficiencies, and patients who are unable to take oral medications. First-line antibiotic therapy generally consists of one of the following antibiotics, guided by antimicrobial susceptibility testing:
  - Azithromycin for 3 days.
  - A fluoroquinolone (eg, ciprofloxacin) for 3 days. Fluoroquinolones should be avoided if the *Shigella* strain has an MIC of ≥0.12 µg/mL for ciprofloxacin, even if the laboratory indicates that the isolate is "susceptible," until more is known about the clinical outcomes of ciprofloxacin treatment when MICs are ≥0.12 µg/mL.
  - Oral ampicillin or trimethoprim-sulfamethoxazole for 5 days are alternative options; amoxicillin is not effective because of its rapid absorption from the gastrointestinal tract.

- Parenteral ceftriaxone for 2 to 5 days. Oral cephalosporins (eg, cefixime) are of unclear efficacy.
- Longer treatment durations may be indicated in patients with invasive infection such as septicemia.
- Antidiarrheal compounds that inhibit intestinal peristalsis are contraindicated, because they can prolong the clinical and bacteriologic course of disease and can increase the rate of complications.
- Nutritional supplementation, including vitamin A (200 000 IU) and zinc (elemental Zn, orally daily for 10–14 days, 10 mg/day for newborn infants to 6 months of age, and 20 mg/day for those older than 6 months), can be given to hasten clinical resolution in geographic areas where children are at risk of malnutrition.

INFECTION PREVENTION AND CONTROL MEASURES IN HEALTH CARE SETTINGS:
In addition to standard precautions, contact precautions are indicated for the duration of illness.

CONTROL MEASURES:

General Control Measures. Strict attention to hand hygiene is essential to limit spread. Other important control measures include improved sanitation, appropriately chlorinating water supplies, proper cooking and storage of food, excluding infected people such as food handlers and child care providers, safe diapering practices, and measures to decrease contamination of food and surfaces by houseflies. People should refrain from recreational water venues (eg, swimming pools, water parks) while they have diarrhea; for children who are incontinent, recreational water activities should be avoided for 1 additional week (or as advised by local public health authorities). (See Prevention of Illness Associated With Recreational Water Use, p 214.) Sexually active people should avoid engaging in sexual activity for at least 1 week (ideally 2 weeks) after resolution of diarrhea. Breastfeeding provides some protection for infants.

Child Care Centers. General measures for interrupting enteric transmission in child care centers are recommended (see Children in Group Child Care and Schools, p 145). Meticulous hand hygiene is the single most important measure to decrease transmission. Waterless hand sanitizers may be effective when access to soap or clean water is limited. Eliminating access to shared water-play areas and contaminated diapers also can limit disease spread. Child care staff members should follow all standard infection control recommendations, specifically enhancing hand hygiene and ensuring that those who change diapers are not responsible for food preparation. When *Shigella* infection is identified in a child care attendee or staff member, stool specimens from symptomatic attendees and staff members should be obtained.

Following this, children may return to child care facilities if stools are contained in the diaper or when toilet-trained children are continent and when stool frequency becomes no more than 2 stools above that child's normal baseline, even if the stools remain loose (see Table 2.3, p 149).

Institutional Outbreaks. Shigella outbreaks that are most difficult to control are those that involve children who are not yet or only recently toilet-trained, adults who are unable to care for themselves (eg, cognitively impaired people and skilled nursing facility residents), or those that occur in areas with an inadequate supply of chlorinated water. A strong emphasis on hand hygiene, infection control, and appropriate antimicrobial therapy is needed to control disease transmission. In residential institutions, ill people should be cohorted in separate areas from those who are not ill to reduce disease spread.

Public Health Reporting. *Shigella* infections are generally a reportable disease to state or local public health authorities. A directory of state and territorial, city and county, and tribal health departments can be found at **www.cdc.gov/publichealthgateway/ healthdirectories/index.html.** At the time of notification, the local health department can assist with additional case finding and management of a possible outbreak. Infected people should be excluded from the child care facility until the state or local health department approves return per state or local child care exclusion regulations. Case reporting to appropriate health authorities (eg, hospital infection control personnel and public health departments) is essential to optimize adherence to inclusion and exclusion policies.

Smallpox (Variola)

In 1980, the World Health Assembly declared that smallpox (caused by variola virus) had been eradicated successfully worldwide, and no subsequent human cases have been confirmed. Following eradication, 2 World Health Organization (WHO) reference laboratories were authorized to maintain stocks of variola virus (Centers for Disease Control and Prevention in Atlanta, Georgia, and VECTOR in Novosibirsk, Russia). The United States discontinued routine childhood immunization against smallpox in 1972 and routine immunization of health care professionals in 1976. As a result of the terrorism events on September 11, 2001 and concern that the virus might be used as a weapon of bioterrorism, the smallpox immunization policy was revisited. In 2002, the United States resumed routine immunization of military personnel deployed to certain areas of the world. During 2003, a civilian smallpox immunization program for first responders in the United States was initiated to facilitate preparedness and response to a possible smallpox bioterrorism event. Such a bioterrorism event has not occurred.

CLINICAL MANIFESTATIONS: People infected with variola major strains develop a severe prodromal illness characterized by high fever (102°F–104°F [38.9°C–40.0°C]) and constitutional symptoms, including malaise, severe headache, backache, abdominal pain, and prostration, lasting for 2 to 5 days. Infected children may suffer from vomiting and seizures during this prodromal period. Most patients with smallpox are severely ill and bedridden during the febrile prodrome. The prodromal period is followed by the development of lesions on the mucosa of the mouth or pharynx, which may not be noticed by the patient. This stage occurs less than 24 hours before onset of rash, which usually is the first recognized manifestation of smallpox. With onset of oral lesions, the patient becomes infectious and remains so until all skin crust lesions have separated. The rash typically begins on the face and rapidly progresses to involve the forearms, trunk, and legs, with the greatest concentration of lesions on the face and distal extremities. The majority of patients will have lesions on the palms and soles. With rash onset, fever decreases but does not resolve. Lesions begin as macules that progress to papules, followed by firm vesicles and then deep-seated, hard pustules described as "pearls of pus." Each stage lasts 1 to 2 days. By the sixth or seventh day of rash, lesions may begin to umbilicate or become confluent. Lesions increase in size for approximately 8 to 10 days, after which they begin to crust. Once all the crusts have separated and a fresh layer of skin has formed, generally 3 to 4 weeks after the onset of rash, the patient no longer is infectious. Variola major in unimmunized people is associated with case fatality rates of approximately 30% during epidemics of small-pox. The mortality rate is highest in pregnant people, children younger than 1 year, and adults older than 40 years. The potential for improved outcomes because of mod-ern supportive therapy and the availability of new antiviral agents is not known.

Variola minor strains cause a disease that is indistinguishable clinically from variola major, except that it causes less severe systemic symptoms and has more rapid rash evolution, reduced scarring, and fewer fatalities.

In addition to the typical presentation of smallpox (90% of cases or greater), there are 2 uncommon severe forms of variola major: hemorrhagic and malignant smallpox. Hemorrhagic smallpox is characterized either by a hemorrhagic diathesis before onset of the typical smallpox rash (early hemorrhagic smallpox) or by hemorrhage into skin lesions and disseminated intravascular coagulation (late hemorrhagic smallpox). In malignant or flat type smallpox, the skin lesions do not progress to the pustular stage but remain flat and soft. Each variant occurs in approximately 5% of cases and is asso-ciated with a 95% to 100% mortality rate. Pregnancy is a risk factor for hemorrhagic variola. Defects in cellular immunity may be responsible for flat type variola major, which is seen more commonly in children than adults.

Varicella (chickenpox) can be mistaken for smallpox. Generally, children with varicella do not have a febrile prodrome, but adults may have a brief, mild prodrome. Although the 2 diseases are confused easily in the first few days of the rash, small-pox lesions develop into pustules that are firm and deeply embedded in the dermis, whereas varicella lesions develop into superficial vesicles. Because varicella erupts in crops of lesions that evolve quickly, lesions on any one part of the body will be in dif-ferent stages of evolution (papules, vesicles, and crusts), whereas all smallpox lesions on any one part of the body are in the same stage of development. The rash distribu-tion of the 2 diseases differs. Varicella most commonly starts on the trunk and moves peripherally with less involvement of the extremities as compared with the trunk (centripetal). Variola lesions can be found distributed on all parts of the body but are generally found in higher numbers on the face and extremities compared with the trunk (centrifugal). Mpox also can be mistaken for smallpox as it produces a clinically similar but milder illness (see Mpox, p 606). Prominent lymphadenopathy can be a dis-tinguishing feature of mpox.

ETIOLOGY: Variola virus, the virus that causes smallpox, is a member of the *Poxviridae* family (genus *Orthopoxvirus*). Other members of this genus that can infect humans include monkeypox virus, cowpox virus, vaccinia virus, and several putative novel spe-cies. Cowpox virus is believed to have been used by Benjamin Jesty in 1774 and by Edward Jenner in 1796 as material for the first smallpox vaccine. Later, cowpox virus was replaced with vaccinia virus.

EPIDEMIOLOGY: Humans are the only natural reservoir for variola virus (smallpox). Smallpox is spread most commonly by large respiratory droplets from the oropharynx of infected people, although rare transmission from aerosol spread has been reported. Infection from direct contact with lesion material or indirectly via fomites, such as clothing and bedding, has also been reported. Because most patients with smallpox are extremely ill and bedridden, spread generally is limited to household contacts, hospital workers, and other health care professionals. Secondary household attack rates for smallpox were considerably lower than for measles and similar to or lower than rates for varicella.

Novel putative orthopox species with clinical presentations similar to cowpox virus and vaccinia virus have been reported in Alaska, Norway, and the country of Georgia.

The **incubation period** for smallpox is 7 to 17 days (mean, 10–12 days).

DIAGNOSTIC TESTS: If smallpox is suspected, consultation should be made immediately with the state or local health department. An algorithm to guide evaluation of smallpox is available at **www.cdc.gov/smallpox/clinicians/algorithm-protocol.html.** Diagnostic work-up should include exclusion of varicella-zoster virus and other common conditions that cause a vesicular/pustular rash illness. Caution is required when collecting specimens from patients in whom a diagnosis of smallpox is considered. Detailed guidelines for safe collection of specimens can be obtained through consultation with the Centers for Disease Control and Prevention (CDC; **www.cdc.gov/smallpox/**; 770-488-7100).

Variola virus can be detected in vesicular or pustular fluid by a number of different methods, including electron microscopy, immunohistochemistry, culture, or nucleic acid amplification test (NAAT). Testing for orthopoxviruses using a NAAT is available through the US Laboratory Response Network, after consultation is made with state or local public health departments. If smallpox is suspected and the orthopoxvirus NAAT result is positive, specimens are sent to CDC for a confirmatory variola-specific NAAT. This is available only at the CDC.

TREATMENT: Tecovirimat (TPOXX or ST-246) was licensed by the US Food and Drug Administration (FDA) in July 2018 as an oral treatment for smallpox for patients weighing 13 kg or more, using the Animal Rule pathway (ie, effectiveness of the drug was based on animal data only). In May 2022, an intravenous formulation was licensed for use in patients weighing 3 kg or more. Dosing information and treatment duration can be found in Table 4.10 (p 1044). Tecovirimat has been shown to be active against monkeypox virus and rabbitpox in animal models. In addition, it was used for mpox treatment in people under an expanded access investigational new drug protocol during the 2022 mpox outbreak. Tecovirimat effectiveness against variola in humans is unknown. It inhibits the function of an envelope protein required for spread of the virus from cell to cell. Tecovirimat is included in the US Strategic National Stockpile that is managed by the US Department of Health and Human Services, Office of the Assistant Secretary for Preparedness and Response.

Brincidofovir is a lipophilic derivative of cidofovir that is administered orally and does not appear to have renal toxicity. It was also approved under the Animal Rule for treatment of smallpox in June 2021. Dosing information can be found in Table 4.10 (p 1044). Brincidofovir has been shown to be active against rabbitpox and mousepox in animal models, although effectiveness against variola virus in humans is unknown. It inhibits viral DNA polymerase-mediated synthesis of viral DNA. Cidofovir inhibits the growth of variola virus in laboratory studies but has not been clinically evaluated in humans for the treatment of smallpox. It is not approved by the FDA for the treatment of smallpox but might be recommended for use during an outbreak using an investigational new drug protocol or emergency use authorization.

INFECTION PREVENTION AND CONTROL MEASURES IN HEALTH CARE SETTINGS:
At the time of admission, a patient suspected of having smallpox should be placed in a private, airborne infection isolation room equipped with negative-pressure ventilation with high-efficiency particulate air filtration. Standard, contact, and airborne precautions plus eye protection should be implemented promptly, and hospital infection control personnel and the state (and/or local) health department should be alerted immediately, even if alternative diagnoses are being evaluated concurrently.

CONTROL MEASURES:

Vaccines. Information on vaccination for orthopoxviruses can be found on the CDC website (**www.cdc.gov/smallpox/clinicians/index.html**). Two vaccines, ACAM2000 and JYNNEOS, are licensed to prevent orthopoxvirus infections, including smallpox. Both are part of the National Strategic Stockpile and are intended for emergency use during a smallpox event. They also are available through CDC for preexposure prophylaxis for select laboratory and health care personnel who are at risk for exposure to orthopoxviruses. In the absence of a smallpox outbreak, preexposure vaccination for smallpox is not recommended for the general US population. Postexposure immunization for smallpox provides some protection against disease and significant protection against a fatal outcome; it should ideally be administered within 3 to 4 days of exposure but may be given later.

ACAM2000 is a live, **replicating** vaccinia virus vaccine licensed to prevent smallpox. The lyophilized vaccine does not contain variola virus but rather the related vaccinia virus. ACAM2000 is grown in tissue culture and elicits an immune response similar to Dryvax, a previously licensed vaccinia virus vaccine (no longer available) that was highly effective in preventing smallpox. Vaccine protection wanes with time, but substantial protection has been observed up to 15 to 20 years after immunization. Administration involves a specialized multiple-puncture technique with a bifurcated needle, but any health care provider can be trained to administer ACAM2000. Inadvertent transmission of the vaccine virus may occur from vaccine recipients to their household contacts. Immunocompromised people and those with atopic skin disease are at increased risk of serious complications following contact transmission including progressive vaccinia and eczema vaccinatum. Detailed information, including information on contraindications and adverse effects, can be found in the ACAM2000 package insert and medication guide (**www.fda.gov/BiologicsBloodVaccines/Vaccines/ApprovedProducts/ucm180810.htm**).

A live, **nonreplicating** vaccinia virus vaccine (JYNNEOS) was approved by the FDA in 2019 for prevention of smallpox and mpox in people 18 years and older who are at high risk for smallpox or mpox infection. Two doses are administered 4 weeks apart. JYNNEOS may be considered for persons with contraindications for receiving ACAM2000 (including individuals with immunocompromising conditions, atopic skin disease, eczema or other exfoliative skin disease, or allergy to a component of ACAM2000). ACIP guidance for JYNNEOS for occupational preexposure prophylaxis has been published.[1]

---

[1] Rao AK, Petersen BW, Whitehill F, et al. Use of JYNNEOS (smallpox and monkeypox vaccine, live, non-replicating) for preexposure vaccination of persons at risk for occupational exposure to orthopoxviruses: recommendations of the Advisory Committee on Immunization Practices—United States, 2022. *MMWR Morb Mortal Wkly Rep.* 2022;71(22);734–742

An investigational vaccinia vaccine similar to ACAM2000 (APSV) is also part of the strategic national stockpile for emergency use during a smallpox event. Guidelines on the use of these vaccines in a smallpox event have been published.[1]

Treatment of Complications of Smallpox Vaccine. Vaccinia immune globulin (VIG) is licensed for certain complications of vaccination with replication competent vaccinia. VIG has no role in treatment of smallpox (**www.cdc.gov/smallpox/clinicians/ vaccine-medical-management6.html**). Tecovirimat and brincidofovir have been used for the treatment of disseminated vaccinia through individual patient expanded access requests. Physicians should consult with their state or local health departments for diagnosis and management of patients with complications of vaccinia vaccination. CDC medical staff can be reached through the CDC emergency operations center at 770-488-7100. The CDC smallpox vaccine adverse events clinical consultation team can discuss need for treatment with VIG or antivirals and arrange shipment when indicated. Physicians at military medical facilities (or physicians treating a US Department of Defense health care beneficiary) can call the Defense Health Agency's 24/7 Immunization Healthcare Support Center at 877-GETVACC (877-438-8222) and select option #1.

Public Health Reporting. Smallpox is a nationally and immediately notifiable condition. Cases of febrile rash illness for which smallpox is considered in the differential diagnosis should be reported immediately to state or local health departments.

Sporotrichosis

CLINICAL MANIFESTATIONS: Three **cutaneous** patterns are described for sporotrichosis. The classic lymphocutaneous process with multiple nodules is seen more commonly in adults. Inoculation occurs at a site of minor trauma, causing a painless papule that enlarges slowly to become a firm, slightly tender, subcutaneous nodule that can develop a violaceous hue or ulcerate. Secondary lesions follow the same evolution and develop along the lymphatic distribution proximal to the initial lesion. A localized cutaneous form of sporotrichosis, also called fixed cutaneous form, is seen more commonly in children and presents as a solitary crusted papule or papuloulcerative or nodular lesion in which lymphatic spread is not observed. The extremities and face are the most common sites of infection. A disseminated cutaneous form with multiple lesions is rare, usually occurring in immunocompromised patients.

Extracutaneous sporotrichosis accounts for 20% of all cases and usually occurs in the setting of unusual areas of trauma or in immunocompromised patients. Osteoarticular infection results from hematogenous spread or local inoculation. The most commonly affected joints are the knees, elbows, wrists, and ankles. Pulmonary sporotrichosis clinically resembles tuberculosis and occurs after inhalation or aspiration of aerosolized conidia. Disseminated disease generally occurs after hematogenous spread from primary skin or lung infection. Disseminated sporotrichosis can involve multiple foci (eg, eyes, pericardium, genitourinary tract, central nervous system) and occurs predominantly in immunocompromised patients. Pulmonary and disseminated forms of sporotrichosis are uncommon in children.

---

[1] Peterson BW, Damon IK, Pertowski CA, et al. Clinical guidance for smallpox vaccine use in a postevent vaccination program. *MMWR Recomm Rep*. 2015;64(RR-2):1-26

ETIOLOGY: *Sporothrix schenckii* is a thermally dimorphic fungus that grows as a mold or mycelial form at room temperature and as a budding yeast at 35°C to 37°C and in host tissues. *S schenckii* is a complex of at least 6 species. Within this complex, *S schenckii sensu stricto* is responsible for most infections, followed by *Sporothrix globosa;* in South America, *Sporothrix brasiliensis* is a major cause of infection.

EPIDEMIOLOGY: *S schenckii* is a ubiquitous organism that has worldwide distribution but is most common in tropical and subtropical regions of Central and South America and parts of North America and Asia. The fungus has been isolated from soil and plant material, including hay, straw, sphagnum moss, and decaying vegetation. Thorny plants such as rose bushes and pine trees commonly are implicated, because pricks from their thorns or needles inoculate the organism from the soil or moss around the bush or tree. *S brasiliensis* is responsible for hyperendemic cutaneous sporotrichosis in Rio de Janeiro. Primarily zoonotic, it is transmitted by direct inoculation through bites or scratches or mucosal exposure to secretions from infected cats.

The **incubation period** is 7 to 30 days after cutaneous inoculation but can be as long as 6 months.

DIAGNOSTIC TESTS: Culture of *Sporothrix* species from a tissue, wound drainage, or sputum specimen is diagnostic. The mold phase of the organism can be isolated on a variety of fungal media, including Sabouraud dextrose agar at 25°C to 30°C. Filamentous colonies generally appear within 1 week. Definitive identification requires conversion to the yeast phase by subculture to enriched media, such as brain-heart infusion agar with 5% blood and incubation at 35°C to 37°C. In some cases, repeated subcultures are required for conversion. Culture of *Sporothrix* species from a blood specimen is definite evidence for disseminated infection, which is associated with immunodeficiency. Histopathologic examination of tissue often is not helpful, because the organism is seldom abundant, but may be useful to exclude clinically similar infections such as cutaneous leishmaniasis. Fungal stains including periodic acid-Schiff or Gomori methenamine silver to visualize this distinctive oval or cigar-shaped organism are required. Antibody tests offered by some reference laboratories have been useful in a few cases of extracutaneous sporotrichosis. Molecular testing on tissue samples is available only in a few reference laboratories and is not standardized.

TREATMENT[1,2]**:** Sporotrichosis usually does not resolve without treatment. Itraconazole is the drug of choice for children with lymphocutaneous and localized cutaneous disease. See Recommended Doses of Parenteral and Oral Antifungal Drugs (p 1026) for dosing. Duration of therapy is 2 to 4 weeks after all lesions have resolved, usually for a total duration of 3 to 6 months. Serum trough concentrations of itraconazole should be 1 to 2 μg/mL. A trough level should be checked 10 days or later following initiation to ensure adequate drug exposure. When measured by high-pressure liquid chromatography, both itraconazole and its bioactive hydroxyitraconazole metabolite are reported, the sum of which should be considered in assessing the trough concentration.

[1] Kauffman CA, Bustamante B, Chapman SW, Pappas PG; Infectious Diseases Society of America. Clinical practice guidelines for the management of sporotrichosis: 2007 update by the Infectious Diseases Society of America. *Clin Infect Dis*. 2007;45(10):1255-1265

[2] Thompson GR III, Le T, Chindamporn A, et al. Global guideline for the diagnosis and management of the endemic mycoses: an initiative of the European Confederation of Medical Mycology in cooperation with the International Society for Human and Animal Mycology. *Lancet Infect Dis*. 2021;21(12):e364-e374

The itraconazole oral solution formulation is preferred over the capsule formulation because of improved absorption and should be taken on an empty stomach. However, a super bioavailable (SUBA) itraconazole is now approved by the Food and Drug Administration for the treatment of pulmonary and extrapulmonary blastomycosis in individuals 18 years or older, with pharmacokinetic studies of this formulation demonstrating less variable absorption than conventional itraconazole capsules and a similar side effect profile; data in children are lacking. Saturated solution of potassium iodide (1 drop taken orally, 3 times daily, increasing as tolerated to a maximum of 1 drop/kg of body weight or 40 to 50 drops, 3 times daily, whichever is lowest) is an alternative therapy for nonsevere forms.

Amphotericin B, preferably as a lipid formulation, is recommended as initial therapy for visceral or disseminated sporotrichosis in children (see Recommended Doses of Parenteral and Oral Antifungal Drugs, p 1026). After clinical response to amphotericin B therapy is documented, itraconazole can be substituted and should be continued for at least 12 months. Itraconazole may be required for lifelong therapy in children with human immunodeficiency virus infection. Pulmonary and disseminated infections respond less well than cutaneous infection, despite prolonged therapy.

Local hyperthermia can be effective in treating cutaneous lesions, as *S schenckii* growth is impaired when temperatures exceed 42°C. Hyperthermia may be considered especially when patients cannot take recommended drugs safely (eg, pregnancy) but may not be well-tolerated by young children.

INFECTION PREVENTION AND CONTROL MEASURES IN HEALTH CARE SETTINGS: Standard precautions are indicated.

CONTROL MEASURES: Use of protective gloves and clothing for occupational and recreational activities that could lead to exposure to *S schenckii* can decrease risk of disease. Interaction with stray cats should be minimized in areas where *S brasiliensis* is endemic or hyperendemic; gloves, clothing, and face shields should be used in these locales if handling a cat with suspected sporotrichosis.

Staphylococcal Food Poisoning

CLINICAL MANIFESTATIONS: Staphylococcal foodborne illness is characterized by abrupt and sometimes violent onset of severe nausea, abdominal cramps, vomiting, and prostration, often accompanied by diarrhea. Low-grade fever or mild hypothermia can occur. The illness typically lasts no longer than 1 day, but symptoms are intense and can require hospitalization. The short incubation period, brevity of illness, and usual lack of fever help distinguish staphylococcal from other infectious causes of food poisoning, with the exception of the vomiting syndrome caused by *Bacillus cereus*. *Clostridium perfringens* food poisoning usually has a longer incubation period, and chemical food poisoning usually has a shorter incubation period. Patients with foodborne *Salmonella*, *Campylobacter*, or *Shigella* infection are more likely to have fever and a longer incubation period (see Appendix VI: Clinical Syndromes Associated With Foodborne Diseases, p 1150).

ETIOLOGY: Enterotoxins produced by strains of *Staphylococcus aureus* and, rarely, *Staphylococcus epidermidis* and *Staphylococcus intermedius* cause the symptoms of staphylococcal food poisoning. More than 20 such enterotoxins have been identified. These are stable in the face of many environmental conditions (freezing, drying, heat treatment, low pH) and resistant to intestinal tract proteolysis. The degree and type of symptoms may vary by toxin type and dose.

EPIDEMIOLOGY: Illness is caused by ingestion of food containing staphylococcal enterotoxins. The most commonly implicated foods are meats, most often pork (including sliced ham) and poultry served after inadequate heating. Food handlers may contaminate foods with enterotoxigenic strains of *S aureus*. When contaminated food remains at room temperature for several hours, the staphylococcal organisms multiply and produce toxins that are heat-stable (ie, not inactivated by reheating). The number of reported outbreaks caused by *S aureus* decreased in the 2000s. Possible reasons include less contamination of raw meat, improved food handling practices, and fewer investigations because of resource constraints.

The **incubation period** is typically 2 to 4 hours (range 30 minutes to 8 hours) after ingestion.

DIAGNOSTIC TESTS: In most cases, given the short duration of illness and rapid recovery with supportive care, diagnostic testing to confirm the diagnosis is not necessary. However, tests for enterotoxin are commercially available. In an outbreak, recovery of large numbers of staphylococci ($\geq 10^5$ *S aureus* organisms/g) from stool or vomitus or detection of enterotoxin in an implicated food can confirm the diagnosis, as can identification of the same subtype of *S aureus* from the stool or vomitus of 2 or more ill people. Guidance for confirming outbreaks of staphylococcal food poisoning can be found online (**www.cdc.gov/foodsafety/outbreaks/investigating-outbreaks/confirming_diagnosis.html**). To aid in outbreak investigations, public health laboratories can determine whether strains are similar using molecular methods. Local public health authorities should be notified about possible outbreaks because they can often determine the source and institute control measures to prevent similar outbreaks.

TREATMENT: Treatment is supportive. Antimicrobial agents are not indicated.

INFECTION PREVENTION AND CONTROL MEASURES IN HEALTH CARE SETTINGS: Staphylococcal food poisoning is not spread from person to person. Standard precautions are recommended.

CONTROL MEASURES: Strict hand hygiene should be enforced for all food handlers. People with boils, abscesses, or other purulent lesions that could be from staphylococcal skin infection should be especially careful to wash hands thoroughly and use gloves or other protective equipment while handling food. Prepared foods should be refrigerated in wide, shallow containers within 2 hours after cooking (within 1 hour if the ambient temperature is higher than 90°F). Information on good food handling practices, including time and temperature recommendations for cooking, storage, and reheating, is available online (**www.foodsafety.gov**).

Staphylococcus aureus

CLINICAL MANIFESTATIONS: *Staphylococcus aureus* causes a variety of localized and invasive suppurative infections and 3 toxin-mediated syndromes: toxic shock syndrome, scalded skin syndrome, and food poisoning (discussed in Staphylococcal Food Poisoning, p 766). Localized infections include cellulitis, skin and soft tissue abscesses, furuncles, carbuncles, pustulosis, impetigo (bullous and nonbullous), paronychia, mastitis, omphalitis, hordeola, orbital cellulitis/abscess, sinusitis, peritonsillar abscesses (Quinsy), parotitis, lymphadenitis, and wound infections. Bacteremia can be associated with focal complications including osteomyelitis; septic arthritis; endocarditis; pneumonia; pleural empyema; septic pulmonary emboli; pericarditis; soft tissue, muscle, or visceral abscesses; and septic thrombophlebitis of small and large vessels. In patients with neutropenia, ecthyma gangrenosum may occur. Primary *S aureus* pneumonia also can occur after aspiration of organisms from the upper respiratory tract and can occur in the context of concurrent or antecedent viral infections from the community (eg, influenza) or in ventilated patients. Meningitis may occur in preterm infants but otherwise is rare unless accompanied by a foreign body (eg, ventriculoperitoneal shunt) or a congenital or acquired defect in the dura. *S aureus* causes a variety of infections with and without bacteremia associated with foreign bodies, including intravascular catheters or grafts, peritoneal catheters, spinal instrumentation or intramedullary rods, pressure equalization tubes, pacemakers and other intracardiac devices, vagal nerve stimulators, and prosthetic joints. *S aureus* infections can be fulminant. Certain chronic diseases, conditions, and events, such as diabetes mellitus, malignancy, prematurity, immunodeficiency, kidney disease, nutritional disorders, dialysis, surgery, and transplantation, increase the risk for severe *S aureus* infections. Metastatic foci and abscesses need to be drained and foreign bodies should be removed when possible. Prolonged antimicrobial therapy for invasive infection often is necessary to achieve cure.

Staphylococcal toxic shock syndrome (TSS), a toxin-mediated disease, usually is caused by strains producing TSS toxin-1 or possibly other related staphylococcal enterotoxins. Characterized by acute onset of fever, generalized erythroderma, rapid-onset hypotension, and signs of multisystem organ involvement, including profuse watery diarrhea, vomiting, conjunctival injection, and severe myalgia (see Table 3.58 for clinical case definition). TSS can occur in menstruating persons using tampons or following childbirth or abortion. TSS also can occur after surgical procedures, in association with cutaneous lesions, or without a readily identifiable focus of infection, and blood cultures are often negative. People with TSS, especially menses-associated illness, are at risk of a recurrent episode.

Prevailing strains (eg, USA300) of methicillin-resistant *S aureus* (MRSA) rarely produce TSS toxin but readily produce other extracellular toxins (eg, leukocidins and enterotoxins) that may lead to clinical presentations that resemble, but do not meet clinical criteria for, TSS. These clinical phenotypes are often referred to as toxin-mediated disease.

Staphylococcal scalded skin syndrome (SSSS) is a toxin-mediated disease caused by circulation of exfoliative toxins A and B. The manifestations of SSSS are age related and include Ritter disease (generalized exfoliation) in the neonate, a tender scarlatiniform eruption and localized bullous impetigo in older children, or a combination of these with thick white/brown flaky desquamation of the entire skin, especially on the face and neck, in older infants and toddlers. The hallmark of SSSS is the toxin-mediated cleavage of the stratum granulosum layer of the epidermis (ie, Nikolsky sign). Proper pain management is a mainstay of therapy for SSSS. Healing occurs without scarring. Bacteremia is rare, but dehydration and superinfection can occur with extensive exfoliation.

ETIOLOGY: Staphylococci are catalase-positive, gram-positive cocci that appear microscopically as grape-like clusters. Staphylococci are ubiquitous and can survive extreme

Table 3.58. *Staphylococcus aureus* Toxic Shock Syndrome: Clinical Case Definition[a]

Clinical Findings
- Fever: temperature 38.9°C (102.0°F) or greater
- Rash: diffuse macular erythroderma
- Desquamation: 1–2 weeks after onset of rash, particularly on palms, soles, fingers, and toes
- Hypotension: systolic pressure 90 mm Hg or less for adults; lower than fifth percentile for age for children younger than 16 years
- Multisystem organ involvement: 3 or more of the following:
  1. Gastrointestinal tract: vomiting or diarrhea at onset of illness
  2. Muscular: severe myalgia or creatinine phosphokinase concentration greater than twice the upper limit of normal
  3. Mucous membrane: vaginal, oropharyngeal, or conjunctival hyperemia
  4. Renal: serum urea nitrogen or serum creatinine concentration greater than twice the upper limit of normal or urinary sediment with 5 white blood cells/high-power field or greater in the absence of urinary tract infection
  5. Hepatic: total bilirubin, aspartate aminotransferase, or alanine aminotransferase concentration greater than twice the upper limit of normal
  6. Hematologic: platelet count 100 000/mm^3 or less
  7. Central nervous system: disorientation or alterations in consciousness without focal neurologic signs when fever and hypotension are absent

Laboratory Criteria
- *Negative* results on the following tests, if obtained:
  1. Blood or cerebrospinal fluid cultures; blood culture rarely may be positive for *S aureus*
  2. Serologic tests for Rocky Mountain spotted fever, leptospirosis, or measles

Case Classification
- ***Probable:*** a case that meets the laboratory criteria and in which 4 of 5 clinical findings are present
- ***Confirmed:*** a case that meets laboratory criteria and all 5 of the clinical findings, including desquamation, unless the patient dies before desquamation occurs.

[a]Adapted from **https://ndc.services.cdc.gov/case-definitions/toxic-shock-syndrome-2011/.**

conditions of drying, heat, and low-oxygen and high-salt environments. *S aureus* has many surface proteins, including the microbial surface components recognizing adhesive matrix molecule (MSCRAMM) receptors, which allow the organism to bind to tissues and foreign bodies coated with fibronectin, fibrinogen, and collagen. This permits a low inoculum of organisms to adhere to sutures, catheters, prosthetic valves, and other devices. They also secrete a robust arsenal of extracellular proteins aimed at nutrient acquisition, host cell destruction, and immune evasion.

EPIDEMIOLOGY: *S aureus* is the most common cause of skin and soft tissue infections and musculoskeletal infections in otherwise healthy children. *S aureus* colonizes the skin and mucous membranes of 30% to 50% of healthy adults and children. The anterior nares, throat, axilla, perineum, vagina, and rectum are usual sites of colonization. *S aureus* is one of the most common causes of health care-associated bacteremia in all age groups and health care-associated pneumonia in children and is the most common pathogen responsible for surgical site infections. Patients with neutrophil dysfunction, such as those with chronic granulomatous disease (CGD), are at increased risk for *S aureus* infections.

S aureus-mediated TSS was first recognized in 1978 by Dr. Jim Todd, and many early cases were associated with tampon use. Although changes in tampon composition and use have resulted in a decreased proportion of cases associated with menses, menstrual and nonmenstrual cases of TSS continue to occur and are reported with similar frequency. Risk factors for TSS include absence of antibody to TSS toxin-1 and focal *S aureus* infection with a TSS toxin-1–producing strain. TSS toxin-1–producing strains can be part of normal flora of the anterior nares or vagina, and colonization at these sites is believed to result in protective antibody in more than 90% of adults.

Transmission of S aureus. Rates of skin carriage of more than 50% occur in children with desquamating skin disorders or burns and in people with frequent needle use (eg, people who have diabetes mellitus, are on hemodialysis, inject drugs, or receive allergy shots). Although domestic animals can be colonized, data suggest that colonization is acquired from other humans. Hospitalized children who are colonized with MRSA on admission or acquire MRSA colonization in the hospital are at increased risk for subsequent MRSA infection compared with noncolonized children.

S aureus is transmitted most often by direct contact in community settings and indirectly from patient to patient via transiently colonized hands of health care professionals in health care settings. Health care professionals and family members who are colonized with *S aureus* in the nares or on skin also can serve as a reservoir for transmission. Contaminated environmental surfaces and objects also can play a role in transmission of *S aureus*. Although not transmitted by the droplet route routinely, *S aureus* can be dispersed into the air over short distances. Dissemination of *S aureus* from people with nasal carriage, including infants, is related to density of colonization, and increased dissemination occurs during viral upper respiratory tract infections. Parental *S aureus* colonization at a variety of body sites has been associated with neonatal colonization.

Health Care-Associated MRSA. MRSA has been endemic in most US hospitals since the 1980s. Risk factors for health care-associated MRSA infections include hospitalization, surgery, dialysis, long-term care stay within the previous year, presence of an indwelling device, presence of wounds, and history of prior MRSA infection or colonization. The incidence of invasive health care-associated MRSA infections has decreased in many communities since the mid-2000s.

Health care-associated MRSA strains (ie, those that historically were responsible for most health care-associated MRSA infections) have often been resistant to more antibiotic classes (including clindamycin) than community-associated strains.

Community-Associated MRSA. Community-associated MRSA infections attributable to strains different from traditional health care-associated MRSA emerged in the 1990s. These strains most commonly cause skin and soft tissue abscesses, although they can also cause more severe infections. Clinical infections are more common in settings where there is crowding; frequent skin-to-skin contact; sharing of personal items, such as towels and clothing; poor personal hygiene; and among those with nonintact skin, including body piercings. Outbreaks have been reported among athletic teams, in correctional facilities, and in military training facilities. Community-associated MRSA strains can also circulate in hospitals and cause health care-associated MRSA infections. Community-associated MRSA strains have tended to be susceptible to a variety of non–beta-lactam antibiotics.

Vancomycin-Intermediately Susceptible S aureus. Vancomycin-intermediately susceptible *S aureus* (VISA) strains (minimum inhibitory concentration [MIC], 4–8 µg/mL) have been isolated from people (historically, dialysis patients) who have received multiple courses of vancomycin. Strains of MRSA can be heterogeneous for vancomycin resistance (see Diagnostic Tests). Extensive vancomycin use allows VISA strains to develop during therapy. Control measures recommended by the Centers for Disease Control and Prevention (CDC) have included using proper methods to detect VISA, using appropriate infection-control measures, and adopting measures to ensure appropriate vancomycin use.

Vancomycin-Resistant S aureus. Vancomycin-resistant *S aureus* (VRSA) infections (MIC >8 µg/mL) are very rare, and in all confirmed cases, reported patients had underlying medical conditions, a history of MRSA infections, and prolonged exposure to vancomycin.

The **incubation period** is variable for staphylococcal disease. A long delay can occur between acquisition of the organism and onset of disease. For SSSS, the **incubation period** usually is 1 to 10 days; for postoperative TSS, the **incubation period** can be as short as 12 hours. Menses-related cases can develop at any time during menstruation.

DIAGNOSTIC TESTS: Gram stains of specimens from skin lesions or pyogenic foci showing gram-positive cocci in clusters can provide presumptive evidence of staphylococcal infection. Isolation of organisms from culture of otherwise sterile body fluid is the method for definitive diagnosis. *S aureus* is almost never a contaminant when isolated from a blood culture or other sterile site.

Molecular assays have been approved by the US Food and Drug Administration for detection of *S aureus* from blood cultures growing gram-positive organisms. These assays include nonamplified molecular assays, such as peptide nucleic acid fluorescent in situ hybridization (PNA-FISH) and Verigene, as well as nucleic acid amplification tests, such as BD GenOhm Staph SR, Xpert MRSA/SA BC, the FilmArray Blood Culture Identification Panel (BCID), and the polymerase chain reaction (PCR)-T2 magnetic resonance sepsis panel. Matrix-assisted laser desorption/ionization–time-of-flight (MALDI-TOF) mass spectrometry can rapidly identify *S aureus* colonies on culture plates or from growth in blood cultures.

S aureus-mediated TSS is a clinical diagnosis (Table 3.58); *S aureus* is isolated from blood cultures in fewer than 5% of patients with TSS. Specimens for culture should be obtained from an identified focus of infection, because these sites usually will yield the organism. Because approximately one third of isolates of *S aureus* from nonmenstrual cases produce toxins other than TSS toxin-1, and TSS toxin-1–producing organisms can be present as normal flora, TSS toxin-1 production by an isolate is not a useful diagnostic test.

Antimicrobial susceptibility testing should be performed for all *S aureus* specimens isolated from normally sterile sites. Laboratory practice includes routine screening (D-testing) to exclude inducible clindamycin resistance. Another phenomenon that has been described is heteroresistance to antibiotics, in which the heterogeneous or heterotypic strains appear susceptible by disk diffusion but contain resistant subpopulations that are only apparent when cultured with antibiotic-containing media. When these resistant subpopulations are cultured on antibiotic-free media, they can continue as stable resistant mutants or revert to susceptible strains (heterogeneous resistance). Bacteria expressing heteroresistance grow more slowly than the susceptible bacteria and can be missed at growth conditions greater than 35°C (95°F). The clinical significance of heteroresistance is not clear, but some have suggested that it could be a cause of some vancomycin treatment failures.

S aureus strain genotyping, in conjunction with epidemiologic information, can facilitate identification of the source, extent, and mechanism of transmission in an outbreak. Several molecular typing methods are available for *S aureus*, including pulsed-field gel electrophoresis, spa typing, multilocus sequence typing, and whole genome sequencing. Choice of method should consider purpose of typing and available resources.

TREATMENT:

Skin and Soft Tissue Infection. Skin and soft tissue infections, such as diffuse impetigo or cellulitis attributable to methicillin-susceptible *S aureus* (MSSA), optimally are treated with oral penicillinase-resistant beta-lactam drugs, such as a first- or second-generation cephalosporin. For the patient with penicillin allergy and in cases in which MRSA is considered, trimethoprim-sulfamethoxazole, doxycycline, or clindamycin can be used if the isolate is susceptible. Topical mupirocin is recommended for localized impetigo.

The most frequent manifestation of community-associated MRSA infection is skin and soft tissue infection, which can range from mild to severe. Drainage is an important component of managing these infections. A randomized placebo-controlled study evaluating treatment strategies for uncomplicated skin infections included children with simple abscesses ≤3 cm (6–11 months of age), ≤4 cm (1–8 years of age), or ≤5 cm (>8 years of age) in diameter and found that drainage plus systemic oral therapy with either clindamycin or trimethoprim-sulfamethoxazole was associated with better outcomes compared with drainage alone.

Invasive Staphylococcal Infections. Empiric therapy for suspected invasive or severe staphylococcal infection, including pneumonia, osteoarticular infection, visceral abscesses, and foreign body-associated infection with bacteremia, is vancomycin plus an antistaphylococcal beta lactam (eg, nafcillin, oxacillin, cefazolin). For children with mild to moderate illness for suspected osteomyelitis attributable to *S aureus*, empiric therapy may be informed by local susceptibility of *S aureus* isolates. When rates of community-associated MRSA are low (<10%), oxacillin, nafcillin, or cefazolin may be initiated; when rates of resistance are higher, empiric therapy should include clindamycin or vancomycin. Subsequent therapy should be based on antimicrobial susceptibility results.

Serious MSSA infections require intravenous therapy with an antistaphylococcal beta-lactam antimicrobial agent, such as nafcillin, oxacillin, or cefazolin, because most *S aureus* strains produce beta-lactamase enzymes and are resistant to penicillin and ampicillin (see Table 3.59). The addition of rifampin may be considered for those with invasive disease associated with an indwelling foreign body, especially if removal of the infected implant or device is not feasible. **Vancomycin is not recommended for treatment of serious MSSA infections (including endocarditis), because outcomes are inferior with vancomycin compared with antistaphylococcal beta lactams.** First- or second-generation cephalosporins (eg, cefazolin) or vancomycin are less effective than nafcillin or oxacillin for treatment of MSSA meningitis.

Table 3.59. Parenteral Antimicrobial Agent(s) for Treatment of Bacteremia and Other Serious *Staphylococcus aureus* Infections

Antimicrobial Agents	Comments
I. Initial empiric therapy (organism of unknown susceptibility)	
Drugs of choice: Vancomycin (15 mg/kg, every 6 h) + nafcillin or oxacillin[a,b]	For life-threatening infections (eg, septicemia, pneumonia, endocarditis, CNS infection); ceftaroline or linezolid are alternatives to vancomycin, but there are limited efficacy data in children
Vancomycin (15 mg/kg, every 6–8 h)[b]	For non–life-threatening infection without signs of sepsis (eg, skin infection, cellulitis, osteomyelitis, septic arthritis) when rates of MRSA colonization and infection in the community are substantial; ceftaroline[e] or linezolid[e] or daptomycin[d] (if no pneumonia) are alternatives
Clindamycin	For non–life-threatening infection without signs of sepsis when rates of MRSA colonization and infection in the community are substantial and prevalence of clindamycin resistance is <15%
II. Methicillin-susceptible *S aureus* (MSSA)	
Drugs of choice: Nafcillin or oxacillin[e]	
Cefazolin	Preferred for meningitis (cefazolin does not penetrate well into central nervous system)
Alternatives: Clindamycin	Only for patients with a serious penicillin allergy and clindamycin-susceptible strain (not for endovascular infections or meningitis)
Vancomycin[a,b,e]	Only for patients with a serious penicillin and cephalosporin allergy infected with a clindamycin-resistant strain (or if there is a serious beta-lactam allergy and endovascular infection or meningitis)
Ampicillin + sulbactam	For patients with polymicrobial infections caused by susceptible isolates

Table 3.59. Parenteral Antimicrobial Agent(s) for Treatment of Bacteremia and Other Serious *Staphylococcus aureus* Infections, continued

Antimicrobial Agents	Comments
III. Methicillin-resistant *S aureus* (MRSA; oxacillin MIC ≥4 µg/mL)	
Drugs of choice: Vancomycin[a,b,e]	For life-threatening infections, including meningitis or endovascular infections including those complicated by venous thrombosis
Clindamycin (if strain susceptible)	For pneumonia,[a] septic arthritis, osteomyelitis, skin or soft tissue infections (not for endovascular infections or meningitis)
Trimethoprim-sulfamethoxazole	For skin or soft tissue infections
Alternative (check susceptibility prior to use): Linezolid[e]	For serious infections caused by clindamycin resistant isolates in patients with renal dysfunction or those intolerant of vancomycin
Ceftaroline[e]	For skin infections, pneumonia, alternative for severe infections
Daptomycin[d]	Bloodstream infections, skin and soft tissue infections, infections other than pneumonia
Dalbavancin[e]	For skin or soft tissue infections
Tedizolid[e]	For skin or soft tissue infections for patients 12 years and over

Table 3.59. Parenteral Antimicrobial Agent(s) for Treatment of Bacteremia and Other Serious *Staphylococcus aureus* Infections, continued

Antimicrobial Agents		Comments
IV. Vancomycin-intermediately susceptible *S aureus* (VISA; MIC 4 to 16 µg/mL)		
Drugs of choice:	Optimal therapy is not known[c]	Consult with an expert in infectious disease; therapy dependent on in vitro susceptibility test results
	Linezolid[c]	
	Ceftaroline[c]	
	Daptomycin[d]	
	Quinupristin-dalfopristin[c]	
	Tigecycline[c]	
Alternatives:	Vancomycin[b] + linezolid ± gentamicin	
	Vancomycin[b] + trimethoprim-sulfamethoxazole	

CNS indicates central nervous system; MIC, minimum inhibitory concentration.

[a] For suspected MRSA pneumonia complicating influenza in critically ill children, add clindamycin, ceftaroline, or linezolid to vancomycin empiric treatment. Empiric selection of antibiotics is highly dependent on the local/regional susceptibility data.

[b] The area-under-the-curve to minimum inhibitory concentration (AUC/MIC) has been identified as the most appropriate pharmacokinetic/pharmacodynamic (PK/PD) target for vancomycin in adult patients with MRSA. Although there are limitations in prospective outcomes data in pediatric patients with serious MRSA infections, the most recent consensus guideline from the American Society of Health-System Pharmacists, the Infectious Diseases Society of America, the Pediatric Infectious Diseases Society, and the Society of Infectious Diseases Pharmacists recommend AUC guided therapeutic monitoring, preferably with Bayesian estimation, for all pediatric age groups receiving vancomycin.[f,g,h] This estimation accounts for developmental changes of vancomycin clearance from newborn to adolescent. Dosing in children should be designed to achieve an AUC of 400 to 600 µg-hour/L (assuming MIC of 1) and/or trough levels <15 µg/mL to minimize acute kidney injury risks. Bayesian estimation can be completed with 2 levels, with 1 level being recommended 1 to 2 hours after end of vancomycin infusion, and the second level being drawn 4 to 6 hours after end of infusion. Levels can be obtained as early as after the second dose. Software to assist with these calculations is available online and for purchase. It is recommended to avoid AUC >800 µg-hour/L and trough levels >15 µg/mL. Most children younger than 12 years will require higher doses to achieve optimal AUC/MIC compared with older children. Consultation with an infectious diseases specialist should be considered to determine which agent to use and duration of use.

Table 3.59. Parenteral Antimicrobial Agent(s) for Treatment of Bacteremia and Other Serious *Staphylococcus aureus* Infections, continued

Antimicrobial Agents	Comments

[c] Linezolid, ceftaroline, dalbavancin, tedizolid, quinupristin-dalfopristin, and tigecycline are agents with activity in vitro and efficacy in adults with multidrug-resistant, gram-positive organisms, including *S aureus*. Because experience with these agents in children is limited, consultation with a specialist in infectious diseases should be considered before use. Further, tigecycline should not be used in children younger than 8 years if there are effective alternatives, because there may be reversible inhibition of bone growth and adverse effects on tooth development. Tigecycline also has a black box warning for an increase in all-cause mortality and should be reserved for situations where alternative agents are not suitable. Tedizolid has not been adequately evaluated in patients with severe neutropenia (neutrophil counts <1000 cells/mm^3).

[d] Daptomycin is active in vitro against multidrug-resistant, gram-positive organisms, including *S aureus*. Daptomycin is approved by the US Food and Drug Administration only for treatment of complicated skin and skin structure infections and for *S aureus* bloodstream infections for patients 1 year and older. Daptomycin is ineffective for treatment of pneumonia. Because experience with these agents in children is limited, consultation with a specialist in infectious diseases should be considered before use.

[e] Gentamicin and rifampin for the first 2 weeks should be added for endocarditis of a prosthetic device. Addition of rifampin is recommended for other device-related infections (spinal instrumentation, prosthetic joint).

[f] Rybak MJ, Le J, Lodise TP, et al. Therapeutic monitoring of vancomycin for serious methicillin-resistant *Staphylococcus aureus* infections: a revised consensus guideline and review by the American Society of Health-System Pharmacists, the Infectious Diseases Society of America, the Pediatric Infectious Diseases Society, and the Society of Infectious Diseases Pharmacists. *Am J Health Syst Pharm.* 2020;77(11):835–864

[g] Rybak MJ, Le J, Lodise TP, et al. Executive summary: Therapeutic monitoring of vancomycin for serious methicillin-resistant *Staphylococcus aureus* infections: a revised consensus guideline and review by the American Society of Health-System Pharmacists, the Infectious Diseases Society of America, the Pediatric Infectious Diseases Society, and the Society of Infectious Diseases Pharmacists. *J Pediatr Infect Dis Soc.* 2020;9(3):281–284

[h] Heil EL, Claeys KC, Mynatt RP, et al. Making the change to area under the curve–based vancomycin dosing. *Am J Health Syst Pharm.* 2018;75(24):1986–1995

Observational data suggest that clindamycin should not be used as the only treatment of persistent bacteremia or endovascular infection.

Guidelines for management of serious skin/soft tissue infection, complicated pneumonia/empyema, central nervous system (CNS) infection, osteomyelitis, and endocarditis caused by MRSA are available.[1] For MRSA pneumonia complicating influenza in children, vancomycin monotherapy in the first 24 hours of treatment was associated with higher mortality compared with vancomycin combined with a second antibiotic (clindamycin, linezolid, or ceftaroline) in a retrospective, multicenter study. Thus, a combination of vancomycin plus one of these agents is recommended for empiric treatment of children with life-threatening pneumonia complicating influenza. Antibiotic therapy can be de-escalated to a single agent if there is clinical improvement and antibiotic susceptibility information to guide treatment.

VISA infection is rare in children. If there is concern for inadequate clinical response or reduced susceptibility to vancomycin, consultation with an infectious disease specialist is recommended. Data on the optimal treatment for VISA infection are limited.

Duration of therapy for serious MSSA or MRSA infections depends on the site and severity of infection but usually is 4 weeks or more for endocarditis, necrotizing pneumonia, or disseminated infection, assuming a documented clinical and microbiologic response. For children with uncomplicated staphylococcal osteoarticular infection, particularly those attributable to MSSA, a 3- to 4-week course of therapy may be adequate.[2,3] For uncomplicated bacteremia, 14 days of therapy is recommended. Overall, in assessing whether modification of therapy is necessary, clinicians should consider whether the patient is improving clinically, should identify and drain sequestered foci of infection and remove foreign material (such as a central catheter) when possible, and for MRSA strains, should consider consultation with an infectious diseases specialist or infection control expert.

Completion of the treatment course with an oral drug can be considered in non-neonates if an endovascular infection (ie, endocarditis or infected thrombus) or CNS infection is not a concern. For endovascular and CNS infections, parenteral therapy is recommended for the entire treatment course. Drainage of large abscesses, often more than once, and removal of foreign bodies are almost always required in addition to medical therapy. In some cases, multiple débridement procedures are necessary for children with complicated *S aureus* osteoarticular infection.

Duration of therapy for *S aureus* central line-associated bloodstream infections is controversial and depends on several factors—the type and location of the catheter, the site of infection (exit site vs tunnel vs line), the feasibility of using an alternative vascular access site at a later date, the presence or absence of a catheter-related

---

[1] Liu C, Bayer A, Cosgrove SE, et al. Clinical practice guidelines by the Infectious Diseases Society of America for the treatment of methicillin-resistant *Staphylococcus aureus* infections in adults and children. *Clin Infect Dis.* 2011;52(3):e18–e55

[2] Woods CR, Bradley JS, Chatterjee A, et al. Clinical practice guideline by the Pediatric Infectious Diseases Society and the Infectious Diseases Society of America: 2021 Guideline on diagnosis and management of acute hematogenous osteomyelitis in pediatrics. *J Pediatr Infect Dis Soc.* 2021;10(8):801-844

[3] Woods CR, Bradley JS, Chatterjee A, et al. Clinical practice guideline by the Pediatric Infectious Diseases Society (PIDS) and the Infectious Diseases Society of America (IDSA): 2023 Guideline on diagnosis and management of acute bacterial arthritis in pediatrics. *J Pediatr Infect Dis Soc.* 2023;Nov 6:piad089

thrombus, and host immunity. Infections are more difficult to treat when associated with a thrombus, thrombophlebitis, or intra-atrial thrombus, and a longer course is suggested if the patient is immunocompromised. Expert opinion differs on recommended treatment duration, but many suggest a minimum of 14 days provided there is no evidence of a metastatic focus, and the patient responds to antimicrobial therapy with rapid sterilization of the blood cultures. If the patient needs a new central line, waiting at least 48 to 72 hours after bacteremia has resolved before insertion, is optimal. If a tunneled catheter is needed for ongoing care, treatment of the infection without removal of the catheter can be attempted but may not always be successful. Vegetations or a thrombus in the heart or great vessels always should be considered when a central line becomes infected and should be suspected more strongly if blood cultures remain positive for more than 2 days on appropriate antimicrobial therapy following removal of the central line or if there are other clinical manifestations associated with endocarditis. Transesophageal echocardiography is the most sensitive technique for identifying vegetations, but transthoracic echocardiography generally is adequate for children younger than 10 years and/or weighing <60 kg.

Management of* S aureus *Toxin-Mediated Diseases. The principles of therapy for TSS include aggressive fluid management (and vasoactive agents, as needed) to maintain adequate venous return and cardiac filling to prevent end organ damage, source control that includes prompt identification and removal of any indwelling foreign body (eg, tampon) or drainable focus, and anticipation and management of the commonly observed multiorgan complications of TSS (eg, acute respiratory distress syndrome, renal dysfunction). Consultation with an expert in infectious diseases is recommended. Initial antimicrobial therapy should include a parentally administered antistaphylococcal beta-lactam antimicrobial agent and a protein synthesis-inhibiting drug, such as clindamycin, at maximum dosages. Vancomycin should be added to the beta-lactam agent in regions where MRSA infections are common, although MRSA-associated TSS is rare in the United States (see Table 3.59, p 773). For TSS with a clindamycin-resistant strain, linezolid may be used as the protein synthesis-inhibiting portion of the therapy. Empiric antibiotic therapy should be modified to targeted therapy once antibiotic susceptibilities are known. Active antimicrobial therapy should be continued for 10 to 14 days. Administration of antimicrobial agents can be changed to the oral route once the patient is tolerating oral alimentation. The total duration of therapy is based on the usual duration for established foci of infection (eg, pneumonia, osteomyelitis). Immune globulin intravenous (IGIV) can be considered in patients with severe staphylococcal TSS unresponsive to other therapeutic measures, because IGIV may neutralize circulating toxin. Although data on the use of IGIV are not robust, it may be considered for critically ill children with shock that is unresponsive to fluid resuscitation, with an undrainable focus of infection, or with persistent oliguria with pulmonary edema. The optimal IGIV regimen is unknown, but 150 to 400 mg/kg per day for 5 days or a single dose of 1 to 2 g/kg has been used. SSSS in infants should be treated with a parenteral antistaphylococcal beta-lactam antimicrobial agent or clindamycin, depending on local susceptibility patterns and the severity of the disease. If MRSA is a consideration, vancomycin or clindamycin (depending on local susceptibility patterns) can be used. Transition to an oral agent is appropriate in nonneonates who have demonstrated excellent clinical response to parenteral therapy.

INFECTION PREVENTION AND CONTROL MEASURES IN HEALTH CARE SETTINGS:
Contact precautions should be added to standard precautions for patients with
abscesses or draining wounds that cannot be covered, regardless of staphylococcal
strain (MSSA versus MRSA), and should be maintained until wound drainage ceases
or can be contained by a dressing. Infants and young children with staphylococcal
furunculosis and patients with SSSS should be placed on contact precautions for the
duration of their illness. Although there has been debate about the practice, the CDC
continues to recommend contact precautions for patients known to be infected or colonized with MRSA (**www.cdc.gov/hai/prevent/staph-prevention-strategies.
html**).

To prevent transmission of VRSA, the CDC has issued specific infection control
recommendations that should be followed (**www.cdc.gov/hai/pdfs/VRSA-
Investigation-Guide-05_12_2015.pdf**).

CONTROL MEASURES: Measures to prevent and control *S aureus* infections can be
considered separately for individual patients and for health care facilities.

Individual Patient. Community-associated *S aureus* infections in immunocompetent hosts
are difficult to prevent in the absence of clearly apparent risk factors or an outbreak,
because the organism is ubiquitous and there is no effective vaccine. Strategies focusing
on hand hygiene, environmental disinfection, and wound care have been effective at
limiting transmission of *S aureus* and preventing spread of infections in community settings. Specific strategies include appropriate wound care, minimizing skin trauma and
keeping abrasions and cuts covered, optimizing hand hygiene and personal hygiene
practices (eg, shower after activities involving skin-to-skin contact), avoiding sharing
of personal items (eg, towels, razors, clothing), cleaning shared equipment between
uses, and regular cleaning of frequently touched environmental surfaces. For patients
who experience recurrent *S aureus* infections or who are predisposed to *S aureus* infections because of disorders of neutrophil function, chronic skin conditions, or obesity,
a variety of techniques have been used to prevent infection, including scrupulous
attention to skin hygiene, dilute bleach baths, and the use of clothing and bed linens
that minimize sweating, but none have shown definitive effectiveness in preventing recurrent infections with community-associated MRSA. Household contacts of
people with *S aureus* infections generally do not need to be tested for colonization. For
patients with multiple recurrent staphylococcal infections, applying mupirocin to the
nares and bathing using chlorhexidine for 5 consecutive days for all family members
have been associated with decreased recurrences (**www.cdc.gov/drugresistance/
microbial-ecology/decolonization.html**).

Measures to prevent health care-associated *S aureus* infections in individual
patients include strict adherence to recommended infection control precautions and
appropriate intraoperative antimicrobial prophylaxis, and in some circumstances, use
of preoperative antimicrobial regimens to attempt to eradicate nasal carriage; use
of chlorhexidine in certain patients also can be considered. Guidelines for prevention of surgical site infections can be found at **www.cdc.gov/infectioncontrol/
guidelines/ssi/index.html.**

Child Care or School Settings. Children with *S aureus* colonization or infection should not
be excluded routinely from child care or school settings. Children with draining or open
abrasions or wounds should have these covered with a clean, dry dressing. Routine
hand hygiene should be emphasized for personnel and children in these facilities.

General Measures. Published recommendations of the CDC Healthcare Infection Control Practices Advisory Committee (HICPAC)[1] for prevention of health care-associated pneumonia should be effective for decreasing the incidence of *S aureus* pneumonia. CDC/HICPAC guidelines for preventing intravascular catheter-related infections include careful preparation of the skin before surgery, including cleansing of skin before placement of intravascular catheters using barrier methods (**www.cdc.gov/infectioncontrol/guidelines/bsi/updates.html**). Meticulous surgical technique with minimal trauma to tissues, maintenance of good oxygenation, and minimal hematoma and dead space formation will minimize risk of surgical site infection. Appropriate hand hygiene, including before and after use of gloves, by health care professionals and strict adherence to contact precautions are of paramount importance.

Intraoperative Antimicrobial Prophylaxis. Most clean surgical procedures do not require antimicrobial prophylaxis. However, antimicrobial prophylaxis is used in surgeries associated with significant rates of infection and in surgeries in which there are severe consequences of infection (eg, insertion of a major prosthetic device, such as a ventriculoperitoneal shunt or a heart valve), or for a known MRSA carrier undergoing a major surgical procedure (see Antimicrobial Prophylaxis in Pediatric Surgical Patients, p 1117). If antimicrobial prophylaxis is used, the agent, usually cefazolin, is administered 30 to 60 minutes before the operation (vancomycin should be administered over a longer period, approximately 60–120 minutes before skin incision, generally as a single dose), and prophylaxis may be stopped at the conclusion of the procedure in most cases. Administering a single preoperative dose of vancomycin in addition to cefazolin is reasonable for patients known to be colonized with MRSA for whom antibiotic prophylaxis is indicated.

Eradication of Nasal Carriage. The combination of preoperative chlorhexidine baths and intranasal mupirocin has been demonstrated to be beneficial in reducing deep surgical site infections in adult MRSA carriers, but data are limited in children. Use of intermittent or continuous intranasal mupirocin for eradication of nasal carriage also has been shown to decrease the incidence of invasive *S aureus* infections in adult patients undergoing long-term hemodialysis or ambulatory peritoneal dialysis. However, long-lasting eradication of nasal carriage of *S aureus* is difficult, and the practice has not been widely adopted for outpatient dialysis because mupirocin-resistant strains can emerge with repeated or widespread use. A controlled trial in high-risk neonates demonstrated that a regimen of 5 days of mupirocin (intranasal, periumbilical, and perianal) was well-tolerated and led to primary *S aureus* decolonization in 94% of active drug recipients (compared with <5% for placebo recipients); however, >50% of infants who remained hospitalized were recolonized after 2 to 3 weeks.[2] Intranasal mupirocin treatment is not recommended for routine use but is considered for those with recurrent skin abscesses or during institutional outbreaks of *S aureus* infection.

---

[1] Centers for Disease Control and Prevention. Guidelines for preventing health-care–associated pneumonia, 2003: recommendations of CDC and the Healthcare Infection Control Practices Advisory Committee. *MMWR Recomm Rep.* 2004;53(RR-3):1–36

[2] Kotloff KL, Shirley DAT, Creech CB, et al. Mupirocin for *Staphylococcus aureus* decolonization of infants in neonatal intensive care units. *Pediatrics.* 2019;143(1):e20181565

Institutions. Measures to control spread of *S aureus* within health care facilities involve use and careful monitoring of adherence to HICPAC guidelines.[1-3] The CDC also recommends strategies for controlling spread of MRSA (**www.cdc.gov/ drugresistance/index.html**). These strategies focus on administrative issues; engagement, education, and training of personnel; judicious use of antimicrobial agents; monitoring of prevalence trends over time; use of standard precautions for all patients; and use of contact precautions when appropriate. The CDC has also published a collection of strategies to prevent hospital-onset *S aureus* bloodstream infections (**www.cdc.gov/hai/prevent/staph-prevention-strategies.html**), which focuses on prevention of device and procedure-associated infections, source control strategies for high-risk patients during high-risk periods, interventions to prevent transmission of MRSA in acute care hospitals, and infrastructure needed for prevention. In addition to those contained in HICPAC guidelines for specific device or procedure associated infections, strategies also include intranasal antistaphylococcal antibiotic/ antiseptic in conjunction with chlorhexidine wash or wipes before high-risk surgery (eg, cardiothoracic, orthopedic, neurologic, especially those with implantable devices). To reduce the risk of central line-associated bloodstream infections, daily chlorhexidine bathing is recommended for intensive care patients who are at least 2 months of age. Some centers use chlorhexidine wash for younger patients being cared for in the pediatric intensive care unit (the package insert recommends using with care in infants younger than 2 months and preterm infants because of concerns about burns). When rates of endemicity are not decreasing despite adherence to these measures, additional interventions, such as use of active surveillance cultures to identify colonized patients and to place them in contact precautions, may be warranted. Decolonization of a health care professional can be considered if the health care professional has been found to be a carrier of *S aureus* and has been epidemiologically linked as a likely source of ongoing transmission to patients. In this situation, attempts to eradicate carriage with topical nasal mupirocin therapy often are made. Both low-level (MIC 8–256 µg/mL) and high-level (MIC ≥512 µg/mL) resistance to mupirocin have been identified in *S aureus*, with high-level resistance associated with failure of decolonization.

Recommendations for investigation and control of VRSA have been published by the CDC (**www.cdc.gov/hai/pdfs/VRSA-Investigation-Guide-05_12_2015. pdf**). The CDC should be contacted for confirmatory testing if *S aureus* isolates with vancomycin MIC of ≥8 µg/mL are identified (generally, notification to the local or state health department should occur first; some initial testing can be performed at

[1] Walters M, Lonsway D, Rasheed K, et al. Investigation and Control of Vancomycin-Resistant *Staphylococcus aureus*: A Guide for Health Departments and Infection Control Personnel. Centers for Disease Control and Prevention; 2015. Available at: **www.cdc.gov/hai/pdfs/VRSA-Investigation-Guide-05_12_2015. pdf**

[2] Siegel JD, Rhinehart E, Jackson M, Chianello L; Healthcare Infection Control Practices Advisory Committee. 2007 Guideline for Isolation Precautions: Preventing Transmission of Infectious Agents in Healthcare Settings. Recommendations of the Healthcare Infection Control Practices Advisory Committee. Centers for Disease Control and Prevention; 2007. Available at: **www.cdc.gov/hicpac/2007IP/2007 isolationPrecautions.html**

[3] Siegel JD, Rhinehart E, Jackwson M, Chiarello L; Healthcare Infection Control Practices Advisory Committee. Management of multidrug-resistant organisms in healthcare settings, 2006. Centers for Disease Control and Prevention; 2006. Available at: **www.cdc.gov/infectioncontrol/guidelines/mdro/ index.html**

many public health laboratories). Ongoing review and restriction of vancomycin use is critical in attempts to control the emergence of VISA and VRSA (see Antimicrobial Resistance and Antimicrobial Stewardship: Appropriate and Judicious Use of Antimicrobial Agents, p 978). To date, the use of catheters impregnated with various antimicrobial agents or metals to prevent health care-associated infections has not been evaluated adequately in children.

Nurseries and Neonatal Intensive Care Units. Outbreaks of *S aureus* infections in newborn nurseries require unique measures of control. Hand hygiene should be emphasized to all personnel and visitors. Standard umbilical cord care currently does not include use of topical products (eg, triple dye). Measures recommended during outbreaks include reinforcement of hand hygiene, alleviating overcrowding and understaffing, surveillance of *S aureus* colonization of newborn infants at admission and periodically thereafter, use of contact precautions for colonized or infected infants, and cohorting of colonized or infected infants and their caregivers. During an outbreak, decolonization measures for infants can be considered. The optimal approach for decolonization of neonates is not yet clear, and some products, such as chlorhexidine, may be associated with risk of caustic cutaneous effects and systemic absorption. A randomized controlled trial of decolonization of high-risk neonates using a mupirocin regimen was well tolerated and was associated with short-term decolonization, although recolonization occurred after 2 to 3 weeks in many neonates who were still hospitalized (see Eradication of Nasal Carriage, p 780). Decolonization of colonized health care professionals who are epidemiologically implicated in *S aureus* transmission can be attempted but may not be successful. The CDC has issued guidance on the prevention and control of *S aureus* infections in neonatal intensive care units (**www.cdc.gov/ infectioncontrol/guidelines/NICU-saureus/),** and the Society for Healthcare Epidemiology of America has issued a white paper on this subject (**https://doi. org/10.1017/ice.2022.53).**

Coagulase-Negative Staphylococcal Infections

CLINICAL MANIFESTATIONS: Coagulase-negative staphylococci (CoNS) are part of normal skin flora and isolates from patient specimens often result from contamination of culture material from skin sites (see Diagnostic Tests). Differentiation between colonization and true infection may be difficult. Of the isolates that do not represent contamination, most come from infections associated with medical devices used in health care, or in patients with obvious disruptions of host defenses caused by surgery, immunosuppression, or prematurity (eg, very low birth weight infants). CoNS cause about 30% of health care-associated bloodstream infections. These organisms are a common cause of late-onset bacteremia and septicemia among preterm infants, typically infants weighing less than 1500 g at birth, and of episodes of health care-associated bacteremia in all age groups. CoNS cause bacteremia in children with intravascular catheters, vascular grafts, intracardiac patches, prosthetic cardiac valves, or pacemaker wires. Infection may also be associated with other indwelling foreign bodies, including cerebrospinal fluid shunts, peritoneal catheters, spinal instrumentation, baclofen pumps, pacemakers, left ventricular assist devices, or prosthetic joints. Mediastinitis after open-heart surgery, endophthalmitis after intraocular trauma, and omphalitis and scalp abscesses in preterm neonates have occurred. CoNS also can enter the bloodstream from the respiratory tract of mechanically ventilated preterm infants or from the gastrointestinal tract of infants with necrotizing enterocolitis. Some species of CoNS are associated with urinary tract infection, including *Staphylococcus saprophyticus* in adolescent and young adult females, often after sexual intercourse, and *Staphylococcus epidermidis* and *Staphylococcus haemolyticus* in hospitalized patients with urinary catheters. *Staphylococcus lugdunensis* is particularly virulent, resulting in infections resembling those caused by *Staphylococcus aureus,* including skin and soft tissue infection and bacteremia with or without endocarditis. *Staphylococcus schleiferi,* like *S lugdunensis,* is a virulent species and has caused pacemaker and osteoarticular infections.

ETIOLOGY: There are more than 50 recognized coagulase-negative *Staphylococcus* species. *Staphylococcus epidermidis, S haemolyticus, S saprophyticus, S schleiferi* (subspecies *schleiferi*), *S lugdunensis, Staphylococcus capitis, Staphylococcus hominis,* and *Staphylococcus simulans* are the CoNS species most frequently associated with human infections. *Staphylococcus saccharolyticus,* the only anaerobic CoNS, has been implicated in a variety of human infections. More recently identified species that have been implicated rarely in clinical disease include S*taphylococcus borealis, Staphylococcus massiliensis,* and *Staphylococcus petrasii* sp nov. Many CoNS produce an exopolysaccharide slime biofilm that enables these organisms to bind to medical devices (eg, catheters) and makes them relatively inaccessible to host defenses and antimicrobial agents.

EPIDEMIOLOGY: CoNS are ubiquitous inhabitants of the skin and mucous membranes. Virtually all neonates are colonized with CoNS at multiple sites by 2 to 4 days of age. The most frequently isolated CoNS organism is *S epidermidis,* which is found widely in most areas of skin. Different species colonize specific areas of the body. *S haemolyticus* is found on areas of skin with numerous apocrine glands, *S capitis* is often isolated from the scalp and forehead, and *S lugdunensis* has a predilection for colonization of the inguinal and groin areas. *S schleiferi* colonizes the mouth of carnivores, can be transferred from pets to owners, and has also been found as a colonizing organism in the preaxillary skin. Infants and children in intensive care units, including neonatal intensive care units, have the highest incidence of CoNS bloodstream infections. CoNS can be introduced at the time of medical device placement, through mucous membrane or skin breaks, through loss of bowel wall integrity (eg, necrotizing enterocolitis in very low birth weight neonates), or during catheter manipulation. Less often, health care professionals with environmental CoNS colonization on their hands transmit the organism.

The **incubation period** is variable for CoNS disease. A long delay can occur between acquisition of the organism and onset of disease.

DIAGNOSTICS TESTS: CoNS are readily isolated in culture using the same media and incubation conditions used for *S aureus.* Tests for coagulase by traditional methods or by latex agglutination are the same as used for *S aureus.* CoNS isolated from a single blood culture are commonly classified as skin contaminants, especially in the absence of risk factors for invasive disease. In this situation, full identification and antimicrobial susceptibility testing are generally not performed in most clinical laboratories. Fluorescent in situ hybridization (FISH) probes or multiplex polymerase chain reaction (PCR) panel assays can rapidly differentiate CoNS and *S aureus* isolated in blood cultures. In a very preterm neonate, an immunocompromised person, or a patient with an indwelling catheter or prosthetic device, repeated isolation of the same species of CoNS from blood cultures or another normally sterile body fluid suggests true infection. When a central line-associated bloodstream infection is present, blood cultures drawn from the catheter generally become positive 2 or more hours before cultures obtained from a peripheral venipuncture. This type of analysis requires that both a peripheral and catheter blood culture be performed at the same time using equal volumes of blood. Typing methods, such as pulsed-field gel electrophoresis or whole genome sequencing may be utilized to define clonality and identify the significance of isolates in outbreak settings or complex clinical scenarios.

Criteria that suggest CoNS as bloodstream pathogens, rather than contaminants, include the following:

- Two or more positive blood cultures with the same *Staphylococcus* species from different collection sites;
- A positive culture from blood and from another sterile site (eg, cerebrospinal fluid, joint) with the same *Staphylococcus* species and identical antimicrobial susceptibility patterns for each isolate;
- Growth in a continuously monitored blood culture system within 15 hours of incubation;
- Clinical findings of infection;
- Presence of an intravascular catheter that has been in place for 3 days or more; and
- Similar or identical genotypes among all isolates collected from the same patient.

TREATMENT: More than 90% of health care-associated CoNS strains are methicillin resistant. Methicillin-resistant strains are resistant to all beta-lactam drugs, including cephalosporins (except ceftaroline), and usually several other drug classes. Intravenous vancomycin is recommended for the treatment of serious infections caused by CoNS strains resistant to beta-lactam antimicrobial agents. Ceftaroline, daptomycin, and linezolid are alternative agents when vancomycin cannot be used. Dalbavancin has received US Food and Drug Administration approval for use in infants and children; other lipoglycopeptides including telavancin and oritavancin have limited data on use in the pediatric population. In noncritical localized infection, antimicrobials such as trimethoprim-sulfamethoxazole, clindamycin, and doxycycline can be considered based on susceptibility data. Unlike most other CoNS species, *S lugdunensis* often is methicillin susceptible, and antistaphylococcal beta lactams can be used as first-line therapy when susceptibility is confirmed. See Tables 4.2 (p 988) and 4.3 (p 993) for dosing and drug monitoring information for neonates and non-neonates, respectively.

Treatment of foreign bodies infected with CoNS often involves removal of the device, in addition to antibiotic therapy. Consultation with an expert in pediatric infectious diseases is advised to assist in the management of these infections. The addition of rifampin to vancomycin or daptomycin therapy in prosthetic joint infections is supported by limited studies. Rifampin and gentamicin are generally added to the primary antistaphylococcal agent in the treatment of prosthetic endocarditis (gentamicin typically for the first 2 weeks). Prolonged therapy is likely necessary when there is endocarditis or if the infected device (eg, spinal hardware) cannot be removed entirely. Adjunctive antimicrobial lock therapy of tunneled central lines may result in a higher rate of catheter salvage in adults with CoNS infections, but experience with this approach is limited in children. If blood cultures remain positive for more than 3 to 5 days after initiation of appropriate antimicrobial therapy for CoNS or if the patient fails to improve, the central line should be removed, parenteral therapy should be continued, and the patient should be evaluated for metastatic foci of infection.

A 5-day course of therapy is generally appropriate for CoNS central line associated blood stream infections in immunocompetent hosts, if the central line is removed, there is no demonstrable thrombus, and bacteremia resolves promptly. If the catheter is retained, a treatment duration of 10 to 14 days is appropriate. For non-neonates, observation without antibiotics could be considered in uncomplicated central line infections if patients are immunocompetent, have no other intravascular device or orthopedic hardware, and there is prompt clearance of bacteremia after the line is removed. The exception is *S lugdunensis*, which should be managed similarly to *S aureus* catheter-related infections regardless of patient age; endocarditis with valvular destruction may require urgent surgical intervention (see *Staphylococcus aureus*, p 767).

INFECTION PREVENTION AND CONTROL MEASURES IN HEALTH CARE SETTINGS: Standard precautions are used.

CONTROL MEASURES: Prevention and control of CoNS infections involves prevention of intraoperative contamination by skin flora and sterile insertion of intravascular and intraperitoneal catheters and other prosthetic devices. Catheter-related bloodstream infections can be markedly reduced with a "bundled" prevention approach, which should include catheter removal as soon as it is no longer needed.

Group A Streptococcal Infections

CLINICAL MANIFESTATIONS: The most common group A streptococcal (GAS) infection is acute pharyngotonsillitis (pharyngitis), which manifests as sore throat with tonsillar inflammation and often tender anterior cervical lymphadenopathy, palatal petechiae, or a strawberry tongue. Purulent complications of pharyngitis include peritonsillar or retropharyngeal abscesses, suppurative cervical adenitis, and rarely, sinusitis and otitis media. Nonsuppurative complications include acute rheumatic fever (ARF) and acute glomerulonephritis (AGN). The goals of antimicrobial therapy for GAS pharyngitis are to reduce acute morbidity, suppurative and nonsuppurative (ARF) complications, and transmission to close contacts. There is insufficient evidence to determine effectiveness of antimicrobials to prevent AGN after pyoderma or pharyngitis.

Scarlet fever occurs most often with pharyngitis and, rarely, with pyoderma or an infected wound. Scarlet fever involves a characteristic confluent erythematous sandpaper-like rash caused by one or more GAS erythrogenic exotoxins. Other than rash, the epidemiologic features, symptoms, signs, sequelae, and treatment of scarlet fever are the same as those of streptococcal pharyngitis.

Acute streptococcal pharyngitis is uncommon in children younger than 3 years. Instead, they may present with rhinitis and a more protracted illness with moderate fever, irritability, and anorexia (streptococcal fever or streptococcosis).

The second most common site of GAS infection is the skin. Streptococcal skin infections (eg, pyoderma or impetigo) can be followed by AGN, occasionally in epidemics. Historically, GAS skin infection has not been proven to lead to ARF; however, emerging evidence from Australia and New Zealand support that ARF can be a complication of GAS skin infection.

Other GAS infections include erysipelas, cellulitis (including perianal), vaginitis, bacteremia, sepsis, pneumonia, endocarditis, pericarditis, septic arthritis, necrotizing fasciitis, purpura fulminans, osteomyelitis, myositis, puerperal sepsis, surgical wound infection, mastoiditis, and neonatal omphalitis. Invasive GAS infections often encompass bacteremia with or without a specific focus of infection and can present as streptococcal toxic shock syndrome (STSS), sepsis, or necrotizing fasciitis. Necrotizing fasciitis can follow minor or unrecognized trauma and uncommonly pharyngitis, often involves an extremity, and manifests as pain out of proportion to examination findings.

STSS is caused by infection with a toxin-producing GAS strain, manifesting as a severe acute illness, which usually has rapid onset. The case definition of STSS (see Table 3.60) requires detection of the GAS organism in a patient with rapid onset of hypotension and signs of multiorgan involvement characterized by 2 or more of the following: acute kidney injury, coagulopathy, liver involvement, acute respiratory distress syndrome, generalized erythematous macular rash, or soft tissue necrosis. Local soft tissue infection (eg, cellulitis, myositis, or necrotizing fasciitis) associated with severe, rapidly increasing pain is common, although STSS can occur without an identifiable focus of infection.

Table 3.60. Streptococcal Toxic Shock Syndrome: Clinical Case Definition[a]

I. Isolation of group A *Streptococcus (Streptococcus pyogenes)*
   A. From a normally sterile site (eg, blood, cerebrospinal fluid, peritoneal, joint, pleural, or pericardial fluid)
   B. From a nonsterile site (eg, throat, sputum, vagina, open surgical wound, or superficial skin lesion)
II. Clinical signs of severity
   A. Hypotension: systolic pressure 90 mm Hg or less in adults or lower than the fifth percentile for age in children <16 years of age

   AND

   B. Two or more of the following signs of multiorgan involvement:
   - Renal impairment: creatinine concentration 177 μmol/L (2 mg/dL) or greater for adults or at least 2 times the upper limit of normal for age[b]
   - Coagulopathy: platelet count 100 000/mm^3 or less and/or disseminated intravascular coagulation defined by prolonged clotting times, low fibrinogen, and presence of fibrin degradation products
   - Hepatic involvement: elevated alanine aminotransferase, aspartate aminotransferase, or total bilirubin concentrations at least 2 times the upper limit of normal for age[b]
   - Acute respiratory distress syndrome defined by acute onset of diffuse pulmonary infiltrates and hypoxemia in absence of cardiac failure or by evidence of diffuse capillary leak
   - A generalized erythematous macular rash that may desquamate
   - Soft tissue necrosis, including necrotizing fasciitis or myositis, or gangrene

Adapted from the 2010 Case Definition from the Council of State and Territorial Epidemiologists (**https://ndc. services.cdc.gov/case-definitions/streptococcal-toxic-shock-syndrome-2010/**) and from: The Working Group on Severe Streptococcal Infections. Defining the group A streptococcal toxic shock syndrome: rationale and consensus definition. *JAMA.* 1993;269(3):390–391

[a] An illness fulfilling criteria IA and IIA and IIB can be defined as a *confirmed* case. An illness fulfilling criteria IB and IIA and IIB can be defined as a *probable* case if no other cause for the illness is identified. Manifestations need not be detected within the first 48 hours of illness or hospitalization.

[b] In patients with preexisting renal or hepatic disease, concentrations twofold or greater over patient's baseline.

An association between GAS infection and sudden onset of obsessive-compulsive behavior, tic disorders, or other unexplained acute neurologic changes—called pediatric autoimmune neuropsychiatric disorders associated with streptococcal infections (PANDAS)—has been proposed. The American Academy of Pediatrics is reviewing PANDAS; it will not be covered in this chapter.

ETIOLOGY: More than 240 distinct serotypes or genotypes of group A streptococci *(Streptococcus pyogenes)* have been identified based on M-protein serotype or M-protein gene sequence (*emm* types). In general, *emm* typing is more discriminating than M-protein serotyping. Epidemiologic studies indicate an association between certain *emm* types (eg, types 1, 3, 5, 6, 14, 18, 19, and 24) and rheumatic fever, but a specific rheumatogenic factor remains unidentified. Several *emm* types (eg, types 2, 49, 55, 57, 59, 60, and 61) are more commonly associated with pyoderma and acute glomerulonephritis. Other serotypes (eg, types 1, 6, and 12) are associated with pharyngitis and acute glomerulonephritis. Although many *emm* types can cause STSS, most cases are caused by *emm* 1 and *emm* 3 strains producing at least 1 pyrogenic exotoxin, most commonly streptococcal pyrogenic exotoxin A (*speA*). These toxins are superantigens, stimulating production of tumor necrosis factor and other inflammatory mediators causing capillary leak and other physiologic changes including hypotension and multiorgan damage. In the United Kingdom, an increase in scarlet fever cases since 2016 has been associated with a new strain of *emm*1 (M1UK lineage).

EPIDEMIOLOGY: Pharyngitis usually results from respiratory droplet transmission but can also occur through contact with respiratory secretions or wound discharge from an infected person. Although environmental transmission via surfaces and fomites was historically not believed to occur, evidence from outbreak investigations indicates that environmental transmission of GAS can occur. Household pets, such as dogs, are not vectors. Pharyngitis and impetigo (and their nonsuppurative complications) can be associated with crowding and often are present in socioeconomically disadvantaged populations. Close contact in schools, child care centers, contact sports (eg, wrestling), boarding schools, and military installations facilitates transmission. Rare foodborne outbreaks of pharyngitis are a consequence of human contamination of food with improper food preparation or refrigeration.

GAS pharyngitis is most common among school-aged children and adolescents, peaking at 7 to 8 years of age. GAS pharyngitis and pyoderma are substantially less common in adults than children.

Geographically, GAS pharyngitis and pyoderma are ubiquitous. Pyoderma is more common in tropical climates and warm seasons, in part because of antecedent insect bites and other minor skin trauma. Streptococcal pharyngitis is more common during late fall, winter, and spring in temperate climates in part because of close contact in schools. Communicability of streptococcal pharyngitis peaks during acute infection and when untreated, then gradually diminishes over a period of weeks.

Throat culture surveys of healthy asymptomatic children during the streptococcal season and during school outbreaks of pharyngitis yield GAS carriage prevalence rates as high as 25%. GAS carriage can persist for many months, but the risks of postinfectious or infectious complications and of transmission are low.

In streptococcal impetigo/pyoderma, the organism usually is acquired by direct contact from another person. GAS colonization of healthy skin usually precedes impetigo.

Impetiginous lesions occur at the site of breaks in skin (eg, insect bites, burns, traumatic wounds, varicella lesions). After development of impetiginous lesions, the upper respiratory tract can become colonized with GAS organisms. Infection of surgical wounds and postpartum (puerperal) sepsis usually result from transmission through direct contact. Health care workers who are pharyngeal, anal, or vaginal GAS carriers and those with skin infection or skin colonization can transmit GAS infection to patients, particularly surgical and obstetrical patients, and long-term care facility residents, sometimes resulting in health care-associated outbreaks. Infections in neonates, uncommon in the United States but common in many low-income countries, result from intrapartum or contact transmission; the latter infection can begin as omphalitis, cellulitis, or necrotizing fasciitis. In the United States, the incidence of invasive GAS infections is highest in the elderly and lowest among children and adolescents. Pregnant people and those in the postpartum period are at increased risk of invasive GAS infection. Fatal cases in children are not common, but they can progress very rapidly (eg, overwhelming sepsis). Before varicella vaccine, varicella infection (chickenpox) was the most commonly identified predisposing factor for invasive GAS infection in children. Other risk factors include exposure to other children and household crowding. The portal of entry is unknown in most invasive GAS infections but presumably relates to skin or mucous membranes. Such infections very rarely follow symptomatic GAS pharyngitis.

STSS can occur at any age. Fewer than 5% of invasive streptococcal infections in children are associated with STSS. Childhood STSS has been reported with focal lesions (eg, varicella, cellulitis, trauma, osteomyelitis, pneumonia), and with bacteremia without a defined focus. Mortality rates are substantially lower for children than for adults with STSS.

ARF is endemic in parts of Africa, Asia, and the Pacific, including the Australian and New Zealand indigenous populations. The United States, Canada, and most of Europe are considered ARF low-risk populations, although sporadic cases continue to occur. During GAS epidemics on military bases in the 1950s, ARF developed in up to 3% of untreated acute GAS pharyngitis. Very rare cases have occurred in treated patients. The current incidence in the United States is not precisely known but is believed to be <0.5%, with much higher rates reported among people of Samoan or Polynesian ancestry living in Hawaii or in residents of American Samoa. Focal outbreaks of ARF in school-aged children occurred in several areas in the United States in the 1990s, and small clusters are reported periodically, most likely related to circulation of particularly rheumatogenic GAS strains.

Poststreptococcal AGN is more common in resource-limited regions, in male individuals, and in children 5 to 12 years of age.[1]

The **incubation period** for streptococcal pharyngitis is 2 to 5 days. For impetigo, a 7- to 10-day period between GAS acquisition on healthy skin and the development of lesions has been demonstrated. The **incubation period** for STSS is not known but can be as short as 14 hours when associated with subcutaneous inoculation of organisms (eg, puerperal sepsis, penetrating trauma). The **incubation period** for ARF is generally 1 to 5 weeks following pharyngitis; chorea occurs 1 to 8 months following pharyngitis. The **incubation period** for poststreptococcal AGN is generally 10 days following pharyngitis and up to 3 weeks following GAS skin infections.

---

[1] The term male refers to sex assigned at birth.

DIAGNOSTIC TESTS[1]:

Testing for Group A Streptococci in Pharyngitis. Children with acute onset of sore throat and clinical signs and symptoms such as pharyngeal exudate, enlarged tonsils, pain on swallowing, fever, and enlarged tender anterior cervical nodes are more likely to have GAS infection and should be tested. Children with pharyngitis and obvious viral features (eg, rhinorrhea, cough, hoarseness, oral ulcers) should not be tested or treated for GAS infection. Testing also is generally not recommended for children younger than 3 years, although testing and treatment may be considered for some symptomatic children younger than 3 years who have other risk factors, such as an older sibling with GAS infection. Laboratory confirmation of GAS before initiation of antimicrobial treatment is required for children with pharyngitis without viral symptoms, because many will not have GAS pharyngitis. A specimen should be obtained by vigorously swabbing both tonsils and the posterior pharynx for rapid antigen testing or other diagnostic test, as discussed below. A second backup swab specimen from a child with a negative rapid antigen test should be submitted for culture or molecular testing. Culture on sheep blood agar can confirm GAS infection, with latex agglutination differentiating group A streptococci from other beta-hemolytic streptococci (eg, group C or G). False-negative culture results occur in <10% of symptomatic patients when an adequate throat swab specimen is obtained and cultured by trained personnel. Recovery of GAS organisms from the pharynx or assessing the density of colonies does not distinguish those patients with acute streptococcal infection from streptococcal carriers with intercurrent viral pharyngitis. Cultures negative for GAS organisms after 18 to 24 hours incubation should be reincubated for a second day to optimize recovery of GAS bacteria.

Several rapid tests for GAS pharyngitis are available. The specificity of these tests generally is high (very few false-positive results), but reported sensitivities vary considerably and generally are 75% to 85% (ie, false-negatives occur). As with throat cultures, the sensitivity of these tests is highly dependent on the quality of the throat swab specimen and the experience of the test performer. Because of the very high specificity of rapid antigen-based tests, a positive result does not require culture confirmation, but a negative result requires a confirmatory test in children. Other diagnostic tests using techniques such as polymerase chain reaction (PCR), chemiluminescent DNA probes, and isothermal nucleic acid amplification tests (NAATs) have been developed. The US Food and Drug Administration has approved some NAATs for detection of group A streptococci from throat swab specimens as stand-alone tests that, because of very high sensitivity, do not require routine culture confirmation of negative test results. Some studies suggest that in addition to providing more timely results, these tests may be even more sensitive than standard cultures of throat swab specimens on sheep blood agar. Additional studies are ongoing to establish the benefits and limitations of these tests.

Testing Contacts for GAS Infection. Indications for testing contacts for GAS infection are few, outside of outbreak investigations. Testing asymptomatic household contacts is not recommended, except when the contacts are at increased risk for sequelae of GAS infection, such as with established ARF or AGN; if test results are positive, contacts should be treated.

---

[1] Shulman ST, Bisno AL, Clegg HW, et al. Clinical practice guideline for the diagnosis and management of group a streptococcal pharyngitis: 2012 update by the Infectious Diseases Society of America. *Clin Infect Dis*. 2012;55(10):e86-e102

In schools, child care centers, or other environments where many people are in close contact, the prevalence of GAS pharyngeal carriage in healthy children can reach 25%, even in the absence of an outbreak of streptococcal disease. Therefore, classroom or more widespread testing generally is not indicated.

Testing asymptomatic household contacts usually is not helpful. However, if multiple household members have pharyngitis or other GAS infections, simultaneous cultures of all household members and treatment of all with positive test results may be of value.

Follow-up Throat Cultures. Post-treatment throat cultures are indicated only for those at particularly high risk of ARF (eg, with previous history of ARF).

Testing for Group A Streptococci in Nonpharyngitis Infections. Cultures of impetigo lesions often yield both streptococci and staphylococci, and determination of the primary pathogen is generally difficult. Culture can be used to determine *S aureus* susceptibility; however, it is generally unnecessary in routine clinical practice. In suspected invasive GAS infections, cultures of blood and focal sites of possible infection are indicated. In necrotizing fasciitis, although imaging studies may be helpful in establishing the diagnosis, surgical exploration should never be delayed for imaging studies. Clinical suspicion of necrotizing fasciitis should prompt urgent surgical evaluation with possible urgent débridement of affected tissues, with Gram stain and culture of surgical specimens. STSS is diagnosed on the basis of clinical findings, laboratory findings, and isolation of GAS organisms (Table 3.60); more than 50% of patients with STSS have blood cultures positive for GAS organisms. Cultures of focal sites of infection are also usually positive and can remain positive for several days after initiation of appropriate antimicrobial agents.

Acute Rheumatic Fever. The Jones criteria for diagnosis of ARF were established in 1944 and revised and modified several times, most recently in 2015.[1] The 2015 Jones criteria revision (Table 3.61) differentiates major and minor criteria on the basis of whether the child is from an area at low or moderate/high risk for ARF. Laboratory evidence of antecedent GAS infection should be confirmed in suspected ARF and includes an elevated or increasing antistreptolysin O or anti-DNAase B titer, a positive rapid antigen test result, or positive streptococcal throat culture (this revision was made prior to widespread availability of molecular tests). Because of the long latency between GAS infection and chorea, laboratory evidence may be lacking when chorea is the only major criterion. See Table 3.61 for the major and minor criteria.

Poststreptococcal Glomerulonephritis. Diagnosis is based on clinical findings of acute nephritis and evidence of a recent GAS infection in the throat or skin, generally by culture or serologic testing.

TREATMENT[2]:

S pyogenes is uniformly susceptible to all beta-lactam antibiotics (penicillins and cephalosporins); thus, susceptibility testing is needed only for non–beta-lactam agents, such as a macrolide or clindamycin, to which some strains of *S pyogenes* are resistant.

---

[1] Gewitz MH, Baltimore RS, Tani LY, et al. Revision of the Jones criteria for the diagnosis of acute rheumatic fever in the era of Doppler echocardiography. *Circulation.* 2015;131(20):1806-1818

[2] Shulman ST, Bisno AL, Clegg HW, et al. Clinical practice guideline for the diagnosis and management of group a streptococcal pharyngitis: 2012 update by the Infectious Diseases Society of America. *Clin Infect Dis.* 2012;55(10):e86-e102

Table 3.61. Revised Jones Criteria (2015)

1. All patients require evidence of antecedent GAS infection for diagnosis of ARF (except in case of isolated chorea, in which evidence of antecedent GAS infection is not required).
2. To confirm an initial diagnosis of ARF, need 2 major OR 1 major and 2 minor criteria.
3. To confirm recurrent ARF diagnosis, need 2 major OR 1 major and 2 minor OR 3 minor criteria.
4. Criteria for diagnosis are dependent on whether patient is from a low-risk or a moderate-/high-risk population. Moderate- and high-risk populations include countries where ARF remains endemic (Africa, Asia-Pacific, indigenous population of Australia and New Zealand). The United States, Canada, and most of western Europe are examples of low-risk areas.
5. Major and minor criteria are listed below, by risk categorization; differences for moderate-/high-risk populations are **bolded.**

Low-Risk Population	Moderate- and High-Risk Population
Major Criteria • Carditis (clinical or subclinical) • Arthritis (polyarthritis only) • Chorea • Subcutaneous nodules • Erythema marginatum	Major Criteria • Carditis (clinical or subclinical) • Arthritis (polyarthritis or **monoarthritis,** or **polyarthralgia**) • Chorea • Subcutaneous nodules • Erythema marginatum
Minor Criteria • Polyarthralgia (unless arthritis is a major criteria) • Fever ≥38.5°C • ESR ≥60 mm/h and/or CRP ≥3 mg/dL • Prolonged PR interval (in absence of carditis)	Minor Criteria • **Monoarthralgia** (unless arthritis is a major criteria) • **Fever ≥38°C** • **ESR ≥30 mm/h** and/or CRP ≥3 mg/dL • Prolonged PR interval (in absence of carditis)

ARF indicates acute rheumatic fever; CRP, C-reactive protein; ESR, erythrocyte sedimentation rate; GAS, group A streptococcal.

Modified from Table 7 in Gewitz MH, Baltimore RS, Tani LY, et al. Revision of the Jones criteria for the diagnosis of acute rheumatic fever in the era of Doppler echocardiography: a scientific statement from the American Heart Association. *Circulation.* 2015;131(20):1806-1818.

Pharyngitis.

- Penicillin V, amoxicillin, or penicillin G benzathine are 3 options for first-line regimens for GAS pharyngitis.
- Administration of penicillin shortens the clinical course (if administered promptly), decreases the risk of transmission and suppurative sequelae, and prevents ARF, even when administered up to 9 days after illness onset. All patients with ARF should receive a complete course of penicillin or another appropriate antimicrobial agent for GAS pharyngitis, even if group A streptococci are not recovered from the throat.
- Amoxicillin, orally as a single daily dose (50 mg/kg; maximum, 1000–1200 mg) for 10 days, is as effective as penicillin V or amoxicillin administered orally multiple times per day for 10 days and is a more palatable suspension than penicillin V. This

regimen is endorsed by the American Heart Association and the Infectious Disease Society of America in their guidelines for the treatment of GAS pharyngitis and the prevention of ARF.[1] Adherence is particularly important for once-daily dosing regimens.

- The dose of oral penicillin V is 400 000 U (250 mg), 2 to 3 times per day, for 10 days for children weighing <27 kg and 800 000 U (500 mg), 2 to 3 times per day, for those weighing ≥27 kg, including adolescents and adults. To prevent ARF, oral penicillin or amoxicillin should be taken for 10 full days, regardless of the promptness of clinical recovery. Treatment failures occur more often with oral penicillin than with intramuscular penicillin G benzathine because of inadequate adherence. Notably, short-course treatment (<10 days) for GAS pharyngitis, particularly with penicillin V, is associated with inferior bacteriologic eradication rates.

- Intramuscular penicillin G benzathine is appropriate therapy, ensuring adequate blood concentrations and avoiding adherence issues, but administration may be painful. See Tables of Antibacterial Drug Dosages (p 987) for dosing. Discomfort is decreased if the preparation of penicillin G benzathine is brought to room temperature before intramuscular injection. Mixtures containing shorter-acting penicillins (eg, penicillin G procaine) in addition to penicillin G benzathine are not more effective than penicillin G benzathine alone but are less painful. Although supporting data are limited, the combination of 900 000 U (562.5 mg) of penicillin G benzathine and 300 000 U (187.5 mg) of penicillin G procaine is satisfactory for most children; however, the efficacy of this combination for heavier patients has not been documented.

- For patients who have a history of nonanaphylactic allergy to penicillin or amoxicillin, a 10-day course of a narrow-spectrum (first-generation) oral cephalosporin (eg, cephalexin) is indicated. Patients with immediate (anaphylactic) or type I hypersensitivity to penicillin or amoxicillin should receive oral clindamycin (20 mg/kg per day in 3 divided doses; maximum, 900 mg/day for 10 days) rather than a cephalosporin.

- An oral macrolide (eg, erythromycin, azithromycin, or clarithromycin) also is acceptable for penicillin–allergic patients. This medication should not be used in patients who can take a beta-lactam agent. Therapy for 10 days is indicated, except for azithromycin, which is given for 5 days. GAS strains resistant to macrolides have resulted in treatment failures.

- In the United States, macrolide and clindamycin (inducible and constitutive) resistance rates of close to 30% have been reported among invasive GAS isolates (**www.cdc.gov/abcs/bact-facts-interactive-dashboard.html**). Testing for macrolide and clindamycin resistance may help in deciding the best antimicrobial agent for a specific patient with penicillin allergy.

- Tetracyclines, sulfonamides, and fluoroquinolones should not be used for treating GAS pharyngitis.

- Children with recurrent GAS pharyngitis shortly after a full course of a recommended oral agent can be retreated with the same antimicrobial agent (if it is a

---

[1] Gerber MA, Baltimore RS, Eaton CB, et al. Prevention of rheumatic fever and diagnosis and treatment of acute streptococcal pharyngitis. A scientific statement from the American Heart Association, Rheumatic Fever, Endocarditis, and Kawasaki Disease Committee, Council on Cardiovascular Disease in the Young, and the Quality of Care and Outcomes Research Interdisciplinary Working Group and endorsed by the American Academy of Pediatrics. *Circulation.* 2009;119(11):1541-1551

beta-lactam), an alternative beta-lactam oral drug (such as cephalexin or amoxicillin-clavulanate), or an intramuscular dose of penicillin G benzathine. Susceptibility testing should be performed when considering a macrolide or clindamycin.

Frequent Acute Pharyngitis With Positive GAS Testing. Patients with repeated episodes of acute pharyngitis at short intervals in whom GAS infection is documented by culture or rapid antigen or NAAT present a special problem. Most often, they are GAS carriers experiencing frequent viral illnesses for whom repeated testing and antimicrobials are unnecessary. In assessing these patients, inadequate adherence to oral treatment also should be considered. To determine whether the patient is a long-term streptococcal pharyngeal carrier who is experiencing repeated episodes of intercurrent viral pharyngitis (the most common situation), it should be determined: (1) whether clinical findings are more suggestive of GAS or viral infection; (2) whether household or community epidemiologic factors support GAS or viral etiology; (3) the nature of the clinical response to antimicrobial therapy (in GAS pharyngitis, response to therapy usually is <24 hours); and (4) whether test results are positive for GAS between episodes of acute pharyngitis (suggesting the patient is a carrier). Measurement of serologic response to GAS extracellular antigens (eg, antistreptolysin O) is discouraged, because interpretation can be very difficult. Typing (M or *emm* typing) of GAS isolates generally is available only in research or public health laboratories, but if performed, repeated isolation of the same type suggests carriage, while isolation of differing types indicates repeated infections.

Pharyngeal Carriers. Antimicrobial therapy is not indicated for most GAS pharyngeal carriers. The few specific situations in which eradication of carriage may be indicated include the following: (1) a local outbreak of ARF, poststreptococcal glomerulonephritis, or severe or invasive GAS disease; (2) an outbreak of GAS pharyngitis in a closed or semiclosed community; (3) a family history of ARF; (4) multiple ("ping-pong") episodes of documented symptomatic GAS pharyngitis occurring within a family for many weeks despite appropriate therapy; or (5) when a patient is being seriously considered for tonsillectomy solely because of frequent GAS isolations.

GAS carriage is difficult to eradicate with conventional antimicrobial therapy. Several agents, including clindamycin, cephalosporins, amoxicillin-clavulanate, azithromycin, or a combination that includes either 10 days of penicillin V or IM penicillin G benzathine with rifampin for the last 4 days of treatment are more effective than penicillin alone in terminating chronic streptococcal carriage. Of these drugs, oral clindamycin, 20 to 30 mg/kg per day in 3 doses (maximum, 900 mg/day) for 10 days, has been reported to be the most effective, although clindamycin resistance is increasingly common in the United States. Documented eradication of carriage is helpful in evaluation of subsequent episodes of acute pharyngitis; however, carriage can recur after reacquisition of GAS infection, as some individuals are "carrier prone."

Nonbullous Impetigo. Topical mupirocin or retapamulin ointment may be useful for limiting person-to-person spread of nonbullous impetigo and for eradicating localized disease. With multiple lesions or nonbullous impetigo in multiple family members, child care groups, or athletic teams, treatment should include oral agents active against both GAS and *S aureus*.

Toxic Shock Syndrome. As outlined in Tables 3.62 and 3.63, most aspects of management are the same for TSS caused by GAS or by *S aureus*. Paramount are prompt

Table 3.62. Management of Streptococcal Toxic Shock Syndrome Without Necrotizing Fasciitis

- Fluid management to maintain adequate venous return and cardiac filling pressures to prevent end-organ damage
- Anticipatory management of multisystem organ failure
- Parenteral antimicrobial therapy at maximum doses with the capacity to:
  - Kill organism with bactericidal cell wall inhibitor (eg, penicillin when group A *Streptococcus* is confirmed)
  - Decrease enzyme, toxin, or cytokine production with protein synthesis inhibitor (eg, clindamycin, or linezolid if clindamycin resistant)
- IGIV often is used as an adjunct, typically at 1 g/kg on day 1, followed by 0.5 g/kg on 1–2 subsequent days

IGIV indicates immune globulin intravenous.

aggressive fluid resuscitation, management of respiratory and cardiac failure, if present, and prompt surgical débridement of any deep-seated infection. Because *S pyogenes* and *S aureus* TSS are difficult to distinguish clinically, initial therapy should include vancomycin, a beta-lactam active *against S aureus*, and a protein synthesis-inhibiting agent, such as clindamycin. The addition of clindamycin is recommended for serious GAS infections, because its antimicrobial activity is unaffected by inoculum size (does not manifest the Eagle effect, the phenomenon in which bacteria exposed to concentrations of antibiotic higher than an optimal bactericidal concentration have paradoxically improved levels of survival, that occurs with beta-lactam antibiotics), it has a long postantimicrobial effect, and it inhibits bacterial protein synthesis, which results in suppression of synthesis of *S pyogenes* antiphagocytic M-protein and bacterial toxins. Clindamycin **should not be used alone** as initial antimicrobial therapy in life-threatening situations because of the potential for resistance, and susceptibility testing should be performed to assess inducible as well as constitutive resistance. In 2020, 29% of invasive GAS case isolates from the Active Bacterial Core surveillance system in the United States were resistant to clindamycin (**www.cdc.gov/abcs/bact-facts-interactive-dashboard.html**).

Once GAS infection is confirmed, antimicrobial therapy should be tailored to penicillin and clindamycin. If the isolate is resistant to clindamycin, linezolid can be used along with penicillin. Intravenous therapy should be continued at least until the patient is afebrile and stable hemodynamically and blood is documented to be sterile. Clindamycin (or linezolid) may be discontinued after a few days if there is adequate source control and clinical improvement, with continuation of the penicillin therapy. The total duration of therapy is based on duration established for the primary site of infection.

Table 3.63. Management of Streptococcal Toxic Shock Syndrome With Necrotizing Fasciitis

- Principles outlined in Table 3.62
- Immediate surgical evaluation
  - Exploration or incisional biopsy for diagnosis and culture
  - Resection of all necrotic tissue
- Repeated resection of tissue may be needed if infection persists or progresses

Aggressive drainage and irrigation of accessible sites of infection should be performed as soon as possible. If necrotizing fasciitis is suspected, immediate surgical exploration or biopsy is crucial to identify and débride deep soft tissue infection.

Immune globulin intravenous (IGIV) should be strongly considered as adjunctive therapy for STSS or necrotizing fasciitis if the patient is moderately to severely ill, although its use is supported by limited data.

Other Infections. Parenteral antimicrobial therapy is required for severe GAS infections, such as endocarditis, pneumonia, empyema, deep abscess, septicemia, meningitis, arthritis, osteomyelitis, erysipelas, necrotizing fasciitis, and neonatal omphalitis. Treatment often is prolonged (2–6 weeks).

Acute Rheumatic Fever. Treatment for ARF includes eradication of GAS with a standard pharyngitis regimen, treatment of acute inflammatory manifestations (eg, arthritis or valvulitis-associated heart failure), education for parents and patient, and initiation of secondary prophylaxis to prevent future GAS infection. Following initial treatment of ARF with a 10-day course of treatment-dose penicillin V or amoxicillin, patients with well-documented history of ARF (including cases manifested solely as Sydenham chorea) and patients with documented rheumatic heart disease (RHD) should be given continuous antimicrobial prophylaxis to prevent recurrent ARF attacks (secondary prophylaxis), because asymptomatic and symptomatic GAS infections can trigger recurrence of ARF. Continuous secondary prophylaxis should be initiated as soon as the diagnosis of ARF or rheumatic heart disease is made, and initial antibiotic therapy is complete. It should be long-term, perhaps for life, for patients with RHD (even after prosthetic valve replacement), because they remain at risk of ARF recurrence. Risk of recurrence decreases as the interval from the most recent acute episode increases, and patients without RHD are at lower risk of recurrence than patients with residual cardiac involvement. These considerations and the estimate of future exposure to GAS infection all influence the duration of secondary prophylaxis in adults but should not alter the duration of secondary prophylaxis for children and adolescents. Secondary prophylaxis for all who have had ARF should be continued for at least 5 years or until the person is 21 years of age, whichever is longer (see Table 3.64). Prophylaxis also should be continued if the risk of contact with people with GAS infection is high (eg, for parents with school-aged children, teachers, and others in frequent contact with children).

The antibiotic regimens in Table 3.65 are effective for secondary prophylaxis. The intramuscular regimen is the most reliable because success of oral prophylaxis depends primarily on patient adherence; however, inconvenience and pain of injection may cause some patients to discontinue intramuscular prophylaxis. In non-US populations in whom risk of ARF is particularly high, administration of penicillin G benzathine every 3 weeks is justified and recommended, because serum penicillin concentrations can decrease below a protective level in the fourth week after a dose. In the United States, administration every 4 weeks is likely adequate, except for those who have developed recurrent ARF despite adherence to an every-4-week regimen. For penicillin-allergic individuals, oral sulfadiazine is as effective as oral penicillin for secondary prophylaxis but may not be as readily available in the United States. By extrapolating from sulfadiazine, sulfisoxazole has been deemed an appropriate alternative; it is available in combination with erythromycin as a generic version.

Allergic reactions to oral penicillin are less common and usually less severe than reactions to parenteral penicillin and occur much more often in adults than in

Table 3.64. Duration of Prophylaxis for People Who Have Had Acute Rheumatic Fever (ARF): Recommendations of the American Heart Association[a]

Category	Duration
Rheumatic fever without carditis	5 years since last episode of ARF or until 21 years of age, whichever is longer
Rheumatic fever with carditis but without residual heart disease (no valvular disease[b])	10 years since last episode of ARF or until 21 years of age, whichever is longer
Rheumatic fever with carditis and residual heart disease (persistent valvular disease[b])	10 years since last episode of ARF or until 40 years of age, whichever is longer; consider lifelong prophylaxis for people with severe valvular disease or likelihood of ongoing exposure to group A streptococcal infection

[a]Modified from Gerber M, Baltimore R, Eaton C, et al. Prevention of rheumatic fever and diagnosis and treatment of acute streptococcal pharyngitis. A scientific statement from the American Heart Association, Rheumatic Fever, Endocarditis, and Kawasaki Disease Committee, Council on Cardiovascular Disease in the Young, and the Quality of Care and Outcomes Research Interdisciplinary Working Group. *Circulation*. 2009;119(11):1541-1551.
[b]Clinical or echocardiographic evidence.

Table 3.65. Chemoprophylaxis for Recurrences of Acute Rheumatic Fever[a]

Drug	Dose	Route
Penicillin G benzathine	1.2 million U, every 4 wk[b]; 600 000 U, every 4 wk for patients weighing less than 27 kg (60 lb)	Intramuscular
OR		
Penicillin V	250 mg, twice a day	Oral
OR		
Sulfadiazine or sulfisoxazole	0.5 g, once a day for patients weighing 27 kg (60 lb) or less	Oral
	1.0 g, once a day for patients weighing greater than 27 kg (60 lb)	
For people who are allergic to penicillin and sulfonamide drugs:		
Macrolide or azalide	Variable (see text)	Oral

[a]Gerber M, Baltimore R, Eaton C, et al. Prevention of rheumatic fever and diagnosis and treatment of acute streptococcal pharyngitis. A scientific statement from the American Heart Association, Rheumatic Fever, Endocarditis, and Kawasaki Disease Committee, Council on Cardiovascular Disease in the Young, and the Quality of Care and Outcomes Research Interdisciplinary Working Group. *Circulation*. 2009;119(11):1541-1551.
[b]In particularly high-risk situations (usually non-US sites), administration every 3 weeks is recommended.

children. Severe allergic reactions rarely occur with intramuscular penicillin G benzathine prophylaxis, but the incidence may be higher in patients older than 12 years with severe RHD. Most severe reactions seem to be vasovagal responses rather than anaphylaxis. A serum sickness-like reaction characterized by fever and joint pains can occur in those receiving prophylaxis and can be mistaken for recurrence of ARF.

Reactions to continuous sulfadiazine or sulfisoxazole prophylaxis are rare and are usually minor; evaluation of blood cell counts may be advisable after 2 weeks of prophylaxis, because leukopenia has been reported. Prophylaxis with a sulfonamide during late pregnancy is contraindicated because of interference with fetal bilirubin metabolism. Febrile mucocutaneous syndromes (erythema multiforme, Stevens-Johnson syndrome, or toxic epidermal necrolysis) rarely have been associated with penicillin and sulfonamides.

When an adverse event occurs with any prophylactic regimen, the drug should be stopped immediately and an alternative drug selected. For the rare patient allergic to both penicillins and sulfonamides, erythromycin is recommended. Other macrolides with less risk of gastrointestinal tract intolerance, such as azithromycin or clarithromycin, are also acceptable.

Poststreptococcal Reactive Arthritis. After an episode of acute GAS pharyngitis, reactive arthritis may develop without sufficient clinical and laboratory findings to fulfill the Jones criteria for diagnosis of ARF. This syndrome has been termed poststreptococcal reactive arthritis (PSRA). The precise relationship of PSRA to ARF is unclear. In contrast to the arthritis of ARF, PSRA does not respond dramatically to nonsteroidal anti-inflammatory agents. Because a very small proportion of patients with PSRA have been reported to develop late valvular heart disease, they should be observed carefully for 1 to 2 years for evidence of cardiac involvement, and some experts recommend secondary prophylaxis during the observation period. If valvular involvement develops, the patient should be considered to have had ARF, and secondary prophylaxis should be initiated (see above).

Poststreptococcal AGN. In addition to management of AGN, the patient should be treated to eradicate the nephritogenic strain with a standard pharyngitis regimen.

INFECTION PREVENTION AND CONTROL MEASURES IN HEALTH CARE SETTINGS: In addition to standard precautions, droplet precautions are recommended for those with GAS pharyngitis or pneumonia until 24 hours after initiation of appropriate antimicrobial therapy. For burns with secondary GAS infection and extensive or draining cutaneous infections that cannot be covered or contained adequately by dressings, contact precautions should be used until at least 24 hours after initiation of appropriate therapy.

CONTROL MEASURES: The most important means of controlling GAS disease and its sequelae is prompt identification and treatment of infections.

School and Child Care. Children with GAS pharyngitis or skin infections should not return to school or child care until well appearing and at least 12 hours after beginning appropriate antimicrobial therapy. In the setting of an outbreak, exclusion for at least 24 hours after treatment has been initiated should be considered, and consultation with the state or local public health department is recommended. Close contact with other children during this time should be avoided if possible.

Care of Exposed People. Symptomatic contacts of a child with documented GAS infection with recent or current clinical evidence of a GAS infection should undergo appropriate laboratory tests and treated if test results are positive. Rates of GAS carriage are higher among sibling contacts of children with GAS pharyngitis than among parent contacts in nonepidemic settings; carriage rates as high as 50% for sibling contacts and 20% for parent contacts are reported during epidemics. Asymptomatic acquisition of GAS infection may pose some low risk of nonsuppurative complications; as many as one third of patients with ARF have no history of recent streptococcal infection and another third have minor respiratory tract symptoms not brought to medical attention. However, routine laboratory evaluation of asymptomatic household contacts is not indicated except during outbreaks or when contacts are at increased risk of developing sequelae of infection. In rare circumstances, such as a large family with documented, repeated, intrafamilial transmission resulting in frequent episodes of GAS pharyngitis over a prolonged period, physicians may elect to treat all family members identified by laboratory tests as harboring GAS organisms.

Household contacts of patients with severe invasive GAS disease, including STSS, are at some increased risk of developing severe invasive GAS disease compared with the general population. However, the risk is not sufficiently high to warrant routine testing for GAS colonization, and a clearly effective regimen has not been identified to justify routine chemoprophylaxis of all household contacts. Because of increased risk of sporadic, invasive GAS disease among certain populations (eg, people with human immunodeficiency virus [HIV] infection) and because of increased risk of death in those 65 years and older who develop invasive GAS disease, physicians may choose to offer targeted chemoprophylaxis to household contacts 65 years and older or to members of other high-risk populations (eg, people with HIV infection, varicella, or diabetes mellitus). Because of the rarity of secondary cases and the low risk of invasive GAS infections in children, chemoprophylaxis is generally not recommended in schools or child care facilities.

Bacterial Endocarditis Prophylaxis.[1] The American Heart Association (AHA) has reaffirmed its 2007 recommendations regarding use of antimicrobial agents to prevent infective endocarditis (see Prevention of Bacterial Endocarditis, p 1127). The AHA no longer recommends prophylaxis for patients with RHD without a prosthetic valve. However, use of oral antiseptic solutions and maintenance of optimal oral health through daily oral hygiene and regular dental visits remain important components of an overall health care program. For individuals with a prosthetic valve, infective endocarditis prophylaxis still is recommended, and current AHA recommendations should be followed. If penicillin is being used for secondary ARF prevention, an agent other than penicillin or amoxicillin should be used for infective endocarditis prophylaxis, because penicillin-resistant alpha-hemolytic streptococci are likely to be present in the mouth.

---

[1] Wilson W, Taubert KA, Gewitz M, et al. Prevention of infective endocarditis. Recommendations by the American Heart Association. A guideline from the American Heart Association Rheumatic Fever, Endocarditis, and Kawasaki Disease Committee, Council on Cardiovascular Disease in the Young, and the Council on Clinical Cardiology, Council on Cardiovascular Surgery and Anesthesia, and the Quality of Care and Outcomes Research Interdisciplinary Working Group. *Circulation.* 2007;116(15):1736–1754

Group B Streptococcal Infections

CLINICAL MANIFESTATIONS: Group B streptococci are a major cause of perinatal infections, including urinary tract infection, bacteremia, intra-amniotic infection (formerly called chorioamnionitis), and endometritis in pregnant and postpartum people, as well as systemic and focal infections in neonates and young infants. In newborn infants, early-onset disease (EOD) usually occurs within the first 24 hours after birth (range, 0 through 6 days), presenting with respiratory distress, apnea, pneumonia, shock and less often, meningitis (5%–10% of cases). Late-onset disease (LOD), which typically occurs at 3 to 4 weeks of age (range, 7 through 89 days), commonly manifests as bacteremia without a focus (60%–65% of cases) or meningitis (approximately 30% of cases); other focal infections, often with concomitant bacteremia, include osteomyelitis, septic arthritis, necrotizing fasciitis, pneumonia, adenitis, and cellulitis. Cases among infants 90 days and older are reported less commonly and typically occur among very preterm infants or infants with immunodeficiency syndromes. Survivors of invasive GBS, particularly cases involving meningitis are at increased risk for neurodevelopmental impairment. A recent study estimated a twofold higher risk for moderate to severe neurodevelopmental impairment by age 10 years for children with invasive neonatal GBS disease in Denmark and a twofold higher risk for the need for educational support compared with uninfected children in the Netherlands.

ETIOLOGY: Group B streptococci *(Streptococcus agalactiae)* are gram-positive diplococci that typically produce a narrow zone of beta hemolysis on 5% sheep blood agar. These organisms are divided into 10 types on the basis of capsular polysaccharides structures. Types Ia, Ib, II, III, IV, and V account for approximately 99% of cases in infants in the United States. Type III causes approximately 30% to 60% of EOD and LOD, respectively.

EPIDEMIOLOGY: Group B streptococci colonize the human gastrointestinal and genitourinary tracts and less commonly the pharynx. The vaginal/rectal colonization rate in pregnant people ranges from 15% to 35% and can be persistent or intermittent. In the 1990s, recommendations were made for prevention of early-onset group B streptococcal (GBS) disease through intrapartum antibiotic prophylaxis (IAP) administered to pregnant people who were found to be colonized or had risk factors for having an infant with EOD (see Control Measures, p 801). As a result of widespread implementation of IAP, the incidence of EOD has decreased by approximately 80% to an estimated 0.22 cases per 1000 live births in 2020. The use of IAP has had no measurable effect on late-onset GBS disease incidence. In 2020, LOD incidence exceeded that of EOD at 0.29 cases per 1000 live births. The case fatality rate for group B streptococcal disease in term infants ranges from 1% to 3% but is higher in preterm neonates (estimated to be 20% for EOD and 8% for LOD). Approximately 70% of EOD and 50% of LOD afflict term neonates.

Transmission from a pregnant person to the infant generally occurs shortly before or during delivery in those who are colonized with GBS organisms. Less commonly, GBS infection may be transmitted in the nursery from health care professionals or visitors or in the community via colonized family members or caregivers. The risk of EOD is increased in preterm infants, infants born 18 hours or more after membrane rupture, and infants born to people with intrapartum fever (temperature ≥38°C [≥100.4°F]), intra-amniotic infection, GBS bacteriuria during the current pregnancy, or a history of a previous infant with invasive GBS disease. A higher incidence of

EOD has also been associated with delivering parents who are younger (age <20 years) and Black. However, the independent contribution of these factors is unclear because each of these has been associated with higher rates of both GBS colonization and preterm birth. Infants can remain colonized for several months despite treatment for systemic infection. Recurrent GBS disease affects an estimated 1% to 3% of appropriately treated infants.

The **incubation period** of EOD is fewer than 7 days. In LOD, the **incubation period** is unknown.

DIAGNOSTIC TESTS: Visualization of gram-positive cocci in pairs or short chains from a normally sterile body fluid provides presumptive evidence of infection, but growth of the organism in culture establishes the diagnosis. Multiplex polymerase chain reaction (PCR) assays are available in many clinical laboratories for direct testing of cerebrospinal fluid (CSF) for GBS and may expedite the diagnosis.

For prenatal GBS screening, swab specimens from lower vaginal and rectal sites are collected (vaginal swab specimens alone underestimate GBS colonization by up to 10%–15%). Culture yield can be increased with the use of commercially available selective broth enrichment media for 18 to 24 hours of incubation before being plated on tryptic soy blood agar or other selective agars for an additional 24 to 48 hours. Alternatively, DNA probe assays, latex agglutination assays, and nucleic acid amplification tests (NAATs) are available to detect GBS in enriched broth specimens. Several NAATs are approved for antepartum or intrapartum detection of GBS organisms from vaginal/rectal swab specimens collected from pregnant people. However, the sensitivity of NAATs may be significantly decreased when used for rapid intrapartum testing, because a preanalysis enrichment incubation step cannot be included in those situations. Cases of neonatal GBS disease have occurred in neonates born to people whose screens were negative during pregnancy.

TREATMENT[1]**:**

- Ampicillin plus an aminoglycoside is the empiric treatment of choice for a **newborn infant ≤7 days of age** with presumptive early-onset GBS infection; this reflects the need for coverage of other pathogens, such as *Escherichia coli*, which is the second-most common cause of EOD. In a critically ill neonate, particularly one with low birth weight, broader-spectrum empiric therapy should be considered when there is concern about non-GBS ampicillin-resistant infection.

- For empiric therapy of late-onset GBS disease in **infants 8 through 28 days of age** who are being admitted from the community and are not critically ill and do not have evidence of meningitis, ampicillin plus either gentamicin or an extended-spectrum cephalosporin (eg, cefotaxime, ceftazidime, cefepime) are recommended. If meningitis is suspected, ampicillin plus an extended-spectrum cephalosporin (eg, cefotaxime, ceftazidime, cefepime) should be used (see also Serious Neonatal Bacterial Infections Caused by *Enterobacterales*, p 365).

- For **infants 29 through 89 days of age**, ceftriaxone is recommended. If there is evidence of meningitis or critical illness, vancomycin should be added to expand empiric coverage.

---

[1] Puopolo KM, Lynfield R, Cummings JJ; American Academy of Pediatrics, Committee on Fetus and Newborn, Committee on Infectious Diseases. Management of infants at risk for group B streptococcal disease. *Pediatrics*. 2019;144(2):e20191881

- For a **preterm infant hospitalized beyond 72 hours**, empiric treatment for sepsis should take into account the potential for health care-associated pathogens as well as coverage for pathogens associated with neonatal sepsis, including group B streptococci.
- When GBS infection is identified definitively, penicillin G or ampicillin is recommended. See Table 4.2 (p 988) in Tables of Antibacterial Drug Dosages for dosing recommendations.
- For meningitis, especially in the neonate, some experts recommend that a second lumbar puncture be performed approximately 24 to 48 hours after initiation of therapy to assist in management and prognosis. If CSF sterility is not achieved or if increasing protein concentration is noted, a complication (eg, cerebral infarcts, cerebritis, ventriculitis, subdural empyema, ventricular obstruction) is more likely. Additional lumbar punctures and intracranial imaging are indicated if neurologic abnormalities persist, or focal neurological deficits occur. A failed hearing screen or abnormal neurologic examination at discharge mandates careful clinical follow-up.
- For infants with **bacteremia without a defined focus** or with an **isolated urinary tract infection** without bacteremia, treatment typically is 10 days of intravenous therapy. On the basis of observational data suggesting that transition to oral therapy for the latter few days of treatment after clinical improvement on intravenous therapy (to complete a total of 10 days) may be effective, some pediatric infectious diseases experts have provided oral antibiotics for the last few days of treatment for low-risk patients with uncomplicated late-onset GBS bacteremia who had rapid clearance and clinical improvement and can be followed closely. For infants with uncomplicated **meningitis**, 14 days of intravenous therapy is recommended, with longer courses of treatment for infants with prolonged or complicated courses. **Septic arthritis or osteomyelitis** requires treatment for 3 to 4 weeks. Patients who have **endocarditis or ventriculitis** require intravenous treatment for at least 4 weeks. Consultation with a specialist in pediatric infectious diseases is recommended for complicated infections.
- Because of the reported increased risk of infection, the birth mates of a multiple-birth index case with EOD or LOD should be observed carefully for signs of infection and evaluated and treated empirically for suspected systemic infection if signs of illness occur. There is no evidence to support full antibiotic treatment courses in the absence of confirmed GBS disease.

INFECTION PREVENTION AND CONTROL MEASURES IN HEALTH CARE SETTINGS: Standard precautions are recommended. Routine cultures to determine whether infants are colonized with group B streptococci are not recommended.

CONTROL MEASURES:

Intrapartum Antibiotic Prophylaxis. Recommendations from the American Academy of Pediatrics[1] (**https://pediatrics.aappublications.org/content/144/2/e20191881**) and the American College of Obstetricians and Gynecology[2] (ACOG)

---

[1] Puopolo KM, Lynfield R, Cummings JJ; American Academy of Pediatrics, Committee on Fetus and Newborn, Committee on Infectious Diseases. Management of infants at risk for group B streptococcal disease. *Pediatrics.* 2019;144(2):e20191881

[2] American College of Obstetricians and Gynecologists. Prevention of group B streptococcal early-onset disease in newborns: ACOG Committee Opinion Number 797. *Obstet Gynecol.* 2020;135(2):e51-e72

(**www.acog.org/clinical/clinical-guidance/committee-opinion/articles/2020/02/prevention-of-group-b-streptococcal-early-onset-disease-in-newborns**) were published in 2019-2020. Components that are directly germane to the management of neonates at risk for GBS include the following:

- All pregnant people should have culture-based screening from vaginal and rectal sites at 36 0/7 to 37 6/7 weeks' gestation unless intrapartum antibiotic prophylaxis (IAP) for GBS infection is already planned because of predelivery risk factors in the pregnant person. For those who are at increased risk for a planned preterm delivery for medical indications, GBS screening within 5 weeks of anticipated delivery can be considered.
- For those who present with preterm labor, baseline GBS screening should be performed before intravenous GBS IAP is initiated.
- Intravenous penicillin G (5 million U initially, then 2.5 to 3.0 million U, every 4 hours, until delivery) is the preferred agent for GBS IAP because of its efficacy and narrow spectrum of antimicrobial activity. Intravenous ampicillin (2 g initially, then 1 g every 4 hours until delivery) can be used as an alternative when penicillin is unavailable. Oral or intramuscular antimicrobial agents should *not* be used as IAP. Pregnant people who report a mild or unknown penicillin allergy should receive intravenous cefazolin for IAP. Those who report penicillin allergies placing them at high risk for anaphylaxis should receive either intravenous clindamycin or vancomycin for IAP, depending on organism susceptibilities, with dosing detailed in the ACOG guidelines (**www.acog.org/clinical/clinical-guidance/committee-opinion/articles/2020/02/prevention-of-group-b-streptococcal-early-onset-disease-in-newborns**).
- Penicillin allergy testing is safe during pregnancy and can be considered for people with a history of allergy to penicillin to optimize the antibiotic choice for GBS IAP.
- For the purpose of newborn evaluation regardless of gestational age, "adequate" GBS IAP is defined as the administration of at least 1 dose of penicillin G, ampicillin, or cefazolin 4 or more hours prior to delivery. Available evidence suggests that administration of penicillin G, ampicillin, or cefazolin for periods of time <4 hours prior to delivery confers some level of protection from GBS EOD. Of note, in the Neonatal Early-Onset Sepsis Risk calculator, "GBS specific antibiotics >2 hours prior to birth" is one of the calculator variables. The 2-hour timing is used because multiple factors in addition to GBS IAP are considered when using these multivariate models.
- The ACOG recommendations updated in 2020 detail the indications for IAP, management of people with penicillin allergy, use of alternative agents, and management of people with preterm prelabor rupture of membranes, taking into account gestational age, presence of labor, and availability of GBS test results. See **www.acog.org/clinical/clinical-guidance/committee-opinion/articles/2020/02/prevention-of-group-b-streptococcal-early-onset-disease-in-newborns** for full discussion.

Management of Neonates at Risk for Early-Onset GBS Disease. Please refer to the AAP clinical report "Management of Infants at Risk for GBS Disease"[1] for detailed discussion. Recommendations include the following:

- Antimicrobial therapy is appropriate only for infants with suspected systemic infection.

[1] Puopolo KM, Lynfield R, Cummings JJ; American Academy of Pediatrics, Committee on Fetus and Newborn, Committee on Infectious Diseases. Management of infants at risk for group B streptococcal disease. *Pediatrics*. 2019;144(2):e20191881

FIG 3.16. RISK ASSESSMENT FOR EARLY-ONSET GROUP B STREPTOCOCCAL DISEASE AMONG INFANTS BORN AT ≥35 WEEKS OF GESTATION

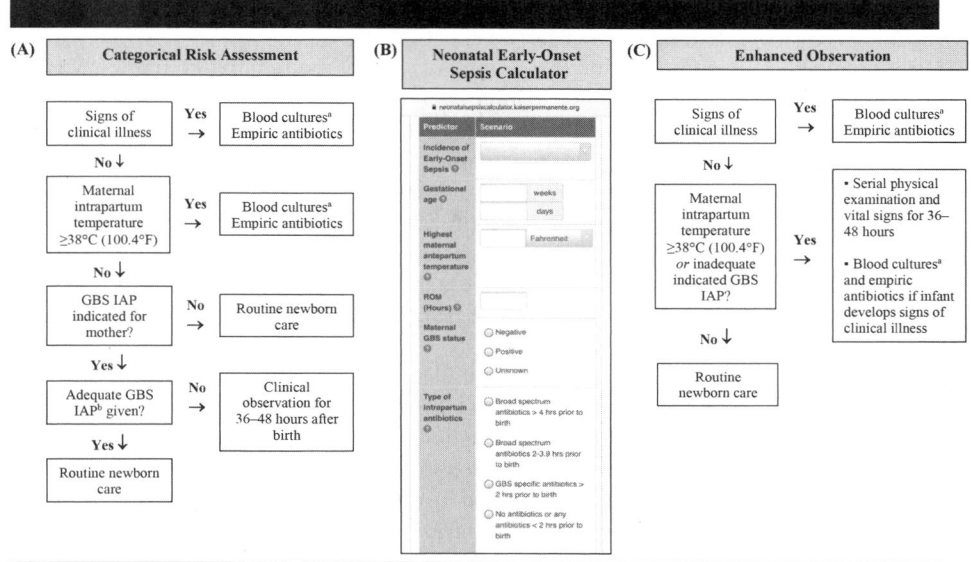

Reproduced from Puopolo KM, Lynfield R, Cummings JJ; American Academy of Pediatrics, Committee on Fetus and Newborn, Committee on Infectious Diseases. Management of infants at risk for group B streptococcal disease. *Pediatrics*. 2019;144(2):e20191881. The screenshot of the Neonatal Early-Onset Sepsis Calculator (**https://neonatalsepsiscalculator.kaiserpermanente.org/**) was used with permission from Kaiser-Permanente Division of Research.
[a]Perform lumbar puncture and CSF culture before initiation of empiric antibiotics for infants who are at the highest risk of infection, especially those with critical illness. Lumbar puncture can be deferred if the infant's clinical condition would be compromised, and antibiotics should be administered promptly and not deferred because of procedure delays.
[b]Adequate GBS IAP is defined as the administration of penicillin G, ampicillin, or cefazolin ≥4 hours before delivery.

- Routine use of antimicrobial chemoprophylaxis for neonates born to people who have received adequate IAP is *not* recommended. Early-onset GBS disease is diagnosed by blood or CSF culture. Lumbar puncture should be performed for culture and analysis of CSF when there is a high suspicion for early onset GBS disease. All cultures should include testing for antibiotic susceptibility. Complete blood cell counts and measurement of C-reactive protein are not accurate enough to reliably identify infected infants. Chest radiography and other studies should be performed as clinically indicated.
- Infants born at ≥35 weeks' gestation can be assessed for risk of early-onset sepsis using 1 of 3 methods: (1) a categorical algorithm, (2) a multivariate risk assessment, or (3) enhanced clinical observation (see Fig 3.16).
  - A categorical approach (Fig 3.16A) uses threshold values to identify infants at increased risk for GBS disease. Because thresholds are used, the risk will vary greatly among newborn infants recommended to undergo laboratory evaluation and receive empiric treatment, and it will include relatively low-risk newborn infants.
  - Multivariate risk assessment (Fig 3.16B, Neonatal Early-Onset Sepsis Calculator, and as an example: **https://neonatalsepsiscalculator.kaiserpermanente. org**) uses the individual infant's combination of risk factors for early-onset sepsis

(including maternal components) and the infant's clinical status to estimate the risk of early-onset sepsis, including risk for GBS disease. It provides recommended clinical actions, such as enhanced clinical observation or laboratory evaluation and empiric antibiotics, on the basis of predicted risk estimates. This tool has been prospectively validated in large newborn cohorts.

- Enhanced clinical observation (Fig 3.16C) is a risk assessment based on newborn clinical conditions. Good clinical condition at birth in term infants is associated with an approximately 60% to 70% reduction in risk for EOD of all infections, including GBS infection. Infants who appear ill at birth and those who develop signs of illness over the first 48 hours after birth will undergo laboratory evaluation and receive empiric antibiotics. This approach can be combined with a categorical or multivariate assessment for risk factors or used on its own for infants born at ≥35 weeks' gestation. Use of this approach requires processes to ensure serial and structured physical assessments and clear criteria for additional evaluation and empiric antibiotic administration.

- Infants born at ≤34 weeks' gestation are at higher risk for early-onset sepsis, including GBS sepsis, than are full-term infants. However, the risk varies and is dependent on several maternal, peripartum, and neonatal factors. Management is outlined in Fig 3.17, with additional summary provided in the bullets below.

  - Infants born preterm because of cervical insufficiency, preterm labor, prelabor rupture of membranes, intra-amniotic infection, and/or acute and otherwise unexplained onset of concerning fetal status are at the highest risk of early-onset sepsis, including from group B streptococci. The administration of GBS IAP can decrease this risk; however, these infants remain at high risk and a laboratory evaluation should be done and empiric antibiotics for pathogens causing early-onset sepsis, including group B streptococci, should be given. The most reasonable approach to these infants is to obtain a blood culture and start empiric antibiotic treatment. Lumbar puncture should be performed for culture and analysis of CSF when there is a high suspicion for early-onset GBS disease, unless the procedure will compromise the neonate's clinical condition.

  - Some infants born at ≤34 weeks' gestation are at much lower risk for early onset sepsis, including GBS sepsis, if they have *all* of the following: (1) delivery for indications in the birthing person (such as pre-eclampsia, other noninfectious medical illness, or placental insufficiency); (2) birthing parent not in labor; (3) no efforts to induce labor occurred; (4) rupture of membranes did not occur prior to delivery, and (5) delivery occurs by cesarean section. Acceptable initial approaches to these infants include (a) no laboratory evaluation and no empiric antibiotic therapy, or (b) blood culture and clinical monitoring. For infants who do not receive empiric antibiotics and do not improve after initial stabilization and/or those who have severe systemic instability, the administration of empiric antibiotics may be reasonable but is not mandatory, because infants can develop instability attributable to noninfectious factors.

  - Infants born at ≤34 weeks' gestation who are delivered for indications in the birthing person but who are ultimately born by vaginal or cesarean delivery after efforts to induce labor and/or with rupture of membranes before delivery are subject to factors associated with the pathogenesis of GBS EOD. If the birthing parent has an indication for GBS IAP, including a positive screen, and adequate IAP is

FIG 3.17. RISK ASSESSMENT FOR EARLY-ONSET GROUP B STREPTOCOCCAL DISEASE AMONG INFANTS BORN AT ≤34 WEEKS' GESTATION

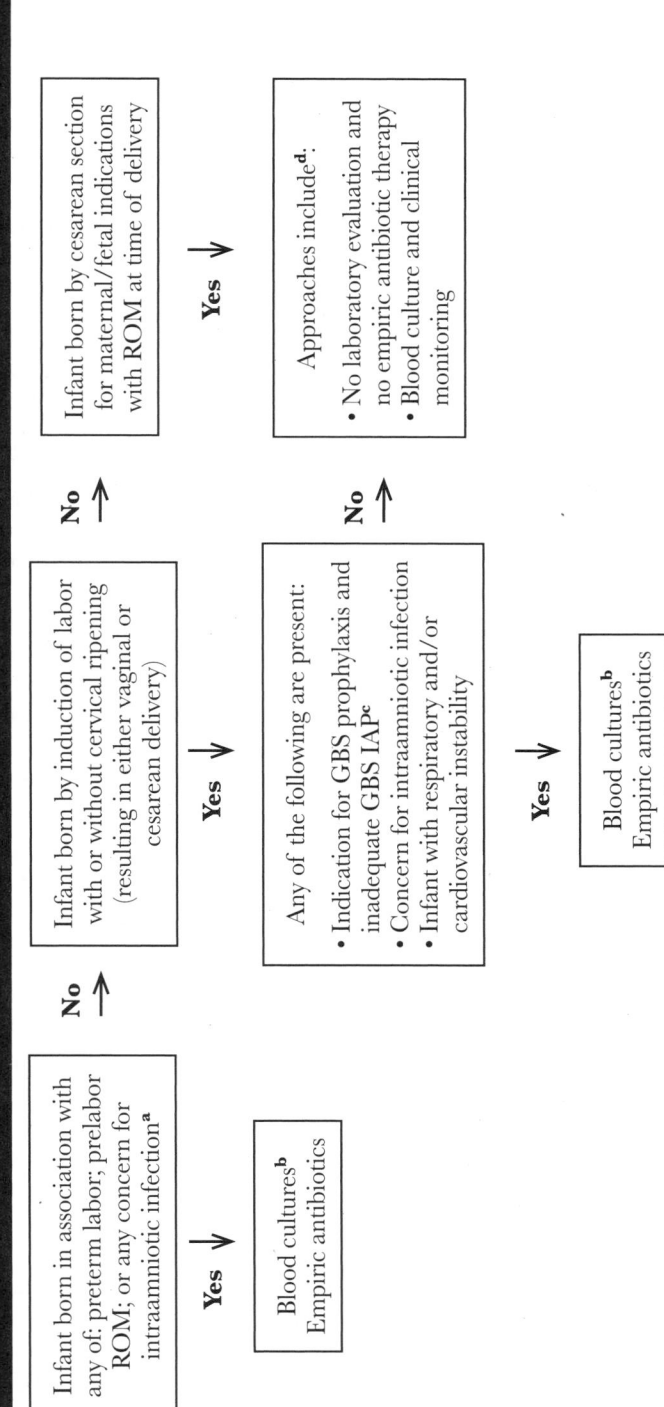

Adapted from Puopolo KM, Lynfield R, Cummings JJ; American Academy of Pediatrics, Committee on Infectious Diseases, Committee on Fetus and Newborn, Committee on Infectious Diseases. Management of infants at risk for group B streptococcal disease. *Pediatrics.* 2019;144(2):e20191881

[a] Intraamniotic infection should be considered when a pregnant person presents with unexplained decreased fetal movement and/or there is sudden and unexplained poor fetal testing.

[b] Lumbar puncture should be performed for culture and analysis of CSF when there is a high suspicion for early onset GBS disease, unless the procedure will compromise the neonate's clinical condition. Antibiotics should be administered promptly and not deferred because of procedural delays.

[c] Adequate GBS IAP is defined as the administration of penicillin G, ampicillin, or cefazolin ≥4 hours before delivery.

[d] For infants who do not improve after initial stabilization and/or those who have severe systemic instability, the administration of empiric antibiotics may be reasonable but is not mandatory.

not given or if any other concerns for infection occur during delivery, the infant should be managed as recommended for infants born at ≤34 weeks' gestation who are at highest risk for early-onset sepsis (see first bullet under "Infants born at ≤34 weeks' gestation"). If there are no concerns for infection based on birthing parent or delivery factors and these preterm infants are clinically well at birth, an acceptable approach is close observation, escalating to laboratory evaluation and empiric antibiotic therapy for infants with respiratory and/or cardiovascular instability after birth.

Late-Onset GBS Disease and Human Milk. Although there are case reports of human milk being a potential source of late-onset GBS disease, a recent multicenter case control study found no increased risk for late onset GBS with breastfeeding. The AAP does not recommend culturing human milk in an infant with late-onset GBS disease.

Non-Group A or B Streptococcal and Enterococcal Infections

CLINICAL MANIFESTATIONS: Streptococci other than Lancefield groups A or B can be associated with invasive disease in infants, children, adolescents, and adults. The principal clinical syndromes of groups C and G streptococci (most belong to the *Streptococcus dysgalactiae* group) are bacteremia, septicemia, upper and lower respiratory tract infections (eg, pharyngitis, sinusitis, and pneumonia), skin and soft tissue infections, septic arthritis, osteomyelitis, meningitis with a parameningeal focus, brain abscess, toxic shock syndrome, pericarditis, and endocarditis with various clinical manifestations. Viridans streptococci are the most common cause of bacterial endocarditis in children, especially children with congenital or valvular heart disease. Viridans streptococci are a common cause of bacteremia in neutropenic patients with cancer, especially following intensive induction chemotherapy for acute myeloid leukemia, after hematopoietic cell transplantation, and as a cause of central line-associated bacteremia. Among the viridans streptococci, group F streptococci (most belong to the *Streptococcus anginosus* group) are implicated in complicated sinus infections but are an infrequent cause of invasive infection. More serious *S anginosus* group infections include brain or dental abscesses or abscesses in other sites, including lymph nodes, liver, pelvis, and lung. These organisms may also cause sinusitis and other head and neck infections, meningitis, spondylodiskitis, spinal epidural abscesses, subdural empyema, peritonitis, complicated intra-abdominal infections, and cholangitis. Enterococci are associated with bacteremia in neonates and immunocompromised hosts, device-associated infections, intra-abdominal abscesses, and urinary tract infections in patients with anatomical anomalies.

ETIOLOGY: Changes in taxonomy and nomenclature of the *Streptococcus* genus have evolved with advances in molecular technology (see Table 3.66). Among gram-positive organisms that are catalase negative and display chains by Gram stain, the genera associated most often with human disease are *Streptococcus* and *Enterococcus.*

With the advent of genome sequencing, the genus *Streptococcus* has been divided, evolutionarily, into 2 major clades (Mitis-Suis and Pyogenes-Equinus-Mutans) and 14 subclades. Members of this genus that are beta-hemolytic on blood agar plates include *Streptococcus pyogenes* (see Group A Streptococcal Infections, p 785), *Streptococcus agalactiae* (see Group B Streptococcal Infections, p 799), groups C and G streptococci (*S dysgalactiae* subspecies *equisimilis* is the group C subspecies most often associated with human

Table 3.66. Classification of Streptococci Most Commonly Associated With Disease, by Lancefield Group and by Hemolysis

Species	Lancefield Group	Hemolysis
Streptococcus pyogenes	A	β
Streptococcus agalactiae	B	β
Streptococcus dysgalactiae subspecies *equisimilis*, *Streptococcus equi* subspecies *zooepidemicus*	C	β
Enterococcus faecalis, *Enterococcus faecium*, *Streptococcus gallolyticus*	D	α or γ[a]
Streptococcus canis	G	β
Streptococcus pneumoniae, viridans streptococci	Not groupable[b]	α

[a] Some *E faecalis* are β-hemolytic on horse blood agar but not sheep (the latter is more commonly used in clinical laboratories).
[b] Occasional viridans streptococci have variable hemolysis and can display Lancefield group A, C, F, or G antigens.

infections), and some members of Groups F and H streptococci. Streptococci that are non-beta–hemolytic (alpha-hemolytic or nonhemolytic) on blood agar plates include: (1) *Streptococcus pneumoniae* (see *Streptococcus pneumoniae* [Pneumococcal] Infections, p 810); (2) the *Streptococcus gallolyticus* (formerly *Streptococcus bovis*) group; and (3) viridans streptococci clinically relevant in humans, which include *S anginosus* group, *Streptococcus mitis* group, *Streptococcus sanguinis* group, *Streptococcus salivarius* group, and *Streptococcus mutans* group. The *anginosus* group (formerly *Streptococcus milleri* group) includes *S anginosus*, *Streptococcus constellatus*, and *Streptococcus intermedius*. This group can have variable hemolysis, and approximately one third possess Lancefield groups A, C, F, or G antigens. Nutritionally variant "streptococci," once believed to be viridans streptococci, now are classified in the genera *Abiotrophia* and *Granulicatella*. Group D streptococci include *S gallolyticus*, *Streptococcus infantarius*, and *Streptococcus pasteurianus*, now classified under the *S gallolyticus* group. Streptococci formerly classified as Lancefield groups R, S, and T are now known as *Streptococcus suis*.

The genus *Enterococcus* contains dozens of species, many of which have not been reported in humans, with *Enterococcus faecalis* and *Enterococcus faecium* accounting for most enterococcal infections in people. Outbreaks and health care-associated spread of intrinsically vancomycin-resistant enterococcal species including *Enterococcus gallinarum*, *Enterococcus casseliflavus*, or *Enterococcus flavescens* have occurred.

EPIDEMIOLOGY: The habitats that non-group A and B streptococci and enterococci occupy in humans include the skin (groups C and G), oropharynx (groups C and G and the *mutans* group), gastrointestinal tract (groups C and G streptococci, *S gallolyticus* group, and *Enterococcus* species), and vagina (groups C, D, and G streptococci and *Enterococcus* species). Typical human habitats of species of viridans streptococci are the oropharynx, epithelial surfaces of the oral cavity, teeth, skin, and gastrointestinal and genitourinary tracts. Intrapartum transmission is responsible for most cases of early-onset neonatal infection caused by non-group A and B streptococci and enterococci. Environmental contamination or transmission via hands of health care professionals can lead to colonization of patients. Groups C and G streptococci can cause food-borne outbreaks of pharyngitis. Zoonotic infection, specifically from *Streptococcus equi* subspecies *zooepidemicus* and rarely *S equi* subspecies *equi*, can result from animal contact or consumption of unpasteurized dairy products or other contaminated food products and has been associated with the development of poststreptococcal glomerulonephritis. *S suis* infections are associated with contact with pigs or raw pork.

The **incubation period** and the period of communicability are unknown.

DIAGNOSTIC TESTS: Diagnosis is established by culture of usually sterile body sites or abscesses with appropriate biochemical testing and serologic analysis for definitive identification. Mass spectrometry is unreliable in differentiation of *S pneumoniae* from viridians streptococci. Genomic methods are being used increasingly, particularly for rapid identification of positive blood cultures. Antimicrobial susceptibility testing of isolates from usually sterile sites should be performed to guide treatment of infections caused by viridans streptococci or enterococci. The proportion of vancomycin-resistant enterococci (VRE), the vast majority of which are *E faecium*, among health care-associated enterococcal infections is about 30%. Selective agars are available for screening of VRE from stool specimens. Molecular assays are available for direct detection of *vanA* and *vanB* genes (which confer vancomycin resistance) from rectal and blood specimens to identify VRE.

TREATMENT: Penicillin G is the drug of choice for groups C and G streptococci. Other agents with good activity include ampicillin, third- and fourth-generation cephalosporins, vancomycin, and linezolid. The combination of gentamicin (when high level resistance is not present) with a beta-lactam antimicrobial agent (eg, penicillin or ampicillin) or vancomycin may enhance the antimicrobial activity needed for treatment of life-threatening infections (eg, endocarditis or meningitis).

Many viridans streptococci remain susceptible to penicillin (minimum inhibitory concentration [MIC] ≤0.12 μg/mL). Infections caused by strains susceptible to penicillin, including endocarditis, can be treated with penicillin or ceftriaxone. Strains with an MIC >0.12 μg/mL and <0.5 μg/mL are considered relatively resistant to penicillin by criteria in the American Heart Association guidelines for treatment of infective endocarditis in childhood.[1] In this situation, penicillin, ampicillin, or ceftriaxone for 4 weeks, combined for the first 2 weeks with gentamicin, is recommended. Strains with a penicillin MIC ≥0.5 μg/mL are considered resistant. Nonpenicillin antimicrobial agents with good activity against viridans streptococci include cephalosporins (especially ceftriaxone), vancomycin, linezolid, and tigecycline, although pediatric experience with tigecycline is limited. Tigecycline also has a black box warning for an increase in all-cause mortality and should be reserved for situations where alternative agents are not suitable. *Abiotrophia* and *Granulicatella* organisms can exhibit relative or high-level resistance to penicillin. The combination of high-dose penicillin or vancomycin and an aminoglycoside can enhance treatment effectiveness. Some species of viridans streptococci (eg, *Streptococcus oralis*, *S mitis*, *S sanguinis*) have shown unexpected, rapid (eg, overnight) in vitro and/or in vivo development of high-level resistance to daptomycin (MIC ≥256 μg/mL), and therefore, daptomycin should be avoided for treatment of infections by these organisms.

---

[1] Baltimore RS, Gewitz M, Baddour LM, et al. Infective endocarditis in childhood: 2015 update. A scientific statement from the American Heart Association. *Circulation.* 2015;132(15):1487-1515

Enterococci exhibit intrinsic resistance to cephalosporins, aztreonam, and anti-staphylococcal penicillins. Most are intrinsically resistant to clindamycin and trime-thoprim-sulfamethoxazole even if in vitro susceptibility indicates otherwise. The vast majority of *E faecalis* strains are susceptible to ampicillin (which can be extrapolated to amoxicillin, piperacillin-tazobactam, and imipenem but not to penicillin). *E faecium* strains may be multidrug resistant. Two types of vancomycin resistance are identified: intrinsic low-level resistance that occurs with *E gallinarum* and *E casseliflavus/E flavescens* (these species are ampicillin susceptible), and acquired resistance, which has been seen in *E faecium* and some *E faecalis* strains but also has been recognized in *Enterococcus raffinosus*, *Enterococcus avium*, and *Enterococcus durans*.

Systemic enterococcal infections, such as endocarditis or meningitis, should be treated with penicillin or ampicillin (if the isolate is susceptible) combined with ceftri-axone or gentamicin (see endocarditis guidelines[1]). Vancomycin plus an aminoglyco-side (with appropriate monitoring of renal function) is suggested for patients unable to tolerate penicillins and who cannot be desensitized. Studies have established ampicillin plus ceftriaxone as equivalent to ampicillin plus gentamicin for *E faecalis* endocarditis. Some experts consider ampicillin plus both ceftriaxone and gentamicin for treatment of enterococcal meningitis, although clinical data are lacking. Gentamicin should not be used if in vitro susceptibility testing demonstrates high-level resistance.

Combination therapy for treating central line-associated bloodstream infections is usually not needed. Options for treatment of other systemic infections caused by vancomycin-resistant *E faecium* include linezolid or daptomycin. Linezolid is approved for use in children, including neonates. Isolates of VRE that are resistant to linezolid have been described, and resistance can develop during prolonged linezolid treatment. Most vancomycin-resistant isolates of *E faecalis* and *E faecium* are daptomycin-suscepti-ble. Data suggest that clearance of daptomycin is more rapid in young children com-pared with adolescents and adults, and dosing may need to be adjusted accordingly. Daptomycin should not be used to treat meningitis or pneumonia, as penetration into cerebrospinal fluid is poor and daptomycin is inactivated by pulmonary surfactants. Microbiologic and clinical cure have been reported in children infected with vanco-mycin-resistant *E faecium* who were treated with quinupristin-dalfopristin. This drug frequently causes phlebitis in peripheral intravenous lines, and pediatric dosing in chil-dren younger than 12 years is unclear. Tigecycline is approved for use in adults with complicated skin and skin structure infections or intra-abdominal infections caused by vancomycin-susceptible *E faecalis*. Tigecycline has activity against both vancomycin-resistant *E faecalis* and vancomycin-resistant *E faecium*, but experience with this drug in children is limited. In children younger than 8 years, there may be reversible inhibition of bone growth and adverse effects on tooth development. Tigecycline has a black box warning for an increase in all-cause mortality and should be reserved for situations where alternative agents are not suitable.

INFECTION PREVENTION AND CONTROL MEASURES IN HEALTH CARE SETTINGS: Standard precautions are recommended. For patients with infection or coloniza-tion attributable to VRE, contact precautions in addition to standard precautions are indicated. Patients harboring vancomycin resistant strains of *E gallinarum* or *E*

---

[1] Baltimore RS, Gewitz M, Baddour LM, et al. Infective endocarditis in childhood: 2015 update. A scientific statement from the American Heart Association. *Circulation*. 2015;132(15):1487-1515

casseliflavus/ E flavescens may be managed using only standard precautions, because these species harbor chromosomally encoded vancomycin resistance genes *(vanC, vanT)* that are not easily exchanged between bacterial populations. Common practice is to maintain precautions until the patient no longer harbors the organism or is discharged from the health care facility. Some experts recommend discontinuation of contact precautions if screening cultures are negative; there is, however, no accepted standard regarding the frequency (1, 2, or 3 cultures), timing (weekly, daily), or preferred site selection (eg, stool, axilla, etc).[1]

CONTROL MEASURES: Use of vancomycin and treatment with broad-spectrum antimicrobial agents are risk factors for colonization and infection with VRE. Hospitals should develop institution-specific guidelines for the appropriate use of vancomycin.

Patients with a prosthetic valve or prosthetic material used for cardiac valve repair, previous infective endocarditis, or congenital heart disease associated with the highest risk of adverse outcome from endocarditis should receive antimicrobial prophylaxis to prevent endocarditis at the time of certain dental procedures (see Prevention of Bacterial Endocarditis, p 1127). For these patients, early instruction in proper diet; oral health, including use of dental sealants and adequate fluoride intake; and prevention or cessation of smoking will aid in prevention of dental caries and potentially will lower their risk of recurrent endocarditis.

Streptococcus pneumoniae (Pneumococcal) Infections[2]

CLINICAL MANIFESTATIONS: *Streptococcus pneumoniae* is a common bacterial cause of acute otitis media, sinusitis, community-acquired pneumonia, and pediatric conjunctivitis; pleural empyema, mastoiditis, and periorbital cellulitis also occur. It is the most common cause of bacterial meningitis in infants and children ages 2 months to 11 years in the United States. *S pneumoniae* also may cause endocarditis, pericarditis, peritonitis, pyogenic arthritis, osteomyelitis, soft tissue infection, and neonatal septicemia. Overwhelming septicemia in patients with splenic dysfunction occurs, and hemolytic-uremic syndrome can accompany pneumococcal infection.

ETIOLOGY: *S pneumoniae* organisms (pneumococci) are lancet-shaped, gram-positive, catalase-negative diplococci. They are α-hemolytic (Table 3.66, p 807). More than 100 pneumococcal serotypes have been identified on the basis of unique polysaccharide capsules.

EPIDEMIOLOGY: Nasopharyngeal carriage rates in children range from 21% in industrialized settings to more than 90% in resource-limited settings. Transmission is from person to person by respiratory droplet contact. Viral upper respiratory tract infections, including influenza and respiratory syncytial virus, can predispose to pneumococcal infection and transmission. Pneumococcal infections are most prevalent during winter months. The period of communicability is unknown and may be as long as the

---

[1] Banach DB, Bearman G, Barnden M, et al. Duration of contact precautions for acute-care settings. *Infect Control Hosp Epidemiol.* 2018;39(2):127-144

[2] Centers for Disease Control and Prevention. Prevention of pneumococcal disease among infants and children—use of 13-valent pneumococcal conjugate vaccine and 23-valent pneumococcal polysaccharide vaccine. *MMWR Recomm Rep.* 2010;59(RR-11):1-18

organism is present in respiratory tract secretions but probably is less than 24 hours after effective antimicrobial therapy is begun.

The incidence and severity of infections are increased in people with congenital or acquired humoral immunodeficiency, human immunodeficiency virus (HIV) infection, absent or deficient splenic function (eg, sickle cell disease, congenital, or surgical asplenia), certain complement deficiencies, diabetes mellitus, chronic liver disease, chronic renal failure, nephrotic syndrome, or abnormal innate immune responses. Children with cochlear implants, particularly those who had placement of an older model that involved a cochlear electrode, have high rates of pneumococcal meningitis, as do children with congenital or acquired cerebrospinal fluid (CSF) leaks.[1] Children at presumed high or moderate risk of developing invasive pneumococcal disease are listed by underlying medical condition in Table 3.67. Infection rates are highest in infants, young children, elderly people, and in Black, Alaska Native, and some American Indian populations. Since introduction of the heptavalent pneumococcal conjugate vaccine (PCV7) in 2000 and the 13-valent pneumococcal conjugate vaccine (PCV13) in 2010, racial disparities in vaccine-type pneumococcal disease have diminished; however, rates of invasive pneumococcal disease (IPD) among some Alaskan Native and American Indian populations remain higher than the rate among children in the general US population. Recent data from Alaska and the southwestern United States indicate that the majority of IPD cases among American Indian/Alaska Native children are now caused by serotypes not contained in the PCV13 vaccine.

By 2019, 9 years after the introduction of PCV13, the incidence of PCV13-type invasive pneumococcal infections decreased by 98% compared with incidence before introduction of PCV7, and the incidence of all IPD decreased by 95% in children younger than 5 years. In adults 65 years and older, IPD caused by PCV13 serotypes decreased 86% compared with pre-PCV7 baseline, and all IPD decreased by 61%. Most of the reduction in cases in this latter group occurred before routine PCV13 use was recommended in 2014 for older adults, indicating the significant indirect (ie, herd effect) benefits of PCV13 immunization achieved by interruption of transmission of pneumococci from vaccinated children to adults. Although *S pneumoniae* strains that are nonsusceptible to penicillin G, ceftriaxone, and other antimicrobial agents have been identified throughout the United States and worldwide, a reduction in the proportion of isolates that are penicillin-nonsusceptible (intermediate or resistant) and ceftriaxone-resistant has been observed since introduction of PCV7 and PCV13.

The **incubation period** varies by type of infection but can be as short as 1 day.

DIAGNOSTIC TESTS: Recovery of *S pneumoniae* from a normally sterile site confirms the diagnosis. The finding of lancet-shaped gram-positive organisms and white blood cells in expectorated sputum (older children and adults) or pleural exudate suggests pneumococcal pneumonia. Recovery of pneumococci by culture of an upper respiratory tract swab specimen is not sufficient to assign an etiologic diagnosis of pneumococcal disease involving the middle ear, upper or lower respiratory tract, or sinus.

There are at least 2 multiplexed nucleic acid amplification tests (NAATs) cleared by the US Food and Drug Administration (FDA) to identify *S pneumoniae* and other

---

[1] American Academy of Pediatrics, Committee on Infectious Diseases. Policy statement: cochlear implants in children: surgical site infections and prevention and treatment of acute otitis media and meningitis. *Pediatrics.* 2010;126(2):381-391

Table 3.67. Underlying Medical Conditions That Are Indications for Immunization With 23-Valent Pneumococcal Polysaccharide Vaccine (PPSV23)[a] or PCV20 Among Children, by Risk Group[b,c,d]

Risk group	Condition
Immunocompetent children	Chronic heart disease[e]
	Chronic kidney disease (excluding maintenance dialysis and nephrotic syndrome)
	Chronic liver disease
	Chronic lung disease[f]
	Diabetes mellitus
	Cerebrospinal fluid leaks
	Cochlear implant
Children with immunocompromising conditions	On maintenance dialysis or nephrotic syndrome
	Congenital or acquired asplenia or splenic dysfunction
	Congenital or acquired immunodeficiencies
	HIV infection
	Diseases and conditions treated with treatment with immunosuppressive drugs or radiation therapy, including malignant neoplasms, leukemias, lymphomas, and Hodgkin disease; or solid organ transplantation
	Sickle cell disease and other hemoglobinopathies
	Congenital immunodeficiency[g]

[a] PPSV23 may be used in people ≥24 months of age.

[b] Centers for Disease Control and Prevention. Licensure of a 13-valent pneumococcal conjugate vaccine (PCV13) and recommendations for use among children. Advisory Committee on Immunization Practices (ACIP). *MMWR Morb Mortal Wkly Rep*. 2010;59(9):258-261; and Centers for Disease Control and Prevention. Use of 13-valent pneumococcal conjugate vaccine and 23-valent pneumococcal polysaccharide vaccine among children aged 6-18 years with immunocompromising conditions: recommendation of the ACIP. *MMWR Morb Mortal Wkly Rep*. 2013;62(25):521-524

[c] Kobayashi M, Farrar JI, Gierke R, et al. Use of 15-valent pneumococcal conjugate vaccine among US children: updated recommendations of the Advisory Committee on Immunization Practices—United States, 2022. *MMWR Morb Mortal Wkly Rep*. 2022;71(4):1174-1181

[d] ACIP Updates: Recommendations for use of 20-valent pneumococcal conjugate vaccine in children—United States, 2023. *MMWR Morb Mortal Wkly Rep*. 2023;72(39):1072

[e] Particularly cyanotic congenital heart disease and cardiac failure.

[f] Including moderate persistent or severe persistent asthma.

[g] Includes B- (humoral) or T-lymphocyte deficiency; complement deficiencies, particularly C_1, C_2, C_3, and C_4 deficiency; and phagocytic disorders (excluding chronic granulomatous disease).

bacterial and fungal pathogens from positive blood culture bottles. At least 1 real-time polymerase chain reaction (PCR) assay is cleared by the FDA for detection of *S pneumoniae* in CSF. The assay is a multiplexed PCR designed to detect a number of agents of bacterial, fungal, and viral meningitis or encephalitis. PCR testing should be accompanied by culture of CSF to obtain an isolate, which is needed for antimicrobial susceptibility testing.

Detection of C-polysaccharide (common to all pneumococci) in urine for diagnosis of pneumococcal pneumonia may have some utility in adults but is generally not useful in children, because asymptomatically colonized children may have positive test results. Similarly, commercially available antigen detection tests performed on CSF or blood are not recommended for routine use because of low sensitivity.

Susceptibility Testing. All *S pneumoniae* isolates from normally sterile body fluids should be tested for antimicrobial susceptibility to determine the minimum inhibitory concentration (MIC) of penicillin, cefotaxime or ceftriaxone, and clindamycin. Susceptibility threshold breakpoints of *S pneumoniae* isolated from blood differ for CSF isolates (Table 3.68) as defined by the Clinical and Laboratory Standards Institute (CLSI). CSF isolates also should be tested for susceptibility to vancomycin, meropenem, and rifampin. Nonsusceptible strains can also be evaluated for susceptibility to erythromycin, trimethoprim-sulfamethoxazole, levofloxacin, and linezolid to treat various pneumococcal infections.

TREATMENT:

Bacterial Meningitis Possibly or Proven to Be Caused by S pneumoniae. For children with bacterial meningitis possibly or known to be caused by *S pneumoniae*, vancomycin should be administered in addition to third-generation cephalosporin because of the possibility of *S pneumoniae* organisms that are nonsusceptible to penicillin and third-generation cephalosporins. In neonates, when cefotaxime is not available then ceftazidime or cefepime can be used in addition to vancomycin. Vancomycin should be stopped if susceptibility to third-generation cephalosporins is documented (using central nervous system [CNS] breakpoints for thresholds of susceptibility, as defined in Table 3.68), if another

Table 3.68. Minimum Inhibitory Concentration Breakpoints (µg/mL) for *Streptococcus pneumoniae*, by Susceptibility Category, as per the Clinical and Laboratory Standards Institute

	Susceptibility category MIC (µg/mL)		
	Susceptible	Intermediate	Resistant
PENICILLIN			
Breakpoints (by clinical syndrome and administered route)			
Nonmeningitis, oral penicillin	≤0.06	0.12–1	≥2
Nonmeningitis, IV penicillin	≤2	4	≥8
Meningitis, IV penicillin	≤0.06	—	≥0.12
CEFOTAXIME OR CEFTRIAXONE			
Breakpoints (by clinical syndrome and administered route)			
Nonmeningitis	≤1	2	≥4
Meningitis	<0.5	1	≥2

IV indicates intravenous; MIC, minimal inhibitory concentration; —, no intermediate category for meningitis.

From Clinical and Laboratory Standards Institute (CLSI). Performance Standards for Antimicrobial Testing; 29th Informational Supplement. Wayne, PA: Clinical and Laboratory Standards Institute; 2019. CLSI document M100-S29.

organism not requiring vancomycin is identified, or if the CSF culture is negative. Antibiotic dosing recommendations for meningitis are included in Tables 4.2, p 988 (neonatal), and 4.3, p 993 (nonneonatal), in Tables of Antibacterial Drug Dosages. If the *S pneumoniae* isolate is nonsusceptible to penicillin or third-generation cephalosporins, treatment options are provided in Table 3.69. Consultation with an infectious diseases specialist should be considered for all children with bacterial meningitis.

For children with serious proven hypersensitivity reactions to third- or fourth-generation cephalosporins, a pediatric infectious diseases specialist should be consulted for consideration of use of vancomycin plus either meropenem or rifampin.

A repeat lumbar puncture should be considered after 48 hours of therapy in the following circumstances:
• The organism is penicillin nonsusceptible by oxacillin disk or quantitative (MIC) testing, and results from cefotaxime and ceftriaxone quantitative susceptibility testing are not yet available or the isolate is cefotaxime and ceftriaxone nonsusceptible; or
• The patient's condition has not improved or has worsened; or
• The child has received dexamethasone, which can interfere with the ability to interpret the clinical response, such as resolution of fever.

Dexamethasone. For infants and children 6 weeks and older, adjunctive therapy with dexamethasone may be considered after weighing the potential benefits and risks. Some experts recommend use of corticosteroids in pneumococcal meningitis, but this

Table 3.69. Antimicrobial Therapy for Infants and Children With Meningitis Caused by *Streptococcus pneumoniae* on the Basis of Susceptibility Test Results, as Defined in Table 3.68

Susceptibility Test Results	Antimicrobial Management[a]
Susceptible to penicillin	Discontinue vancomycin **AND EITHER** Continue cefotaxime or ceftriaxone alone[b] **OR** Begin penicillin (and discontinue cephalosporin)
Nonsusceptible to penicillin (*intermediate* or *resistant*) **AND** *Susceptible* to cefotaxime and ceftriaxone	Discontinue vancomycin **AND** Continue cefotaxime or ceftriaxone
Nonsusceptible to penicillin (*intermediate* or *resistant*) **AND** *Nonsusceptible* to cefotaxime and ceftriaxone (*intermediate* or *resistant*) **AND** *Susceptible* to rifampin	Continue vancomycin and high-dose cefotaxime or ceftriaxone **AND** Rifampin may be added in selected circumstances (see text)

[a]Initial empiric therapy of nonallergic children older than 1 month of age with presumed bacterial meningitis should be vancomycin and cefotaxime or ceftriaxone. For dosages, see Tables 4.2, p 988 (neonatal), and 4.3, p 993 (nonneonatal), in Tables of Antibacterial Drug Dosages. Some experts recommend the maximum dosages.
[b]Some physicians may choose this alternative for convenience but only in treatment of meningitis.

issue is controversial and data are not sufficient to make a routine recommendation for children. The Infectious Diseases Society of America recommends use of dexamethasone in adults with suspected or proven pneumococcal meningitis. If used, dexamethasone should be administered before or concurrently with the first dose of parenteral antimicrobial agents.

Nonmeningeal Invasive Pneumococcal Infections Requiring Hospitalization. For nonmeningeal invasive infections in previously healthy children who are not critically ill, antimicrobial agents that treat infections with *S pneumoniae* and other potential pathogens should be initiated at the usually recommended dosages (see Tables 4.2, p 988 [neonatal], and 4.3, p 993 [nonneonatal], in Tables of Antibacterial Drug Dosages).

For critically ill infants and children with invasive infections potentially attributable to *S pneumoniae*, vancomycin, in addition to empiric antimicrobial therapy (eg, cefotaxime or ceftriaxone or others), can be considered. Such patients include those with presumed septic shock, severe pneumonia with empyema, or significant hypoxia or myopericardial involvement. If vancomycin is administered, it should be discontinued as soon as antimicrobial susceptibility test results demonstrate effective alternative agents.

If the organism has in vitro nonsusceptibility to penicillin, cefotaxime, and ceftriaxone according to guidelines of the CLSI (see Table 3.68), therapy should be modified on the basis of clinical response, susceptibility to other antimicrobial agents, and results of follow-up cultures of blood and other infected body fluids. Consultation with an infectious diseases specialist should be considered.

For children with severe hypersensitivity to beta-lactam antimicrobial agents (ie, penicillins and cephalosporins), initial management should include vancomycin or clindamycin, in addition to antimicrobial agents for other potential pathogens, as indicated. Vancomycin should not be continued if the organism is susceptible to other appropriate non–beta-lactam antimicrobial agents. Consultation with an infectious diseases specialist should be considered.

Acute Otitis Media.[1] According to clinical practice guidelines of the American Academy of Pediatrics (AAP) and the American Academy of Family Physicians (AAFP) on acute suppurative otitis media (AOM), amoxicillin (80–90 mg/kg/day) is recommended for infants younger than 6 months, for those 6 through 23 months of age with bilateral disease, and for those older than 6 months with severe signs and symptoms (see *Haemophilus influenzae* Infections, p 400, and Appropriate and Judicious Use of Antimicrobial Agents, p 978). A watch-and-wait option can be considered for older children and those with nonsevere disease. Optimal duration of therapy is uncertain. For younger children and children with severe disease at any age, a 10-day course is recommended; for children 6 years and older with mild or moderate disease, a duration of 5 to 7 days is appropriate. Otalgia should be treated symptomatically.

Patients who fail to respond to initial management should be reassessed at 48 to 72 hours to confirm the diagnosis of AOM and exclude other causes of illness. If AOM is confirmed in the patient managed initially with observation, amoxicillin should be administered. If initial antibacterial therapy has failed, a change in antibacterial agent is indicated. Suitable alternative agents should be active

---

[1] Lieberthal AS, Carroll AE, Chonmaitree T, et al. Clinical practice guideline: diagnosis and management of acute otitis media. *Pediatrics.* 2013;131(3):e964-e999

against penicillin-nonsusceptible pneumococci as well as beta-lactamase–producing *Haemophilus influenzae* and *Moraxella catarrhalis*. Such agents include high-dose oral amoxicillin-clavulanate; oral cefdinir, cefpodoxime, or cefuroxime; or once-daily doses of intramuscular ceftriaxone for 3 consecutive days. Macrolide resistance in *S pneumoniae* is common, so clarithromycin and azithromycin are not considered appropriate alternatives for initial therapy even in patients with a type I (immediate, anaphylactic) reaction to a beta-lactam agent. In such cases, treatment with clindamycin (if susceptibility is known) or levofloxacin is preferred. For patients with a history of non-type I allergic reaction to penicillin, agents such as cefdinir, cefuroxime, or cefpodoxime can be used orally.

Myringotomy or tympanocentesis should be considered for children failing to respond to second-line therapy, for severe cases to obtain cultures to guide therapy, and for patients with invasive pneumococcal infection. For multidrug-resistant strains of *S pneumoniae*, use of levofloxacin or other agents should be considered in consultation with an infectious diseases specialist and based on the specific susceptibility profile.

Sinusitis. Antimicrobial agents effective for treatment of AOM also are likely to be effective for acute sinusitis and are recommended when a child meets clinical criteria for diagnosis.

Pneumonia.[1] Oral amoxicillin at a dose of 45 mg/kg/day in 3 equally divided doses or 90 mg/kg/day in 2 divided portions is likely to be effective in ambulatory children with pneumonia caused by susceptible and relatively resistant pneumococci, respectively. Intravenous ampicillin by intermittent dosing or penicillin by continuous infusion is recommended for therapy of hospitalized cases caused by penicillin-susceptible strains. Cefotaxime or ceftriaxone is recommended for treatment of inpatients infected with pneumococci suspected or proven to be penicillin-nonsusceptible strains, for serious infections including empyema, or in those not fully immunized with PCV13 or the more recently licensed 15-valent or 20-valent pneumococcal conjugate vaccines (PCV15 and PCV20, respectively). Vancomycin should be included in those with life-threatening infection. For patients with isolates nonsusceptible to penicillin (MICs of 4.0 µg/mL or higher; see Table 3.68) or significant allergy to beta-lactam antimicrobials, treatment with clindamycin (if susceptible) or levofloxacin should be considered, assuming that concurrent meningitis has been excluded.

INFECTION PREVENTION AND CONTROL MEASURES IN HEALTH CARE SETTINGS: Standard precautions are recommended, including for patients with infections caused by drug-resistant *S pneumoniae*.

CONTROL MEASURES:

Active Immunization. Four pneumococcal vaccines are available for use in children in the United States: 3 pneumococcal conjugate vaccines (PCV13, PCV15, and PCV20), and 1 pneumococcal polysaccharide vaccine (the 23-valent PPSV23). PCV13, PCV15, and PCV20 are licensed for use in infants and children 6 weeks and older as well as in adults. PCV13 is composed of 13 purified capsular polysaccharide serotypes (1, 3, 4, 5, 6A, 6B, 7F, 9V, 14, 18C, 19A, 19F, and 23F). PCV15 contains all PCV13 serotypes plus serotypes 22F and 33F. PCV20 contains all PCV15 serotypes plus serotypes 8,

---

[1] Bradley JS, Byington CL, Shah SS, et al. The management of community-acquired pneumonia in infants and children older than 3 months of age: clinical practice guidelines by the Pediatric Infectious Diseases Society and the Infectious Diseases Society of America. *Clin Infect Dis.* 2011;53(7):e25–e76

10A, 11A, 12F, and 15B. PPSV23 is licensed for use in children 2 years and older and adults. PPSV23 is composed of 23 capsular polysaccharides, including all of those in PCV13, PCV15, and PCV20 except 6A. PPSV23 is available in single or multidose vials and single-dose prefilled syringes that do not contain latex. Each available vaccine is recommended in a dose of 0.5 mL to be administered intramuscularly. In contrast to immunization with PCV13, PCV15, and PCV20, immunization with PPSV23 does not induce immunologic memory or boosting with subsequent doses, has no effects on nasopharyngeal carriage, and therefore, does not interrupt transmission and indirectly protect unimmunized people.

Routine Immunization With Pneumococcal Conjugate Vaccine. PCV15 or PCV20 is recommended for all infants and children 2 through 59 months of age. There is no preference for one of these vaccines over the other. For infants, the vaccine should be administered at 2, 4, 6, and 12 through 15 months of age; catch-up immunization is recommended for all children 59 months of age or younger (Table 3.70). Infants should begin the PCV15 or PCV20 immunization series in conjunction with other recommended vaccines at the time of the first regularly scheduled health maintenance visit after 6 weeks of age. Infants of very low birth weight (1500 g or less) should be immunized when they attain a chronologic age of 6 to 8 weeks, regardless of their gestational age at birth. PCV15 or PCV20 can be administered concurrently with all other age-appropriate childhood immunizations (except PPSV23 and MenACWY-D [Menactra], see General Recommendations for Use of Pneumococcal Vaccines, below) using a separate syringe and a separate injection site.

Immunization of Children Under 6 Years of Age Who Are Unimmunized or Incompletely Immunized With PCV13, PCV15, or PCV20. For healthy children 2 through 59 months of age with an incomplete PCV vaccination status, use of either PCV15 or PCV20 according to the currently recommended dosing and schedules is recommended (see Table 3.70). For all children 2 through 71 months who are at high risk or presumed high risk of acquiring invasive pneumococcal infection, as defined in Table 3.67 (p 812), the recommended use of PCV15, PCV20, and PPSV23 is outlined in Table 3.71 (p 819).

Immunization of Children 6 Through 18 Years of Age With High-Risk Conditions Who Have Not Received Any Dose of PCV.[1-3]
For children 6 through 18 years of age who previously have not received PCV13, PCV15, or PCV20 and who are at increased risk of IPD because of a high-risk condition (defined in Table 3.67, p 812), administration of a single PCV15 or PCV20 dose is recommended. When PCV15 is used, it should be followed by either a dose of PCV20 or a dose of PPSV23 at least 8 weeks later.

---

[1] Centers for Disease Control and Prevention. Use of 13-valent pneumococcal conjugate vaccine and 23-valent pneumococcal polysaccharide vaccine among children aged 6–18 years with immunocompromising conditions: recommendations of the Advisory Committee on Immunization Practices (ACIP). *MMWR Morb Mortal Wkly Rep.* 2013;62(25):521-524

[2] Kobayashi M, Farrar JI, Gierke R, et al. Use of 15-valent pneumococcal conjugate vaccine among U.S. children: updated recommendations of the Advisory Committee on Immunization Practices—United States, 2022. *MMWR Morb Mortal Wkly Rep.* 2022;71(4):1174-1181

[3] ACIP Updates: Recommendations for use of 20-valent pneumococcal conjugate vaccine in children—United States, 2023. *MMWR Morb Mortal Wkly Rep.* 2023;72(39):1072

Table 3.70. Recommended Schedule for Doses of PCV15 or PCV20, Including Catch-up Immunizations, for Previously Unimmunized and Partially Immunized Children 2 Through 59 Months of Age

Age at Examination	Immunization History	Recommended Regimen[a,b,c,d]
2 through 6 mo	0 doses	4 doses: 3 doses, 8 wk apart; fourth dose at age 12–15 mo
	1 dose	3 additional doses: 2 doses, 8 wk apart; last dose at age 12–15 mo
	2 doses	2 additional doses: 1 dose 8 wk after most recent dose; last dose ≥8 wk later at age 12–15 mo
	3 doses	1 additional dose at age 12–15 mo
7 through 11 mo	0 doses	3 doses: 2 doses, ≥4 wk apart; third dose ≥8 wk later at age 12–15 mo
	1 or 2 doses (at age <7 mo)	2 additional doses: 1 dose 8 wk after most recent dose; last dose ≥8 wk later at age 12–15 mo
	3 doses (at age <7 mo)	1 additional dose at age 12–15 mo
	1 dose (at age ≥7 mo)	2 additional doses: 1 dose 8 wk after most recent dose; last dose ≥8 wk later at age 12–15 mo
	2 doses (at age ≥7 mo)	1 additional dose at age 12–15 mo
12 through 23 mo	0 doses	2 doses, ≥8 wk apart
	1 dose (at age <12 mo)	2 additional doses: 1 dose ≥8 wk after most recent dose; last dose ≥8 wk later
	1 dose (at ≥12 mo)	1 additional dose, ≥8 wk after most recent dose
	2 or 3 doses (at <12 mo)	1 additional dose, ≥8 wk after most recent dose
24 through 59 mo[e] Healthy children	Any incomplete schedule	1 dose, ≥8 wk after the most recent dose[e]

PCV15 indicates 15-valent pneumococcal conjugate vaccine. PCV20 indicates 20-valent pneumococcal conjugate vaccine.

[a]For children immunized at younger than 12 months, the minimum interval between doses is 4 weeks. Doses administered at 12 months or older should be at least 8 weeks apart.

[b]Centers for Disease Control and Prevention. Licensure of a 13-valent pneumococcal conjugate vaccine (PCV13) and recommendations for use among children. Advisory Committee on Immunization Practices (ACIP). *MMWR Morb Mortal Wkly Rep.* 2010;59(RR-11):1-18.

[c]Kobayashi M, Farrar JI, Gierke R, et al. Use of 15-valent pneumococcal conjugate vaccine among US children: updated recommendations of the Advisory Committee on Immunization Practices—United States, 2022. *MMWR Morb Mortal Wkly Rep.* 2022;71(4):1174-1181.

[d]ACIP Updates: Recommendations for use of 20-valent pneumococcal conjugate vaccine in children—United States, 2023. *MMWR Morb Mortal Wkly Rep.* 2023;72(39):1072

[e]A single dose should be administered to all healthy children 24 through 59 months of age with any incomplete schedule.

Table 3.71. Recommendations for Pneumococcal Immunization With PCV15, PCV20, and/or PPSV23 Vaccine for Children at High Risk or Presumed High Risk of Pneumococcal Disease, as Defined in Table 3.67 (p 812)

Age	Previous Dose(s) of Any Pneumococcal Vaccine	Recommendations
23 mo or younger	None	PCV15 or PCV20, as in Table 3.70.
24 through 71 mo	4 doses of PCV13, PCV15, or PCV20	If none of the prior 4 doses were PCV20: 1 dose of PPSV23 or PCV20, ≥8 wk after last dose of PCV13 or PCV15.
		If ≥1 of the prior 4 doses was PCV20: no additional doses of any pneumococcal vaccine are indicated.
24 through 71 mo	Incomplete series of 3 previous doses of PCV13, PCV15, or PCV20 before 24 mo of age	1 dose of PCV15 or PCV20.
		If PCV15 is used for this dose and there are no prior doses of PCV20, 1 dose of PPSV23 ≥8 wk after the last dose of PCV15.
		If PCV20 is used for this or any prior dose, no additional doses of any pneumococcal vaccine are indicated.
24 through 71 mo	Incomplete series of <3 doses of PCV13, PCV15, or PCV20 before 24 mo of age	2 doses of PCV15 or PCV20, ≥8 wk after last dose of PCV13, PCV15, or PCV20 (if applicable).
		If PCV15 is used for this dose, 1 dose of PPSV23 vaccine, ≥8 wk after the last dose of PCV13 or PCV15.
		If PCV20 is used for this dose, no additional doses of any pneumococcal vaccine are indicated.
24 through 71 mo	1 dose of PPSV23	2 doses of PCV15 or PCV20, 8 wk apart, beginning at 8 wk after last dose of PPSV23.
6 years through 18 years with immunocompromising conditions[a,b,c,d]	No previous doses of PCV13, PCV15, PCV20, or PPSV23	1 dose of PCV15 followed by 1 dose of PPSV23 at least 8 weeks later and a second dose of PPSV23 5 years after the first[e]; OR 1 dose of PCV20 with no additional doses of any pneumococcal vaccine indicated thereafter

Table 3.71. Recommendations for Pneumococcal Immunization With PCV15, PCV20, and/or PPSV23 Vaccine for Children at High Risk or Presumed High Risk of Pneumococcal Disease, as Defined in Table 3.67 (p 812), continued

Age	Previous Dose(s) of Any Pneumococcal Vaccine	Recommendations
	1 dose of PCV13, PCV15, or PCV20	If prior dose was with PCV13 or PCV15: 1 dose of PPSV23 and a second dose of PPSV23 5 years after the first.[e] If prior dose was with PCV20: no additional doses of any pneumococcal vaccine are indicated.
	≥1 dose of PPSV23 and no previous dose of PCV13, PCV15, or PCV20	1 dose of PCV15 or PCV20 (even if PCV7 previously administered) ≥8 weeks after the last PPSV23 dose; if a second PPSV23 dose is indicated,[e] it should be administered ≥5 years after the first PPSV23 dose

PCV13 indicates 13-valent pneumococcal conjugate vaccine; PCV15 indicates 15-valent pneumococcal conjugate vaccine; PCV20 indicates 20-valent pneumococcal conjugate vaccine; PPSV23, 23-valent pneumococcal polysaccharide vaccine.

[a] Includes anatomic or functional asplenia, human immunodeficiency virus (HIV) infection, cochlear implant, cerebrospinal fluid (CSF) leak, nephrotic syndrome, chronic renal failure, or other immunocompromising conditions.

[b] American Academy of Pediatrics, Committee on Infectious Diseases. Policy statement: Immunization for *Streptococcus pneumoniae* infections in high-risk children. *Pediatrics*. 2014;134(6):1230–1233

[c] Kobayashi M, Farrar JI, Gierke R, et al. Use of 15-valent pneumococcal conjugate vaccine among US children: updated recommendations of the Advisory Committee on Immunization Practices—United States, 2022. *MMWR Morb Mortal Wkly Rep*. 2022;71(4):1174-1181.

[d] ACIP Updates: Recommendations for use of 20-valent pneumococcal conjugate vaccine in children—United States, 2023. *MMWR Morb Mortal Wkly Rep*. 2023;72(39):1072.

[e] A second dose of PPSV23 5 years after the first dose is recommended only for children who have functional or anatomic asplenia, HIV infection, or other immunocompromising conditions (Table 3.67, p 812). No more than 2 doses of PPSV23 are recommended.

A second dose of PPSV23 or a first dose of PCV20 (if no prior PCV20 has been administered) is recommended 5 years after the first dose of PPSV23 in children with sickle cell disease or functional or anatomic asplenia, HIV infection, or other immunocompromising conditions, but no more than a total of 2 PPSV23 doses should be administered before 65 years of age.

Immunization of Children 2 Through 18 Years of Age Who Are at Increased Risk of IPD With PPSV23 After PCV13, PCV15, or PCV20.[1–3] Children 2 years or older with an underlying medical condition increasing the risk of IPD should receive a dose of PPSV23 at least

[1] American Academy of Pediatrics, Committee on Infectious Diseases. Immunization for *Streptococcus pneumoniae* infections in high-risk children. *Pediatrics*. 2014;134(6):1230–1233

[2] Kobayashi M, Farrar JI, Gierke R, et al. Use of 15-valent pneumococcal conjugate vaccine among U.S. children: updated recommendations of the Advisory Committee on Immunization Practices–United States, 2022. *MMWR Morb Mortal Wkly Rep*. 2022;71(37):1174-1181

[3] ACIP Updates: Recommendations for use of 20-valent pneumococcal conjugate vaccine in children—United States, 2023. *MMWR Morb Mortal Wkly Rep*. 2023;72(39):1072

8 weeks after completing all recommended doses of PCV13 or PCV15. However, if they have received one or more doses of PCV20, no additional doses of any pneumococcal vaccine, including PPSV23, are indicated. In children who are candidates for solid organ transplantation and in cases when a splenectomy is planned for a patient older than 2 years, a dose of PPSV23 (if they previously had received only PCV13 or PCV15) or one dose of PCV20 should be administered at least 2 weeks before transplant or splenectomy. In candidates for solid organ transplantation not previously vaccinated with PCV13 or PCV15, a dose of PCV15 or PCV20 should be administered, even for those older than 6 years.

A second dose of PPSV23 or a first dose of PCV20 (if no prior PCV20 has been administered) is recommended 5 years after the first dose of PPSV23 in children with sickle cell disease or functional or anatomic asplenia, HIV infection, or other immunocompromising conditions, but no more than a total of 2 PPSV23 doses should be administered before 65 years of age.

General Recommendations for Use of Pneumococcal Vaccines.
- PPSV23 should not be given together with a conjugate pneumococcal vaccines (PCV15 or PCV20) but can be administered concurrently with other childhood vaccines, with 1 exception. For children for whom quadrivalent meningococcal conjugate vaccine is indicated, MenACWY-D (Menactra) should not be administered concomitantly OR within 4 weeks of administration of PCV15 or PCV20 immunization to avoid potential interference with the immune response to PCV15 or PCV20. Because of their high risk for IPD, children with functional or anatomic asplenia should not be immunized with MenACWY-D (Menactra) before 2 years of age so that they can complete their PCV15 or PCV20 series; only MenACWY-CRM (Menveo]) should be used in this age group because it has been shown to not interfere with the immune response to PCV15 or PCV20 and because the only other alternative, MenACWY-TT (MenQuadfi), is only approved in children ≥2 years of age (see Table 3.40, p 594).
- When elective splenectomy is performed for any reason, immunization with PCV15 or PCV20 should be completed at least 2 weeks before splenectomy. Immunization also should precede initiation of immune-compromising therapy or placement of a cochlear implant by at least 2 weeks. PPSV23 should be administered 8 or more weeks after PCV15, but should not be administered if one or more doses of PCV20 has already been given (see Immunization and Other Considerations in Immunocompromised Children, p 93).
- Generally, pneumococcal vaccines should be deferred during pregnancy. However, pregnant people with underlying conditions that warrant pneumococcal immunization may be vaccinated when the benefit of the vaccination is considered to outweigh any potential risks.

Adverse Reactions to Pneumococcal Vaccines. Adverse reactions after administration of polysaccharide or conjugate vaccines generally are mild to moderate. The most commonly reported adverse reactions are local reactions of injection site, pain, redness, or swelling in addition to irritability, decreased appetite, or impaired sleep. Fever may occur within the first 1 to 2 days after injections, particularly after use of conjugate vaccine. Other systemic reactions include fatigue, headache, generalized muscle pain, decreased appetite, and chills.

Chemoprophylaxis. Daily antimicrobial prophylaxis is recommended for certain children with functional or anatomic asplenia, regardless of their immunization status, for prevention of pneumococcal disease on the basis of results of a large, multicenter study (see Asplenia and Functional Asplenia, p 108). Oral penicillin V (125 mg, twice a day, for children younger than 3 years; 250 mg, twice a day, for children 3 years and older) is recommended. The study, performed before routine use of any of the conjugate pneumococcal vaccines in the United States, demonstrated that oral penicillin V administered to infants and young children with sickle cell disease decreased the incidence of pneumococcal bacteremia by 84% compared with the placebo control group. Although overall incidence of IPD is decreased after penicillin prophylaxis, cases of penicillin-nonsusceptible IPD and nasopharyngeal carriage of penicillin-nonsusceptible strains in patients with sickle cell disease have increased since these studies were conducted. Parents should be informed that penicillin prophylaxis may not be effective in preventing all cases of IPD. In children with suspected or proven penicillin allergy, erythromycin is an alternative agent for prophylaxis.[1]

The age at which prophylaxis is discontinued is an empiric decision. Most children with sickle cell disease who have received all recommended pneumococcal vaccines for age and who had received penicillin prophylaxis for prolonged periods, who are receiving regular medical attention, and who have not had a previous severe pneumococcal infection or a surgical splenectomy may discontinue prophylactic penicillin safely at 5 years of age. However, they must be counseled to seek medical attention promptly for all febrile events. The duration of prophylaxis for children with asplenia attributable to other causes is unknown. Some experts continue prophylaxis throughout childhood or longer.

Control of Transmission of Pneumococcal Infection and Invasive Disease Among Children Attending Out-of-Home Child Care. Antimicrobial chemoprophylaxis is not recommended for contacts of children with IPD, regardless of their immunization status.

Public Health Reporting. Cases of IPD should be reported according to state standards. The majority of cases of invasive disease are caused by non-PCV13 serotypes. Therefore, the overwhelming majority of invasive pneumococcal disease cases occurring among immunized children do not represent vaccine failures. To differentiate PCV13 (or PCV15 or PCV20) failure in an immunized child from disease caused by a serotype not included in PCV13 (or PCV15 or PCV20), the isolate should be serotyped. If the invasive isolate is a serotype included in the vaccine, an evaluation of the patient's HIV status and immunologic function should be considered if the child had received an age-appropriate regimen of PCV13, PCV15, or PCV20 at least 2 weeks before the onset of the invasive infection.

Strongyloidiasis
(Strongyloides stercoralis)

CLINICAL MANIFESTATIONS: Most infections with *Strongyloides stercoralis* are asymptomatic. When symptoms occur, they are related most often to larval tissue migration and/or the presence of adult worms in the intestine. Infective (filariform) larvae are acquired from skin contact with contaminated soil, which may produce transient pruritic papules

---

[1] American Academy of Pediatrics, Committee on Genetics. Health supervision for children with sickle cell disease. *Pediatrics.* 2002;109(3):526-535 (Reaffirmed January 2011, February 2016)

at the site of penetration. Larvae then migrate to the lungs, where they may cause a transient pneumonitis or Löffler-like syndrome characterized by a dry cough. After ascending the tracheobronchial tree, larvae are swallowed and mature into adult forms within the gastrointestinal tract. Symptoms of intestinal infection may include non-specific abdominal pain (epigastric), vomiting, intermittent constipation, and diarrhea. Presentation rarely may resemble inflammatory bowel disease. Larval migration may produce migratory serpiginous pruritic erythematous skin lesions that advance rapidly (centimeters in hours). These tracks are referred to as "larva currens" and are pathognomonic for *Strongyloides*. Other dermatologic findings include urticaria and pruritus.

The most feared complication is *Strongyloides* hyperinfection syndrome and disseminated disease. Hyperinfection refers to increased larval migration within the gastrointestinal and pulmonary tracts; dissemination refers to migration of larva to distant organs such as the brain, liver, kidney, heart, and skin. Dissemination is associated with septicemia believed to occur when large numbers of larvae penetrate the intestinal wall, seeding the bloodstream with gram-negative bacteria. Hyperinfection/dissemination syndrome typically occurs in the immunocompromised host, most often those receiving immunosuppressive agents, particularly corticosteroids, for underlying disease (eg, malignancy or autoimmunity) but also in recipients of solid organ or hematopoietic cell transplants (through either reactivation of prior asymptomatic infection in the recipient or donor-derived infection). Hyperinfection/dissemination also is associated closely with human T-lymphotropic virus 1 (HTLV-1) coinfection, which is most common among persons from the Caribbean, East Asia (particularly southwest Japan), Latin America, and West Africa. *Strongyloides* hyperinfection/dissemination syndrome may be characterized by fever, abdominal pain, diffuse pulmonary infiltrates, and septicemia or meningitis caused by enteric gram-negative bacilli. Left untreated, mortality rates can approach 90%. For unknown reasons, it is extremely rare during childhood.

ETIOLOGY: *S stercoralis*, a nematode (roundworm), is the major causative agent in humans, although other species, including zoonotic species, are reported rarely.

EPIDEMIOLOGY: Strongyloidiasis is endemic in the tropics and subtropics, including parts of the United States, wherever suitable moist soil and improper disposal of human waste coexist. Humans are the principal hosts, but dogs, cats, and other animals can serve as reservoirs. Transmission involves penetration of skin by filariform larvae from contact with soil contaminated by human feces. Infections also can be acquired via the fecal-oral route with ingestion of food contaminated with human feces containing larvae or from inadvertent coprophagy. Adult female worms release eggs in the small intestine, where they hatch as first-stage (rhabditiform) larvae that are excreted in feces. A small percentage of larvae molt to the infective (filariform) stage during intestinal transit and can penetrate the bowel mucosa or perianal skin, thus maintaining the life cycle within a single person (autoinfection). This capacity for autoinfection is unique among soil-transmitted infections and allows for infection to persist for decades (eg, in immigrants from or travelers to endemic regions many years before).

The **incubation period** in humans can range from weeks for acute strongyloidiasis to decades for chronic infection.

DIAGNOSTIC TESTS: Strongyloidiasis can be difficult to diagnose. Testing generally is performed on stool or serologically. Visualization of larvae (rhabditiform, or less often, filariform) with direct microscopy of stool (or from duodenal biopsy or fluid obtained using the string test [Entero-Test] or a direct aspirate through a flexible endoscope) confirms the diagnosis. At least 3 consecutive stool specimens should be examined microscopically for characteristic larvae (not eggs) using a concentration method (eg, sedimentation techniques), but a negative test result does not exclude infection, because larvae excretion can be intermittent and of low intensity. Other techniques that provide greater sensitivity but are not available routinely in the United States include stool polymerase chain reaction (PCR) assay, stool agar culture, or other specialized tests on stool specimens. Filariform larvae may be identified in disseminated strongyloidiasis from other specimens such as sputum or bronchoalveolar lavage fluid, spinal fluid, pleural fluid, or peritoneal fluid or in skin biopsies.

Serologic tests, including enzyme-linked immunosorbent assays (ELISAs) that detect immunoglobulin (Ig) G to filariform larvae, are highly sensitive, but cross-reactivity may occur in patients with filariasis and other nematode infections. Serologic tests using recombinant antigens have similar high sensitivity but greater specificity for strongyloidiasis. Serologic testing has several limitations. Detection does not confirm active infection, because antibodies may remain positive for a period of time following infection resolution. False-negative results may occur, and therefore a negative test result does not eliminate the possibility of ongoing infection. Quantitative serologic monitoring may be useful in following treatment in immunocompetent patients, because antibody concentrations decline over time with successful treatment, although the timing of seroconversion following treatment, and how often it occurs, is unknown. The Centers for Disease Control and Prevention (CDC) performs reference serologic testing to confirm equivocal results (**www.cdc.gov/parasites/strongyloides/ health_professionals/index.html**).

Eosinophilia (blood eosinophil count greater than $400-500/\mu L$) is associated with acute and chronic infection, but may be absent in up to 50% of infected individuals. Eosinophilia often is absent in patients with hyperinfection/dissemination syndrome, which predicts a poor outcome.

TREATMENT: Ivermectin is the treatment of choice for all forms of strongyloidiasis and is approved by the US Food and Drug Administration for the treatment of intestinal strongyloidiasis. Ivermectin is contraindicated in people with confirmed or suspected coinfection with *Loa loa* and a high microfilarial load. An alternative agent is albendazole, although it is associated with lower cure rates (see Drugs for Parasitic Infections, p 1068). Prolonged or repeated treatment may be necessary in people with hyperinfection/disseminated strongyloidiasis, and relapse can occur.

Treatment for suspected or confirmed hyperinfection/dissemination syndrome is immediate ivermectin, continued until stool or sputum examinations are negative for 2 weeks. Rectal and subcutaneous routes have been used when oral or enteral tube administration was not possible. Suspected or confirmed hyperinfection/dissemination syndrome should be managed in consultation with an expert.

INFECTION PREVENTION AND CONTROL MEASURES IN HEALTH CARE SETTINGS: Standard precautions are recommended. Hospital transmission has never been reported.

CONTROL MEASURES: Sanitary disposal of human waste is effective at interrupting transmission of *S stercoralis*. Eligible refugees who arrive in the United States through the US Refugee Resettlement Program receive presumptive treatment with ivermectin before arrival, but other immigrants, including internationally adopted children, may not. Any individual at risk epidemiologically for strongyloidiasis who will undergo a solid organ or hematopoietic cell transplant or immunosuppressant therapy, particularly with corticosteroids or tumor necrosis factor alpha inhibitors, either should be treated presumptively for strongyloidiasis or tested serologically and treated if the serologic test result is positive before initiation of immunosuppression. Providers should screen for *Strongyloides* in organ donors from areas with endemic infection and consider the diagnosis in select patients with hematologic malignancies, people on corticosteroids or other immune suppressants, people with HTLV-1 infection, people with persistent or unexplained eosinophilia, household contacts with shared risk factors, and people who traveled recently or remotely to areas with endemic disease.

Syphilis

CLINICAL MANIFESTATIONS:

Congenital Syphilis. Intrauterine infection with *Treponema pallidum* can result in stillbirth, hydrops fetalis, or preterm birth or may be asymptomatic at birth. Infected infants can have hepatosplenomegaly; snuffles (copious nasal secretions); lymphadenopathy; mucocutaneous lesions; pneumonia; osteochondritis, periostitis, and pseudoparalysis; edema; rash (maculopapular consisting of small dark red-copper spots that is most severe on the hands and feet); hemolytic anemia; or thrombocytopenia at birth or within the first 4 to 8 weeks of age. Untreated infants, including those asymptomatic at birth, may develop late manifestations, which usually appear after 2 years of age and involve the central nervous system (CNS), bones and joints, teeth, eyes, and skin. Some findings may not become apparent until many years after birth, such as interstitial keratitis, eighth cranial nerve deafness, Hutchinson teeth (peg-shaped, notched central incisors), anterior bowing of the shins, frontal bossing, mulberry molars, saddle nose, rhagades (perioral fissures), and Clutton joints (symmetric, painless swelling of the knees). Late manifestations can be prevented by treatment of early infection.

Acquired Syphilis. Acquired disease can be divided into 3 stages. The **primary stage** (or **"primary syphilis"**) can appear as painless or painful indurated ulcers (chancres) of the skin or mucous membranes at the site of inoculation. These lesions appear, on average, 3 weeks after exposure and heal spontaneously in a few weeks. Adjacent lymph nodes frequently are enlarged but are nontender. The **secondary stage** (or **"secondary syphilis"**), beginning 1 to 2 months later, is characterized by fever, sore throat, muscle aches, rash, mucocutaneous lesions, hepatitis, and generalized lymphadenopathy. The polymorphic maculopapular rash is generalized and typically includes the palms and soles. In moist areas of the perineum, hypertrophic papular lesions (condyloma lata) can be confused with condyloma acuminata secondary to human papillomavirus (HPV) infection. Malaise, splenomegaly, headache, alopecia, and arthralgia can be present. This stage resolves spontaneously without treatment in approximately 3 to 12 weeks. A variable asymptomatic latent period follows but may be interrupted during the first few years by recurrences of symptoms of secondary syphilis. **Latent syphilis** is the period after infection when patients are seroreactive but demonstrate no clinical manifestations of disease. Development of latent syphilis within the preceding year is referred to as **early latent syphilis;** if >1 year in duration, it is known as **late latent syphilis.** If the duration of infection is unknown, the patient should be considered to have late latent syphilis for the purposes of management. The **tertiary stage** of syphilis occurs 15 to 30 years after the initial infection and can include gumma formation (soft, noncancerous, granulomatous growths that can destroy tissue) or cardiovascular involvement (including aortitis). Neurosyphilis, defined as infection of the central nervous system (CNS), can occur at any stage of infection, especially in people with advanced or poorly controlled human immunodeficiency virus (HIV) disease and in neonates with congenital syphilis; manifestations include meningitis, uveitis, seizures, optic atrophy, hearing loss, and (typically years after infection) dementia and posterior spinal cord degeneration (tabes dorsalis, including a characteristic high-stepping gait with the feet slapping the ground because of loss of proprioception).

ETIOLOGY: *T pallidum* subspecies *pallidum* *(T pallidum)* is a thin, motile spirochete that is extremely fastidious, surviving only briefly outside the host. It is very closely related to 3 other organisms causing nonvenereal human disease in distinct geographic regions of the world: *T pallidum* subspecies *pertenue,* which causes yaws; *T pallidum* subspecies *endemicum,* which causes endemic syphilis; and *Treponema carateum,* which causes pinta. The genus *Treponema* is classified in the family *Spirochaetaceae.*

EPIDEMIOLOGY: From 2016 to 2020, the primary and secondary syphilis rate increased 52% nationally, from 8.6 to 12.7 cases per 100 000 population. Rates increased among both male and female individuals and in most regions of the United States (Midwest, Northeast, South).[1] Rates of primary and secondary syphilis also increased in most racial and ethnic groups, with the greatest increases observed among non-Hispanic American Indian/Alaska Native persons as well as non-Hispanic multiracial persons.

In 2020, men who have sex with men (MSM) only and men who have sex with both men and women accounted for 43% of all primary and secondary syphilis cases among male patients when sex of the partner was known.

In 2020, a total of 2148 cases of congenital syphilis were reported, including 149 stillbirths and infant deaths. The 2020 national rate of 57 cases per 100 000 live births represents a 15% increase relative to 2019 (49.9 cases per 100 000 live births) and a 254% increase relative to 2016 (16.2 cases per 100 000 live births). This trend mirrors the increase in primary and secondary syphilis cases seen in women of reproductive age. From 2016 to 2020, rates of primary and secondary syphilis among women of reproductive age (15–44 years) increased 147%, from 1.9 to 4.7 per 100 000 female individuals.

Congenital syphilis may be contracted at any stage of the pregnant person's infection via transplacental transmission, at any time during pregnancy, or via contact with the birthing parent's lesions at the time of delivery. Among pregnant people with untreated early syphilis, up to 40% of their pregnancies will result in spontaneous abortion, stillbirth, or perinatal death. The rate of perinatal transmission is 60% to 100% in the setting of primary and secondary syphilis and decreases with later stages of infection of the birthing parent (approximately 40% with early latent infection and <8% with late latent infection). Among people who acquire syphilis during pregnancy, the risk of transmission to the infant increases directly with the gestational age at the time the pregnant person becomes infected. People with HIV, in particular, have a higher prevalence of untreated or inadequately treated syphilis during pregnancy; therefore, their newborn infants may be at higher risk of congenital syphilis.

---

[1] Unless otherwise noted, the terms male, female, men, and women refer to sex assigned at birth.

In addition, syphilis coinfection during pregnancy may also increase the rate of vertical transmission of HIV.

T pallidum is not transmitted through human milk, but transmission may occur if the breastfeeding person has an infectious lesion (chancre) on the breast.

Acquired syphilis almost always is contracted through direct sexual contact with ulcerative lesions of the skin or mucous membranes of infected people. Open, moist lesions of the primary or secondary stages are highly infectious. Syphilis acquired beyond the neonatal period should be considered diagnostic of sexual abuse in infants and young children once vertical transmission is excluded (see Sexual Assault and Abuse in Children and Adolescents/Young Adults, p 182).

The **incubation period** for acquired primary syphilis typically is 3 weeks but ranges from 10 to 90 days.

DIAGNOSTIC TESTS: Definitive diagnosis is made by molecular tests for detecting *T pallidum* or when spirochetes are identified by microscopic darkfield examination of lesion exudate, nasal discharge, or tissue, such as placenta, lymph node, umbilical cord, or autopsy specimens. Darkfield microscopy, however, no longer is routinely available in most clinics and laboratories because of its complexity. Although no *T pallidum* direct-detection molecular nucleic acid amplification test (NAAT) is available commercially, certain laboratories provide locally developed and validated polymerase chain reaction (PCR) tests.

Presumptive diagnosis requires the use of both nontreponemal and treponemal serologic tests. Nontreponemal tests for syphilis include the Venereal Disease Research Laboratory (VDRL) slide test and the rapid plasma reagin (RPR) test. These tests are inexpensive, can be performed across a range of laboratory levels of complexity with fairly rapid turnaround times for analysis, and provide semiquantitative results that can both help define disease activity and monitor response to therapy. Nontreponemal test results may be falsely negative (ie, nonreactive) in early primary syphilis, latent acquired syphilis of long duration, and late congenital syphilis. Occasionally, a nontreponemal test performed on serum containing high concentrations of antibody will be weakly reactive or falsely negative, a reaction termed the prozone phenomenon; diluting the serum being tested will then result in a positive test result. The prozone phenomenon may be observed more often in HIV-coinfected individuals. When nontreponemal tests are used serially to monitor treatment response, the same test (RPR or VDRL), ideally analyzed in the same laboratory, must be used throughout the follow-up period to ensure comparability of results.

Except with congenital infection, a reactive nontreponemal test result should be confirmed by a specific treponemal test to exclude a false-positive test result. False-positive nontreponemal results can be caused by certain viral infections (eg, Epstein-Barr virus infection, hepatitis, HIV, varicella, measles), lymphoma, tuberculosis, malaria, endocarditis, connective tissue disease, older age, abuse of injection drugs, or laboratory or technical error. A non-cord neonatal blood sample is preferred for testing. Cord blood samples are not recommended for testing a newborn infant's RPR or VDRL status, because blood from the birthing parent can contaminate the specimen and yield a false-positive result, and Wharton's jelly can yield a false-negative result.

Treponemal tests in use include the *T pallidum* particle agglutination (TP-PA) test (which is the preferred treponemal test), *T pallidum* enzyme immunoassay (TP-EIA), *T pallidum* chemiluminescence assay (TP-CIA), and fluorescent treponemal antibody absorption (FTA-ABS) test. The Centers for Disease Control and Prevention (CDC) has assessed the performance characteristics of seven of the treponemal tests that are commercially available.[1] Generally, immunoassays have similar performance to manual treponemal assays, although certain immunoassays may be less specific. Most people who have reactive treponemal test results remain reactive for life, even after successful therapy. However, 15% to 25% of patients treated during primary syphilis revert to being serologically nonreactive on treponemal testing after 2 to 3 years. Treponemal test results may be variably positive in patients with other spirochetal diseases, such as yaws, pinta, leptospirosis, rat-bite fever, relapsing fever, and Lyme disease.

In most cases, if a patient has a positive RPR or VDRL result in low titer and has a negative treponemal test result, the nontreponemal test result will be a false positive. However, because false-negative test results can occur in early syphilis, retesting in 2 to 4 weeks and again later if clinically indicated should be considered in people at increased risk for syphilis, especially in pregnant people and those with HIV.

The CDC[2] and the US Preventive Services Task Force[3] recommend syphilis serologic screening with a nontreponemal test; this screening is followed by confirmation using one of the several available treponemal tests ("conventional diagnostic" approach). Some clinical laboratories and blood banks, however, screen samples using treponemal tests first rather than beginning with a nontreponemal test. This is known as "reverse-sequence screening" and may result in false-positive results, especially in low-prevalence populations. When the reverse-sequence algorithm is used, people with a positive treponemal test result and a negative nontreponemal test result (eg, EIA positive, RPR negative) should have a second treponemal test targeting a different *T pallidum* antigen performed to confirm the results of the original test. If the second treponemal-specific test result is negative (eg, EIA-positive, RPR-negative, then TP-PA-negative) and the person is at low risk for syphilis, the original treponemal test result likely was a false positive. However, in individuals at high-risk for infection, retesting in 2 to 4 weeks and again later if clinically indicated should be considered.

Cerebrospinal Fluid Tests. Cerebrospinal fluid (CSF) abnormalities in adolescents and adults with neurosyphilis can include increased protein concentration, increased white blood cell (WBC) count, and/or a reactive CSF-VDRL test result. The CSF leukocyte count usually is elevated in neurosyphilis (>5 WBCs/mm^3). Interpretation of CSF test results requires a nontraumatic lumbar puncture (ie, a CSF sample not contaminated with blood). The CSF-VDRL is highly specific but insensitive; therefore, a negative result does not exclude a diagnosis of neurosyphilis. A positive CSF FTA-ABS or TP-PA result can support the diagnosis of neurosyphilis but does not establish the diagnosis definitively.

Conversely, a reactive CSF-VDRL test in a neonate or infant from a nontraumatic lumbar puncture confirms the diagnosis of neurosyphilis. CSF cell count and protein can be difficult to interpret during the neonatal period; normal values differ by gestational age and are higher in preterm infants. Studies suggest that 95% of healthy

[1] Park IU, Fakile YF, Chow JM, et al. Performance of treponemal tests for the diagnosis of syphilis. *Clin Infect Dis.* 2019;68(6):913–918

[2] Centers for Disease Control and Prevention. Sexually transmitted infections treatment guidelines, 2021. *MMWR Recomm Rep.* 2021;70(RR-4):1-185

[3] US Preventive Services Task Force. Screening for syphilis infection in non-pregnant adults and adolescents. *JAMA.* 2016;315(21):2321-2327

neonates have values ≤16 to 19 white blood cells (WBCs)/mm^3 and/or protein ≤115 to 118 mg/dL on CSF examination. During the second month of life, 95% of healthy infants have ≤9 to 11 WBCs/mm^3 and/or protein of ≤89 to 91 mg/dL. Lower values (ie, 5 WBCs/mm^3 and protein of 40 mg/dL) might be considered the upper limits of normal in older infants. Other causes of elevated CSF values should be considered when an infant is being evaluated for congenital syphilis.

Testing During Pregnancy. Prevention of congenital syphilis requires that pregnant people be screened serologically early in pregnancy. False-negative test results are possible in recent infection, and syphilis may be acquired later in pregnancy. In communities and populations in which the prevalence of syphilis is high and for people at high risk for infection, serologic testing at the first prenatal visit, with repeat serologic testing at 28 weeks' gestation and again at delivery, is recommended. A nontreponemal test (RPR or VDRL) is recommended for screening, followed by a treponemal test (eg, TP-PA) if the screening result is positive. In most cases, if the treponemal antibody test result is negative, the nontreponemal test result is falsely positive and no further evaluation is necessary. However, retesting in 2 to 4 weeks, and again later if clinically indicated, should be considered for pregnant people who are at high risk of syphilis, such as those living in communities with high rates of syphilis or those who have been at risk for syphilis acquisition during pregnancy (eg, sex with multiple partners, sex in conjunction with drug use or transactional sex, late or no prenatal care, incarceration of the pregnant person or partner, or unstable housing or homelessness).

If the reverse-sequence screening algorithm is used, pregnant people with reactive treponemal screening test results should have confirmatory testing with a quantitative nontreponemal test. If the nontreponemal test result is negative (eg, EIA positive, RPR negative), a second treponemal-specific test using a different *T pallidum* antigen should be obtained to determine whether the initial treponemal test result was a false positive (TP-PA preferred). If the second treponemal test result is negative (eg, EIA positive, RPR negative, then TP-PA negative) and the person is at low risk for syphilis, the original treponemal test result likely was a false positive. However, retesting in 2 to 4 weeks and again later if clinically indicated should be considered for pregnant people who are at high risk of syphilis.

Ultrasonographic evaluation of the fetus from the second trimester onward should be performed when syphilis is diagnosed at any time during pregnancy, even if appropriate treatment has been administered to the pregnant person. Pathologic examination of the placenta and/or umbilical cord at delivery also should be performed.

Evaluation of Infants for Congenital Infection During the Newborn Period to 1 Month of Age.
No newborn infant should be discharged from the hospital without confirmation of the birthing parent's serologic status for syphilis. This may prolong infant hospitalization, because a confirmatory maternal TP-PA for a birthing parent who is TP-CIA or TP-EIA positive and RPR or VDRL negative usually is performed off-site and takes several days to result. All infants born to seropositive persons require a careful examination and nontreponemal testing. A negative RPR or VDRL test result for the birthing parent at delivery does not rule out the possibility of the infant having congenital syphilis, although such a situation is rare. The diagnostic approach to infant evaluation for congenital syphilis is presented in Fig 3.18. In addition to the blood and CSF tests noted, infants in whom congenital syphilis is proven or highly probable should have long-bone radiographs as should those with possible congenital syphilis, for whom

FIG 3.18. ALGORITHM FOR DIAGNOSTIC APPROACH OF INFANTS BORN TO MOTHERS WITH REACTIVE SEROLOGIC TESTS FOR SYPHILIS

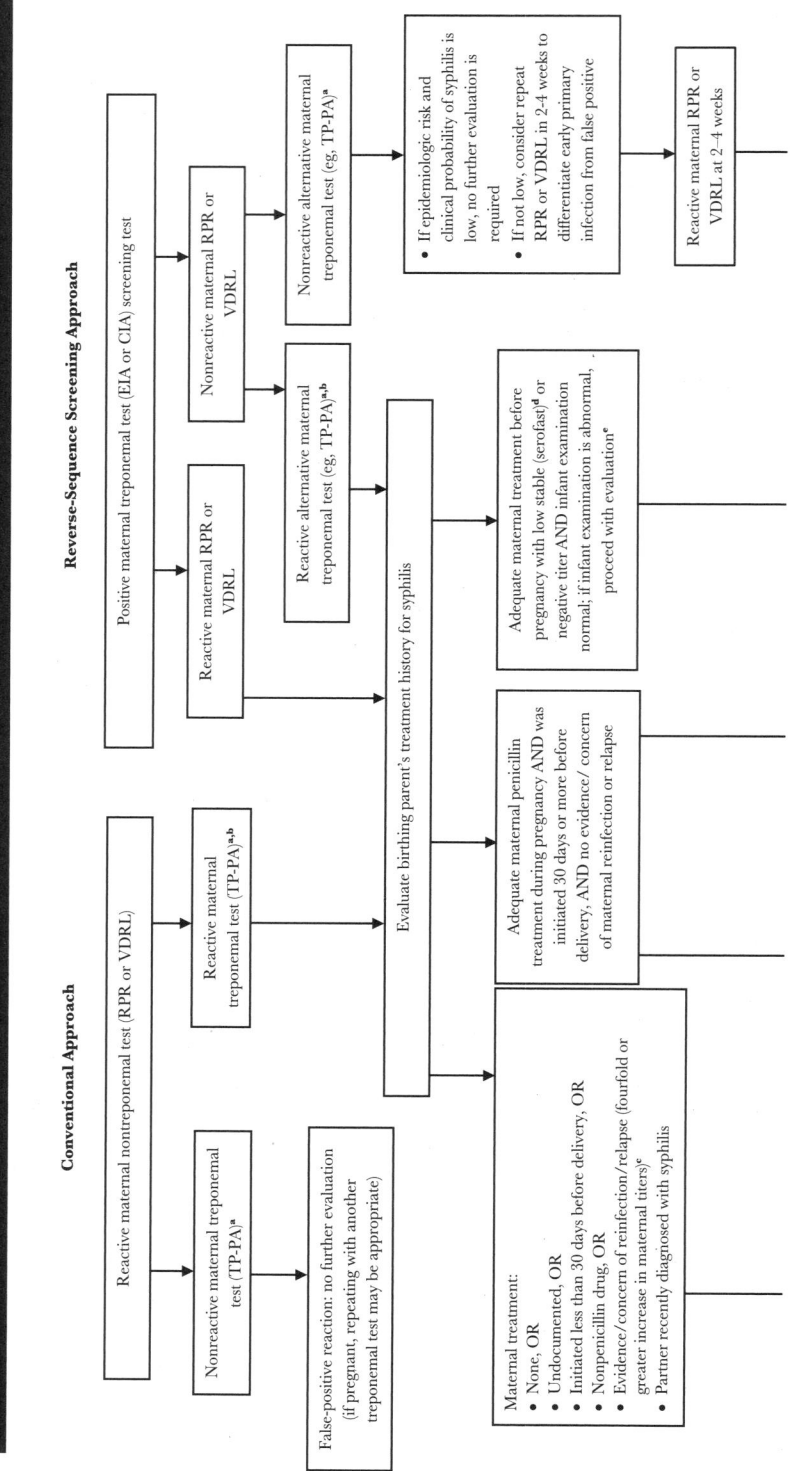

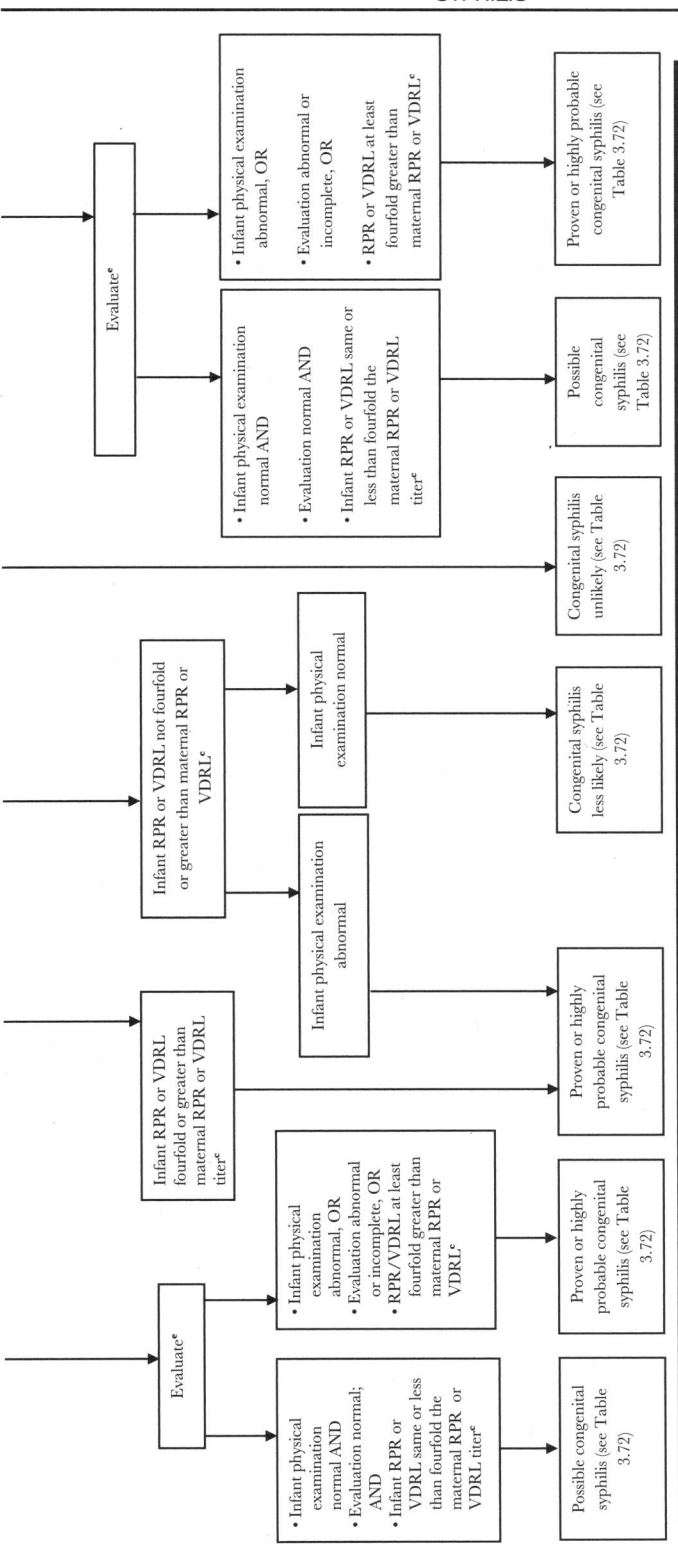

RPR indicates rapid plasma reagin; VDRL, Venereal Disease Research Laboratory.

[a] *Treponema pallidum* particle agglutination (TP-PA) (which is the preferred treponemal test) or fluorescent treponemal antibody absorption (FTA-ABS).

[b] Test for human immunodeficiency virus (HIV) antibody. Infants of HIV-infected mothers do not require different evaluation or treatment for syphilis.

[c] A fourfold change in titer is the same as a change of 2 dilutions. For example, a titer of 1:64 is fourfold greater than a titer of 1:16, and a titer of 1:4 is fourfold lower than a titer of 1:16. When comparing titers, the same type of nontreponemal test should be used (eg, if the initial test was an RPR, the follow-up test should also be an RPR).

[d] Stable VDRL titers 1:2 or less or RPR 1:4 or less beyond 1 year after successful treatment are considered low serofast.

[e] Complete blood cell (CBC) and platelet count; cerebrospinal fluid (CSF) examination for cell count, protein, and quantitative VDRL; other tests as clinically indicated (eg, chest radiographs, long-bone radiographs, eye examination, liver function tests, neuroimaging, and auditory brainstem response). For neonates, pathologic examination of the placenta or umbilical cord with specific fluorescent antitreponemal antibody staining, if possible.

long-bone radiographs can further support the diagnosis. Neonates known to be exposed to syphilis at delivery should not have delayed bathing.[1]

Evaluation of Infants >1 Month of Age and Children. For the infant or child identified as having reactive serologic tests for syphilis, the birthing parent's serologic test results and records should be reviewed to assess whether the infant or child has congenital or acquired syphilis. Evaluation for congenital syphilis after 1 month of age includes: (1) CSF analysis for VDRL, cell count, and protein; (2) complete blood cell count with differential and platelet count; (3) if clinically indicated, long-bone radiographs, chest radiograph, liver function tests, ophthalmologic examination, neuroimaging, and auditory brain-stem response); and (4) testing for HIV infection.

TREATMENT[2]: Parenteral penicillin G is the preferred drug for treatment of syphilis at any stage. The type and duration of penicillin G therapy varies depending on the stage of disease and clinical manifestations. Parenteral penicillin G is the only documented effective therapy for patients who have neurosyphilis, congenital syphilis, or syphilis during pregnancy and also is recommended for people with HIV.

Penicillin Allergy. Infants and children with a history of penicillin allergy or who develop presumed penicillin allergy during treatment should be desensitized and then treated with penicillin whenever possible. Data to support the use of alternatives to penicillin are limited, but options for nonpregnant patients who are allergic to penicillin may include doxycycline, tetracycline, and ceftriaxone. Ceftriaxone also can be considered as an alternative therapy for neurosyphilis. These therapies should be used with close clinical and laboratory follow-up to ensure expected serologic response and cure. In pregnant people with penicillin allergy, desensitization and treatment with doses of intramuscular penicillin G benzathine, guided by the stage of syphilis diagnosed, is the only appropriate therapy. Erythromycin and azithromycin, which have been suggested as extended-course alternatives in nonpregnant adults with penicillin allergy, are not appropriate for treatment in pregnancy because they may suboptimally treat the pregnant person and will not cross the placenta adequately to treat the fetus. Similarly, doxycycline is not appropriate for use in the second and third trimesters of pregnancy.

Congenital Syphilis: Newborn Period to 1 Month of Age. The management of congenital syphilis is based on whether the infant has proven or probable congenital syphilis, has possible congenital syphilis, or is considered less likely or unlikely to have syphilis, as detailed in Fig 3.18 and Table 3.72. If more than 1 day of therapy is missed, the entire course should be restarted. Data supporting use of other antimicrobial agents (eg, ampicillin) for treatment of congenital syphilis are not available. When possible, a full 10-day course of penicillin is preferred, even if ampicillin initially was provided for possible sepsis. Use of agents other than penicillin requires close serologic follow-up to assess adequacy of therapy. Expert advice for evaluation and management of neonates, infants, or children with suspected or confirmed congenital syphilis is available within 1 to 5 business days from the National Network of STD Clinical Prevention Training Centers (NNPTC) STD Clinical Consultation Network, which is supported by the CDC Division of STD Prevention, at **www.stdccn.org.**

[1] Nolt D, O'Leary ST, Aucott SW; American Academy of Pediatrics, Committee on Infectious Diseases, Committee on Fetus and Newborn. Risks of infectious diseases in newborns exposed to alternative perinatal practices. *Pediatrics.* 2022;149(2):e2021055554

[2] Centers for Disease Control and Prevention. Sexually transmitted infections treatment guidelines, 2021. *MMWR Recomm Rep.* 2021;70(RR-4):1-187

Table 3.72. Evaluation and Treatment of Infants *Up To 1 Month of Age* With Possible, Probable, or Confirmed Congenital Syphilis[a]

Category	Findings	Recommended Evaluation	Treatment
Proven or highly probable congenital syphilis	Abnormal physical examination consistent with congenital syphilis OR A serum quantitative nontreponemal serologic titer fourfold (or greater) higher than the birthing parent's titer at delivery (eg, maternal titer = 1:2, neonatal titer ≥1:8; or maternal titer = 1:8, neonatal titer ≥1:32) OR A positive result of darkfield test or PCR assay of lesions or body fluid(s)	CSF analysis (CSF VDRL, cell count, and protein) CBC with differential and platelet count Long-bone radiography Other tests (as clinically indicated): Chest radiography Aminotransferases Neuroimaging Ophthalmologic examination Auditory brain stem response HIV testing	Aqueous crystalline penicillin G, 50 000 U/kg, IV, every 12 hours (1 wk or younger), then every 8 h for infants older than 1 wk, for a total of 10 days of therapy[b] (**preferred**) OR Penicillin G procaine, 50 000 U/kg, IM, as single daily dose for 10 days

Table 3.72. Evaluation and Treatment of Infants *Up To 1 Month of Age* With Possible, Probable, or Confirmed Congenital Syphilis,[a] continued

Category	Findings	Recommended Evaluation	Treatment
Possible congenital syphilis	Normal infant examination AND A serum quantitative nontreponemal serologic titer less than fourfold the birthing parent's titer at delivery (eg, maternal titer = 1:8, neonatal titer ≤1:16) AND ONE OF THE FOLLOWING: Birthing parent was not treated, was inadequately treated, or had no documentation of receiving treatment; OR Birthing parent was treated with a regimen other than recommended in the guideline (ie, a nonpenicillin G regimen) OR Birthing parent received recommended regimen but treatment was initiated <30 days before delivery	CSF analysis (CSF VDRL, cell count, and protein) CBC with differential and platelet count Long-bone radiography	Aqueous crystalline penicillin G, 50 000 U/kg, IV, every 12 h (1 wk or younger), then every 8 h for infants older than 1 wk, for a total of 10 days of therapy[b] **(preferred)** OR Penicillin G procaine, 50 000 U/kg, IM, as single daily dose for 10 days OR Penicillin G benzathine, 50 000 U/kg, IM, single dose (recommended by some experts, but **only** if all components of the evaluation are obtained and are normal[e] and follow-up is certain)

Table 3.72. Evaluation and Treatment of Infants *Up To 1 Month of Age* With Possible, Probable, or Confirmed Congenital Syphilis,[a] continued

Category	Findings	Recommended Evaluation	Treatment
Congenital syphilis less likely	Normal infant examination AND A serum quantitative nontreponemal serologic titer less than fourfold the birthing parent's titer at delivery (eg, maternal titer = 1:8, neonatal titer ≤1:16) AND Birthing parent was treated during pregnancy, treatment was appropriate for stage of infection, and treatment was initiated ≥30 days before delivery AND Birthing parent has no evidence of reinfection or relapse	Not recommended	Penicillin G benzathine, 50 000 U/kg, IM, single dose (**preferred**) Alternatively, infants whose birthing parent's nontreponemal titers decreased at least fourfold after appropriate therapy for early syphilis or remained stable at low titer (eg, VDRL ≤1:2; RPR ≤1:4) may be followed every 2–3 mo without treatment until the nontreponemal test becomes nonreactive Nontreponemal antibody titers should decrease by 3 mo of age and should be nonreactive by 6 mo of age; patients with increasing titers or with persistent stable titers 6 to 12 mo after initial treatment should be reevaluated, including a CSF examination, and treated with a 10-day course of parenteral penicillin G, even if they were treated previously

Table 3.72. Evaluation and Treatment of Infants *Up To 1 Month of Age* With Possible, Probable, or Confirmed Congenital Syphilis,[a] continued

Category	Findings	Recommended Evaluation	Treatment
Congenital syphilis is unlikely	Normal infant examination AND A serum quantitative nontreponemal serologic titer less than fourfold the birthing parent's titer at delivery AND Birthing parent was treated adequately before pregnancy AND Birthing parent's nontreponemal serologic titer remained low and stable (ie, serofast) before and during pregnancy and at delivery (eg, VDRL ≤1:2 or RPR ≤1:4)	Not recommended	None, but infants with reactive nontreponemal tests should be followed serologically to ensure test result returns to negative Penicillin G benzathine, 50 000 U/kg, IM, single dose can be considered if follow-up is uncertain and infant has a reactive test (some experts) Neonates with a negative nontreponemal test result at birth and whose birthing parent was seroreactive at delivery should be retested at 3 mo to rule out incubating congenital syphilis

CBC indicates complete blood cell count; CSF, cerebrospinal fluid; IM, intramuscularly; IV, intravenously; PCR, polymerase chain reaction; RPR, rapid plasma reagin VDRL, Venereal Disease Research Laboratory.

Adapted and modified from Centers for Disease Control and Prevention. Sexually transmitted diseases treatment guidelines, 2021. *MMWR Recomm Rep.* 2021;70(RR-4):52-54.

[a] For treatment of infants ≥1 month of age with congenital syphilis, see text on p 832.

[b] If 24 hours or more of therapy is missed, the entire course must be restarted.

[c] If CSF is not obtained or uninterpretable (eg, bloody tap), a 10-day course is recommended.

Congenital Syphilis: Infants ≥1 Month of Age and Children. Infants older than 1 month who possibly have congenital syphilis and children older than 2 years who have late and previously untreated congenital syphilis should be treated with intravenous aqueous crystalline penicillin (200 000–300 000 U/kg/day, intravenously, administered as 50 000 U/kg, every 4–6 hours for 10 days). Some experts suggest giving such patients a single dose of penicillin G benzathine (50 000 U/kg, intramuscularly, not to exceed 2.4 million U) after the 10-day course of intravenous aqueous crystalline penicillin. If the patient has no clinical manifestations of disease, the CSF examination is normal, and the CSF-VDRL test result is negative, some experts would treat with 3 weekly doses of penicillin G benzathine (50 000 U/kg, intramuscularly, not to exceed 2.4 million U).

Congenital Syphilis: Penicillin Shortage. During periods when the availability of aqueous crystalline penicillin G is compromised, check local sources for aqueous crystalline penicillin G (potassium or sodium) and notify the CDC and US Food and Drug Administration of the limited supply. Information on current drug shortages in the United States can be found at **www.ashp.org/shortages.**

For infants with proven or highly probable congenital syphilis, if intravenous penicillin G is limited, then substitution of some or all daily doses with penicillin G procaine (50 000 U/kg/dose intramuscularly a day in a single daily dose for 10 days), if available, can be used; as of July 2023, however, penicillin G procaine production in the United States has been discontinued by the manufacturer. If aqueous crystalline penicillin G or penicillin G procaine is not available, ceftriaxone (50 to 75 mg/kg/day intravenously every 24 hours) can be considered with careful clinical and serologic follow-up and in consultation with a pediatric infectious diseases specialist, as evidence is insufficient to support the use of ceftriaxone for the treatment of congenital syphilis. In neonates ≤28 days of age, ceftriaxone is contraindicated if they have hyperbilirubinemia or if they require treatment with calcium-containing intravenous solutions because of the risk of precipitation of ceftriaxone-calcium.

For term infants with possible congenital syphilis or in whom congenital syphilis is less likely, penicillin G procaine (50 000 U/kg/dose intramuscularly in a single daily dose for 10 days) or penicillin G benzathine (50 000 U/kg intramuscularly as a single dose) should be used. If any part of the evaluation for congenital syphilis is abnormal or was not performed, CSF examination is not interpretable, or follow-up is uncertain, penicillin G procaine is recommended. A single dose of ceftriaxone is inadequate therapy.

For preterm infants with possible congenital syphilis or in whom congenital syphilis is less likely, who might not tolerate intramuscular injections because of decreased muscle mass, intravenous ceftriaxone can be considered with careful clinical and serologic follow-up and in consultation with a pediatric infectious diseases specialist; ceftriaxone dosing must be adjusted according to birth weight, and has the contraindications listed above for jaundice or if calcium-containing intravenous solutions are being administered concomitantly.

Syphilis in Pregnancy. Regardless of stage of pregnancy, pregnant people should be treated with penicillin according to the dosage schedules appropriate for the stage of syphilis as recommended for nonpregnant patients (see Table 3.73). Nonpenicillin treatment of syphilis during pregnancy cannot be considered reliable to cure infection in the pregnant person and will not cross the placenta adequately to ensure fetal treatment.

Acquired Primary, Secondary, Early Latent Syphilis; Late Latent Syphilis; Tertiary Syphilis; and Neurosyphilis. Treatment recommendations for children and adults are detailed in Table 3.73.

Table 3.73. Recommended Treatment for Acquired Primary, Secondary, Early Latent Syphilis; Late Latent Syphilis; Tertiary Syphilis; and Neurosyphilis[a]

Status	Children	Adults
Primary, secondary, and early latent syphilis[b]	Penicillin G benzathine,[c] 50 000 U/kg, IM, up to the adult dose of 2.4 million U in a single dose *If allergic to penicillin and not pregnant,* Doxycycline, 4.4 mg/kg per day, orally, twice a day for max 200 mg per day, orally, twice a day for 14 days **OR** Tetracycline, 25–50 mg/kg divided in 4 doses, max 2 g per day, orally, for 14 days **(for age ≥8 years)**	Penicillin G benzathine, 2.4 million U, IM, in a single dose **OR** *If allergic to penicillin,* Doxycycline, 100 mg, orally, twice a day for 14 days (avoid in the second and third trimesters of pregnancy) **OR** Tetracycline, 500 mg, orally, 4 times/day for 14 days (avoid in the second and third trimesters of pregnancy) **OR** Ceftriaxone, 1 g daily either IM or IV for 10 days
Late latent syphilis[d]	Penicillin G benzathine, 50 000 U/kg, IM, up to the adult dose of 2.4 million U, administered as 3 single doses at 1-wk intervals (total 150 000 U/kg, up to the adult dose of 7.2 million U) *If allergic to penicillin and not pregnant,* Doxycycline, 4.4 mg/kg divided in 2 doses, max 200 mg per day, orally, twice a day for 4 wk	Penicillin G benzathine, 7.2 million U total, administered as 3 doses of 2.4 million U, IM, each at 1-wk intervals; pregnant people who have delays in any dose of therapy beyond 9 days between doses should repeat the full course of therapy **OR** *If allergic to penicillin,* Doxycycline, 100 mg, orally, twice a day for 4 wk (avoid in the second and third trimesters of pregnancy) **OR** Tetracycline, 500 mg, orally, 4 times/day for 4 wk (avoid in the second and third trimesters of pregnancy)

Table 3.73. Recommended Treatment for Acquired Primary, Secondary, Early Latent Syphilis; Late Latent Syphilis; Tertiary Syphilis; and Neurosyphilis,[a] continued

Status	Children	Adults
	OR	Penicillin G benzathine, 7.2 million U total, administered as 3 doses of 2.4 million U, IM, at 1-wk intervals
	Tetracycline, 25–50 mg/kg divided in 4 doses, max 2 g per day, orally, for 4 wk **(for age ≥8 years)**	*If allergic to penicillin and not pregnant, consult an infectious diseases expert*
Tertiary	…	Aqueous crystalline penicillin G, 18–24 million U per day, administered as 3–4 million U, IV, every 4 h or as a continuous infusion for 10–14 days[f]
		OR
		Penicillin G procaine,[c] 2.4 million U, IM, once daily **PLUS** probenecid, 500 mg, orally, 4 times/day, both for 10–14 days[f]
		OR
Neurosyphilis[e]	Aqueous crystalline penicillin G, 200 000–300 000 U/kg/day, IV, administered as 50 000 U/kg every 4–6 h or as a continuous infusion for 10–14 days, in doses not to exceed the adult dose	*If allergic to penicillin,* Ceftriaxone, 1–2 g daily either IM or IV for 10–14 days

IM indicates intramuscularly; IV, intravenously.

[a] Excludes patients with either early or late recognition of congenital syphilis.

[b] Early latent syphilis is defined as being acquired within the preceding year.

[c] Penicillin G benzathine and penicillin G procaine are approved for intramuscular administration only.

[d] Late latent syphilis is defined as syphilis beyond 1 year's duration.

[e] Patients who are allergic to penicillin should be desensitized.

[f] Penicillin G benzathine, 2.4 million U, IM, once per week for up to 3 weeks after completion of these neurosyphilis treatment regimens can be considered.

Other Considerations.

- Outside of the neonatal period, all patients with syphilis should be tested for other sexually transmitted infections (STIs), including *Neisseria gonorrhoeae*, *Chlamydia trachomatis*, HIV, hepatitis B, and hepatitis C. Patients who have syphilis should be retested for HIV infection after 3 months if the first HIV test result is negative. Immunization status for hepatitis B and HPV should be reviewed and vaccines should be administered if not up to date.
- All recent sexual contacts of people with acquired syphilis should be evaluated for other STIs as well as syphilis (see Control Measures, p 841).
- Children with acquired primary, secondary, or latent syphilis should be evaluated for possible sexual assault or abuse (see Sexual Assault and Abuse in Children and Adolescents/Young Adults, p 182).

Follow-up and Management.

Congenital Syphilis. All infants who have reactive serologic tests for syphilis or were born to a person who was seroreactive at delivery should receive careful follow-up evaluations during well-child care visits at 2, 4, 6, and 12 months of age. Serologic nontreponemal tests should be performed every 2 to 3 months until the test becomes nonreactive. Nontreponemal antibody titers typically decrease by 3 months of age and should be nonreactive by 6 months of age, whether the infant was infected and adequately treated or was not infected and initially seropositive because of transplacentally acquired maternal antibody. The serologic response after therapy may be slower for infants treated after the neonatal period. Patients with increasing titers or with persistent stable titers 6 to 12 months after initial treatment should be reevaluated, including a CSF examination. Retreatment with a 10-day course of parenteral penicillin G may be indicated, even if they were treated previously. Neonates with a negative nontreponemal test at birth whose birthing parent was seroreactive at delivery should be retested at 3 months to rule out incubating congenital syphilis.

Treponemal tests should not be used to evaluate treatment response, because results can remain positive despite effective therapy. Transplacentally acquired treponemal antibodies can persist in an infant until 15 months of age. A reactive treponemal test after 18 months of age is diagnostic of congenital syphilis and should be followed by evaluation and, if necessary, treatment for congenital syphilis. If the treponemal test is nonreactive at this time, no further evaluation or treatment is necessary.

Neonates whose initial CSF evaluations are abnormal do not need repeat lumbar puncture unless they exhibit persistent nontreponemal serologic test titers at age 6 to 12 months. After 2 years of follow-up, a reactive CSF VDRL test or abnormal CSF indices that cannot be attributed to another ongoing illness at the 6-month interval are indications for retreatment.

Acquired Syphilis. People with acquired primary or secondary syphilis should have clinical and serologic evaluations at 6 and 12 months after treatment. More frequent evaluation might be necessary if adherence to follow-up or reinfection is a concern. If signs or symptoms persist or recur, or a fourfold or greater increase in nontreponemal titers occurs, treatment failure or reinfection may be responsible. CSF analysis, HIV testing, and retreatment based on CSF findings are indicated. Failure of nontreponemal titers to decline fourfold within 6 to 12 months may also indicate treatment failure.

Following treatment, people with acquired latent syphilis should have serologic evaluation at 6, 12, and 24 months after treatment; people with HIV should have serologic testing at 3, 6, 9, 12, and 24 months. Patients should experience a fourfold or greater decline in nontreponemal titers within 12 to 24 months. If titers increase at least fourfold or initial high titers fail to fall fourfold, or symptoms of syphilis develop, reevaluation, including a CSF examination, is warranted. Additional guidance can be found in the current CDC guidelines for the management of STIs.[1]

Patients with neurosyphilis associated with acquired syphilis must have periodic serologic testing and clinical evaluation at 6-month intervals. Among immunocompetent persons and persons with HIV who are receiving effective antiretroviral treatment, normalization of the serum RPR titer predicts normalization of abnormal CSF parameters after neurosyphilis treatment, and repeated CSF examinations are not necessary. CSF abnormalities may persist for extended periods of time in people with combined HIV and neurosyphilis infections.

INFECTION PREVENTION AND CONTROL MEASURES IN HEALTH CARE SETTINGS:
Standard precautions are recommended for all patients, including infants with suspected or proven congenital syphilis. Because moist open lesions, secretions, and possibly blood are contagious in all patients with syphilis, gloves should be worn when caring for patients with congenital, primary, and secondary syphilis with skin and mucous membrane lesions until 24 hours of treatment has been completed.

CONTROL MEASURES:
- All recent sexual contacts of a person with acquired syphilis should be identified, examined, serologically tested, and treated as needed. Sexual contacts of people with primary, secondary, or early latent syphilis exposed within the preceding 90 days may be infected even if seronegative and should be treated for early-acquired syphilis. Sexual contacts exposed >90 days previously who have negative serologic tests do not require treatment; however, contacts should be treated presumptively if serologic test results are not available immediately and follow-up is uncertain. For identification of at-risk sexual partners, the periods before treatment are as follows: (1) 3 months plus duration of symptoms for primary syphilis; (2) 6 months plus duration of symptoms for secondary syphilis; and (3) 1 year for early latent syphilis.
- All people who have had close unprotected contact with a patient with early congenital syphilis before identification of the disease or during the first 24 hours of therapy should be examined clinically for the presence of lesions 2 to 3 weeks after contact. Serologic testing should be performed and repeated 3 months after contact or sooner if symptoms occur. If the degree of exposure is considered substantial, immediate treatment should be considered.
- Doxycycline, 200 mg, administered within 24 to 72 hours of condomless sex (doxy-PEP) has been shown in studies to reduce the incidence of syphilis, chlamydia, and gonorrhea among cisgender men who have sex with men (MSM) and transgender women with a recent history of these infections.

Public Health Reporting. Congenital syphilis is a nationally notifiable disease in the United States.

---

[1] Centers for Disease Control and Prevention. Sexually transmitted infections treatment guidelines, 2021. *MMWR Recomm Rep.* 2021;70(RR-4):1-187

Tapeworm Diseases
(Taeniasis and Cysticercosis)

CLINICAL MANIFESTATIONS:

Taeniasis. Infection with adult tapeworms often is asymptomatic. The most common sign is noting tapeworm segments passing from the anus or in feces. Other mild gastrointestinal tract symptoms, such as nausea or diarrhea, can occur.

Cysticercosis. Cysticercosis, caused by larval pork tapeworm (*Taenia solium*) infection, can have serious consequences. Manifestations depend on the location and number of pork tapeworm larval cysts (cysticerci) and on the host response. Cysticerci may be found anywhere in the body. The most common and serious clinical manifestations are caused by cysticerci in the central nervous system. Larval cysts of *T solium* in the brain (neurocysticercosis) can result in seizures, headache, obstructive hydrocephalus, and other neurologic signs and symptoms. Neurocysticercosis is the leading infectious cause of epilepsy in low- and middle-income countries. Most symptoms result from the host reaction to degenerating cysticerci. Cysts in the spinal column can cause gait disturbance, pain, or transverse myelitis. Subcutaneous cysticerci produce palpable nodules, and ocular involvement can cause visual impairment.

ETIOLOGY: Taeniasis is caused by intestinal infection by the adult tapeworm, *Taenia saginata* (beef tapeworm) or *T solium* (pork tapeworm). *Taenia asiatica* causes taeniasis in Asia. Human cysticercosis is caused only by the larvae of *T solium*.

EPIDEMIOLOGY: Tapeworm diseases have worldwide distribution. Prevalence is high in areas with poor sanitation and human fecal contamination in areas where cattle graze or swine are fed. Most cases of *T solium* infection in the United States are imported from Latin America, although the disease is prevalent in parts of Asia and sub-Saharan Africa as well. *T saginata* infection occurs at high rates in East Africa and the Middle East and also is prevalent in Latin America, much of Asia, and eastern Europe. *T asiatica* is common in China, Taiwan, and Southeast Asia. Taeniasis is acquired by eating undercooked beef *(T saginata),* pork *(T solium),* or pig viscera *(T asiatica)* that contain encysted larvae.

Cysticercosis in humans is acquired by ingesting eggs of the pork tapeworm *(T solium).* Transmission is fecal-oral from a person harboring the adult tapeworm — for example, eating food or drinking water contaminated with pork tapeworm eggs from an infected person. Studies in endemic areas show household clustering, suggesting increased risk of exposure for those residing with or near tapeworm carriers. Autoinfection, in which tapeworm carriers infect themselves, also occurs. Humans are the obligate definitive host and the only host to shed eggs. Pigs act as an intermediate host, developing cysts upon acquisition of eggs from human stool contaminating their feeding, and developing cysts in their muscles. Humans who eat undercooked pork swallow cysts in the meat, and larvae come out of these cysts to complete the infection cycle. Eating of undercooked infected pork does not directly cause cysticercosis, but can spread cysticercosis through release of eggs from an infected person and can lead to cysticercosis in the person who eats the undercooked pork through autoinfection. Eggs liberate oncospheres in the intestine that migrate through the blood and lymphatics to tissues throughout the body, including the central nervous system, where the oncospheres develop into cysticerci. Although nearly all cases of cysticercosis in the United States are imported, cysticercosis can be acquired in the United States from tapeworm carriers who emigrated from an area with endemic infection and still have *T solium* intestinal-stage infection. *T saginata* and *T asiatica* do not cause cysticercosis.

The **incubation period** for taeniasis (the time from ingestion of the larvae until segments are passed in the feces) is 2 to 3 months. For cysticercosis, the **incubation period** between infection and onset of symptoms is typically several years.

DIAGNOSIS[1]: Diagnosis of taeniasis (adult tapeworm infection) is based on demonstration of the proglottids or ova in feces or the perianal region, although these techniques are insensitive, so 3 tests on different days are recommended for evaluation. Antigen detection, nucleic acid tests, and immunoblot assays for tapeworm stage-specific antibody are more sensitive but are not commercially available. Species identification of the parasite is based on the different structures of gravid proglottids and scolex or on a nucleic acid amplification test (NAAT).

Diagnosis of neurocysticercosis typically depends on clinical presentation and imaging of the central nervous system. Serologic testing also can be helpful in certain cases. Computed tomography (CT) scanning or magnetic resonance imaging (MRI) of the brain or spinal cord are used to demonstrate lesions compatible with cysticerci. CT scans are helpful in identifying calcifications. MRI is better at identifying extraparenchymal cysts (eg, in ventricles or the subarachnoid space) and the invaginated scolex within the parasite cysticercus. Antibody assays that detect specific antibodies to larval *T solium* in serum can be useful to confirm the diagnosis. Commercially available antibody tests that use crude antigen in an enzyme-linked immunosorbent assay (ELISA) format lack adequate sensitivity and specificity and are not reliable diagnostic techniques. In the United States, immunoblot assays (including the Enzyme-linked ImmunoTransfer Blot [EITB]) are available through the Centers for Disease Control and Prevention and a few commercial laboratories and are the antibody tests of choice. In general, immunoblot assays are more sensitive with serum specimens than with cerebrospinal fluid specimens. Even immunoblot tests can have limited sensitivity if only 1 cysticercus or only calcified cysticerci are present. Thus, results often are negative in children with solitary parenchymal lesions. A negative serologic test result does not exclude the diagnosis of neurocysticercosis when clinical suspicion is high. A serologic test result could be positive in patients who have *T solium* cysticerci in parts of the body other than the central nervous system. Antigen-detection assays are available commercially in Europe. NAATs have been used in diagnosis and follow-up of selected cases. Antigen-detection and NAATs are available from the National Institutes of Health for selected cases.

TREATMENT[1]:

Taeniasis. Praziquantel is highly effective for eradicating infection with the adult tapeworm (see Drugs for Parasitic Infections, p 1068). Praziquantel is not approved for this indication, but dosing recommendations are available for children 4 years and older.

[1] White AC Jr, Coyle CM, Rajshekhar V, et al. Diagnosis and treatment of neurocysticercosis: 2017 clinical practice guidelines by the Infectious Diseases Society of America (IDSA) and the American Society of Tropical Medicine and Hygiene (ASTMH). *Clin Infect Dis.* 2018;66(8):1159-1163

Safety is not established in children younger than 4 years, but this drug has been used successfully to treat cases of *Dipylidium caninum* infection in children as young as 6 months. Praziquantel is detected in the milk of lactating people, and people should not breastfeed on the day of treatment or during the subsequent 72 hours. Niclosamide is an alternative agent for treatment of taeniasis but is not available commercially in the United States. Albendazole has been used successfully for taeniasis in a small number of individuals and is an alternative treatment if praziquantel and niclosamide are not available.

Cysticercosis. Neurocysticercosis treatment should be individualized based on the number, location, and viability of cysticerci as assessed by neuroimaging studies (MRI and CT scan) and clinical manifestations. Symptomatic therapy is critical and should include antiseizure medications for patients with seizures and surgery for patients with hydrocephalus. Two antiparasitic drugs—albendazole and praziquantel—are available (see Drugs for Parasitic Infections, p 1068). Praziquantel is not approved by the US Food and Drug Administration for this indication. Both drugs are cysticercidal and hasten radiologic resolution of cysts, but symptoms resulting from host inflammatory response may be exacerbated by treatment. In symptomatic patients with a single cyst within brain parenchyma, controlled studies demonstrate that clinical resolution and seizure recurrence rates are improved slightly when children are treated with albendazole along with corticosteroids. Two studies have demonstrated that in individuals with more than 2 lesions, the response rate was better when albendazole was coadministered with praziquantel and corticosteroids. When a single agent is used, albendazole is preferred over praziquantel, because it has fewer drug-drug interactions with anticonvulsants and steroids. Patients with calcified cysts do not benefit from antiparasitic treatment. An ophthalmic examination should be performed before antiparasitic treatment to rule out intraocular cysticerci (see below). Coadministration of corticosteroids during antiparasitic therapy decreases adverse effects during treatment and is recommended for all patients with viable intraparenchymal neurocysticercosis who are treated with antiparasitic drugs, starting before antiparasitic therapy is initiated. See footnote 61 of Drugs for Parasitic Infections, p 1112, for steroid dosing. Duration of corticosteroid therapy is longer in patients with subarachnoid disease, vasculitis, or encephalitis. Arachnoiditis, vasculitis, or diffuse cerebral edema (cysticercal encephalitis) are treated with corticosteroid therapy until cerebral edema is controlled. Corticosteroids can affect tissue concentrations of albendazole. Patients requiring steroids may need screening for strongyloidiasis, latent tuberculosis, and vitamin D deficiency.

Medical and surgical management of cysticercosis can be highly complex and often needs to be conducted in consultation with a neurologist or neurosurgeon and an infectious diseases or other specialist with experience treating neurocysticercosis. Seizures may recur for months or years. Anticonvulsant therapy is recommended until there is neuroradiologic evidence of resolution and seizures have not occurred for 6 months (for a single lesion) or 2 years (for multiple lesions). Calcification of cysts may require prolonged or indefinite use of anticonvulsants. Subarachnoid cysticercosis does not respond well to the regimens used for parenchymal disease and generally should be treated with prolonged courses of antiparasitic and anti-inflammatory medications, monitoring radiologic resolution and NAAT or antigen assay results. Methotrexate and/or tumor necrosis factor inhibitors have been used as steroid-sparing agents. Intraventricular cysticerci and hydrocephalus usually should be treated surgically. Surgical removal of intraventricular cysticerci is the treatment of choice when possible and often can be accomplished by endoscopic surgery (lateral, third, and sometimes fourth ventricles) or open surgery (fourth ventricle). If cysticerci cannot be removed, hydrocephalus should be corrected with placement of intraventricular shunts. Adjunctive chemotherapy with antiparasitic agents and corticosteroids may decrease the rate of subsequent shunt failure. Ocular cysticercosis is treated by surgical excision of the cysticerci. Ocular cysticercosis generally is not treated with anthelmintic drugs, which can exacerbate inflammation. Spinal cysticercosis may be treated with medical and/or surgical therapy as there is not adequate evidence to guide the choice of therapy.

INFECTION PREVENTION AND CONTROL MEASURES IN HEALTH CARE SETTINGS: Standard precautions are recommended.

CONTROL MEASURES: Eating raw or undercooked beef or pork should be avoided. Whole cuts of meat should be cooked to at least 145°F (63°C) and then allowed to rest for 3 minutes before consuming, and ground meat and wild game meat should be cooked to at least 160°F (71°C). Freezing pork or beef below −5°C (23°F) for more than 4 days kills cysticerci. People known to harbor the adult tapeworm of *T solium* should be treated immediately. Careful attention to hand hygiene and appropriate disposal of fecal material are important preventive measures. People traveling to resource-limited countries with high endemic rates of cysticercosis should avoid eating uncooked vegetables and fruits that cannot be peeled. If someone in a household is found to have cysticercosis, household members should be screened for taeniasis (see Diagnosis), and people with compatible neurologic signs and symptoms should be evaluated for cysticercosis.

Other Tapeworm Infections
(Including Hydatid Disease)

Most intestinal tapeworm (cestode) infections are asymptomatic, but nausea, abdominal pain, and diarrhea have been observed in people who are heavily infected.

ETIOLOGIES, DIAGNOSIS, AND TREATMENT

Hymenolepis nana. This tapeworm, also called the dwarf tapeworm because it is the smallest of the adult human tapeworms (about 3 to 4 cm long), can complete its entire life cycle within humans. Transmission occurs by inadvertent ingestion of eggs present in feces of infected people or rarely by ingestion of infected arthropods (certain species of beetles and fleas) present in food. Autoinfection, in which eggs can hatch within the intestine and reinitiate the life cycle, leads to development of new worms and increases the worm burden. Most infections are asymptomatic. Young children may develop abdominal cramps, diarrhea, and anemia with heavy infection. Anal pruritus and difficulty sleeping mimic pinworm infections. Diagnosis is by identification of the characteristic eggs in stool. Praziquantel is the treatment of choice, with nitazoxanide as an alternative drug; niclosamide is another therapeutic option but is not available commercially in the United States (see Drugs for Parasitic Infections, p 1068). Praziquantel and nitazoxanide are not approved for this indication, but these drugs have been used safely and effectively in children as young as 6 months (praziquantel) and 1 year (nitazoxanide) for other indications. Stools should be reexamined 1 month after treatment to document cure. If infection persists, retreatment with praziquantel is indicated.

Dipylidium caninum. This is the most common tapeworm of dogs and cats and has a wide geographic distribution. Children develop infection with *D caninum* after inadvertently swallowing a dog or cat flea (the intermediate host). Most cases are asymptomatic and come to attention when motile proglottids are passed in stool. Some children have abdominal pain, diarrhea, and anal pruritus. Diagnosis is made by finding the characteristic eggs or motile proglottids in stool. Proglottids resemble rice kernels and may be mistaken for maggots (fly larvae) or pinworms. Infection is self-limiting in the human host and typically clears spontaneously by 6 weeks. Therapy with praziquantel is effective. Niclosamide is an alternative therapeutic option but is not available commercially in the United States (see Drugs for Parasitic Infections, p 1068). Praziquantel and niclosamide are not approved for this indication. These drugs have been used safely and effectively in children as young as 6 months (praziquantel) and 2 years (niclosamide) (**www.cdc.gov/parasites/dipylidium/health_professionals/index.html**).

Diphyllobothriid *species (Dibothriocephalus and Related Species).* These are the largest tapeworms that infect humans and are also known as fish tapeworm or broad tapeworm. Fish are intermediate hosts of the diphyllobothriid tapeworms, which were previously all known as *Diphyllobothrium* species. Consumption of infected raw or undercooked freshwater (including trout and pike), saltwater (at least 17 species including one shark), or anadromous (salmon) fish may lead to infection with these tapeworms. Three to 6 weeks after ingestion, the adult tapeworm matures and begins to lay eggs. The most common symptom is the passage of proglottids. Abdominal pain and diarrhea may occur. The worm rarely may cause mechanical obstruction of the bowel or gallbladder, diarrhea, or abdominal pain. Megaloblastic anemia secondary to vitamin B_{12} deficiency has been noted only with the species *Dibothriocephalus latus* (formerly *Diphyllobothrium latum*) found in trout and pike in northern Europe and North America. Other common species include *Dibothriocephalus nihonkaiense,* found in salmon in Northeast Asia (Japan, Korea) and the North Pacific of North America, and *Adenocephalus pacificus,* found in marine fish off the Pacific coast of South America. Diagnosis is made by recognition of the characteristic proglottids or eggs passed in stool. Therapy with praziquantel is effective; niclosamide is an alternative but is not available commercially in the United States (see Drugs for Parasitic Infections, p 1068). Praziquantel and niclosamide are not approved for this indication. These drugs have been used safely and effectively in children as young as 6 months (praziquantel) and 2 years (niclosamide).

Echinococcus granulosus *and* Echinococcus multilocularis.[1] The larval forms of these tapeworms cause human echinococcosis. *Echinococcus granulosus* causes the disease cystic echinococcosis, also known as hydatid disease. The distribution of *E granulosus* is related to areas where sheep or cattle are raised and dogs, the definitive host, are used for herding. Areas of high prevalence include parts of South America, East Africa, Eastern Europe, the Middle East, the Mediterranean region, China, and Central Asia. The parasite also is endemic in Australia and New Zealand. In the United States, small foci of endemic transmission have been reported in Arizona, California, New Mexico, and Utah, and a strain of the parasite has adapted to wolves, moose, and caribou in Alaska, northern New England, and Canada. Dogs, coyotes, wolves, dingoes, and

[1] Brunetti E, Kern P, Vuitton DA; Writing Panel for the WHO-Informal Working Group on Echinococcosis. Expert consensus for the diagnosis and treatment of cystic and alveolar echinococcosis in humans. *Acta Trop.* 2010;114(1):1-16

jackals can become infected by swallowing protoscolices of the parasite within hydatid cysts in the organs of slaughtered sheep or other intermediate hosts. Dogs pass embryonated eggs in their feces, and humans become infected by ingesting the viable parasite eggs. Humans then develop cysts in various organs, such as the liver, lungs, kidneys, and spleen. Cysts caused by larvae of *E granulosus* usually grow slowly (1 cm in diameter per year in the liver) and eventually can contain several liters of fluid. If a cyst ruptures, anaphylaxis and multiple secondary cysts from seeding of protoscolices can result. Clinical diagnosis often is difficult. A history of contact with dogs in an area with endemic infection is helpful. Cystic lesions can be demonstrated by radiography, ultrasonography, or computed tomography of various organs. Serologic testing is helpful, but false-negative results occur. Treatment depends on ultrasonographic staging and may include antiparasitic therapy, PAIR (**p**uncture, **a**spiration, **i**njection of protoscolicidal agents, and **r**easpiration), surgical excision, or no treatment but with watchful waiting. Optimal therapy varies with the location, size, and stage of the parasite (**www.cdc.gov/parasites/echinococcosis/health_professionals/index. html#tx**). Small cysts in the liver may respond to antiparasitic drugs alone. For larger, uncomplicated liver cysts, treatment of choice is PAIR. Contraindications to PAIR include communication of the cyst with the biliary tract (eg, bile staining after initial aspiration), superficial cysts, and heavily septated cysts. Surgical therapy is indicated for complicated cases and requires meticulous care to prevent spillage, including preparations such as soaking of surgical drapes in hypertonic saline. In general, the cyst should be removed intact, because leakage of contents is associated with a higher rate of complications, including anaphylactic reactions to cyst contents. Treatment with albendazole (or mebendazole) alone or with praziquantel generally should be initiated days to weeks before surgery or PAIR and continued for several weeks to months thereafter (see Drugs for Parasitic Infections, p 1068). Degenerating cysts can be managed by watchful waiting with follow-up imaging studies. For lung lesions, small cysts often resolve with antiparasitic drugs alone. Larger cysts are best removed surgically. Many surgeons prefer to avoid preoperative antiparasitic drugs for lung cysts.

Echinococcus multilocularis, the causative agent for alveolar echinococcosis, also has definitive hosts (foxes, coyotes, other wild canines) and intermediate hosts (rodents). Alveolar echinococcosis is characterized by invasive growth of the larvae in the liver (which may mimic neoplasm) with occasional metastatic spread. Alveolar echinococcosis is limited to the Northern Hemisphere and usually is diagnosed in people 50 years or older. The disease has been reported frequently from western China and also is endemic in central Europe. More recently, a focus was identified in western Canada. Diagnosis can be confirmed by imaging and serologic testing. The preferred treatment is surgical removal of the entire larval mass followed by treatment with albendazole. In nonresectable cases, continuous treatment with albendazole has been associated with clinical improvement (see Drugs for Parasitic Infections, p 1068). Two other species, *Echinococcus vogeli* and *Echinococcus oligarthrus*, rarely infect humans; they cause polycystic echinococcosis.

INFECTION PREVENTION AND CONTROL MEASURES IN HEALTH CARE SETTINGS: Standard precautions are recommended.

CONTROL MEASURES: Preventive measures for *H nana* include educating the public about personal hygiene and sanitary disposal of feces.

Infection with *D caninum* is prevented by keeping dogs and cats free of fleas and worms. Children should wash their hands after playing with dogs and cats and after playing in areas soiled with pet feces.

To protect against diphyllobothriid infections, fish should be cooked thoroughly to an internal temperature of 63°C (145°F) or should be frozen per the following recommendations:

- At −4°F (−20°C) or below for 7 days (total time), or
- At −31°F (−35°C) or below until solid, and storing at −31°F (−35°C) or below for 15 hours, or
- At −31°F (−35°C) or below until solid and storing at −4°F (−20°C) or below for 24 hours.

Control measures for prevention of *E granulosus* and *E multilocularis* include educating the public about hand hygiene and avoiding exposure to dog and wild canid feces. Prevention and control of infection in dogs (preventing dogs from feeding on rodents or carcasses of sheep, treating dogs for parasitic infections) decreases the risk of subsequent human infection.

Tetanus
(Lockjaw)

CLINICAL MANIFESTATIONS: Tetanus is caused by neurotoxin produced by the anaerobic bacterium *Clostridium tetani* in a contaminated wound and can manifest in 3 overlapping clinical forms: generalized, local, and cephalic.

Generalized tetanus (lockjaw) is a neurologic disease manifesting as trismus and severe muscular spasms, including risus sardonicus, which is a facial expression characterized by raised eyebrows and grinning distortion of the face resulting from spasm of facial muscles. Onset is gradual, occurring over 1 to 7 days, and symptoms progress to severe painful generalized muscle spasms, which often are aggravated by any external stimulus. Autonomic dysfunction, manifesting as diaphoresis, tachycardia, labile blood pressure, and arrhythmias, often is present. Other potential complications include fractures associated with muscle spasms, laryngospasm, pulmonary embolism, and aspiration pneumonia. Severe spasms persist for 1 week or more and subside over several weeks in people who recover. Neonatal tetanus is a form of generalized tetanus occurring in newborn infants lacking protective passive immunity because their birthing parent was not immune. Early symptoms include inability to suck or breastfeed and excessive crying that then progress to findings typical of generalized tetanus.

Local tetanus manifests as local muscle spasms in areas contiguous to a wound. **Cephalic tetanus** is the rarest form of tetanus and usually causes flaccid cranial nerve palsies, although trismus can occur. It is associated with infected wounds on the head and neck including, rarely, suppurative otitis media. Local and cephalic tetanus can precede generalized tetanus.

ETIOLOGY: *C tetani* is a spore-forming, obligate anaerobic, gram-positive bacillus. This organism is a wound contaminant that causes neither tissue destruction nor an inflammatory response. The vegetative form of *C tetani* produces a potent plasmid-encoded exotoxin (tetanospasmin). The heavy chain of tetanospasmin binds to the presynaptic motor neuron and facilitates entry of the light chain, a zinc-dependent protease, into the cytosol. As a result, gamma-aminobutyric acid- and glycine-containing vesicles are not released, and inhibitory action on motor and autonomic neurons is lost.

EPIDEMIOLOGY: Tetanus occurs worldwide and is more common in warmer climates and during warmer months, in part because of higher frequency of contaminated wounds associated with those locations and seasons. The organism, a normal inhabitant of soil and animal and human intestines, is ubiquitous in the environment, especially where contamination by excreta is common. Organisms multiply in wounds, recognized or unrecognized, and elaborate toxins in the presence of anaerobic conditions. Contaminated wounds, especially wounds with devitalized tissue and deep-puncture trauma, are at greatest risk. Neonatal tetanus is common in many resource-limited countries where pregnant people are not immunized appropriately against tetanus and nonsterile practices for umbilical cord care are followed. Globally, activities are ongoing to eliminate tetanus in pregnant people and neonates by improving vaccination coverage among pregnant people and promoting safe delivery practices. In December 2020, only 12 countries had not yet achieved tetanus elimination in pregnant people and neonates; globally, the estimated burden of neonatal tetanus has declined by more than 90% since the 1980s.[1]

Widespread active immunization against tetanus has modified the epidemiology of disease in the United States, where it is now rare. Tetanus is not transmissible from person to person.

In the United States, nearly all cases of tetanus occur in individuals who have never received a tetanus vaccine or who have not received their 10-year booster vaccine. At particular risk are people with immune-compromising conditions, people with diabetes mellitus, or people who use intravenous drugs.

The **incubation period** ranges from 3 to 21 days, with most cases occurring within 8 days. In general, the farther the injury site from the central nervous system, the longer the incubation period. Shorter incubation periods have been associated with more heavily contaminated wounds, more severe disease, and a worse prognosis. In neonatal tetanus, the **incubation period** from birth to onset of symptoms is usually 4 to 14 days, averaging 7 days. Cephalic tetanus may have an **incubation period** as short as 1 to 2 days.

DIAGNOSTIC TESTS: The diagnosis of tetanus is made clinically by excluding other causes of tetanic spasms, such as hypocalcemic tetany, phenothiazine reaction, strychnine poisoning, and conversion disorder. Attempts to culture *C tetani* are associated with poor yield, and a negative culture does not rule out disease. A protective serum antitoxin concentration should not be used to exclude the diagnosis of tetanus, because tetanus disease has been known to occur rarely despite adequate antibody concentrations.

TREATMENT: Human tetanus immune globulin (TIG) binds circulating unbound toxin and prevents further progression of disease, but it does not reverse the effects of already bound toxin. A single dose of human TIG is recommended for treatment. However, the optimal therapeutic dose has not been established. Most experts recommend 500 IU, which appears to be as effective as higher doses ranging from 3000 to 6000 IU and causes less discomfort. Available preparations must be administered intramuscularly. Infiltration of part of the dose locally around the wound is recommended, although the efficacy of this approach has not been proven. Results of studies on the benefit from intrathecal administration of TIG are conflicting. The TIG preparation

[1] GBD 2019 Diseases and Injuries Collaborators. Global burden of 369 diseases and injuries in 204 countries and territories, 1990-2019: a systematic analysis for the Global Burden of Disease Study 2019. *Lancet.* 2020;396(10258):1204-1222

in use in the United States is not licensed or formulated for intrathecal or intravenous use. If TIG is not available (as is the case in some countries), immune globulin intravenous (IGIV) can be used at a dose of 200 to 400 mg/kg. IGIV is not approved by the US Food and Drug Administration for this use, and antitetanus antibody concentrations can vary from lot to lot. In some countries, equine tetanus antitoxin may be considered if TIG is not available and the patient is tested for sensitivity and desensitized as necessary. Additional management is as follows:

- All wounds should be cleaned and débrided properly, especially if extensive necrosis is present. In neonatal tetanus, wide excision of the umbilical stump is not indicated.
- Supportive care and pharmacotherapy to control tetanic spasms and autonomic instability are of major importance.
- Oral (or intravenous) metronidazole is effective in decreasing the number of vegetative forms of *C tetani* and is the antimicrobial agent of choice. Parenteral penicillin G is an alternative treatment. Therapy for 7 to 10 days is recommended.
- Active immunization against tetanus always should be undertaken during convalescence from tetanus. Because of the extreme potency of tiny amounts of toxin, tetanus disease may not result in immunity.

INFECTION PREVENTION AND CONTROL MEASURES IN HEALTH CARE SETTINGS: Standard precautions are recommended.

CONTROL MEASURES:

Care of Exposed People (see Fig 3.19). Risk of tetanus disease depends on the type of wound and immune status of the patient. Depending on the clinical scenario, there are 3 potential interventions to prevent tetanus: wound care, active immunization, and passive immunization. Antimicrobial prophylaxis has not been shown to prevent tetanus and is not recommended.

- Wound care: Although any open wound is a potential source of tetanus, wounds contaminated with dirt, feces, soil, or saliva (eg, animal bites) are at increased risk. Punctures and wounds containing devitalized tissue, including necrotic or gangrenous wounds, frostbite, crush and avulsion injuries, and burns, are particularly conducive to *C tetani* infection. Wounds with devitalized tissue should be débrided and have dirt removed. It is not necessary or appropriate to débride puncture wounds extensively.
- Active immunization: Immunization status should be assessed for all wounds, and age-appropriate vaccine should be administered (see Immunization) if not contraindicated on the basis of clinical scenario (Fig 3.19). For infants younger than 6 months, prior infant doses and maternal tetanus toxoid immunization history at time of delivery should be considered in determining need for infant immunization (and need for TIG, if clinically indicated).
- Passive immunization: Patients with tetanus-prone wounds who have not completed a primary series of tetanus vaccine should be considered nonimmune and should receive passive immunization with TIG (in addition to active immunization with tetanus toxoid vaccine, as clinically appropriate). In patients with human immunodeficiency virus (HIV) or other severe immunodeficiency, TIG should be administered for tetanus-prone wounds regardless of the history of tetanus toxoid immunization. When TIG is required for wound prophylaxis, it is administered intramuscularly in a dose of 250 U (regardless of age or weight). If tetanus toxoid vaccine and TIG are administered concurrently, separate syringes and sites should be used. Administration of tetanus toxoid vaccine simultaneously with or at an interval after receipt of TIG

FIG 3.19. SUMMARY GUIDE TO TETANUS PROPHYLAXIS IN ROUTINE WOUND MANAGEMENT

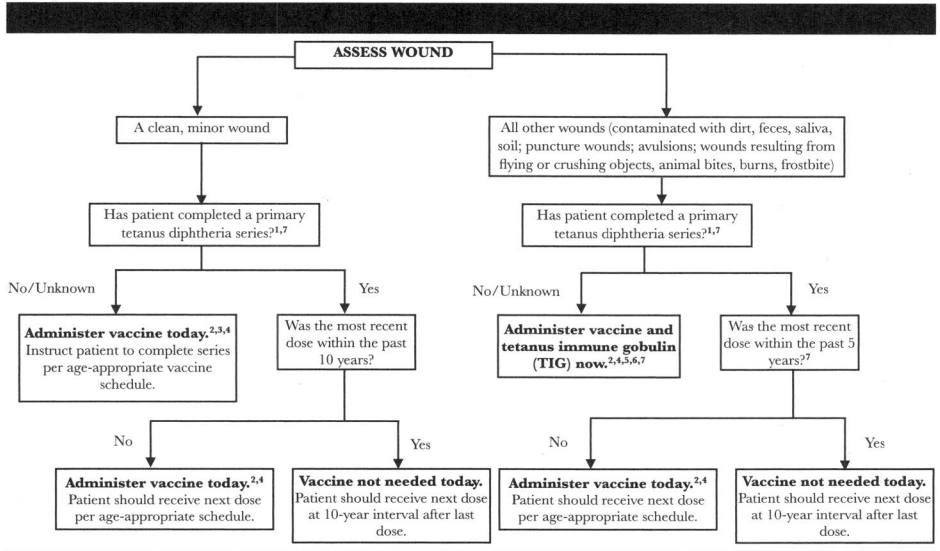

[1] A primary series consists of a minimum of 3 doses of tetanus- and diphtheriacontaining vaccine (DTaP/DTP/Tdap/DT/Td).

[2] Age-appropriate vaccine:
- DTaP for infants and children 6 weeks up to 7 years of age.
- Tetanus-diphtheria (Td) toxoid for persons 7 through 9 years of age and 65 years of age and older.
- Tdap for persons 11 through 64 years of age if using Adacel* or 10 years of age and older if using Boostrix*, unless the person has received a prior dose of Tdap.*

[3] No vaccine or TIG is recommended for infants younger than 6 weeks of age with clean, minor wounds. (And no vaccine is licensed for infants younger than 6 weeks of age.)

[4] Tdap* is preferred for persons 11 through 64 years of age if using Adacel* or 10 years of age and older if using Boostrix* who have never received Tdap. Td is preferred to tetanus toxoid (TT) for persons 7 through 9 years, 65 years and older, or who have received a Tdap previously. If TT is administered, and adsorbed TT product is preferred to fluid TT. (All DTaP/DTP/Tdap/Td products contain adsorbed tetanus toxoid.)

[5] Give TIG 250 U IM for all ages. It can and should be given simultaneously with the tetanus-containing vaccine.

[6] For infants younger than 6 weeks of age, TIG (without vaccine) is recommended for "dirty" wounds (wounds other than clean, minor).

[7] Persons who are HIV positive should receive TIG regardless of tetanus immunization history.

*Brand names are used for the purpose of clarifying product characteristics and are not an endorsement of either product. Tdap vaccines:
    Boostrix (GSK) is licensed for persons 10 years of age and older.
    Adacel (sanofi) is licensed for persons 11 through 64 years of age.

Courtesy of the Minnesota Department of Health (**www.health.state.mn.us/diseases/tetanus/hcp/tetwdmgmt. html**), with modifications.

does not impair development of protective antibody substantially. Efforts should be made to initiate active immunization and arrange for its completion.

Immunization. Antibody to tetanus toxoid is detectable 4 to 7 days after a dose of tetanus vaccine, and its concentration peaks at 2 to 4 weeks. Protective antibody is not reliably achieved following a first dose of vaccine to prevent tetanus disease. After completing a vaccination series, circulating antitoxin usually lasts at least 10 years and for a longer time after a booster dose.

Active immunization against tetanus always should be undertaken during convalescence from tetanus, because this exotoxin-mediated disease usually does not confer immunity.

Active immunization with tetanus toxoid vaccine is recommended for all people. For all appropriate indications, tetanus immunization is administered with diphtheria toxoid-containing vaccines or with diphtheria toxoid- and acellular pertussis-containing vaccines. Vaccine is administered intramuscularly and may be administered concurrently with other vaccines (see Simultaneous Administration of Multiple Vaccines, p 63). Conjugate vaccines containing tetanus toxoid (eg, *Haemophilus influenzae* type b) are not substitutes for tetanus toxoid immunization. Recommendations for use of tetanus toxoid-containing vaccines (**https://publications.aap.org/redbook/pages/Immunization-Schedules**) are as follows:

- Immunization for children from 6 weeks through 6 years (up to the seventh birthday) of age:
  - Recommended schedule: should consist of 5 doses of tetanus- and diphtheria toxoid-containing vaccine. All doses are administered as DTaP (or DTaP-containing vaccines) at 2, 4, and 6 months of age, then a dose at 15 through 18 months of age, and another dose at 4 through 6 years of age (recommended before kindergarten or elementary school entry). DTaP can be administered concurrently with other vaccines (see Simultaneous Administration of Multiple Vaccines, p 63). If a dose of Tdap is administered inadvertently instead of DTaP as any one of the primary 3 dose series, then it should not be counted as valid. DTaP can be administered at any interval after the Tdap dose and remaining DTaP doses can be administered as per the recommended schedule. If Tdap is inadvertently administered as the 4th or 5th dose in the series, the Tdap dose is counted as valid toward the 5-dose DTaP series.
  - Catch up vaccination: the 5-dose DTaP series can be administered with a minimum of 4 weeks between each of the first 3 doses and 6 months between dose 3 and 4 as well as dose 4 and 5. If the fourth dose is administered at 4 years or older, the fifth dose is not needed.
  - Pertussis vaccination contraindicated: Contraindications to DTaP and Tdap occur only very rarely, and in questioning about them providers should probe whether a true contraindication actually exists. DTaP and Tdap contraindications are limited to severe allergic reactions (eg, anaphylaxis) and encephalopathy (eg, coma, decreased level of consciousness, or prolonged seizures) not attributable to another identifiable cause within 7 days after administration of a previous dose of diphtheria and tetanus toxoids and pertussis vaccine (see Pertussis [Whooping Cough], p 656). Note that as of 2023, DT is no longer available in the United States (**www.cdc.gov/vaccines/vpd/dtap-tdap-td/hcp/recommendations.html** and **www.cdc.gov/vaccines/vpd/dtap-tdap-td/hcp/td-offlabel.html**; see Diphtheria p 357, and Pertussis p 656). For young children with a contraindication to pertussis-containing vaccines, vaccine providers may administer Td for all recommended remaining doses in place of DTaP. Td contains a lower dose (approximately 1/12th the amount) of diphtheria toxoid compared with DT. The impact of this lower dose on the protection provided against diphtheria in young children is uncertain. Available evidence suggests young children who receive Td in place of DTaP may have suboptimal protection against diphtheria.
  - Series was started with DT, but pertussis vaccination is desired and is not contraindicated: doses of DTaP should be administered to complete the recommended pertussis immunization schedule (see Pertussis, p 656); however, the total number

of doses of diphtheria and tetanus toxoid vaccines (as DT, DTaP, or DTwP) should not exceed 6 before the seventh birthday.

- Immunization for children ≥7 years (see **https://publications.aap.org/ redbook/pages/Immunization-Schedules** and Pertussis [Whooping Cough], p 656)[1]:
  - ◆ Adolescents 11 years and older should receive a single dose of Tdap instead of Td for booster immunization against tetanus, diphtheria, and pertussis. The preferred age for Tdap immunizations is 11 through 12 years of age.
  - ◆ Adolescents who received Td but not Tdap should receive a single dose of Tdap to provide protection against pertussis regardless of time since receipt of Td.
  - ◆ Simultaneous administration of Tdap and all other recommended vaccines is recommended when feasible.
  - ◆ Inadvertent administration of DTaP instead of Tdap in people 7 years and older is counted as a valid dose of Tdap.
  - ◆ Children 7 through 10 years of age who have not completed their immunization schedule with DTaP before 7 years of age or who have an unknown vaccine history should receive at least 1 dose of Tdap. If further dose(s) of tetanus and diphtheria toxoids are needed in a catch-up schedule, either Td or Tdap can be used. The preferred schedule is Tdap followed by Td or Tdap at 2 months and 6 to 12 months (if needed).
  - ◆ Children 7 through 9 years of age who receive Tdap or DTaP for any reason should receive the adolescent Tdap booster at 11 through 12 years of age.
  - ◆ A Tdap or DTaP dose received by a 10 year-old for any reason can count as the adolescent Tdap booster dose.
- If more than 5 years have elapsed since the last dose, a booster dose of a tetanus-containing vaccine should be considered for people at risk of occupational exposure in locations where tetanus boosters may not be available readily. Tdap is preferred over Td if the person has not received Tdap previously.
- Tdap is approved for use by the US Food and Drug Administration (FDA) for use in the third trimester of pregnancy to prevent pertussis in infants younger than 2 months of age. Pregnant people should receive Tdap during each pregnancy, preferably between 27 and 36 weeks' gestation, but the vaccine may be administered at any time during the pregnancy. Pregnant people who have not completed their primary tetanus series should receive 3 vaccinations containing tetanus and reduced diphtheria toxoids, if time permits. The recommended schedule is 0, 4 weeks, and 6 months or later. The risk of neonatal tetanus is minimal if a previously unimmunized person receives at least 2 properly spaced doses of tetanus toxoid-containing vaccines. If there is insufficient time, 2 doses of Td or Tdap should be administered at least 4 weeks apart, and the second dose should be administered at least 2 weeks before delivery. Tdap should be used for at least one of the tetanus-containing doses, preferably early in the interval between 27 and 36 weeks' gestation (see Pertussis [Whooping Cough], p 656).

Adverse Events, Precautions, and Contraindications. Severe anaphylactic reactions, Guillain-Barré syndrome (GBS), and brachial neuritis attributable to tetanus toxoid have been reported but are rare. No increased risk of GBS has been observed with use of DTaP in children. For a child with a history of GBS, the decision to administer

---

[1] Havers FP, Moro PL, Hunter P, Hariri S, Berstein H. Use of tetanus toxoid, reduced diphtheria toxoid, and acellular pertussis vaccines: updated recommendations of the Advisory Committee on Immunization Practices—United States, 2019. *MMWR Morb Mortal Wkly Rep.* 2020;69(3):77-83

additional doses of DTaP should be made on the basis of consideration of the benefit of further immunization versus the risk of recurrence of GBS.

An immediate anaphylactic reaction to tetanus- and diphtheria toxoid-containing vaccines (ie, DTaP, Tdap, DT, Td, or conjugate vaccine containing diphtheria or tetanus toxoid) is a contraindication to further doses unless the component responsible is determined and the patient can be desensitized to that component. Because of the importance of tetanus vaccination, people who experience anaphylactic reactions should be referred to an allergist to determine whether they have a specific allergy to tetanus toxoid and can be desensitized to tetanus toxoid.

Injection site pain and erythema are common. Fever may occur, and rarely, whole limb swelling occurs (with or without pain and erythema). Repeat vaccination, as age appropriate, appears to be safe in children who had whole limb swelling.

Arthus-type hypersensitivity reaction has been reported in adults who received excessive doses of Td over a short period and usually is associated with high concentrations of tetanus antitoxin. Arthus reactions are rare in children and did not occur in clinical trials of Tdap vaccines. People who experienced an Arthus-type hypersensitivity reaction after a previous dose of a tetanus toxoid-containing preparation should not receive dose(s) of tetanus toxoid-containing preparation more frequently than every 10 years, even if they have a wound that is neither clean nor minor.

Other Control Measures. Sterilization of hospital supplies will prevent the rare instances of tetanus that may occur in a hospital from contaminated sutures, instruments, or plaster casts.

For prevention of neonatal tetanus, preventive measures (in addition to immunization of pregnant people) include community immunization programs for people capable of becoming pregnant and appropriate training of obstetric providers (including midwives) in recommendations for immunization and sterile technique.

Tinea Capitis
(Ringworm of the Scalp)

CLINICAL MANIFESTATIONS: Dermatophytic fungal infections of the scalp usually present with an area of localized alopecia and scaling but may include subtle findings of mild hair loss with faint scaling or a large hairless, boggy erythematous area (kerion). Other manifestations include a common "black dot" pattern reflecting stubs of broken-off hairs at the scalp surface; a less common "grey patch" seborrheic dermatitis-like pattern with or without hair loss and prominent, well-demarcated areas of scaling and erythema; or a vesiculopustular pattern resembling bacterial folliculitis. Regional lymphadenopathy may be present.

The differential diagnosis for tinea capitis depends on the clinical presentation. In the classic scaling presentation, clinicians should consider atopic dermatitis, seborrheic dermatitis, and psoriasis. Alopecia should raise the possibility of trichotillomania and alopecia areata, although these disorders usually are not associated with scaling. When vesiculopustular in nature, lice infestation and bacterial infection should be considered. A boggy fluctuant mass likely represents a kerion, but primary (or secondary) bacterial infection can be considered. Although scalp scarring can result from tinea, particularly when a kerion suppurates, presence of scalp scarring should raise the possibility of an autoimmune disorder, such as discoid lupus.

An associated skin eruption, known as a dermatophytic or "id" reaction, can occur as a hypersensitivity reaction to the infecting fungus and can manifest as diffuse, pruritic, papular, vesicular, and/or eczematous lesions occurring at sites distant from the fungal infection including the trunk and extremities. Id reactions often begin after starting therapy but do not represent a drug allergy and should not prompt discontinuation of treatment.

Tinea capitis can occur in association with tinea corporis. Examination of the body (face, trunk, and limbs) should be performed, particularly in wrestlers and others engaged in contact sports.[1] Close contacts including parents, siblings, and other close contacts should be examined for clinical findings consistent with tinea capitis.

ETIOLOGY: Tinea capitis develops when dermatophyte fungal elements invade the scalp hair follicle and shaft. The specific pathogen varies by geographic region and mode of transmission. The primary causes are fungi of the genus *Trichophyton*, including *Trichophyton tonsurans* and *Trichophyton violaceum*, as well as *Microsporum*, including *Microsporum canis* and *Microsporum audouinii*.

EPIDEMIOLOGY: Tinea capitis primarily occurs in prepubertal children but may occur in children of all ages and in adults. In the United States, *T tonsurans* is responsible for up to 95% of tinea capitis and is most common in school-aged children. Infection with *T tonsurans* is contracted from direct contact with an infected individual, animal, or contaminated object such as hat or brush. *T violaceum* is the dominant organism in eastern Europe and south Asia and is seen more frequently in immigrant populations in the United States.

M canis is associated with less than 5% of infections in the United States. *M canis* infection almost always results from contact with infected pets, particularly kittens or puppies. *M canis* outbreaks in schools and child care facilities have followed visits from infected animals. Unlike infections caused by *Trichophyton* species, infections caused by *M canis* are often associated with inflammatory lesions early in the course.

The dermatophyte organism remains viable for prolonged periods on fomites (eg, brushes, combs, hats, towels), and the rate of asymptomatic carriage and infected individuals among family members of index cases is high. Asymptomatic carriers almost certainly serve as a reservoir of infection within families, schools, and communities.

Immunocompromised people and those with trisomy 21 have an increased susceptibility to dermatophyte infections.

The **incubation period** is unknown but is believed to be 1 to 3 weeks. Dermatophyte infections have been reported as early as 3 days of age.

DIAGNOSTIC TESTS: The presence of alopecia, pruritus, scale, and posterior cervical lymphadenopathy makes the diagnosis of tinea capitis almost certain. Treatment can be initiated based on clinical findings, but fungal culture should be obtained to confirm the diagnosis. Diagnosis can also be confirmed at the time of initial evaluation by dermatoscopic examination of the affected area and by microscopic evaluation of a potassium hydroxide wet mount of cutaneous scrapings. Dermatoscopic evaluation of areas of alopecia with a lighted magnifier may show comma, corkscrew, or elbow-shaped hairs. Potassium hydroxide wet mount microscopy may be used to

---

[1] Davies HD, Jackson MA, Rice SG; American Academy of Pediatrics, Committee on Infectious Diseases, Council on Sports Medicine and Fitness. Infectious diseases associated with organized sports and outbreak control. *Pediatrics.* 2017;140(4):e20172477

examine hairs and scale obtained by gentle scraping of an area of the scalp with a blunt scalpel or scalpel blade, hairbrush, toothbrush, or cotton swab or by plucking with tweezers. Visualization of spores filling the interior of the hair shaft indicates an endothrix infection caused by *T tonsurans*, while coating of the outside of the hair shaft with spores indicates an ectothrix infection, such as from *M canis*. In both forms, septate hyphae may be visualized in scrapings from the scalp surface. Clinicians should obtain a fungal culture to establish a diagnosis, in conjunction with microscopy. To obtain a fungal culture, a cotton-tipped applicator can be used to swab an affected area. The sample is transported to a mycology laboratory for processing; 2 to 4 weeks of incubation on Sabouraud dextrose agar are required for results. Nucleic acid amplification tests (NAATs) are very useful and increasingly available. Under Wood lamp, tinea lesions are not fluorescent unless the etiologic agent is of the *Microsporum* genus, in which blue-green fluorescence is noted, because it is an ectothrix infection.

TREATMENT: Tinea capitis always requires systemic medication, because the fungal infection is found within the hair follicles, where topical agents do not reach. Optimal treatment of tinea capitis includes consideration of drug tolerability, availability, and cost. Current treatment options are summarized in Table 3.74.

Griseofulvin is approved by the US Food and Drug Administration (FDA) for children 2 years and older, is available in either liquid or tablet form, can be administered on a daily basis, and should be taken with fatty foods. Experts generally use higher doses of griseofulvin than have been approved by the FDA or that were used in clinical trials. Laboratory testing of serum hepatic enzymes is not required if duration of griseofulvin therapy is less than 8 weeks (but treatment of longer than 8 weeks is often required for resolution of infection). High-dose griseofulvin is considered standard of care for *M canis* infection.

Terbinafine granules are approved by the FDA for tinea capitis in children 4 years and older but are no longer available in the United States. Terbinafine clearance is higher in children than adults; pharmacokinetic data derived from studies of the granule formulation are the best information available regarding terbinafine clearance in children, and some experts extrapolate this "higher dosing" when utilizing tablets. Advantages of terbinafine for treatment of *T tonsurans* infection include the possibility of shorter treatment duration (Table 3.74) and equal or superior effectiveness compared with griseofulvin.

Two triazole agents can be considered in therapy. Fluconazole is the only oral antifungal agent approved by the FDA for children younger than 2 years, albeit not for tinea capitis. It had lower cure rates than other oral agents in a large randomized controlled trial. Accumulating evidence supports that itraconazole (currently not FDA approved for use in children or for tinea capitis) can be effective and safe for this disease. Liver function testing need not be assessed at baseline unless the child has preexisting liver disease or is on concomitant hepatotoxic medications.

Topical treatment, such as shampoos containing selenium sulfide, ketoconazole, or ciclopirox, may be useful as an adjunct to systemic therapy to decrease carriage of viable conidia for all forms of tinea capitis. Shampoo can be applied 2 to 3 times per week and left in place for 5 to 10 minutes. Treatments should continue for at least 2 weeks, and some experts recommend continuing topical treatments until clinical and mycologic cure occurs.

Table 3.74. Recommended Systemic Therapy for Tinea Capitis

Drug	Dosage	Duration	FDA Approved for Tinea Capitis
Griseofulvin microsize (liquid, 125 mg/5 mL)	15–25 mg/kg/day (max 1 g/day)	6–8 wk; continue until clinically clear	Yes (children ≥2 y)
Griseofulvin ultramicrosize (tablets of varying size)	10–15 mg/kg/day (max 750 mg/day)		
Terbinafine tablets (250 mg)[a]	4–6 mg/kg/day (max: 250 mg); or 10–20 kg: 62.5 mg 20–40 kg: 125 mg >40 kg: 250 mg	*T tonsurans*: 4–6 wk *M canis*: 8–12 wk	No
Terbinafine granules (125 mg and 187.5 mg)[b]	<25 kg: 125 mg 25–35 kg: 187.5 mg >35 kg: 250 mg	*T tonsurans*: 4–6 wk *M canis*: 8–12 wk	Yes (children ≥4 y)
Fluconazole[c] (liquid, 10 mg/mL; suspension, 40 mg/mL; tablet, 50 mg, 100 mg 150 mg, and 200 mg)	6 mg/kg/day (max 400 mg/day)	3–6 wk, depending on severity	No
Itraconazole[c] solution (10 mg/mL)	3 mg/kg/day (max 600 mg/day)	2–4 wk or longer, depending on severity	No
Itraconazole capsule (65 mg, 100 mg)	5 mg/k/day (max 600 mg/day)		

[a] Some experts use "higher" dosing listed for terbinafine granules instead.
[b] Terbinafine granules have been discontinued in the United States.
[c] See Antifungal Drugs for Systemic Fungal Infections, p 1017, and Recommended Doses of Parenteral and Oral Antifungal Drugs, p 1026, for adverse reactions and therapeutic drug monitoring recommendations.

Affected patients receiving therapy should be reassessed in 1 month for clinical response. Fungal cultures may be obtained to evaluate for a mycologic response. Poor response may prompt retreatment with a different agent if compliance with the initial drug is confirmed.

Kerion is managed by systemic antifungal treatment as outlined previously. Removal of crusts with wet compresses is thought to decrease the risk of secondary bacterial infection. Combined antifungal and corticosteroid therapy (either oral or intralesional) has not been shown to be superior to antifungal therapy alone. Nonetheless, if the condition is unresponsive to traditional therapy, many experts will add systemic prednisone, 1 mg/kg/day for 2 weeks, to decrease likelihood of scarring. Treatment with antibacterial agents is unnecessary unless secondary bacterial infection occurs.

INFECTION PREVENTION AND CONTROL MEASURES IN HEALTH CARE SETTINGS: Standard precautions apply.

CONTROL MEASURES: If discovered while at school, the affected student need not be sent home early. Once therapy is initiated, children should not be excluded from school. Family members and close contacts should be questioned regarding symptoms, and anyone with symptoms should be evaluated. Some experts recommend topical antifungal shampoo therapy for asymptomatic family members, but evidence is lacking regarding efficacy of this intervention. Sharing of items such as hats and combs/brushes should be avoided in households with an affected person. If pets are suspected as a source of *M canis* infection, evaluation and appropriate treatment of the affected animal should be implemented.

Tinea Corporis
(Ringworm of the Body)

CLINICAL MANIFESTATIONS: Superficial fungal infections (superficial mycoses) are called tinea corporis when involving the skin of the trunk and extremities, and tinea faciei when involving the face. Lesions often are ring-shaped or circular (hence, the lay term "ringworm") and are sharply marginated. Involved skin is slightly erythematous and scaly, with color variations from red to brown. The classic eruption displays a scaly, vesicular, or pustular border (often serpiginous) with central clearing. Small confluent plaques or papules as well as multiple lesions can occur, particularly in wrestlers (tinea gladiatorum).[1] Although tinea faciei may have the above clinical features, the findings may be more variable in this location.

The differential diagnosis for tinea corporis includes pityriasis rosea (particularly the herald patch), candidiasis, psoriasis, other dermatitides (seborrheic, atopic, irritant or allergic, generally caused by therapeutic agents applied to the area), pityriasis versicolor (tinea versicolor), nummular eczema, granuloma annulare, erythema annulare centrifugum, impetigo and erythrasma (an eruption of reddish brown patches resulting from superficial bacterial skin infection caused by *Corynebacterium minutissimum*).

The typical appearance of the lesions is altered in patients who have been treated erroneously with topical corticosteroids. Known as tinea incognito, this altered appearance includes diminished erythema and absence of typical scaling borders. Such patients also can develop Majocchi granuloma, a fungal invasion of the hair shaft and surrounding dermis, which causes a granulomatous dermal reaction that can extend into the surrounding subcutaneous fat. Majocchi granuloma also can occur without prior use of corticosteroids.

An associated dermatophytic or "id" reaction can be present as a hypersensitivity reaction to the infecting fungus, manifesting as diffuse, pruritic, papular, vesicular, or eczematous lesions, which can occur at sites distant from the fungal infection. Sometimes id reactions first appear following institution of therapy, but they do not represent a drug allergy.

Skin lesions can occur as grouped papules or pustules without erythema or scaling in patients with diminished T-lymphocyte function (eg, human immunodeficiency virus infection). Tinea corporis presenting with rapidly progressive lesions that include vesicles, pus-filled bullae, nonindurated, nontender erythema-mimicking cellulitis is

---

[1] Davies HD, Jackson MA, Rice SG; American Academy of Pediatrics, Committee on Infectious Diseases, Council on Sports Medicine and Fitness. Infectious diseases associated with organized sports and outbreak control. *Pediatrics.* 2017;140(4):e20172477

called inflammatory tinea. Tinea corporis can occur in association with tinea capitis. The scalp should be examined, particularly in wrestlers and others engaged in contact sports.

ETIOLOGY: Tinea corporis develops when dermatophytic fungi (dermatophytes) invade the outer skin layers at the affected body region. Primary etiologic agents are *Trichophyton* species, especially *Trichophyton tonsurans, Trichophyton rubrum,* and *Trichophyton mentagrophytes; Microsporum* species, especially *Microsporum canis;* and *Epidermophyton floccosum.*

EPIDEMIOLOGY: Causative fungi occur worldwide and are transmissible by direct contact with infected humans, animals, soil, or fomites (eg, brushes, combs, hats, towels), where organisms can remain viable for prolonged periods. Drug-resistant strains of *Trichophyton* have been reported globally and are considered endemic in India and Iran. *Trichophyton indotineae* is antifungal-resistant, including to terbinafine, and has caused epidemics in South Asia. It is highly transmissible and characterized by widespread, inflamed, pruritic plaques on the body (tinea corporis), the crural fold, pubic region, and adjacent thigh (tinea cruris), or the face (tinea faciei). *T indotineae* isolates have recently been reported in the United States.[1]

Immunocompromised people have an increased susceptibility to dermatophyte infections.

The **incubation period** is believed to be 1 to 3 weeks but can be shorter, as reported cases have occurred at 3 days of age.

DIAGNOSTIC TESTS: Tinea corporis is diagnosed by clinical manifestations and can be confirmed by microscopic examination of a potassium hydroxide wet mount of skin scrapings or fungal culture. Skin scrapings, ideally at the scaly edges of lesions for best recovery of organisms, are obtained by gentle scraping of a cleansed, moistened area with a scalpel blade or blunt scalpel, glass microscope slide or brush such as a toothbrush. If fungal culture is desired, a cotton-tipped applicator can be premoistened with sterile saline or water and used to swab an affected area gently. The sample is transported to a mycology laboratory for processing; 2 to 4 weeks of incubation on Sabouraud dextrose agar are required for results. Nucleic acid amplification tests (NAATs) are available but generally are not necessary. Under Wood lamp, tinea is not fluorescent unless the etiologic agent is of the genus *Microsporum,* in which case a blue-green fluorescence can be seen because it is an ectothrix infection. For recurrent tinea infections, especially those associated with international travel, consideration should be given to obtaining culture for species identification and antifungal susceptibility testing.

TREATMENT: A myriad of topical antifungal options are available for treatment and should be applied on the lesions and 1 to 2 cm beyond the borders. Some topical agents are approved by the US Food and Drug Administration (FDA) only for certain lesion locations and age groups and with applications specified as once or twice daily (Table 3.75). Any of the following products (applied twice daily) are reasonable first-line therapies if appropriate for age: miconazole, clotrimazole, tolnaftate, or ciclopirox. Any of the following products also can be used (applied once daily) if appropriate for age: ketoconazole, terbinafine, econazole, naftifine, luliconazole, or butenafine.

---

[1] Caplan AS, Chaturvedi S, Zhu Y, et al. Notes from the field: first reported U.S. cases of tinea caused by *Trichophyton indotineae*—New York City, December 2021–March 2023. *MMWR Morb Mortal Wkly Rep.* 2023;72(19):536–537

Table 3.75. Products for Topical Treatment of Tinea Corporis, Cruris, and Pedis

Topical Product	Age for Use	Daily Application
Miconazole (cream, 2%)	Age ≥2 y	Twice
Clotrimazole (cream or solution, 1%)	All ages	Twice
Tolnaftate (cream or solution, 1%)	Age ≥2 y	Twice
Ciclopirox (cream or lotion, 0.77%)	Age ≥10 y	Twice
Ciclopirox (gel, 0.77%)	Age ≥16 y for tinea corporis or pedis	Twice
Ketoconazole (cream, gel, and foam 2%)[a]	Seborrheic dermatitis, age ≥12 y	Once
Terbinafine (cream, 1%)	Age ≥12 y	Once for tinea corporis and cruris Twice for tinea pedis
Econazole (cream, foam 1%)	Foam for tinea pedis, age ≥12 y	Once
Naftifine (cream and gel, 1% and 2%)	2% products for tinea cruris/pedis: Age ≥12 y Tinea corporis: Age ≥2 y	Once or twice
Luliconazole (cream, 1%)	Age ≥2 y for tinea corporis Age ≥12 y for tinea cruris and pedis	Once
Butenafine (cream, 1%)	Age ≥12 y	Once for tinea corporis and tinea cruris Twice for tinea pedis
Oxiconazole (cream, lotion 1%)	All ages	Once or twice
Sulconazole (cream or solution, 1%)	Adults only	Once or twice
Sertaconazole (cream, 2%)	Age ≥12 y, for tinea pedis only	Twice

[a] Safety and effectiveness in children have not been established for ketoconazole 2% cream.

Oxiconazole and sulconazole can be used (once or twice daily) if appropriate for age (also see Topical Drugs for Superficial Fungal Infections, p 1037).

Although clinical resolution may be evident within 2 weeks of therapy, continuing therapy for another 2 to 4 weeks generally is recommended. If significant clinical improvement is not observed after 2 weeks of treatment, an alternate diagnosis and/or systemic therapy should be considered. Topical preparations of antifungal medication combined with a corticosteroid should not be used because of inferior effectiveness, the possibility of leading to Majocchi granuloma, and increase in the rate of relapse, higher cost, and potential for adverse corticosteroid effects.

If lesions are extensive or unresponsive to topical therapy or involving a hair-bearing area such as the beard, griseofulvin (for children ≥2 years) or terbinafine (for children ≥4 years) may be administered orally for 4 to 6 weeks (see Tinea Capitis, p 854). Terbinafine granules are no longer available in the United States. Griseofulvin may be preferred over terbinafine in cases known to be caused by *Microsporum* species. Oral itraconazole and fluconazole do not have FDA indications for treatment of many tinea conditions. There are reports of successful treatment of terbinafine-resistant *Trichophyton* infections with itraconazole. If a Majocchi granuloma is present, oral antifungal therapy is recommended, because topical therapy is unlikely to penetrate adequately to eradicate infection.

Dermatophyte infections in other locations, if present, should be treated concurrently.

INFECTION PREVENTION AND CONTROL MEASURES IN HEALTH CARE SETTINGS: Standard precautions apply. Recent outbreaks of tinea infection in both acute and chronic care facilities among patients and caregivers illustrate the need for education regarding clinical manifestations of tinea and infection control procedures in the care of infected individuals.

CONTROL MEASURES[1]: Infections should be treated promptly. Direct contact with known or suspected sources of infection should be avoided. Periodic inspections of contacts for early lesions and prompt therapy are recommended. Pet rodents, including guinea pigs, may carry dermatophytes in their claws. Scratches by these animals should be washed immediately. Athletic mats and equipment should be cleaned frequently, and actively infected athletes in sports with person-to-person contact must be excluded from competitions. Athletes with tinea corporis may resume participation in contact sports a minimum of 72 hours after initiation of topical therapy and when the affected area can be covered. Prophylaxis of wrestling team members is controversial. Fluconazole, 100 mg per day for 3 days, given prophylactically before initiation of competitive interscholastic high school wrestling and given again 6 weeks into the season, has been reported to reduce the incidence of *T corporis* significantly, from 67.4% to 3.5%. The risk-benefit analysis of giving fluconazole prophylactically in this manner has not been determined, however, and its use should be in consultation with an infectious diseases expert. Infected pets also should receive antifungal treatment.

Tinea Cruris
(Jock Itch)

CLINICAL MANIFESTATIONS: Tinea cruris is a common superficial fungal disorder of the groin, pubic/perianal area, suprapubic abdomen, and upper thighs. It is more common in male adults and adolescents and uncommon in prepubertal children.[2] The

---

[1] Davies HD, Jackson MA, Rice SG; American Academy of Pediatrics, Committee on Infectious Diseases, Council on Sports Medicine and Fitness. Infectious diseases associated with organized sports and outbreak control. *Pediatrics.* 2017;140(4):e20172477

[2] The term male refers to sex assigned at birth.

lesions often are ring-shaped or circular (hence, the lay term "ringworm"), are sharply marginated, and can be intensely pruritic (jock itch). The involved skin is slightly erythematous and scaly, with color variations from red to brown. Lesions can display a scaly, vesicular, or pustular border (often serpiginous) with central clearing. Maceration may also develop. Scaling is less prominent in the presence of maceration. The disorder usually spares the scrotum unless candidiasis also is present. The margins can be subtle in chronic infections, and lichenification may be present.

The differential diagnosis for tinea cruris includes intertrigo, candidiasis, psoriasis (particularly inverse psoriasis), other dermatitides (seborrheic, atopic, irritant or allergic contact, generally caused by therapeutic agents applied to the area), pityriasis versicolor (tinea versicolor), nummular eczema, erythema annulare centrifugum, and erythrasma (an eruption of reddish brown patches resulting from superficial bacterial skin infection caused by *Corynebacterium minutissimum*).

An altered appearance known as tinea incognito can occur in patients who have been treated erroneously with topical corticosteroids, which includes diminished erythema and absence of typical scaling borders. Such patients also can develop Majocchi granuloma when fungi invade the hair shaft and surrounding dermis, causing a granulomatous dermal reaction that can extend into the surrounding subcutaneous fat. Majocchi granuloma also can occur without prior use of topical corticosteroid.

An associated skin eruption, known as a dermatophytic or "id" reaction, can occur as a hypersensitivity reaction to the infecting fungus and manifests as diffuse, pruritic, papular, vesicular, or eczematous lesions at sites distant from the fungal infection. An id reaction can first occur following institution of therapy but does not represent a drug allergy.

Concomitant tinea pedis, tinea unguium, and tinea corporis have been reported in patients with tinea cruris.

ETIOLOGY: Tinea cruris develops when dermatophyte fungi invade the outer skin layers of the affected body region. The fungi *Epidermophyton floccosum*, *Trichophyton rubrum*, and *Trichophyton mentagrophytes* are the most common causes. *Trichophyton tonsurans*, *Trichophyton verrucosum*, and *Trichophyton interdigitale* also have been identified as causes.

EPIDEMIOLOGY: Tinea cruris occurs predominantly in male adolescents and adults and is acquired principally through indirect contact with desquamated epithelium or hair. Direct person-to-person transmission also occurs. Moisture, close-fitting garments, noncotton underwear, friction, and obesity are predisposing factors. Recurrence is common.

Immunocompromised patients have increased susceptibility to dermatophyte infections. In patients with diminished T-lymphocyte function (eg, human immunodeficiency virus infection), skin lesions can appear as grouped papules or pustules unaccompanied by scaling or erythema.

The **incubation period** is unknown but is thought to be approximately 1 to 3 weeks.

DIAGNOSTIC TESTS: Confirmatory diagnostic modalities for tinea cruris are similar to that for tinea corporis (see Tinea Corporis, p 858).

TREATMENT: Treatment is similar to that for tinea corporis (see Tinea Corporis, Table 3.75, p 860). Treatment of concurrent onychomycosis (tinea unguium) and tinea pedis may reduce recurrence. Recurrence is common, particularly if predisposing factors such as moisture and friction are not minimized. Loose-fitting clothing and use of antifungal powders, such as tolnaftate and miconazole, should aid in recovery and prevent recurrence.

Oral terbinafine, itraconazole, and fluconazole are options but do not have a US Food and Drug Administration indication for tinea cruris. Griseofulvin, administered orally for 4 to 6 weeks, may be effective if lesions are unresponsive to topical therapy (see Tinea Capitis, p 854). Oral antifungal therapy is recommended if a Majocchi granuloma (deep folliculitis) is present, because topical therapy is unlikely to penetrate adequately to eradicate infection. Dermatophyte infections in other locations, if present, should be treated concurrently, and may be an indication for oral therapy.

Topical steroids are not recommended, even in formulations coupled with antifungal agents, as these may exacerbate the infection.

INFECTION PREVENTION AND CONTROL MEASURES IN HEALTH CARE SETTINGS: Standard precautions apply.

CONTROL MEASURES: Infections should be treated promptly. Involved areas should be kept dry to prevent recurrences, and antifungal powders and wearing loose fitting undergarments may be useful. Patients should be advised to dry the groin area before drying their feet to avoid inoculating dermatophytes of tinea pedis into the groin area. When infection is present, towel sharing should be avoided.

Tinea Pedis and Tinea Unguium (Onychomycosis)
(Athlete's Foot, Ringworm of the Feet)

CLINICAL MANIFESTATIONS: Tinea pedis can have a variety of clinical manifestations in children. Lesions can involve all areas of the foot but usually are patchy in distribution, with a predisposition to cause fissures, macerated areas, and scaling between toes. A pruritic, fine scaly, or vesiculopustular eruption is most common and can be associated with a confluent, hyperkeratotic, dry scaling of the soles. Recurrence of tinea pedis is common, and it can be a chronic infection. Toenails can be infected (onychomycosis or tinea unguium) and become distorted, discolored, and thickened with accumulation of subungual debris. A superficial white form of toenail fungal infection can occur in children. Toenails may be the source for recurrent tinea pedis.

Tinea pedis must be differentiated from dyshidrotic eczema, atopic dermatitis, psoriasis, contact dermatitis, juvenile plantar dermatosis, palmoplantar keratoderma, and erythrasma (reddish brown patches that can affect the feet and axillae resulting from superficial bacterial skin infection caused by *Corynebacterium minutissimum*).

An associated skin eruption, known as a dermatophytid or "id" reaction, can occur as a hypersensitivity reaction to the infecting fungus and manifests as diffuse, pruritic, papular, vesicular, or eczematous lesions at sites distant from the fungal infection. An id reaction can occur first following institution of therapy but does not represent a drug allergy. Id reaction lesions may appear as grouped papules or pustules unaccompanied by erythema or scaling in patients with diminished T-lymphocyte function (eg, human immunodeficiency virus infection).

The differential diagnosis of tinea unguium includes trauma (particularly if only 1 nail is involved), psoriasis, congenital malalignment of the great toenails (if only great toenails are involved), twenty nail dystrophy (trachyonychia), and subungual exostosis if only 1 nail is involved.

Concomitant tinea in other body sites has been reported in patients with tinea pedis and tinea unguium.

ETIOLOGY: Tinea pedis and unguium develop when dermatophytic fungi invade the skin layers and nails of the affected body region. The fungi *Trichophyton rubrum*, *Trichophyton mentagrophytes*, and *Epidermophyton floccosum* are the most common causes of tinea pedis.

EPIDEMIOLOGY: Tinea pedis is a common infection worldwide in adolescents and adults but is less common in young children. Fungi are acquired by contact with infected skin scales or organisms present in damp areas, such as swimming pools, locker rooms, and showers. Tinea pedis may spread among family members in the household; this may represent enhanced genetic susceptibility as well as increased exposure to the organism. The incidence of onychomycosis, which is more common in toenails, increases with age, with worldwide prevalence in children estimated to be from 0.1% to 0.87%. The increased use of occlusive footwear earlier in childhood and exposure to high-risk areas (eg, swimming pools, gyms) earlier in life may be associated with an increase of tinea pedis in children. Childhood onychomycosis is associated with a history of tinea pedis, a history of family member infection, increased number of siblings, and male sex.[1]

Immunocompromised people and those with trisomy 21 have increased susceptibility to dermatophyte infections.

The **incubation period** is unknown.

DIAGNOSTIC TESTS: Confirmatory diagnostic tests for tinea pedis are similar to those for tinea corporis (see Tinea Corporis, p 858). Fungal infection of the nail (tinea unguium or onychomycosis) can be verified by direct microscopic examination with potassium hydroxide, fungal culture of desquamated subungual material, or fungal stain of nail clippings fixed in formalin. Nucleic acid amplification tests (NAATs) are a useful and increasingly used tool.

TREATMENT: A myriad of topical options are available for treatment of tinea pedis (see Tinea Corporis, Table 3.75, p 860; also see Topical Drugs for Superficial Fungal Infections, p 1037). Therapy duration of 2 weeks usually is sufficient for milder cases of tinea pedis in children. Acute vesicular lesions can be treated with intermittent use of open wet compresses (eg, with Burow solution, diluted 1:80). Tinea pedis that is severe, chronic, or refractory to topical treatment can be treated with oral therapy similar to that for tinea capitis (see Tinea Capitis, Table 3.74, p 857).

Recurrence of tinea pedis is prevented by proper foot hygiene, which includes keeping the feet dry and cool, cleaning gently, drying between the toes, use of absorbent antifungal foot powder, exposing affected areas to air frequently, and avoidance of occlusive footwear, nylon socks, and other fabrics that interfere with dissipation of moisture. Wearing protective footwear in public facilities such as pools and gyms may prevent transmission.

Topical antifungal lacquers and solutions that are effective for distal toenail infections that do not involve the nail matrix now are available. Despite lower cure rates, topical agents are preferred because of substantially lower adverse effects, lack of drug-drug interactions, and avoidance of need for laboratory test monitoring for toxicity.

---

[1] The term male refers to sex assigned at birth.

Topical ciclopirox 8% lacquer, with a US Food and Drug Administration (FDA) indication for tinea unguium for patients 12 years and older, can be applied to affected toenail(s) once daily for up to 48 weeks, or twice daily for shorter durations, in combination with a comprehensive nail management program. Efinaconazole 10% solution and tavaborole 5% solution are indicated for onychomycosis for patients 6 years and older, applied once daily for up to 48 weeks; both have higher cure rates in adults than ciclopirox. Topical therapies appear to show a higher cure rate in children than in adults, possibly because of thinner nail plates and faster nail growth rate in children. Most of these agents are expensive and not usually covered by insurance.

Studies in adults have demonstrated the best cure rates for onychomycosis (tinea unguium) are with oral terbinafine or itraconazole. Although oral therapies are more likely to lead to cure, they also require laboratory monitoring and can induce drug–drug interactions. Guidelines for dosing of terbinafine for children are based on studies for treatment of tinea capitis and are weight based (see Table 3.74, p 857). The duration of therapy is the same as for adults (6 weeks for fingernail infection, 12 weeks for toenail infection). Pediatric dosing of oral itraconazole is not established for superficial mycoses, although a suggested dosing may follow that for tinea capitis (see Table 3.74, p 857, Antifungal Drugs for Systemic Fungal Infections, p 1017, and Recommended Doses of Parenteral and Oral Antifungal Drugs, p 1026, for dosing, adverse reactions, and therapeutic drug monitoring recommendations). Griseofulvin, although approved by the FDA for treatment of tinea unguium, is rarely used for this indication.

Factors that influence choice of therapy include severity of infection, results of fungal culture or potassium hydroxide preparation (if performed), prior treatments, concomitant drug therapy for other illnesses, patient preference, and cost. Topical and systemic therapy may be used concurrently to increase therapeutic response. Cure rates following oral or combined therapy approach 80% in children. Mechanical and chemical débridement of the nail, using 40% urea ointment daily under occlusion for 10 days to soften the nail, should be performed in refractory cases or when severe thickening of the nail is likely to decrease absorption and response to therapy.

Dermatophyte infections in other locations, if present, should be treated concurrently.

INFECTION PREVENTION AND CONTROL MEASURES IN HEALTH CARE SETTINGS: Standard precautions apply.

CONTROL MEASURES: Treatment of patients with active infections should decrease transmission. Using public areas conducive to transmission (eg, swimming pools) is discouraged in those with untreated, active infection. Chemical foot baths can facilitate spread of infection. Because recurrence after treatment is common, proper foot hygiene is important (as described in Treatment). Patients should be advised to dry the groin area before drying the feet to avoid inoculating dermatophytes from tinea pedis into the groin area. Prevention of tinea unguium includes keeping nails short and not sharing nail clippers.

Toxocariasis

CLINICAL MANIFESTATIONS: Clinical disease is caused by migration of parasitic nematode larvae through tissues. Signs and symptoms differ depending on the affected organ and host inflammatory response. Toxocariasis can be of following types: covert toxocariasis, visceral larva migrans, neurotoxocariasis, or ocular larva migrans. Most infected children are asymptomatic. Covert disease presents with nonspecific symptoms and may be accompanied by eosinophilia. Symptoms of visceral toxocariasis include fever, cough, wheezing, abdominal pain, anorexia, and malaise, with myocarditis and rash less common. Hepatomegaly or pneumonia may be present, along with eosinophilia. Neurotoxocariasis may manifest with an eosinophilic meningoencephalitis, space-occupying lesions, myelitis, or cerebral vasculitis, and may present with change in mental status or seizures. Laboratory abnormalities include leukocytosis, eosinophilia, and hypergammaglobulinemia. Ocular invasion (resulting in uveitis, endophthalmitis, or retinal granulomas) most often manifests as unilateral vision loss (with subsequent strabismus), frequently without other systemic signs or eosinophilia.

ETIOLOGY: Toxocariasis is caused by *Toxocara* species, which are nematode (roundworm) parasites of dogs and cats, specifically *Toxocara canis* and *Toxocara cati*, respectively; most cases are caused by *T canis*.

EPIDEMIOLOGY: Toxocariasis is most common in the tropics. In the United States, 5% of the population 6 years and older have serologic evidence of *Toxocara* infection. Visceral toxocariasis typically occurs in children 2 to 7 years of age but can occur in older children and adults. Ocular toxocariasis usually occurs in older children and adolescents. Infection is more likely among people who own dogs and people living in poverty and is more prevalent in hot and humid regions (in the United States, the southern states) where eggs can remain viable in soil for years. Humans are infected by ingestion of soil containing infective eggs of the parasite. Eggs may be found wherever dogs and cats defecate, often in sandboxes and playgrounds. Eggs become infective after 2 to 4 weeks in the environment and may persist long-term in the soil. Direct contact with dogs or cats does not typically lead to infection, because eggs are not infectious immediately when shed in the feces.

The **incubation period** cannot be determined accurately.

DIAGNOSTIC TESTS: Laboratory findings include marked leukocytosis with eosinophilia and occasionally anemia and hypergammaglobulinemia (elevated serum concentrations of immunoglobulin [Ig] G and IgE). Patients with visceral disease frequently have increased titers of isohemagglutinin to the A and B blood group antigens. Diagnosis is made most commonly by enzyme-linked immunosorbent assay (ELISA) for *Toxocara* antibodies in serum or vitreous fluid. A positive antibody test result does not distinguish between past and current infection, and the test is less sensitive for diagnosis of ocular toxocariasis. For visceral disease, imaging of the liver using ultrasonography, computed tomography, or magnetic resonance imaging may reveal diffuse nodular lesions measuring less than 2 cm in diameter. Microscopic identification of larvae in a liver biopsy specimen is diagnostic, but this test is not sensitive or specific and therefore rarely indicated.

TREATMENT: Albendazole is recommended for treatment of visceral and ocular toxocariasis (see Drugs for Parasitic Infections, p 1068). The drug has been approved by the US Food and Drug Administration but not for this indication. Mebendazole is an alternative. In severe cases with myocarditis or involvement of the central nervous system, corticosteroid therapy administered concurrently with albendazole is warranted. Control of inflammation of the eye with oral or topical corticosteroids may be required; surgical therapy may be helpful in complicated ophthalmic cases.

INFECTION PREVENTION AND CONTROL MEASURES IN HEALTH CARE SETTINGS: Standard precautions are recommended. There is no person-to-person spread.

CONTROL MEASURES: Proper disposal of cat and dog feces is essential. Regular veterinary care and periodic deworming of dogs and cats, and especially puppies and kittens, decreases environmental contamination with *Toxocara* eggs and has public health benefit. Covering sandboxes when not in use is helpful. No specific management following exposure is recommended.

Toxoplasma gondii Infections[1]
(Toxoplasmosis)

CLINICAL MANIFESTATIONS: Up to 50% of patients with acute *Toxoplasma* infection are asymptomatic. When present, common signs and symptoms of acute *Toxoplasma* infection can include influenza-like symptoms, lymphadenopathy with atypical lymphocytosis, fever, myalgia, arthralgia, sweats, chills, fatigue, headache, chorioretinitis, hepatic dysfunction, pneumonitis, meningoencephalitis, myocarditis, myositis, acute disseminated encephalomyelitis (ADEM), and myelitis. Reactivation of chronic *Toxoplasma* infection in immunocompromised patients may result in fever, pneumonia, septic shock, brain abscesses, diffuse encephalitis without brain-space occupying lesions, seizures, chorioretinitis, myocarditis, myelitis, and polymyositis.

Congenital Infection. People are not screened routinely for toxoplasmosis during pregnancy in the United States. Clinically apparent signs and symptoms of congenital toxoplasmosis are found on routine physical examination in a minority of infected infants at birth, but more specific testing (of cerebrospinal fluid [CSF], dilated eye examination, or central nervous system imaging) can reveal evidence of infection. Visual or hearing impairment, learning disabilities, or severe developmental delay will become apparent later in life in a large proportion of congenitally infected infants. Chorioretinitis occurs in approximately 70% of congenitally infected infants whose birthing parents were not treated during pregnancy and in up to 25% of those whose birthing parents were treated.

Clinical illness is more likely to be severe when infection occurs in the first trimester and is not treated during pregnancy. The classic triad of chorioretinitis, cerebral calcifications, and hydrocephalus is highly suggestive of congenital toxoplasmosis. Additional signs at birth include microcephaly, seizures, hearing loss, strabismus, petechial rash, jaundice, generalized lymphadenopathy, hepatomegaly, splenomegaly, pneumonia, thrombocytopenia, and anemia. Meningoencephalitis may be associated with CSF abnormalities including high protein concentrations, hypoglycorrhachia, and eosinophilia. Some severely affected fetuses/infants with disseminated congenital toxoplasmosis die in utero or within a few days of birth. Cerebral calcifications can be demonstrated by plain radiography, ultrasonography, computed tomography (CT), or magnetic resonance imaging (MRI) of the head. CT is the radiologic technique most sensitive for intracranial calcifications and can reveal them when ultrasonographic studies are normal.

[1] Maldonado YA, Read JS; American Academy of Pediatrics, Committee on Infectious Diseases. Diagnosis, treatment, and prevention of congenital toxoplasmosis in the United States. *Pediatrics.* 2017;139(2):e20163860

Postnatally Acquired Primary Infection. Postnatally acquired *Toxoplasma gondii* infections in immunocompetent patients usually are asymptomatic. When symptoms develop, they may be nonspecific and can include malaise, fever, headache, sore throat, arthralgia, and myalgia. Lymphadenopathy, frequently cervical, is the most common sign. Patients occasionally have a mononucleosis-like illness associated with a maculopapular rash, hepatosplenomegaly, hepatic dysfunction, and atypical lymphocytosis. The clinical course usually is benign and self-limited.

In a subset of patients, primary infection may be severe and/or persistent, including fever, myocarditis, pericarditis, myositis, hepatitis, pneumonia, encephalitis with and without brain abscesses, and skin lesions (maculopapular rash). These severe syndromes are especially common in patients who acquired primary *T gondii* infections with high parasite loads and/or in areas where atypical, more virulent strains are present (eg, Mexico, French Guiana, Brazil, and Colombia).

Chorioretinitis. Toxoplasmic chorioretinitis can occur: (a) with congenital infection; (b) from a postnatally acquired acute infection; and (c) from reactivation of a congenital or postnatally acquired infection. Acute onset of blurred vision, eye pain, decreased visual acuity, floaters, scotoma, photophobia, epiphora, nystagmus, or strabismus are noted. Ocular findings in toxoplasmic eye disease include white focal retinitis with overlying vitreous inflammation ("headlight in the fog"), nearby prior pigmented retinochoroidal scar, retinal vasculitis, vitreous inflammation, cataracts, iridocyclitis and stellate keratic precipitates (accompanying chorioretinitis), and elevated intraocular pressure. Complications can include retinal detachment, cystoid macular edema, optic atrophy, chronic iridocyclitis, cataract formation, secondary glaucoma, or band keratopathy.

Reactivation of Chronic Infection in Immunocompromised Patients. Reactivation of latent infection may occur in immunosuppressed patients. Reactivation can result in encephalitis, brain abscesses, seizures, pneumonia, myocarditis, hepatitis, skin lesions, posterior uveitis or panuveitis with chorioretinitis, fever of unknown origin, and disseminated disease and death. Toxoplasmic encephalitis (TE) can present as a single or multiple brain lesions on MRI or as a "diffuse form" with a rapidly progressive clinical course leading to death despite apparently normal brain imaging. MRI is superior to CT for the diagnosis of TE. In patients with acquired immunodeficiency syndrome (AIDS), TE is the most common cause of space-occupying brain lesions and typically presents with acute to subacute neurologic or psychiatric symptoms and multiple ring-enhancing brain lesions. In these patients, a clear improvement in the neurologic examination within 7 to 10 days of beginning empiric anti-*Toxoplasma* therapy is considered diagnostic of TE. Lack of radiographic response 2 weeks after initiation of anti-*Toxoplasma* therapy is an indication to consider alternative diagnoses. Patients without AIDS who have multiple brain lesions should not be treated empirically for only toxoplasmosis, and other etiologies should be considered for diagnostic and empiric treatment purposes.

Seropositive hematopoietic cell transplant and solid organ transplant recipients are at risk of reactivation of latent infection in the absence of appropriate prophylaxis. Transmission occurs in ≥50% of seronegative recipients who receive hearts from seropositive donors unless appropriate prophylaxis is prescribed. Toxoplasmosis in this setting presents as pneumonia, unexplained fever or seizures, myocarditis, hepatitis, hepatosplenomegaly, lymphadenopathy, skin lesions, or brain abscesses and diffuse encephalitis. Transplant donors and recipients should be screened pretransplant for *Toxoplasma* infection.

ETIOLOGY: *T gondii* is a protozoan and obligate intracellular parasite. The infectious forms include tachyzoites, tissue cysts containing bradyzoites, and oocysts containing sporozoites. The tachyzoite and the corresponding host immune reaction are responsible for observed symptoms. The tissue cyst is responsible for latent infection and usually is present in brain, eye, cardiac tissue, and skeletal muscle.

EPIDEMIOLOGY: Seroprevalence of *T gondii* infection varies by geographic locale and socioeconomic strata of the population. The overall *T gondii* seropositivity rate in the United States (according to the National Health and Nutrition Examination Survey 2011–2014) in people older than 6 years was 11.1% and among women 15 to 44 years of age was 7.5%.

Individuals become infected through foodborne, zoonotic, or person-to-person modes of transmission (eg, vertical transmission). Congenital transmission occurs in most cases as a result of acute primary infection acquired during pregnancy or within 3 months before conception. In utero infection rarely can occur as a result of reactivated parasitemia in a latently infected immunocompromised person in the absence of prophylaxis. Rarely, congenital toxoplasmosis is acquired from an immunocompetent pregnant person reinfected with a different *T gondii* strain. Incidence of acute primary *T gondii* infection during pregnancy in the United States is estimated to be 0.2 to 1.1/1000 pregnant people on the basis of data from Massachusetts and New Hampshire, which are the only 2 states in the United States with universal toxoplasmosis newborn screening. Transmission through organ donation or blood transfusions is rare.

The **incubation period** of postnatally acquired infection is approximately 7 days, with a range of 4 to 21 days. Parasites can be detected in the blood for up to 2 weeks after acute infection; prolonged parasitemia also has been reported.

DIAGNOSTIC TESTS: Serologic tests are the primary means of diagnosis. *Toxoplasma* immunoglobulin (Ig) G and IgM can be performed by commercial laboratories in most situations; exceptions are testing of pregnant people with suspected acute *Toxoplasma* infections during gestation and neonates with suspected congenital toxoplasmosis, for whom testing should be performed at a reference laboratory (see below). *Toxoplasma* IgM results from commercial laboratories can be falsely positive; confirmation should be obtained from reference laboratories with special expertise such as the Palo Alto Medical Foundation Toxoplasma Serology Laboratory (PAMF-TSL; Palo Alto, CA; **www.sutterhealth.org/RemingtonLab;** telephone: 650-853-4828; email: **RemingtonLab@sutterhealth.org**). Confirmatory testing at the reference laboratory may include IgM, IgA, IgE, IgG avidity, and the differential agglutination (of acetone [AC]-fixed versus that of formalin [HS]-fixed tachyzoites) test (AC/HS test).

IgG-specific antibodies achieve a peak concentration 3 to 5 months after infection and remain positive indefinitely. IgM-specific antibodies can be detected 1 to 2 weeks after infection (IgG-specific antibodies usually are negative during this period), achieve peak concentrations in 1 month, and usually become undetectable within 6 to 9 months, but may also persist for years without apparent clinical significance. The lack of *T gondii*-specific IgM antibodies in a person with low-positive titers of IgG antibodies (eg, a dye test at PAMF-TSL ≤1:512) indicates infection of at least 6 months' duration. In contrast, detectable *T gondii*-specific IgM antibodies can indicate recent infection, chronic (latent) infection, or a false-positive reaction. If timing of infection is clinically important (eg, in a pregnant person), sera with positive *T gondii* IgM test results can be sent to PAMF-TSL to establish acute versus chronic infection using an additional panel of tests such as IgG avidity, AC/HS, and IgA- and IgE-specific antibody tests.

Polymerase chain reaction (PCR) detection has been applied to body fluid or tissue, and *T gondii*-specific immunoperoxidase staining can be performed with any tissue, depending on the clinical scenario. A positive PCR test result in tissue must be interpreted with caution, because it may amplify tachyzoite or bradyzoite DNA and cannot distinguish between tachyzoites with acute infection or reactivation or bradyzoites with chronic latent infection. CSF PCR for *T gondii* has high specificity (96%–100%), but sensitivity is only 50%. CSF PCR results can also be negative because of anti-*Toxoplasma* therapy.

Congenital Toxoplasmosis. During pregnancy, PCR assay of amniotic fluid is the method of choice to confirm fetal infection. Fetal ultrasonography can assess for anatomical abnormalities. Examination of the placenta by histologic testing and PCR assay may provide additional information but is not sufficiently sensitive or specific for diagnostic purposes. At birth or postnatally, serologic tests for IgG, IgM, and IgA should be performed. Neonates who are born to persons with primary infection during pregnancy, or in whom there is high suspicion for congenital toxoplasmosis, should have a lumbar puncture for CSF analysis and toxoplasma PCR. Urine and whole blood should be sent for *T gondii* PCR assay. Positive neonatal serum *Toxoplasma* IgM (after 5 days of life) and/or IgA (after 10 days of life), along with a positive IgG, is considered diagnostic of congenital toxoplasmosis. IgM immunosorbent agglutination assay (ISAGA) test results can be falsely positive after transfusion of blood products but usually become negative 14 days after transfusion. Occasionally, false-positive results for IgG, IgM, and IgA can be observed as a result of platelet transfusions or immune globulin intravenous infusions. Diagnosis of congenital toxoplasmosis also can be made definitively in an infant who remains *Toxoplasma* IgG positive at 12 months of life.

Newborn infants being evaluated for toxoplasmosis also should have a complete blood cell count (CBC) with differential, liver function tests, and cerebrospinal fluid cell count, differential, protein, and glucose performed (in addition to *T gondii* PCR, above). Ophthalmologic and audiologic assessments should be conducted, and head ultrasonography (readily available but does not detect calcifications well), brain MRI (allows avoidance of radiation but may require sedation), or brain CT (the best modality for detecting calcifications) should be performed. Abdominal ultrasonography can be considered to evaluate for hepatosplenomegaly or intrahepatic calcifications.

Asymptomatic newborn infants with low suspicion for congenital toxoplasmosis but who were initially IgG positive but IgM and IgA negative should have follow-up serologic testing with IgG only at 4- to 6-week intervals until complete disappearance of transplacentally acquired IgG antibodies, usually within 6 to 12 months. In the absence of postnatal treatment, disappearance of IgG antibodies in the infant safely excludes the diagnosis of congenital toxoplasmosis.

Expert advice for evaluation and management of neonates/infants with suspected or confirmed congenital toxoplasmosis is available at: (a) the PAMF-TSL (**www.sutterhealth.org/RemingtonLab;** telephone 650-853-4828; email

RemingtonLab@sutterhealth.org) and (b) the Toxoplasmosis Center, University of Chicago, Chicago, IL (**www.uchicagomedicine.org/conditions-services/ophthalmology/toxoplasmosis-center;** telephone 773-834-4131; email **rmcleod@bsd.uchicago.edu**).

TREATMENT: Most cases of acquired acute *T gondii* infections in immunocompetent hosts do not require specific therapy unless: (a) infection occurs during pregnancy; (b) there is ocular involvement; or (c) symptoms are severe or persistent. Treatment of acute *T gondii* infections in immunocompromised patients is always recommended.

Neonates and infants with confirmed/strongly suspected congenital toxoplasmosis should receive oral therapy with pyrimethamine, sulfadiazine, and folinic acid (P/S/FA), usually for 12 months, as outlined in Table 3.76. While receiving pyrimethamine, neonates/infants should be monitored for development of neutropenia weekly for 4 weeks; if the absolute neutrophil count (ANC) is stable, then a CBC should be obtained every 2 weeks for 2 to 3 months and then every 3 to 4 weeks for the remainder of treatment. If the ANC decreases to <750 cells/mm^3, the frequency of folinic acid administration should be increased to daily dosing and pyrimethamine therapy should be held temporarily.

Ophthalmologic evaluations should be continued at least every 3 to 6 months during the first 3 years of life for children with confirmed/probable congenital toxoplasmosis, even if the initial evaluation at or near birth was normal. Long-term neurodevelopmental evaluation also is required.

Infected neonates/infants with asymptomatic congenital toxoplasmosis with normal fetal ultrasonography and normal findings in all postnatal evaluations, including head ultrasonography or head CT/MRI, abdominal ultrasonography, eye examination, hearing test, CBC, and liver function tests, should be managed with the regimen used for symptomatic infants (P/S/FA). Treatment duration may be shorter than 12 months (but should be at least 3 months) and should be discussed with a congenital toxoplasmosis expert. Ophthalmologic and neurodevelopmental follow-up should be performed as detailed above.

Older children with active toxoplasmic chorioretinitis represent a medical emergency, and treatment should be initiated as soon as possible, as outlined in Table 3.77. Close monitoring by a retinal specialist with expertise in management of toxoplasmic eye disease and a toxoplasmosis infectious diseases expert is recommended. Treatment for eye disease usually is given for 1 to 2 weeks beyond complete resolution of all clinical signs and symptoms and usually is approximately 4 to 6 weeks total. Treatment courses up to 3 months total are required occasionally.

Immunocompetent and immunocompromised children with severe primary (acute) toxoplasmosis and *immunocompromised children with reactivation of latent (chronic)* **Toxoplasma infection** should receive oral therapy with P/S/FA, as outlined in Table 3.78. In patients for whom P/S/FA is not immediately available, who are allergic or unable to take P or S, or who have significant issues with absorption of oral medications, see alternative regimens listed in Table 3.78.

While children are receiving pyrimethamine, weekly monitoring with CBC and differential is recommended. If neutropenia is detected, the dose of folinic acid (leucovorin) should be increased.

Table 3.76. Treatment of Neonates/Infants With Confirmed or Strongly Suspected Congenital Toxoplasmosis

Regimen	Dosing and Duration
Pyrimethamine PLUS Sulfadiazine PLUS Folinic acid[a]	Doses: Pyrimethamine[b]: 1 mg/kg every 12 hours orally for 2 days, followed by 1 mg/kg once daily for 2–6 months (6 months should be considered for symptomatic cases), followed by 1 mg/kg once per day every Monday, Wednesday, Friday to complete a total course of 12 months PLUS Sulfadiazine: 50 mg/kg every 12 hours orally for 12 months PLUS Folinic acid (leucovorin): 10 mg/dose 3 times per week orally (during and up to 1 week after completing pyrimethamine) Duration: Treatment usually is recommended for 1 year[c] Prednisone (if CSF protein ≥1 g/dL or severe chorioretinitis in vision threatening area): 0.5 mg/kg (maximum 20 mg/dose) every 12 hours orally until CSF protein <1 g/dL or resolution of severe chorioretinitis (if prednisone is used, it should be started 48–72 hours after the initiation of anti-*Toxoplasma* therapy)

CSF indicates cerebrospinal fluid.

[a] Folic acid should not be used as a substitute for folinic acid (leucovorin).

[b] In some centers in Europe, the regimen of pyrimethamine/sulfadoxine (Fansidar) every 10 days, plus folinic acid, is used for subclinical/mild forms of congenital toxoplasmosis and/or for poor compliance and/or frequent hematologic adverse effects. This regimen is used after the first 2 months of daily therapy with pyrimethamine/sulfadiazine (plus folinic acid 2 to 3 times per week). No other alternative medications have been studied adequately for treatment of congenital toxoplasmosis.

[c] For infants with delayed diagnosis of congenital toxoplasmosis (several months after birth), optimal duration of treatment should be discussed with a toxoplasmosis expert.

Primary and Secondary Prophylaxis. Current treatment recommendations and recommendations for primary and secondary toxoplasmosis prophylaxis in children and adolescents with human immunodeficiency virus (HIV) infection are available at **https:// clinicalinfo.hiv.gov/en/guidelines/pediatric-opportunistic-infection/ toxoplasmosis.**

INFECTION PREVENTION AND CONTROL MEASURES IN HEALTH CARE SETTINGS: Standard precautions are recommended.

Table 3.77. Treatment of Older Children With Active Toxoplasmic Chorioretinitis

- Active toxoplasmic chorioretinitis, particularly in patients with severe eye disease in vision-threatening areas, is a medical emergency and treatment should begin as soon as possible.
- Duration: Treatment is usually given for 1 to 2 weeks beyond resolution of clinical manifestations, and usually is approximately 4–6 weeks total; prolonged treatment courses up to 3 months sometimes may be needed.
- Consultation with a retinal specialist (with experience in management of patients with toxoplasmic chorioretinitis) AND with a toxoplasmosis infectious diseases expert should be requested to assist with optimal medication dosing, duration of therapy, and necessary monitoring.

Doses:

Pyrimethamine[a,b,c]:

Loading dose: 1 mg/kg once every 12 hours orally (maximum 50 mg/day) for 2 days, followed by maintenance dose: 1 mg/kg once per day orally (maximum 25 mg/day)

PLUS

Sulfadiazine:

Loading dose: 75 mg/kg (first dose), followed (12 hours later) by maintenance dose: 50 mg/kg every 12 hours orally (maximum 4 g/day)

PLUS

Folinic acid (leucovorin)[d]:

10–20 mg/dose daily orally (during and 1 week after therapy with pyrimethamine)

Prednisone (for severe eye disease in vision-threatening areas [eg, fovea/macula]): 0.5 mg/kg every 12 hours orally (maximum 40 mg/day). If steroids are used, they should be started after 48–72 hours of anti-*Toxoplasma* therapy, with rapid taper. Use steroids at the lowest possible dose and for the shortest possible duration.

Suppressive therapy for recurrent toxoplasmic chorioretinitis:

Although there are no pediatric clinical trials for primary or secondary prophylaxis (suppressive therapy), 2 adult randomized trials in Brazil for secondary prophylaxis showed that after recurrent active toxoplasmic chorioretinitis, initiation of chronic suppressive anti-*Toxoplasma* therapy (1 double strength TMP/SMX every 2–3 days, for 12–20 months) significantly decreased the incidence of recurrences.[e]

[a] If pyrimethamine tablets cannot be obtained immediately, compounded pyrimethamine can be obtained by calling Imprimis Rx at: 844-446-6979. Treatment should change back to pyrimethamine tablets as soon as they are acquired.

[b] Trimethoprim-sulfamethoxazole (TMP/SMX) can also be used when the first-line therapy (pyrimethamine/sulfadiazine) is not readily available, but ONLY until the first-line therapy with pyrimethamine/sulfadiazine/folinic acid becomes available. In those cases, the highest doses should be used (15–20 mg/kg TMP, 75–100 mg/kg SMX per day, divided every 6–8 h).

[c] While on pyrimethamine therapy, a complete blood cell count should be performed weekly. Screening for glucose-6-phosphate dehydrogenase (G6PD) deficiency before starting sulfadiazine or TMP/SMX should be performed for patients from regions with high prevalence of severe G6PD deficiency.

[d] Folic acid should not be used as a substitute for folinic acid (leucovorin).

[e] Silveira C, Belfort R Jr, Muccioli C, et al. The effect of long-term intermittent trimethoprim-sulfamethoxazole treatment on recurrences of toxoplasmic retinochoroiditis. *Am J Ophthalmol*. 2002;134(1):41-46; and Fernandez Felix JP, Cavalcanti Lira RP, Santos Zacchia R, et al. Trimethoprim-sulfamethoxazole versus placebo to reduce the risk of recurrences of toxoplasma gondii retinochoroiditis: randomized controlled clinical trial. *Am J Ophthalmol*. 2014;157(4):762-766.e1.

Table 3.78. Treatment Regimens for Children and Adolescents With Severe Primary (Acute) Toxoplasmosis[a] and Immunocompromised Children and Adolescents With Severe Toxoplasmosis Attributable to Reactivation[b]

Regimen	Dose
PREFERRED REGIMEN Pyrimethamine[c,d] (PO)	Loading dose: 1 mg/kg every 12 hours (maximum 100 mg/day) for 2 days; followed by 1 mg/kg once per day (up to 50 mg/day [if <60 kg] or up to 75 mg/day [if ≥60 kg] in older patients with severe disease)
PLUS Folinic acid[e] (PO)	10–20 mg/dose once per day (up to 50 mg/day) (during and 1 week after therapy with pyrimethamine)
PLUS Sulfadiazine (PO)	100–200 mg/kg/day divided every 6 hours (maximum 4–6 g/day for severe disease)
PREFERRED ALTERNATIVE REGIMEN Trimethoprim-sulfamethoxazole[d] (IV or PO)	
ALTERNATIVE REGIMENS (WITH LIMITED DATA) Pyrimethamine + Folinic acid + Clindamycin Pyrimethamine + Folinic acid + Atovaquone Pyrimethamine + Folinic acid + Clarithromycin Pyrimethamine + Folinic acid + Azithromycin Atovaquone + Sulfadiazine	

IV intravenous; PO, oral.

[a] Includes immunocompetent or immunocompromised children with severe acute *Toxoplasma gondii* infection, particularly in the setting of myocarditis, myositis, hepatitis, pneumonia, brain lesions, and lymphadenopathy accompanied by severe or persisting symptoms **(for drug dosing for ocular toxoplasmosis, see Table 3.77)**. For toxoplasmic encephalitis in HIV patients, treatment should be continued for 6 weeks, assuming clinical improvement, followed by suppressive therapy. Longer courses of treatment may be required for extensive disease or poor response after 6 weeks **(https://clinicalinfo. hiv.gov/en/guidelines/pediatric-opportunistic-infection/toxoplasmosis)**.

[b] Expert advice is available at the PAMF-TSL **(www.sutterhealth.org/RemingtonLab;** telephone 650-853-4828; email **RemingtonLab@sutterhealth.org**) and the Toxoplasmosis Center, University of Chicago, Chicago, IL (**www. uchicagomedicine.org/conditions-services/ophthalmology/toxoplasmosis-center;** telephone 773-834-4131; email **rmcleod@bsd.uchicago.edu**).

[c] If pyrimethamine tablets cannot be obtained immediately, compounded pyrimethamine can be obtained by calling Imprimis Rx at: 844-446-6979. Treatment should change back to pyrimethamine tablets as soon as they are acquired. Refer to **www.daraprimdirect.com** regarding access to pyrimethamine in the United States.

[d] Trimethoprim-sulfamethoxazole (TMP/SMX) can also be used when the first-line therapy (pyrimethamine/sulfadiazine) is not readily available, and ONLY until the first-line therapy with pyrimethamine/sulfadiazine/folinic acid becomes available. In those cases, the highest doses of TMP/SMX should be used (10–15 mg/kg/day of the TMP component, divided every 8–12 hours).

[e] Folinic acid = leucovorin; folic acid must not be used as a substitute for folinic acid.

CONTROL MEASURES: Testing household or close family members of individuals diagnosed with acute *Toxoplasma* infection should be considered in settings in which there are individuals at high risk (eg, pregnant people, immunocompromised individuals, and young children in whom visual impairment associated with acute infection may be missed). HIV-infected, immunocompromised, and pregnant individuals should be counseled about avoidance of sources of *Toxoplasma* infection (see below). Pregnant people and immunocompromised patients whose serostatus for *T gondii* is negative or unknown should avoid activities that may expose them to cat feces by avoiding changing litter boxes, gardening, and landscaping or wearing gloves while doing so and washing hands immediately thereafter. If it must be done, changing of cat litter daily decreases risk of infection, because oocysts are not infective during the first 1 to 2 days after passage. Domestic cats can be protected from infection by feeding them commercially prepared cat food and preventing them from eating undercooked meat and hunting wild rodents and birds.

Oral ingestion of viable *T gondii* can be prevented by the following:
- Avoiding consumption of raw or undercooked meat and cooking meat—particularly pork, lamb, and venison—to an internal temperature of 65.5°C to 76.6°C (150°F–170°F), whole cuts of meat (excluding poultry) to at least 145°F (63°C), ground meat (excluding poultry) to at least 160°F (71°C), and all poultry to at least 165°F (74°C) before consumption;
- Avoiding consumption of smoked meat and meat cured in brine;
- Freezing meat to −20°C for 48 hours before consumption;
- Washing fruits and vegetables;
- Washing hands and cleaning kitchen surfaces after handling fruits, vegetables, and raw meat;
- Washing hands after gardening or other contact with soil;
- Preventing contamination of food with raw or undercooked meat or soil;
- Avoiding ingestion of raw shellfish such as oysters, clams, and mussels;
- Avoiding ingestion of raw goat milk; and
- Avoiding ingestion of untreated water, particularly in resource-limited countries.

Additional resources for health care personnel can be found at **www.cdc.gov/ parasites/toxoplasmosis/health_professionals/index.html.**

Trichinellosis
(*Trichinella spiralis* and Other Species)

CLINICAL MANIFESTATIONS: The clinical spectrum of *Trichinella* infection ranges from inapparent infection to fulminant and fatal illness; most infections are asymptomatic. Severity of disease is proportional to the infective dose and varies with the causative species of *Trichinella*. During the first week after ingesting infected meat, a person may experience abdominal discomfort, nausea, vomiting, and/or diarrhea as excysted larvae penetrate the intestinal mucosa. Two to 8 weeks later, as progeny larvae migrate into tissues, fever, myalgia, periorbital edema, urticarial rash, and conjunctival and subungual hemorrhages may develop. Other findings may correlate with organ system involvement, for example arrhythmia and myocarditis (cardiac), meningitis and encephalitis (central nervous system), myositis (musculoskeletal), and proteinuria or hematuria (renal). Larvae may remain viable in tissues for years; calcification of some larvae in skeletal muscle usually occurs within 6 to 24 months and may be detected using various imaging modalities.

ETIOLOGY: Infection is caused by nematodes (roundworms) of the genus *Trichinella*. *Trichinella spiralis* is the most common of the 7 species that cause human infection.

EPIDEMIOLOGY: Animal infections occur worldwide in carnivores and omnivores, especially scavengers. Humans acquire the infection following ingestion of raw or insufficiently cooked meat containing larvae of *Trichinella* species. Commercial and home-raised pork remain a source of human infections, but meats other than pork, such as venison, horse meat, and particularly meats from wild carnivorous or omnivorous game (especially bear, boar, seal, and walrus) now are the most common sources of infection. US cases have occurred after ingestion of homemade jerky and sausage. The disease is not transmitted from person to person.

The **incubation period** usually is less than 1 month.

DIAGNOSTIC TESTS: Eosinophilia of up to 70% in the setting of compatible symptoms and dietary history suggests the diagnosis. Increases in concentrations of muscle enzymes, such as creatinine phosphokinase and lactic dehydrogenase, may occur but are not always present. Larvae can be detected in suspect meat, but this is not often feasible. Encapsulated larvae in a skeletal muscle biopsy specimen (particularly deltoid and gastrocnemius) are visible under light microscopy beginning 2 weeks after infection by examining hematoxylin-eosin–stained slides or sediment from digested muscle tissue. Serologic testing is available through the Centers for Disease Control and Prevention, some state reference laboratories, and commercial laboratories. Serum antibodies are detectable at 3 or more weeks postinfection and may remain for years. Testing of paired acute and convalescent serum specimens showing an increase in titer is diagnostic, but a single positive test result in the appropriate clinical setting makes the diagnosis likely.

TREATMENT: Albendazole and mebendazole are each recommended for treatment of acute trichinellosis (see Drugs for Parasitic Infections, p 1068), although anthelmintics typically do not kill larvae that have already encysted within muscles. Administration of corticosteroids with or without anthelmintics is recommended when systemic symptoms are severe. Corticosteroids can be lifesaving when the central nervous system or heart is involved.

INFECTION PREVENTION AND CONTROL MEASURES IN HEALTH CARE SETTINGS: Standard precautions are recommended. There is no person-to-person spread.

CONTROL MEASURES: Transmission to pigs can be prevented by not feeding them garbage, by preventing cannibalism among animals, and by effective rat control. The public should be educated about the importance of cooking pork and wild game meat thoroughly. Curing, drying, smoking, and microwaving do not kill *Trichinella* worms reliably. Specific recommendations include the following:

- For whole cuts of meat (excluding poultry and wild game): cook to at least 145°F (63°C) as measured with a food thermometer placed in the thickest part of the meat, then allow the meat to rest for 3 minutes before carving or consuming.
- For ground meat (including wild game, excluding poultry): cook to at least 160°F (71°C); ground meats do not require a rest time. Clean meat grinders thoroughly after each use.

- For all wild game (whole cuts and ground): cook to at least 160°F (71°C). Freezing pork less than 6 inches thick at 5°F (−15°C) for 20 days kills *T spiralis*. *Trichinella* organisms in wild animals, such as bears and raccoons, are resistant to freezing. For people who have ingested undercooked meat known to be contaminated with *Trichinella* organisms, preemptive therapy with albendazole or mebendazole may be considered if initiated within 6 days of exposure.

Public Health Reporting. Trichinellosis is a notifiable disease (see Appendix III: Nationally Notifiable Infectious Diseases in the United States, p 1141).

Trichomonas vaginalis Infections
(Trichomoniasis)

CLINICAL MANIFESTATIONS: A *Trichomonas vaginalis* (TV) infection, which has been described as the most common nonviral sexually transmitted infection (STI) affecting approximately 3.7 million people in the United States, is asymptomatic in 70% to 85% of infected individuals. Untreated infections may persist for months to years. Clinical manifestations in symptomatic pubertal or postpubertal females may include a diffuse vaginal discharge, odor, and vulvovaginal pruritus and irritation.[1] Dysuria and, less often, lower abdominal pain can occur. Vaginal discharge may be any color but classically is yellow-green, frothy, and malodorous. The vulva and vaginal mucosa can be erythematous and edematous. The cervix can be inflamed and sometimes is covered with numerous punctate cervical hemorrhages and swollen papillae, referred to as "strawberry" cervix. This finding occurs in fewer than 5% of infected female patients, is most often seen on colposcopy, and is highly suggestive of trichomoniasis. Clinical manifestations in symptomatic male individuals include urethritis and, rarely, epididymitis or prostatitis. Reinfection is common, and resistance to treatment is uncommon but increasing. Rectal and oral infections are uncommon.

TV infections in pregnant people have been associated with increased risks of premature rupture of the membranes and preterm delivery, although direct causation has not been clearly established. Perinatal infection may occur in up to 5% of neonates born to infected individuals. TV in female newborn infants may cause vaginal discharge during the first weeks of life but usually is self-limited. Respiratory infections in newborn infants may occur as well.

ETIOLOGY: *T vaginalis* is a flagellated protozoan approximately the size of a leukocyte. It requires adherence to host cells for survival.

EPIDEMIOLOGY: Among sexually active female participants in the 2013–2016 cycles of the National Health and Nutrition Examination Survey, the estimated prevalence was 0.7% among 14- through 19-year-olds and 2.7% and 20- through 29-year-olds. Unlike chlamydia and gonorrhea, TV prevalence rates were low among female participants 14 through 19 years of age and high among female participants 20 through 29 years and did not differ significantly among women 30 through 39 years of age or 40 through 49 years of age. Overall prevalence was almost 4-fold higher among female than male individuals and almost 11-fold higher among non-Hispanic Black female individuals than non-Hispanic white female individuals. Prevalence was higher among people with lower family income, those with less education, and

---

[1] The terms female, male, women, and men refer to sex assigned at birth.

those who were unmarried. Among female participant, younger age at coitarche and higher number of sex partners were associated with higher TV prevalence. Female individuals with bacterial vaginosis (BV) are at higher risk for TV. Male partners of female individuals with TV are likely to have infection, although the prevalence of trichomoniasis in men who have sex with men is low. Transmission results almost exclusively from sexual contact. The presence of TV in a child or preadolescent beyond the perinatal period is considered indicative of sexual abuse (see STI Evaluation After Sexual Assault of a Prepubertal Child, p 184, and Table 2.5, p 183). TV infection can increase both the acquisition and transmission of human immunodeficiency virus (HIV).

The **incubation period** averages 1 week but ranges from 5 to 28 days.

DIAGNOSTIC TESTS[1]: Wet mount microscopy of vaginal discharge traditionally has been used as the preferred diagnostic test for TV among female individuals, but its sensitivity is low (44%–68%) compared with culture. TV culture in Diamond media or other trichomonas-specific culture systems is a specific method of diagnosis in female patients with a sensitivity of 44% to 75% and specificity of nearly 100%. In female patients, vaginal secretions are the preferred specimen type for culture, because urine culture is less sensitive. In male patients, culture specimens require a urethral swab, urine sediment, and/or semen specimen.

In contrast, nucleic acid amplification tests (NAATs) are highly sensitive, detecting more TV infections than wet-mount microscopy among women. Sensitivities and specificities generally are in the 95% to 100% range. TV NAATs can be used on various specimens including vaginal swab (self- or provider-collected), endocervical swab, urine, and liquid Pap smear specimens from female patients and urine specimens from male patients. Some TV NAAT platforms also test for chlamydia or gonorrhea. Other TV NAATs test for pathogens causing vaginitis, such as BV-associated bacteria and *Candida* species. The GeneXpert TV (Cepheid) is a moderately complex rapid test that can be performed in less than 1 hour as a point-of-care (POC) test with a sensitivity and specificity of 99.5% to 100% and 99.4% to 99.9%, respectively.

There are also antigen-detection tests that use immunochromatographic capillary flow dipstick technology that have high sensitivity and specificity.

TREATMENT[1]: The recommended treatment for TV infection in female patients is metronidazole, 500 mg, orally, twice daily for 7 days. In male patients, the recommended treatment is metronidazole 2 g, orally in a single dose. An alternative regimen in both female and male individuals is tinidazole 2 g, orally, in a single dose. Tinidazole is generally more expensive, reaches higher concentrations in serum and the genitourinary tract, has a longer half-life than metronidazole (12.5 hours versus 7.3 hours), and has fewer gastrointestinal adverse effects. Metronidazole gel does not reach therapeutic concentrations in the urethra and perivaginal glands. Because it is less efficacious than oral metronidazole, it is not recommended. Secnidazole is also approved by the US Food and Drug Administration for treatment of TV in people 12 years and older.

---

[1] Centers for Disease Control and Prevention. Sexually transmitted infections treatment guidelines, 2021. *MMWR Recomm Rep.* 2021;70(RR-4):1-187. Available at: **www.cdc.gov/std/treatment-guidelines/ trichomoniasis.htm**

A recurrent infection can result from reinfection from an untreated sex partner, treatment failure because of antimicrobial resistance, or lack of adherence to therapy. In cases of persistent or recurrent trichomoniasis, retesting with culture is preferred. If NAAT is used, it should not be conducted before 3 weeks after treatment completion because of possible detection of residual nucleic acid from the prior infection that is not clinically relevant.

If treatment failure occurs in a female patient after completing a 7-day course of metronidazole and the patient has been reexposed to an untreated partner, a repeat course of the same regimen is recommended. If there has been no reexposure, the female patient should be treated with 2 g of metronidazole or tinidazole, once daily, for 7 days. If a male patient is still infected with TV after a single dose of 2 g of metronidazole and has been reexposed to an untreated partner, the patient should be given another single dose of 2 g of metronidazole. If there has been no reexposure, the male patient should be given a course of metronidazole, 500 mg, twice daily for 7 days. Nitroimidazole-resistant TV is concerning, because few alternatives to standard therapy exist. For people who are experiencing persistent infection not attributable to reexposure, clinicians should request a kit from the Centers for Disease Control and Prevention (CDC) to perform drug susceptibility testing (**www.cdc.gov/laboratory/specimen-submission/detail. html?CDCTestCode=CDC-10239**). Treatment can then be determined based on the test results. The CDC can perform susceptibility testing for people with clinical treatment failure and can provide guidance regarding treatment in cases of nitroimidazole resistance. Treatments for infections caused by antimicrobial-resistant TV strains can include metronidazole or tinidazole 2 g daily for 7 days. If a person has treatment failure after the 7-day regimen of high-dose oral metronidazole or tinidazole, high-dose oral tinidazole, 2 g daily, plus intravaginal tinidazole, 500 mg, 2 times/day for 14 days, has been successful among female patients. If this regimen fails, high-dose oral tinidazole (1 g, 3 times/day) plus intravaginal paromomycin (4 g of 6.25% intravaginal paromomycin cream nightly) for 14 days should be considered.

Pregnancy and Lactation. TV infection in pregnant people has been associated with adverse pregnancy outcomes, particularly premature rupture of membranes, preterm delivery, and delivery of an infant with low birth weight. In symptomatic infected pregnant people, regardless of pregnancy stage, consideration should be given to treatment with metronidazole. Although metronidazole crosses the placenta, data indicate that it poses a low risk to the developing fetus. No evidence of teratogenicity or mutagenic effects among infants has been found in multiple cross-sectional and cohort studies among pregnant people examining single-dose (2 g) and multidose metronidazole regimens. Metronidazole is secreted in human milk. With oral therapy of the lactating parent, breastfed infants receive metronidazole in doses that are lower than those used to treat infections in infants, although the active metabolite adds to the total infant exposure. Multiple reported case series identified no evidence of metronidazole-associated adverse effects for breastfed infants. Data from studies involving human subjects are limited regarding use of tinidazole in pregnancy; however, animal data suggest this drug poses moderate risk. Thus, tinidazole should be avoided in pregnant people, and breastfeeding should be deferred for 72 hours following a single 2-g dose of tinidazole.

Neonatal. For newborn infants, infection with TV acquired perinatally is self-limited, and treatment generally is not recommended.

INFECTION PREVENTION AND CONTROL MEASURES IN HEALTH CARE SETTINGS: Standard precautions are recommended.

CONTROL MEASURES: Measures to prevent STIs, particularly the consistent and correct use of condoms, are indicated. Patients should be instructed to avoid sexual activity until they and their sexual partners are treated and there is resolution of symptoms. Testing for other STIs including HIV, syphilis, gonorrhea, and chlamydia should be performed.

Follow-up. Because of the high rate of trichomoniasis reinfection among female individuals, retesting for TV is recommended for all sexually active female patients within 3 months following initial treatment, regardless of whether they are symptomatic or believe their sex partners were treated. If retesting at 3 months is not possible, clinicians should retest at the next presentation for medical care within 12 months following initial treatment. Data are insufficient to support retesting male patients.

Routine Screening Tests.[1] Although routine TV screening of asymptomatic adolescents is not recommended, screening can be considered for people receiving care in high-prevalence settings (eg, STI clinics and correctional facilities) and for asymptomatic women at high risk of infection. Risk factors that may put female individuals at higher risk of TV include new or multiple partners, exchanging sex for payment, illicit drug use, or an STI history. The CDC recommends screening for TV in all female individuals with HIV infection at least annually and at their first prenatal visit.

Management of Sexual Partners. All people with a known exposure to TV infection should be treated routinely, regardless of a diagnostic test result. Expedited partner therapy might have a role in partner management for trichomoniasis and may be used in states where this approach is permissible.

Trichuriasis
(Whipworm Infection)

CLINICAL MANIFESTATIONS: Disease caused by the whipworm *Trichuris trichiura* generally is proportional to the intensity of the infection. Most infected children are asymptomatic, but those with heavy infestations may develop colitis that mimics inflammatory bowel disease, with signs and symptoms that include chronic abdominal pain and diarrhea, physical growth restriction, and clubbing. A more serious condition is *Trichuris* dysentery syndrome, which is characterized by severe abdominal pain, tenesmus, bloody diarrhea, and occasionally rectal prolapse. Children may have anemia and peripheral eosinophilia.

ETIOLOGY: *T trichiura*, the human whipworm, is the causative agent of trichuriasis. Adult worms are 30 to 50 mm long with a large, thread-like anterior end that embeds in the mucosa of the large intestine. Adult worms typically reside in the cecum and ascending colon; with heavy infection, worms may extend further into the colon and rectum.

---

[1] American Academy of Pediatrics, Committee on Adolescence; Society for Adolescent Health and Medicine. Screening for nonviral sexually transmitted infections in adolescents and young adults. *Pediatrics.* 2014;134(1):e302-e311

EPIDEMIOLOGY: *T trichiura* is the second most prevalent soil-transmitted helminth in the world, with approximately 600 to 800 million people infected worldwide, most in tropical regions that lack proper sanitation infrastructure. It is frequently coendemic with *Ascaris* and hookworm species. Humans are the natural reservoir. Eggs excreted in moist soil require a range of 10 days to 4 weeks of incubation, depending on temperature, before they are infectious. Children become infected by accidental ingestion of infective eggs in food or on hands contaminated with soil. The disease is not communicable directly from person to person.

The time between infection and appearance of eggs in the stool (**incubation period**) is approximately 12 weeks; worms may live 1 to 3 years or more.

DIAGNOSTIC TESTS: Quantitative techniques like the Kato-Katz, McMaster, and FLOTAC methods are used typically in research settings to quantify fecal egg excretion as a measure of infection intensity. Direct microscopic visualization of eggs using stool concentrating techniques is recommended in routine clinical settings, and for screening at-risk populations such as immigrants, refugees, and international adoptees. Adult worms may be seen on proctoscopy or colonoscopy.

TREATMENT: Mebendazole and albendazole are considered first-line therapies in the treatment of trichuriasis, although cure rates for both are low. Combination therapy with albendazole plus ivermectin is also a reasonable treatment approach. The recommended duration of therapy is 3 days, although a longer course (5–7 days) of albendazole may be warranted for heavy infections (see Drugs for Parasitic Infections, p 1068).

Stool specimens should be reexamined approximately 2 weeks after therapy to document cure. Those in whom therapy fails should be retreated, with consideration of combination therapy (albendazole plus ivermectin). Iron supplements should be prescribed to patients with severe or symptomatic anemia.

INFECTION PREVENTION AND CONTROL MEASURES IN HEALTH CARE SETTINGS: Standard precautions are recommended; there is no direct person-to-person transmission.

CONTROL MEASURES: Proper disposal of contaminated feces is the most effective means of control for whipworm and other soil-transmitted helminths. Depending on prevalence, annual or biannual administration of anthelmintics in communities with endemic *Trichuris* burden is currently recommended by the World Health Organization for control of soil-transmitted helminth infections, including *T trichiura*.

African Trypanosomiasis
(Sleeping Sickness)

CLINICAL MANIFESTATIONS: The clinical course of human African trypanosomiasis has 2 stages: the hemolymphatic stage, in which the parasite multiplies in subcutaneous tissues, lymph, and blood; and the neurologic stage, after the parasite crosses the blood-brain barrier and infects the central nervous system (CNS). The rapidity of disease progression and clinical manifestations vary with the infecting subspecies. With *Trypanosoma brucei gambiense* infection (found in western and central Africa), initial symptoms may be mild and include intermittent fever, headaches, muscle and joint aches, and malaise. Pruritus, rash, hepatosplenomegaly, weight loss, and lymphadenopathy (mainly posterior cervical [Winterbottom sign] but also possible in axillary, inguinal, and epitrochlear areas) can occur. CNS involvement typically develops after 1 to 2 years with development of confusion, behavioral changes, cachexia, headache, sensory disturbances, poor coordination and movement disorders, seizures, tremors, speech disorders (eg, dysarthria, logorrhea), hallucinations, delusions, and daytime somnolence followed by night-time insomnia. Trypanosome infiltration of endocrine organs (mainly thyroid and adrenal glands) and the heart may lead to disruptions of hormonal secretions and mild perimyocarditis.

Symptoms of *Trypanosoma brucei rhodesiense* infection (found in eastern and southern Africa) are similar to those of *T brucei gambiense* infection. An inoculation chancre may develop at the site of the tsetse fly bite. Initial manifestations include high fever, headaches, pruritis, lymphadenopathy (more often submandibular, axillary, and inguinal), rash, and muscle and joint aches. Thyroid dysfunction, adrenal insufficiency, and hypogonadism are found more frequently in *T brucei rhodesiense* infection and myoperi-carditis may be earlier and more severe. Edema is reported more frequently in *T brucei rhodesiense* infection, and liver involvement with hepatomegaly is usually moderate, sometimes with ascites.

Clinical meningoencephalitis can develop after onset of the untreated systemic illness caused by both *Trypanosoma* subspecies. As the disease progresses, severe but less frequent complications can include renal failure requiring dialysis, multiorgan failure, disseminated intravascular coagulopathy, and coma. Both forms of African trypanoso-miasis have high fatality rates; without treatment, infected patients usually die within 6 months after clinical onset of disease caused by *T brucei rhodesiense* and within 2 to 3 years from disease caused by *T brucei gambiense.*

ETIOLOGY: Human African trypanosomiasis (sleeping sickness) is caused by *Trypanosoma brucei* subspecies, which are protozoan parasites transmitted by blood-feeding tsetse flies. The west and central African (Gambian) form is caused by *T brucei gambiense,* and the east and southern African (Rhodesian) form is caused by *T brucei rhodesiense.* Both are extracellular protozoan hemoflagellates that live in blood and tissue of the human host.

EPIDEMIOLOGY: The number of cases of human African trypanosomiasis is decreasing, with 663 cases reported to the World Health Organization (WHO) in 2020, a 98% reduction since 2000. Most reported cases worldwide (>95%) are caused by *T brucei gambiense.* There are occasional reported cases of African trypanosomiasis in the United States, typically in returning travelers who became infected with *T brucei rhodesiense* in East Africa. Transmission of *T brucei* subspecies is confined to an area in Africa between the latitudes of 14° north and 29° south, corresponding to the distribution of the tsetse fly vector (*Glossina* species), although many tsetse-infested areas are free of disease risk. Humans are the main reservoir of *T brucei gambiense* in West and Central Africa, although the parasite sometimes can be found in domestic animals, such as dogs and pigs. In East Africa, wild animals, such as antelope, bush buck, and hartebeest, constitute the major reservoirs for sporadic infections with *T brucei rhod-esiense,* although cattle serve as reservoir hosts in local outbreaks. *T brucei* subspecies also can be transmitted congenitally. Accidental infections in laboratories have occurred as a result of pricks with contaminated needles.

The **incubation period** for acute disease symptoms from *T brucei rhodesiense* infection ranges from 3 to 21 days, and for most cases is 5 to 14 days. For *T brucei gam-biense* infection, the **incubation period** for acute disease symptoms usually is longer but is not well defined; it is generally <1 month for travelers from countries without endemic disease.

DIAGNOSTIC TESTS: Diagnosis is made by identification of trypanosomes in specimens of blood, cerebrospinal fluid (CSF), or fluid aspirated from a chancre or lymph node, or by inoculation of susceptible laboratory animals (mice) with heparinized blood in the case of *T brucei rhodesiense* infection. Examination of CSF is critical to management, and all patients diagnosed in the United States should undergo lumbar puncture; concentration methods (such as the double centrifugation or modified single centrifugation techniques) typically should be used. Concentration and Giemsa staining of the buffy coat layer of peripheral blood are easier for *T brucei rhodesiense*, because the density of organisms in circulating blood is higher than for *T brucei gambiense*. Wet preparations of the buffy coat and of concentrated CSF sediment should be examined within a few minutes for motile trypanosomes. *T brucei gambiense* is more likely to be found in lymph node aspirates than in blood. The most widely used criteria for stage determination to assess CNS involvement include identification of trypanosomes in CSF or a CSF white blood cell count of 6 cells/μL or higher; elevated CSF neopterin and an increase in intrathecal immunoglobulin M also may suggest second-stage disease. Serologic testing for antibodies to *T brucei gambiense* is available outside the United States and typically is used only for screening purposes to help identify suspect cases; there is no comparable serologic screening test for *T brucei rhodesiense*.

TREATMENT: The choice of drug(s) used for treatment depends on the type and stage of African trypanosomiasis (**www.cdc.gov/parasites/sleepingsickness/index. html**). When no evidence of CNS involvement is present, the drugs of choice for the acute hemolymphatic stage of infection are pentamidine for *T brucei gambiense* infection and suramin for *T brucei rhodesiense* infection (pentamidine is also effective, although less well documented). For treatment of *T brucei gambiense* infection with CNS involvement, the drug of choice is eflornithine in combination with nifurtimox, or eflornithine alone if nifurtimox is not available or contraindicated; for *T brucei rhodesiense* infection with CNS involvement, the drug of choice is melarsoprol (eflornithine is not effective for CNS treatment of *T brucei rhodesiense* infection). Melarsoprol encephalopathy may be reduced in severity by pretreatment with corticosteroids. Eflornithine is not approved by the US Food and Drug Administration (FDA) but is available through the Centers for Disease Control and Prevention (CDC) under an individual provider investigational new drug application from the FDA. Oral fexinidazole, a nitroimidazole adapted for use in rural health facilities in Africa to be administered under directly observed therapy in selected patients, was approved recently (including by the FDA, in 2021) for children ≥6 years of age and ≥20 kg for the treatment of both first-stage (hemolymphatic) and second-stage (meningoencephalitic) gambiense trypanosomiasis. Because of decreased efficacy observed in patients with severe second-stage human African trypanosomiasis (CSF white blood cell count >100 cells/μL) attributable to *T brucei gambiense* disease, fexinidazole tablets should be used only if there are no other available treatment options. Suramin, eflornithine, and melarsoprol can be obtained from the CDC (phone: 404-718-4745). As of 2023, fexinidazole is not available commercially or through the CDC in the United States. Consultation with a specialist familiar with the disease and its treatment is recommended. Patients who have had CNS involvement should undergo repeated follow-up CSF examinations every 6 months for 2 years because of the risk of relapse. The optimal approach to treatment of relapse is uncertain. The WHO has developed interim updated guidelines for the treatment of human African trypanosomiasis caused by *T brucei gambiense* (**apps.who.int/iris/ bitstream/handle/10665/326178/9789241550567-eng.pdf?ua=1**). These guidelines allow for certain patients (older children and adults without clinically apparent severe disease) to forego a lumbar puncture when oral fexinidazole is an option and certain conditions are met by the patient.

INFECTION PREVENTION AND CONTROL MEASURES IN HEALTH CARE SETTINGS: Standard precautions are recommended.

CONTROL MEASURES: Travelers to areas with endemic infection should avoid known foci of sleeping sickness and tsetse fly infestation and should minimize fly bites by wearing long-sleeved shirts and pants of medium-weight material in neutral colors. Avoid light-weight cloth that tsetse flies can bite through and bright or dark colors that attract the flies (especially blue and black). Newborn infants whose birthing parent is infected should be examined clinically and their blood should be tested for trypanosomes; breastfeeding may continue during treatment.

American Trypanosomiasis
(Chagas Disease)

CLINICAL MANIFESTATIONS: The acute phase of *Trypanosoma cruzi* infection (Chagas disease) lasts 2 to 3 months, followed by the chronic phase that, in the absence of successful antiparasitic treatment, is lifelong. The acute phase commonly is asymptomatic or characterized by mild, nonspecific symptoms. When disease is acquired by oral transmission, patients are more likely to exhibit symptoms of febrile illness with higher morbidity and mortality. In the minority of patients with symptomatic acute-phase infection, fever, edema, cutaneous rash, myalgia, pallor, malaise, lymphadenopathy, and hepatosplenomegaly may develop. Meningoencephalitis and/or acute myocarditis are rare manifestations. Unilateral edema of the eyelids, known as the Romaña sign, may occur if the portal of entry is the conjunctiva. The edematous skin may be violaceous and associated with conjunctivitis and enlargement of the ipsilateral preauricular lymph node. In some patients, a red, indurated nodule known as a chagoma develops at the site of the original inoculation, usually on the face or arms.

Symptoms of acute Chagas disease can resolve without treatment within 3 months, and patients pass into the chronic phase of the infection. Most people with chronic *T cruzi* infection have no signs or symptoms and are said to have the indeterminate form of chronic Chagas disease. Serious progressive sequelae affecting the heart and/ or gastrointestinal tract develop in an estimated 20% to 30% of cases years to decades after the initial infection (called determinate forms of chronic Chagas disease). Chagas cardiomyopathy is characterized by conduction system abnormalities, especially right bundle branch block and ventricular arrhythmias, and may progress to dilated cardiomyopathy and congestive heart failure. Patients with Chagas cardiomyopathy may die suddenly from ventricular arrhythmias, complete heart block, or embolic phenomena; death also may occur from intractable congestive heart failure. Less commonly, patients with chronic Chagas disease may develop digestive disease with dilatation of the colon and/or esophagus with swallowing difficulties accompanied by severe weight loss.

Congenital Chagas disease occurs in an estimated 1% to 5% of infants born to infected people in the United States and may be characterized by low birth weight, hepatosplenomegaly, and anemia. Myocarditis, pneumonitis, and/or meningoencephalitis with seizures and tremors are rare. Most infants with congenital *T cruzi* infection have no signs or symptoms of disease.

Reactivation of chronic *T cruzi* infection with parasitemia may be life threatening and may occur in immunocompromised people, including people infected with human immunodeficiency virus and those who are immunosuppressed after transplantation.

ETIOLOGY: *Trypanosoma cruzi*, a protozoan hemoflagellate, causes American trypanosomiasis (Chagas disease). Chagas disease is named after the Brazilian physician Carlos Chagas, who discovered it in 1909.

EPIDEMIOLOGY: Parasites are transmitted in feces of infected triatomine insects (sometimes called "kissing bugs," a type of reduviid; local Spanish/Portuguese names include vinchuca, chinche picuda, or barbeiro). When found indoors, they tend to be located in pet areas, under bedding, and in areas of rodent infestation. The bugs defecate during or after taking a blood meal. The bitten person is inoculated through inadvertent rubbing of insect feces containing the parasite into the site of the bite through the harmed skin or mucous membranes of the eye. The parasite also can be transmitted congenitally, during solid organ transplantation, through blood transfusion, and by ingestion of food or drink contaminated by the vector's excreta. Accidental laboratory infections can result from handling parasite cultures or blood from infected people or laboratory animals, usually through needlestick injuries. Vector-borne transmission of the disease is limited to the Western Hemisphere, predominantly Mexico and Central and South America.

In the United States, 11 species of kissing bugs have been identified, and most have been found to be infected naturally with *T cruzi*. Triatomines have been found throughout the southern half of the United States, from California to Florida and as far north as Illinois and Pennsylvania. Significant numbers of wild animals are infected, including opossums, armadillos, wood rats, and raccoons. Animals usually acquire the parasite by eating infected triatomines. Rare vector-borne cases of Chagas disease have been noted in the United States. Most *T cruzi*-infected individuals in the United States are immigrants from areas of Latin America with endemic infection.

It is estimated that more than 300 000 individuals with *T cruzi* infection live in the United States, including about 40 000 people capable of becoming pregnant. Assuming a 1% to 5% risk of congenital transmission, based on estimates of infection in pregnant people, approximately 63 to 315 infants are born with Chagas disease in the United States every year. Transfusion- and transplantation-associated cases have been documented in the United States.

The disease is an important cause of morbidity and death in Latin America, where as many as 6 million people may be infected, of whom approximately 20% to 30% either have or will develop cardiomyopathy and/or gastrointestinal tract disorders (**www.paho.org/en/topics/chagas-disease**). Many individuals with the disease remain undiagnosed, with some estimates as high as 95%.

The **incubation period** for the acute phase of disease is 1 to 2 weeks or longer. Chronic manifestations do not appear for years to decades.

DIAGNOSTIC TESTS: During the acute phase of disease, the parasite is demonstrable in blood specimens by Giemsa staining after a concentration technique or in direct wet-mount or buffy coat preparations. Molecular detection techniques (available at the Centers for Disease Control and Prevention [CDC]) also have high sensitivity in the acute phase. Next-generation diagnostic techniques using cell-free pathogen DNA are commercially available. The chronic phase of *T cruzi* infection is characterized by low-level intermittent parasitemia. Diagnosis in the chronic phase relies on serologic tests to demonstrate immunoglobulin (Ig) G antibodies against *T cruzi*. Serologic tests include indirect immunofluorescence, enzyme-linked immunosorbent assays, immunochromatographic testing, hemagglutination inhibition, and chemiluminescence microparticle immunoassays (CMIA); no single serologic test is sufficiently sensitive or specific to confirm a diagnosis of chronic *T cruzi* infection. The Pan American Health Organization and the World Health Organization recommend that samples be tested using 2 diagnostic assays of different formats before treatment decisions are made.

The diagnosis of congenital Chagas disease can be made during the first 3 months of life by identification of motile trypomastigotes by direct microscopy of fresh anticoagulated blood specimens or by a nucleic acid amplification test (NAAT), which is a useful tool in infants and has higher sensitivity than serologic testing. If an infant is not tested before 3 months of age, serologic testing should be performed after 9 months of age once serum immunoglobulin (Ig) G measurements are expected to reflect infant response rather than transplacentally acquired antibody. The CDC has developed algorithms for evaluation of Chagas disease in infants <3 months (Fig 3.20) and ≥3 months (Fig 3.21).

FIG 3.20. EVALUATION OF CONGENITAL CHAGAS DISEASE (CCD): INFANT <3 MONTHS OF AGE[a]

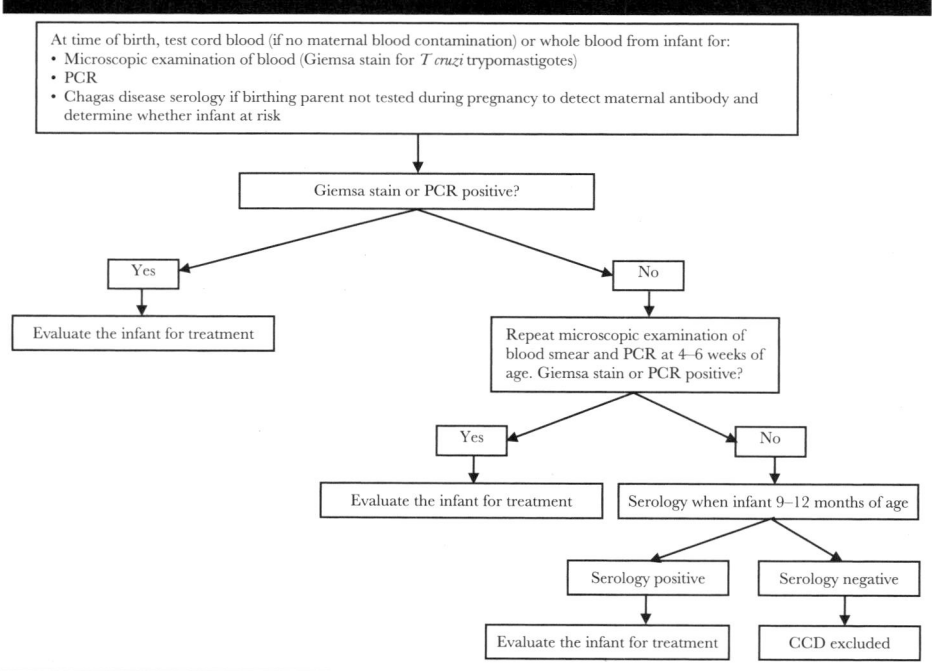

[a] Infant whose birthing parent has suspected or confirmed Chagas disease **OR** infant with symptoms of congenital Chagas disease in at-risk birthing parent whose serologic status is unknown.

Adapted from: **www.cdc.gov/parasites/chagas/health_professionals/congenital_chagas.html.**

FIG 3.21. EVALUATION OF CONGENITAL CHAGAS DISEASE (CCD): INFANT ≥3 MONTHS OF AGE

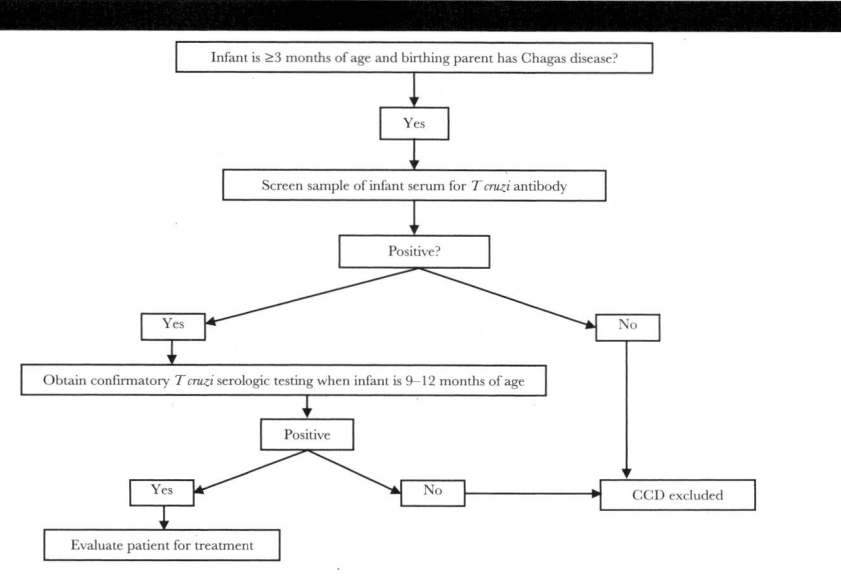

Adapted from: **www.cdc.gov/parasites/chagas/health_professionals/congenital_chagas.html.**

Some countries have congenital Chagas disease screening programs that combine (1) screening of the birthing parent; and (2) microscopic examination of cord blood from infants whose birthing parent is seropositive.

Low sensitivity of some screening tests and low rates of follow-up likely lead to underestimation of infection rates. Diagnostic testing and consultation are available from the CDC Division of Parasitic Diseases and Malaria (phone: 404-718-4745; email: **parasites@cdc.gov;** CDC Emergency Operator [after business hours and on weekends]: 770-488-7100).

TREATMENT: The only drugs with proven efficacy are benznidazole and nifurtimox (see Drugs for Parasitic Infections, p 1068). Benznidazole was approved in 2017 by the US Food and Drug Administration (FDA) for use in children 2 to 12 years of age and nifurtimox in 2020 for treatment of Chagas disease in children from birth to 18 years of age. The recommended treatment courses are 60 days.

Antitrypanosomal treatment is recommended for all cases of acute and congenital Chagas disease, reactivated infection attributable to immunosuppression, and chronic *T cruzi* infection in children younger than 18 years. Treatment of chronic *T cruzi* infection in adults without advanced cardiomyopathy generally is recommended. The efficacy of either agent appears high if given soon after infection, but wanes in the setting of longer infection or advancing age, during which adverse medication effects are also more common.

Trypanocidal therapy with benznidazole in patients with established Chagas cardiomyopathy significantly reduces serum parasite detection by NAAT but does not reduce cardiac clinical deterioration or death significantly through 5 years of follow-up and, therefore, is not recommended. Both drugs have significant adverse event profiles. The only currently recognized test of cure is reversion to negative serologic status, which may take years in chronic infection. Careful consideration of potential risks and benefits in consultation with an expert in treatment of the disease or with CDC may be necessary, especially for patients in whom chronic infection is diagnosed and/or who do not fall under a clearly recommended treatment category.

INFECTION PREVENTION AND CONTROL MEASURES IN HEALTH CARE SETTINGS: Standard precautions should be followed.

CONTROL MEASURES: Risk to travelers is low. Travelers to areas with endemic infection should avoid contact with triatomine bugs by avoiding habitation in buildings vulnerable to infestation, particularly those constructed of mud, palm thatch, or adobe brick. The use of insecticide-impregnated bed nets, tucked under the mattress on all sides, also may be beneficial. Camping or sleeping outdoors in areas with endemic transmission is not recommended. Travelers to regions with endemic infection also should avoid ingestion of unpasteurized juices, such as sugar cane, guava, or açaí palm fruit juice, which have been linked to oral transmission of Chagas disease. Diagnostic testing should be performed on members of households with an infected patient if they have had exposure to the vector similar to that of the patient. All children of a birthing parent with *T cruzi* infection should be tested for Chagas disease.

Education about the mode of spread and methods of prevention is warranted in areas with endemic infection. Homes should be examined for the presence of the vectors, and if found, measures to eliminate the vector should be taken.

People with known *T cruzi* infection should not donate blood. Most US blood collection agencies started screening for *T cruzi* infection in 2007; final guidance to all blood collection agencies for appropriate use of serologic tests to screen blood donors for *T cruzi* infection was issued by the FDA in December 2010.

Tuberculosis

CLINICAL MANIFESTATIONS: Tuberculosis (TB) disease is caused by organisms of the *Mycobacterium tuberculosis* complex. Most infections caused by *M tuberculosis* complex in children and adolescents are asymptomatic. When pulmonary TB occurs, clinical manifestations most often appear 1 month to 2 years after infection and include fever, weight loss or poor weight gain, cough, night sweats, and chills. Chest radiographic findings rarely are specific for TB and include lymphadenopathy of the hilar, subcarinal, paratracheal, or mediastinal nodes; atelectasis or infiltrate of a segment or lobe; pleural effusion that can conceal small interstitial lesions; interstitial cavities; or miliary-pattern infiltrates. In selected instances, computed tomography or magnetic resonance imaging of the chest can clarify nonspecific or subtle radiographic findings. Although cavitation is a typical presentation of TB in adults (and sometimes in adolescents), cavitation is uncommon in childhood TB. Necrosis and cavitation, however, can result from a progressive primary focus in very young or immunocompromised patients and in patients with lymphobronchial disease. Extrapulmonary manifestations include meningitis and granulomatous inflammation of the lymph nodes, bones, joints, skin, and middle ear and mastoid. Gastrointestinal tract TB can mimic inflammatory bowel disease. Renal TB is unusual in younger children but can occur in adolescents. In addition, chronic abdominal pain with peritonitis and intermittent partial intestinal obstruction can be present in disease caused by *Mycobacterium bovis.* Congenital TB can mimic neonatal sepsis, or the infant may come to medical attention in the first 90 days of life with bronchopneumonia and/or hepatosplenomegaly. Clinical findings in patients with drug-resistant TB disease are indistinguishable from manifestations in patients with drug-susceptible disease.

ETIOLOGY: The causative agent is *M tuberculosis* complex, a group of closely related acid-fast bacilli: *M tuberculosis, M bovis, Mycobacterium africanum,* and a few additional species infrequently associated with human infection. *M africanum* is rare in the United States, so clinical laboratories do not distinguish it routinely, and treatment recommendations are the same as for *M tuberculosis. M bovis* can be distinguished from *M tuberculosis* in reference laboratories, and although the spectrum of illness caused by *M bovis* is similar to that of *M tuberculosis,* the epidemiology, treatment, and prevention are different, as detailed later in the chapter.

Definitions:
- **Bacille Calmette-Guérin (BCG)** is a live attenuated vaccine strain of *M bovis.* BCG vaccine rarely is administered to children in the United States but is one of the most widely used vaccines in the world. An isolate of BCG can be distinguished from wild-type *M bovis* only in a reference laboratory.
- **Positive tuberculin skin test (TST) result.** A positive TST result (see Table 3.79) indicates possible infection with *M tuberculosis* complex. Tuberculin reactivity appears 2 to 10 weeks after initial infection; the median interval is 3 to 4 weeks (see Tuberculin Skin Test, p 892). BCG immunization can produce a positive TST result (see Diagnostic Tests, Testing for *M tuberculosis* Infection, p 892).
- **Positive interferon-gamma release assay (IGRA) result.** A positive IGRA result indicates possible infection with *M tuberculosis* complex. IGRAs measure ex vivo interferon-gamma production from T lymphocytes in response to stimulation with antigens mostly specific to *M tuberculosis* complex, including *M tuberculosis* and *M bovis.* The antigens used in IGRAs are not found in BCG or most pathogenic nontuberculous mycobacteria (eg, are not found in *Mycobacterium avium* complex, but are found in *Mycobacterium kansasii, Mycobacterium szulgai,* and *Mycobacterium marinum).*
- **TB infection (TBI)** is defined as *M tuberculosis* complex bacteria present in the body. Most commonly, TBI is used to describe infection in a person who has no symptoms or signs of disease and chest radiograph findings that are normal or reveal evidence of healed infection (eg, calcification in the lung, lymph nodes, or both) and a positive TST or IGRA result. This situation is also referred to as latent TB infection.
- **TB disease** is illness in a person with infection attributable to *M tuberculosis* complex in whom symptoms, signs, or radiographic manifestations caused by *M tuberculosis* complex are apparent; disease can be pulmonary, extrapulmonary, or both.
- **Multidrug-resistant (MDR) *M tuberculosis*** is a strain of *M tuberculosis* that is resistant to at least isoniazid and rifampin.
- **Extensively drug-resistant (XDR) *M tuberculosis*** is a strain of *M tuberculosis* that is resistant to isoniazid, rifampin, any fluoroquinolone, and either bedaquiline or linezolid (or both).
- **Pre-XDR *M tuberculosis*** is defined by the Centers for Disease Control and Prevention (CDC) as a strain of *M tuberculosis* that fulfills the definition of multidrug resistant and that is resistant to any fluoroquinolone.

Table 3.79. Definitions of Positive Tuberculin Skin Test (TST) Results in Infants, Children, and Adolescents[a,b]

Induration 5 mm or greater

Children in close contact with known or suspected contagious people with tuberculosis (TB) disease

Children suspected to have TB disease:
- Findings on chest radiograph consistent with active or previous TB disease
- Clinical evidence of TB disease[c]

Children receiving immunosuppressive therapy[d] or with immunosuppressive conditions, including human immunodeficiency (HIV) infection

Induration 10 mm or greater

Children at increased risk of disseminated TB disease:
- Children younger than 4 y
- Children with other medical conditions, including Hodgkin disease, lymphoma, diabetes mellitus, chronic renal failure, or malnutrition (see Table 3.80)
- Children born in high-prevalence regions of the world
- Children with significant travel to high-prevalence regions of the world[e]
- Children frequently exposed to adults who are living with HIV, lacking housing, or incarcerated, or to people who inject or use drugs

Induration 15 mm or greater

Children without any risk factors

[a] See www.cdc.gov/tb/publications/guidelines/pdf/ciw778.pdf.

[b] These definitions apply regardless of previous bacille Calmette-Guérin (BCG) immunization (see Testing for *M tuberculosis* Infection, p 892); erythema alone at TST site does not indicate a positive test result. Tests should be read at 48 to 72 hours after placement.

[c] Evidence by physical examination or laboratory assessment that would include tuberculosis in the working differential diagnosis (eg, meningitis).

[d] Including immunosuppressive doses of corticosteroids (see Corticosteroids, p 913) or tumor necrosis factor-alpha antagonists or blockers (see Biologic Response-Modifying Drugs Used to Decrease Inflammation, p 104) or immunosuppressive drugs used in transplant recipients (see Solid Organ Transplantation, p 107).

[e] Some experts define significant travel as travel or residence in a country with an elevated TB rate for at least 1 month.

- **Drug-resistant (DR)** *M tuberculosis* is a strain of *M tuberculosis* that is resistant to any drug used to treat drug-susceptible tuberculosis and includes isoniazid-resistant, rifampin-resistant, MDR, pre-XDR, and XDR strains.
- **Directly observed therapy (DOT)** is an intervention by which medications are taken by the patient while a health care professional or trained third party (not a relative or friend) observes and documents that the patient ingests each dose of medication and assesses for possible adverse drug effects. DOT can be in person or via video.
- **Exposed person** is anyone who has had contact with another person with suspected or confirmed contagious TB disease (ie, pulmonary, laryngeal, tracheal, or endobronchial disease). Recently (<3 months) exposed people may have an initially negative TST or IGRA result, normal physical examination findings, and chest radiographic findings that are normal or not compatible with TB. Some recently exposed people are or become infected (and subsequently develop a positive TST or IGRA result), and others do not become infected after exposure; the 2 groups cannot be distinguished initially.
- **Source person** is the person who has transmitted *M tuberculosis* complex to another person who subsequently develops TB infection or disease.

EPIDEMIOLOGY: Case rates of TB in all ages in North America are higher in urban, low-income areas. In recent years, more than 70% of all US cases have occurred in people born outside the United States. Almost 80% of childhood TB disease in the United States is associated with some form of foreign contact of the child, parent, or a household member. Specific groups with greater rates of TB include immigrants, international adoptees, refugees from or travelers to high-prevalence regions (eg, Asia, Africa, Latin America, and countries of the former Soviet Union), people lacking housing or those with unstable housing, people who inject or use drugs, and residents of some correctional facilities and other congregate settings. Secondhand smoke exposure increases the risk of TB disease developing in infected children.

Infants and postpubertal adolescents are at increased risk of progression from TBI to TB disease. Other predictive factors for development of disease include recent infection (within the past 2 years); immunodeficiency, especially from uncontrolled human immunodeficiency virus (HIV) infection; use of immunosuppressive drugs, such as prolonged or high-dose corticosteroid therapy or chemotherapy and drugs for preventing transplant organ rejection (see Solid Organ Transplantation, p 107); and certain diseases or medical conditions, including Hodgkin disease, lymphoma, diabetes mellitus, chronic renal failure, and malnutrition. Patients with TBI who are being treated with tumor necrosis factor (TNF)-alpha antagonists or blocking agents (see Biologic Response-Modifying Drugs Used to Decrease Inflammation, p 104) are at higher risk of progressing to TB disease. A positive TST or IGRA result should be accepted as indicative of infection in individuals receiving or soon to receive immunosuppressive medications,[1,2] and the patient should be evaluated and treated accordingly.

A diagnosis of TBI or TB disease in a young child is a public health sentinel event often representing recent transmission. Transmission of *M tuberculosis* is airborne, with inhalation of droplet nuclei usually produced by an adult or adolescent with contagious pulmonary, endobronchial, or laryngeal TB disease. The probability of transmission increases if the person has a positive acid-fast sputum smear, productive cough, or pulmonary cavities or is a household contact. Although contagiousness usually lasts only a few days to weeks after initiation of effective drug therapy, it can last longer if the source patient does not adhere to medical therapy or is infected with a drug-resistant strain. If the sputum smear becomes negative for acid-fast bacilli (AFB) on 3 separate specimens at least 8 hours apart after treatment is initiated and the patient has improved clinically, the treated patient can be considered at low risk of transmitting *M tuberculosis*. Children younger than 10 years with only adenopathy in the chest or small pulmonary lesions (paucibacillary disease) and nonproductive cough are not contagious. Rare cases of pulmonary disease in young children, particularly with lung cavities or presence of AFB on sputum microscopy, and infants with congenital TB disease can be contagious.

M bovis is transmitted most often by unpasteurized dairy products, but airborne human-to-human transmission can occur.

---

[1] Starke JR; American Academy of Pediatrics, Committee on Infectious Diseases. Technical report: Interferon-γ release assays for diagnosis of tuberculosis infection and disease in children. *Pediatrics*. 2014;134(6): e1763-e1773 (Reaffirmed July 2018)

[2] Nolt D, Starke JR; American Academy of Pediatrics, Committee on Infectious Diseases. Clinical report. Tuberculosis infection in children: testing and treatment. *Pediatrics*. 2021;148(6):e2021054663

The **incubation period** from infection to development of a positive TST or IGRA result is 2 to 10 weeks. The risk of developing TB disease is highest during the 12 months after infection and remains high for 2 years; however, many years can elapse between initial *M tuberculosis* infection and subsequent disease.

DIAGNOSTIC TESTS:

Testing for M tuberculosis *Infection*

Tuberculin Skin Test. The TST is one of two indirect methods for detecting *M tuberculosis* complex infection, the other method being IGRA (p 893). Both methods rely on specific lymphocyte sensitization after infection. Conditions that decrease lymphocyte numbers or function, including severe TB disease, can reduce the sensitivity of these tests. Tuberculin is a purified protein derivative (PPD) from heat-inactivated *M tuberculosis*. The routine (ie, Mantoux) technique of administering the skin test consists of 5 tuberculin units of solution (PPD; 0.1 mL) injected intradermally using a 27-gauge needle and a 1.0-mL syringe into the volar aspect of the forearm. Creation of a palpable wheal 6 to 10 mm in diameter is crucial to accurate testing.

Administration of TSTs and interpretation of results should be performed by trained and experienced health care personnel because administration and interpretation by unskilled people or family members are unreliable. The standardized time for assessing the TST result is 48 to 72 hours after administration. The **induration** is measured transversely at its widest diameter and the result should be recorded in millimeters. Positive TST results, as defined in Table 3.79 (p 890), can persist for several weeks.

Lack of reaction to a TST does not exclude TBI or TB disease. Approximately 10% to 40% of immunocompetent children with culture-documented TB disease do not react initially to a TST. Host factors, such as young age, poor nutrition, immunosuppression, viral infections (especially measles, varicella, and influenza), and disseminated TB disease, can decrease TST reactivity.

Classification of TST results is based on epidemiologic and clinical factors. Interpretation of the size of induration (mm) as a positive result varies with the person's epidemiologic risk of TBI and likelihood of progression to TB disease. Current guidelines from the CDC, the American Thoracic Society, and the American Academy of Pediatrics (AAP) recommend interpretation of TST findings on the basis of an individual's risk stratification and are summarized in Table 3.79 (p 890). Prompt clinical and radiographic evaluation of all children and adolescents with a positive TST result is recommended (see Assessing for *M tuberculosis* Disease, p 896).

BCG immunization, because of cross-reacting antigens present in the PPD, can result in induration of a TST. Distinguishing between a positive TST result caused by *M tuberculosis* complex infection and that caused by BCG requires a qualitative assessment of several factors. Reactivity of the TST (ie, mm of induration) attributable to prior BCG immunization may be absent or variable and depends on many factors, including age at BCG immunization, quality and strain of BCG vaccine used, number of doses of BCG vaccine received, nutritional and immunologic status of the vaccine recipient, frequency of TST administration, and time between immunization and TST. Evidence that increases the probability that a positive TST result is attributable to TBI or TB disease includes known contact with a person with contagious TB disease, a family history of TB disease, more than 2 years since neonatal BCG immunization, and a TST reaction 15 mm or greater. Generally, interpretation of TST results in BCG recipients who are known contacts of a person with TB disease or who are at high risk of developing TB disease is the same as for people who have not received BCG vaccine.

Blood-Based Testing With IGRAs.[1-3] IGRAs measure ex vivo interferon-gamma production from T lymphocytes in response to stimulation with proprietary polypeptide mixtures that simulate antigens specific to *M tuberculosis* complex. The IGRA antigens used are not found in BCG or most pathogenic nontuberculous mycobacteria (eg, *M avium* complex) but are found in the nontuberculous mycobacteria *M kansasii*, *M szulgai,* and *M marinum.* Examples of IGRAs are the T-SPOT.TB assay and the QuantiFERON-TB Gold Plus assay. As with TSTs, IGRAs cannot distinguish between TBI and TB disease, and a negative IGRA result cannot exclude infection with *M tuberculosis* complex or the possibility of TB disease in a patient with suggestive clinical findings. The sensitivity of IGRA tests is similar to that of TSTs in adults and children who have untreated culture-confirmed TB disease. In many clinical settings, the specificity of IGRAs is higher than that for the TST, because the antigens used are not found in BCG or most pathogenic nontuberculous mycobacteria. The published experience on testing children with IGRAs demonstrates that IGRAs consistently perform well in children of all ages. The negative predictive value of IGRAs is not clear, but in general, if the IGRA result is negative and the TST result is positive in an asymptomatic child with no known TB exposure, the diagnosis of TBI is unlikely, especially if the child has received a BCG vaccine.

TST Versus IGRA. Either TST or IGRA testing is acceptable for children of any age. IGRA is preferred for children who have received a BCG vaccine or who are unlikely to return for the TST reading. Low-grade, false-positive IGRA results occur in some individuals. For children without specific TB risk factors other than foreign birth or travel who have an unexpected low-level positive IGRA result (QuantiFERON-TB Gold Plus <1.00 IU/mL, T-SPOT.TB with 5–7 spots), a second diagnostic test, either an IGRA or a TST, should be performed; the child is considered infected only if both tests are positive. Indeterminate or invalid IGRA results have several possible causes that could be related to the patient, the assay itself, or its performance; these results do not exclude *M tuberculosis* infection and may necessitate repeat testing, possibly with a different test. Indeterminate/invalid IGRA results should not be used to make clinical decisions.

Specific recommendations for TST and IGRA use are provided in Table 3.80 (p 894).

Use of Tests for M tuberculosis *Infection.* The most reliable strategies for identifying TBI and preventing TB disease in children are based on identification of known risk factors for TBI or progression to TB disease and thorough and expedient contact tracing associated with cases of TB disease, rather than nonselective testing of large populations.

---

[1] Centers for Disease Control and Prevention. Updated guidelines for using interferon gamma release assays to detect *Mycobacterium tuberculosis* infection—United States. *MMWR Recomm Rep.* 2010;59(RR-5):1-26

[2] Starke JR; American Academy of Pediatrics, Committee on Infectious Diseases. Technical report: Interferon-γ release assays for diagnosis of tuberculosis infection and disease in children. *Pediatrics.* 2014;134(6): e1763-e1773 (Reaffirmed July 2018)

[3] Nolt D, Starke JR; American Academy of Pediatrics, Committee on Infectious Diseases. Clinical report Tuberculosis infection in children: testing and treatment. *Pediatrics.* 2021;148(6):e2021054663

Table 3.80. Tuberculin Skin Test (TST) and IGRA Recommendations for Infants, Children, and Adolescents[a]

Children for whom immediate TST or IGRA is indicated[b]:
- Contacts of people with confirmed or suspected contagious tuberculosis (contact tracing)
- Children with radiographic or clinical findings suggesting TB disease
- Children immigrating from countries with endemic infection (eg, Asia, Middle East, Africa, Latin America, countries of the former Soviet Union), including international adoptees
- Children with history of significant[c] travel to countries with endemic infection who have substantial contact with the resident population[d]

Children who should have annual TST or IGRA:
- Children living with HIV

Children at increased risk of progression of TB infection to TB disease: Infants (age <1 year) and children with other medical conditions, including diabetes mellitus, chronic renal failure, malnutrition, congenital or acquired immunodeficiencies, and children receiving tumor necrosis factor (TNF) antagonists, deserve special consideration. Underlying immune deficiencies associated with these conditions theoretically would enhance the possibility for rapid progression to severe disease. Initial histories of potential exposure to tuberculosis should be included for all these patients. If these histories or local epidemiologic factors suggest a possibility of exposure, immediate and periodic TST or IGRA should be considered.

A TST or IGRA should be performed before initiation of immunosuppressive therapy, including prolonged systemic corticosteroid administration, organ transplantation, use of TNF-alpha antagonists or blockers, or other immunosuppressive therapy in any child requiring these treatments.

IGRA indicates interferon-gamma release assay; HIV, human immunodeficiency virus; TBI, *M tuberculosis* infection.
[a]Bacille Calmette-Guérin (BCG) immunization is not a contraindication to a TST; IGRA is generally preferred for BCG-vaccinated children.
[b]Beginning as early as 3 months of age for TST; IGRA may be used at all ages.
[c]Some experts define significant travel as birth, travel, or residence in a country with an elevated tuberculosis rate for at least 1 month.
[d]If the child is well and has no history of exposure, the TST or IGRA should be delayed for 8 to 10 weeks after return.

Contact tracing is an intervention that should be coordinated through the local public health department. Universal testing with TST or IGRA, including programs based at schools, child care centers, and camps that include populations at low risk, is discouraged because it results in either a low yield of positive results or a large proportion of false-positive results, leading to an inefficient use of health care resources. However, using a questionnaire to determine risk factors for infection with *M tuberculosis* and identifying who should have a TST or IGRA performed can be useful (see Table 3.81). Risk assessment for TB should be performed at the first medical home encounter with a child and then annually if possible. Testing children for infection with *M tuberculosis* and clinical evaluation for possible TB disease is indicated whenever a TST or IGRA result of a household member converts from a negative to positive result (indicating recent infection) or after travel for >1 month to a country with endemic disease.

HIV Infection. In the United States, annual testing for infection with *M tuberculosis* is recommended for children living with HIV beginning at ages 3 to 12 months and annually thereafter for those who test negative, depending on the local epidemiology

Table 3.81. Validated Questions for Determining Risk of Infection with *M tuberculosis* in Children in the United States

- Has a family member or contact had tuberculosis disease?
- Has a family member had a positive tuberculin skin test result?
- Was your child born in a high-prevalence country (countries other than the United States, Canada, Australia, New Zealand, or Western and North European countries)?
- Has your child traveled to a high-prevalence country? How much contact did your child have with the resident population?

and the child's region of birth and travel history. Conversely, children who have TB disease should be tested for HIV infection. The clinical manifestations and radiographic appearance of TB disease in children living with HIV tend to be similar to those in immunocompetent children, but manifestations in these children can be more severe, unusual, and more often include extrapulmonary involvement of multiple organs. In people living with HIV, a TST induration of ≥5 mm is considered a positive result (see Table 3.79, p 890); however, a false-negative TST or IGRA result attributable to HIV-related immunosuppression also can occur. Confirming TB disease in a child living with HIV using microbiological specimens is challenging, given the paucibacillary nature of TB in this population. Antituberculosis therapy for children living with HIV must be selected with careful consideration of antiretroviral drug interactions, which are very common with the rifamycins.

Organ Transplant Recipients. The risk of TB disease in organ transplant recipients is several-fold greater than in the general population. A careful history should be taken from all transplant candidates, including details about previous TST or IGRA results and exposure to individuals with TB disease. All transplant candidates should undergo evaluation by TST or IGRA before the initiation of immunosuppressive therapy. A positive result of either test should be taken as evidence of infection with *M tuberculosis* complex. In addition, donor-derived TB disease can be transmitted via an infected organ and should be considered as a possible cause of post-transplant fever and related symptoms.

Patients Receiving Immunosuppressive Therapies Including Biologic Response Modifiers. In addition to a detailed history of risk factors for infection with *M tuberculosis*, all patients should have a TST or IGRA performed before the initiation of therapy with high-dose systemic corticosteroids, antimetabolite agents, TNF antagonists or blockers, and some other biologic response-modifying drugs (see Biologic Response-Modifying Drugs Used to Decrease Inflammation, p 104). Some experts recommend that if the child has at least 1 TB risk factor, both a TST and an IGRA should be performed to maximize sensitivity; a positive result of either test should be taken as evidence of *M tuberculosis* infection.

Other Considerations. Testing for infection with *M tuberculosis* complex at any age is not required before administration of live-virus vaccines. Live attenuated measles, mumps, and rubella vaccines temporarily can suppress tuberculin reactivity for at least 4 to 6 weeks, and data suggest a similar suppression with varicella and yellow fever vaccines. The effect of live attenuated influenza vaccines on TST reactivity is not known. If indicated, a TST can be performed or blood drawn for an IGRA at the same visit during which these vaccines are administered (ie, before substantial replication of the vaccine virus). The effects of live-virus vaccination on IGRA characteristics have not been determined; the same precautions as for TST should be followed.

Sensitivity to PPD tuberculin antigen persists for years in most instances, even after effective treatment. The durability of positive IGRA results has not been determined but is likely similar. Repeat testing with either TST or IGRA has no known clinical utility for assessing the effectiveness of treatment or for diagnosing newly acquired infection in patients who previously were infected with *M tuberculosis*.

Assessing for M tuberculosis *Disease.* Although both IGRA and TST provide evidence for infection with *M tuberculosis* complex, they cannot distinguish TBI from TB disease. Therefore, patients testing positive for *M tuberculosis* infection by IGRA or TST should be assessed for TB disease before therapeutic intervention is undertaken. This assessment should include: (1) asking about symptoms of TB disease and exposure to a possible source person; (2) physical examination for signs of TB disease; and (3) a chest radiograph. If radiographic signs of TB disease (eg, airspace opacities, pleural effusions, cavities, or changes on serial radiographs) are seen, then sputum, gastric aspirate, or nasopharyngeal aspirate sampling should then be performed, as described below. Most experts recommend that children younger than 12 months who are suspected of having pulmonary or extrapulmonary TB disease (eg, have a positive TST result **and** symptoms, physical examination signs, or chest radiograph abnormalities consistent with TB disease), with or without neurologic symptoms, should have a lumbar puncture to evaluate for tuberculous meningitis. Children 12 months and older with TB disease require a lumbar puncture only if they have neurologic signs or symptoms.

Laboratory Confirmation of M tuberculosis. Laboratory isolation of *M tuberculosis* complex by culture from a specimen of sputum (expectorated or induced), gastric aspirate, nasopharyngeal aspirate, bronchial washing, pleural fluid, cerebrospinal fluid (CSF), urine or other body fluid, or a tissue biopsy specimen confirms the diagnosis of TB disease. Positive results from a rapid molecular method (eg, nucleic acid amplification tests [NAATs]) increasingly are also considered confirmatory, but culture isolation of the organism is still required for phenotypical susceptibility testing, genotyping, most rapid molecular detection of drug-resistance genes, and species identification with the *M tuberculosis* complex. Children older than 2 years and adolescents frequently produce sputum spontaneously or by induction with aerosolized hypertonic saline. Studies have demonstrated successful collection of induced sputum from infants with pulmonary TB disease, but this requires special expertise. The best specimen for diagnosis of pulmonary TB disease in any child or adolescent in whom cough is absent or nonproductive and sputum cannot be induced is an early-morning gastric aspirate, which is best obtained with a nasogastric tube on awakening the child and before ambulation or feeding. Aspirates collected on 3 separate mornings should be submitted for AFB staining and culture. Nasopharyngeal aspirates (multiple specimens or in addition to other specimen types) are an acceptable specimen for children particularly when gastric aspirates are difficult to obtain, but sensitivity may be lower compared to gastric aspirate samples. Stool has been recommended by the World Health Organization (WHO) as a specimen for young children because it is easier to obtain than gastric aspirates, and swallowed sputum passes through the gastrointestinal tract. The WHO has released guidance on processing stool for NAAT for the diagnosis of pulmonary TB disease in young children (**www.who.int/publications/i/item//9789240042650**).

Fluorescent staining methods for specimen smears are more sensitive than the traditional Kinyoun acid fast smears and are preferred. The overall diagnostic yield of microscopy of gastric aspirates, induced sputum, or nasopharyngeal aspirates is low in children with clinically suspected pulmonary TB disease, and false-positive stain results caused by the presence of nontuberculous mycobacteria occur rarely. Histologic examination for and demonstration of AFB and granulomas in biopsy specimens from lymph node, pleura, mesentery, liver, bone marrow, or other tissues can be useful, but *M tuberculosis* complex organisms cannot be distinguished reliably from other mycobacteria in stained specimens. The CDC and several reference laboratories offer molecular species identification of mycobacteria including *M tuberculosis* in fixed tissues. Regardless of results of the AFB smears, each specimen should be cultured.

Because *M tuberculosis* complex organisms are slow growing, detection of these organisms may take as long as 10 weeks using solid media; use of liquid media and continuous monitoring systems allows detection within 1 to 6 weeks and usually within 3 weeks. Even with optimal culture techniques, *M tuberculosis* complex organisms are isolated from fewer than 75% of infants and less than 50% of children with pulmonary TB disease diagnosed by clinical criteria; the culture yields for most forms of extrapulmonary TB disease are even lower. Current methods for species identification of isolates from culture include molecular probes, NAATs, genetic sequencing, mass spectrometry, and biochemical tests. *M bovis* usually is suspected because of isolated pyrazinamide resistance, which is characteristic of almost all *M bovis* isolates, but further biochemical or molecular testing is required to distinguish *M bovis* from *M tuberculosis*.

For a child with clinically suspected TB disease, finding the culture-positive source person supports the child's presumptive diagnosis and provides the likely drug susceptibility of the child's organism. Culture material should be collected from children with evidence of TB disease, especially when (1) an isolate from a source person is not available; (2) the presumed source person has drug-resistant TB; (3) the child is immunocompromised or ill enough to require hospital admission; or (4) the child has extrapulmonary disease. Traditional methods of determining drug susceptibility require bacterial isolation. Several molecular methods that rapidly detect drug resistance directly from clinical samples are available.

NAATs cleared by the US Food and Drug Administration (FDA) are available for rapid detection of *M tuberculosis* complex organisms from smear-positive and smear-negative sputum specimens, and other laboratory-developed tests for rapid molecular detection are available locally. Some tests have been validated for specimens other than sputum; expert consultation is recommended for test availability and interpretation of results. Molecular methods, such as Xpert MTB/RIF that find *M tuberculosis* genetic markers associated with drug resistance, are supplementing the culture-based (ie, phenotypic) methods for drug susceptibility testing as they decrease the time to detection of drug resistance from weeks to hours, and in some instances the results could be more reliable for patient care decisions. Some of the methods are verified for direct testing of patient specimens. It is recommended that results from molecular susceptibility testing are confirmed through culture-based testing. Molecular methods continue to evolve and consultation with an expert is useful to determine a testing strategy when drug resistance is suspected.

TREATMENT (SEE TABLE 3.82)[1]:

Specific Drugs. Regimen and dosage recommendations and the more commonly reported adverse reactions of first-line antituberculosis drugs are summarized in Tables 3.82, 3.83 (p 902), and 3.84 (p 904). The less commonly used antituberculosis drugs, their doses, and adverse effects are listed in Table 3.85 (p 906). Some of these drugs have less effectiveness and greater toxicity or they are reserved for treating MDR, pre-XDR, or XDR TB disease; they should be used only in consultation with a specialist familiar with treatment of childhood TB disease. For treatment of TB disease, drugs always must be used in recommended combination and dosage to minimize emergence of drug-resistant strains. Use of nonstandard regimens for any reason (eg, drug allergy, drug resistance) should be undertaken only by an expert in treating TB disease.

Occasionally, a patient cannot tolerate oral medications. Isoniazid, rifampin, linezolid, fluoroquinolones, and aminoglycosides can be administered parenterally.

Treatment Regimens for Tuberculosis Infection (TBI). Several regimens are recommended for TBI (without evidence of TB disease), depending on the circumstances for individual patients. Dosages and intervals are provided in Table 3.83.

Isoniazid-Rifapentine Therapy for TBI.[2] A 3-month course, comprising a once-weekly dose of isoniazid and rifapentine, is a regimen that is safe, well tolerated, and at least as efficacious as 9 months of isoniazid taken daily. Extensive published and unpublished experience with this combination in children has demonstrated excellent results. Isoniazid-rifapentine is a preferred regimen for treatment of TBI for children ≥2 years of age, although the pill burden in younger children is substantial and sometimes not well tolerated. Isoniazid-rifapentine should not be used in children <2 years of age because of a lack of pharmacokinetic data in this age group.

Rifampin Therapy for TBI. A 4-month course of rifampin given daily also is a preferred regimen for the treatment of TBI, and especially when isoniazid resistance is present or likely, as judged from the exposure history. The data supporting the efficacy and safety of this regimen are from randomized controlled trials and case control studies in adults, and several studies that included children. The regimen has been as effective as 9 months of daily isoniazid, the rates of adverse effects have been low, and the completion rates of therapy have been much higher than for 9 months of isoniazid. There has been extensive published and unpublished experience with this regimen in children demonstrating safety, tolerability, and high rates of completion.

Isoniazid-Rifampin Therapy for TBI. An additional possible regimen for treatment of TBI is 3 months of daily isoniazid and rifampin, with no age restriction on it use. This regimen is quite similar in principle to the isoniazid-rifapentine option; however, the medications are given daily because of the relatively short half-life of rifampin compared with rifapentine. Efficacy and rates of completion are comparable or better when compared with isoniazid monotherapy.

Isoniazid Therapy for TBI. Isoniazid monotherapy has been the most widely recommended and utilized treatment for pediatric TBI. The efficacy of isoniazid

---

[1] Nolt D, Starke JR; American Academy of Pediatrics, Committee on Infectious Diseases. Clinical report. Tuberculosis infection in children: testing and treatment. *Pediatrics.* 2021;148(6):e2021054663

[2] Sterling TR, Njie G, Zenner D, et al. Guidelines for the treatment of latent tuberculosis infection: recommendations from the National Tuberculosis Controllers Association and CDC, 2020. *MMWR Recomm Rep.* 2020;69(1):1-11

Table 3.82. Recommended Usual Treatment Regimens for Drug-Susceptible TB Infection and TB Disease in Infants, Children, and Adolescents

Infection or Disease Category	Regimen	Remarks
TB infection (positive TST or IGRA result, no disease)[a]		
• Isoniazid susceptible	3 mo of isoniazid plus rifapentine, once a week	Isoniazid-rifapentine is a preferred regimen for treatment of TBI for children ≥2 years.
	OR	
	4 mo of rifampin, once a day	Continuous daily therapy is required. Intermittent therapy even by DOT is not recommended.
	OR	
	3 mo of isoniazid plus rifampin, once a day	To be considered if above 2 regimens are not feasible.
	OR	
	6 or 9 mo of isoniazid, once a day	9 months preferred (see text for discussion, Isoniazid Therapy for TBI, p 898). If daily therapy is not possible, DOT twice a week can be used; medication doses differ with daily and twice-weekly regimens.
• Isoniazid resistant	4 mo of rifampin, once a day	Continuous daily therapy is required. Intermittent therapy even by DOT is not recommended.
• Isoniazid-rifampin resistant	Consult a tuberculosis specialist	Moxifloxacin or levofloxacin, with consideration of a second drug based on drug susceptibility testing of presumed source isolate and consultation with a tuberculosis specialist.

Table 3.82. Recommended Usual Treatment Regimens for Drug-Susceptible TB Infection and TB Disease in Infants, Children, and Adolescents, continued

Infection or Disease Category	Regimen	Remarks
Pulmonary and extrapulmonary TB disease (except meningitis and osteoarticular disease)[b,c]	If nonsevere pulmonary disease,[d] 2 mo of rifampin, isoniazid, pyrazinamide, and ethambutol (RIPE) daily, followed by 2 mo of isoniazid and rifampin daily for drug-susceptible *M tuberculosis*	Some experts recommend a 3-drug initial regimen (isoniazid, rifampin, and pyrazinamide) if the risk of drug resistance is low.
		DOT is highly desirable and, in many jurisdictions, DOT is required for all regimens.
	If severe pulmonary disease, 2 mo of rifampin, isoniazid, pyrazinamide, and ethambutol (RIPE) daily, followed by 4 mo of isoniazid and rifampin daily for drug-susceptible *M tuberculosis*	In many public health jurisdictions, DOT is recommended for all regimens.
		If a cavity is present, or sputum culture takes longer than 2 months to become negative, treatment should be extended to 9 months.
	If severe or nonsevere pulmonary disease in a patient ≥12 years of age (and ≥40 kg), an alternative is a 4 month regimen with isoniazid, rifapentine, moxifloxacin and pyrazinamide (8 weeks of the 4 drugs given daily, followed by 9 weeks of isoniazid, rifapentine, and moxifloxacin given daily by DOT)[e]	DOT is required for 4-month regimen containing isoniazid, rifapentine, moxifloxacin and pyrazinamide.
		Patients with a positive culture at completion of 2 months of therapy, with or without ongoing symptoms, should be evaluated to identify cause of delayed response.
	For *Mycobacterium bovis* disease, at least 9 mo of isoniazid and rifampin, with or without ethambutol, when the organism is susceptible to these drugs	

Table 3.82. Recommended Usual Treatment Regimens for Drug-Susceptible TB Infection and TB Disease in Infants, Children, and Adolescents, continued

Infection or Disease Category	Regimen	Remarks
Meningitis	2 mo of isoniazid, rifampin, pyrazinamide, and ethionamide or a fluoroquinolone (levofloxacin or moxifloxacin)[f] followed by 4–10 mo of isoniazid and rifampin, once a day or 3 times per week (6–12 mo total) for drug-susceptible *M tuberculosis*[g]	See text for information on corticosteroids (Corticosteroids, p 913). High-dose rifampin (30 mg/kg/day) for TB meningitis is recommended.
	At least 9 mo of therapy without pyrazinamide for *M bovis* susceptible to isoniazid and rifampin	

TST indicates tuberculin skin test; IGRA, interferon-gamma release assay; DOT, directly observed therapy.

[a] See text for comments and additional acceptable/alternative regimens.

[b] Duration of therapy may be longer for people living with HIV, and additional drugs and dosing intervals may be indicated (see Tuberculosis Disease and HIV Infection, p 913).

[c] Consultation with an expert is recommended. Susceptible osteoarticular tuberculosis is generally treated with a 4- drug regimen of isoniazid, rifampin, pyrazinamide, and ethambutol for 2 months and isoniazid and rifampin for another 10 months.

[d] Nonsevere pulmonary disease is defined as tuberculosis confined to one lobe with no cavities or isolated intrathoracic adenopathy, no signs of miliary tuberculosis, no complex pleural effusion, and no clinically significant airway obstruction.

[e] For patients 12 and older receiving isoniazid, rifapentine, pyrazinamide, and moxifloxacin for treatment of susceptible pulmonary tuberculosis, the daily dose for patients 40 kg and over of isoniazid is 300 mg, rifapentine 1200 mg, and moxifloxacin 400 mg. Dosing for pyrazinamide in patients weighing 40 to <55 kg is 1000 mg; for patients weighing 55 to 75 kg is 1500 mg, and for patients weighing >75 kg is 2000 mg daily. Isoniazid, rifapentine, moxifloxacin, and pyrazinamide are administered by DOT daily for 8 weeks followed by isoniazid, rifapentine, and moxifloxacin daily by DOT for another 9 weeks (**www.cdc.gov/mmwr/volumes/71/wr/mm7108a1.htm**).

[f] Consultation with an expert in tuberculosis is recommended. When susceptibility to first-line drugs is established, the ethionamide or fluoroquinolone can be discontinued.

[g] In children and adolescents with TB meningitis presumed to be drug susceptible, the WHO states that 6 months of isoniazid, rifampin, pyrazinamide, and ethionamide daily may be used, but the longer treatment regimen in this table is preferred.

Table 3.83. Regimens and Dosages Used in Pediatric Patients With TB Infection (TBI)

Agent(s)	Dose and Age Group	Administration	Duration (months)	Age Restriction	Comments
INH + Rifapentine (3HP)	**Age ≥12 y** INH: 15 mg/kg, rounded up to nearest 50 or 100 mg (max 900 mg) Rifapentine (by weight): 10–14 kg: 300 mg 14.1–25 kg: 450 mg 25.1–32 kg: 600 mg 32.1–49.9 kg: 750 mg ≥50.0 kg: 900 mg **Age 2–11 y** INH: 25 mg/kg, rounded up to nearest 50 or 100 mg (max 900 mg) Rifapentine: see above	Weekly (SAT or DOT)	3	Not for children <2 y	Take with food, containing fat if possible; pyridoxine for selected patients[a]

Table 3.83. Regimens and Dosages Used in Pediatric Patients With TB Infection (TBI), continued

Agent(s)	Dose and Age Group	Administration	Duration (months)	Age Restriction	Comments
Rifampin (4R)	**Adult:** 10 mg/kg (max 600 mg) **Child:** 15–20 mg/kg (max 600 mg)	Daily (SAT)	4	None	Drug-drug interactions
INH + Rifampin	Same doses as when drugs are used individually for SAT	Daily (SAT)	3	None	Not considered unless 3HP or 4R are not feasible
INH	**Adult:** 5 mg/kg (max dose 300 mg) **Child:** 10–20 mg/kg (max 300 mg)	Daily (SAT)	6 or 9	None	Seizures with overdose; pyridoxine for selected patients[a]
	Adult: 15 mg/kg (max dose 900 mg) **Child:** 20–40 mg/kg (max 900 mg)	Twice weekly (DOT)			

INH indicates isoniazid; DOT, directly observed therapy; SAT, self-administered therapy.

[a] Exclusively breastfed infants and for children and adolescents on meat- and milk-deficient diets; children with nutritional deficiencies, including all symptomatic children living with HIV infection; and pregnant adolescents and pregnant adults.

Adapted from Nolt D, Starke JR; American Academy of Pediatrics, Committee on Infectious Diseases. Clinical report. Tuberculosis infection in children: testing and treatment. *Pediatrics.* 2021;148(6):e2021054663

Table 3.84. Drugs for Treatment of Drug-Susceptible Pulmonary TB Disease in Infants, Children, and Adolescents[a]

Drugs	Dosage Forms	Daily Dosage (Range), mg/kg	Three Times per Week Dosage, mg/kg per Dose	Maximum Dose	Most Common Adverse Reactions
Ethambutol	Tablets 100 mg 400 mg	20 (15–25)	50	Daily, 1 g Twice a week, 2.5 g	Optic neuritis (usually reversible), decreased red-green color discrimination, gastrointestinal tract disturbances, hypersensitivity
Isoniazid[b]	Scored tablets 100 mg 300 mg	10 (10–15)[b]	20–30	Daily, 300 mg Twice a week, 900 mg	Mild hepatic enzyme elevation, hepatitis,[c] peripheral neuritis, hypersensitivity
Pyrazinamide	Scored tablets 500 mg	35 (30–40)	50	2 g	Hepatotoxic effects, hyperuricemia, arthralgia, gastrointestinal tract upset, pruritus, rash
Rifampin	Capsules 150 mg 300 mg Syrup formulated from capsules	15–20[d] 30[e]	15–20[d]	600 mg	Orange discoloration of secretions or urine, staining of contact lenses, vomiting, hepatitis, hyperbilirubinemia, influenza-like reaction, thrombocytopenia, pruritus; oral contraceptives may be ineffective
Rifapentine	Tablets 150 mg			1200 mg dose for age ≥12 years as part of a multidrug 4-month regimen for pulmonary tuberculosis disease[f]	Orange discoloration of secretions or urine, staining of contact lenses, vomiting, hepatitis, hyperbilirubinemia, influenza-like reaction, anemia, lymphopenia, pruritus; oral contraceptives may be ineffective

Table 3.84. Drugs for Treatment of Drug-Susceptible Pulmonary TB Disease in Infants, Children, and Adolescents,[a] continued

Drugs	Dosage Forms	Daily Dosage (Range), mg/kg	Three Times per Week Dosage, mg/kg per Dose	Maximum Dose	Most Common Adverse Reactions
Moxifloxacin[g]	Tablet: 400 mg Intravenous: 400 mg/ 250 mL	Adults: 400 mg (once daily) Children: 10 mg/kg (once daily)		400 mg	Hypersensitivity reactions; theoretical effect on growing cartilage; tendonitis, gastrointestinal tract disturbances, cardiac disturbances, peripheral neuropathy, rash, headache, restlessness, confusion; can prolong QTc interval

[a] Rifamate is a capsule containing 150 mg of isoniazid and 300 mg of rifampin. Two capsules provide the usual adult (greater than 50 kg) daily doses of each drug. Rifater, in the United States, is a capsule containing 50 mg of isoniazid, 120 mg of rifampin, and 300 mg of pyrazinamide. Isoniazid and rifampin also are available for parenteral administration.

[b] Concomitant administration of pyridoxine is recommended for breastfeeding infants and for children or adolescents at risk for nutritional deficiency

[c] When isoniazid in a dosage exceeding 10 mg/kg/day is used in combination with rifampin, the incidence of hepatotoxic effects may be increased.

[d] Many experts recommend using a daily rifampin dose of 20–30 mg/kg/day for infants and toddlers and for serious forms of tuberculosis, such as disseminated disease.

[e] A dose of 30 mg/kg/day of rifampin is recommended for TB meningitis and has been shown to improve mortality and neurodevelopmental outcomes.

[f] 4-drug therapy for susceptible pulmonary tuberculosis disease in ≥12 years includes isoniazid, rifapentine, pyrazinamide, and moxifloxacin daily by DOT for 8 weeks followed by isoniazid, rifapentine, and moxifloxacin daily by DOT for 9 weeks (see www.cdc.gov/mmwr/volumes/71/wr/mm7108a1.htm).

[g] Moxifloxacin does not have an FDA indication for the treatment of TB infection or disease and is not approved for use in children younger than 18 years; its use in younger children necessitates assessment of the potential risks and benefits (see Antimicrobial Agents and Related Therapy, p 973). The Centers for Disease Control and Prevention recommends moxifloxacin use for drug susceptible pulmonary TB disease in persons ≥12 years, with body weight of ≥40 kg.

Table 3.85. Additional Drugs for Treatment of Drug-Resistant TB Disease in Infants, Children, and Adolescents[a]

Drugs	Dosage, Forms	Daily Dosage	Maximum Daily Dose	Adverse Reactions
Amikacin[b,c]	Vials, 500 mg and 1 g	15–20 mg/kg (intravenous or intramuscular administration)	1 g	Auditory and vestibular toxic effects, nephrotoxic effects.
Bedaquiline[d]	Tablets, 100 mg Dispersible tablets, 20 mg	Children age ≥5 years: 15 kg <30 kg: 200 mg daily for first 2 wk, then 100 mg 3 times/wk with 48 h between doses for wk 3–24	200 mg	Can prolong QTc interval, hepatotoxicity, arthralgia, nausea, abdominal pain, headache. Bedaquiline has an FDA "black box warning" regarding unexplained mortality imbalance noted in placebo-controlled trial in adults (based on the 120-week visit window).
		≥30 kg: 400 mg daily for first 2 wk, then 200 mg 3 times/wk with 48 h between doses for wk 3–24	400 mg	Bedaquiline is metabolized by CYP3A4, and its systemic exposure and therapeutic effect may be reduced during coadministration with inducers of CYP3A4 such as rifamycins and efavirenz.
Clofazimine[e]	Capsules, 50 mg	2–5 mg/kg given in 1 daily dose	300 mg	Investigational in United States. Limited data in children. Photosensitivity, skin discoloration, ichthyosis; can prolong QTc interval; gastrointestinal tract disturbance; avoid in pregnancy; cross-resistance with bedaquiline.
Cycloserine	Capsules, 250 mg	10–20 mg/kg/day; given in 1 dose or in 2 divided doses	1 g	Psychosis, personality changes, seizures, rash.
Delamanid	Tablets, 50 mg Dispersible tablet, 25 mg	<7 kg consult a specialist 7–23 kg: 50 mg/day in 2 divided doses 24–34 kg: 100 mg/day given in 2 divided doses ≥35 kg: 200 mg/day given in 2 divided doses	200 mg	Investigational in United States; gastrointestinal tract disturbances; can prolong QTc interval; paresthesia, tremor, anxiety, depression, insomnia, tinnitus, blurred vision; nightmares and hallucinations in children.

Table 3.85. Additional Drugs for Treatment of Drug-Resistant TB Disease in Infants, Children, and Adolescents,[a] continued

Drugs	Dosage, Forms	Daily Dosage	Maximum Daily Dose	Adverse Reactions
Ethionamide[f]	Tablets, 250 mg	15–20 mg/kg/day, given in 1 dose or in 2–3 divided doses	1 g	Gastrointestinal tract disturbances, hepatotoxic effects, hypersensitivity reactions, hypothyroidism.
Levofloxacin[b,g]	Tablets 250 mg 500 mg 750 mg Oral solution 25 mg/mL Vials 5 mg/mL 25 mg/mL	Adults: 750–1000 mg (once daily) Children: 15–20 mg/kg (for those 6 months and older, but <50 kg given in 2 divided doses)	1 g	Hypersensitivity reactions; theoretical effect on growing cartilage, tendonitis, gastrointestinal tract disturbances, cardiac disturbances, peripheral neuropathy, rash, headache, restlessness, confusion; can prolong QTc interval.
Linezolid[b,h]	Tablets, 600 mg Oral suspension, 20 mg/mL	Adults: 600 mg (once daily) Children <15 kg: 15 mg/kg given once daily Children ≥15 kg: 10–12 mg/kg given once daily	600 mg	Bone marrow suppression, peripheral neuropathy.

Table 3.85. Additional Drugs for Treatment of Drug-Resistant TB Disease in Infants, Children, and Adolescents,[a] continued

Drugs	Dosage, Forms	Daily Dosage	Maximum Daily Dose	Adverse Reactions
Para-aminosalicylic acid (PAS)	Packets, 3 g	200–300 mg/kg/day (given in 2–4 divided doses)	12 g	Gastrointestinal tract disturbances, hypersensitivity, hepatotoxic effects, hypothyroidism.

[a] These drugs should be used in consultation with a TB specialist.

[b] These drugs do not have an indication from the US Food and Drug Administration (FDA) for treatment of TB infection or disease.

[c] Dose adjustment needed with renal insufficiency.

[d] Bedaquiline is not FDA-approved for use in children <5 years, but the World Health Organization has suggested dosing for children <5 years of age (**www.who.int/publications/i/item/9789240055193**). Use with caution in end-stage renal impairment. Refer to product information and consult with pharmacist regarding drug interactions with CYP3A4 inhibitors.

[e] Avoid if hepatic impairment present unless benefits outweigh risks. May administer higher dose every other day if needed based on dosage form constraints (particularly an issue for children weighing <10 kg; 50-mg capsule is difficult to manipulate). Clofazimine is not commercially available, and the healthcare provider needs to contact manufacturer (Novartis: 1-888-NOW-NOVA). Subsequently, health care provider will need to obtain single-patient expanded access investigational new drug approval from the Center for Drug Evaluation and Research, Division of Anti-Infective Products at the FDA (301-796-1400) and **www.fda.gov/drugs/investigational-new-drug-ind-application/physicians-how-request-single-patient-expanded-access-compassionate-use.**

[f] When ethionamide is used, concomitant administration of pyridoxine (vitamin B₆) is recommended.

[g] Levofloxacin is not approved for use in children younger than 18 years; its use in younger children necessitates assessment of the potential risks and benefits (see Antimicrobial Agents and Related Therapy, p 973).

[h] Linezolid pharmacokinetics have not been well established in children. The doses listed will yield a drug exposure approximately equal to that in adults taking 600 mg daily.

monotherapy reaches 98% against development of TB disease, but many studies have shown that the long duration of isoniazid monotherapy results in poor adherence and low completion rates. The WHO recommends a treatment duration of 6 months to provide high coverage of the population in countries with a high disease burden. A 9-month regimen gives an additional 20% to 30% increase in efficacy. The CDC and National TB Controllers Association recommend 6-month or 9-month durations of isoniazid monotherapy for adults, if shorter-course rifamycin-based regimens cannot be used. This option may be very unattractive to patients and families because of its long duration. Many TB care providers and clinics use this regimen only when a rifamycin-containing regimen cannot be used because of drug interactions or rifamycin intolerance.

For infants, children, and adolescents, including those living with HIV or other immunocompromising conditions, the recommended duration of isoniazid therapy in the United States is 9 months for those for whom isoniazid is selected for treatment of TBI. Although there have been no formal trials of interrupted 9-month courses, many experts in North America accept 6 months of uninterrupted treatment as adequate. When adherence with daily therapy with isoniazid cannot be ensured, twice-a-week DOT on the basis of expert opinion and published experience can be considered, but each dose should be observed. Determination of serum aminotransferase concentrations before or during therapy is not indicated except in patients with underlying liver or biliary disease, during pregnancy or the first 12 weeks postpartum, with concurrent use of other potentially hepatotoxic drugs (eg, anticonvulsant or HIV agents), or if there is clinical concern of possible hepatotoxicity.

Therapy for TBI and Contacts of Patients With Isoniazid-Resistant M tuberculosis *and When Isoniazid Cannot Be Administered.* The incidence of isoniazid resistance among *M tuberculosis* complex isolates from US patients in 2020 was 4.8% among cases born in the United States and 9.5% among cases born outside the United States. Risk factors for drug resistance are listed in Table 3.86. If the source person is found to have isoniazid-resistant, rifampin-susceptible organisms, isoniazid should be discontinued, and rifampin should be administered daily to contacts with TBI for a total course of 4 months.

Table 3.86. People at Increased Risk of Drug-Resistant Tuberculosis Infection or Disease[a]

- People with a history of prior treatment for tuberculosis disease (or whose source person for the contact received prior treatment)
- Contacts of a patient with drug-resistant contagious tuberculosis disease
- People who resided in countries or areas with high prevalence of drug-resistant tuberculosis, such as Russia and certain nations of the former Soviet Union, Asia, Africa, and Latin America[a,b]
- Infected people whose source person has positive smears for acid-fast bacilli or cultures after 2 months of appropriate antituberculosis therapy and patients who do not respond to a standard treatment regimen

[a]See wwwnc.cdc.gov/travel/page/yellowbook-home.
[b]For current information on countries with high prevalence of drug resistant tuberculosis disease refer to the most recent WHO Global Tuberculosis Report (eg, www.who.int/publications/i/item/9789240037021).

Optimal therapy for children with TBI caused by organisms with resistance to isonia-zid and rifampin (ie, MDR) is not known. In these circumstances, a fluoroquinolone alone and multidrug regimens have been used in observational studies, but the safety and the efficacy of these empiric regimens have not been assessed in controlled clinical trials. A common approach is to give 6 to 12 months of treatment with a later-genera-tion fluoroquinolone (levofloxacin or moxifloxacin), alone or with a second drug, based on the drug susceptibility of the source person's *M tuberculosis* isolate. On the basis of evidence of increased toxicity, adverse events, and discontinuations, pyrazinamide should not be routinely used as the second drug. Consultation with a TB specialist is indicated.

Treatment of Tuberculosis Disease.[1-6] The goal of treatment is to achieve killing of replicat-ing organisms in the tuberculous lesions in the shortest possible time. Achievement of this goal minimizes the possibility of development of resistant organisms. The major problem limiting successful treatment is poor adherence to prescribed treatment regi-mens. The use of DOT decreases the rates of relapse, treatment failures, and drug resistance; therefore, DOT is strongly recommended for treatment of all children and adolescents with TB disease in the United States. Intervals and dosages are provided in Tables 3.82, 3.84, and 3.85.

Therapy for Presumed or Known Drug-Susceptible Pulmonary Tuberculosis Disease. Recent clinical trials have shown efficacy of shorter treatment regimens for children with pul-monary tuberculosis disease. For nonsevere pulmonary disease in children 3 months to 16 years of age, defined as tuberculosis confined to 1 lobe with no cavities or iso-lated intrathoracic adenopathy, no signs of miliary tuberculosis, no complex pleural effusion, and no clinically significant airway obstruction, a 4-month, 4-drug regimen consisting initially of rifampin, isoniazid, pyrazinamide, and ethambutol (RIPE) daily for the first 2 months and isoniazid and rifampin daily for the remaining 2 months is recommended.

If criteria are not met for the 4-month course of RIPE (ie, patient has severe pul-monary disease or extrapulmonary TB disease other than peripheral lymph node TB), at least 6 months of treatment should be given. RIPE should be administered daily for the first 2 months, followed by isoniazid and rifampin daily for 4 months. For either the 4- or 6-month regimen, some experts administer 3 drugs (isoniazid, rifampin, and

[1] Turkova A, Wills GH, Wobudeya E, et al. Shorter treatment for nonsevere tuberculosis in African and Indian children. *N Engl J Med*. 2022;386(10):911-922

[2] Dorman SE, Nahid P, Kurbatova EK. Four-month rifapentine regimens with or without moxifloxacin for tuberculosis. *N Engl J Med*. 2021;384(18):1705-1718

[3] World Health Organization. Consolidated Guidelines on Tuberculosis. Module 5: Management of tuber-culosis in children and adolescents. World Health Organization; 2022. Available at: **www.who.int/publications/i/item/9789240046764**

[4] World Health Organization. Consolidated Guidelines on Tuberculosis. Module 4: Treatment drug susceptible tuberculosis treatment. World Health Organization; 2022. Available at: **www.who.int/publications/i/item/9789240048126**

[5] Nahid P, Dorman SE, Alipanah N, et al. Official American Thoracic Society/Centers for Disease Control and Prevention/Infectious Diseases Society of America Clinical Practice Guidelines: Treatment of Drug-Susceptible Tuberculosis. *Clin Infect Dis*. 2016;63(7):e147-e195

[6] Nahid P, Mase SR, Migliori GB, et al. Treatment of drug-resistant tuberculosis. An Official ATS/CDC/ERS/IDSA Clinical Practice Guideline. *Am J Respir Crit Care Med*. 2019;200(10):e93-e142

pyrazinamide) as the initial regimen if a presumed source person has been identified with known pansusceptible *M tuberculosis* or has no risk factors for drug-resistant *M tuberculosis*.

If the chest radiograph shows one or more pulmonary cavities and/or the sputum culture result remains positive after 2 months of therapy, the duration of therapy should be extended to at least 9 months.

An alternative regimen for patients ≥12 years of age (and ≥40 kg) with nonsevere or severe, susceptible pulmonary disease is a 4-month regimen with isoniazid, rifapentine, moxifloxacin, and pyrazinamide; all 4 drugs are given daily for 8 weeks, followed by daily isoniazid, rifapentine, and moxifloxacin for 9 weeks (**www.cdc.gov/ mmwr/volumes/71/wr/mm7108a1.htm**).

Therapy for Drug-Resistant Pulmonary Tuberculosis Disease. Consultation with an expert is strongly recommended when drug-resistant TB disease is suspected or confirmed. Guidance is also available from the WHO (**https://apps.who.int/iris/rest/ bitstreams/1280998/retrieve**), the Sentinel Project (**http://sentinel- project.org/wp-content/uploads/2022/04/DRTB-Field-Guide-2021_ v5.1.pdf**), and the CDC (**www.cdc.gov/tb/topic/drtb/default.htm**). Drug resistance is more common in certain groups (Table 3.86). When resistance to drugs other than isoniazid is likely (see Table 3.86), initial therapy should be adjusted by adding at least 2 drugs to match the presumed drug susceptibility pattern until drug susceptibility results are available. If an isolate from the child under treatment is not available, drug susceptibilities can be inferred by the drug susceptibility pattern of isolates from the presumed source person. Data for guiding drug selection may not be available for foreign-born children or in circumstances of international travel or adoption. If this information is not available, consultation with an expert should occur to determine a multidrug oral regimen that includes close monitoring for clinical response.

Most pulmonary TB disease in children that is caused by an isoniazid-resistant but rifampin- and pyrazinamide-susceptible strain of *M tuberculosis* complex can be treated with a 6-month regimen of rifampin, pyrazinamide, and ethambutol. If disease is extensive, many experts add a fluoroquinolone to this regimen. For MDR TB disease, the treatment regimen needed for cure should include multiple antituberculosis drugs to which the organism is susceptible, and consultation with an expert is strongly recommended as new regimens are being evaluated and new guidance developed. There is now a strong emphasis on the use of all-oral regimens whenever possible to avoid the toxicity of the injectable drugs. Bedaquiline is approved by the US Food and Drug Administration as part of combination therapy in the treatment for children ages 5 years and older with MDR pulmonary TB disease. Currently, there are limited safety, tolerability, efficacy, and pharmacokinetic data on its use in children <5 years of age. However, the WHO has recommended its use in children of all ages and has made provisional dosing recommendations for children of all weights, based on preliminary data from pediatric trials and other emerging evidence (**www.who. int/publications/i/item/9789240055193**). Delamanid is another new oral drug for treatment of MDR, pre-XDR, and XDR TB disease; this drug is available in the United States under a compassionate use protocol. Regimens in which drugs are administered intermittently are not recommended for drug-resistant disease; daily DOT is critical to prevent emergence of additional resistance.

Extrapulmonary Tuberculosis Disease.[1] In general, extrapulmonary TB disease, with the exception of meningitis and osteoarticular TB, can be treated with the same regimens as used for pulmonary TB disease. Peripheral lymph node TB disease has been successfully treated with the 4-month, 4-drug regimen used for nonsevere pulmonary TB disease (rifampin, isoniazid, pyrazinamide, and ethambutol daily for the first 2 months, and isoniazid and rifampin daily for the remaining 2 months). For suspected drug-susceptible tuberculous meningitis, daily treatment with isoniazid, rifampin, pyrazinamide, and ethionamide or a fluoroquinolone (levofloxacin or moxifloxacin) should be initiated. For CNS TB disease, rifampin should be given at a dose of 30 mg/kg/day to ensure adequate CNS penetration and because this dose has been shown to improve neurodevelopmental outcomes. When susceptibility to first-line drugs is established, ethionamide or fluoroquinolone can be discontinued. Pyrazinamide is given for a total of 2 months, and isoniazid and rifampin are given for a total of 6 to 12 months (the longer therapy is preferred by many experts). In children and adolescents with TB meningitis presumed to be drug susceptible, the WHO now states that 6 months of isoniazid, rifampin, pyrazinamide, and ethionamide daily may be used, but the longer treatment regimen of at least 9 months is preferred. Osteoarticular tuberculosis is generally treated with a 4- drug regimen of isoniazid, rifampin, pyrazinamide, and ethambutol for 2 months and isoniazid and rifampin for an additional 10 months (sensitivities should be obtained and treatment adjusted if needed). Consultation with an expert in tuberculosis is advised for treatment of meningitis and osteoarticular disease.

Evaluation and Monitoring of Therapy in Children and Adolescents. Careful monthly monitoring of clinical and bacteriologic responses to therapy is important. With DOT, clinical evaluation is an integral component of each visit (which may be accomplished virtually by video) for drug administration. For patients with pulmonary TB disease, chest radiographs often are obtained after 2 months of therapy to evaluate response. After initiation of treatment, alveolar or interstitial infiltrates may start to decrease within 1 to 2 weeks but take much longer to resolve completely. Pleural effusions are slower to resolve and may require drainage for symptom relief; partial reaccumulation is common as an isolated finding but does not indicate treatment failure. Even with successful 4- to 6-month treatment regimens, hilar adenopathy can persist for 2 to 3 years; normal radiographic findings are not necessary to discontinue therapy. Follow-up chest radiography beyond termination of successful therapy usually is not necessary unless clinical deterioration occurs.

If therapy has been interrupted, the date of completion should be extended. Although guidelines cannot be provided for every situation, factors to consider when establishing the date of completion include the following: (1) length of interruption of therapy; (2) time during therapy (early or late) when interruption occurred; and (3) the patient's clinical, radiographic, and bacteriologic status before, during, and after interruption of therapy. The total doses administered by DOT should be calculated to guide the duration of therapy.

Untoward effects of TB therapy, including severe hepatitis in otherwise healthy infants, children, and adolescents, are rare. Routine determination of serum

---

[1] World Health Organization. Consolidated Guidelines on Tuberculosis. Module 5: Management of tuberculosis in children and adolescents. World Health Organization; 2022. Available at: **www.who.int/publications/i/item/9789240046764**

aminotransferase concentrations is not recommended (see Isoniazid Therapy for TBI, p 898) during treatment of TBI or in most cases of TB disease unless the child develops symptoms suggestive of hepatotoxicity or has additional risks for hepatotoxicity such as preexisting liver disease or coadministration of other potentially hepatotoxic drugs. For most children, monthly clinical evaluations to observe for signs or symptoms of hepatitis and other adverse effects of drug therapy without routine monitoring of aminotransferase concentrations is appropriate follow-up. Regular patient contact to assess drug adherence, effectiveness, and adverse effects is an important aspect of management. DOT encounters also are opportunities for checking on well-being and treatment tolerance. Patients should be provided with written instructions and advised to call a physician or clinic immediately if symptoms of adverse events, in particular hepatotoxicity (ie, nausea, vomiting, abdominal pain, jaundice), develop.

Other Treatment Considerations

Corticosteroids. Corticosteroids are given when the host inflammatory response is contributing significantly to organ dysfunction or tissue damage. The evidence supporting adjuvant treatment with corticosteroids for children with TB disease is incomplete. Corticosteroids are definitely indicated for children with tuberculous meningitis, because corticosteroids decrease rates of mortality and long-term neurologic impairment. Corticosteroids can be considered for children with pleural and pericardial effusions (to hasten reabsorption of fluid), severe miliary disease (to mitigate alveolocapillary block), endobronchial disease (to relieve obstruction and atelectasis), and abdominal TB (to decrease the risk of strictures). Corticosteroids should be given only when accompanied by appropriate antituberculosis drug therapy. Most experts give 2 mg/kg per day of prednisone (maximum, 60 mg/day) or its equivalent for 4 to 6 weeks followed by tapering.

Tuberculosis Disease and HIV Infection.[1] Most adults living with HIV with drug-susceptible TB disease respond well to standard treatment regimens. However, optimal therapy for TB disease in children living with HIV has not been established. Treating TB disease in a child living with HIV is complicated by antiretroviral drug interactions with the rifamycins and overlapping toxicities. Therapy always should include at least 4 drugs initially, should be administered daily via DOT, and should be continued for at least 6 months unless it is nonsevere pulmonary disease (defined as tuberculosis confined to 1 lobe with no cavities or isolated intrathoracic adenopathy, no signs of miliary tuberculosis, no complex pleural effusion, and no clinically significant airway obstruction), in which case a 4-month treatment course is acceptable. Rifampin, isoniazid, pyrazinamide, and ethambutol (RIPE) should be administered for at least the first 2 months. Ethambutol can be discontinued once drug-resistant TB disease is excluded. Coadministration of rifampin and antiretroviral therapy may be contraindicated or require antiretroviral therapy dose adjustments, depending on the antiretroviral agents used. Rifabutin is substituted for rifampin in some circumstances. Consultation with a specialist who has experience in managing patients living with HIV with TB disease is strongly advised. If pulmonary disease TB is diagnosed in a person living with HIV

---

[1] Panel on Opportunistic Infections in Children with and Exposed to HIV. Guidelines for the Prevention and Treatment of Opportunistic Infections in Children with and Exposed to HIV. Department of Health and Human Services. Available at: **https://clinicalinfo.hiv.gov/en/guidelines/ pediatric-opportunistic-infection**

who is not yet receiving antiretroviral therapy, even in the presence of severe immune suppression, antiretroviral therapy can be safely initiated within 2 weeks of antituberculosis therapy, despite the risk of inciting immune reconstitution syndrome.

Immunizations. Patients who are receiving treatment for TB disease can receive measles and other age-appropriate attenuated live-virus vaccines unless they are receiving high-dose systemic corticosteroids, are severely ill, or have other specific contraindications to immunization.

Tuberculosis During Pregnancy and Breastfeeding. Pregnant people who have a positive TST or IGRA result, are asymptomatic, have a normal chest radiograph, and have had recent contact with a contagious person should be considered for TBI therapy with isoniazid, which usually should begin after the first trimester; consultation with an expert in TB is recommended. If there has been no recent contact with a contagious person, TBI therapy can be delayed until after delivery. Pyridoxine supplementation is indicated for all pregnant and breastfeeding people receiving isoniazid.

If TB disease is diagnosed during pregnancy, a standard 6-month regimen for drug-susceptible TB is usually initiated; however, 9 months of therapy is indicated if pyrazinamide is not used initially. Prompt initiation of therapy is mandatory to protect the pregnant person and fetus.

There are few adequate and well-controlled studies evaluating the adverse effects of isoniazid, rifampin, ethambutol, and pyrazinamide on the fetus. Isoniazid, ethambutol, and rifampin are believed (based on extensive clinical experience) to be relatively safe for the fetus. The benefit of ethambutol and rifampin for therapy of TB disease in the pregnant person outweighs the risk to the infant. Because aminoglycosides (streptomycin, kanamycin, amikacin) or capreomycin may cause ototoxic effects in the fetus, they should not be used unless administration is essential for effective treatment. Ethionamide has been demonstrated to be teratogenic, so its use during pregnancy is contraindicated. The effects of other antituberculous drugs on the fetus are unknown.

Although isoniazid is secreted in human milk, no adverse effects of isoniazid on breastfeeding infants have been demonstrated. Breastfed infants do not require pyridoxine supplementation unless they are receiving isoniazid, but breastfeeding people who are taking isoniazid should take pyridoxine. The isoniazid dosage of a breastfed infant whose lactating parent is taking isoniazid does not require adjustment for the small amount of drug in the milk.

Congenital Tuberculosis. Congenital TB disease is rare, but in utero infections can occur after bacillemia in the pregnant person and have been reported following in vitro fertilization of persons from countries with endemic disease in whom infertility likely was related to subclinical genitourinary tract TB disease. The affected neonate is rarely ill at birth, more often becoming ill at 2 to 4 weeks of life.

None of the possible signs of congenital TB disease, such as fever, tachypnea, lethargy, organomegaly, or pulmonary infiltrates, distinguish it from other systemic infections of the newborn infant. The prognosis is poor without prompt treatment. If a newborn infant is suspected of having congenital TB disease, a TST and IGRA test (both are recommended in order to increase sensitivity), chest radiography, abdominal ultrasound, lumbar puncture, and appropriate cultures and radiography should be performed promptly. The TST result usually is negative in newborn infants with congenital or perinatally acquired infection; IGRA sensitivity in this context is not known but is likely to be low. Regardless of the TST or IGRA results, treatment of the infant should be initiated promptly with rifampin, isoniazid, pyrazinamide, and ethambutol (RIPE). If meningitis is confirmed, corticosteroids should be added (see Corticosteroids, p 913). The placenta should be examined histologically for granulomata and AFB, and a specimen should be cultured for *M tuberculosis* complex. The parent who gave birth should be evaluated for presence of pulmonary or extrapulmonary disease, including genitourinary tuberculosis. HIV testing of the birth parent is essential.

Management of the Newborn Infant Whose Birth Parent Has TBI or TB Disease. Management of the newborn infant is based on categorization of the infection in the parent who gave birth to the newborn. Although protection of the infant from exposure and infection is of paramount importance, contact between infant and birth parent should be allowed when possible. Differing circumstances and resulting recommendations are as follows:

- **Birthing parent has a positive TST or IGRA result and normal chest radiographic findings.** If the birthing parent is asymptomatic, no separation is required. The birthing parent usually is a candidate for treatment of TBI during the postpartum period. The newborn infant needs no special evaluation or therapy. Because of the young infant's high susceptibility for TB disease and because the birthing parent's positive TST or IGRA result could be a marker of an unrecognized person with contagious TB disease within the household, other household members should be questioned about having symptoms of TB and have a TST or IGRA and further evaluation as indicated; this should not delay the infant's discharge from the hospital. These birthing parents can breastfeed their infants.

- **Birthing parent has clinical signs and symptoms or abnormal findings on chest radiograph consistent with TB disease.** Birthing parents with suspected or proven TB disease should be reported immediately to the local health department, and evaluation of all household members should be initiated as soon as possible. If the birthing parent has TB disease, the infant should be evaluated for congenital TB (see Congenital Tuberculosis, p 914), and the birthing parent should be tested for HIV infection. The birthing parent and the infant should be separated until the birthing parent has completed TB evaluation and, if TB disease is suspected, until the birthing parent and infant are receiving appropriate antituberculosis therapy, the birthing parent wears a mask, the birthing parent understands and is willing to adhere to infection control measures, and contact is in a well-ventilated space. A birthing parent with proven or likely drug-susceptible TB disease who has been treated appropriately for 2 or more weeks and who is not considered contagious (smear-negative sputum) may breastfeed; a birthing parent with TB disease suspected of being contagious or with risk factors for drug-resistant TB disease should refrain from breastfeeding and from other close contact with the infant because of potential spread of *M tuberculosis* through respiratory tract droplets or airborne transmission (see Tuberculosis During Pregnancy and Breastfeeding, p 914). During separation, expressed human milk can be fed to the infant unless the birthing parent has signs of tuberculous mastitis, which is rare. Once the infant is receiving isoniazid or rifampin (see next paragraph), separation is not necessary unless the birthing parent has possible drug-resistant TB disease or has poor adherence to treatment and DOT is not possible. If the birthing parent is suspected of having isoniazid-resistant TB disease, an expert in TB disease management should be consulted.

If congenital TB is excluded, isoniazid or rifampin is administered until the infant is 3 or 4 months of age (or adjusted age if the infant was born prematurely), when a TST or IGRA should be performed. If the result is negative at 3 to 4 months of age and the birthing parent has good adherence and response to treatment and no longer is contagious, the treatment can be discontinued in the infant. If the result is positive, the infant should be reassessed for TB disease. If TB disease is excluded, isoniazid should be continued for a total of 9 months, or a 4-month course of rifampin can be completed. The infant should be evaluated monthly during treatment for signs of illness or poor growth.

- **Birthing parent has a positive TST or IGRA result and abnormal findings on chest radiography but no evidence of TB disease.** If the chest radiograph of the birthing parent appears abnormal but is not suggestive of TB disease and the history, physical examination, and sputum smear indicate no evidence of TB disease, the infant can be assumed to be at low risk of *M tuberculosis* infection and need not be separated from the birthing parent. The birthing parent and infant should receive follow-up care, and the birthing parent should be treated for TBI. Other household members should have a TST or IGRA and further evaluation.

TUBERCULOSIS CAUSED BY *M BOVIS*: Infections with *M bovis* account for approximately 1% to 2% of TB cases in the United States, with higher rates along the border with Mexico. Children who come from countries where *M bovis* is prevalent in cattle or whose parents come from those countries are more likely to be infected. Most infections in humans are transmitted from cattle by unpasteurized milk and its products, such as fresh cheese,[1] although human-to-human transmission by the airborne route has been documented rarely. In children, *M bovis* more commonly causes cervical lymphadenitis, intestinal TB disease and peritonitis, and meningitis. In adults, *M bovis* infection can progress to advanced pulmonary disease with a risk of transmission to others.

The TST result typically is positive in a person infected with *M bovis*; IGRAs have not been studied systematically for diagnosing *M bovis* infection in particular, but theoretically they should have acceptable test characteristics (see Blood-Based Testing With IGRAs, p 893). The definitive diagnosis of *M bovis* infection requires an isolate. The commonly used methods for identifying a microbial isolate as *M tuberculosis* complex do not distinguish *M bovis* from *M tuberculosis, M africanum,* and BCG, which is a live attenuated vaccine strain of *M bovis*; *M bovis* is suspected in clinical laboratories by its typical resistance to pyrazinamide. This approach can be unreliable, and species confirmation at a reference laboratory should be requested when *M bovis* is suspected. Molecular genotyping through the state health department may assist in identifying *M bovis*. BCG rarely is isolated from pediatric clinical specimens in the United States; however, it should be suspected from localized BCG suppuration or draining lymphadenitis in children who recently (within several months) received BCG vaccine, or in infants with selected congenital immunodeficiency syndromes who received a BCG vaccine. Only a reference laboratory can distinguish an isolate of BCG from an isolate of *M bovis*.

---

[1] American Academy of Pediatrics, Committee on Infectious Diseases and Committee on Nutrition. Consumption of raw or unpasteurized milk and milk products by pregnant women and children. *Pediatrics.* 2014;133(1):175-179 (Reaffirmed November 2019)

Therapy for* M bovis *Disease. Controlled clinical trials for treatment of *M bovis* disease have not been conducted, and treatment recommendations for *M bovis* disease in adults and children are based on results from treatment trials for *M tuberculosis* disease. Although most strains of *M bovis* are pyrazinamide-resistant and resistance to other first-line drugs has been reported, MDR strains are rare. Initial therapy for disease caused by *M bovis* should include 3 or 4 drugs, excluding pyrazinamide, that would be used to treat disease attributable to *M tuberculosis*. For isoniazid- and rifampin-susceptible strains, a total treatment course of at least 9 months is recommended.

Parents should be counseled about the many infectious diseases transmitted by unpasteurized milk and its products,[1] and parents who might import traditional, unpasteurized dairy products from countries where *M bovis* infection is prevalent in cattle should be advised against giving those products to their children. When people are exposed to an adult who has pulmonary disease caused by *M bovis* infection, they should be evaluated by the same methods as for *M tuberculosis*.

INFECTION PREVENTION AND CONTROL MEASURES IN HEALTH CARE SETTINGS: Most children with TB disease, especially children younger than 10 years, are not contagious. Possible exceptions are the following: (1) children with pulmonary cavities; (2) children with positive sputum AFB smears; (3) children with laryngeal involvement; (4) children with extensive pulmonary disease; or (5) neonates or infants with congenital TB disease undergoing procedures that involve the oropharyngeal airway (eg, endotracheal intubation). In these instances, airborne infection isolation precautions for TB are indicated until effective therapy has been initiated, specimen smears are negative, and coughing has abated. Additional criteria apply to suspected or known MDR TB disease.

Children with no cough and smear-negative sputum AFB smears can be hospitalized in an open ward. Infection prevention measures for hospital personnel and visitors exposed to contagious patients should include the use of personally "fit tested" and "sealed" N95 or higher respirators for all patient contacts (see Infection Prevention and Control for Hospitalized Children, p 163). If the patient has or is suspected to have drug-resistant TB disease, consultation regarding infection prevention and control should be made with public health authorities.

The major concern in infection control relates to adult household members and contacts who can be the source of infection. Visitation should be limited to people who have been evaluated by symptom screening and chest radiograph and do not have TB disease.

CONTROL MEASURES[2,3]: Control of TB disease in the United States requires collaboration between health care providers and health department personnel, obtaining a thorough history of exposure(s) to people with contagious TB disease, timely and

---

[1] American Academy of Pediatrics, Committee on Infectious Diseases and Committee on Nutrition. Consumption of raw or unpasteurized milk and milk products by pregnant women and children. *Pediatrics.* 2014;133(1):175-179 (Reaffirmed November 2019)

[2] American Thoracic Society, Centers for Disease Control and Prevention, and Infectious Diseases Society of America. Controlling tuberculosis in the United States. Recommendations from the American Thoracic Society, CDC, and the Infectious Diseases Society of America. *MMWR Recomm Rep.* 2005;54(RR-12):1–81

[3] Nolt D, Starke JR; American Academy of Pediatrics, Committee on Infectious Diseases. Clinical report. Tuberculosis infection in children: testing and treatment. *Pediatrics.* 2021;148(6):e2021054663

effective contact tracing, proper interpretation of TST or IGRA results, and appropriate antituberculosis therapy, including DOT services. A plan to control and prevent XDR TB disease has been published.[1] Eliminating ingestion of unpasteurized dairy products will prevent most *M bovis* infection.[2]

Management of Contacts, Including Epidemiologic Investigation.[3,4] Children with a positive TST or IGRA result or TB disease ideally should be the starting point for epidemiologic investigation by the local health department. Close contacts of a TST- or IGRA-positive child, if the test was performed because the child has 1 or more risk factors, should have a TST or IGRA, and people with a positive TST or IGRA result or with symptoms consistent with TB disease should be investigated further. Because children with TB disease usually are not contagious unless they have an adult-type multibacillary form of pulmonary or laryngeal disease, their contacts are not likely to be infected unless they also have been in contact with an adult source person. After the presumptive adult source of the child's TBI or TB disease is identified, other contacts of that adult should be evaluated.

Therapy for Contacts. Children and adolescents recently exposed to a contagious person with TB disease should have a TST or IGRA test performed and should be evaluated for TB disease (history and physical examination, as well as chest radiography if symptomatic or positive TST or IGRA results). For exposed contacts with impaired immunity (eg, HIV infection) and all contacts younger than 5 years, treatment for presumptive TBI should be initiated with either isoniazid or rifampin, even if the initial TST or IGRA result is negative, once TB disease is excluded (see Treatment Regimens for TBI, p 898). Children with TBI can have a negative TST or IGRA result because a cellular immune response has not yet developed or because of anergy. Children with a negative TST or IGRA result should be retested 8 to 10 weeks after the last exposure to a source of infection. If the TST or IGRA result still is negative in an immunocompetent person, treatment can be discontinued. If the contact is immunocompromised and TBI cannot be excluded, after an evaluation for TB disease, treatment should be continued to the completion of the regimen. If a TST or IGRA result of a contact becomes positive, the regimen for TBI should be completed after an evaluation for TB disease.

Child Care and Schools. Children with TB disease can attend school or child care if they are receiving therapy (see Children in Group Child Care and Schools, p 145). They can return to regular activities as soon as effective therapy has been instituted, adherence to therapy has been documented, and clinical symptoms have diminished. Children with TBI can participate in all activities whether they are receiving treatment or not.

---

[1] Centers for Disease Control and Prevention. Plan to combat extensively drug-resistant tuberculosis: recommendations of the Federal Tuberculosis Task Force. *MMWR Recomm Rep.* 2009;58(RR-3):1–43

[2] American Academy of Pediatrics, Committee on Infectious Diseases and Committee on Nutrition. Consumption of raw or unpasteurized milk and milk products by pregnant women and children. *Pediatrics.* 2014;133(1):175-179 (Reaffirmed November 2019)

[3] National Tuberculosis Controllers Association and Centers for Disease Control and Prevention. Guidelines for the investigation of contacts of persons with infectious tuberculosis. Recommendations from the National Tuberculosis Controllers Association and CDC. *MMWR Recomm Rep.* 2005;54(RR-15):1–47

[4] Nolt D, Starke JR; American Academy of Pediatrics, Committee on Infectious Diseases. Clinical report. Tuberculosis infection in children: testing and treatment. *Pediatrics.* 2021;148(6):e2021054663

BCG Vaccines. BCG vaccine is a live vaccine originally prepared from attenuated strains of *M bovis*. Use of BCG vaccine[1] is recommended by the Expanded Programme on Immunization of the World Health Organization for administration at birth in countries with endemic TB (see Table 1.7, p 40). BCG is used in more than 100 countries to reduce the incidence of disseminated and other life-threatening manifestations of TB disease in infants and young children. Although BCG immunization decreases the risk of serious complications of TB disease in young children, the various BCG vaccines used throughout the world differ in composition and efficacy.

Two meta-analyses of published clinical trials and case-control studies concerning the efficacy of BCG vaccines concluded that BCG vaccine has relatively high protective efficacy (approximately 80%) against meningeal and miliary TB disease in children. The protective efficacy against pulmonary TB disease differed significantly among the studies, precluding a specific conclusion. Protection against pulmonary TB disease by BCG vaccine in one meta-analysis was estimated to be 50%. Comparative evaluations of the BCG vaccine that is licensed in the United States (TICE strain) for the prevention of TB disease versus other BCG vaccines globally have not been performed.

Indications. In the United States, administration of BCG vaccine should be considered only in limited and select circumstances, such as unavoidable risk of exposure to *M tuberculosis* and failure or unfeasibility of other control methods. Recommendations for use of BCG vaccine for control of TB disease among children and health care personnel have been published by the Advisory Committee on Immunization Practices of the CDC and the Advisory Council for the Elimination of Tuberculosis.[2] For infants and children, BCG immunization should be considered only for those who have a negative TST result and who do not have contraindications in the following circumstances:

* The child is exposed continually to a person or people with contagious pulmonary TB disease arising from a strain that is resistant to isoniazid and rifampin and the child cannot be removed from this exposure; OR
* The child is exposed continually to a person or people with untreated or ineffectively treated contagious pulmonary TB disease and the child cannot be removed from such exposure or given antituberculosis therapy.

Careful assessment of the potential risks and benefits of BCG vaccine and consultation with personnel in local TB control programs are strongly recommended before use of BCG vaccine.

Adverse Reactions. Uncommonly (1%–2% of immunizations), BCG vaccine can result in local adverse reactions, such as subcutaneous abscess and regional lymphadenopathy, which generally are not serious. One rare complication, osteitis affecting the epiphysis of long bones, can occur as long as several years after BCG immunization. Disseminated fatal infection occurs rarely (approximately 2 per 1 million people), primarily in people who are severely immunocompromised, such as children with poorly controlled HIV infection or severe combined immunodeficiency. Antituberculosis

---

[1] **www.bcgatlas.org**

[2] Centers for Disease Control and Prevention. The role of BCG vaccine in the prevention and control of tuberculosis in the United States: a joint statement by the Advisory Committee for the Elimination of Tuberculosis and the Advisory Committee on Immunization Practices. *MMWR Recomm Rep.* 1996;45(RR-4):1–18

therapy is recommended to treat osteitis and disseminated disease caused by BCG vaccine.

Children with complications caused by BCG vaccine should be referred for management by a TB expert and should be evaluated for an underlying immune deficiency.

Contraindications. People with burns, skin infections, and most primary or secondary immunodeficiencies should not receive BCG vaccine. Children living with HIV who are vaccinated with BCG at birth in the absence of antiretroviral therapy (ART) are at increased risk for disseminated disease attributable to BCG. BCG vaccine should not routinely be administered to infants and children with HIV in the United States. Use of BCG vaccine is contraindicated for people receiving immunosuppressive medications including high-dose corticosteroids (see Corticosteroids, p 913). Although no untoward effects of BCG vaccine on the fetus have been observed, immunization of people during pregnancy is not recommended.

Public Health Reporting. Reporting of suspected and confirmed cases of TB disease is mandated by law in all states. TB disease is a nationally notifiable condition. TBI (latent tuberculosis) is reportable in some states.

Nontuberculous Mycobacteria
(Environmental Mycobacteria, Mycobacteria Other Than *Mycobacterium tuberculosis*)

CLINICAL MANIFESTATIONS: Several syndromes are caused by nontuberculous mycobacteria (NTM).
- In children, the most common of these syndromes is cervical lymphadenitis.
- Cutaneous infection may follow soil- or water-contaminated traumatic wounds, surgeries, or cosmetic procedures (eg, tattoos, pedicures, body piercings).
- Less common syndromes include skin and soft tissue infection, osteomyelitis, otitis media, central catheter-associated bloodstream infections, and pulmonary infections, especially in adolescents with cystic fibrosis.
- NTM, especially *Mycobacterium avium* complex (MAC [including *Mycobacterium avium* and *Mycobacterium avium-intracellulare*]) and *Mycobacterium abscessus,* can be recovered from sputum in 10% to 20% of adolescents and young adults with cystic fibrosis and can be associated with fever and declining clinical status.
- Disseminated infections almost always are associated with impaired cell-mediated immunity, as found in children with congenital immune defects (eg, interleukin-12 deficiency, cytokine–JAK–STAT pathways abnormalities, NF-kappa-B essential modulator [NEMO] mutation and related disorders, and interferon-gamma receptor defects), hematopoietic cell transplants, or advanced human immunodeficiency virus (HIV) infection. Disseminated NTM infection, most commonly MAC, is rare in children living with HIV during the first year of life. The frequency of disseminated MAC increases with increasing age and declining CD4+ T-lymphocyte counts, typically less than 50 cells/mm^3, in children 6 years or older.[1] Manifestations of disseminated NTM infections depend on the species and route of infection and

---

[1] Panel on Opportunistic Infections in Children with and Exposed to HIV. Guidelines for the Prevention and Treatment of Opportunistic Infections in Children with and Exposed to HIV. Department of Health and Human Services. Available at: **https://clinicalinfo.hiv.gov/en/guidelines/pediatric-opportunistic-infection**

include fever, night sweats, weight loss, abdominal pain, fatigue, diarrhea, and anemia. These signs and symptoms also are found in advanced immunosuppressed children living with HIV infection without disseminated MAC. For children living with HIV infection who have disseminated MAC, respiratory symptoms and isolated pulmonary disease are uncommon. In patients living with HIV infection who develop immune restoration with initiation of antiretroviral therapy, local NTM symptoms can worsen temporarily. This immune reconstitution syndrome usually occurs 2 to 4 weeks after initiation of antiretroviral therapy. Symptoms can include worsening fever, swollen lymph nodes, local pain, and laboratory abnormalities.

ETIOLOGY: Of the close to 200 species of NTM that have been identified, only a few species cause most human infections. The species most commonly infecting children in the United States are MAC, *Mycobacterium fortuitum*, *M abscessus*, and *Mycobacterium marinum* (Table 3.87). Several new species, which can be detected by nucleic acid amplification tests (NAATs) but cannot be grown by routine culture methods, have been identified in lymph nodes of children with cervical adenitis. NTM disease in patients living with HIV infection usually is caused by MAC. *M fortuitum*, *Mycobacterium chelonae*, *Mycobacterium smegmatis*, and *M abscessus* are referred to as "rapidly growing" mycobacteria, because visible growth can be detected in subculture usually within 7 days on solid media, whereas MAC, *M marinum*, and *Mycobacterium szulgai* require several weeks before sufficient growth occurs and are referred to as "slow growing" mycobacteria. Rapidly growing mycobacteria have been implicated most often in wound, soft tissue, bone, pulmonary, central venous catheter, and middle-ear infections. Other mycobacterial species that usually are not pathogenic have caused infections in immunocompromised hosts or have been associated with the presence of a foreign body.

EPIDEMIOLOGY: NTM are ubiquitous in nature, being found in soil, food, water, and animals. Tap water is the major reservoir for *M avium* (included in MAC), *Mycobacterium chimaera* (belonging to MAC), *Mycobacterium kansasii*, *Mycobacterium lentiflavum*, *Mycobacterium xenopi*, *Mycobacterium simiae*, and health care-associated infections attributable to *M abscessus* and *M fortuitum*. Outbreaks have been associated with contaminated water used for acupuncture and pedicures and inks used for tattooing. Health care-associated outbreaks have occurred among children undergoing pulpotomy or other dental procedures associated with improperly maintained dental unit water lines. Outbreaks of otitis media caused by *M abscessus* have been associated with polyethylene ear tubes and use of contaminated equipment or water. Health care-associated outbreaks of *M chelonae* have been associated with the use of commercial-grade misting humidifiers and nonsterile ice for invasive procedures. For *M marinum*, water in a fish tank or aquarium or an injury in a salt-water environment are the major sources of infection. A waterborne route of transmission has been implicated for MAC infection in some immunocompromised hosts. A variety of other outbreaks associated with contaminated medical equipment, inoculation through injections, surgery, and other procedures have been reported, particularly in settings of poor infection control practices. Pseudo-outbreaks associated with contamination of specimens or reagents have also been reported.

An international outbreak of *M chimaera* infection (including prosthetic valve endocarditis, vascular graft infection, and disseminated infection) has been associated with heater-cooler devices used in heart surgery requiring cardiopulmonary bypass and is

Table 3.87. Diseases Caused by Nontuberculous Mycobacteria Species

Clinical Disease	Species
Cutaneous infection	*Mycobacterium marinum* *Mycobacterium chelonae* *Mycobacterium fortuitum* *Mycobacterium abscessus* *Mycobacterium ulcerans*[a]
Lymphadenitis	*Mycobacterium avium* complex (MAC) *Mycobacterium haemophilum* *Mycobacterium lentiflavum* *Mycobacterium kansasii* *M fortuitum* *M abscessus* *Mycobacterium malmoense*[b]
Otologic infection	*M abscessus* *M fortuitum*
Pulmonary infection	MAC *M kansasii* *M abscessus* *Mycobacterium xenopi* *M malmoense*[b] *Mycobacterium szulgai* *M fortuitum* *Mycobacterium simiae*
Catheter-associated infection	*M chelonae* *M fortuitum* *M abscessus*
Prosthetic valve endocarditis	*M chelonae* *M fortuitum* *Mycobacterium chimaera*
Skeletal infection	MAC *M kansasii* *M fortuitum* *M chelonae* *M marinum* *M abscessus* *M ulcerans*[a]
Disseminated	MAC *M kansasii* *Mycobacterium genavense* *M haemophilum* *M chelonae*

[a] Not endemic in the United States.
[b] Found primarily in Northern Europe.

attributable to aerosolization of *M chimaera* from contaminated devices. Clinical presentation is indolent and includes fever, myalgia, arthralgia, fatigue, and weight loss, with diagnosis in patients often occurring up to several years after exposure. The US Food and Drug Administration (FDA) has determined that all heater-cooler devices have common design features that could lead to bioaerosol formation.

Although many people are exposed to NTM, it is unknown why some exposures result in acute or chronic infection. Usual portals of entry for NTM infection are believed to be abrasions in the skin, such as cutaneous lesions caused by *M marinum;* penetrating trauma such as needles and organic material most often associated with *M abscessus* and *M fortuitum;* surgical sites, especially for cosmetic surgery and central vascular or peritoneal dialysis catheters; oropharyngeal mucosa, which is the presumed portal of entry for cervical lymphadenitis; tooth eruption, which is the presumed portal of entry for submandibular lymphadenitis; gastrointestinal or respiratory tract, for disseminated MAC; and respiratory tract, including tympanostomy tubes for otitis media. Pulmonary disease and rare cases of mediastinal adenitis and endobronchial disease occur. NTM are important pathogens in patients with cystic fibrosis and are emerging pathogens in individuals receiving biologic response modifiers, such as anti-tumor necrosis factor-alpha agents (see Biologic Response-Modifying Drugs Used to Decrease Inflammation, p 104). Most infections remain localized at the portal of entry or in regional lymph nodes. Dissemination to distal sites primarily occurs in severely immunocompromised hosts.

No definitive evidence of person-to-person transmission of NTM exists outside of reports of possible occurrence in cystic fibrosis care centers.

Buruli ulcer disease is a skin and bone infection caused by *Mycobacterium ulcerans,* an emerging disease causing significant morbidity and disability in tropical areas such as Africa, Asia, South America, Australia, and the western Pacific.

The **incubation periods** for NTM are variable.

DIAGNOSTIC TESTS: Routine screening of respiratory or gastrointestinal tract specimens for NTM is not recommended except in the setting of cystic fibrosis, where respiratory specimens should be cultured for mycobacteria annually in those with a stable course who are spontaneously expectorating. Definitive diagnosis of NTM disease generally requires isolation of the organism, although molecular diagnostic tests are becoming more widely available. Consultation with the laboratory should occur to ensure that cultures and other specimens are handled correctly. For example, isolation of *Mycobacterium haemophilum* requires that the culture is maintained at 30°C and that heme-containing medium is added for isolation. Because NTM commonly are found in the environment, contamination of cultures or transient colonization can occur. Caution must be exercised in interpretation of cultures obtained from nonsterile sites, such as gastric washing specimens, endoscopy material, a single expectorated sputum sample, or urine specimens, and when the species cultured usually is nonpathogenic (eg, *Mycobacterium terrae* complex or *Mycobacterium gordonae*). An acid-fast bacilli smear-positive sample and repeated isolation on culture media of a single species from any site are more likely to indicate disease rather than culture contamination or transient colonization. Diagnostic criteria for NTM lung disease in adults include 2 or more separate sputum samples or 1 bronchial alveolar lavage or bronchial wash specimen that grows NTM. These criteria have not been validated in children and apply best to MAC, *M kansasii,* and *M abscessus.* NTM isolates from draining sinus tracts or wounds almost always are clinically significant. Recovery of NTM from sites that usually are sterile, such as cerebrospinal fluid, pleural fluid, bone marrow, blood, lymph node aspirates, middle ear or mastoid aspirates, or surgically excised tissue, is very likely to be clinically significant. However, rare instances of sample or laboratory contamination leading to a false-positive culture result have been reported. With radiometric or nonradiometric broth techniques, blood cultures are highly sensitive in recovery of MAC and other bloodborne NTM species. If disseminated MAC disease is confirmed, the patient should be evaluated for underlying immunodeficiency conditions. Polymerase chain reaction-based assays for some NTM have been developed but are not yet widely available in commercial diagnostic laboratories. Matrix-assisted laser desorption/ionization–time-of-flight (MALDI-TOF) instruments have been approved for the identification of mycobacteria species and may allow for more NTM isolates to get species identification faster than traditional methods.

Patients with NTM infections can have positive tuberculin skin test (TST) result, because the purified protein derivative preparation, derived from *Mycobacterium tuberculosis*, shares a number of antigens with these NTM species. These TST reactions usually measure less than 10 mm of induration but can measure more than 15 mm (see Tuberculosis, p 888). The interferon-gamma release assays (IGRAs) use 2 or 3 antigens more specific to *M tuberculosis* complex and result in less cross-reactivity from MAC and most other NTM species compared with TST. However, cross-reactions can occur with infection caused by *M kansasii*, *M marinum*, and *M szulgai* (see Tuberculosis, p 888).

TREATMENT[1,2]: NTM are relatively resistant in vitro to antimycobacterial drugs, but this does not necessarily correlate with clinical response, especially with MAC infections. Only limited controlled trials of drug treatment have been performed in adults with NTM infections, and none have been conducted in children. The approach to initial therapy for an NTM infection should be directed by the following: (1) the species causing the infection; (2) the results of drug-susceptibility testing, especially to macrolides and amikacin; (3) the site(s) of infection; (4) the patient's immune status; and (5) the need to treat a patient presumptively for tuberculosis while awaiting culture reports that subsequently reveal NTM.

For NTM lymphadenitis in otherwise healthy children, especially when the disease is caused by MAC, complete surgical excision is curative and limits scar formation. Published reports of antimicrobial therapy without surgical incision have had variable success rates. Therapy with azithromycin or clarithromycin combined with either a rifamycin (eg, rifampin or rifabutin) or ethambutol may be beneficial for children in whom surgical excision is not possible or is incomplete and for children with recurrent disease; use of a 3-drug regimen consisting of a macrolide, a rifamycin, and ethambutol can be considered for children with more extensive disease (see Table 3.88).

---

[1] Daley CL, Iaccarino JM, Lange C, et al. Treatment of nontuberculous mycobacterial pulmonary disease: an official ATS/ERS/ESCMID/IDSA clinical practice guideline: executive summary. *Clin Infect Dis.* 2020;71(4):e1-e36

[2] Floto RA, Olivier KN, Saiman L, et al. US Cystic Fibrosis Foundation and European Cystic Fibrosis Society consensus recommendations for the management of non-tuberculous mycobacteria in individuals with cystic fibrosis. *Thorax.* 2016;71:i1-i22. Available at: **https://thorax.bmj.com/content/thoraxjnl/71/Suppl_1/i1.full.pdf**

Table 3.88. Treatment of Nontuberculous Mycobacteria Infections in Children[a]

Organism	Disease	Initial Treatment
Slowly Growing Species[a]		
Mycobacterium avium complex (MAC); *Mycobacterium haemophilum; Mycobacterium lentiflavum*	Lymphadenitis	Complete excision of lymph nodes; if excision incomplete or disease recurs, azithromycin or clarithromycin plus either a rifamycin (rifampin or rifabutin) or ethambutol; children with more extensive disease may require a 3-drug regimen consisting of a macrolide, a rifamycin, and ethambutol.
	Pulmonary infection	Azithromycin or clarithromycin plus ethambutol and rifampin (or rifabutin); pulmonary resection may be needed in some patients who fail to respond to drug therapy. For severe disease, an initial course of amikacin or streptomycin often is included. Clinical data in adults with mild to moderate disease support that 3-times-weekly therapy is as effective as daily therapy, with less toxicity. For patients with advanced or cavitary disease, or those with cystic fibrosis drugs should be given daily.
Mycobacterium chimaera (belonging to MAC)	Prosthetic valve endocarditis	Valve removal, prolonged antimicrobial therapy based on susceptibility testing, but generally azithromycin or clarithromycin, ethambutol, and rifampin (or rifabutin). Additional drugs including amikacin and/or clofazimine are often used.
	Disseminated	See text.
Mycobacterium kansasii	Pulmonary infection	Azithromycin or clarithromycin plus rifampin and ethambutol daily or three times a week. Alternatively, isoniazid plus rifampin and ethambutol daily. If rifampin resistance is detected, a 3-drug regimen based on drug susceptibility testing should be used.
	Osteomyelitis	Surgical débridement and prolonged antimicrobial therapy using the regimen above.
Mycobacterium marinum	Cutaneous infection	None, if minor; rifampin, trimethoprim-sulfamethoxazole, clarithromycin, or doxycycline[b] for moderate disease; extensive lesions may require surgical débridement. Susceptibility testing not routinely required.
Mycobacterium ulcerans	Cutaneous and bone infections	Rifampin and clarithromycin for 8 weeks; excision to remove necrotic tissue, if present; potential response to thermotherapy.

Table 3.88. Treatment of Nontuberculous Mycobacteria Infections in Children,[a] continued

Organism	Disease	Initial Treatment
Rapidly Growing Species[a]		
Mycobacterium fortuitum complex	Cutaneous infection	Initial therapy for serious disease is amikacin plus imipenem (or meropenem), IV. When starting oral therapy, options often include doxycycline,[b] trimethoprim-sulfamethoxazole, or ciprofloxacin.[c] Antimicrobial selection should be based on in vitro susceptibility testing. May require surgical excision.
	Catheter infection	Catheter removal; amikacin plus meropenem, IV; oral options often include trimethoprim-sulfamethoxazole or ciprofloxacin.[c] Antimicrobial selection should be based on in vitro susceptibility testing.
Mycobacterium abscessus	Otitis media; cutaneous infection	For macrolide-susceptible isolates, 3 or more drugs guided by drug susceptibility test results. Example regimen include azithromycin or clarithromycin plus initial course of amikacin, imipenem or meropenem, cefoxitin, or tigecycline[d] for at least 2 months, followed by 2 or more oral drugs guided by drug susceptibility test results. For macrolide resistant (mutational or inducible) isolates, 4 or more drugs guided by drug susceptibility test results. May require surgical débridement; expert consultation is advised.
	Pulmonary infection (in cystic fibrosis)	Regimen options as above; may include inhaled drugs; may require surgical resection although rarely performed in people with cystic fibrosis; expert consultation advised.
Mycobacterium chelonae	Catheter infection, prosthetic valve endocarditis	Catheter removal; débridement, removal of infected foreign material; valve replacement; and tobramycin (initially), imipenem or meropenem, plus azithromycin or clarithromycin, and linezolid or clofazimine.
	Disseminated cutaneous infection	Tobramycin (initially), imipenem or meropenem, plus azithromycin or clarithromycin, and linezolid or clofazimine.

IV indicates intravenously; MIC, minimum inhibitory concentration.

[a] Treatment always includes 2 or more drugs.

[b] Doxycycline can be used without regard to patient age.

[c] See Fluoroquinolones, p 973.

[d] Experience with using tigecycline in children is limited; it should not be used in children younger than 8 years if there are effective alternatives, because there may be reversible inhibition of bone growth and adverse effects on tooth development. Tigecycline also has a black box warning for an increase in all-cause mortality and should be reserved for situations where alternative agents are not suitable.

The natural history of NTM lymphadenitis without curative surgical excision is slow resolution but with a high risk of spontaneous drainage through the skin and resulting scarring, even when antimicrobial management is used. Joint decision making with the parent(s) and possibly the child depending on age, and the surgeon and pediatric infectious disease consultant are important in developing the best treatment plan for each patient.

The choice of drugs, dosages, and duration should be reviewed with a consultant experienced in the management of NTM infections but always includes 2 or more drugs to which the organism is susceptible (see Table 3.88). Infected indwelling foreign bodies must be removed, and surgical débridement for serious localized disease is optimal, especially for infections caused by *M abscessus*. Clinical isolates of MAC usually are resistant to many of the approved antituberculosis drugs, including isoniazid but generally are susceptible to azithromycin and clarithromycin with variable susceptibility to ethambutol, rifabutin or rifampin, amikacin, or streptomycin. Secondary agents include moxifloxacin and linezolid; susceptibility testing to these other agents has not been correlated with clinical outcomes, so they are not recommended routinely. Isolates of rapidly growing mycobacteria (*M fortuitum, M abscessus,* and *M chelonae*) should be tested in vitro against drugs to which they commonly are susceptible and that have been used with some therapeutic success (eg, amikacin, imipenem, sulfamethoxazole or trimethoprim-sulfamethoxazole, cefoxitin, ciprofloxacin, clarithromycin, linezolid, clofazimine, doxycycline, and tigecycline, although tigecycline has a black box warning for an increase in all-cause mortality and should be reserved for situations in which alternative agents are not suitable). Additionally, evidence of inducible macrolide resistance should be investigated by extending the culture incubation to 14 days or identifying the *erm* gene with sequencing or line-probe assay.

Patients receiving therapy should be monitored for evidence of treatment response and adverse drug reactions. Patients receiving clarithromycin plus rifabutin or high-dose rifabutin (with another drug) should be observed for rifabutin-related development of leukopenia, uveitis, polyarthralgia, and pseudojaundice.

The duration of therapy for NTM infections depends on host status, site(s) of involvement, severity of disease, and response to therapy. Most patients who respond ultimately show substantial clinical improvement in the first 4 to 6 weeks of therapy. Elimination of the organisms from blood cultures can take longer, often up to 12 weeks. Most experts recommend a minimum treatment duration of 3 to 6 months, but longer therapy is often required. In patients with cystic fibrosis who have NTM pulmonary disease, the duration of therapy is 12 months beyond achievement of culture negativity.

For patients with cystic fibrosis and isolation of MAC species, treatment is suggested only for those with clinical symptoms not attributable to other causes, worsening lung function, and chest radiographic progression. The decision to initiate therapy should take into consideration susceptibility testing results and should involve consultation with a specialist in cystic fibrosis care.

In children with living with HIV infection and in other immunocompromised patients with disseminated MAC infection, multidrug therapy is recommended. Treatment of disseminated MAC infection should be undertaken in consultation with an expert because the infections are life threatening and drug-drug interactions may occur between medications used to treat disseminated MAC and HIV.

The optimal time to initiate antiretroviral therapy in a child in whom HIV infection and disseminated MAC are newly diagnosed is not established. Many experts provide treatment of disseminated MAC for 2 weeks before initiating antiretroviral therapy in an attempt to minimize occurrence of the immune reconstitution syndrome and minimize confusion relating to the cause of drug-associated toxicity.

Chemoprophylaxis. The most effective way to prevent disseminated MAC in children living with HIV infection is to preserve their immune function through use of antiretroviral therapy. Children living with HIV infection who have advanced immunosuppression should be offered prophylaxis against disseminated MAC with azithromycin or clarithromycin based on their CD4+ T-lymphocyte counts, provided disseminated MAC has been excluded by a negative blood culture in AFB-specific blood culture bottles.[1] Combination therapy for prophylaxis should be avoided in children, if possible, because it has not been shown to be cost-effective and increases rates of adverse events. Children with a history of disseminated MAC and continued immunosuppression should receive lifelong prophylaxis to prevent recurrence. Prophylaxis can be discontinued in some children living with HIV infection after immune reconstitution as detailed in the guidelines for opportunistic infections in children.[1] For adolescents who are diagnosed with HIV infection, MAC prophylaxis does not need to be started if antiretroviral therapy is immediately started after the HIV diagnosis. Adolescents who are not receiving antiretroviral therapy or are viremic on antiretroviral therapy with no current options for a fully suppressive antiretroviral therapy regimen should receive MAC prophylaxis if they have CD4+ T-lymphocyte counts <50 cells/mm^3. MAC prophylaxis can be discontinued for adolescents after immune reconstitution, as detailed in the HIV guidelines for opportunistic infections.[2]

INFECTION PREVENTION AND CONTROL MEASURES IN HEALTH CARE SETTINGS: Standard precautions are recommended. For patients with cystic fibrosis see recommendations from the Cystic Fibrosis Foundation.[3]

CONTROL MEASURES: Control measures include chemoprophylaxis for high-risk patients living with HIV infection (see Treatment, p 924) and avoidance of tap water contamination of central venous catheters, dental procedures, surgical procedures and

---

[1] Panel on Opportunistic Infections in Children with and Exposed to HIV. Guidelines for the Prevention and Treatment of Opportunistic Infections in Children with and Exposed to HIV. Department of Health and Human Services. Available at: **https://clinicalinfo.hiv.gov/en/guidelines/pediatric-opportunistic-infection**

[2] Panel on Guidelines for the Prevention and Treatment of Opportunistic Infections in Adults and Adolescents with HIV. Guidelines for the Prevention and Treatment of Opportunistic Infections in Adults and Adolescents with HIV. National Institutes of Health, Centers for Disease Control and Prevention, HIV Medicine Association, and Infectious Diseases Society of America. Available at: **https://clinicalinfo.hiv.gov/en/guidelines/adult-andadolescent-opportunistic-infection**

[3] The Cystic Fibrosis Foundation has additional recommendations for infection prevention and control in patients with cystic fibrosis, regardless of respiratory tract culture results: Saiman L, Seigel JD, LiPuma JJ, et al. Infection prevention and control guideline for cystic fibrosis: 2013 update. *Infect Control Hosp Epidemiol.* 2014;35(Suppl 1): S1-S67. Available at: **www.cff.org/Care/Clinical-Care-Guidelines/Infection-Prevention-and-Control-Clinical-Care-Guidelines/Infection-Prevention-and-Control-Clinical-Care-Guidelines/**

wounds, injections and injectable medications, skin, or endoscopic equipment and other medical devices.

FDA instructions are available regarding the use of filtered water (not tap water) for heater-cooler devices and other recommendations related to these devices (**www.fda.gov/medical-devices/what-heater-cooler-device/recommendations-use-any-heater-cooler-device**). If heater-cooler devices are implicated in *M chimaera* infection or have been or are to be used in cardiac surgeries, patients should be informed (preferably before their surgery) of the risk and monitored after surgery for signs and symptoms suggestive of infection. These devices are also used for extracorporeal membrane oxygenation (ECMO), but to date no cases related to use in this setting have been reported. If *M chimaera* or any NTM is suspected or documented to be potentially associated with a device, an FDA medical device report should be filed with MedWatch (see MedWatch – the FDA Safety Information and Adverse Event-Reporting Program, p 1113).

Tularemia

CLINICAL MANIFESTATIONS: There are several common presentations of tularemia in children, with ulceroglandular disease being the most frequently identified. Characterized by a maculopapular lesion at the entry site with subsequent ulceration and slow healing, the ulceroglandular variant is associated with tender regional lymphadenopathy that can drain spontaneously. The glandular variant (regional lymphadenopathy with no ulcer) also is common. Less common disease variants include oculoglandular (severe conjunctivitis with preauricular lymphadenopathy), oropharyngeal (exudative stomatitis, painful pharyngitis, or tonsillitis with cervical lymphadenopathy), typhoidal (high fever, septicemia, possible splenomegaly or hepatomegaly), and meningitis. Secondary skin eruptions, which can include vesicular skin lesions, can be mistaken for herpes simplex virus or varicella zoster virus cutaneous infections. Pneumonic tularemia presents with fever, dry or productive cough, chest pain, and hilar adenopathy with or without chest abnormalities. Pneumonic tularemia is normally caused by inhalation of contaminated dust or aerosols often associated with farming or lawn maintenance activities; it can also occur when other forms of tularemia remain untreated and spread through the bloodstream to the lungs. Pneumonic tularemia would be the anticipated variant after intentional release of aerosolized organisms.

ETIOLOGY: *Francisella tularensis* is a small, weakly staining, gram-negative pleomorphic coccobacillus. Two subspecies cause human infection in North America: *F tularensis* subspecies *tularensis* (type A), and *F tularensis* subspecies *holarctica* (type B). Type A is generally considered more virulent, especially if inhaled. In the absence of effective chemotherapy, inhalation of small numbers of type A bacteria has a mortality rate of >30%. Therefore, in this situation, rapid diagnosis and chemotherapy is critical.

EPIDEMIOLOGY: *F tularensis* can infect more than 100 animal species; the vertebrate species considered most important in enzootic cycles are lagomorphs (rabbits and hares) and rodents (especially muskrats, voles, beavers, and prairie dogs). Domestic cats and dogs are an additional but uncommon source of infection. In the United States, most human cases are attributed to tick bites but may also result from bites of other arthropod vectors, such as deer flies, or direct contact with any of the aforementioned animal species. Infections attributable to tick and deer fly bites usually take the form of ulceroglandular or glandular tularemia. *F tularensis* bacteria can be transmitted to humans via the skin when handling infected animal tissue, as can occur when hunting or skinning infected rabbits, muskrats, prairie dogs, and other rodents. Infection has been reported in commercially traded hamsters and prairie dogs. Infection also can be acquired following ingestion of contaminated water (including contaminated well water) or inadequately cooked meat, or by inhalation of contaminated aerosols generated during lawn mowing, brush cutting, or certain farming activities (eg, baling contaminated hay). At-risk people have occupational or recreational exposure to infected animals or their habitats; this includes rabbit hunters and trappers, people exposed to certain ticks or biting insects, and laboratory technicians working with *F tularensis,* which is highly infectious and may be aerosolized when grown in culture. In the United States, most cases occur from May through September. Approximately two thirds of cases occur in male individuals, and one quarter of cases occur in children younger than 15 years of age.

Tularemia has been reported in all US states except Hawaii. It is most common in central and western states and parts of Massachusetts (particularly Martha's Vineyard). In 2019, a total of 274 cases in the United States were reported.

Organisms can be present in blood during the first 2 weeks of disease and in cutaneous lesions for as long as 1 month if untreated. Person-to-person transmission has not been reported.

The **incubation period** usually is 3 to 5 days, with a range of 1 to 21 days.

DIAGNOSTIC TESTS: Because of its propensity for causing laboratory-acquired infections, laboratory personnel should be alerted immediately when *F tularensis* infection is suspected. Isolation of *F tularensis* confirms infection and is most successful from specimens of ulcers, lymph node aspirates or biopsies, pleural fluid and/or other respiratory tract specimens, pharyngeal swabs, or blood depending on the form of illness, and is best achieved by inoculation of cysteine-enriched media. Blood cultures are often negative. Biosafety level 2 practices are recommended for initial activities involving clinical specimens. If tularemia is suspected on the basis of clinical and epidemiological history or Gram stain identification of tiny gram-negative coccobacilli, biological safety level (BSL)-3 practices, containment equipment, and facilities are recommended for all manipulations of suspect cultures. All isolates suspected to be *F tularensis* should be discussed with the state public health agency and forwarded for confirmation to local reference laboratories (usually the state laboratory) that are part of the Laboratory Response Network.

F tularensis in clinical samples can be identified by a laboratory-developed and validated nucleic acid amplification test (NAAT). Immunohistochemical staining is specific for detection of *F tularensis* in fixed tissues; however, this method is not available in most clinical laboratories.

Diagnosis is established most often by serologic testing. Patients do not develop antibodies until the second week of illness. Serologic assays include microagglutination, tube agglutination, enzyme-linked immunosorbent assay, and indirect immunofluorescence assy. Confirmatory serologic laboratory evidence includes a fourfold or greater change in serum antibody titer to *F tularensis* antigen between acute and convalescent specimens. Seroconversion from negative to positive immunoglobulin (Ig) M and/or IgG antibodies in paired sera is also indicative of infection. A single elevated serum antibody titer to *F tularensis* antigen, collected at least 14 days after illness onset, is supportive of the diagnosis, but can also occur with past infection. Additional information on confirmatory and supportive laboratory diagnosis is available at **www.cdc. gov/tularemia/clinicians/index.html.**

TREATMENT: Gentamicin (2.5 mg/kg/dose, administered 3 times daily, intravenously or intramuscularly, with the dose adjusted to maintain the desired peak serum concentrations of at least 5 µg/mL) is the drug of choice for the treatment of tularemia in children because of the limited availability of streptomycin and the fewer adverse effects of gentamicin. Gentamicin administered as a once daily dose, rather than divided, may be considered in consultation with an expert in infectious diseases. The usual duration of therapy is 10 to 14 days. A 7-day course may be sufficient in mild disease, but a longer course is required for more severe illness (eg, meningitis). Because of the difficulty in achieving adequate cerebrospinal fluid concentrations of gentamicin, combination therapy of gentamicin plus ciprofloxacin or gentamicin plus doxycycline may be considered for patients with tularemia meningitis (see Tables of Antibacterial Drug Dosages, p 987, and **www.cdc.gov/tularemia/clinicians/ index.html**). Suppuration of lymph nodes can occur despite antimicrobial therapy.

Oral ciprofloxacin is an alternative for mild to moderate disease, but it is not approved by the US Food and Drug Administration for the treatment of tularemia. Doxycycline is associated with a higher rate of relapse compared with other therapies and is not recommended for definitive treatment; if doxycycline is used, some experts recommend extending treatment to 21 days. *F tularensis* is not susceptible to beta-lactam drugs, including carbapenems.

Because treatment delay is associated with therapeutic failure, treatment should be initiated as soon as tularemia is suspected. Clinically relevant resistance to antimicrobials recommended for treatment of tularemia has not been identified in the United States; when treatment failures occur, they are likely related to delays in treatment or inadequate antimicrobial penetration of infected tissue.

INFECTION PREVENTION AND CONTROL MEASURES IN HEALTH CARE SETTINGS: Standard precautions are recommended.

CONTROL MEASURES:
- People should protect themselves against arthropod bites by wearing protective clothing, by frequent inspection for and removal of ticks from the skin and scalp, and by using insect repellents (see Prevention of Mosquito-borne and Tick-borne Infections, p 207).
- Drinking untreated surface water should be avoided.
- Gloves should be worn by those handling the carcasses of wild rabbits, muskrats, prairie dogs, and other potentially infected animals. Children should not handle sick or dead animals, including pets.
- People should avoid mowing over live or dead animals because this may aerosolize infective material.
- Game meats should be cooked thoroughly.
- Primary clinical specimens may be handled in the laboratory using BSL-2 precautions. BSL-3 precautions are recommended for all manipulations of suspect cultures. Note that *F tularensis* is a tier 1 select agent and must be handled as such after it has been identified. Additional information on laboratory safety can be found in the Centers for

Disease Control and Prevention (CDC) Biosafety in Microbiological and Biomedical Laboratories manual (**www.cdc.gov/biosafety/publications/bmbl5/**).

- Standard precautions should be used for handling clinical materials.
- Oral doxycycline or ciprofloxacin for 10 to 14 days is recommended for children and adults after exposure to an intentional release of tularemia (eg, a bioterrorism attack) and for laboratory workers with inadvertent exposure to *F tularensis*.

Public Health Reporting. Tularemia is a nationally notifiable condition; a suspected case should be reported immediately to the state or local health department.

Louse-borne Typhus
(Epidemic or Sylvatic Typhus)

CLINICAL MANIFESTATIONS: Louse-borne or epidemic typhus is an uncommon disease that is spread through contact with infected human body lice. Patients develop abrupt onset of high fever, chills, and myalgia accompanied by severe headache and malaise. A rash often develops by day 4 to 7 after the start of illness but may not always be present and should not be relied on for diagnosis. When present, the rash usually begins on the trunk and axilla, spreads centrifugally to the limbs, and generally spares the face, palms, and soles. The rash typically is macular to maculopapular but in advanced stages can become petechial or hemorrhagic. The rash can be difficult to observe on patients with darkly pigmented skin and is absent in up to 40% of patients. There is no eschar, as might be present in many other rickettsial diseases. Abdominal complaints (stomach pain, nausea) and changes in mental status are common, including delirium, drowsiness, seizures, and coma. Cough and tachypnea may be present. Myocardial and renal failure can occur when disease is severe. The fatality rate in untreated people can exceed 30%, particularly among persons who are malnourished and those without access to supportive care. Mortality is less common in children and increases with advancing age. Untreated patients who recover typically have an illness lasting 2 weeks.

Brill-Zinsser disease is a recrudescent form of epidemic typhus that is unrelated to louse infestation. It can occur years after the initial episode, and generally occurs when the body's immune system is weakened from illness, medications, advanced age, or stress. The symptoms of Brill-Zinsser disease generally are milder in nature and shorter in duration than the initial infection.

Laboratory abnormalities in epidemic typhus may include thrombocytopenia, increased hepatic enzymes, hyperbilirubinemia, and elevated blood urea nitrogen.

ETIOLOGY: Epidemic typhus is caused by *Rickettsia prowazekii*, which are gram-negative obligate intracellular bacteria.

EPIDEMIOLOGY: Epidemic typhus is transmitted by the human body louse (*Pediculus humanus corporis*), which is infected through feeding on patients with acute typhus fever. Humans are the primary reservoir of the organism. Infected lice generally defecate during feeding and excrete the bacteria in their feces. Disease transmission can occur when infected louse feces are rubbed into broken skin or mucous membranes or are inhaled. All ages can be affected. Poverty, crowding, and poor sanitary conditions such as those found in war, famine, drought, and other natural disasters contribute to the spread of body lice and, hence, the disease. Cases have occurred throughout the world, including the colder, mountainous areas of Asia, Africa, some parts of Europe, and Central and South America, particularly in refugee camps and jails in resource-limited countries. Epidemic typhus is most common during winter months, when conditions favor person-to-person transmission of the vector. The last known epidemic of louse-borne typhus in the United States occurred in 1921. Sporadic human cases associated with close contact with infected flying squirrels *(Glaucomys volans)*, their nests, or their ectoparasites occasionally are reported in the eastern United States. Cases have been reported in people who reside or work in flying squirrel-infested dwellings, even when direct contact is not reported. Flying squirrel-associated disease, called sylvatic typhus, typically presents with a similar but generally milder illness to that observed with body louse-transmitted infection. Untreated illness can be severe, although no fatal cases of sylvatic typhus have been reported; the later development of Brill-Zinsser disease has been confirmed in at least 1 case of untreated sylvatic typhus.

People with Brill-Zinsser disease harbor active *R prowazekii* and, therefore, may pose a risk for reintroduction of the organism and new outbreaks. Rickettsiae are present in the blood and tissues of patients during the early febrile phase but are not found in secretions. Direct person-to-person spread of the disease does not occur in the absence of the louse vector.

The **incubation period** is 1 to 2 weeks.

DIAGNOSTIC TESTS: Louse-borne typhus may be diagnosed via indirect immunofluorescence antibody (IFA) assay; immunohistochemistry (IHC); a nucleic acid amplification test (NAAT) of blood, plasma, or tissue samples; or isolation by culture. Serologic tests are the most common means of confirmation and can be used to detect either immunoglobulin (Ig) G or IgM antibodies. The specimen preferably should be obtained within the first week of symptoms and before (or within 24 hours of) doxycycline administration. Detectable levels of IgG and IgM antibodies generally do not appear until around 7 to 10 days after onset of symptoms, so a negative test result early in the disease does not rule out infection. The gold standard for serologic diagnosis of louse-borne typhus is a fourfold increase in IgG antibody titer by the IFA test between acute sera obtained in the first week of illness and convalescent sera obtained 2 to 4 weeks later. Low-level antibody titers may persist in persons for years; therefore, only a change in titer in paired samples is diagnostic of recent infection. People with Brill-Zinsser disease generally show an elevation in their IgG but not IgM antibody concentrations to *R prowazekii*. Cross-reactivity may be observed to antibodies to *Rickettsia typhi* (the agent of endemic typhus) and, to a lesser degree, *Rickettsia rickettsii* (the etiologic agent of Rocky Mountain spotted fever) and other spotted fever group rickettsiae. *R prowazekii* also may be cultured and identified through submission to specific reference laboratories that are equipped to culture and identify epidemic typhus. Cell culture cultivation of the organism must be confirmed by molecular methods. NAATs can detect *Rickettsia prowazekii* in acute whole blood, serum, or tissue specimens, but sensitivity is lower during the first few days of the illness or following 48 hours of doxycycline therapy. Treatment should never be withheld pending results of diagnostic tests. Because epidemic typhus is not common in the United States, testing generally is not available at commercial laboratories but can be performed at the Centers for Disease Control and Prevention through submission by state health departments.

TREATMENT: Because of the rapid progression of louse-borne typhus, treatment should not be delayed pending diagnostic results in patients who present with clinically and epidemiologically compatible disease. Doxycycline is the drug of choice to treat louse-borne typhus, regardless of patient age. The recommended dosage of doxycycline for adults is 100 mg, twice per day, intravenously or orally, and for children weighing less than 45 kg (100 lb) is 2.2 mg/kg per dose, administered twice a day (maximum 100 mg/dose [see Tetracyclines, p 975]). Treatment should be continued for at least 3 days after clinical defervescence and evidence of clinical improvement is documented; the total treatment course usually is 7 to 10 days. Some patients may relapse if not treated for the full 7 to 10 days. Patients treated early may experience less severe illness and shorter recovery time. Chloramphenicol, where available, may be used in cases of absolute contraindication of doxycycline (life-threatening allergy) but also carries significant risks (ie, aplastic anemia). In epidemic situations in which antimicrobial agents have limited availability (eg, refugee camps), a single 200-mg dose of doxycycline in adults (or 4.4 mg/kg, maximum dose 200 mg, as a single dose for children) may provide effective treatment and facilitate outbreak control when combined with delousing efforts.

INFECTION PREVENTION AND CONTROL MEASURES IN HEALTH CARE SETTINGS: Standard precautions are recommended after delousing has been completed. Precautions should be taken when delousing hospitalized patients infected with *R prowazekii* using pediculicide, because aerosolized louse feces associated with these patients pose an exposure risk. Therefore, health care providers initially caring for these patients and handling potentially contaminated clothing should consider wearing an N95 or higher respirator (or similar respiratory protection) and eye protection.

CONTROL MEASURES: Thorough delousing in epidemic situations, particularly among exposed contacts of cases, is recommended. Several applications of pediculicides may be needed, because lice eggs are resistant to most insecticides. Washing clothes in hot water kills lice and eggs. During epidemics, insecticides dusted onto clothes of louse-infested populations are effective. In situations involving outbreaks of epidemic typhus in prisons and refugee settings, active surveillance for fever is important to assess efficacy of control measures and to ensure rapid and effective treatment. To halt the spread of disease to other people, louse-infested patients should be treated with cream or gel pediculicides containing pyrethrins or permethrin; malathion is prescribed most often when pyrethroids fail. Prevention and control of flying squirrel-associated typhus requires application of insecticides and precautions to prevent contact with these animals and their ectoparasites and to exclude them from nesting in, or entering into, human dwellings. No prophylaxis is recommended for people exposed to flying squirrels.

Public Health Reporting. *R prowazekii* is considered a select agent and a category B potential biological terrorism agent requiring additional regulation and oversight for its storage, use, and transfer. Cases should be reported to local, state, regional, or national public health departments.

Murine Typhus
(Endemic or Flea-borne Typhus)

CLINICAL MANIFESTATIONS: Murine typhus, also known as endemic typhus or flea-borne typhus, resembles epidemic (louse-borne) typhus but usually has a less abrupt onset with less severe systemic symptoms. The disease can be mild in young children. Fever, present in almost all patients, can be accompanied by myalgia and a persistent, usually severe, headache. Nausea, vomiting, anorexia, and abdominal pain and tenderness also develop in approximately half of patients. A macular or maculopapular rash appears by day 4 to 7 of illness in approximately 50% of patients and lasts 4 to 8 days. The rash often is distributed on the patient's trunk, although extremities also can be involved. Untreated illness seldom lasts longer than 2 weeks. The clinical course is usually uncomplicated, but severe manifestations, such as sepsis or central nervous system abnormalities (eg, meningitis), are possible. Laboratory findings can include thrombocytopenia, elevated liver aminotransferases, hypoalbuminemia, hypocalcemia, and hyponatremia. Fatal outcome is rare but has been reported in up to 4% of hospitalized patients.

ETIOLOGY: Murine typhus is caused by *Rickettsia typhi,* which are gram-negative obligate intracellular bacteria.

EPIDEMIOLOGY: Rats, in which infection is inapparent, are the natural reservoirs for *R typhi*. The disease is worldwide in distribution and tends to occur most commonly in male adults; male and female children are affected equally. Outside the United States, the primary vector for transmission among rats and transmission to humans is the rat flea, *Xenopsylla cheopis,* although other fleas and mites have been implicated. A suburban cycle has emerged in the United States involving primarily cat fleas *(Ctenocephalides felis),* mouse fleas *(Leptopsylla segnis),* and fleas from opossums (often cat fleas) and other peridomestic species. Infection occurs when infected flea feces are rubbed into broken skin or mucous membranes or are inhaled. Murine typhus is uncommon in most of the United States; most diagnosed cases occur during spring to early fall and in southern California, southern Texas, the southeastern Gulf Coast, and Hawaii.

The **incubation period** is 6 to 14 days.

DIAGNOSTIC TESTS: Serologic testing for *R typhi* by an indirect immunofluorescence antibody (IF) assay is the most common means of diagnosis. Enzyme immunoassay or latex agglutination tests also are available. Antibody concentrations peak at around 4 weeks after infection, but results of antibody tests may be negative early in the course of illness. A fourfold increase in immunoglobulin (Ig) G titer between acute and convalescent serum specimens obtained 2 to 4 weeks apart is confirmatory for laboratory diagnosis. Use of IgM assays alone is not recommended. Because of cross-reactivity, standard serologic tests might not differentiate murine typhus caused by *R typhi* from epidemic (louse-borne) typhus (*Rickettsia prowazekii*) or from infection with spotted fever rickettsiae, such as *Rickettsia rickettsii*. More specific testing with antibody cross-adsorption assay or western blot analyses is not available routinely. Routine hospital blood cultures are not suitable for culture of *R typhi*. Nucleic acid amplification tests (NAATs) can detect *R typhi* and distinguish murine and epidemic typhus and other rickettsioses in acute whole blood, serum, and skin biopsies, but sensitivity is lower during the first few days of illness or following 48 hours of antibiotic treatment. Because murine typhus is not common in many regions of the United States, testing may not be available at commercial labs but can be performed at the Centers for Disease Control and Prevention through submission by state health departments.

TREATMENT: Doxycycline is the treatment of choice for murine typhus, regardless of patient age. The recommended dosage of doxycycline for children weighing less than 45 kg (100 lb) is 2.2 mg/kg per dose, administered intravenously or orally, twice a day (maximum 100 mg/dose) and for adults is 100 mg/dose, twice daily (see Tetracyclines, p 975). Early diagnosis should be based on clinical suspicion and epidemiology. In a patient with disease that is clinically compatible with murine typhus, treatment should not be withheld because of a negative laboratory result or while awaiting laboratory confirmation, because severe or fatal infection can develop when treatment is delayed. Treatment should be continued for at least 3 days after defervescence and evidence of clinical improvement is documented. The total treatment course usually is 7 to 14 days. Fluoroquinolones or chloramphenicol are alternative medications but may not be as effective; fluoroquinolones are not approved for this use in children younger than 18 years (see Fluoroquinolones, p 973).

INFECTION PREVENTION AND CONTROL MEASURES IN HEALTH CARE SETTINGS: Standard precautions are recommended.

CONTROL MEASURES: Fleas should be controlled by appropriate insecticides before use of rodenticides because fleas will seek alternative hosts, including humans. Suspected animal populations should be controlled by species-appropriate means, such as avoiding leaving food out for stray or wild animals, flea control on pets, and keeping pets indoors. No prophylaxis is recommended for exposed individuals.

Public Health Reporting. Patients infected with murine typhus should be reported to local or state public health departments.

Ureaplasma urealyticum and *Ureaplasma parvum* Infections

CLINICAL MANIFESTATIONS: The role of *Ureaplasma* species in human disease is controversial. There has been an inconsistent association between presence of *Ureaplasma urealyticum* and nongonococcal urethritis (NGU). Without treatment, the urethritis usually resolves within 1 to 6 months. There also has been an inconsistent relationship of infection by *Ureaplasma* species with prostatitis and epididymitis in male individuals and upper genital tract syndromes in female individuals, including salpingitis, endometritis, and pelvic inflammatory disease.[1] *Ureaplasma* organisms commonly are detected in placentas with histologic chorioamnionitis (now known as intra-amniotic infection), and studies suggest that there is an association of upper genital tract infection by *Ureaplasma* species and adverse pregnancy outcomes. Some reports also describe an association between the presence of *Ureaplasma* in the vaginal flora and preterm birth.

Ureaplasma urealyticum and *Ureaplasma parvum* are frequently isolated from the lower respiratory tract and from lung biopsy specimens of preterm infants, and studies have demonstrated an association of *Ureaplasma* species with the development of bronchopulmonary dysplasia in preterm infants. These organisms also have been recovered from respiratory tract secretions of infants 3 months or younger with pneumonia, but their role in development of lower respiratory tract disease in otherwise healthy young infants is unclear. *Ureaplasma* species have been isolated from the bloodstream of newborn infants and from cerebrospinal fluid of infants with meningitis, intraventricular hemorrhage, and hydrocephalus. The contribution of *U urealyticum* to the outcome of infants with infections of the central nervous system is unclear given the confounding effects of preterm birth and intraventricular hemorrhage.

Cases of *U urealyticum* or *U parvum* arthritis, osteomyelitis, pneumonia, pericarditis, meningitis, and progressive sinopulmonary disease have been reported, almost

---

[1] The terms male, female, men, and women refer to sex assigned at birth.

exclusively in immunocompromised patients. Patients with primary antibody deficiency and solid organ transplants appear to be the major risk groups. A recently described syndrome of *Ureaplasma* sepsis with hyperammonemia (caused by rapid hydrolysis of host urea by the organism) in lung transplant patients appears to be attributable to the introduction of the organism from the transplanted lung into naïve recipients who are immunosuppressed.

ETIOLOGY: *Ureaplasma* organisms are small pleomorphic bacteria that lack a cell wall. The genus contains 2 species capable of causing human infection, *U urealyticum* and *U parvum*. At least 14 serotypes have been described, 4 for *U parvum* and 10 for *U urealyticum*.

EPIDEMIOLOGY: The principal reservoir of human *Ureaplasma* species is the genital tract of sexually active adults. Colonization occurs in more than half of sexually active female individuals; the incidence in sexually active male individuals is lower. Colonization is uncommon in prepubertal children and adolescents who are not sexually active, but a positive genital tract culture is not clearly definitive of sexual abuse. *Ureaplasma* species may colonize the throat, eyes, umbilicus, and perineum of newborn infants and may persist for several months after birth. *U parvum* generally is more common than *U urealyticum* as a colonizer in pregnant people and their offspring.

Because *Ureaplasma* species commonly are isolated from the female lower genital tract and neonatal respiratory tract in the absence of disease, a positive culture does not establish its causative role in acute infection. However, recovery of these organisms from an upper genital tract or lower respiratory tract specimen in the appropriate host who has evidence of clinical disease is much more indicative of true infection.

The **incubation period** after sexual transmission is 10 to 20 days.

DIAGNOSTIC TESTS: Specimens for culture require *Ureaplasma* compatible transport media, with refrigeration at 4°C (39°F). If the specimen cannot be transported to the reference laboratory within 24 hours, the sample should be frozen at −70° C (not −20° C). If a vaginal or urethral swab is used for collection, Dacron or calcium alginate swabs should be used to collect and inoculate transport media; cotton swabs should be avoided. Several rapid, sensitive real-time polymerase chain reaction assays for detection of *U urealyticum* and *U parvum* have been developed. Many of these assays have greater sensitivity than culture, but they are not widely available outside of reference laboratories. Transport medium is not necessary for urine to be tested only by polymerase chain reaction (PCR) assay. Such specimens can be concentrated 10-fold and frozen at −70°C immediately after collection and shipped on dry ice. *Ureaplasma* species can be cultured in urea-containing broth and agar in 2 to 4 days. Serologic testing is of limited value for diagnostic purposes and is not available commercially.

TREATMENT: A positive *Ureaplasma* culture or PCR assay result does not indicate need for therapy if the patient is asymptomatic. *Ureaplasma* species generally are susceptible to macrolides, tetracyclines, and quinolones, but because they lack a cell wall they are not susceptible to penicillins or cephalosporins. They also are not susceptible to trimethoprim-sulfamethoxazole or clindamycin. For symptomatic children, adolescents, and adults, doxycycline can be used for treatment. Doxycycline can be used without regard to patient age; azithromycin is the preferred antimicrobial agent for children younger than 8 years or people who are allergic to tetracyclines. Persistent urethritis after doxycycline treatment may be attributable to doxycycline-resistant *U urealyticum* or *Mycoplasma genitalium*. Recurrences are common, and tetracycline resistance may occur in up to 50% of *Ureaplasma* isolates in some patient populations. If tetracycline resistance is likely, azithromycin is indicated; a quinolone is an option if azithromycin resistance also is possible. On the basis of very limited data, quinolone and macrolide coresistance remains uncommon, at less than 5% in the United States, but up to 10% elsewhere including Australia and Southeast Asia. Such infections are difficult to treat, but pristinamycin (not approved by the US Food and Drug Administration) has proven effective.

In neonates, antimicrobial treatment with erythromycin has generally failed to prevent chronic pulmonary disease in small randomized trials, possibly because erythromycin does not eliminate *Ureaplasma* organisms from the airways in a large proportion of infants. One small randomized trial suggests that bronchopulmonary dysplasia or death may be reduced by azithromycin (10 mg/kg/day for 7 days followed by 5 mg/kg/day for a maximum of 6 weeks). Another recent randomized clinical trial of azithromycin in mechanically ventilated preterm neonates showed significant benefit with respect to death or oxygen requirement at 28 days in infants who received the drug regardless of the presence of *Ureaplasma* species, highlighting the difficulty in defining a possible pathogenic role for *Ureaplasma* species in preterm infants, given that azithromycin has anti-inflammatory as well as antimicrobial properties. Pharmacokinetic studies suggest that a 3-day course of 20 mg/kg/day of intravenous azithromycin may be more effective in clearance of *Ureaplasma* organisms from preterm infants, although efficacy in improving clinical outcomes needs to be demonstrated. Definitive evidence of efficacy of antimicrobial agents in the treatment of central nervous system infections caused by *Ureaplasma* species in infants and children also is lacking. There are reports of preterm infants with *Ureaplasma* species identified in cerebrospinal fluid who have or have not received antimicrobial therapy and who have had documentation of sterilization of cerebrospinal fluid.

INFECTION PREVENTION AND CONTROL MEASURES IN HEALTH CARE SETTINGS: Standard precautions are recommended.

CONTROL MEASURES: None recommended.

Varicella-Zoster Virus Infections

CLINICAL MANIFESTATIONS: Primary infection results in varicella (chickenpox), manifesting in unvaccinated people as a generalized, pruritic, erythematous vesicular rash typically consisting of 250 to 500 lesions in varying stages of development (papules, vesicles) and resolution (crusting), low-grade fever, and other systemic symptoms. Complications include bacterial superinfection of skin lesions with or without bacterial sepsis, pneumonia, central nervous system involvement (acute cerebellar ataxia, encephalitis, stroke/vasculopathy), thrombocytopenia, and rarer complications such as glomerulonephritis, arthritis, and hepatitis. Primary viral pneumonia is uncommon among immunocompetent children but is the most common complication in adults. Varicella tends to be more severe in adults, infants, and adolescents than in other children. Breakthrough cases can occur in immunized children, as described in Active Immunization (p 947), but usually are mild and rash presentation is modified. Reye syndrome may follow varicella, although this outcome has become very rare with the recommendation not to use salicylate-containing compounds (eg, aspirin, bismuth-subsalicylate) in children with chickenpox. In immunocompromised children, progressive, severe varicella may occur with continuing eruption of lesions (sometimes including hemorrhagic skin lesions) along with high fever persisting into the second week of illness and visceral dissemination (ie, encephalitis, hepatitis, and pneumonia). Severe and even fatal varicella has been reported in otherwise healthy children on high-dose corticosteroids (greater than 2 mg/kg/day of prednisone or equivalent) for treatment of asthma and other illnesses.

Varicella-zoster virus (VZV) establishes latency in sensory (dorsal root, cranial nerve, and autonomic including enteric) ganglia during primary VZV infection. This latency occurs with both wild-type VZV and the varicella vaccine strain. Reactivation results in herpes zoster (shingles), typically characterized by grouped vesicular skin lesions on an erythematous base in the unilateral distribution of 1 to 3 contiguous sensory dermatomes, most commonly in the thoracic and lumbar regions, frequently accompanied by localized pain and/or itching. Zoster may also result in cranial neuropathy, particularly in the fifth, seventh, and eighth cranial nerve distributions. Postherpetic neuralgia (PHN), pain that persists after resolution of the zoster rash, may last for weeks to months but is unusual in children. Zoster occasionally becomes disseminated in immunocompromised patients, with lesions appearing outside the primary dermatomes and/or visceral complications. Uncommonly, VZV reactivation occurs in the absence of skin rash (zoster sine herpete); these patients may present with aseptic meningitis, encephalitis, stroke, acute retinal necrosis, or gastrointestinal tract involvement (visceral zoster). Recurrent zoster is rare and should prompt a consideration for an evaluation for immunodeficiency or consideration of an alternative diagnosis. A vesicular rash, especially in the distribution of the trigeminal ganglion or sacral sensory roots, may represent herpes simplex virus infection (so-called zosteriform HSV) and should be assessed virologically (eg, by a nucleic acid amplification test [NAAT] of swabbed material from the base of an unroofed vesicle) to distinguish this from zoster attributable to VZV.

Fetal infection after a pregnant person is infected with varicella during the first or early second trimester of pregnancy occasionally results in fetal death or varicella embryopathy, characterized by limb hypoplasia, cutaneous scarring, eye abnormalities, and damage to the central nervous system (congenital varicella syndrome. The incidence of the congenital varicella syndrome among infants born to persons who experience gestational varicella is approximately 2% when infection occurs between 8 and 20 weeks of gestation. Rarely, cases of congenital varicella syndrome have been reported in infants born to persons infected after 20 weeks of pregnancy, the latest occurring at 28 weeks' gestation. Children infected with VZV in utero may develop zoster early in life without having had extrauterine varicella.

Varicella infection has a higher case fatality rate in infants when varicella infection occurs in the birthing parent from 5 days before to 2 days after delivery, because there is little opportunity for development and transfer of antibody across the placenta prior to delivery, and the infant's cellular immune system is immature.

ETIOLOGY: VZV (also known as human herpesvirus 3) is a member of the *Herpesviridae* family, the subfamily *Alphaherpesvirinae*, and the genus *Varicellovirus*.

EPIDEMIOLOGY: Humans are the only source of infection for this highly contagious virus. Infection occurs when the virus comes in contact with the mucosa of the upper respiratory tract or the conjunctiva of a susceptible person. Person-to-person transmission occurs from contact with lesions from varicella or herpes zoster or from airborne spread. Varicella is more contagious than herpes zoster. There is no evidence of VZV spread from fomites; the virus is extremely labile and is unable to survive for long in the environment. Varicella infection in a household member usually results in infection of almost all susceptible people in that household. Children who acquire their infection at home (secondary family cases) often have more skin lesions than the index case. Health care-associated transmission is well documented.

In temperate climates in the prevaccine era, varicella was a disease with a marked seasonal distribution, with peak incidence during winter and spring mainly among children younger than 10 years. In tropical climates, acquisition of varicella often occurs later, resulting in a significant proportion of susceptible adults. High rates of vaccine coverage in the United States have eliminated discernible seasonality of varicella. Following implementation of universal immunization in the United States in 1995, varicella incidence declined by approximately 98% in all age groups as a result of personal and herd immunity.

The age of peak varicella incidence has shifted from children younger than 10 years to children 10 through 14 years of age. Immunity to wild-type varicella generally is lifelong. Symptomatic reinfection is uncommon. Asymptomatic primary infection is unusual.

Immunocompromised people with primary (varicella) or reactivated (herpes zoster) infection are at increased risk of severe disease. Severe varicella and disseminated zoster are more likely to develop in children with congenital T-lymphocyte defects or acquired immunodeficiency syndrome (AIDS) than in people with B-lymphocyte abnormalities. Other groups of pediatric patients who may experience more severe or complicated varicella include infants, adolescents, patients with chronic cutaneous or pulmonary disorders, and patients receiving systemic corticosteroids or other immunosuppressive therapy or long-term salicylate therapy.

Patients are considered contagious from 1 to 2 days before onset of the rash until all lesions have dried/crusted.

The **incubation period** usually is 14 to 16 days, with a range of 10 to 21 days after exposure to rash. The **incubation period** may be prolonged for as long as 28 days after receipt of varicella-zoster immune globulin or immune globulin intravenous (IGIV) and may be shortened in immunocompromised patients. Varicella can develop after birth in infants born to people with active varicella around the time of delivery; the usual interval from onset of rash in a birthing parent to onset in the neonate is 9 to 15 days.

DIAGNOSTIC TESTS: Diagnostic tests for VZV are summarized in Table 3.89. Vesicular fluid or a scab can be used to identify VZV using a NAAT, which currently is the diagnostic method of choice. During the acute phase of illness, VZV also can be identified by a NAAT of saliva or buccal swab specimens, although viral DNA is more likely to be detected in vesicular fluid or scabs. VZV can be demonstrated by direct fluorescent antibody (DFA) assay, using scrapings of a vesicle base early in the eruption, or by viral isolation in cell culture from vesicular fluid. Viral culture and DFA assay both are much less sensitive than a NAAT. NAATs that discriminate between vaccine-strain and wild-type VZV are available free of charge through the specialized reference laboratory at the Centers for Disease Control and Prevention (CDC), through a safety research program sponsored by Merck & Co, and through the Association of

Table 3.89. Diagnostic Tests for Varicella-Zoster Virus (VZV) Infection

Test	Specimen	Comments
NAAT	Vesicular swabs or scrapings, scabs from crusted lesions, biopsy tissue, CSF	Very sensitive method. Specific for VZV. Methods have been designed that distinguish vaccine strain from wild-type (see text).
DFA	Vesicle scraping, swab of lesion base (must include cells)	Specific for VZV. More rapid and more sensitive than culture, less sensitive than NAAT.
Viral culture	Vesicular fluid, CSF, biopsy tissue	Distinguishes VZV from HSV. Limited availability, requires up to a week for result. Least sensitive.
Serology (IgG)[a]	Acute and convalescent serum specimens for IgG	Specific for VZV. Commercial assays generally have low sensitivity to reliably detect vaccine-induced immunity.
Serology (IgM)	Acute serum specimens for IgM	IgM serology is less specific than IgG serology. IgM inconsistently detected. Not reliable method for routine confirmation.

CSF indicates cerebrospinal fluid; DFA, direct fluorescent antibody; HSV, herpes simplex virus; IgG, immunoglobulin G; IgM, immunoglobulin M; NAAT, nucleic acid amplification test.
[a]See Table 1.19, p 122.

Public Health Laboratories/CDC Vaccine Preventable Diseases Reference Centers (**www.aphl.org/programs/infectious_disease/Pages/VPD.aspx**).

A significant increase (fourfold rise in titer) in serum varicella immunoglobulin (Ig) G antibody between acute and convalescent samples by any standard serologic assay can confirm a diagnosis retrospectively, but this may not reliably occur in immunocompromised people (see Care of Exposed People, p 944). However, diagnosis of varicella by serologic testing seldom is indicated. Commercially available enzyme immunoassay (EIA) tests usually are not sufficiently sensitive to reliably demonstrate a vaccine-induced antibody response, and therefore, routine postvaccination serologic testing is not recommended (see Table 1.19, p 122). Commercial IgM tests are not reliable for routine confirmation or ruling out of acute infection because of potential false-negative and false-positive results.

TREATMENT: Nonspecific therapies for varicella include keeping fingernails short to prevent trauma and secondary bacterial infection from scratching, frequent bathing, application of lotion to reduce pruritus, and acetaminophen for fever. Children with varicella should not receive salicylates or salicylate-containing products (eg, aspirin, bismuth-subsalicylate), because these products increase the risk of Reye syndrome. Salicylate therapy should be stopped, if possible, in an unimmunized child who is exposed to varicella. Treatment with ibuprofen is controversial, because some data suggest an association with life-threatening streptococcal skin infections, perhaps because of delays in recognition, and should be avoided if possible.

The decision to use antiviral therapy and the route and duration of therapy should be determined by host factors and extent of infection. Antiviral drugs have a limited window of opportunity to affect the outcome of VZV infection. In immunocompetent hosts, most virus replication has stopped by 72 hours after onset of rash; the duration of replication may be extended in immunocompromised hosts. Oral acyclovir and valacyclovir are not routinely recommended for otherwise healthy younger children with varicella, because their use results in only a modest decrease in symptoms. Antiviral therapy should be considered for otherwise healthy people at increased risk of moderate to severe varicella, such as unvaccinated people older than 12 years, those with chronic cutaneous or pulmonary disorders, those receiving long-term salicylate therapy, or those receiving short or intermittent courses of corticosteroids. Some experts also recommend use of oral acyclovir or valacyclovir for secondary household cases in which the disease usually is more severe than in the primary case or in children who have immunocompromised household contacts. Acyclovir or valacyclovir therapy should also be considered for children with zoster and the continuing development of new lesions. For recommendations on dosage and duration of therapy, see Non-HIV Antiviral Drugs (p 1044).

The American College of Obstetricians and Gynecologists recommends that pregnant people with varicella should be considered for treatment to minimize morbidity. No controlled data are available that treatment will impact the likelihood or severity of congenital varicella syndrome. Intravenous acyclovir is recommended for pregnant people with serious complications of varicella.

Intravenous acyclovir therapy is recommended for immunocompromised patients, including patients being treated with high-dose corticosteroid therapy for more than 14 days. Therapy initiated early in the course of the illness, especially within 24 hours of rash onset, maximizes benefit. Oral acyclovir should not be used to treat immunocompromised children with varicella because of poor oral bioavailability. In the event of national shortages of intravenous acyclovir (as occurred in 2011–2012 and 2019), intravenous ganciclovir or foscarnet may be reasonable alternatives. Information on current drug shortages in the United States can be found at **www.ashp.org/ shortages**. Valacyclovir (20 mg/kg per dose, with a maximum dose of 1000 mg, administered orally 3 times daily for 5 days) is licensed for treatment of varicella in children 2 through 17 years of age. Some experts have used valacyclovir, with its improved bioavailability compared with oral acyclovir, in selected immunocompromised patients perceived to be at low to moderate risk of developing severe varicella, such as human immunodeficiency virus (HIV)-infected patients with relatively normal concentrations of CD4+ T-lymphocytes and children with leukemia in whom careful follow-up is ensured. Famciclovir is available for treatment of VZV infections in adults, but its efficacy and safety have not been established for children. Although varicella-zoster immune globulin or IGIV, administered shortly after exposure, can prevent or modify the course of disease, immune globulin preparations are not effective treatment once disease is established (see Care of Exposed People, p 944).

Antiviral susceptibility testing is not validated but can be considered in cases of poor response to standard therapy; susceptibility testing requires growth of the virus in cell culture, however, which is challenging with VZV. Infections caused by acyclovir-resistant VZV strains, which generally are rare and limited to immunocompromised hosts with prior prolonged exposure to antiviral therapy or prophylaxis, have been successfully treated with parenteral foscarnet.

CONTROL MEASURES:

Evidence of Immunity to Varicella. Evidence of immunity to varicella includes any of the following:
1. Documentation of age-appropriate immunization
   - Preschool-aged children (ie, age 12 months through 3 years): 1 dose
   - School-aged children, adolescents, and adults: 2 doses
2. Laboratory evidence of immunity or laboratory confirmation of disease[1]
3. Birth in the United States before 1980 (should not be considered evidence of immunity for health care personnel, pregnant people, and immunocompromised people)
4. Diagnosis or verification of a history of varicella or zoster by a health care provider

Isolation and Exclusions

Child Care and School. Children with uncomplicated varicella who have been excluded from school or child care may return when the rash has crusted or, in immunized people without crusts, until no new lesions appear within a 24-hour period. Exclusion of children with zoster whose lesions cannot be covered is based on similar criteria. Zoster lesions that are covered pose little risk to susceptible people, although transmission has been reported.

Hospitalized Patients.

VARICELLA. In addition to standard precautions, airborne and contact precautions are recommended for patients with varicella until all lesions are dry and crusted, typically at least 5 days after onset of rash but a week or longer in immunocompromised patients. In patients with varicella pneumonia, precautions are maintained for the duration of illness. For previously immunized patients with breakthrough varicella with only maculopapular lesions, isolation is recommended until no new such lesions appear within a 24-hour period, even if lesions have not resolved completely. For exposed patients without evidence of immunity (see Evidence of Immunity to Varicella, above), airborne and contact precautions from 8 until 21 days after exposure to the index patient also are indicated; these precautions should be maintained until 28 days after exposure for those who received varicella-zoster immune globulin or IGIV.

ZOSTER. Airborne and contact precautions are recommended for both immunocompetent and immunocompromised patients with disseminated zoster for the duration of illness. Immunocompromised patients with localized disease require airborne and contact precautions until disseminated infection is ruled out. For immunocompetent patients with localized zoster, standard precautions and complete covering of the lesions (if possible) are indicated until all lesions are crusted.

NEWBORN INFANTS. For neonates born to persons with varicella or disseminated zoster, airborne and contact precautions are recommended until 21 days of age or until 28 days of age if varicella-zoster immune globulin or IGIV was administered to the infant. To minimize risk of transmission to the infant, the birthing parent and the infant should be isolated separately until the parent's vesicles have dried, even if the infant has received varicella-zoster immune globulin. Neither wild-type VZV nor Oka vaccine-strain virus has been shown to be transmitted by human milk; expressed/pumped milk from a parent with varicella or zoster can be fed to the infant, provided no lesions are evident on the breast. If the infant develops clinical varicella, the birthing parent may care for the infant. If the neonate is born with varicella, the parent and her newborn infant should be isolated together and discharged home when clinically

---

[1] Commercial assays can be used to assess disease-induced immunity, but they lack sensitivity to detect vaccine-induced immunity (ie, they might yield false-negative results).

stable. Infants whose birthing parent has localized zoster may be in contact with the parent as long as the lesions can be covered. The birthing parent should be advised to practice good hand hygiene before holding the infant.

If an infant is clinically stable for discharge during the potential incubation period and has not yet developed varicella, quarantine to complete the 21- or 28-day period may continue at home after ensuring that all relatives and contacts have evidence of immunity to varicella. If the infant needs to see the health care provider during that period, the office should be notified of the need for airborne and contact precautions.

Infants with congenital varicella do not require isolation if they do not have active skin lesions.

Care of Exposed People. Potential interventions for people without evidence of immunity exposed to a person with varicella or herpes zoster include: (1) varicella vaccine, administered ideally within 3 days but up to 5 days after exposure; (2) when indicated, varicella-zoster immune globulin; or (3) if the child cannot be immunized, preemptive oral valacyclovir or acyclovir starting day 7 after exposure. These options and their use in different settings are discussed in detail below.

Postexposure Immunization. Varicella vaccine should be administered to healthy people without evidence of immunity who are 12 months or older, including adults, as soon as possible, preferably within 3 days and up to 5 days after exposure. This approach may prevent or modify disease. Patients should be counseled that not all close exposures result in infection, so vaccination even after 3 to 5 days following exposure is still warranted.

Passive Immunoprophylaxis. The decision to administer varicella-zoster immune globulin depends on 3 factors: (1) the likelihood that the exposed person is susceptible to varicella; (2) the probability that a given exposure to varicella or zoster will result in infection; (3) the likelihood that complications of varicella will develop if the person is infected. Fig 3.22 identifies what constitutes a significant exposure and people without evidence of immunity who should receive varicella-zoster immune globulin if exposed, including immunocompromised people, pregnant people, and certain newborn infants. Varicella-zoster immune globulin is commercially available in the United States from a broad network of specialty distributors (list available at **www.varizig.com**).

Data are not available regarding the sensitivity and specificity of serologic tests in immunocompromised patients. Detection of VZV IgG after 1 dose of varicella vaccine might not correspond to adequate protection in immunocompromised people, and false-positive results can occur. Therefore, regardless of serologic test results, careful questioning of the child and parents about potential past disease or exposure to disease can be helpful in determining immunity. Administration of varicella-zoster immune globulin is recommended as soon as possible within 10 days to immunocompromised children without evidence of immunity (see Fig 3.22 for dosing). However, the degree and type of immunosuppression should be considered in making this decision, and consultation with pediatric infectious diseases or immunology specialists can assist in decision making.

Patients receiving monthly high-dose IGIV (400 mg/kg or greater) at regular intervals are likely to be protected if the last dose of IGIV was administered 3 weeks or less before exposure.

Any patient to whom varicella-zoster immune globulin is administered to prevent varicella subsequently should receive age-appropriate varicella vaccine, provided that receipt of live vaccines is not contraindicated. Administration of varicella vaccine; measles, mumps, and rubella (MMR) vaccine; and measles, mumps, rubella,

FIG 3.22. MANAGEMENT OF EXPOSURES TO VARICELLA-ZOSTER VIRUS

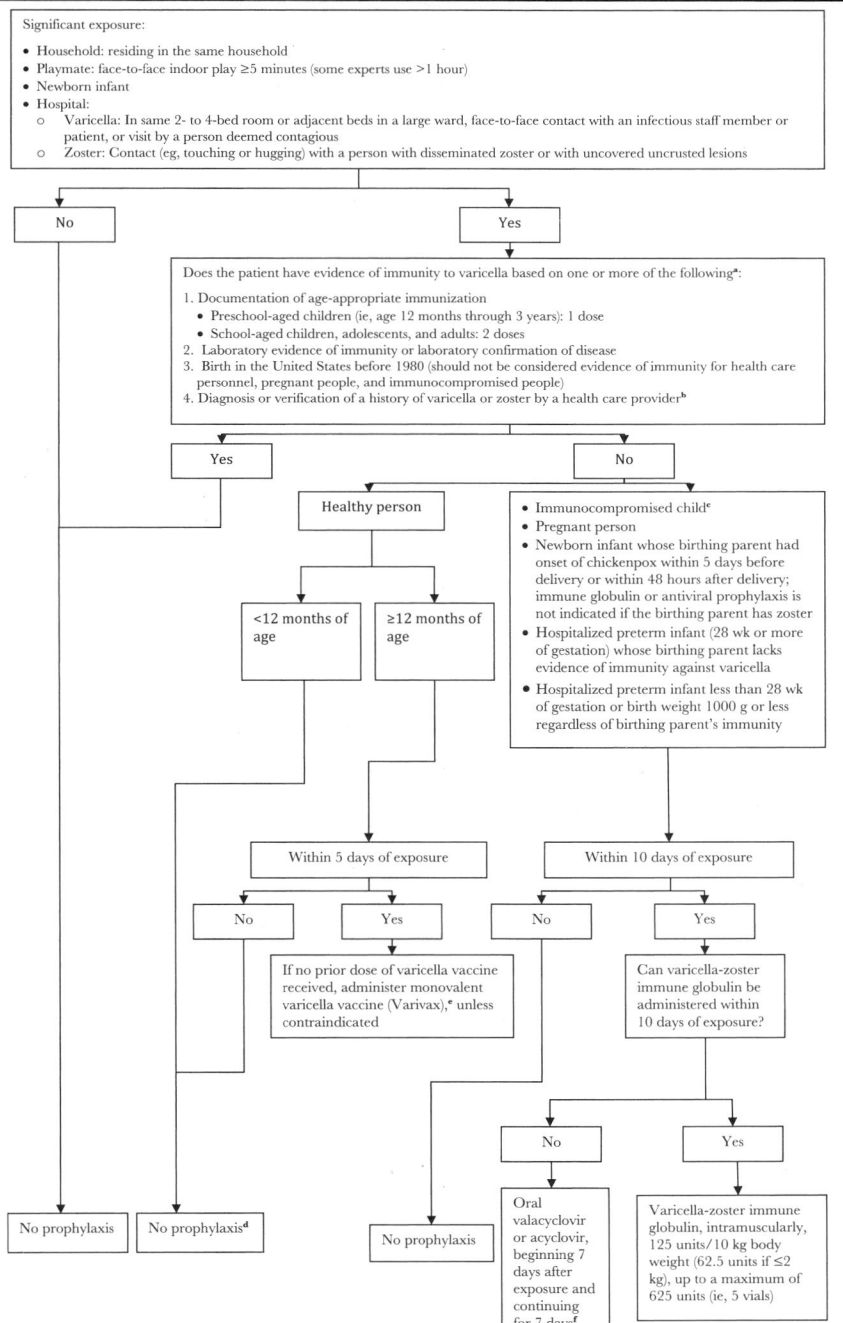

FIG 3.22. MANAGEMENT OF EXPOSURES TO VARICELLA-ZOSTER VIRUS, CONTINUED

IGIV indicates immune globulin intravenous.

[a] People who receive hematopoietic cell transplants should be considered nonimmune regardless of previous history of varicella disease or varicella vaccination in themselves or in their donors.

[b] To verify a history of varicella in an immunocompromised child, health care providers should inquire about an epidemiologic link to another typical varicella case or to a laboratory confirmed case, or evidence of laboratory confirmation. Immunocompromised children who have neither an epidemiologic link nor laboratory confirmation of varicella should not be considered as having a valid history of disease.

[c] Immunocompromised children include those with congenital or acquired T-lymphocyte immunodeficiency, including leukemia, lymphoma, and other malignant neoplasms affecting the bone marrow or lymphatic system; children receiving immunosuppressive therapy, including ≥2 mg/kg/day of systemic prednisone (or its equivalent) for ≥14 days, and certain biologic response modifiers; all children with human immunodeficiency virus (HIV) infection regardless of CD4+ T-lymphocyte percentage; and all hematopoietic cell transplant patients regardless of pretransplant immunity status.

[d] If the exposed person is an adolescent or adult, has chronic illness, or there are other compelling reasons to try to avert varicella, some experts recommend preemptive therapy with oral valacyclovir or acyclovir (see Chemoprophylaxis, below, for dosing). For exposed people ≥12 months of age, vaccination is recommended for protection against subsequent exposures.

[e] If 1 prior dose of varicella vaccine has been received, a second dose should be administered at ≥4 years of age. If the exposure occurred during an outbreak, a second dose is recommended for preschool-aged children younger than 4 years for outbreak control if at least 3 months have passed after the first dose.

[f] See Chemoprophylaxis, below, for dosing. If varicella-zoster immune globulin and either valacyclovir or acyclovir are not available, IGIV may be administered (400 mg/kg).

and varicella (MMRV) vaccine should be delayed until 5 months after varicella-zoster immune globulin administration (see Table 1.11, p 69). Varicella vaccine is not needed if the patient develops varicella despite receipt of varicella-zoster immune globulin.

Chemoprophylaxis. For immunocompromised patients without evidence of immunity or for immunocompetent patients for whom varicella prevention is desired (eg, healthy older adolescent or adult contacts for whom vaccination is not possible) who have been exposed to varicella or herpes zoster (Fig 3.22), valacyclovir (20 mg/kg per dose, administered orally 3 times per day, with a maximum daily dose of 3000 mg), if available and dosage form is tolerable, or acyclovir (20 mg/kg per dose, administered orally 4 times per day, with a maximum daily dose of 3200 mg) may be used as chemoprophylaxis if passive immunoprophylaxis is not utilized. Antiviral treatment should begin 7 days after exposure and should continue for a total of 7 days. No studies of oral prophylaxis have been performed for adults. VZV-seropositive patients receiving intensive and/or myeloablative chemotherapy should routinely receive antiviral prophylaxis; children receiving antiviral prophylaxis or treatment with valganciclovir, ganciclovir, or foscarnet do not require additional antiviral prophylaxis against VZV.

Postexposure Passive Immunization of Children Living With HIV. Children living with HIV who lack evidence of immunity to varicella (eg, serologic evidence of immunity to varicella, or documentation of receipt of 2 doses of varicella vaccine after initiation of ART, or health care provider-confirmed clinical diagnosis of varicella), **or** who have severe immune suppression (for people ≤5 years of age, defined as a CD4+ T-lymphocyte percentage <15%; for people >5 years of age, defined as a CD4+ T-lymphocyte percentage <15% or a CD4+ T-lymphocyte count <200 lymphocytes/mm^3) should receive varicella-zoster immune globulin, if available, ideally within 96 hours but potentially beneficial up to 10 days, after close contact with a person who has chickenpox or shingles (see Human Immunodeficiency Virus Infection, p 489). An alternative to varicella-zoster immune globulin for passive immunization is oral valacyclovir or acyclovir beginning 7 days after exposure, and if this is not available, then IGIV, 400 mg/kg, administered once within 10 days after exposure (see Fig 3.22, p 945). Children who have received IGIV for other reasons within 3 weeks of exposure do not require additional passive immunization.

Hospital Exposures. The CDC recommends health care institutions evaluate employees proactively for evidence of immunity to varicella and establish protocols and recommendations for vaccinating and managing health care personnel following workplace exposures. If exposure to an infected person occurs in the hospital, the following control measures are recommended:

- Health care professionals, patients, and visitors who have been exposed (see Fig 3.22, p 945) and who lack evidence of immunity to varicella should be identified.
- Varicella immunization is recommended for people without evidence of immunity, provided there are no contraindications to vaccine use.
- Varicella-zoster immune globulin should be administered to appropriate candidates (see Fig 3.22, p 945) up to day 10 after exposure.
- If vaccine cannot be administered, varicella-zoster immune globulin or preemptive oral valaciclovir or acyclovir can be considered.
- All exposed patients without evidence of immunity should be discharged as soon as possible. Patients who remain hospitalized should be isolated from day 8 through 21 after exposure or through day 28 if they received varicella-zoster immune globulin.
- Health care professionals who have received 2 doses of vaccine and who are exposed to VZV should self-monitor or be monitored daily during days 8 through 21 after exposure through the employee health program or by infection-control staff to determine clinical status. They should be restricted from work immediately if symptoms such as fever, headache, other constitutional symptoms, or any suspicious skin lesions occur.
- Health care professionals who have received only 1 dose of vaccine and who are exposed to VZV should receive the second dose with a single-antigen live attenuated varicella vaccine (ie, not given in combination as in MMRV vaccine), preferably within 3 to 5 days of exposure, provided at least 4 weeks have elapsed after the first dose. After immunization, management is similar to that of 2-dose vaccine recipients.
- Health care professionals who lack evidence of immunity should receive varicella vaccine as soon as possible and be restricted from work from day 8 through 21 after exposure or through day 28 if they received varicella-zoster immune globulin.
- Previously immunized health care professionals who develop breakthrough infection should be considered infectious until vesicular lesions have crusted or, if they had maculopapular lesions, until no new lesions appear within a 24-hour period.

Exposure of Newborn Infants. Preterm infants and term infants whose birthing parent had varicella in the immediate peripartum period may need varicella-zoster immune globulin (see Fig 3.22, p 945). For healthy term infants exposed postnatally to varicella or zoster outside of the immediate perinatal period, varicella-zoster immune globulin is not indicated. However, some experts advise use of varicella-zoster immune globulin for exposed newborn infants within the first 2 weeks of life whose birthing parent does not have evidence of immunity to varicella.

Active Immunization.[1]

Vaccine. Varicella vaccine is a live attenuated vaccine developed in Japan in the early 1970s by Professor Michiaki Takahashi and licensed in 1995 by the US Food and

---

[1] Centers for Disease Control and Prevention. Prevention of varicella: recommendations of the Advisory Committee on Immunization Practices (ACIP). *MMWR Recomm Rep.* 2007;56(RR-4):1–40

Drug Administration (FDA) for use in healthy people 12 months or older who have not had varicella illness. Quadrivalent MMRV vaccine was licensed in September 2005 by the FDA for use in healthy children 12 months through 12 years of age.

Dose and Administration. The recommended dose of monovalent or quadrivalent varicella-containing vaccines is 0.5 mL, administered subcutaneously or intramuscularly.

Immunogenicity. Approximately 76% to 85% of immunized healthy children older than 12 months develop a humoral immune response to VZV at levels considered associated with protection after a single dose of varicella vaccine. Seroresponse rates and cell-mediated immune responses approach 100% after 2 doses.

Effectiveness. The effectiveness of 1 dose of varicella vaccine is about 82% against any clinical varicella and 98% against severe disease. Two doses of vaccine demonstrated 92% to 95% effectiveness against any clinical varicella.

Simultaneous Administration With Other Vaccines or Antiviral Agents. Varicella-containing vaccines may be administered simultaneously with other childhood immunizations recommended for children 12 through 15 months of age and 4 through 6 years of age (**https://publications.aap.org/redbook/pages/Immunization-Schedules**). If not administered at the same visit or as MMRV vaccine, the interval between administration of a varicella-containing vaccine and MMR vaccine should be at least 28 days (see Table 1.9, p 60). The minimal interval between MMRV vaccine doses is 3 months. Because of susceptibility of vaccine virus to acyclovir, valacyclovir, or famciclovir, these antiviral agents may interfere with immunogenicity and, thus, should be avoided from 1 day before to 21 days (the outer limit of likely viral replication) after receipt of a varicella-containing vaccine.

Adverse Events. Reactions to varicella vaccine generally are mild and occur with an overall frequency of approximately 5% to 35%. Approximately 20% to 25% of immunized children will experience minor injection site reactions (eg, pain, redness, swelling). In approximately 1% to 3% of immunized children, a localized rash develops, and in an additional 3% to 5%, a generalized varicella-like rash develops. These rashes typically consist of 2 to 5 lesions and may be maculopapular rather than vesicular; lesions usually appear 5 to 26 days after immunization, usually at or near the injection site when localized. After MMRV or monovalent varicella vaccine plus MMR, a measles-like rash was reported in 2% to 3% of recipients. Fever was reported in a higher proportion after the first dose of MMRV than after the first dose of monovalent varicella vaccine plus MMR (22% vs 15%, respectively) in young children. Both fever and measles-like rash usually occurred within 5 to 12 days of immunization, were of short duration, and resolved without sequelae.

A slightly increased risk of febrile seizures is associated with the higher likelihood of fever following the first dose of MMRV compared with MMR and monovalent varicella vaccine. One additional febrile seizure is expected to occur per approximately 2300 to 2600 young children immunized with a first dose of MMRV compared with a first dose of MMR and monovalent varicella vaccine. After the second vaccine dose administered in older children (4 to 6 years of age), there were no differences in incidence of fever, rash, or febrile seizures among recipients of MMRV vaccine compared with recipients of simultaneous MMR and varicella vaccines.[1]

---

[1] Centers for Disease Control and Prevention. Use of combination measles, mumps, rubella, and varicella vaccine: recommendations of the Advisory Committee on Immunization Practices (ACIP). *MMWR Recomm Rep.* 2010;59(RR-3):1-12

Breakthrough Disease. Breakthrough disease is defined as a case of infection with wild-type VZV occurring more than 42 days after immunization. Varicella in vaccine recipients usually is very mild, with rash frequently atypical (predominantly maculopapular) with a median of fewer than 50 lesions), a lower rate of fever, and faster recovery than disease in unimmunized children. It may be mistaken for other conditions, such as insect bites or poison ivy.

Herpes Zoster After Immunization. Vaccine-strain VZV can cause herpes zoster in immunocompetent and immunocompromised people. However, data from postlicensure surveillance indicate that the age-specific risk of herpes zoster is much lower among immunocompetent children immunized with varicella vaccine than among children who have had natural varicella infection.

Transmission of Vaccine-Strain VZV. Vaccine-strain VZV transmission to contacts is rare. In all cases in which transmission has occurred, the immunized person had a rash following vaccine. Some experts believe that immunocompromised people with skin lesions that are presumed to be attributable to vaccine virus should receive acyclovir or valacyclovir treatment.

Recommendations for Immunization.

Children 12 Months Through 12 Years of Age. Both monovalent varicella vaccine and MMRV have been licensed for use for healthy children 12 months through 12 years of age.[1] Children in this age group should receive two 0.5-mL doses of monovalent varicella vaccine or MMRV administered subcutaneously or intramuscularly, separated by at least 3 months. However, provided the second dose is administered a minimum 28 days after the first dose, it does not need to be repeated.

All healthy children should receive the first dose of varicella-containing vaccine at 12 through 15 months of age. The second dose of vaccine is recommended routinely when children are 4 through 6 years of age (ie, before a child enters kindergarten or first grade) but can be administered at an earlier age. The American Academy of Pediatrics expresses no preference between MMR plus monovalent varicella vaccine or MMRV for toddlers receiving their first immunization of this kind. Parents should be counseled about the rare possibility of their child developing a febrile seizure 1 to 2 weeks after immunization with MMRV for the first immunizing dose. For the second dose at 4 through 6 years of age, MMRV generally is preferred over MMR plus monovalent varicella to minimize the number of injections. A catch-up second dose of varicella vaccine should be offered to all children 7 years and older who have received only 1 dose.

People 13 Years or Older. Immunocompetent individuals 13 years or older without evidence of varicella immunity should receive two 0.5-mL doses of monovalent varicella vaccine, separated by at least 28 days. For people who previously received only 1 dose of varicella vaccine, a second dose is necessary. Only monovalent varicella vaccine is licensed for use in this age group.

Contraindications and Precautions.

Allergy to Vaccine Components. Varicella vaccine should not be administered to people who have had an anaphylactic or severe allergic reaction to any component of the vaccine, including gelatin and neomycin, or to a previous dose of a varicella-containing vaccine.

---

[1] Centers for Disease Control and Prevention. Use of combination measles, mumps, rubella, and varicella vaccine: recommendations of the Advisory Committee on Immunization Practices (ACIP). *MMWR Recomm Rep.* 2010;59(RR-3):1-12

Immunization of Immunocompromised Patients.

GENERAL RECOMMENDATIONS.[1] Varicella vaccine (as a 2-dose regimen if there is sufficient time) should be administered to immunocompetent patients without evidence of varicella immunity, if it can be administered ≥4 weeks before initiating immunosuppressive therapy. Varicella vaccine should not be administered to highly immunocompromised patients. This includes persons receiving certain immune response mediators (eg, monoclonal antibodies, interleukins, tumor necrosis factor-alpha inhibitors), who either should be immunized before starting therapy or should wait at least 3 months after such therapies to be immunized. Given the increasing number of such therapies, decisions about immunization with live-virus vaccines should be made in consultation with an infectious disease or immunology specialist.

Certain categories of patients (eg, patients with HIV without severe immunosuppression [see HIV Infection, below] or with a primary immune deficiency disorder without defective T-lymphocyte–mediated immunity, such as primary complement component deficiency disorder, isolated impairment of humoral immunity, or chronic granulomatous disease [CGD]) should receive varicella vaccine. Immunodeficiency should be excluded before immunization in children with a family history of hereditary immunodeficiency.

In people with possible altered immunity, only monovalent varicella vaccine (not MMRV) should be used for immunization against varicella. The Oka vaccine strain remains susceptible to acyclovir, and if a high-risk patient develops vaccine-related rash then acyclovir or valacyclovir may be used as treatment.

MALIGNANCY.[1] The interval until immune reconstitution varies with the intensity and type of immunosuppressive therapy, radiation therapy, underlying disease, and other factors, complicating the ability to make a broadly applicable recommendation for an interval after cessation of immunosuppressive therapy when live-virus vaccines can be administered safely and effectively. Current recommendations are for patients to be vaccinated with varicella vaccine when in remission and at least 3 months after cancer chemotherapy, with evidence of restored immunocompetence. In regimens that included anti–B-lymphocyte antibodies, vaccinations should be delayed at least 6 months.

TRANSPLANT RECIPIENTS.[1] A 2-dose series of varicella vaccine should be administered a minimum of 24 months after hematopoietic cell transplant to varicella-seronegative patients who do not have graft-versus-host disease, are considered immunocompetent, and whose last dose of IGIV was 8 to 11 months previously (see Table 1.11, p 69). Varicella reimmunization generally is not recommended for solid organ transplant recipients after transplantation, although this is an evolving area, especially for certain organs.[2,3]

[1] Rubin LG, Levin MJ, Ljungman P, et al. 2013 IDSA clinical practice guideline for vaccination of the immunocompromised host. *Clin Infect Dis.* 2014;58(3):e44-e100

[2] Danziger-Isakov L, Kumar D, AST ID Community of Practice. Vaccination of solid organ transplant candidates and recipients: guidelines from the American Society of Transplantation Infectious Diseases Community of Practice. *Clin Transplant.* 2019;33(9):e13563

[3] Suresh S, Upton J, Green M, et al. Live vaccines after solid organ transplant: proceedings of a consensus meeting, 2018. *Pediatr Transplant.* 2019;23(7):e13571

HIV INFECTION.[1] The live-virus MMR vaccine and monovalent varicella vaccine can be administered to children and adolescents living with HIV without severe immunosuppression. Severely immunocompromised infants, children, adolescents, and young adults living with HIV (for people ≤5 years of age, defined as a CD4+ T-lymphocyte percentage <15%; for people >5 years of age, defined as a CD4+ T-lymphocyte percentage <15% **or** a CD4+ T-lymphocyte count <200 lymphocytes/ mm^3) should not receive measles virus-containing vaccine, because vaccine-related pneumonia has been reported. Eligible children should receive 2 doses of single-antigen varicella vaccine at the appropriate intervals. The quadrivalent MMRV vaccine should not be administered to any infant or child living with HIV, regardless of degree of immunosuppression, because of lack of safety data in this group.

CHILDREN RECEIVING CORTICOSTEROIDS. Varicella vaccine should not be administered to people who are receiving high doses of systemic corticosteroids (2 mg/kg per day or more of prednisone or its equivalent or 20 mg/day of prednisone or its equivalent) for 14 days or more. The recommended interval between discontinuation of high-dose corticosteroid therapy and immunization with varicella vaccine is at least 1 month. Varicella vaccine may be administered to individuals receiving only inhaled, nasal, or topical steroids.

HOUSEHOLDS WITH POTENTIAL CONTACT WITH IMMUNOCOMPROMISED PEOPLE. Household contacts of immunocompromised people should be immunized if they have no evidence of immunity to decrease the likelihood that wild-type VZV will be introduced into the household. No precautions are needed following immunization of healthy people who do not develop a rash. Immunized people in whom a postimmunization rash develops should avoid direct contact with an immunocompromised host who lacks evidence of immunity for the duration of the rash.

Pregnancy and Lactation. Varicella vaccine should not be administered to pregnant people, because the possible effects on fetal development are unknown, although no cases of congenital varicella syndrome or patterns of malformation have been identified after inadvertent immunization of pregnant people. Pregnancy should be avoided for at least 1 month after immunization. A pregnant person or other household member is not a contraindication for immunization of a child in the household. Breastfeeding is not a contraindication to immunization.

Immune Globulin. Whether immune globulin (IG) can interfere with varicella vaccine-induced immunity is unknown, although IG can interfere with immunity induction by measles vaccine. Pending additional data, varicella vaccine should be withheld for the same intervals after receipt of any form of IG or other blood product as for measles vaccine (see Measles, p 570; and Table 1.11, p 69). Additionally, IG should be withheld for at least 2 weeks after receipt of varicella vaccine.

Salicylates. No cases of Reye syndrome have been reported following varicella vaccination, with more than 140 million doses distributed in the United States. However, because use of salicylates during varicella infection is associated with Reye syndrome, the vaccine manufacturer recommends that salicylates be avoided for 6 weeks after administration of varicella vaccine.

---

[1] Panel on Opportunistic Infections in Children with and Exposed to HIV. Guidelines for the Prevention and Treatment of Opportunistic Infections in Children with and Exposed to HIV. Department of Health and Human Services. Available at: **https://clinicalinfo.hiv.gov/en/guidelines/ pediatric-opportunistic-infection**

VIBRIO INFECTIONS

Cholera
(*Vibrio cholerae*)

CLINICAL MANIFESTATIONS: Cholera is characterized by voluminous watery diarrhea and rapid onset of life-threatening dehydration. Hypovolemic shock may occur within hours of the onset of diarrhea. Stools have a characteristic rice-water appearance, are white-tinged with small flecks of mucus, and contain high concentrations of sodium, potassium, chloride, and bicarbonate. Vomiting is a common feature of cholera. Fever and abdominal cramps usually are absent. In addition to dehydration and hypovolemia, common complications of cholera include hypokalemia, metabolic acidosis, and hypoglycemia, particularly in children. Although severe cholera is a distinctive illness characterized by profuse diarrhea and rapid dehydration, people infected with toxigenic *Vibrio cholerae* may have no symptoms or mild to moderate diarrhea lasting 3 to 7 days.

ETIOLOGY: *V cholerae* is a curved or comma-shaped motile gram-negative rod. There are more than 200 *V cholerae* serogroups, some of which carry the cholera toxin (CT) gene and other virulence factors. Although those serogroups with the CT gene and others without the CT gene can cause acute watery diarrhea, only toxin-producing serogroups O1 and O139 have caused epidemic cholera, with the currently circulating 7th pandemic strain of O1 causing the vast majority of cases worldwide. *V cholerae* O1 is classified into 2 biotypes, classical and El Tor, and 2 major serotypes, Ogawa and Inaba. All other serogroups of *V cholerae* are known collectively as *V cholerae* non-O1/non-O139. Toxin-producing strains of *V cholerae* non-O1/non-O139 can cause sporadic cases of severe dehydrating diarrheal illness but have not caused large outbreaks of cholera. Non–toxin-producing strains of *V cholerae* non-O1/non-O139 are associated with sporadic cases of gastroenteritis, sepsis, and rare cases of wound infection (discussed in Other Vibrio Infections, p 955).

EPIDEMIOLOGY: Cholera is an underreported infection, and estimates of the global burden are imprecise. In areas where the disease is endemic, cholera disproportionately affects young children. Cholera also causes explosive epidemics across all age groups in vulnerable populations. These outbreaks occur frequently in the setting of natural or manmade humanitarian disasters. Examples include large epidemics that occurred after the introduction of pandemic *V cholerae* into Haiti in 2010 and into Yemen in 2017. In the United States, cholera is a sporadic disease. Cases resulting from travel to or ingestion of contaminated food transported from regions with endemic cholera have been reported. Domestically acquired cases in the United States have been reported from eating Gulf Coast seafood.

Humans are the only documented natural host, but free-living *V cholerae* organisms can persist in the aquatic environment. Infection primarily is acquired by ingestion of large numbers of organisms from contaminated water or food (particularly raw or undercooked shellfish, raw or partially dried fish, or moist grains or vegetables held at ambient temperature). People with low gastric acidity and those with blood group O are at increased risk of severe cholera infection.

The **median incubation period** usually is 1 to 2 days, with a range of a few hours to 5 days.

DIAGNOSTIC TESTS: *V cholerae* can be cultured from fecal specimens (preferred) or vomitus plated on thiosulfate citrate bile salts sucrose agar. Because most laboratories in the United States do not culture routinely for *V cholerae* or other *Vibrio* organisms, clinicians should request appropriate cultures for clinically suspected cases. Isolates of *V cholerae* should be sent to a state health department laboratory for confirmation and then forwarded to the Centers for Disease Control and Prevention (CDC) for species identification using DNA-based methods, serotyping, and detection of the cholera toxin gene (**www.cdc.gov/laboratory/specimen-submission/detail. html?CDCTestCode=CDC-10119**). Tests to detect serum antibodies to *V cholerae*, such as the vibriocidal assay and an anticholera toxin enzyme-linked immunoassay, are available at the CDC, subject to preapproval. Both assays require submission of acute and convalescent serum specimens and, thus, provide a retrospective diagnosis. A fourfold increase in vibriocidal antibody titers between acute and convalescent sera suggests the diagnosis of cholera. Several commercial tests for rapid antigen detection of *V cholerae* O1 and O139 in stool specimens have been developed. These *V cholerae* O1 and O139 rapid diagnostic tests have sensitivities ranging from approximately 80% to 97% and specificities of approximately 70% to 90% compared with culture on thiosulfate citrate bile salts sucrose agar. Rapid diagnostic tests are not a substitute for stool culture but might provide an indication of a suspect cholera outbreak in regions where stool culture is not immediately available. Multiplex molecular panels have been cleared by the US Food and Drug Administration for detection of various bacteria, parasites, and viruses associated with gastrointestinal tract infections, and some can specifically detect *V cholerae* from unpreserved stool specimens and/or stool specimens preserved in Cary Blair transport media. Culture confirmation is recommended following a positive result from these culture-independent diagnostic testing panels, as low levels of contaminating nucleic acid from media have been reported.

TREATMENT: Timely and appropriate rehydration therapy is the cornerstone of management of cholera and reduces the mortality of severe cholera from more than 10% to less than 0.5%. Rehydration therapy should be based on World Health Organization (WHO) standards, with the goal of replacing the estimated fluid deficit within 3 to 4 hours of initial presentation. In patients with severe dehydration, isotonic intravenous fluids should be used, and lactated Ringer solution is the preferred commercially available option.[1] For patients without severe dehydration, oral rehydration therapy using the WHO's reduced-osmolality oral rehydration solution (ORS) has been the standard, but data suggest that rice-based ORS or amylase-resistant starch ORS are more effective.

Antimicrobial therapy decreases the duration and volume of diarrhea as well as the shedding of viable bacteria. Antimicrobial therapy should be considered for people who are moderately to severely ill. The choice of antimicrobial therapy should be made based on the age of the patient (Table 3.90) as well as prevailing patterns of antimicrobial resistance. When local patterns of resistance are unknown, antimicrobial susceptibility testing should be performed on isolates and monitored. Zinc supplementation should be considered as an adjunct to rehydration in children (**www.cdc.gov/ cholera/treatment/zinc-treatment.html**).

---

[1] World Health Organization. *The Treatment of Diarrhoea, a Manual for Physicians and Other Senior Health Workers.* 4th Rev. World Health Organization; 2005

Table 3.90. Antibiotics for Suspected Cholera

Antibiotic	Pediatric Dose[a]	Adult Dose	Comment(s)
Doxycycline	4.4 mg/kg, single dose	300 mg, single dose	Use should be in epidemics caused by susceptible isolates. Can be used without regard to patient age, but is not recommended for pregnant people.
Ciprofloxacin[b]	15 mg/kg, twice daily for 3 days (single dose 20 mg/kg has been used)	500 mg, twice daily for 3 days	Decreased susceptibility to fluoroquinolones is associated with treatment failure.
Azithromycin	20 mg/kg, single dose	1 g, single dose	
Erythromycin	12.5 mg/kg, 4 times/day for 3 days	250 mg, 4 times/day for 3 days	
Tetracycline[c]	12.5 mg/kg, 4 times/day for 3 days	500 mg, 4 times/day for 3 days	

[a] Not to exceed adult dose.
[b] Fluoroquinolones are not approved for children younger than 18 years for this indication.
[c] For use in children ≥8 y.

INFECTION PREVENTION AND CONTROL MEASURES IN HEALTH CARE SETTINGS:
In addition to standard precautions, contact precautions are indicated for diapered children or incontinent people for the duration of illness.

CONTROL MEASURES:

Hygiene. Disinfection of drinking water through chlorination or boiling prevents waterborne transmission of *V cholerae*. Thoroughly cooking crabs, oysters, and other shellfish from the Gulf Coast before eating is recommended to decrease the likelihood of illness. Foods such as fish, rice, or grain gruels should be refrigerated promptly and thoroughly reheated before eating, and fruits and vegetables should be peeled before eating. The use of latrines or burying feces is recommended, and defecation should be avoided near any body of water. Appropriate hand hygiene after defecating and before preparing or eating food is important for preventing transmission.

Treatment of Contacts. Although administration of appropriate antimicrobial agents within 24 hours of identification of the index case may prevent additional cases of cholera among household contacts, chemoprophylaxis of contacts currently is not recommended.

Vaccine. A single-dose, live attenuated monovalent oral vaccine (CVD 103-HgR; Vaxchora), has been approved by the US Food and Drug Administration and is available in the United States for use for travelers 2 through 64 years of age who are traveling to areas where cholera is a risk. In addition to following safe food and water precautions, the Advisory Committee on Immunization Practices of the CDC recommends cholera vaccine for immunocompetent pediatric and adult travelers 2 through 64 years of age to an area of active cholera transmission.[1] No data exist on use of the currently licensed CVD 103-HgR formulation in immunocompromised populations. An area of active cholera transmission is defined as a province, state, or other administrative subdivision within a country with endemic or epidemic cholera caused by toxigenic *V cholerae* and includes areas with cholera activity within the past year that are prone to recurrence of cholera epidemics; it does not include areas where only rare sporadic cases have been reported. Information about destinations with active cholera transmission is available at **wwwnc.cdc.gov/travel/.**

Three non-live oral vaccines are approved by the WHO and available outside the United States. Dukoral is a monovalent inactivated vaccine based on heat-killed whole cells of serogroup O1 plus recombinant cholera toxin B subunit. The vaccine also may provide some protection against heat-labile enterotoxigenic *Escherichia coli* infection and is primarily used by travelers to areas with endemic cholera. Children between 2 and 6 years of age require 3 doses, and adults and children 6 years and older require 2 doses at least 1 week apart. Two bivalent (O1 and O139) vaccines, ShanChol and Euvichol, provide durable protection in older children and adults but do not provide significant protection in young children. In 2011, the WHO initiated a global oral cholera vaccine stockpile, comprised of bivalent vaccine, to allow for its rapid deployment during cholera epidemics and other emergencies. Instructions regarding access to the stockpile are available at **www.who.int/groups/Icg/cholera/stockpiles.**

Cholera immunization is not required for travelers entering the United States from cholera-affected areas, and the WHO no longer recommends immunization for travel to or from areas with cholera transmission. No country requires cholera vaccine for entry.

Public Health Reporting. Confirmed cases of cholera must be reported to health authorities in any country in which they occur and were contracted. Local and state health departments should be notified immediately of presumed or known cases of cholera.

Other *Vibrio* Infections

CLINICAL MANIFESTATIONS: Vibriosis is illness attributable to more than 20 species of the *Vibrionaceae* family. Species commonly isolated from clinical samples include: (1) *Vibrio parahaemolyticus, Vibrio vulnificus, Vibrio alginolyticus,* and other *Vibrio* species; (2) nontoxigenic *Vibrio cholerae;* (3) toxigenic *Vibrio cholerae* O75 and O141; and (4) members of the *Vibrionaceae* family that are not in the genus *Vibrio* (eg, *Grimontia, Photobacterium*). Associated clinical syndromes include gastroenteritis, wound infection, and septicemia. Gastroenteritis is the most common syndrome and is characterized by acute onset of watery, nonbloody stools and crampy abdominal pain. Approximately half of affected people will have low-grade fever, headache, and chills; approximately 30% will have vomiting. Spontaneous recovery occurs in 2 to 5 days. Wound infections typically start as cellulitis with vesicles and can progress to hemorrhagic bullae, necrosis, and/or necrotizing fasciitis. Septicemia can be primary or follow gastroenteritis or wound infection and often is fulminant and accompanied by development of metastatic skin lesions

---

[1] Collins JP, Ryan ET, Wong KK, et al. Cholera vaccine: recommendations of the Advisory Committee on Immunization Practices, 2022. *MMWR Recomm Rep.* 2022;71(RR-2):1–8

within 36 hours. Risk factors for severe wound infections and for septicemia include liver disease, iron overload, hemolytic anemia, chronic renal failure, diabetes mellitus, low gastric acidity, and immunosuppression. Various otolaryngologic manifestations attributable to *V alginolyticus* have been linked to swimming in salt water.

ETIOLOGY: *Vibrio* organisms are facultatively anaerobic, motile, gram-negative bacilli that are tolerant of salt. The most commonly reported nontoxigenic *Vibrio* species associated with diarrhea are *V parahaemolyticus* and *V cholerae* non-O1/non-O139. *V vulnificus* typically causes primary septicemia and severe wound infections, but the other species also can cause these syndromes. *V alginolyticus* typically causes wound and ear infections, with ear infections more commonly seen in children.

EPIDEMIOLOGY: *Vibrio* species are natural inhabitants of marine and estuarine environments. In temperate climates, most noncholera *Vibrio* infections occur during summer and fall months, when *Vibrio* populations in seawater are highest due to favorable growth conditions in warm temperatures. Following trends in climate change, global *Vibrio* infections are expected to continue increasing. Gastroenteritis usually follows ingestion of raw or undercooked seafood, especially oysters, clams, crabs, and shrimp. Wound infections usually are attributable to *V vulnificus* and can result from exposure of a preexisting wound to contaminated seawater or from punctures resulting from handling of contaminated fish or shellfish. Exposure to contaminated water during natural disasters, such as hurricanes, has resulted in wound infections. Person-to-person transmission has not been reported. National surveillance for infections associated with noncholera *Vibrio* organisms has been in place since 1997 (**www.cdc.gov/vibrio/surveillance.html**). It is estimated that 80 000 cases, 500 hospitalizations, and 100 deaths from vibriosis occur each year in the United States.

The **incubation period** is typically 24 hours (with a range of 5 to 92 hours) for gastroenteritis and is 1 to 7 days for wound infections and septicemia.

DIAGNOSTIC TESTS: Depending on the clinical syndrome, *Vibrio* organisms can be isolated from stool, wound exudates, or blood. Because identification of the organism requires special techniques, laboratory personnel should be notified when infection with *Vibrio* species is suspected. Multiplex molecular panels are available, but the specificity of some diagnostic tests is poor. Infection should be confirmed by culture, and isolates (or clinical specimens if isolates are not available on a positive nonculture diagnostic test) should be forwarded as required to the local or state public health laboratory for characterization, outbreak investigation, and surveillance.

TREATMENT: Diarrhea typically is mild and self-limited, and oral rehydration is recommended as treatment. Wound infections require prompt surgical débridement of necrotic tissue, if present. Antimicrobial therapy is recommended for severe diarrhea, wound infection, or septicemia. Septicemia, with or without hemorrhagic bullae, and wound infections should be treated with a third-generation cephalosporin plus either doxycycline or ciprofloxacin. Severe diarrhea should be treated with doxycycline or ciprofloxacin. Doxycycline can be used without regard to patient age. A combination of trimethoprim-sulfamethoxazole and an aminoglycoside is an alternative regimen.

INFECTION PREVENTION AND CONTROL MEASURES IN HEALTH CARE SETTINGS: In addition to standard precautions, contact precautions are recommended for diapered or incontinent children.

CONTROL MEASURES: Seafood should be cooked fully and refrigerated if not consumed immediately. Cross-contamination of cooked seafood by contact with surfaces and containers contaminated by raw seafood should be avoided. Uncooked mollusks and crustaceans should be handled with care, and gloves can be worn during preparation. Abrasions suffered by ocean bathers should be rinsed with clean fresh water. All children, immunocompromised people, and people with chronic liver disease should avoid eating raw oysters or clams, and all individuals should be advised of risks associated with seawater exposure if a wound is present or likely to occur.

Public Health Reporting. Vibriosis is a nationally notifiable disease, and cases should be reported to local or state health departments immediately.

West Nile Virus

CLINICAL MANIFESTATIONS: West Nile virus (WNV) is the leading cause of mosquito-borne illness in the United States. An estimated 80% of people infected with WNV are asymptomatic. Most of the 20% of people who are symptomatic experience an acute systemic febrile illness that often includes headache, myalgia, arthralgia, vomiting, diarrhea, or a transient maculopapular rash. Less than 1% of infected people (1 in 150) develop neuroinvasive disease, which typically manifests as meningitis, encephalitis, or acute flaccid myelitis. WNV meningitis is indistinguishable clinically from aseptic meningitis caused by other viruses. Patients with WNV encephalitis usually present with fever, headache, seizures, mental status changes (including disorientation, stupor, or coma), focal neurologic deficits, or movement disorders (including tremor). WNV acute flaccid myelitis often is clinically and pathologically identical to poliovirus-associated poliomyelitis, with damage of anterior horn cells and resulting weakness and paralysis of one or more limbs; this may progress to respiratory paralysis requiring mechanical ventilation. WNV-associated Guillain-Barré syndrome also has been reported and can be distinguished from WNV acute flaccid myelitis by clinical manifestations, findings on cerebrospinal fluid analysis, and electrophysiologic testing. Cardiac dysrhythmias, myocarditis, rhabdomyolysis, optic neuritis, uveitis, chorioretinitis, orchitis, pancreatitis, and hepatitis have been described rarely after WNV infection.

Routine clinical laboratory results are nonspecific in WNV infections. In patients with neuroinvasive disease, cerebrospinal fluid (CSF) examination generally shows lymphocytic pleocytosis, but neutrophils may predominate early in the illness. Brain magnetic resonance imaging frequently is normal, but signal abnormalities may be seen in the basal ganglia, thalamus, and brainstem with WNV encephalitis and in the spinal cord with WNV acute flaccid myelitis.

Most patients with WNV nonneuroinvasive disease or meningitis recover completely, but fatigue, malaise, and weakness can linger for weeks or months. Recovery from WNV encephalitis or acute flaccid myelitis often takes weeks to months, and patients commonly have residual neurologic deficits. Among patients with neuroinvasive disease, the overall case fatality rate is approximately 10% but is significantly higher in WNV encephalitis and acute flaccid myelitis than in WNV meningitis.

Most people known to have been infected with WNV during pregnancy have delivered infants without evidence of infection or clinical abnormalities. Rare cases of congenital infection and probable transmission via human milk (see Breastfeeding and Human Milk, p 135) have been reported. If WNV disease is diagnosed during pregnancy, a detailed examination of the fetus and of the newborn infant should be performed.[1]

ETIOLOGY: WNV is an RNA virus of the *Flaviviridae* family (genus *Flavivirus*) that is related antigenically to St. Louis encephalitis and Japanese encephalitis viruses.

EPIDEMIOLOGY: WNV is an arthropod-borne virus (arbovirus) that is transmitted in an enzootic cycle between mosquitoes and amplified in vertebrate hosts, primarily birds. WNV is transmitted to humans primarily through bites of infected *Culex* mosquitoes. Humans usually do not develop a level or duration of viremia sufficient to infect mosquitoes and, therefore, are dead-end hosts. Person-to-person WNV transmission can occur rarely through blood transfusion and solid organ transplantation. Congenital and perinatal transmission during pregnancy, delivery, or via breastfeeding has been described. Transmission through percutaneous and mucosal exposure has occurred in laboratory workers and occupational settings.

WNV transmission has been documented on every continent except Antarctica. Since the 1990s, the largest outbreaks of WNV neuroinvasive disease have occurred in the Middle East, Europe, and North America. WNV first was detected in the Western Hemisphere in New York City in 1999 and subsequently spread across the continental United States and Canada. From 1999 through 2020, 52 532 cases of WNV infection were reported in the United States, of which 26 683 were nonneuroinvasive disease and 25 849 were neuroinvasive disease, with peaks in national incidence in 2002, 2003, and 2012. WNV is the leading cause of neuroinvasive arboviral disease in the United States. In 2020 (latest finalized data available from the Centers for Disease Control and Prevention [CDC]), there were 559 cases of WNV neuroinvasive disease reported. Although the lower number of cases reported in 2020 likely was associated with the COVID-19 pandemic, WNV caused 4 times more neuroinvasive disease cases than the number reported for all other domestic arboviruses combined (eg, La Crosse [88], Powassan [20], St. Louis encephalitis viruses [14], eastern equine encephalitis [13], and Jamestown Canyon [10]). WNV human cases have been reported from all US states; the states with the highest average annual incidence (>1.0 case per 100 000) of human WNV disease over the period 1999-2020 were Colorado, Louisiana, Mississippi, Nebraska, North Dakota, South Dakota, and Wyoming. Preliminary data from 2021 has shown Arizona to have nearly 10 times the number of cases reported in other states. A map of the distribution of WNV neuroinvasive disease across the United States can be found on the CDC website (**www.cdc.gov/westnile/statsmaps/final.html**). Climate change likely is one factor associated with the expanded range of mosquito vectors and, therefore, WNV disease.

Most human WNV infections occur in summer or early fall in temperate and subtropical regions. All age groups are susceptible to WNV infection, but incidence of severe disease (eg, neuroinvasive disease and death) is highest among older adults. Overall incidence is 0.05/100 000 in those <20 years of age compared with 1.2/100 000 in those ≥70 years of age. Chronic renal failure, history of cancer, alcohol use disorder, diabetes mellitus, and hypertension have been associated with developing severe WNV disease.

---

[1] Centers for Disease Control and Prevention. Interim guidelines for the evaluation of infants born to mothers infected with West Nile virus during pregnancy. *MMWR Morb Mortal Wkly Rep*. 2004;53(7):154-157

The **incubation period** usually is 2 to 6 days but ranges from 2 to 14 days and can be up to 21 days in immunocompromised people and up to 37 days in solid organ transplant recipients.

DIAGNOSTIC TESTS: Detection of anti-WNV immunoglobulin (Ig) M antibodies in serum or cerebrospinal fluid (CSF) is the most common method for diagnosis of WNV infection. Presence of anti-WNV IgM usually is good evidence of recent WNV infection but may indicate infection with another closely related flavivirus. WNV IgM antibodies are detectable in most WNV-infected patients within 3 to 8 days of symptom onset and typically remain detectible for months and, in some individuals, years after the acute illness. For patients from whom serum collected within 8 days of illness lacks detectable IgM, testing should be repeated on a convalescent-phase sample. Because anti-WNV IgM can persist in the serum of some patients for longer than 1 year, a positive test result may reflect past infection. Detection of WNV IgM in CSF generally is indicative of recent neuroinvasive infection. IgG antibody generally is detectable shortly after IgM and usually persists for years. Plaque-reduction neutralization tests can be performed to measure virus-specific neutralizing antibodies and to discriminate between cross-reacting antibodies from closely related flaviviruses. A fourfold or greater increase in virus-specific neutralizing antibodies between acute- and convalescent-phase serum specimens collected 2 to 3 weeks apart may be used to confirm recent WNV infection. State and local health departments can assist with diagnostic testing and with determination of whether additional testing is indicated via the CDC Arbovirus Diagnostic Laboratory (**www.cdc.gov/ncezid/dvbd/specimensub/ arboviral-shipping.html**).

Viral culture and WNV nucleic acid amplification tests (including reverse transcriptase-polymerase chain reaction) can be performed on acute-phase serum, CSF, or tissue specimens. By the time most immunocompetent patients present with clinical symptoms, WNV RNA usually no longer is detectable; therefore, polymerase chain reaction assay is not recommended for diagnosis in immunocompetent hosts. Sensitivity of these tests is likely higher in immunocompromised patients. Immunohistochemical staining can detect WNV antigens in fixed tissue, but negative results are not definitive.

WNV disease should be considered in the differential diagnosis of febrile or acute neurologic illnesses associated with recent exposure to mosquitoes, blood transfusion, or solid organ transplantation and of illnesses in neonates whose birthing parent was infected with WNV during pregnancy or while breastfeeding. WNV and other arboviruses should be considered in the differential diagnosis of aseptic meningitis and encephalitis along with other causes such as herpes simplex virus and enteroviruses.

TREATMENT: No specific therapy is available; management of WNV disease is supportive. Although various therapies have been evaluated or used empirically for WNV disease, none has shown specific benefit thus far. A review summarizing potential treatments (including immune globulin intravenous with or without a high titer of WNV antibody, WNV recombinant humanized monoclonal antibody, interferon, corticosteroids, and ribavirin) is available online at **www.cdc.gov/westnile/healthcareproviders/healthCareProviders-TreatmentPrevention.html.**

INFECTION PREVENTION AND CONTROL MEASURES IN HEALTH CARE SETTINGS: Standard precautions are recommended.

CONTROL MEASURES: Candidate WNV vaccines are being evaluated, but none are licensed for use in humans. Prevention of WNV disease depends on community-level mosquito control programs to reduce vector densities, personal protective measures to decrease exposure to infected mosquitoes, and screening of blood and organ donors. Successful community-level integrated pest-management strategies combine removing mosquito habitats by eliminating standing water, using structural barriers, and controlling both larval stage and adult mosquitos (**www.epa.gov/mosquitocontrol/ success-mosquito-control-integrated-approach** and **www.epa.gov/insect-repellents/using-repellent-products-protect-against-mosquito-borne-illnesses**). Personal protective measures include use of mosquito repellents, wearing long-sleeved shirts and long pants, and limiting outdoor exposure from dusk to dawn (see Prevention of Mosquito-borne and Tick-borne Infections, p 207). Using air conditioning, installing window and door screens, and reducing peridomestic mosquito breeding sites can decrease the risk of WNV exposure further. Blood donations in the United States are screened for WNV infection, but physicians should remain vigilant for the possible transmission of WNV through blood transfusion or organ transplantation. Any suspected WNV infections temporally associated with blood transfusion or organ transplantation should be reported promptly to the appropriate state health department and to the United Network for Organ Sharing in the case of suspected organ transmission.

Pregnant people should take precautions to avoid mosquito bites. Products containing N,N-diethyl-meta-toluamide (DEET) can be used in pregnancy without adverse effects. Pregnant people who develop meningitis, encephalitis, acute flaccid myelitis, or unexplained fever in areas of ongoing WNV transmission should be tested for WNV infection. Confirmed WNV infections should be reported to local or state health departments, and infected pregnant people should be followed to determine the outcomes of their pregnancies. Although WNV probably has been transmitted through human milk, such transmission appears rare, and no adverse effects on infants have been described. Because the benefits of breastfeeding outweigh the risk of WNV disease in breastfeeding infants, people should be encouraged to breastfeed even in areas with ongoing WNV transmission.

Yersinia enterocolitica and *Yersinia pseudotuberculosis* Infections
(Enteritis and Other Illnesses)

CLINICAL MANIFESTATIONS: *Yersinia enterocolitica* causes several age-specific syndromes and a variety of other less commonly reported clinical illnesses. Infection with *Y entero-colitica* typically manifests as fever, diarrhea, and abdominal pain in children younger than 5 years; stool often contains leukocytes, blood, and mucus. Symptoms of *Y entero-colitica* generally resolve within 7 days but diarrhea may persist for more than 2 weeks. Relapsing disease and, rarely, necrotizing enterocolitis and protein-losing enteropathy also have been described. In older children and adults, a pseudoappendicitis syndrome attributable to mesenteric lymphadenitis (fever, abdominal pain, tenderness in the right lower quadrant of the abdomen, and leukocytosis) is common. Bacteremia is the major complication of *Y enterocolitica* infection occurring mostly in children younger than 1 year and in older children with predisposing conditions, such as excessive iron storage (eg, deferoxamine use, sickle cell disease, and beta-thalassemia) and immuno-suppressive states. Extraintestinal manifestations of *Y enterocolitica* are uncommon but include pharyngitis, meningitis, osteomyelitis, pyomyositis, conjunctivitis, pneumonia, empyema, endocarditis, acute peritonitis, abscesses of the liver and spleen, urinary tract infection, and primary cutaneous infection. Postinfectious sequelae with *Y enterocolitica* infection include erythema nodosum, reactive arthritis, uveitis, and glomerulo-nephritis. These sequelae occur most often in older children and adults, particularly people with HLA-B27 antigen.

Major manifestations of *Y pseudotuberculosis* infection include fever, scarlatiniform rash, acute gastroenteritis, and abdominal symptoms. Acute pseudoappendiceal abdominal pain is common, resulting from ileocecal mesenteric adenitis or terminal ileitis. Other uncommon findings reported have been intestinal intussusception; erythema nodosum; septicemia, mainly among individuals with underlying conditions; acute renal failure with nephritis; and sterile pleural and joint effusions. *Y pseudotuberculosis* infection may cause a severe systemic inflammatory disease called Far East scarlet-like fever (FESLF), which has been reported sporadically and in outbreaks in Russia and Japan.

Although not common, recent case reports suggest that infection with *Y enterocolitica* and *Y pseudotuberculosis* may mimic or contribute to the pathogenesis of Kawasaki disease. In Japan, nearly 10% of children with a diagnosis of Kawasaki disease have serologic or culture evidence of *Y pseudotuberculosis* infection. These patients often require more than 1 dose of intravenous immune globulin (IVIG) and are more likely to develop cardiac sequelae than Kawasaki disease patients without *Y pseudotuberculosis* infection.

ETIOLOGY: The genus *Yersinia* consists of 17 species of gram-negative bacilli belonging to the family *Yersiniaceae*. *Y enterocolitica*, *Y pseudotuberculosis*, and *Yersinia pestis* (see Plague, p 671) are the 3 most recognized human pathogens; however, other *Yersinia* species also have been isolated from clinical specimens. Isolates of *Y enterocolitica* involved in human infections belong to several serotypes (O:3, O:8, O:9, and O:5.27) and are divided into 3 groups according to their pathogenic potential: nonpathogenic biotype 1A, weakly pathogenic biotypes 2 through 5, and highly pathogenic biotype 1B. Strains from biotype 1A can induce infections only in immunocompromised individuals. Serotype O:8, from biotype 1B, is the most virulent and has been responsible for several food poisoning outbreaks in the United States. At present, carriage of pathogenic *Y enterocolitica* serotype O:3, found primarily in pigs, is the most frequent cause of yersiniosis in Europe and North America. The 3 *Yersinia* species have in common a tropism for lymphoid tissue and share factors that promote serum resistance, coordinate gene expression, and facilitate iron acquisition. Differences in virulence gene distribution exist among *Yersinia* species.

EPIDEMIOLOGY: *Y enterocolitica* and *Y pseudotuberculosis* are isolated most often during the cool months of temperate climates because of favorable growth conditions at cooler temperatures (4°C to 43°C). The Foodborne Disease Active Surveillance Network (FoodNet) conducts active surveillance for infections caused by *Yersinia* (see Appendix V: Prevention of Infectious Disease From Contaminated Food Products, p 1145). During 2019, FoodNet identified 681 *Yersinia* cases of infection (21% were hospitalized and 0.6% died), with an average incidence of 1.4 per 100 000 population, which represents a 153% increase in comparison to 2016-2018.[1] This increased incidence likely resulted from increased use of culture-independent diagnostic tests that detect bacterial antigens and genes for *Y enterocolitica*. *Yersinia* incidence is highest in children younger than 5 years and in Black people; however, in recent years, a significant declining incidence among Black children has been observed. FoodNet data from 1996–2007 indicate that compared with *Y enterocolitica* infection, the average annual incidence of *Y pseudotuberculosis* infection is much lower (0.04 cases per 1 million population), occurs in older people (median age was 47 years), and is more severe and invasive (72% were hospitalized, 11% died, and two thirds of isolates were recovered from blood).

The principal reservoir of *Y enterocolitica* is swine, although it can be isolated from a variety of domestic and wildlife animals; *Y pseudotuberculosis* has been isolated from ungulates (deer, elk, goats, sheep, cattle), rodents (rats, squirrels, beaver), rabbits, and many bird species. Infection with *Y enterocolitica* is reported to be transmitted by ingestion of contaminated food (raw or incompletely cooked pork products, tofu, and unpasteurized or inadequately pasteurized milk[2]), by contaminated surface or well water, by direct or indirect contact with animals, and rarely by transfusion with contaminated packed red blood cells and by person-to-person transmission. Cross-contamination has been documented to lead to infection in infants if their caregivers handle raw pork intestines (ie, chitterlings) and do not clean their hands or food preparation surfaces adequately before handling the infant or the infant's toys, bottles, or pacifiers. *Y pseudotuberculosis* can follow exposure to well and mountain waters contaminated with animal feces. Household pets can be source of infection for children.

The **incubation period** typically is 4 to 6 days, with a range of 1 to 14 days. Organisms typically are excreted for 2 to 3 weeks and up to 2 to 3 months in untreated cases. Prolonged asymptomatic carriage is possible.

DIAGNOSTIC TESTS: *Y enterocolitica* and *Y pseudotuberculosis* can be recovered from stool, mesenteric lymph nodes, and blood. Stool cultures generally yield bacteria during the first 2 weeks of illness, regardless of the nature of gastrointestinal tract manifestations. Laboratory personnel should be notified when *Yersinia* infection is suspected so that stool can be appropriately stored (eg, Cary-Blair transport media) and cultured on suitable media (eg, blood, chocolate, and MacConkey agars incubated at 25°C to 35°C for 24 to 48 hours in ambient air). Because of relatively slow growth conditions of *Yersinia*, isolation from nonsterile sources (eg, stool) is recommended using selective media.

DNA-based gastrointestinal syndrome panels are commercially available but typically target only *Y enterocolitica* and may cross-react with other *Yersinia* species. In 2018, 68% of yersiniosis cases reported to FoodNet were diagnosed using such culture-independent panels. Reliable species identification using matrix-assisted laser desorption/ionization–time-of-flight (MALDI-TOF) mass spectrometry, DNA-based methods, biotyping, and serotyping of pathogenic strains isolated from clinical, food, and environmental samples are available through public health reference laboratories.

---

[1] Tack DM, Ray L, Griffin PM, et al. Preliminary incidence and trends of infections with pathogens transmitted commonly through food - Foodborne Diseases Active Surveillance Network, 10 U.S. Sites, 2016-2019. *MMWR Morb Mortal Wkly Rep.* 2020;69(17):509-514

[2] American Academy of Pediatrics, Committee on Infectious Diseases, Committee on Nutrition. Consumption of raw or unpasteurized milk and milk products by pregnant women and children. *Pediatrics.* 2014;133(1):175-179 (Reaffirmed November 2019)

Infection also can be confirmed by demonstrating increases in serum antibody titer after infection, but these tests generally are available only in reference or research laboratories. Cross-reactions of these antibodies with *Brucella, Vibrio, Salmonella,* and *Rickettsia* organisms and *Escherichia coli* can lead to false-positive *Y enterocolitica* and *Y pseudotuberculosis* titers. In patients with thyroid disease, persistently increased *Y enterocolitica* antibody titers can result from antigenic similarity of the organism with antigens of the thyroid epithelial cell membrane. Characteristic ultrasonographic features demonstrating edema of the wall of the terminal ileum and cecum with normal appendix help to distinguish pseudoappendicitis from appendicitis and can help avoid exploratory surgery.

TREATMENT: In immunocompetent hosts, yersiniosis is typically self-limited and does not require antibiotic treatment. Although a clinical benefit of antimicrobial therapy for immunocompetent patients with enterocolitis, pseudoappendicitis syndrome, or mesenteric adenitis has not been established, some clinicians consider treatment because it can decrease the duration of shedding of *Yersinia* organisms. Antibiotic treatment is recommended for neonates, immunocompromised hosts, and all patients with severe manifestations like septicemia or extraintestinal disease. Parenteral therapy with a third-generation cephalosporin is appropriate in these situations, and evaluation of cerebrospinal fluid should be performed for infected neonates. In addition to third-generation cephalosporins, trimethoprim-sulfamethoxazole, aminoglycosides, fluoroquinolones, chloramphenicol, tetracycline, and doxycycline may be used. *Y enterocolitica* isolates are usually resistant to first-generation cephalosporins and most penicillins. Antibiotic therapy has no beneficial effect on postinfectious syndromes.

INFECTION PREVENTION AND CONTROL MEASURES IN HEALTH CARE SETTINGS: In addition to standard precautions, contact precautions are indicated for diapered or incontinent children for the duration of diarrheal illness.

CONTROL MEASURES: Ingestion of uncooked or undercooked meat (especially pork), unpasteurized milk,[1] or contaminated water should be avoided. People who handle raw meat products should minimize contact with young children and their possessions while handling raw products. Meticulous hand hygiene and proper sanitization of food preparation surfaces should be practiced before and after handling and preparation of uncooked products. No vaccines against *Y enterocolitica* and *Y pseudotuberculosis* are available, although several candidates are under evaluation.

Public Health Reporting. *Yersinia* infections are not nationally notifiable but are reportable in many states (a directory of state and territorial, city and county, and tribal health departments can be found at **www.cdc.gov/publichealthgateway/healthdirectories/index.html**).

Zika

CLINICAL MANIFESTATIONS: Most Zika virus infections are asymptomatic or result in mild clinical disease with symptoms lasting a few days to a week. Commonly reported signs and symptoms include fever, pruritic maculopapular rash, arthralgia, and conjunctival hyperemia. Other findings include myalgia, headache, edema of the

---

[1] American Academy of Pediatrics, Committee on Infectious Diseases and Committee on Nutrition. Consumption of raw or unpasteurized milk and milk products by pregnant women and children. *Pediatrics.* 2014;133(1):175-179 (Reaffirmed November 2019)

extremities, vomiting, retro-orbital pain, and lymphadenopathy. Clinical laboratory abnormalities are observed uncommonly in symptomatic patients but can include thrombocytopenia, leukopenia, and increased liver aminotransferase concentrations. Severe disease requiring hospitalization and deaths are rare. However, Guillain-Barré syndrome and rare reports of other neurologic complications (eg, meningoencephalitis, myelitis, and uveitis) have been associated with Zika virus infection.

Congenital Zika virus infection can cause fetal loss, intrauterine growth restriction, premature delivery, microcephaly, and other serious neurologic anomalies. Clinical findings most specific for congenital Zika syndrome include severe microcephaly with partially collapsed skull, cortical hypoplasia with abnormal gyral patterns, intracranial calcifications between the cortex and subcortex), congenital contractures (arthrogryposis), and ocular abnormalities (eg, chorioretinal scarring and pigmentary mottling). Other abnormalities have been reported among infants with congenital infection including other structural brain abnormalities (eg, ventriculomegaly, corpus callosum agenesis, cerebellar hypoplasia, mild microcephaly), other structural eye abnormalities (eg, microphthalmia, cataracts, chorioretinal atrophy, or optic nerve hypoplasia), and neurologic sequelae associated with structural brain abnormalities (eg, hypertonia, dystonia, swallowing dysfunction, seizures, hearing loss). Approximately 5% of infants in the US Zika Pregnancy and Infant Registry had any Zika-associated brain or eye defect; one third of those infants had more than 1 defect reported. The frequency of Zika-associated birth defects in infants was similar among those born to symptomatic (5.3%) and asymptomatic (4.2%) pregnant people. Among pregnancies with confirmed Zika infection, the frequency of any Zika-associated birth defect was higher among those with first (8.0%) and second (6.0%) trimester infections compared with third trimester infections (3.8%). Rare cases of perinatal transmission from birthing parents who were viremic at delivery have been reported. These perinatal transmissions generally result in asymptomatic or mildly symptomatic illness in the neonate.

ETIOLOGY: Zika virus is a single-stranded, RNA virus in the genus *Flavivirus* that is most closely related antigenically to dengue. Two major lineages, African and Asian, have been identified through phylogenetic analyses.

EPIDEMIOLOGY: Zika virus is transmitted to humans primarily by *Aedes aegypti* mosquitoes and less commonly by *Aedes albopictus* and possibly other *Aedes* (*Stegomyia*) species (eg, *Aedes polynesiensis* and *Aedes hensilli)*. In the United States, *Ae aegypti* mosquitoes are found primarily in southern states. *Ae albopictus* mosquitoes have a wider distribution (see map at **www.cdc.gov/zika/vector/range.html**). Both *Aedes* species bite humans primarily during the daytime hours. These are the same vectors that transmit dengue, chikungunya, and yellow fever viruses. Human and nonhuman primates are the main reservoirs of the virus, with humans acting as the primary host in which the virus multiplies, allowing spread to additional mosquitoes and then other humans. Additional modes of transmission have been identified, including perinatal, in utero, sexual, blood transfusion, and laboratory exposure. Although Zika virus has been detected in human milk, and a few possible cases of transmission of Zika virus by breastfeeding have been reported, to date there is no consistent evidence that infants acquire Zika virus through breastfeeding.

Prior to 2007, only sporadic human Zika virus disease cases were reported from countries in Africa and Asia. In 2007, the first documented Zika virus disease outbreak was reported in the Federated States of Micronesia. In subsequent years, outbreaks of Zika virus disease were identified in countries in Southeast Asia and the Western Pacific. In 2015, Zika virus was identified for the first time in the Western hemisphere and subsequently spread throughout much of the Americas, with 48 countries and territories in the Americas reporting local transmission. During 2016, large outbreaks occurred in Puerto Rico and the US Virgin Islands, and limited local transmission was identified in parts of Florida and Texas. In 2017, Zika virus disease cases started to decline worldwide. Since 2018, there have been no locally acquired cases reported from US states. Current information on Zika virus transmission and travel guidance can be found at **www.cdc.gov/zika/geo/index.html** and **wwwnc.cdc.gov/travel/page/zika-travel-information,** respectively.

The **incubation period** is 3 to 14 days after the bite of an infected mosquito.

DIAGNOSTIC TESTS: Zika virus infection should be considered in patients with acute onset of fever, maculopapular rash, arthralgia, or conjunctivitis who live in or have traveled to or had sex with someone who lived in or recently traveled to an area with ongoing transmission in the 2 weeks preceding illness onset. Because dengue and chikungunya virus infections share a similar geographic distribution and symptoms with Zika virus infection, patients with suspected Zika virus infection also should be evaluated and managed for possible dengue or chikungunya virus infection. Other considerations in the differential diagnosis include malaria, rubella, measles, parvovirus, adenovirus, enterovirus, leptospirosis, rickettsiosis, group A streptococcal infections, and COVID-19.

Nucleic acid amplification tests (NAATs) are the preferred method of diagnosis. Zika virus RNA is likely to be detected in serum from approximately 2 days before to 1 week after illness onset; RNA also can be detected in other body fluids (eg, whole blood, urine, saliva, amniotic fluid, semen, and breast milk). Immunoglobulin (Ig) M and neutralizing antibody testing also can be used to identify Zika virus infections, particularly in patients who present after viral nucleic acid is no longer detectable. IgM antibody assays can be conducted on serum, plasma, whole blood, or cerebrospinal fluid (CSF). IgM antibodies develop during the first week of illness and may be detectable for months to years following infection, making it difficult to distinguish the timing of Zika virus infection. Cross-reactivity of the Zika virus IgM antibody tests with other flaviviruses can result in a false-positive test result making it difficult to differentiate between flavivirus infections. Recent epidemiologic data indicate a declining prevalence of Zika virus infection in the Americas; this lower prevalence will result in a lower pretest probability of infection and a higher probability of false-positive test results for both molecular and serologic testing.

Although neutralizing antibody titers can yield cross-reactive results in people with previous flavivirus infections or who were vaccinated against a related flavivirus, they may differentiate flavivirus infections, particularly in individuals who were flavivirus-naïve before their infection. Testing guidance is updated as new information is obtained; for the most recent guidance, visit **www.cdc.gov/Zika.**

Zika Laboratory Testing in Nonpregnant Symptomatic Individuals. Given the current global arboviral epidemiology, Zika virus testing is currently not recommended for this group unless people live in or have traveled to a country with a current Zika outbreak (**wwwnc.cdc.gov/travel/page/zika-travel-information**). For individuals traveling to or living in an area with a current Zika virus outbreak, both Zika and dengue virus NAATs should be performed as soon as possible on serum collected ≤7 days after onset of symptoms (Fig 3.23). IgM antibody testing for Zika and dengue should be performed in NAAT-negative serum specimens and serum collected >7 after onset of symptoms. For individuals traveling to or living in areas not experiencing a Zika virus outbreak, refer to testing guidance for dengue.

Zika Laboratory Testing in Pregnant People. Current recommendations from the Centers for Disease Control and Prevention (CDC; **www.cdc.gov/zika/hc-providers/ testing-guidance.html**) take into account the decreasing prevalence of Zika virus

FIG 3.23. DENGUE AND ZIKA VIRUS TESTING RECOMMENDATIONS FOR NONPREGNANT PERSONS WITH A CLINICALLY COMPATIBLE ILLNESS AND RISK FOR INFECTION WITH BOTH VIRUSES[a]

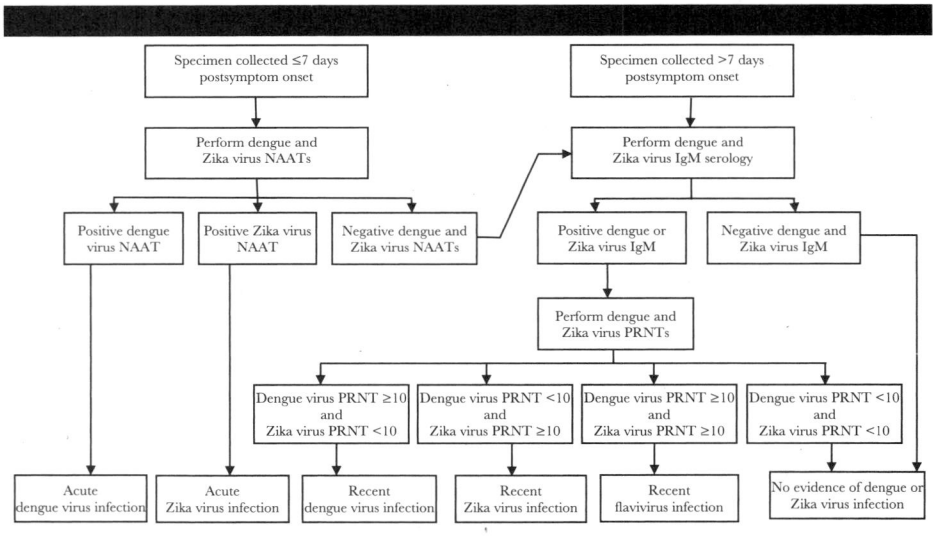

IgM indicates immunoglobulin M; NAAT, nucleic acid amplification test; PRNT, plaque-reduction neutralization test.

[a]*Specimen and test selection:* Dengue and Zika virus NAATs, IgM antibody testing, and PRNTs should be performed on serum. Some NAATs also can be performed on plasma, whole blood, cerebrospinal fluid, or urine, and some antibody tests can be performed on plasma, whole blood, or cerebrospinal fluid. Laboratories might choose to perform dengue and Zika virus NAATs and IgM antibody testing simultaneously rather than sequentially, or to perform dengue virus nonstructural protein-1 testing instead of dengue virus NAAT.

Indications to repeat assay(s): If the patient's illness has epidemiologic or clinical significance (eg, first case of local transmission in area, new transmission mode, or unusual clinical syndrome), repeat a positive NAAT on newly extracted RNA from the same specimen. For indeterminate IgM antibody test results, repeat IgM antibody testing or perform PRNT on the same specimen. In areas where PRNTs are not performed, report the indeterminate results and request a second serum specimen for IgM antibody testing.

Interpretation of results: Dengue and Zika virus IgM antibodies can be detected in serum for months following infection. The specific timing of infection cannot be determined. Data on the epidemiology of viruses known to be circulating at the location of exposure and clinical findings should be considered when interpreting the results of serologic diagnostic testing. Figure illustrates dengue and Zika virus testing recommendations for nonpregnant persons with a clinically compatible illness and risk for infection with both viruses. Diagnostic testing recommendations include immunoglobulin M assays, nucleic acid amplification tests, and plaque reduction neutralization tests.

From: Sharp TM, Fischer M, Muñoz-Jordán JL, et al. Dengue and Zika virus diagnostic testing for patients with a clinically compatible illness and risk for infection with both viruses. *MMWR Recomm Rep.* 2019;68(1):1-10.

disease cases globally, current dengue outbreaks in many areas of the world, and current knowledge of diagnostic limitations.[1,2] For asymptomatic pregnant people with recent travel to areas with risk of Zika (**wwwnc.cdc.gov/travel/page/zika-travel-information**), Zika virus testing is not routinely recommended because of its inability to differentiate between recent and remote infections and risk of false-positive results. Testing recommendations for symptomatic pregnant people who had recent travel to areas with active dengue transmission and risk of Zika virus transmission can be found at **www.cdc.gov/zika/hc-providers/testing-guidance.html.**

Zika Laboratory Testing for Congenital Infection. Zika virus testing is recommended for infants with clinical findings consistent with congenital Zika syndrome and possible in utero Zika virus exposure, regardless of the birthing parent's testing results, and for infants without clinical findings consistent with congenital Zika syndrome who are born to persons with laboratory evidence of possible infection during pregnancy. Recommended laboratory testing for possible congenital Zika virus infection includes evaluation for Zika virus RNA in infant serum, urine and CSF, if available. Zika virus IgM antibodies testing should be performed in serum and CSF, if available.

Laboratory testing of infants should be performed as soon as possible after birth (within the first few days of life), although testing specimens within the first few weeks to months after birth might still be useful. Diagnosis of congenital Zika virus infection is confirmed by a positive Zika virus NAAT or by a positive Zika virus IgM and neutralizing antibody result. If neither Zika virus RNA nor Zika IgM antibodies are detected on the appropriate specimens obtained within the first few days after birth, congenital Zika virus infection is unlikely (Table 3.91).

If the infant's initial sample is IgM nonnegative (nonnegative serologic terminology varies by assay and might include "positive," "equivocal," "presumptive positive," or "possible positive") and the NAAT result is negative, and PRNT was not performed on the birthing parent's sample, PRNTs for Zika and dengue viruses should be performed on the infant's initial sample. If the Zika virus PRNT result is negative, this suggests that the infant's Zika virus IgM test result is a false positive. For infants with clinical findings consistent with congenital Zika syndrome or evidence in the birthing parent of possible Zika virus infection during pregnancy but with no testing near the time of delivery, a PRNT at age ≥18 months (after transplacentally acquired antibodies have dissipated from the infant's system) might help confirm or rule out congenital Zika virus infection.

Fig 3.24 (p 969) outlines the current recommended evaluation of infants with possible congenital Zika virus from exposure during pregnancy.[3]

TREATMENT: No specific antiviral treatment currently is available for Zika virus disease. Supportive care is indicated, including rest, fluids, and symptomatic treatment

---

[1] Oduyebo T, Polen KD, Walke HT, et al. Update: Interim guidance for health care providers caring for pregnant women with possible zika virus exposure—United States (including U.S. territories), July 2017. *MMWR Morb Mortal Wkly Rep.* 2017;66(29):781-793

[2] Sharp TM, Fischer M, Muñoz-Jordán JL, et al. Dengue and Zika virus diagnostic testing for patients with a clinically compatible illness and risk for infection with both viruses. *MMWR Recomm Rep.* 2019;68(1):1-10

[3] Adebanjo T, Godfred-Cato S, Viens L, et al. Update: interim guidance for the diagnosis, evaluation, and management of infants with possible congenital Zika virus infection—United States, October 2017. *MMWR Morb Mortal Wkly Rep.* 2017;66(41):1089–1099

Table 3.91. Interpretation of Results of Laboratory Testing of Infant's Blood, Urine, and/or Cerebrospinal Fluid for Evidence of Congenital Zika Virus Infection[a]

Infant Test Result[b]			
NAAT	IgM	Interpretation	Comments
Positive	Any result	Confirmed congenital Zika virus infection	Distinguishing between congenital and postnatal infection is difficult in infants who live in areas where there is ongoing transmission of Zika virus and who are not tested soon after birth. If the timing of infection cannot be determined, infants should be evaluated as if they had congenital Zika virus infection.
Negative	Nonnegative[c]	Probable congenital Zika virus infection[d]	If Zika virus PRNT result is negative, this suggests that the infant's Zika virus IgM test is a false positive.
Negative	Negative	Congenital Zika virus infection unlikely[d]	Congenital Zika virus infection is unlikely if specimens are collected within the first few days after birth and the clinical evaluation is normal; however, health care providers should remain alert for any new findings of congenital Zika virus infection.

NAAT indicates nucleic acid amplification test; IgM, immunoglobulin M, PRNT, plaque-reduction neutralization test.

[a]Adapted from: Adebanjo T, Godfred-Cato S, Viens L, et al. Update: interim guidance for the diagnosis, evaluation, and management of infants with possible congenital Zika virus infection—United States, October 2017. *MMWR Morb Mortal Wkly Rep.* 2017;66(41):1089–1099.

[b]Infant serum, urine, or cerebrospinal fluid.

[c]Nonnegative serologic terminology varies by assay and might include "positive," "equivocal," "presumptive positive," or "possible positive."

[d]Laboratory results should be interpreted in the context of timing of infection during pregnancy, serology results in birthing parent, clinical findings consistent with congenital Zika syndrome, and any confirmatory testing with PRNT.

(acetaminophen to relieve fever and antihistamines to treat pruritus). Aspirin and nonsteroidal anti-inflammatory drugs (NSAIDs) should be avoided until dengue can be ruled out to reduce the risk of hemorrhagic complications.

Clinical Management of Infants With Clinical Findings Consistent With Congenital Zika Infection. Zika virus testing is recommended (see Zika Laboratory Testing for Congenital Infection, p 967), ultrasonography of the head should be performed, and a comprehensive ophthalmologic examination should be performed by age 1 month by an ophthalmologist experienced in assessment of infants. Referrals to a developmental specialist and early intervention are recommended. Additional consultation should be considered by infectious diseases (for evaluation of other congenital infections and assistance with Zika virus diagnosis and testing), clinical genetics (for evaluation for other causes of microcephaly or congenital anomalies), and neurology by age 1 month (for comprehensive neurologic examination and consideration for other evaluations, such as advanced neuroimaging and electroencephalography [EEG]). Infants should be referred for automated brainstem response (ABR) testing by age 1 month

FIG 3.24. RECOMMENDATIONS FOR THE EVALUATION OF INFANTS WITH POSSIBLE CONGENITAL ZIKA VIRUS INFECTION BASED ON INFANT CLINICAL FINDINGS,[a,b] TEST RESULTS IN BIRTHING PARENT,[c,d] AND INFANT TEST RESULTS[e,f]

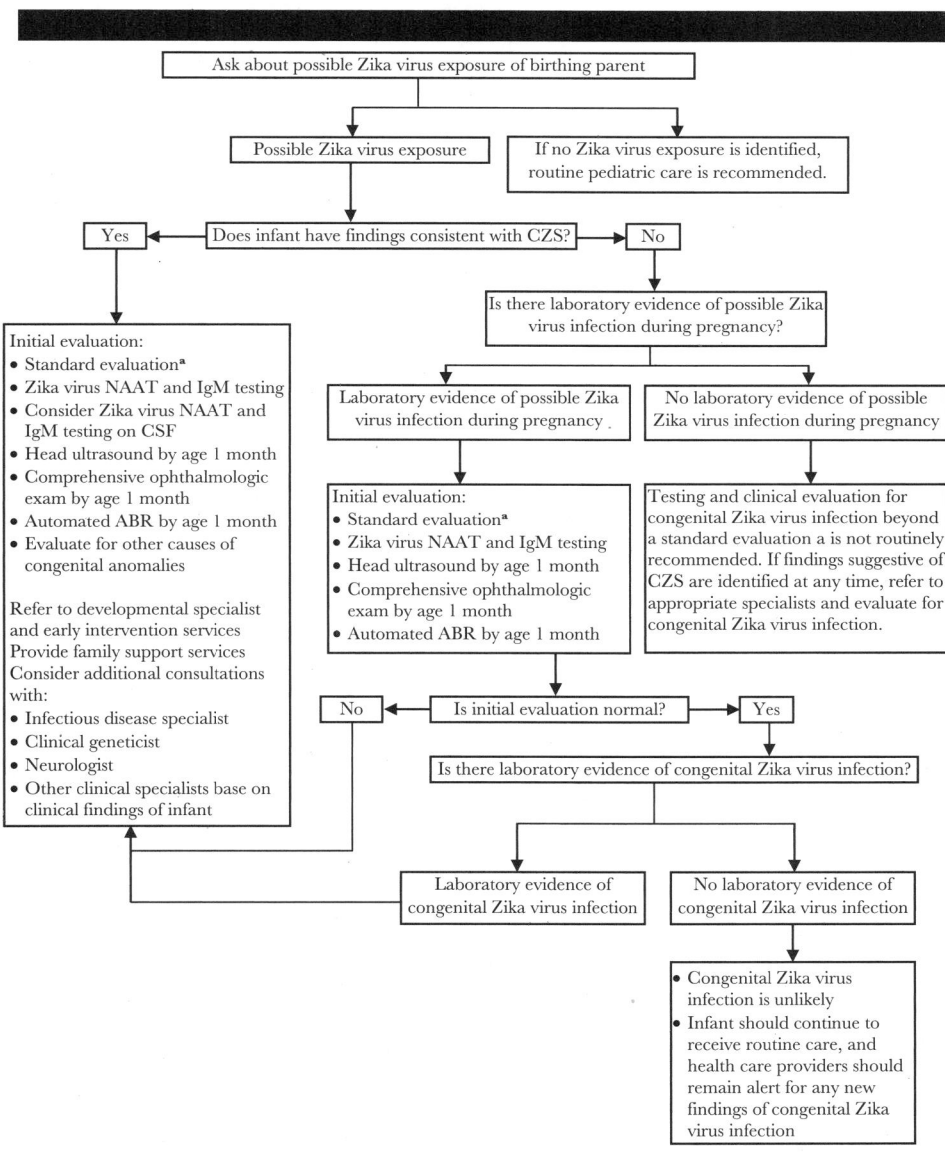

ABR indicates auditory brainstem response; CSF, cerebrospinal fluid; CZS, congenital Zika syndrome; IgM, immunoglobulin M; NAAT, nucleic acid amplification test; PRNT, plaque-reduction neutralization test.

Adapted from Adebanjo T, Godfred-Cato S, Viens L, et al. Update: interim guidance for the diagnosis, evaluation, and management of infants with possible congenital Zika virus infection—United States, October 2017. *MMWR Morb Mortal Wkly Rep.* 2017;66(41):1089–1099

Fig 3.24. Recommendations for the Evaluation of Infants with Possible Congenital Zika Virus Infection Based on Infant Clinical Findings,[a,b] Test Results in Birthing Parent,[c,d] and Infant Test Results,[e,f] Continued

[a]All infants should receive a standard evaluation at birth and at each subsequent well-child visit by their health care providers, including (1) comprehensive physical examination, including growth parameters; and 2) age-appropriate vision screening and developmental monitoring and screening using validated tools. Infants should receive a standard newborn hearing screen at birth, preferably using auditory brainstem response (ABR).

[b]Automated ABR by age 1 month if newborn hearing screen passed but performed with otoacoustic emission methodology.

[c]Laboratory evidence of possible Zika virus infection during pregnancy is defined as 1) Zika virus infection detected by a Zika virus RNA NAT on any maternal, placental, or fetal specimen (referred to as NAAT-confirmed), or 2) diagnosis of Zika virus infection, timing of infection cannot be determined or unspecified flavivirus infection, timing of infection cannot be determined by serologic tests on a maternal specimen (ie, positive/equivocal Zika virus IgM and Zika virus PRNT titer ≥10, regardless of dengue virus PRNT value; or negative Zika virus IgM, and positive or equivocal dengue virus IgM, and Zika virus PRNT titer ≥10, regardless of dengue virus PRNT titer). The use of PRNT for confirmation of Zika virus infection, including in pregnant people, is not routinely recommended in Puerto Rico (**www.cdc.gov/zika/laboratories/lab-guidance.html**).

[d]This group includes people who were never tested during pregnancy as well as those whose test result was negative because of issues related to timing or sensitivity and specificity of the test. Because the latter issues are not easily discerned, all birthing parents with possible exposure to Zika virus during pregnancy who do not have laboratory evidence of possible Zika virus infection, including those who tested negative with currently available technology, should be considered in this group.

[e]Laboratory testing of infants for Zika virus should be performed as early as possible, preferably within the first few days after birth, and includes concurrent Zika virus NAAT in infant serum and urine, and Zika virus IgM testing in serum. If CSF is obtained for other purposes, Zika virus NAAT and Zika virus IgM testing should be performed on CSF.

[f]Laboratory evidence of congenital Zika virus infection includes a positive Zika virus NAAT or a nonnegative Zika virus IgM with confirmatory neutralizing antibody testing, if PRNT confirmation is performed.

if the newborn hearing screen was passed using only otoacoustic emission (OAE) methodology.

Clinical Management of Infants Without Clinical Findings Consistent With Congenital Zika Infection but Laboratory Evidence of Possible Zika Virus Infection of the Birthing Parent During Pregnancy. Zika virus testing is recommended (see Zika Laboratory Testing for Congenital Infection, p 967), and ultrasonography of the head should be performed by age 1 month to detect subclinical brain findings. All infants should have a comprehensive ophthalmologic examination by age 1 month to detect subclinical eye findings. Infants should be referred for automated ABR testing by 1 month of age if newborn screen was passed using only OAE methodology. Infants should be monitored for findings consistent with congenital Zika syndrome that could develop over time (eg, impaired visual acuity/function, hearing problems, developmental delay, delay in head growth).

Clinical Management of Infants Without Clinical Findings Consistent With Congenital Zika Infection Whose Birthing Parent Had Possible Zika Virus Infection During Pregnancy but Without Laboratory Evidence of Zika Virus During Pregnancy. Zika virus testing is not routinely recommended, and specialized clinical evaluation or follow-up is not routinely indicated. Health care providers can consider additional evaluation in consultation with families. If findings suggestive of congenital Zika virus disease are identified at any time, referrals to the appropriate specialists should be made.

INFECTION PREVENTION AND CONTROL MEASURES IN HEALTH CARE SETTINGS:
Standard precautions are recommended. People infected with Zika virus should be protected from further mosquito exposure, especially during the first week of illness, to reduce the risk of local transmission to others.

CONTROL MEASURES: No vaccines or preventive drugs are available, but a number of candidate vaccines are under evaluation in clinical trials. Prevention and control measures rely on personal prevention measures to avoid mosquito bites and community-level programs to reduce vector densities in areas with endemic infection. Personal measures include using insect repellent; wearing long pants, socks, and long-sleeved shirts while outdoors; and staying in air-conditioned buildings or buildings with window and door screens. Permethrin-treated clothing and gear can repel mosquitoes. Travelers returning to the United States from an area with risk of Zika, even if asymptomatic, should take steps to prevent mosquito bites for 3 weeks to minimize spread to local mosquito populations (**www.cdc.gov/zika/prevention/prevent-mosquito-bites.html**).

Insect repellents registered by the US Environmental Protection Agency (EPA) can be used according to directions on the product labels. Products containing N,N-diethyl-meta-toluamide (DEET), picaridin, oil of lemon eucalyptus, IR3535, para-menthane-diol (PMD), and 2-undecanone provide protection from mosquito bites (see Prevention of Mosquito-borne and Tick-borne Infections, p 207). More information about these ingredients can be found at **www.epa.gov/insect-repellents/skin-applied-repellent-ingredients.** All travelers should take precautions to avoid mosquito bites to prevent Zika virus infection and other mosquito-borne diseases.

Sexual Transmission. Zika virus can be transmitted sexually. Couples in which the man or woman has had possible Zika virus exposure who want to maximally reduce their risk for sexually transmitting Zika virus to the uninfected partner should use condoms or abstain from sex for at least 3 months for men or 2 months for women after symptom onset (if symptomatic) or last possible Zika virus exposure (if asymptomatic) (**www.cdc.gov/zika/prevention/sexual-transmission-prevention.html**).[1] Sperm should not be donated for at least 3 months from infection or last exposure.

People Who Are Pregnant or Seeking to Become Pregnant. Pregnant people should not travel to areas with ongoing Zika outbreaks (**wwwnc.cdc.gov/travel/page/zika-travel-information**). Before traveling to areas with current or past transmission of Zika, pregnant people should discuss their travel plans with their health care provider. In deciding whether to travel, pregnant people should consider the destination, reasons for traveling, and ability to prevent mosquito bites. There is no restriction on the use of insect repellents by pregnant women if used in accordance with the instructions on the product label. Male partners of pregnant people who have traveled to areas with local transmission of Zika virus should abstain from sex or use condoms for the duration of the pregnancy to avoid sexual transmission to their pregnant partners (**www.cdc.gov/zika/prevention/sexual-transmission-prevention.html**).

For couples who have possible Zika virus exposure and who are considering pregnancy, the CDC recommends postponing pregnancy for 3 months following potential exposure or diagnosis of Zika infection (**www.cdc.gov/zika/prevention/sexual-transmission-prevention.html**).

---

[1] The terms man, men, male, woman, and women refer to sex assigned at birth.

Blood and Tissue Donation. Following the decrease in incidence of Zika virus in the United States and its territories, the US Food and Drug Administration (FDA) removed the requirement for routine Zika virus NAAT screening of blood donations. However, it is recommended that individuals who were infected with Zika virus infection defer blood donations for 120 days following symptom resolution or their last positive test, whichever is longer, to reduce the risk for transfusion-associated transmission of Zika virus. It is also recommended that individuals should be ineligible to donate human cells, tissues, and cellular and tissue-based products if they had a diagnosis of Zika virus infection within the past 6 months. Individuals suspected of having Zika virus infection at any point during a pregnancy should not be eligible to donate umbilical cord blood, placenta tissue, or other gestational tissues.

Breastfeeding. The World Health Organization and Centers for Disease Control and Prevention (CDC) recommend infants born to a person with suspected, probable, or confirmed Zika virus infection, or to a person who lives in or has traveled to areas with Zika virus, should be fed according to local infant feeding guidelines. Breastfeeding is encouraged even in areas where Zika virus is found because of the benefits of breastfeeding.

Public Health Reporting. Health care professionals should report suspected Zika virus infection to their state or local health departments to facilitate diagnosis and mitigate the risk of local transmission. Zika virus disease and congenital infections were added to the list of nationally notifiable diseases in 2016. State health departments should then report cases to the CDC through ArboNET, the national surveillance system for arboviral diseases.

Antimicrobial Agents and Related Therapy

....

INTRODUCTION

Initial studies evaluating the efficacy and safety of new antimicrobial agents are usually conducted in adults, with pediatric studies occurring later. The product label (package insert) approved by the US Food and Drug Administration (FDA) for a given antimicrobial drug provides information on indications based on clinical trial data reviewed by the FDA. Virtually all current antimicrobial product labels are available at **https://dailymed.nlm.nih.gov/dailymed/.** The FDA also maintains a website (**www.accessdata.fda.gov/scripts/cder/daf/**) of approved drug products with therapeutic equivalence evaluations, an online repository of labels for approved drugs (**https://labels.fda.gov/**), and information about drug shortages (**www.accessdata.fda.gov/scripts/drugshortages/default.cfm**). Additional information from the American Society of Health System Pharmacists on current drug shortages in the United States can be found at **www.asph.org/shortages.**

An FDA-approved indication usually means that adequate and well-controlled studies were conducted, presented to, and reviewed by the FDA for use in the populations in which the drug was investigated. However, accepted medical practice often includes use of drugs that are not reflected in approved indications found in the drug label ("off-label" use). These additional clinical uses of antimicrobial agents may become apparent and investigated years after initial approval of an agent. Oftentimes, because of high cost, additional trials are not performed or presented to the FDA to allow for a change in the package label. For this reason, lack of FDA approval may not necessarily mean lack of effectiveness. Unapproved use also does not imply improper use, provided that reasonable supporting medical evidence exists and that use of the drug is deemed to be in the best interest of the patient. The decision to prescribe a drug is the responsibility of the medical provider, who must weigh the risks and benefits of using the drug for a specific situation.

Some antimicrobial agents with proven therapeutic benefit in adults are not approved by the FDA for use in pediatric patients or, rarely, are considered contraindicated in children because of possible toxicity. The following information delineates general principles for use of fluoroquinolones, tetracyclines, and other approved agents.

Fluoroquinolones

Fluoroquinolones (eg, ciprofloxacin, levofloxacin, moxifloxacin, delafloxacin) should not be used routinely as first-line agents in children younger than 18 years except when specific indications exist or in specific conditions for which there are no alternative agents (including oral agents) and the drug is known to be effective for the specific situation. Use of fluoroquinolones in adults and children is a driver of fluoroquinolone resistance and, therefore, using fluoroquinolones judiciously is an important strategy to combat antibiotic resistance as well as to improve patient safety. Information on the safety of fluoroquinolones for children was reviewed and published by the American Academy of Pediatrics.[1]

Rare risks related to fluoroquinolones are summarized as follows:

- *Clostridioides difficile* (formerly called *Clostridium difficile*) disease: Fluoroquinolones are among the most common antimicrobials to be associated with *C difficile* disease.
- Tendinopathy: Fluoroquinolones are associated in adults with an increased risk of tendon rupture (with a predilection for the Achilles tendon) and tendonitis, with further increased risk in people older than 60 years; in those who have received renal, heart, kidney, or lung transplants; and in those with concurrent use of corticosteroids. To date, there have been no reports of Achilles tendon rupture in children in association with fluoroquinolone use.
- QT interval prolongation: Certain fluoroquinolones (moxifloxacin, levofloxacin, ciprofloxacin) can prolong the QT interval and should be avoided, if possible, in patients with long QT syndrome, those with hypokalemia or hypomagnesemia, those with organic heart disease including congestive heart failure, those receiving an antiarrhythmic agent from class Ia (particularly quinidine) or class III (see **www.ncbi. nlm.nih.gov/books/NBK482322/**), those who are receiving a concurrent drug that prolongs the QTc interval independently, and those with hepatic insufficiency-related metabolic derangements that may promote QT prolongation.
- Central nervous system toxicity: Neurologic complications associated with fluoroquinolone use, although very uncommon in children, include peripheral neuropathy, seizures, lightheadedness, sleep disorders, hallucinations, dizziness, headaches, disturbances in attention, disorientation, agitation, nervousness, memory impairment, delirium, and pseudotumor cerebri.
- Myasthenia gravis: Fluoroquinolones may unmask or worsen muscle weakness in people with myasthenia gravis.
- Arthralgia: Transient arthralgia has been reported in patients treated with fluoroquinolones. However, arthralgia has not been confirmed by clinical examination and controlled trials have not yet proven direct causal effect of fluoroquinolones. Some pediatric studies have observed an increased incidence of reversible adverse events involving joints or surrounding tissues with fluoroquinolones compared with other agents. For some fluoroquinolones, cartilage damage in some animal models occurs at doses that approximate therapeutic doses in humans. The mechanism of damage remains speculative, but there are emerging in vitro data to suggest direct collagen effects. Long-term safety data have been reported for both levofloxacin and moxifloxacin. To date, there is no compelling evidence of long-term sequelae related to fluoroquinolone bone or joint toxicity in children.
- Thrombocytopenia, immune-mediated hemolytic anemia, hepatic dysfunction, renal dysfunctions (interstitial nephritis and crystal nephropathy), hyperglycemia/hypoglycemia, hypersensitivity, and photosensitivity reactions have also been reported.

The FDA has issued a Drug Safety Communication for the fluoroquinolone class, advising that health care providers should not prescribe systemic fluoroquinolones to patients who have other treatment options for acute bacterial sinusitis, acute bacterial

---

[1] Jackson MA, Schutze GE; American Academy of Pediatrics, Committee on Infectious Diseases. The use of systemic and topical fluoroquinolones. *Pediatrics*. 2016;138(5):e20162706

exacerbation of chronic bronchitis, and uncomplicated urinary tract infections, because the risks outweigh the benefits in these patients.[1] Although ciprofloxacin is approved for use in children 1 year and older with complicated urinary tract infection or pyelonephritis, it should not be a first-line agent, and other agents should be used preferentially if the pathogens are suspected or documented to be susceptible to other agents with a more favorable safety profile. The significant exceptions in which ciprofloxacin may be used as a first-line agent in children are for postexposure prophylaxis for inhalation anthrax (ciprofloxacin primarily, with levofloxacin and moxifloxacin considered equivalent alternatives; see Anthrax, p 232) and treatment of plague (ciprofloxacin, levofloxacin, or moxifloxacin; see Plague, p 671).

Circumstances in which use of systemic fluoroquinolones may be justified in children include the following: (1) parenteral therapy is not practical, and no other safe and effective oral agent is available (eg, tularemia); and (2) infection is caused by a multidrug-resistant pathogen for which there is no other effective intravenous or oral agent available. Clinical situations for the use of systemic or topical fluoroquinolones may include the following:

- Urinary tract, bone, or other invasive infections, including chronic suppurative otitis media or malignant otitis externa caused by *Pseudomonas aeruginosa* or other multidrug-resistant, gram-negative bacteria resistant to beta-lactams and other classes of antimicrobial agents.
- Multidrug-resistant (beta-lactam, carbapenem, macrolide, and trimethoprim-sulfamethoxazole resistant) pneumococcal infections.
- Gastrointestinal tract infection or bacteremia caused by suspected or documented multidrug-resistant *Shigella* species, *Salmonella* species, *Vibrio cholerae*, *Campylobacter jejuni*, or *Campylobacter coli* or *Enterobacterales*.
- Mycobacterial infections that are multidrug resistant for which no other oral drug is available or appropriate.
- Serious infections attributable to fluoroquinolone-susceptible pathogen(s) in children with severe allergy to alternative agents.
- Otorrhea associated with tympanic membrane perforation as well as tympanostomy tube otorrhea, for which topical fluoroquinolone-containing agents are considered as safer alternatives to aminoglycoside-containing agents.

Tetracyclines

Use of tetracyclines as a class of drugs in pediatric patients historically has been limited because of reports that this class could cause permanent dental discoloration in children younger than 8 years, because their degradation products are incorporated in tooth enamel. The period of odontogenesis to completion of formation of enamel in permanent teeth appears to be the critical time for effects of these drugs, and it is now known that the calcification stage of tooth development starts at the sixth week of development in utero and is usually completed at 3 to 4 months of life. The degree of teeth staining from tetracyclines appears to depend on dosage, duration of therapy, and which drug in the tetracycline class is used.

[1] US Food and Drug Administration. FDA Drug Safety Communication: FDA advises restricting fluoroquinolone antibiotic use for certain uncomplicated infections; warns about disabling side effects that can occur together. Available at: **www.fda.gov/Drugs/DrugSafety/ucm500143.htm**

Doxycycline binds less readily to calcium compared with other members of the tetracycline class. The use of doxycycline was previously limited largely to patients 8 years and older due to historical concern for a drug class effect with tetracyclines. However, data from the United States and Europe suggest that doxycycline is not likely to cause visible teeth staining or enamel hypoplasia in children younger than 8 years. These reassuring data support the current recommendation by the American Academy of Pediatrics that doxycycline can be administered without regard to the patient's age or the duration of therapy. When used, patients of all skin tones and colors should be careful to avoid excess sun exposure because of photosensitivity associated with doxycycline.

Antimicrobial Agents Approved for Use in Adults but Not Children

Antimicrobial agents in a variety of classes have been studied and approved by the FDA for use in adults for certain indications, particularly for infections caused by methicillin-resistant *Staphylococcus aureus* and multidrug-resistant gram-negative bacilli but still are under investigation for pharmacokinetics and safety in children. For some agents that the pharmaceutical sponsor wishes to market for children, additional investigation for clinical and microbiologic efficacy in children are required to obtain FDA approval. These agents include but are not limited to oritavancin, telavancin, imipenem/relebactam, meropenem/vaborbactam, lefamulin, plazomicin, and for older children, tetracycline-class agents eravacycline and omadacycline. These drugs should be used in children only when no other safe and effective agents that are FDA approved for use in children are available and when benefits are expected to exceed risks for that patient. For these agents with relatively undefined or emerging safety and efficacy in pediatrics, consultation with an expert in pediatric infectious diseases should be considered.

· ·

BETA-LACTAM AND MONOBACTAM ALLERGIES[1,2]

Although true penicillin allergy (immunoglobulin [Ig] E mediated) occurs in only 1% of the population, a full 10% of patients are labeled as penicillin allergic. Penicillin allergy is often unconfirmed and reported by patients and families because of a history of rash (urticarial or nonurticarial), other adverse events (eg, diarrhea), or even family history. Labeling a patient as penicillin allergic complicates treatment of many infections (eg, acute otitis media, sinusitis, and skin and soft tissue infections), leading to alternative antibiotic therapies that often are more broad spectrum, increase antibiotic resistance, and are less efficacious. To reduce antibiotic allergy overlabeling, investigation of the type of reaction and timing of the penicillin allergy should be undertaken. For patients who do not report potential IgE-mediated reactions (eg, anaphylaxis,

---

[1] Joint Task Force on Practice Parameters representing the American Academy of Allergy, Asthma and Immunology; American College of Allergy, Asthma and Immunology; Joint Council of Allergy, Asthma and Immunology. Drug allergy: an updated practice parameter. *Ann Allergy Asthma Immunol.* 2010;105(4):259-273

[2] Kahn DA, Banerji A, Blumenthal KG, et al. Drug allergy: a 2022 practice parameter update. *J Allergy Clin Immunol.* 2022;150(6):1333-1393

wheezing, lightheadedness, bronchospasm, angioedema/swelling, flushing/redness) or more severe reactions (eg, Stevens-Johnson syndrome), penicillin allergy delabeling should be considered.

Most (80%) patients with a history of true IgE-mediated penicillin allergy lose their sensitivity after 10 years. Therefore, in patients with a remote history of allergy (>10 years ago) or a history of benign reactions (eg, nonspecific rash or delayed urticarial rash), oral challenge testing should be undertaken to remove the penicillin allergy label without the need for skin testing. In patients with a recent history of a

FIG 4.1. CEPHALOSPORIN CROSS-REACTIVITY MATRIX[a]

[a]This matrix describes the risk of cross-reactivity between 2 beta-lactam antibiotics. Boxes with a symbol indicate either a similar (light gray) or an identical (dark gray) side chain and, therefore, higher risk for an allergic reaction. Empty boxes indicate a lack of side-chain similarity and decreased risk of allergic reaction.

Reproduced with permission from Blumenthal KG, Shenoy ES, Wolfson AR, et al. Addressing inpatient beta-lactam allergies: a multihospital implementation. *J Allergy Clin Immunol Pract.* 2017;5(3):616-625.

suspected IgE-mediated reaction (eg, immediate urticaria), skin testing should be performed prior to oral challenge testing. In patients who report other adverse events from penicillin (eg, headache, abdominal pain) or a family history of penicillin allergy, delabeling procedures are not necessary; the penicillin allergy label may be removed and penicillin antibiotics may be used as needed.

Studies have shown that the risk of beta-lactam cross-reactivity with cephalosporins is lower than previously reported and is believed to be related to beta-lactam ring R group side chains (see Fig 4.1). Patients with unconfirmed nonanaphylactic penicillin allergy can safely receive any cephalosporin without any testing or precautions. Patients with a history of penicillin anaphylaxis may receive a non–cross-reactive cephalosporin (eg, cefazolin) without prior testing.

Patients with cephalosporin allergy should be categorized by severity of reaction and whether the reaction is confirmed or not. In patients with nonanaphylactic and unconfirmed reactions to cephalosporins, penicillin antibiotic agents may be prescribed without testing or precautions. For example, amoxicillin may be safely prescribed in patients with history of urticaria to cephalexin without testing. However, patients with previous anaphylaxis to a cephalosporin should undergo penicillin skin testing prior to receipt of a penicillin agent.

Patients with a history of penicillin or cephalosporin allergy, even anaphylaxis, may receive carbapenems and/or aztreonam without prior testing or precautions (with the exception of ceftazidime because of identical R1 side chain).

A cephalosporin cross-reactivity matrix has been published (Fig 4.1) that quantifies the likelihood of cross-reactivity. This figure indicates side-chain cross-reactivity only; when considering cross-reactivity between penicillins and cephalosporins, cross-reactivity is also possible with the core beta-lactam ring.

···

Antimicrobial Resistance and Antimicrobial Stewardship: Appropriate and Judicious Use of Antimicrobial Agents

Antimicrobial Resistance

The Centers for Disease Control and Prevention (CDC), World Health Organization (WHO), and other international agencies have identified antimicrobial resistance as one of the world's most pressing public health threats. In the United States, more than 2.8 million people are infected with antimicrobial-resistant bacteria, and at least 35 000 deaths occur annually as a direct result of these infections.[1] Highly resistant gram-negative pathogens (eg, carbapenemase-producing *Enterobacterales* and *Acinetobacter* species, multidrug-resistant *Pseudomonas aeruginosa*, and extended-spectrum beta-lactamase–producing *Enterobacterales*), gram-positive pathogens (eg, methicillin-resistant *Staphylococcus aureus* and *Enterococcus* species resistant to ampicillin and vancomycin),

[1] Centers for Disease Control and Prevention. Antibiotic Resistance Threats in the United States 2019. Available at: **www.cdc.gov/drugresistance/pdf/threats-report/2019-ar-threats-report-508.pdf**

and drug-resistant *Candida* species are increasingly associated with invasive infections. *Clostridioides difficile* disease is the most common cause of diarrhea acquired in a health care facility and an infection that usually results from antimicrobial exposure. *C difficile* causes approximately 223 900 infections and at least 12 800 deaths annually in the United States. The CDC has ranked the antimicrobial-resistant bacteria and fungi that have the most impact on human health in categories of urgent, serious, and concerning threats (Table 4.1).

The presence of resistant pathogens complicates patient management, increases morbidity and mortality, and increases medical expenses for patients and the health care system. Studies have estimated that antimicrobial resistance in the United States adds as much as $20 billion in excess costs to the health care system each year, and the costs to society from lost productivity are as high as $35 billion.

Factors Contributing to Resistance

The use of antimicrobial agents is a key driver of antimicrobial resistance. Antimicrobial agents are among the most commonly prescribed drugs used in human medicine. Many studies have measured the extent of inappropriate or unnecessary antibiotic use, which has been observed in 25% to 50% of hospitalized adults and children. The problem of inappropriate antibiotic use extends to outpatient settings, where the bulk of antibiotics are prescribed. In the United States, it is estimated that one-third of outpatient antibiotic prescriptions are inappropriate, including half of those prescribed for respiratory tract infections, millions of which are for children.

Table 4.1. Antimicrobial-Resistant Bacteria and Fungi Posing Health Threats

Urgent Threats	Serious Threats	Concerning Threats	Watch List
Carbapenem-resistant *Acinetobacter* *Candida auris* *Clostridioides difficile* Carbapenem-resistant *Enterobacterales* Drug-resistant *Neisseria gonorrhoeae*	Drug-resistant *Campylobacter* Drug-resistant *Candida* ESBL-producing *Enterobacterales* Vancomycin-resistant enterococci (VRE) Multidrug-resistant *Pseudomonas aeruginosa* Drug-resistant nontyphoidal *Salmonella* Drug-resistant *Salmonella* serotype Typhi Drug-resistant *Shigella* Methicillin-resistant *Staphylococcus aureus* (MRSA) Drug-resistant *Streptococcus pneumoniae* Drug-resistant tuberculosis	Erythromycin-resistant group A *Streptococcus* Clindamycin-resistant group B *Streptococcus*	Azole-resistant *Aspergillus fumigatus* Drug-resistant *Mycoplasma genitalium* Drug-resistant *Bordetella pertussis*

Adapted from **www.cdc.gov/drugresistance/biggest-threats.html.**

The number of antibiotic-resistant bacteria and the diversity of molecular mechanisms of resistance continue to increase, while the development of newer, effective antimicrobial agents has dwindled. The loss of effective antimicrobial agents will hamper clinicians' efforts to treat potentially life-threatening infections. Compounding this problem, advances in medical treatment involving immunosuppression have expanded the population of immunocompromised people, who rely on the receipt of effective antimicrobial agents to prevent or control infection. When first- and second-line treatment options are rendered ineffective against antimicrobial resistant pathogens, clinicians are forced to use agents that may be more toxic, costly, and/or less effective.

The overuse of antimicrobial agents in animal agriculture also contributes substantially to the problem of antimicrobial resistance.[1] The CDC has determined that antimicrobial use in animals is linked to resistance in humans. The US Food and Drug Administration has described a pathway toward reducing inappropriate antimicrobial use in animals, and major medical and public health organizations, including the American Academy of Pediatrics (AAP), have called for stronger action.[2]

Actions to Prevent or Slow Antimicrobial Resistance

Antimicrobial resistance can only be addressed through concerted and collaborative efforts. The CDC's Antibiotic Resistance Solutions initiative invests in US infrastructure to detect, respond to, contain, and prevent antimicrobial resistant infections (**www.cdc.gov/drugresistance/solutions-initiative/index.html**). Actions to combat antimicrobial resistance include:

1. **Prevent infections and reduce the spread of resistance.** Antimicrobial-resistant infections can be prevented by immunization, infection prevention in health care settings, safe food preparation and handling, and handwashing. The CDC has also provided guidance on the containment of highly resistant pathogens of public health concern (**www.cdc.gov/hai/containment/**).

2. **Track antimicrobial resistant infections.** The CDC, in collaboration with health care facilities and state and local health departments, gathers data on antimicrobial-resistant infections to help inform strategies and interventions for prevention. The CDC Antibiotic Resistance Laboratory Network (**www.cdc. gov/drugresistance/solutions-initiative/ar-lab-network.html**) provides regional capacity to detect and characterize resistant pathogens.

3. **Improve antimicrobial use and promote antimicrobial stewardship.** It is critical to modify the way antimicrobial agents are used in humans and animals. Unnecessary and inappropriate use of antimicrobial agents is common across the continuum of care. Inappropriate use of antimicrobial agents often is a result of

---

[1] Katz SE, Banerjee R; American Academy of Pediatrics, Committee on Infectious Diseases, Council on Environmental Health and Climate Change. Technical report: Antimicrobial agents in animals: One Health perspectives and implications for pediatrics. *Pediatrics.* 2024; in press

[2] Pediatric Infectious Diseases Society. Pediatric ASP Toolkit. Advocacy Addressing Antibiotic Overuse in Animal Agriculture and the Environment. Available at: **https://pids.org/pediatric-asp-toolkit/advocacy-addressing-antibiotic-overuse-in-animal-agriculture-and-the-environment/**

errors in antimicrobial selection, dosing, or duration of therapy. Unnecessary exposure to antimicrobial agents results in adverse drug reactions, subsequent treatment challenges related to the development of antimicrobial resistance, and complications including *C difficile* disease. Every health care facility should have a formal antimicrobial stewardship program (ASP) built on the CDC's Core Elements of Antimicrobial Stewardship (see next section). Outpatient antimicrobial stewardship also is important to combat inappropriate antibiotic prescribing and antibiotic resistance.

4. **Develop drugs and improve diagnostic tests.** Discovery of new antimicrobial agents is needed to keep pace with the emergence of pathogen resistance. Unfortunately, the number of antimicrobial agents in late-phase clinical development is low. In particular, few agents are being developed with new mechanisms of action to treat resistant gram-negative infections. In addition, new diagnostic tests are needed to guide antimicrobial therapy and to track the development of resistance.

Antimicrobial Stewardship

The primary goal of antimicrobial stewardship is to optimize antimicrobial use with the aim of decreasing inappropriate use that leads to unwarranted toxicity and spread of resistant organisms. The CDC's Core Elements of Antibiotic Stewardship provides a framework for implementing stewardship across the spectrum of health care and includes guidance for hospitals, including small and critical access hospitals; nursing homes; outpatient settings; and resource-limited settings outside the United States (**www.cdc.gov/antibiotic-use/core-elements/index.html**). The AAP and Pediatric Infectious Diseases Society have developed a toolkit to aid in the implementation of inpatient stewardship programs (**https://pids.org/pediatric-asp-toolkit/**).

For inpatient facilities, the CDC describes 7 core elements needed for a successful ASP (**www.cdc.gov/antibiotic-use/healthcare/implementation/core-elements.html**):

• *Hospital leadership commitment.* Hospital administration should support and provide dedicated time to a stewardship program leader and a pharmacist co-leader as well as financial and technologic resources needed to accomplish the programmatic goals.

• *Accountability.* A program leader (often a physician) should work collaboratively with a pharmacy leader and other core members of the ASP team (infectious diseases specialists, clinical pharmacists, nurses, clinical microbiologists, hospital epidemiologists, infection prevention professionals, and information systems specialists). This leader should ensure that other core elements of a successful program are implemented.

• *Pharmacy expertise.* A pharmacy leader should work collaboratively with the physician leader to implement the key actions and other core elements.

• *Action.* Numerous actions have been described to successfully improve antibiotic use. Requiring **prior authorization** for select antimicrobials and/or prolonged durations of therapy (eg, beyond 48–72 hours) and **prospective audit with feedback** are evidence-based approaches proven to reduce unnecessary antimicrobial use, adverse drug effects, and costs. Additional actions include development of clinical practice guidelines, clinical decision support, clinician and patient education, conversion from intravenous to oral agents, and dose optimization. Supplementation of these interventions with face-to-face interactions is recommended when possible, and stewardship of antimicrobial prescribing at the point of hospital discharge is an emerging target.

- *Tracking.* Antibiotic use data should be monitored and reported as days of therapy per 1000 patient days or days present. The CDC has developed the Antimicrobial Use and Resistance module within the National Healthcare Safety Network that provides a standardized antimicrobial administration ratio for a specific institution. The standardized antimicrobial administration ratio can be used in benchmarking with other institutions. (**www.cdc.gov/nhsn/pdfs/pscmanual/11pscaurcurrent. pdf**). Other data to be monitored may include hospital-onset *C difficile* disease rates, length of stay, adverse drug events, and rates of concerning antibiotic-resistant pathogens (eg, carbapenem-resistant *Enterobacterales*, methicillin-resistant *S aureus*), and hospital costs.
- *Reporting.* Regular updates on key process and outcome metrics, including antimicrobial use, resistance, adverse effects, and cost, should be given to prescribers, pharmacists, nurses, and senior administrators.
- *Education.* All health care workers should receive annual education regarding current antimicrobial stewardship practices and additional methods to improve use. Furthermore, efforts are needed to educate patients, families, and caregivers about antimicrobial stewardship and the impact of inappropriate antimicrobial use.

As part of the Choosing Wisely campaign, the AAP and the Pediatric Infectious Diseases Society (**www.pids.org**) have published "Five Things Physicians and Patients Should Question" about antimicrobial therapy:

- Don't initiate empiric antibiotic therapy in a patient with suspected invasive bacterial infection without first confirming that blood, urine, or other appropriate cultures have been obtained, excluding exceptional cases.
- Don't use a broad-spectrum antimicrobial agent for perioperative prophylaxis or continue prophylaxis after the incision is closed for uncomplicated clean and clean-contaminated procedures.
- Don't treat uncomplicated community-acquired pneumonia in otherwise healthy, immunized, hospitalized patients with antibiotic therapy broader than ampicillin.
- Don't use vancomycin or carbapenems empirically for neonatal intensive care patients unless an infant is known to have a specific risk for pathogens resistant to narrower-spectrum agents.
- Don't place peripherally inserted central catheters and/or use prolonged intravenous antibiotics in otherwise healthy children with infections that can be transitioned to an appropriate oral agent.

Although inpatients are frequently exposed to broad-spectrum and potentially toxic antimicrobial agents, the vast majority of antibiotic exposure occurs in the outpatient setting. The CDC has developed the Core Elements of Outpatient Antibiotic Stewardship to help improve the use of antibiotics in this setting (**www.cdc.gov/ antibiotic-use/core-elements/outpatient.html**). These core elements include commitment, action for policy and practice, tracking and reporting, education, and expertise. Actions that have been successful in the outpatient setting include clinician audit and feedback with peer comparisons, commitment "nudge" posters, communications training, clinical decision support, patient education about viral and bacterial infections or adverse events associated with antibiotic use, and clinician education. Interventions that incorporate a combination of approaches tend to be most effective. In addition, pediatricians should seek understanding of parent expectations for antibiotics, which can influence clinician antibiotic prescribing.

The AAP, along with the Pediatric Infectious Diseases Society, has developed pediatric toolkits for implementing antibiotic stewardship in both inpatient and outpatient settings (**https://pids.org/pediatric-asp-toolkit/**).

Role of the Clinician

Clinicians can integrate key recommendations that focus on antibiotic prescribing for common infections in children. These include the following:

1. Confirm the diagnosis of urinary tract infection by documenting that the patient is symptomatic and has a properly obtained urinalysis and positive quantitative culture. When the infection is confirmed and susceptibility tests are completed, choose an appropriate agent with the narrowest spectrum of activity to target the isolated organism. If cultures are negative and alternative diagnoses are found, contact families to recommend discontinuing antibiotics.

2. Before treating a patient for bacterial pneumonia, ensure that there is not an alternate diagnosis. Respiratory syncytial virus infections in infants are rarely complicated by bacterial infection, but migratory atelectasis is common. For infants with bronchiolitis, antibiotics are not indicated unless a concomitant bacterial infection is present.[1]

3. Standardize processes to ensure that appropriate cultures and other diagnostic tests are obtained before antimicrobial agents are administered.

4. Know how to access local antibiograms and be aware of antimicrobial resistance patterns.

5. Initiate antimicrobial therapy promptly for suspected or proven infection, and document indication, dose, timing, and anticipated duration.

6. Perform an "antibiotic timeout" in hospitalized patients to reassess response to therapy within 48 hours, considering new clinical and laboratory data. Adjust therapy to use the most appropriate agent with the narrowest spectrum and to discontinue antibiotic therapy when a treatable bacterial infection is excluded.

7. Collaborate with the local antimicrobial stewardship team and request formal infectious diseases consultation for complicated cases, such as those with immune deficiency, severe or prolonged illness, difficult to treat organisms, or uncertain diagnosis.

In addition, clear and effective communication is critical for antibiotic stewardship across settings. A study implementing an online intervention (Dialogue Around Respiratory Tract Illness Treatment) demonstrated improvement in antibiotic prescribing for respiratory tract infection when clinicians followed 4 consecutive communication steps: (1) review your findings for a viral infection with the family;

---

[1] Ralston SL, Lieberthal AS, Meissner HC, et al. Clinical practice guideline: the diagnosis, management, and prevention of bronchiolitis. *Pediatrics.* 2015;136(4):2015-2862

(2) provide a specific diagnosis that is nonbacterial in origin; (3) offer positive treatment recommendations like hydration and fever control; and (4) offer a contingency plan if the child does not get better. The CDC has also developed a communication training module for clinicians to improve outpatient antibiotic prescribing (**www.train.org/cdctrain/course/1076989/**). Additional information for health care professionals and parents on judicious use of antimicrobial agents and antimicrobial resistance is available on the CDC website (**www.cdc.gov/antibiotic-use/community/materials-references/index.html and www.cdc.gov/drugresistance**).

Principles of Appropriate Use of Antimicrobial Therapy for Upper Respiratory Tract Infections

More than three-quarters of outpatient antibiotic prescriptions for children are given for 5 conditions: otitis media, sinusitis, cough illness/bronchitis, pharyngitis, and nonspecific upper respiratory tract infection (the common cold). Antibiotics are often prescribed even though most of these illnesses are caused by viruses. Children treated with antibiotics for respiratory tract infections are at increased risk of becoming colonized with resistant respiratory tract flora, including *Streptococcus pneumoniae* and *Haemophilus influenzae*. These same children are more likely to experience failure of subsequent antimicrobial therapy and are likely to spread resistant bacteria to close contacts. In addition, antibiotics are the most common cause of emergency department visits for adverse drug events in children. The following principles can assist pediatricians in prescribing antibiotic agents appropriately and only when needed for these common pediatric conditions.

OTITIS MEDIA

- The decision to initiate antibiotic therapy versus observation for children diagnosed with acute otitis media (AOM) should incorporate information about illness severity, laterality of infection, age, and assurance of follow-up. **Immediate antibiotic treatment** is indicated for children <6 months of age, those with otorrhea or severe signs and symptoms (temperature ≥39°F [102.2°F], ear pain for ≥48 hours, or moderate to severe ear pain), and children 6 through 23 months of age with bilateral AOM (regardless of severity). **Observation and pain management** for 48 to 72 hours with close follow-up can be offered (on the basis of shared decision making with the parent or caregiver) to children 6 through 23 months of age without severe symptoms and unilateral AOM and for children 24 months and older without severe symptoms (with unilateral or bilateral AOM).
- When antibiotics are used for AOM, a narrow-spectrum agent (eg, amoxicillin, 80–90 mg/kg per day in 2 divided doses) should be used for most children. For children younger than 24 months or those with severe symptoms at any age, a 10-day course is recommended. For children 2 through 5 years of age without severe symptoms, a 7-day course may be used. For children 6 years and older without severe symptoms, a 5- to 7-day course may be used. Microbiologic and clinical failure with high-dose amoxicillin has been associated with highly penicillin-resistant pneumococci (uncommon currently with widespread use of pneumococcal conjugate

vaccine) and with beta-lactamase–producing *Haemophilus* species and *Moraxella* species, which might be increasing as the proportion of cases of AOM caused by pneumococci decreases. Including beta-lactamase coverage by using amoxicillin-clavulanate when treating a child for AOM is indicated if the child has received amoxicillin in the last 30 days, has concurrent purulent conjunctivitis, or has a history of recurrent AOM unresponsive to amoxicillin.

- Children with underlying medical conditions, craniofacial abnormalities, chronic or recurrent otitis media, or perforation of the tympanic membrane represent a more complicated and diverse population. Initial therapy with a 10-day antibiotic course is likely to be more effective than shorter courses for many of these children.

- Persistent middle ear effusion (MEE) is common and can be detected by pneumatic otoscopy (with or without verification by tympanometry) after resolution of acute symptoms. Two weeks after successful antibiotic treatment of AOM, 60% to 70% of children have MEE, decreasing to 40% at 1 month and 10% to 25% at 3 months after successful antibiotic treatment. The presence of MEE without clinical symptoms is defined as otitis media with effusion (OME). OME must be differentiated clinically from AOM and requires infrequent additional monitoring and no antibiotic therapy.

ACUTE SINUSITIS

- Clinical practice guidelines from the AAP[1] and the Infectious Diseases Society of America[2] outline evidence-based criteria for the diagnosis and treatment of acute bacterial sinusitis. Existing clinical criteria are limited in their ability to differentiate bacterial from viral acute rhinosinusitis. A clinical diagnosis of acute bacterial sinusitis requires the presence of at least one of the following criteria: (1) persistent nasal discharge (of any quality) or daytime cough (which may be worse at night) without evidence of clinical improvement for ≥10 days; (2) a worsening course (worsening or new onset of nasal discharge, daytime cough, or fever after initial improvement); or (3) body temperature of ≥39°C (≥102.2°F) with either purulent nasal discharge and/or facial pain concurrently for at least 3 consecutive days in a child who appears ill. Findings on sinus imaging correlate poorly with disease and should not be used for diagnosing acute uncomplicated bacterial sinusitis or to distinguish acute bacterial sinusitis from viral upper respiratory infection. Computed tomography and/or magnetic resonance imaging of sinuses is indicated when complications (eg, orbital or central nervous system complications) are suspected.

- Antibiotic therapy is indicated for all children with severe onset or a worsening course. For children with nonsevere, persistent illness with ≥10 days of symptoms, either observation for an additional 3 days or antibiotic therapy is indicated.

- When antibiotic therapy is initiated, amoxicillin alone or with clavulanate is preferred. Amoxicillin may be used in standard dose (45 mg/kg/day in 2 divided doses);

[1] Wald ER, Applegate KE, Bordley C, et al; American Academy of Pediatrics. Clinical practice guideline for the diagnosis and management of acute bacterial sinusitis in children aged 1 to 18 years. *Pediatrics*. 2013;132(1):e262-e280

[2] Chow AW, Benninger MS, Brook I, et al; Infectious Disease Society of America. IDSA clinical practice guideline for acute bacterial rhinosinusitis in children and adults. *Clin Infect Dis*. 2012;54(8):e72-e112

in areas with high prevalence (>10%) of nonsusceptible *S pneumoniae*, a high dose (80–90 mg/kg/day in 2 divided doses) should be used. Amoxicillin-clavulanate (80–90 mg/kg/day of amoxicillin with 6.4 mg/kg/day of clavulanate [14:1 formulation] in 2 divided doses) may be indicated for children with moderate-to-severe illness, children younger than 2 years, children attending child care, or when antimicrobial resistance is likely (eg, recent treatment with amoxicillin). Five days of therapy is often sufficient.

COUGH ILLNESS/BRONCHITIS

- Nonspecific cough illness/bronchitis in children typically does not warrant antimicrobial treatment.
- Prolonged cough is most often caused by a viral pathogen, but may be caused by *Bordetella pertussis, Bordetella parapertussis, Mycoplasma pneumoniae* and other *Mycoplasma* species, or *Chlamydia pneumoniae.* When infection caused by one of these organisms is suspected clinically or is confirmed, appropriate antimicrobial therapy is indicated (see Pertussis, p 656, *Mycoplasma pneumoniae* and Other *Mycoplasma* Infections, p 616, and Chlamydial Infections, p 298).

PHARYNGITIS

(See Group A Streptococcal Infections, p 785.)
- Diagnosis of group A streptococcal pharyngitis should be made based on results of appropriate laboratory tests in conjunction with clinical and epidemiologic findings.
- Group A streptococcal testing should only be performed in patients with signs and symptoms of pharyngitis without evidence of a viral upper respiratory infection. Testing is not recommended for children younger than 3 years.
- Most cases of pharyngitis are caused by viruses. Antibiotics should not be prescribed to children with pharyngitis without positive group A streptococcal testing. Rarely, other bacteria may cause pharyngitis (eg, *Arcanobacterium haemolyticum, Corynebacterium diphtheriae, Francisella tularensis,* groups G and C hemolytic streptococci, *Neisseria gonorrhoeae, Fusobacterium* species), and treatment should be provided according to recommendations in disease-specific chapters in Section 3.
- Penicillin (intramuscular injection or 10 days orally) remains the treatment of choice for group A streptococcal pharyngitis. Amoxicillin suspension (once daily dosing for 10 days) may be more palatable to children than penicillin and is equally as effective.

THE COMMON COLD

- Antimicrobial agents should not be given for the common cold.
- Mucopurulent rhinitis (thick, opaque, or discolored nasal discharge that begins a few days into a viral upper respiratory tract infection) commonly accompanies the common cold and is not an indication for antibiotic treatment.
- Symptomatic therapies like ibuprofen, acetaminophen, humidified air, and honey in children older than 12 months can be recommended for symptomatic relief.

TABLES OF ANTIBACTERIAL DRUG DOSAGES

Recommended dosages for antibacterial agents commonly used for neonates (see Table 4.2, p 988) and for infants and children (see Table 4.3, p 993) are provided separately because of the pharmacokinetic and dosing differences between these 2 groups.

Table 4.2 is organized by variables such as gestational age (GA), postnatal age (PNA), and postmenstrual age (PMA) that best guide neonatal dosing for a given group of antimicrobial agents. Aminoglycosides and vancomycin are listed in separate tables to highlight their target serum concentration. For agents used to treat *Bacillus anthracis*, see Fluoroquinolones (p 973) and Anthrax (p 232).

Recommended dosages are not absolute and are intended only as a guide. When a dosage range is provided, the high dose generally is intended for severe infections. Clinical judgment about the disease, predicted drug concentration at the site of infection, alterations in renal or hepatic function, drug interactions, patient response, and laboratory test results may dictate modifications of these dosage recommendations in an individual patient. In some cases, monitoring of serum drug concentrations is recommended to avoid toxicity and to achieve concentrations associated with therapeutic efficacy. For vancomycin, this includes a recent consensus recommendation to utilize area under the curve (AUC)-guided therapeutic monitoring, preferably with Bayesian estimation, for all pediatric age groups based on developmental changes of vancomycin clearance documented from the newborn to the adolescent to reduce the risk of nephrotoxicity, as explained in the tables' footnotes. Trough-only monitoring is no longer recommended.

Product label information or a pediatric pharmacist should be consulted for guidance on the appropriate methods of preparation and administration, measures to be taken to avoid drug interactions, and other precautions. US Food and Drug Administration (FDA)-approved drug labels can be found online at the FDA website (**https://labels.fda.gov/**), Drugs@FDA (**www.accessdata.fda.gov/scripts/cder/daf/**), and DailyMed (**https://dailymed.nlm.nih.gov/dailymed/**).

For antimicrobial agents under investigation and not yet approved for use in children by the FDA, their indications under study and dosages can be found at **http://clinicaltrials.gov.**

Table 4.2. Antibacterial Drugs for Neonates (≤28 Postnatal Days of Age)[a]

Penicillins

Drug	Route	GA ≤34 wk 6 d		GA ≥35 wk 0 d	
		PNA ≤7 d	PNA >7 d	PNA ≤7 d	PNA >7 d
Bacteremia					
Ampicillin	IV, IM	50 mg/kg every 12 h	75 mg/kg every 12 h	50 mg/kg every 8 h	50 mg/kg every 8 h
Penicillin G aqueous	IV, IM	50 000 U/kg every 12 h	50 000 U/kg every 8 h	50 000 U/kg every 12 h	50 000 U/kg every 8 h
Meningitis					
Ampicillin	IV, IM	100 mg/kg every 8 h	75 mg/kg every 6 h	100 mg/kg every 8 h	75 mg/kg every 6 h
Penicillin G aqueous	IV, IM	150 000 U/kg every 8 h	125 000 U/kg every 6 h	150 000 U/kg every 8 h	125 000 U/kg every 6 h

Drug	Route	GA ≤34 wk 6 d		GA ≥35 wk 0 d	
		PNA ≤7 days	PNA >7 days	PNA ≤7 days	PNA >7 days
Nafcillin, oxacillin[b]	IV, IM	25 mg/kg every 12 h	25 mg/kg every 8 h	25 mg/kg every 8 h	25 mg/kg every 6 h

Drug	Route	PNA ≤7 days	PNA >7 days
Penicillin G procaine	IM only	50 000 U/kg every 24 h	50 000 U/kg every 24 h
Penicillin G benzathine	IM only	50 000 U/kg once	50 000 U/kg once

Drug	Route	PMA ≤30 wk	PMA >30 wk
Piperacillin-tazobactam	IV	100 mg/kg every 8 h	80 mg/kg every 6 h

Table 4.2. Antibacterial Drugs for Neonates (≤28 Postnatal Days of Age),ᵃ continued

Cephalosporins

Drug	Route	GA ≤31 wk 6 d		GA ≥32 wk 0 d	
		PNA <7 days	PNA ≥7 days	PNA ≤7 days	PNA >7 days
Cefazolinᶜ	IV, IM	25 mg/kg every 12 h	25 mg/kg every 12 h	25 mg/kg every 8 h	25 mg/kg every 8 h
Cefotaximeᵈ	IV, IM	50 mg/kg every 12 h	50 mg/kg every 8 h	50 mg/kg every 12 h	50 mg/kg every 8 h
Ceftazidime	IV, IM	50 mg/kg every 12 h	50 mg/kg every 8 h	50 mg/kg every 12 h	50 mg/kg every 8 h
Cefuroxime	IV, IM	50 mg/kg every 12 h	50 mg/kg every 8 h	50 mg/kg every 12 h	50 mg/kg every 8 h

Drug	Route	GA ≤31 wk 6 d		GA ≥32 wk 0 d
		PNA ≤7 days	PNA >7 days	
Cefoxitin	IV, IM	35 mg/kg every 12 h	35 mg/kg every 8 h	35 mg/kg every 8 h
Ceftolozane/tazobactam	IV	--	--	20 mg ceftolozane/kg every q8h

Drug	Route	All neonates
Ceftriaxoneᵉ	IV, IM	50 mg/kg every 24 h

Drug	Route	GA ≤35 wk 6 d	GA ≥36 wk 0 d
Cefepime	IV	30 mg/kg every 12 h	50 mg/kg every 12 hᶠ

Drug	Route	GA ≥34 wk 0 d and PNA ≥12 d
Ceftaroline	IV	6 mg/kg every 8 h

Table 4.2. Antibacterial Drugs for Neonates (≤28 Postnatal Days of Age),[a] continued

Carbapenems

Drug	Route	GA ≤31 wk 6 d		GA ≥32 wk 0 d	
		PNA <14 days	PNA ≥14 days	PNA <14 days	PNA ≥14 days
Meropenem (non-meningitic dosing)	IV	20 mg/kg every 12 h	20 mg/kg every 8 h	20 mg/kg every 8 h	30 mg/kg every 8 h
Meropenem (meningitic dosing)	IV	40 mg/kg every 12 h	40 mg/kg every 8 h	40 mg/kg every 8 h	40 mg/kg every 8 h

Drug	Route	PNA ≤7 days	PNA >7 days
Imipenem-cilastatin	IV	25 mg/kg every 12 h	25 mg/kg every 8 h

Other agents

Drug	Route	All neonates
Azithromycin[g,h]	IV, PO	10 mg/kg every 24 h
Erythromycin[g]	IV, PO	12.5 mg/kg every 6 h
Rifampin[i]	IV, PO	10–15 mg/kg every 24 h

Drug	Route	GA ≤33 wk 6 d		GA ≥34 wk 0 d	
		PNA ≤7 days	PNA >7 days	PNA ≤7 days	PNA >7 days
Aztreonam[b]	IV	30 mg/kg every 12 h	30 mg/kg every 8 h	30 mg/kg every 8 h	30 mg/kg every 6 h

Drug	Route	PMA ≤32 wk	PMA 33–40 wk	PMA >40 wk
Clindamycin	IV, PO	5 mg/kg every 8h	7 mg/kg every 8 h	9 mg/kg every 8 h

Table 4.2. Antibacterial Drugs for Neonates (≤28 Postnatal Days of Age),ᵃ continued

Drug	Route	GA ≤33 wk 6 d		GA ≥34 wk 0 d	
		PNA ≤7 days	PNA >7 days	PNA ≤7 days	PNA >7 days
Linezolid	IV, PO	10 mg/kg every 12 h	10 mg/kg every 8 h	10 mg/kg every 8 h	10 mg/kg every 8 h

Drug	Route	PMA ≤34 wk	PMA 35–40 wk	PMA >40 wk
Metronidazoleʲ	IV	7.5 mg/kg every 12 h	7.5 mg/kg every 8 h	10 mg/kg every 8 h

Aminoglycosides

Drug	Route	GA ≤29 wk 6 d		GA 30 wk 0 d – 34 wk 6 d		GA ≥35 wk 0 d	
		PNA ≤14 days	>14 days	≤10 days	>10 days	≤7 days	>7 days
Amikacinᵏ	IV, IM	15 mg/kg every 48 h	15 mg/kg every 36 h	15 mg/kg every 36 h	15 mg/kg every 24 h	15 mg/kg every 24 h	18 mg/kg every 24 h
Gentamicinˡ	IV, IM	5 mg/kg every 48 h	5 mg/kg every 36 h	5 mg/kg every 36 h	5 mg/kg every 24 h	4 mg/kg every 24 h	5 mg/kg every 24 h
Tobramycinˡ	IV, IM	5 mg/kg every 48 h	5 mg/kg every 36 h	5 mg/kg every 36 h	5 mg/kg every 24 h	4 mg/kg every 24 h	5 mg/kg every 24 h

Vancomycinᵐ

Begin with a 20-mg/kg loading dose followed by a maintenance dose, according to the table

GA ≤28 wk 6 d		GA ≥29 wk 0 d	
Creatinine (mg/dL)	Dosage	Creatinine (mg/dL)	Dosage
<0.5	15 mg/kg every 12 h	<0.7	15 mg/kg every 12 h
0.5–0.7	20 mg/kg every 24 h	0.7–0.9	20 mg/kg every 24 h
0.8–1	15 mg/kg every 24 h	1–1.2	15 mg/kg every 24 h
1.1–1.4	10 mg/kg every 24 h	1.3–1.6	10 mg/kg every 24 h
>1.4	15 mg/kg every 48 h	>1.6	15 mg/kg every 48 h

Table 4.2. Antibacterial Drugs for Neonates (≤28 Postnatal Days of Age),[a] continued

Other glycopeptides

Drug	Route	All Neonates
Dalbavancin	IV	22.5 mg/kg, one time

GA, gestational age; IM, intramuscular; IV, intravenous; PNA, postnatal age; PO, oral.

[a] Dosages are given as per dose and the per dose frequency.

[b] Higher (double) doses than those listed may be required for meningitis, although safety and efficacy data for dosing of neonates with central nervous system (CNS) infection are lacking for these agents.

[c] Higher or more frequent dosing required for systemic, non-CNS, intermediately susceptible *Enterobacterales* infections.

[d] Cefotaxime is available by importation from Canada. See **www.fda.gov/media/152896/download** for details.

[e] Given dose also appropriate for meningitis. Neonates should not receive IV cefotaxime if they also are receiving IV calcium in any form, including parenteral nutrition. Use in hyperbilirubinemic neonates should be undertaken thoughtfully, especially for those who were born preterm. In vitro studies have shown that cefotaxime can displace bilirubin from its binding to serum albumin.

[f] May give 30 mg/kg, every 12 h, if target pathogen minimum inhibitory concentration (MIC) is ≤4 mg/L, such as *E coli*.

[g] An association between orally administered erythromycin and azithromycin and infantile hypertrophic pyloric stenosis (IHPS) has been reported in infants younger than 6 weeks. Infants treated with either of these antimicrobials should be followed for signs and symptoms of IHPS. Because of antibiotic resistance, these agents are not recommended to treat congenital *Mycoplasma hominis* infections.

[h] 20 mg/kg, every 24 hours for 3 days, for *Ureaplasma* or *Chlamydia trachomatis* infection.

[i] See *Haemophilus influenzae* Infections, p 400, and Meningococcal Infections, p 585, for alternate dosing in special situations.

[k] Begin with a 15-mg/kg loading dose.

[l] Desired serum or plasma concentrations: 20–40 mg/L or 10 x MIC (peak), <7 mg/L (trough).

[l] Desired serum or plasma concentrations: 6–12 mg/L or 10 x MIC (peak), <2 mg/L (trough).

[m] The maintenance dose should begin at the same number of hours after the loading dose as the maintenance interval. Creatinine concentrations normally fluctuate and are partly influenced by transplacental maternal creatinine in the first week of postnatal age. Cautious use of creatinine-based dosing strategy with frequent reassessment of renal function and vancomycin serum concentrations is recommended in neonates ≤7 days of age. The area-under-the-curve (AUC) to MIC has been identified as the most appropriate pharmacokinetic/pharmacodynamic (PK/PD) target vancomycin in adult patients with methicillin-resistant *Staphylococcus aureus* (MRSA) infections and is preferred over trough monitoring to prevent unnecessary overexposure to vancomycin. Although there are limitations in prospective outcomes data in pediatric patients with serious MRSA infections, the most recent consensus guideline from the American Society of Health-System Pharmacists, the Infectious Diseases Society of America, the Pediatric Infectious Diseases Society, and the Society of Infectious Diseases Pharmacists recommends AUC-guided therapeutic monitoring, preferably with Bayesian estimation, for all pediatric age groups receiving vancomycin.[n] This estimation accounts for developmental changes of vancomycin clearance from newborn to adolescent. Dosing in children should be designed to achieve an AUC of 400–600 mg-hour/L (assuming MIC of 1 mg/L) and/or trough levels <15 mg/L to minimize acute kidney injury risks. Bayesian estimation can be completed with 2 levels, with 1 level being recommended 1–2 hours after end of vancomycin infusion, and the second level being drawn 4–6 hours after end of infusion. Levels can be obtained as early as after the second dose. Software to assist with these calculations is available online and for purchase. It is challenging to avoid AUC >800 mg-hour/L and trough concentrations >15 mg/L. In situations in which AUC calculation is not feasible, a trough concentration ≥10 mg/L is very highly likely (>90%) to achieve the AUC target in neonates and children when the MIC is 1 mg/L. Trough concentrations as low as 7 mg/L can still achieve an AUC ≥400 mg-hour/L in some preterm neonates because of their slower clearance. For centers where invasive MRSA infection is relatively common or where MRSA with MIC of 1 mg/L is common, an online dosing tool is available that may improve the likelihood of empirically achieving AUC ≥400 mg-hour/L, compared with doses given in Table 4.2 **(https://connect.insight-rx.com/neovanco).**

[n] Rybak MJ, Le J, Lodise TP, et al. Executive summary: Therapeutic monitoring of vancomycin for serious methicillin-resistant *Staphylococcus aureus* infections: a revised consensus guideline and review by the American Society of Health-System Pharmacists, the Infectious Diseases Society of America, the Pediatric Infectious Diseases Society, and the Society of Infectious Diseases Pharmacists. *J Pediatric Infect Dis Soc*. 2020;9(3):281-284

Adapted from American Academy of Pediatrics. *2024 Nelson's Pediatric Antimicrobial Therapy*. 30th ed. Itasca, IL: American Academy of Pediatrics; 2024.

Table 4.3. Antibacterial Drugs for Pediatric Patients Beyond the Newborn Period

Drug Generic (Trade Name)	Generic Available	Route	Dosage per kg per Day Absolute Maximum Dosage Provided, If Known	Comments[a]
Aminoglycosides				Not ideal for CNS infections. See Table 4.2 footnotes for serum concentration targets.
Amikacin[b]	Y	IV, IM	15–22.5 mg, divided in 2–3 doses or once daily	Higher doses than those given are appropriate for cystic fibrosis.
Gentamicin[b]	Y	IV, IM	6–7.5 mg, divided in 3 doses, or 5–7.5 mg once daily	
Neomycin	Y	PO	100 mg, divided in 4 doses, max 12 g per day	For some enteric infections.
Tobramycin[b]	Y	IV, IM	6–7.5 mg, divided in 3–4 doses, or 5–7.5 mg once daily	Higher doses than those given are appropriate for cystic fibrosis.
		Inhaled	300 mg, inhaled every 12 h	
Aztreonam (Azactam)	Y	IV, IM	90–120 mg, divided in 3 or 4 doses, max 8 g per day	A monobactam. Can be used for CNS infections.
Carbapenems[c]				
Imipenem/cilastatin (Primaxin)	Y	IV	60–100 mg, divided in 4 doses, max 4 g per day	Caution when treating CNS infections because of increased risk of seizures. High end of dose range for *Pseudomonas aeruginosa* infections.

Table 4.3. Antibacterial Drugs for Pediatric Patients Beyond the Newborn Period, continued

Drug Generic (Trade Name)	Generic Available	Route	Dosage per kg per Day Absolute Maximum Dosage Provided, If Known	Comments[a]
Meropenem (Merrem)	Y	IV	60 mg, divided in 3 doses, max 3 g per day 120 mg, divided in 3 doses for meningitis, max 6 g per day	Extended infusion over 3 to 4 hours may be needed for susceptible infections in critically ill children.
Ertapenem (Invanz)	N	IV/IM	30 mg, divided in 2 doses, max 1 g per day ≥13 y and adults, 1 g, once daily	Poor activity against Pseudomonas and Acinetobacter. Should not be used for CNS infections.
Cephalosporins[c]				The generation of each agent is listed as a guide to antimicrobial spectrum.
Cefaclor (Ceclor)	Y	PO	20–40 mg, divided in 2 or 3 doses, max 1 g per day	Second generation.
Cefadroxil (Duricef)	Y	PO	30 mg, divided in 2 doses, max 2 g per day	First generation.
Cefazolin (Ancef)	Y	IV, IM	25–75 mg, divided in 3 doses, max 6 g per day Up to 150 mg, divided in 3–4 doses for bone/joint infections, max 12 g per day	First generation. Limited data on dosages above 100 mg/kg/day. Should not be used for CNS infections.
Cefdinir (Omnicef)	Y	PO	14 mg, divided in 1 or 2 doses, max 600 mg/day	Third generation. Inadequate activity against penicillin-resistant Streptococcus pneumoniae.
Cefepime (Maxipime)	Y	IV, IM	100 mg, divided in 2 doses, max 4 g per day 150 mg, divided in 3 doses for Pseudomonas infections or febrile neutropenia, max 6 g per day	Fourth generation. Extended infusion over 3 to 4 hours may be needed for susceptible infections in critically ill children. Can be used for CNS infections.

Table 4.3. Antibacterial Drugs for Pediatric Patients Beyond the Newborn Period, continued

Drug Generic (Trade Name)	Generic Available	Route	Dosage per kg per Day Absolute Maximum Dosage Provided, If Known	Comments[a]
Cefixime (Suprax)	Y	PO	8 mg, divided in 1 or 2 doses, max 400 mg per day	Third generation. Inadequate activity against penicillin-resistant *Streptococcus pneumoniae*.
Cefotaxime (Claforan)[d]	Y	IV, IM	150–180 mg, divided in 3 doses, max 8 g per day 200–225 mg, divided in 4 doses for meningitis, max 12 g per day	Third generation. Up to 300 mg, divided in 4 or 6 doses. May be used for CNS infections.
Cefotetan (Cefotan)	Y	IV, IM	60–100 mg, divided in 2 doses, max 6 g per day	Second generation. A cephamycin, active against anaerobes. Should not be used for CNS infections.
Cefoxitin (Mefoxin)	Y	IV, IM	80–160 mg, divided in 3–4 doses, max 12 g per day	Second generation. A cephamycin, active against anaerobes. Should not be used for CNS infections.
Cefpodoxime (Vantin)	Y	PO	10 mg, divided in 2 doses, max 400 mg per day 800 mg (not per kg), divided in 2 doses for severe non-MRSA skin infections and ≥40 kg	Third generation.
Cefprozil (Cefzil)	Y	PO	15–30 mg, divided in 2 doses, max 1 g per day	Second generation.

Table 4.3. Antibacterial Drugs for Pediatric Patients Beyond the Newborn Period, continued

Drug Generic (Trade Name)	Generic Available	Route	Dosage per kg per Day Absolute Maximum Dosage Provided, If Known	Comments[a]
Ceftaroline (Teflaro)	N	IV	1 mo to <2 mo: 18 mg, divided in 3 doses 2 mo to <2 y: 24 mg, divided in 3 doses ≥2 y: ≤33 kg: 36 mg, divided in 3 doses >33 kg: 1200 mg (not per kg), divided in 2–3 doses	Fifth generation with anti-MRSA activity. No activity against *Pseudomonas* species. Adult dose: 400 mg/dose, every 8 h, or 600 mg/dose, every 12 h (max 1200 mg/day). Potentially useful for CNS infections, based on limited data.
Ceftazidime (Fortaz)	Y	IV, IM	90–150 mg, divided in 3 doses 200–300 mg, divided in 3 doses for serious *Pseudomonas* infections	Third generation. Max 6 g per day (12 g per day for serious *Pseudomonas* infections). Can be used for CNS infections.
Ceftazidime/avibactam (Avycaz)	N	IV	<6 mo: 120 mg, divided in 3 doses 6 mo–18 y: 150 mg, divided in 3 doses, max 6 g per day	Dose based on ceftazidime component. Used for certain multidrug-resistant gram-negative bacterial infections. Can be used for CNS infections.
Ceftolozane/tazobactam (Zerbaxa)	N	IV	90 mg, divided in 3 doses, max 4.5 g per day	Used for complicated intra-abdominal infections and complicated urinary tract infections

Table 4.3. Antibacterial Drugs for Pediatric Patients Beyond the Newborn Period, continued

Drug Generic (Trade Name)	Generic Available	Route	Dosage per kg per Day Absolute Maximum Dosage Provided, If Known	Comments[a]
Ceftriaxone (Rocephin)	Y	IV, IM	50–75 mg, once daily; max 1 g per day (for non-CNS, non-endocarditis infections) 100 mg, divided in 1 or 2 doses, max 4 g per day (for CNS or endocarditis infections) 50 mg/kg, IM, once daily for 1–3 days for AOM, max 1 g per day	Third generation.
Cefuroxime (Zinacef)	Y	IV, IM	100–150 mg, divided in 3 doses, max 6 g per day	Second-generation. Limited activity against penicillin-resistant *Streptococcus pneumoniae.* Other agents preferred for CNS infections.
Cefuroxime axetil (Ceftin)	Y	PO	20–30 mg, divided in 2 doses, max 1 g per day Up to 100 mg, divided in 3 doses for bone or joint infections, max 3 g per day	Second-generation. Limited activity against penicillin-resistant *Streptococcus pneumoniae.*
Cephalexin (Keflex)	Y	PO	25–50 mg divided in 2 doses 75–100 mg divided in 3–4 doses for bone or joint infections, max 4 g per day	First-generation.
Clindamycin (Cleocin)	Y	IM, IV	20–40 mg, divided in 3–4 doses, max 2.7 g per day	Often active against *Streptococcus pneumoniae, Streptococcus pyogenes,* and *Staphylococcus aureus* (including some MRSA) and many anaerobes of the respiratory tract. Penetrates into brain but not CSF.
	Y	PO	10–25 mg, divided in 3 doses 30–40 mg, divided in 3–4 doses for AOM or CA-MRSA, max 1.8 g per day	

Table 4.3. Antibacterial Drugs for Pediatric Patients Beyond the Newborn Period, continued

Drug Generic (Trade Name)	Generic Available	Route	Dosage per kg per Day Absolute Maximum Dosage Provided, If Known	Comments[a]
Daptomycin (Cubicin)	N	IV	For *Staphylococcus aureus* bacteremia: 1–6 y: 12 mg, once daily 7–11 y: 9 mg, once daily 12–17 y: 7 mg, once daily For skin and skin structure infections: 1–2 y: 10 mg, once daily 2–6 y: 9 mg, once daily 7–11 y: 7 mg, once daily 12–17 y: 5 mg, once daily	Neuromuscular toxicity in neonatal and juvenile canine model. FDA warns to avoid use in infants <12 mo. Not used for CNS infections.

Fluoroquinolones see also p 973, and Anthrax, p 232.

Drug Generic (Trade Name)	Generic Available	Route	Dosage per kg per Day Absolute Maximum Dosage Provided, If Known	Comments[a]
Ciprofloxacin (Cipro)	Y	PO	30 mg, divided in 2 doses, max 1.0 g per day	Can be used to treat CNS infections.
		IV	20–30 mg, divided in 2 or 3 doses, max 1.2 g per day	
Levofloxacin (Levaquin)	Y	PO	<50 kg: 16 mg, divided in 2 doses, max 500 mg per day ≥50 kg: 500 mg per dose (not per kg), once daily	For empiric therapy or therapy of penicillin-resistant strains of anthrax, the benefits of fluoroquinolones for pediatric anthrax are far greater than potential toxicities.
		IV	<50 kg: 20 mg, divided in 2 doses, max 500 mg per day ≥50 kg: 500 mg per dose (not per kg), once daily	

Table 4.3. Antibacterial Drugs for Pediatric Patients Beyond the Newborn Period, continued

Drug Generic (Trade Name)	Generic Available	Route	Dosage per kg per Day Absolute Maximum Dosage Provided, If Known	Comments[a]
Macrolides				
Azithromycin (Zithromax, Zmax)	Y	PO	5–10 mg, once daily for the immediate-release products 60 mg as a single dose for the extended-release (ER) formulation Respiratory tract infection dosages (per kg, interval is once daily): AOM: 10 mg for 3 days; or 30 mg for 1 day; or 10 mg for 1 day then 5 mg for 4 days Pharyngitis: 12 mg for 1 day, then 6 mg for 4 days Sinusitis: 10 mg for 3 days CAP: 10 mg for 1 day, then 5 mg for 4 days	Per dose max 250 mg for 6 mg/kg, 500 mg for 10–12 mg/kg, 1.5 g for 30 mg/kg. Normal adult total course is 1.5–2 g. Total course max 2.5 g. Multiple additional indications. See relevant chapters in Section 3.
	Y	IV	10 mg, once daily, max 500 mg per day	See *Legionella* Infections, p 531. Can be used for some CNS infections.
Clarithromycin (Biaxin)	Y	PO	15 mg, divided in 2 doses, max 1 g per day	Similar activity to erythromycin; more activity against *Mycobacterium avium* and *Helicobacter pylori.*
Erythromycin (numerous)	Y	PO	40–50 mg, divided in 3–4 doses, max 4 g per day	
	N	IV	20 mg, divided in 4 doses, max 4 g per day	Administer over at least 60 minutes to potentially prevent cardiac arrhythmias. Not used for CNS infections.

Table 4.3. Antibacterial Drugs for Pediatric Patients Beyond the Newborn Period, continued

Drug Generic (Trade Name)	Generic Available	Route	Dosage per kg per Day Absolute Maximum Dosage Provided, If Known	Comments[a]
Fidaxomicin (Dificid)	N	PO	≥6 mo (per day, not per kg/day, divided twice a day): 4–<7 kg: 160 mg 7–<9 kg: 240 mg 9–<12.5 kg: 320 mg ≥12.5 kg: 400 mg	For treatment of *Clostridioides difficile* infection.
Metronidazole (Flagyl)	Y	PO	Range: 15–50 mg, divided in 3 doses, max 2.25 g per day 30 mg, divided in 3 doses for anaerobic bacterial infections including *Clostridioides difficile* (maximum 500 mg per dose) For bacterial vaginosis, see Table 4.4 (p 1007) and Table 4.5 (p 1014) For *Trichomonas vaginalis*, see Table 4.4 (p 1007) and Table 4.5 (p 1014) For Amebiasis, see Table 4.11 (p 1036)	Can be used for CNS infections.
		IV	22.5–40 mg, divided in 3 or 4 doses, max 4 g per day	Can be used for CNS infections.
Nitrofurantoin (Furadantin, Macrodantin, Macrobid)	Y	PO	UTI prophylaxis: 1–2 mg, once daily Cystitis treatment: <12 y: 5–7 mg divided in 4 doses, max 200 mg per day ≥12 y: 200 mg total daily dosage (not per kg), divided in 2 doses	For treatment of cystitis; not appropriate for pyelonephritis. Macrobid form for twice daily dosing.

Table 4.3. Antibacterial Drugs for Pediatric Patients Beyond the Newborn Period, continued

Drug Generic (Trade Name)	Generic Available	Route	Dosage per kg per Day Absolute Maximum Dosage Provided, If Known	Comments[a]
Oxazolidinones				
Linezolid (Zyvox)	Y	PO, IV	≤11 y: 30 mg divided in 3 doses, max 1200 mg per day >11 y: 1200 mg total daily dose (not per kg) divided in 2 doses	Myelosuppression increases with duration of therapy over 10 days. Can be used for CNS infections (IV or PO).
Tedizolid (Sivextro)	N	PO, IV	≥ 12 y: 200 mg (not per kg) once daily	Not known if effective for CNS infections.
Penicillins[e]				
Amoxicillin (Amoxil)	Y	PO	Standard dose: 40–45 mg, divided in 3 doses High dose: 80–90 mg, divided in 2 doses, max 4 g per day Streptococcal pharyngitis: 50 mg once daily (see Group A Streptococcal Infections, p 785). *Bacillus anthracis* exposure: 75 mg, divided in 3 doses, max 3 g per day, for prophylaxis and empiric treatment (see Anthrax, p 232). See fluoroquinolones row above for empiric or therapy of penicillin-resistant strains of anthrax.	Higher doses may be needed for some penicillin-resistant *Streptococcus pneumoniae* infections (see p 810).

Table 4.3. Antibacterial Drugs for Pediatric Patients Beyond the Newborn Period, continued

Drug Generic (Trade Name)	Generic Available	Route	Dosage per kg per Day Absolute Maximum Dosage Provided, If Known	Comments[a]
Amoxicillin-clavulanic acid (Augmentin)	Y	PO	14:1 Formulation: 90 mg, divided in 2 doses 7:1 Formulation: 25–45 mg, divided in 2 doses, max 1750 mg per day 4:1 Formulation: 30 mg, divided in 2 doses for <3 months of age	Dosed on amoxicillin component. 14:1 Formulation – Augmentin ES-600 7:1 Formulation – Augmentin 400 4:1 Formulation – Augmentin 250
Ampicillin	Y	IV, IM	50–200 mg, divided in 4 doses, max 8 g per day 300–400 mg, divided in 6 doses for meningitis, endocarditis, max 12 g per day	Can be used for CNS infections.
	Y	PO	50–100 mg, divided in 4 doses, max 2 g per day	
Ampicillin-sulbactam (Unasyn)	Y	IV	100–200 mg, divided in 4 doses, max 8 g per day 400 mg, divided in 4 doses for meningitis	Dosed on ampicillin component. Can be used for CNS infections.
Dicloxacillin (Dynapen)	Y	PO	12–25 mg, divided in 4 doses, max 1 g per day 100 mg, divided in 4 doses for bone or joint infections, max 2 g per day	Oral suspension not commercially available.
Nafcillin (Nallpen)	Y	IV, IM	100–200 mg, divided in 4–6 doses, max 12 g per day	Can be used for CNS infection.
Oxacillin (Bactocill)	Y	IV, IM	100–200 mg, divided in 4–6 doses, max 12 g per day	Can be used for CNS infection.
Penicillin G, crystalline potassium or sodium	Y	IV, IM	100 000–300 000 U, divided in 4–6 doses, 300 000–400 000 U, divided in 6 doses for CNS infection	Max 24 million U per day.

Table 4.3. Antibacterial Drugs for Pediatric Patients Beyond the Newborn Period, continued

Drug Generic (Trade Name)	Generic Available	Route	Dosage per kg per Day Absolute Maximum Dosage Provided, If Known	Comments[a]
Penicillin G procaine	Y	IM	50 000 U, divided in 1–2 doses, max 1.2 million U	Not safe for IV administration. Should not be used for CNS infection. As of July 2023, no longer manufactured in the United States.
Penicillin G benzathine (Bicillin LA)	N	IM	<27 kg (60 lb): 600 000 U (not per kg), one time >27 kg (60 lb): 1.2 million U (not per kg), one time See Table 4.2 for congenital syphilis dosing	Not safe for IV administration. Main use is treatment of group A streptococcal infections (see p 785). Should not be used for acute CNS infection (see Syphilis, p 825).
Penicillin G benzathine/procaine (Bicillin CR)	N	IM	<14 kg (30 lb): 600 000 U (not per kg), one time 14–27 kg (30–60 lb): 1.2 million U (not per kg), one time ≥27 kg (60 lb): 2.4 million U (not per kg), one time	Not safe for IV administration. Main use is treatment of group A streptococcal infections (see p 785).
Penicillin V	Y	PO	25–50 mg, divided in 4 doses, max 2 g per day	50–75 mg, divided in 4 doses for group A streptococcal pneumonia.
Piperacillin-tazobactam (Zosyn)	Y	IV	240–300 mg, divided in 3–4 doses, max 16 g per day	Dosed on piperacillin component. Extended infusion may be needed for susceptible-dose dependent infections. 400–600 mg, divided in 6 doses, max 24 g per day, may be appropriate in some patients with cystic fibrosis. Other agents preferred for CNS infections.

Table 4.3. Antibacterial Drugs for Pediatric Patients Beyond the Newborn Period, continued

Drug Generic (Trade Name)	Generic Available	Route	Dosage per kg per Day Absolute Maximum Dosage Provided, If Known	Comments[a]
Polymyxins				
				Not ideal for CNS infections; local (intraventricular) administration required to achieve therapeutic concentrations.
Colistimethate (Colymycin M)	Y	IV, IM	2.5–5 mg base, divided in 3 doses	Up to 7 mg base/kg/day may be required. 1 mg base = 2.7 mg colistimethate.
Polymyxin B	Y	IV	2.5 mg, divided in 2 doses	>3 mg/kg/day not well studied. 1 mg = 10 000 U.
Rifamycins				
Rifampin (Rifadin)	Y	IV, PO	15–20 mg, divided in 1–2 doses, max 600 mg per day See p 902–905 for *Mycobacterium tuberculosis* dosing	Should not be used routinely as monotherapy because of rapid emergence of resistance. Many experts recommend using a daily rifampin dose of at least 20 mg/kg/day for infants and toddlers. Can be used for CNS infections (IV or PO).
Rifaximin (Xifaxan)	N	PO	20–30 mg, divided in 3 doses, max 600 mg per day	For travelers' diarrhea
Sulfonamides				
Sulfadiazine	Y	PO	120–150 mg, divided in 4 doses, max 6 g per day Rheumatic fever secondary prevention: 500 mg (not per kg), once daily in children <30 kg; 1 g, once daily in bigger children and adults	G6PD deficiency should be evaluated when using this drug.

Table 4.3. Antibacterial Drugs for Pediatric Patients Beyond the Newborn Period, continued

Drug Generic (Trade Name)	Generic Available	Route	Dosage per kg per Day Absolute Maximum Dosage Provided, If Known	Comments[a]
Trimethoprim-Sulfamethoxazole (TMP-SMX) (Bactrim, Septra)	Y	PO, IV	8–12 mg, divided in 2 doses, max 640 mg per day 2 mg, once daily for UTI prophylaxis 15–20 mg, divided in 3–4 doses for *Pneumocystis jirovecii* treatment, no max; 5 mg, divided in 2 doses 3 times/wk for prophylaxis	Dosed on TMP component. See also *Pneumocystis jirovecii* Infections (p 676). Can be used for CNS infections.
Tetracyclines see also p 975				
Doxycycline (Vibramycin)	Y	PO, IV	2.2–4.4 mg, divided in 2 doses, max 200 mg per day	Can be used for CNS infections (IV or PO). Higher doses reported (max 400 mg per day) in adults with Lyme neuroborreliosis.
Minocycline (Minocin)	Y	PO, IV	4 mg, divided in 2 doses, max 200 mg per day	Other agents preferred for CNS infections.
Tetracycline	Y	PO	25–50 mg, divided in 4 doses, max 2 g per day	Tetracycline limited to ≥8 y of age.
Vancomycin and other glycopeptides				
Vancomycin (Vancocin)	Y	IV	45–60 mg, divided in 3–4 doses 60–70 mg, divided in 4 doses, may be necessary in some patients to achieve target serum concentrations for invasive MRSA infections	Measured serum concentrations should guide ongoing therapy.[e] Can be used for CNS infections.
		PO	40 mg, divided in 4 doses, up to 500 mg per day	For treatment of *Clostridioides difficile* infection (see Table 3.3, p 317). Up to 2 g per day divided in 4 doses for severe, complicated cases.

Table 4.3. Antibacterial Drugs for Pediatric Patients Beyond the Newborn Period, continued

Drug Generic (Trade Name)	Generic Available	Route	Dosage per kg per Day Absolute Maximum Dosage Provided, If Known	Comments[a]
Dalbavancin (Dalvance)	N	IV	<6 y: 22.5 mg, one time ≥6 y: 18 mg, one time, max 1500 mg (not per kg)	Should not be used for CNS infections.

AOM indicates acute otitis media; CAP, community-acquired pneumonia; CA-MRSA, community-associated methicillin-resistant *Staphylococcus aureus*; CDI, *Clostridioides difficile* infection; CNS, central nervous system; eGFR, estimated glomerular filtration rate; ER, extended-release; FDA, US Food and Drug Administration; G6PD, glucose-6-phosphate dehydrogenase; IBD, inflammatory bowel disease; IM, intramuscular; IV, intravenous; MRSA, methicillin-resistant *Staphylococcus aureus*; PO, oral; SBBO, small bowel bacterial overgrowth; SSTI, skin and soft tissue infection; UTI, urinary tract infection.

[a] Comments regarding CNS infections are based on FDA-approved indication or evidence from clinical studies in children or adults and apply to administration by the intravenous route unless otherwise specified.

[b] Extended interval ("once daily") dosing may provide equal efficacy with reduced toxicity.

[c] Children with a history of an IgE-mediated, immediate hypersensitivity reaction to penicillins (urticaria, angioedema, bronchospasm, anaphylaxis) who require treatment with an alternate beta-lactam should be considered for skin testing (if available) to confirm the allergy, and/or undergo supervised graded clinical challenge or desensitization with the alternate beta-lactam agent under the supervision of an expert in drug allergy and desensitization. See Beta-lactam and Monobactam Allergies (p 976) and Fig 4.1 (p 979).

[d] Cefotaxime is available by importation from Canada. See **www.fda.gov/media/152896/download** for details.

[e] The area-under-the-curve to minimum inhibitory concentration (AUC/MIC) has been identified as the most appropriate pharmacokinetic/pharmacodynamic (PK/PD) target vancomycin in adult patients with methicillin-resistant *Staphylococcus aureus* (MRSA). Although there are limitations in prospective outcomes data in pediatric patients with serious MRSA infections, the most recent consensus guideline from the American Society of Health-System Pharmacists, the Infectious Diseases Society of America, the Pediatric Infectious Diseases Society, and the Society of Infectious Diseases Pharmacists recommends AUC-guided therapeutic monitoring, preferably with Bayesian estimation, for all pediatric age groups receiving vancomycin.[f] This estimation accounts for developmental changes of vancomycin clearance from newborn to adolescent, and is preferred over trough monitoring to prevent unnecessary overexposure to vancomycin. Dosing in children should be designed to achieve an AUC of 400–600 mg-hour/L (assuming MIC of 1 mg/L) and/or trough levels <15 mg/L to minimize acute kidney injury risks. Bayesian estimation can be completed with 2 levels, with 1 level being recommended 1–2 hours after end of vancomycin infusion, and the second level being drawn 4–6 hours after end of infusion. Levels can be obtained as early as after the second dose. Software to assist with these calculations is available online and for purchase. It is recommended to avoid AUC >800 mg-hour/L and troughs >15 mg/L. Most children younger than 12 years will require higher doses to achieve optimal AUC/MIC compared with older children.

[f] Rybak MJ, Le J, Lodise TP, et al. Executive summary: Therapeutic monitoring of vancomycin for serious methicillin-resistant *Staphylococcus aureus* infections: a revised consensus guideline and review by the American Society of Health-System Pharmacists, the Infectious Diseases Society of America, the Pediatric Infectious Diseases Society, and the Society of Infectious Diseases Pharmacists. *J Pediatric Infect Dis Soc.* 2020;9(3):281-284

Adapted from American Academy of Pediatrics. *2024 Nelson's Pediatric Antimicrobial Therapy.* 30th ed. Itasca, IL: American Academy of Pediatrics; 2024.

SEXUALLY TRANSMITTED INFECTIONS

Table 4.4. Guidelines for Treatment of Sexually Transmitted Infections in Children ≥45 kg, Adolescents, and Young Adults According to Syndrome

For further information concerning other acceptable regimens and diseases not included, see recommendations in disease-specific chapters in Section 3. In addition, recommendations on treatment of sexually transmitted infections have been issued by the Centers for Disease Control and Prevention at **www.cdc.gov/std/treatment.**[a]

	Organisms/ Diagnoses	Treatment of Children Weighing ≥45 kg, Adolescents, and Young Adults[a]
Urethritis and Cervicitis: Inflammation of urethra and/or cervix with erythema and/or mucoid, mucopurulent, or purulent discharge	*Neisseria gonorrhoeae*	45–150 kg: Ceftriaxone, 500 mg, IM, in a single dose[b] >150 kg: Ceftriaxone, 1 g, IM, in a single dose[b] If chlamydial infection has not been excluded, also treat for *Chlamydia trachomatis* (see next row)
	Chlamydia trachomatis	Recommended: Doxycycline, 100 mg, orally, 2 times daily for 7 days Alternative: Azithromycin, 1 g, orally, in a single dose **OR** Levofloxacin, 500 mg, orally, once daily for 7 days
	Nongonoccal urethritis[c] or cervicitis	Recommended: Doxycycline, 100 mg, orally, 2 times daily day for 7 days Alternative: Azithromycin, 1 g, orally, in a single dose **OR** Azithromycin, 500 mg, orally, as a single dose, followed by 250 mg, orally once daily for 4 additional days

Table 4.4. Guidelines for Treatment of Sexually Transmitted Infections in Children ≥45 kg, Adolescents, and Young Adults According to Syndrome, continued

	Organisms/ Diagnoses	Treatment of Children Weighing ≥45 kg, Adolescents, and Young Adults[a]
Persistent and Recurrent Nongonococcal Urethritis: Persistent symptoms after treatment with objective signs of urethral inflammation	The most common cause of persistent or recurrent NGU is *Mycoplasma genitalium*, especially following doxycycline therapy	*M genitalium* treatment If macrolide sensitive: Doxycycline, 100 mg, orally, 2 times daily for 7 days, followed by azithromycin, 1 g, orally, initial dose, followed by 500 mg, orally, once daily for 3 additional days (2.5 g total) If macrolide resistant or no resistance testing available: Doxycycline, 100 mg, orally, 2 times daily for 7 days, followed by moxifloxacin, 400 mg, orally, once daily for 7 days
	Trichomonas vaginalis (in males who only have sex with females[d])	Recommended: Metronidazole, 2 g, orally, in a single dose[e] Alternative: Tinidazole, 2 g, orally, in a single dose[e]
Vulvovaginitis	*T vaginalis*	Recommended: Metronidazole, 500 mg, orally, 2 times daily for 7 days Alternative: Tinidazole, 2 g, orally, in a single dose[f]
	Bacterial vaginosis	Recommended: Metronidazole, 500 mg, orally, 2 times daily for 7 days **OR** Metronidazole gel, 0.75%, 1 full applicator (5 g), intravaginally, once daily for 5 days **OR** Clindamycin cream 2%, 1 full applicator (5 g), intravaginally at bedtime, for 7 days[g] Alternative: Clindamycin, 300 mg, orally, 2 times daily for 7 days[g] **OR** Clindamycin ovules, 100 mg, intravaginally, once at bedtime for 3 days[g] **OR** Secnidazole, 2-g oral granule in a single dose[h]

Table 4.4. Guidelines for Treatment of Sexually Transmitted Infections in Children ≥45 kg, Adolescents, and Young Adults According to Syndrome, continued

Organisms/ Diagnoses	Treatment of Children Weighing ≥45 kg, Adolescents, and Young Adults[a]
Bacterial vaginosis	**OR** Tinidazole, 2 g, orally, once daily for 2 days[f] **OR** Tinidazole, 1 g, orally, once daily for 5 days[f]
Candida albicans (and occasionally other *Candida* species or yeasts)	See Table 4.6, Recommended Regimens for Vulvovaginal Candidiasis (p 1016)

Pelvic inflammatory disease (PID)[i]

Recommended Parenteral Regimens:

Ceftriaxone, 1 g, IV, every 24 h
PLUS
Doxycycline, 100 mg, orally or IV, every 12 h
PLUS
Metronidazole, 500 mg, orally or IV, every 12 h

OR

Cefotetan, 2 g, IV, every 12 h
OR
Cefoxitin, 2 g, IV, every 6 h
PLUS
Doxycycline, 100 mg, orally or IV, every 12 h

Alternative Parenteral Regimens:

Ampicillin-sulbactam, 3 g, IV, every 6 h
PLUS
Doxycycline, 100 mg, orally or IV, every 12 h

OR

Clindamycin, 900 mg, IV, every 8 h
PLUS
Gentamicin loading dose, IV or IM (2 mg/kg body weight), followed by a maintenance dose (1.5 mg/kg body weight) every 8 h; single daily dosing (3–5 mg/kg body weight) can be substituted

Table 4.4. Guidelines for Treatment of Sexually Transmitted Infections in Children ≥45 kg, Adolescents, and Young Adults According to Syndrome, continued

Organisms/ Diagnoses	Treatment of Children Weighing ≥45 kg, Adolescents, and Young Adults[a]
	Recommended Intramuscular/ Oral Regimens[j,k]: One of the following: Ceftriaxone, 500 mg, IM, once **OR** Cefoxitin, 2 g, IM, **and** Probenecid, 1 g, orally, in a single dose concurrently **OR** Other parenteral third-generation Cephalosporin (eg, Ceftizoxime, Cefotaxime) **PLUS** Doxycycline, 100 mg, orally, 2 times daily for 14 days **PLUS** Metronidazole, 500 mg, orally, 2 times daily for 14 days
	Alternative Intramuscular/ Oral Regimens: Levofloxacin, 500 mg, orally, once daily for 14 days **OR** Moxifloxacin, 400 mg, orally, once daily for 14 days **PLUS** Metronidazole, 500 mg, orally, 2 times daily for 14 days[l] **OR** Azithromycin, 500 mg, IV, daily for 1–2 doses, followed by 250 mg, orally, daily **PLUS** Metronidazole, 500 mg, 3 times daily for 12–14 days[l]
Genital ulcer disease	*Treponema pallidum* (primary or secondary syphilis)	Benzathine penicillin G, 2.4 million U, IM, in a single dose

Table 4.4. Guidelines for Treatment of Sexually Transmitted Infections in Children ≥45 kg, Adolescents, and Young Adults According to Syndrome, continued

Organisms/ Diagnoses	Treatment of Children Weighing ≥45 kg, Adolescents, and Young Adults[a]
Genital herpes simplex virus (HSV)—1st clinical episode[m]	Acyclovir, 400 mg, orally, 3 times daily for 7–10 days **OR** Valacyclovir, 1 g, orally, twice daily for 7–10 days **OR** Famciclovir, 250 mg, orally, 3 times daily for 7–10 days
Genital HSV— episodic treatment of recurrences	Acyclovir, 800 mg, orally, 2 times daily for 5 days **OR** Acyclovir, 800 mg, orally, 3 times daily for 2 days **OR** Famciclovir, 1 g, orally, 2 times daily for 1 day **OR** Famciclovir, 500 mg, orally, once, followed by 250 mg, orally, 2 times daily for 2 days **OR** Famciclovir, 125 mg, orally, 2 times daily for 5 days **OR** Valacyclovir, 500 mg, orally 2 times daily for 3 days **OR** Valacyclovir, 1 g, orally, once daily for 5 days
Genital HSV— suppressive therapy	Acyclovir, 400 mg, orally, 2 times daily **OR** Valacyclovir, 500 mg, orally, once daily[n] **OR** Valacyclovir, 1 g, orally, once daily **OR** Famciclovir, 250 mg, orally, 2 times daily
Haemophilus ducreyi (chancroid)	Azithromycin, 1 g, orally, in a single dose **OR** Ceftriaxone, 250 mg, IM, in a single dose **OR** Ciprofloxacin, 500 mg, orally, 2 times daily for 3 days[o] **OR** Erythromycin base, 500 mg, orally, 3 times daily for 7 days

Table 4.4. Guidelines for Treatment of Sexually Transmitted Infections in Children ≥45 kg, Adolescents, and Young Adults According to Syndrome, continued

	Organisms/ Diagnoses	Treatment of Children Weighing ≥45 kg, Adolescents, and Young Adults[a]
	Klebsiella granulomatis (granuloma inguinale [Donovanosis])	Recommended: Azithromycin, 1 g, orally, once/wk, or 500 mg, orally, daily, for at least 3 weeks[p] Alternatives Doxycycline, 100 mg, orally, 2 times daily for at least 3 weeks[p] **OR** Erythromycin base, 500 mg, orally, 4 times daily for at least 3 weeks[p] **OR** Trimethoprim-sulfamethoxazole, 1 double-strength (160 mg/800 mg) tablet, orally, 2 times daily for >3 weeks[p]
	C trachomatis serovars L1, L2, or L3 (Lymphogranuloma venereum [LGV])	Recommended: Doxycycline, 100 mg, orally, 2 times daily for 21 days Alternative: Azithromycin, 1 g, orally, once weekly for 3 weeks[q] **OR** Erythromycin base, 500 mg, orally 4 times daily for 21 days
Epididymitis	*C trachomatis, N gonorrhoeae*	Ceftriaxone, 500 mg, IM, in a single dose If >150 kg: Ceftriaxone, 1 g, IM in a single dose **PLUS** Doxycycline, 100 mg, orally, 2 times daily for 10 days
	Enteric organisms (eg, *Escherichia coli*), *C trachomatis, N gonorrhoeae* among males who practice insertive anal sex	Ceftriaxone, 500 mg, IM, in a single dose If >150 kg: Ceftriaxone, 1 g, IM in a single dose **PLUS** Levofloxacin, 500 mg, orally, once daily for 10 days
Proctitis	*C trachomatis, N gonorrhoeae*, HSV	Ceftriaxone, 500 mg, IM, in a single dose If >150 kg: Ceftriaxone, 1 g, IM in a single dose

Table 4.4. Guidelines for Treatment of Sexually Transmitted Infections in Children ≥45 kg, Adolescents, and Young Adults According to Syndrome, continued

Organisms/ Diagnoses	Treatment of Children Weighing ≥45 kg, Adolescents, and Young Adults[a]
	PLUS Doxycycline, 100 mg, orally, 2 times daily for 7 days; extend to 21 days for presence of bloody discharge, perianal or mucosal ulcers, or tenesmus and a positive rectal *C trachomatis* test **PLUS** in the presence of rectal ulcers, one of the following: Valacyclovir, 1 g, orally, 2 times daily **OR** Acyclovir, 400 mg, orally, 3 times daily **OR** Famciclovir, 250 mg, orally, 3 times daily for 7–10 days
External anogenital warts (ie, penis, groin, scrotum, vulva, perineum, external anus, and perianus) Human papillomavirus	*Patient-applied:* Imiquimod 3.75% or 5% cream[o,r] **OR** Podofilox 0.5% solution or gel[o] **OR** Sinecatechins 15% ointment[o] *Provider-administered:* Cryotherapy with liquid nitrogen or cryoprobe **OR** Surgical removal either by tangential scissor excision, tangential shave excision, curettage, laser, or electrosurgery **OR** Trichloroacetic acid or bichloroacetic acid 80%–90% solution

IM indicates intramuscularly; STI, sexually transmitted infection.

[a] For additional information and recommendations, see Centers for Disease Control and Prevention. Sexually transmitted infections treatment guidelines, 2021. *MMWR Recomm Rep.* 2021;70(RR-4):1-187. Available at: **www.cdc.gov/std/ treatment-guidelines/toc.htm**

[b] If ceftriaxone is not available or feasible, may substitute cefixime, 800 mg, orally, in a single dose.

[c] Nongonococcal urethritis (NGU) is diagnosed when microscopy indicates inflammation without evidence of diplococci by Gram, methylene blue, or gentian violet staining on microscopy. If microscopy is unavailable, urine testing for leukocyte esterase can be performed on first-void urine, and microscopic examination of sediment from a spun first-void urine demonstrating ≥10 white blood cells/high-powered field has a high negative predictive value.

[d] The terms male and female refer to sex assigned at birth.

[e] In areas where *T vaginalis* is prevalent, males who have sex with females and have persistent or recurrent urethritis should be presumptively treated for *T vaginalis.*

[f] Breastfeeding should be deferred for 72 hours after lactating person has received a 2-g dose of tinidazole.

Table 4.4. Guidelines for Treatment of Sexually Transmitted Infections in Children ≥45 kg, Adolescents, and Young Adults According to Syndrome, continued

[g]Intravaginal clindamycin might weaken latex or rubber products (eg, condoms and diaphragms), and their use within 72 hours after intravaginal clindamycin treatment is not recommended.
[h]Oral granules should be sprinkled onto unsweetened applesauce, yogurt, or pudding before ingestion. A glass of water can be taken after administration to aid in swallowing.
[i] Hospitalization and parenteral treatment is recommended if patient has severe illness such as tubo-ovarian abscess, is pregnant, or is unable to tolerate or follow ambulatory regimens.
[j] Patients with inadequate response to outpatient therapy after 72 hours should be reevaluated for possible misdiagnosis and may require parenteral therapy.
[k]The recommended third-generation cephalosporins are limited in the coverage of anaerobes. Therefore, the addition of metronidazole to treatment regimens with third-generation cephalosporins should be considered.
[l] Can consider if the patient has cephalosporin allergy, gonorrhea community prevalence and individual risk are low, and follow-up is likely.
[m]Treatment can be extended if healing is incomplete after 10 days of therapy.
[n]Valacyclovir, 500 mg, once a day, might be less effective than other valacyclovir or acyclovir dosing regimens for persons with frequent recurrences (ie, ≥10 episodes/year).
[o]Avoid in pregnancy or while breastfeeding.
[p]Treat for at least 3 weeks and until all lesions have completely healed.
[q]Because this regimen has not been validated, a test of cure with a *C trachomatis* nucleic acid amplification test 4 weeks after completion of treatment can be considered.
[r]Wash treatment area with soap and water 6–10 hours after application.

Adapted from Centers for Disease Control and Prevention. Sexually transmitted infections treatment guidelines, 2021. *MMWR Recomm Rep*. 2021;70(RR-4):1-187. Available at: **www.cdc.gov/std/treatment-guidelines/toc.htm**

Table 4.5. Guidelines for Treatment of Sexually Transmitted Infections in Infants and Children <45 kg According to Syndrome

Preferred regimens are listed. For further information concerning other acceptable regimens and diseases not included, see recommendations in disease-specific chapters in Section 3. In addition, recommendations on treatment of sexually transmitted infections have been issued by the Centers for Disease Control and Prevention in 2021[a] (**www.cdc.gov/std/treatment-guidelines/toc.htm**).

Syndrome	Organisms/ Diagnoses	Treatment of Infants and Children <45 kg[a,b]
Urethritis: Inflammation of urethra with erythema and/or mucoid, mucopurulent, or purulent discharge Note: Cervicitis occurs rarely in prepubertal children	*Neisseria gonorrhoeae*, *Chlamydia trachomatis* Other causes include *Mycoplasma genitalium*, possibly *Ureaplasma urealyticum*, and sometimes *Trichomonas vaginalis* and herpes simplex virus (HSV)	Ceftriaxone, 25–50 mg/kg, IV or IM, in a single dose, not to exceed 250 mg, IM[c] **PLUS** Erythromycin base or ethylsuccinate, 50 mg/kg per day, orally, in 4 divided doses for 14 days

Table 4.5. Guidelines for Treatment of Sexually Transmitted Infections in Infants and Children <45 kg According to Syndrome, continued

Syndrome	Organisms/ Diagnoses	Treatment of Infants and Children <45 kg[a,b]
Prepubertal vaginitis (STI related):	*N gonorrhoeae*	Ceftriaxone, 25–50 mg/kg, IV or IM, in a single dose, not to exceed 250 mg, IM[c]
	C trachomatis	Erythromycin base or ethylsuccinate, 50 mg/kg per day, orally, in 4 divided doses for 14 days
	T vaginalis	Metronidazole, 45 mg/kg per day, orally, in 3 divided doses (max 2 g/day) for 7 days
	Bacterial vaginosis	Metronidazole, 15–25 mg/kg per day, orally, in 3 divided doses (max 2 g/day) for 7 days
Genital ulcer disease	*Treponema pallidum* (primary syphilis)[d]	Benzathine penicillin G, 50 000 U/kg, IM, up to the adult dose of 2.4 million U in a single dose
	HSV—1st clinical episode	Acyclovir, 80 mg/kg per day, orally, in 4 divided doses (max 3.2 g/day) for 7–10 days **OR** Valacyclovir, 40 mg/kg per day (max 2 g/day), orally, in 2 divided doses for 7–10 days
	Haemophilus ducreyi (chancroid)	Ceftriaxone, 50 mg/kg, IM, in a single dose (max 250 mg) **OR** Azithromycin, 20 mg/kg, orally, in a single dose (max 1 g)
Anogenital warts	Human papillomavirus	Same as for adolescents. See Table 4.4.

IM indicates intramuscularly; STI, sexually transmitted infection.

[a] For additional information and recommendations, see Centers for Disease Control and Prevention. Sexually transmitted infections treatment guidelines, 2021. *MMWR Recomm Rep.* 2021;70(RR-4):1-187. Available at: **www.cdc.gov/std/ treatment-guidelines/toc.htm.**

[b] Infants and children aged ≥1 month with a sexually transmitted infection should be evaluated for sexual abuse (eg, through consultation with child-protection services). See Table 2.5, p 183.

[c] Providers treating patients with a severe cephalosporin allergy should consult an infectious disease specialist (see also Beta-lactam and Monobactam Allergies, p 976).

[d] Infants and children >1 mo of age who receive a diagnosis of syphilis should have medical records from their birthing parent and delivery reviewed to assess whether they have congenital or acquired syphilis. Infants and children ≥1 mo of age with primary syphilis should be managed by a pediatric infectious disease specialist.

Table 4.6. Recommended Treatment Regimens for Vulvovaginal Candidiasis[a]

Over-the-Counter Intravaginal Agents[b]

Clotrimazole 1% cream, 5 g, intravaginally, for 7–14 days

OR

Clotrimazole 2% cream, 5 g, intravaginally, for 3 days

OR

Miconazole 2% cream, 5 g, intravaginally, for 7 days

OR

Miconazole 4% cream, 5 g, intravaginally, for 3 days

OR

Miconazole, 100-mg vaginal suppository, 1 suppository for 7 days

OR

Miconazole, 200-mg vaginal suppository, 1 suppository for 3 days

OR

Miconazole, 1200-mg vaginal suppository, 1 suppository for 1 day

OR

Tioconazole, 6.5% ointment, 5 g, intravaginally, in a single application

Prescription Intravaginal Agents[b]

Butoconazole 2% cream (single-dose bioadhesive product), 5 g, intravaginally, in a single application

OR

Terconazole 0.4% cream, 5 g, intravaginally, daily for 7 days

OR

Terconazole 0.8% cream, 5 g, intravaginally, for 3 days

OR

Terconazole, 80-mg vaginal suppository, 1 suppository for 3 days

Prescription Oral Agent

Fluconazole, 150-mg oral tablet, 1 tablet in single dose

[a]Adapted from Centers for Disease Control and Prevention. Sexually transmitted infections treatment guidelines, 2021. *MMWR Recomm Rep*. 2021;70(RR-4):1-187. Available at: **www.cdc.gov/std/treatment-guidelines/candidiasis. htm.**

[b]These creams and suppositories are oil-based and might weaken latex condoms and diaphragms.

ANTIFUNGAL DRUGS FOR SYSTEMIC FUNGAL INFECTIONS

Table 4.7 (p 1021) provides data on the relative in vitro susceptibilities of specific fungal species with amphotericin B, azoles, echinocandins, and flucytosine.

Polyenes

Amphotericin B is a fungicidal agent that is effective against a broad array of fungal species. Amphotericin B, especially the "conventional" deoxycholate formulation, is associated with multiple adverse reactions, particularly acute and chronic renal toxicity, so its use is limited to certain patients, primarily neonates. Lipid-associated formulations of amphotericin B, especially liposomal amphotericin B, limit renal toxicity but also are associated with multiple other adverse effects and do not achieve optimal concentrations in some sites of infection (eg, kidneys).

Amphotericin B deoxycholate is the preferred formulation for treatment of neonates with systemic candidiasis because of better penetration into the central nervous system, urinary tract, and eye, which often are involved in neonatal *Candida* infections; lipid-associated formulations do not penetrate as well into many of these body sites. Amphotericin B deoxycholate is generally administered intravenously in a single daily dose of 1 mg/kg in 5% dextrose in water at a concentration of 0.1 mg/mL and delivered through a central or peripheral venous catheter. Infusion times of 1 to 2 hours have been shown to be well tolerated in adults and older children and theoretically increase the blood-to-tissue gradient, thereby improving drug delivery. Total duration of therapy depends on the type and extent of the specific fungal infection.

Amphotericin B deoxycholate is eliminated by a renal mechanism for approximately 2 weeks after therapy is discontinued. No adjustment in dose is required for neonates or for children with impaired renal function, because serum concentrations are not increased significantly in these patients. Because of concentration-dependent killing, if renal toxicity occurs, it is recommended to maintain the dose but switch to alternate-day dosing. Neither hemodialysis nor peritoneal dialysis significantly decreases serum concentrations of the drug.

Infusion-related reactions to amphotericin B deoxycholate include fever, chills, and sometimes nausea, vomiting, headache, generalized malaise, hypotension, and arrhythmias; these reactions are rare in neonates. Onset usually is within 1 to 3 hours after starting the infusion; duration typically is less than an hour. Hypotension and arrhythmias are idiosyncratic reactions that are unlikely to occur if not observed after the initial dose but also can occur in association with rapid infusion. Multiple regimens have been used to prevent infusion-related reactions, but few have been studied in controlled clinical trials. Pretreatment with acetaminophen, alone or combined with diphenhydramine, may alleviate febrile reactions; these reactions appear to be less common in children than in adults. Hydrocortisone (25–50 mg in adults and older children) also can be added to the infusion to decrease febrile and other systemic reactions. Tolerance to febrile reactions develops with time, allowing tapering and eventual discontinuation of the hydrocortisone and often diphenhydramine and antipyretic agents. Meperidine and ibuprofen have been effective in preventing or treating fever and chills in some patients who are refractory to the conventional premedication regimen.

Toxicity from amphotericin B deoxycholate can include nephrotoxicity, hepatotoxicity, anemia, or neurotoxicity. Nephrotoxicity is caused by decreased renal blood flow and can be prevented or ameliorated by hydration, saline solution loading (0.9% saline solution over 30 minutes) before infusion of amphotericin B, and avoidance of diuretic drugs. Hypokalemia is common and can be exacerbated by sodium loading. Renal tubular acidosis can occur but usually is mild. Permanent nephrotoxicity is related to cumulative dose. Nephrotoxicity is increased by concomitant administration of amphotericin B and aminoglycosides, cyclosporine, tacrolimus, cisplatin, nitrogen mustard compounds, or acetazolamide. Anemia is secondary to inhibition of erythropoietin production. Neurotoxicity occurs rarely and can manifest as confusion, delirium, obtundation, psychotic behavior, seizures, blurred vision, or hearing loss.

Lipid preparations of amphotericin B, such as amphotericin B lipid complex (ABLC [Abelcet]) and liposomal amphotericin B (L-AmB [AmBisome]), are the preferred formulation in all patient populations except neonates. Lipid formulations of amphotericin B achieved higher central nervous system concentrations than other formulations of amphotericin B in a rabbit model. Acute infusion-related reactions occur with both formulations but are less frequent with AmBisome. Nephrotoxicity is less common with lipid-associated products than with amphotericin B deoxycholate. Liver toxicity, which generally is not associated with amphotericin B deoxycholate, has been reported with the lipid formulations.

Pyrimidines

Among pyrimidine antifungal agents, only flucytosine (5-fluorocytosine) is approved by the US Food and Drug Administration (FDA) for use in children. Flucytosine has a limited spectrum of activity against fungi (*Cryptococcus* and *Candida* species) and has potential for toxicity and should be avoided in the setting of renal dysfunction. When flucytosine is used as a single agent, resistance often emerges rapidly. Flucytosine should be used in combination with amphotericin B for cryptococcal meningitis. It is important to monitor complete blood cell counts and serum concentrations of flucytosine to avoid bone marrow toxicity, reported to frequently occur with flucytosine serum trough concentrations ≥100 µg/mL. Flucytosine is only available in oral formulation in the United States.

Azoles

Six oral azoles are available in the United States: ketoconazole, fluconazole, itraconazole, voriconazole, posaconazole, and isavuconazonium sulfate (the prodrug for isavuconazole). All have relatively broad activity against common fungi but differ in their in vitro activity (see Table 4.7, p 1021), bioavailability, adverse effects, and potential for drug interactions. Fewer data are available regarding safety and efficacy of azoles in pediatric than in adult patients. Azoles are easy to administer and have little toxicity, but their use can be limited by the frequency of their interactions with coadministered drugs. These drug interactions can result in decreased serum concentrations of the azole potentially leading to therapeutic failure or unexpected toxicity from the coadministered drug (caused by increased serum concentrations of the coadministered drug). When considering use of azoles, the patient's concurrent medications should be reviewed to avoid potential adverse clinical outcomes. The FDA reaffirmed in 2016 that it strongly discourages use of systemic ketoconazole for uncomplicated skin and nail infections because of significant risks of liver toxicity, adrenal insufficiency, and interactions with multiple medications that have resulted in at least 1 fatality.

Another potential limitation of azoles is emergence of resistant fungi, especially *Candida* species resistant to fluconazole and *Aspergillus fumigatus* resistant to itraconazole, posaconazole, and voriconazole. *Candida krusei* are intrinsically resistant to fluconazole, and strains of *Candida glabrata* and *Candida parapsilosis* increasingly are resistant to fluconazole. Itraconazole is approved by the FDA for treatment of blastomycosis and histoplasmosis (nonmeningeal) and for empiric therapy of febrile neutropenic patients with suspected fungal infection. Efficacy and safety have not been established in pediatric patients. Itraconazole does not cross the blood-brain barrier and should not be used for infections of the central nervous system. Itraconazole formulations are not interchangeable; when taken on an empty stomach, the oral solution has greater bioavailability and is preferred over the capsule formulation. A super bioavailable (SUBA) itraconazole formulation was approved by the FDA in 2018 for individuals ≥18 years of age for the treatment of aspergillosis, blastomycosis, and histoplasmosis in individuals intolerant of amphotericin. Voriconazole has been approved by the FDA for individuals 2 years and older for primary treatment of invasive *Aspergillus* species, for candidemia in nonneutropenic patients, for esophageal candidiasis, and for refractory infection with *Fusarium* species and some *Scedosporium* species, such as *Scedosporium apiospermum*. Intravenous and oral formulations are available. Posaconazole is approved for use in adults (all formulations), children ≥13 years of age (delayed-release tablets and oral suspension), and children ≥2 years of age and weighing ≤40 kg (powder for delayed-release oral suspension) for prophylaxis of invasive aspergillosis and candidiasis in patients who are high risk of developing these infections. In addition, the oral suspension is approved for treatment of oropharyngeal candidiasis. Strategies to enhance absorption are necessary (eg, administration with high-fat meal, avoidance of proton pump inhibitors) when using the oral suspension. Isavuconazole, available in oral and intravenous forms, has been approved by the FDA for patients 18 years or older for invasive aspergillosis and invasive mucormycosis. Dose adjustments for most azoles are required in patients with renal and/or hepatic insufficiency. Posaconazole renal clearance is negligible; therefore, in patients with renal impairment as well as in patients on intermittent hemodialysis, no dose adjustment is required. Therapeutic monitoring of azole drugs, especially itraconazole, voriconazole, and posaconazole, with measurement of serum trough concentrations is critical in patients with invasive fungal infections (see Table 4.7, p 1021). Drugs with a narrow therapeutic window that are P-glycoprotein substrates, such as digoxin, may require dose adjustment when administered concomitantly with isavuconazole.

Echinocandins

Caspofungin, micafungin, and anidulafungin are the only echinocandins approved by the FDA. Caspofungin is approved for treatment of pediatric patients 3 months of age and older with invasive candidiasis and esophageal candidiasis; for empiric therapy for presumed fungal infections in febrile neutropenic patients; and for treatment of aspergillosis in patients who are refractory to or intolerant of other antifungal drugs. Clinical trials have demonstrated safety and efficacy in pediatric patients as young as 3 months of age Although efficacy and safety of caspofungin has not specifically been evaluated in neonates, in retrospective studies of immunocompromised pediatric patients that included neonates, the safety and tolerability of caspofungin was favorable. Micafungin is approved by the FDA for intravenous treatment of pediatric patients 4 months and older with candidemia without meningoencephalitis, acute disseminated candidiasis, *Candida* peritonitis and abscesses, and esophageal candidiasis and for prophylaxis of invasive *Candida* infections in patients undergoing hematopoietic cell transplantation. Although micafungin is not FDA approved for aspergillosis, data are available to support its use in the treatment of refractory disease, preferably in combination with another antifungal agent.[1] Anidulafungin is not approved by the FDA for use in children but is FDA approved for the treatment of candidemia, *Candida* infections, and esophageal candidiasis in adults.

Triterpenoids

Ibrexafungerp was approved for adults with vulvovaginal candidiasis following 2 phase 3 studies and is the first new class of antifungals approved since 2001. Similar to the echinocandins, ibrexafungerp noncompetitively inhibits beta-1,3-glucan synthase and is also fungicidal against *Candida* species and *Aspergillus* species. Ibrexafungerp is the first orally available glucan synthase inhibitor and has a long half-life, suggesting once daily dosing for clinical use. Similar to the echinocandins, initial studies show limited to no distribution to the central nervous system and variable distribution to the eye. Dose adjustment is required when used concomitantly with strong CYP3A inhibitors or inducers to avoid systemic toxicity or therapeutic failure. In a phase 2 study for invasive candidiasis, ibrexafungerp as step-down therapy following initial echinocandin therapy was well-tolerated and achieved a favorable global response similar to the standard of care. It currently is not approved for use in children.

---

[1] Patterson TF, Thompson GR, Denning DW, et al. Practice guidelines for the diagnosis and management of aspergillosis: 2016 update by the Infectious Diseases Society of America. *Clin Infect Dis.* 2016;63(4):e1-e60

Table 4.7. Fungal Species, Antifungal Drugs, Activity, Route, Clearance, CSF Penetration, Drug Monitoring Targets, and Adverse Events

Fungal Species	Amphotericin B Formulations	Fluconazole	Itraconazole	Voriconazole	Posaconazole	Isavuconazole	Flucytosine	Echinocandins[a]
Candida albicans	+	++	+	++	+	+	+	++
Candida tropicalis	+	++	+	++	+	+	+	++
Candida parapsilosis	++	++	+	++	+	+	+	+
Candida glabrata	+	–	–	–	+/-	+/-	+	+/-
Candida krusei	+	–	–	+	+	+	+	++
Candida lusitaniae	–	++	+	++	+	+	+	+
Candida guilliermondii	+	+	+	+	+	+	+	+/-
Candida auris	+/-	–	+/-	+/-	+	+	+/-	++
Cryptococcus species	++	++	+	+	+	+	++	–
Trichosporon species	+	+	+	++	+	+	–	–

Table 4.7. Fungal Species, Antifungal Drugs, Activity, Route, Clearance, CSF Penetration, Drug Monitoring Targets, and Adverse Events, continued

Fungal Species	Amphotericin B Formulations	Fluconazole	Itraconazole	Voriconazole	Posaconazole	Isavuconazole	Flucytosine	Echinocandins[a]
Aspergillus fumigatus[b]	+	–	+	++	+	++	–	+
Aspergillus terreus[b]	–	–	+	++	+	++	–	+
Aspergillus calidoustus[b]	++	–	–	–	–	–	–	++
Fusarium species[b]	+	–	–	++	+	+	–	–
Mucor species[b]	++	–	+/–	–	+	++	–	–
Rhizopus species[b]	++	–	–	–	+	++	–	–
Scedosporium apiospermum[b]	–	–	+	++	+	+	–	–
Scedosporium prolificans[b]	–	–	+/–	+/–	+/–	+/–	–	–
Penicillium (Talaromyces) species[b]	+/–	–	++	+	+	+	–	–

Table 4.7. Fungal Species, Antifungal Drugs, Activity, Route, Clearance, CSF Penetration, Drug Monitoring Targets, and Adverse Events, continued

Fungal Species	Amphotericin B Formulations	Fluconazole	Itraconazole	Voriconazole	Posaconazole	Isavuconazole	Flucytosine	Echinocandins[a]
Histoplasma capsulatum[e]	++	+	++	+	+	+	–	–
Coccidioides immitis[e]	++	++	++	+	+	+	–	–
Blastomyces dermatitidis[e]	++	+	++	+	+	+	–	–
Paracoccidioides species[e]	+	+	++	+	+	+	–	–
Sporothrix species[e]	+	+	++	+	+	+	–	–
IV/PO	IV only	IV and PO	PO only	IV and PO	IV and PO	IV and PO	PO only	IV only
Clearance	Renal	Renal/hepatic	Hepatic	Hepatic	Hepatic	Hepatic	Renal	Hepatic (micafungin)
CSF penetration	Good	Good	Limited	Good	Minimal	Good	Good	Minimal

Table 4.7. Fungal Species, Antifungal Drugs, Activity, Route, Clearance, CSF Penetration, Drug Monitoring Targets, and Adverse Events, continued

Fungal Species	Amphotericin B Formulations	Flucona-zole	Itraconazole	Voriconazole	Posacona-zole	Isavucona-zole	Flucytosine	Echi-nocandins[a]
Therapeutic drug monitoring (treatment)	No	No	Obtain trough after at least 10 days of therapy. Therapeutic trough 1–2 µg/mL (when measured by high-pressure liquid chromatography; both itraconazole and its bioactive hydroxy-itraconazole metabolite are reported, the sum of which should be considered in assessing drug levels). The itraconazole oral solution formulation is preferred over the capsule formulation because of improved absorption, and should be taken on an empty stomach.	Obtain trough after at least 3 days of therapy. Therapeutic trough 2–6 µg/mL. It is important to individualize dosing in patients following initiation of voriconazole therapy; because there is high interpatient variability in metabolism.	IV and PO tablets: Obtain trough after at least 3 days of therapy. Therapeutic trough 1–4 µg/mL, with a target of 1.25 µg/mL. PO suspension: Obtain trough after at least 10 days of therapy. Therapeutic trough 1–4 µg/mL, with a target of 1.25 µg/mL.	Unknown.	Obtain 2 h post-peak levels after 3–5 doses. Peak 40–80 µg/mL.	No

Table 4.7. Fungal Species, Antifungal Drugs, Activity, Route, Clearance, CSF Penetration, Drug Monitoring Targets, and Adverse Events, continued

Fungal Species	Amphotericin B Formulations	Flucona-zole	Itraconazole	Voriconazole	Posacona-zole	Isavucona-zole	Flucytosine	Echi-nocandins[a]
Common adverse reactions	Infusion reaction, nephrotoxicity (watch potassium, magnesium); liposomal: hepatotoxicity	Hepatotoxicity; increased QTc, headache, gastrointestinal tract effects	Hepatotoxicity; increased QTc; negative inotrope (avoid in congestive heart failure).	Hepatotoxicity; increased QTc; central nervous system effects, vision changes, phototoxicity.	Hepatotoxicity; increased QTc, headache, gastrointestinal tract effects.	Headache, hypokalemia, abdominal pain, nausea, diarrhea, conjunctivitis, flu-like illness, hepatotoxicity, cough.	Neutropenia, hepatotoxicity (avoid in decreased renal function), gastrointestinal.	Usually well tolerated; gastrointestinal tract effects, headache, hepatotoxicity.

CSF indicates cerebrospinal fluid; IV, intravenous; PO, oral.

NOTE: ++, more active; scenario dependent; +, usually active; +/−, variably active; −, usually not active.

[a] Caspofungin, anidulafungin, and micafungin.

[b] Mold.

[c] Endemic fungi where mold/yeast phase is temperature dependent.

RECOMMENDED DOSES OF PARENTERAL AND ORAL ANTIFUNGAL DRUGS

Table 4.8. Recommended Doses of Parenteral and Oral Antifungal Drugs

Drug	Route	Dose (per day)	Adverse Reactions[a,b]
Amphotericin B deoxycholate (see Antifungal Drugs for Systemic Fungal Infections, p 1017, for detailed information)	IV	0.8 mg/kg/day to 1.0 mg/kg per day (or 1.5 mg/kg every other day) (max 1.5 mg/kg/day); infuse as a single dose over 2–4 h.	Fever, chills, phlebitis, gastrointestinal tract symptoms, headache, hypotension, renal dysfunction, hypokalemia, anemia, cardiac arrhythmias, neurotoxicity, anaphylaxis.
	IT	0.01–0.025 mg, slow increase to 0.5 mg, twice/wk.	Headache, gastrointestinal tract symptoms, arachnoiditis/radiculitis.
Amphotericin B lipid complex (Abelcet)[c]	IV	3–5 mg/kg per day, infused over 2 h.	Fever, chills, other reactions associated with amphotericin B deoxycholate, but less nephrotoxicity; hypokalemia, hepatotoxicity has been reported with lipid complex.
Liposomal amphotericin B (AmBisome)[c]	IV	3–5 mg/kg, infused over 1–2 h. IFI prophylaxis[d]: 1 mg/kg/dose every other day or 2.5 mg/kg/dose twice/wk. Doses up to 10 mg/kg have been used in patients with mucormycosis or central nervous system infection.	Fever, chills, fewer infusion reactions and less nephrotoxicity than associated with amphotericin B deoxycholate; hypokalemia, hepatotoxicity has been reported.

Table 4.8. Recommended Doses of Parenteral and Oral Antifungal Drugs, continued

Drug	Route	Dose (per day)	Adverse Reactions[a,b]
Anidulafungin[c,e]	IV	For adults and adolescents 12 y and older: Candidemia and other forms of *Candida* infections: 200 mg on day 1, followed by 100-mg daily dose thereafter for at least 14 days after the last positive culture. Esophageal candidiasis: 100 mg on day 1, followed by 50-mg daily dose thereafter for a minimum of 14 days and for at least 7 days following resolution of symptoms. Dosage in pediatric patients (2 y through 11 y): Candidemia and other forms of *Candida* infections: 3-mg/kg loading dose on day 1, followed by 1.5 mg/kg once daily thereafter. Maximum loading dose 200 mg and daily dose 100 mg. Esophageal candidiasis: 1.5-mg/kg loading dose on day 1, followed by 0.75 mg/kg once daily thereafter.	Fever, headache, nausea, vomiting, diarrhea, leukopenia, hypokalemia, hepatitis, hepatic enzyme elevations, hypersensitivity, and phlebitis. Because of high alcohol content of solution, the rate of infusion should not exceed 1.1 mg/minute.
Caspofungin[e]	IV	Dosage in adults (18 y and older): 70-mg loading dose on day 1, followed by 50 mg once daily for all indications except esophageal candidiasis. For esophageal candidiasis, use 50 mg once daily with no loading dose. Dosage in pediatric patients (3 mo through 17 y of age): For all indications, 70-mg/m² loading dose on day 1, followed by 50 mg/m² once daily thereafter. Maximum dose should not exceed 70 mg, regardless of the patient's weight and calculated dose. Dosage in neonates: 25 mg/m² daily.	Adults: Diarrhea, pyrexia, hepatic enzymes elevations, and hypokalemia. Pediatric: diarrhea, rash, hepatic enzymes elevations, hypokalemia, infusion-related reactions. Isolated cases of hepatic dysfunction, hepatitis, or hepatic failure have been reported.

Table 4.8. Recommended Doses of Parenteral and Oral Antifungal Drugs, continued

Drug	Route	Dose (per day)	Adverse Reactions[a,b]
Clotrimazole	PO	Oropharyngeal candidiasis: 10-mg lozenge, 5 times per day for 14 consecutive days (dissolved slowly in mouth).	Gastrointestinal tract symptoms, unpleasant mouth sensations, hepatotoxicity. .
Fluconazole	IV, PO	Neonatal candidiasis[f]: 25 mg/kg on day 1, followed by 12 mg/kg/dose once daily Oropharyngeal and esophageal candidiasis: 6 mg/kg (adult dose: 200 mg) on the first day, followed by 3–6 mg/kg (adult dose: 100 mg) once daily. Doses up to 12 mg/kg/day have been used based on clinical judgment. Systemic *Candida* infections: 12 mg/kg/day. Prophylaxis in children (when indicated)[d]. : 6 mg/kg once daily (max 400 mg/day). Cryptococcal meningitis (children)[g]: Following induction therapy with amphotericin B plus flucytosine for at least 2 weeks, fluconazole 10–12 mg/kg/day (max 800 mg per day) in 2 divided doses for at least 8 weeks; for suppression of relapse in children with AIDS, use 6 mg/kg (max 200 mg per day) once daily.	Rash, gastrointestinal tract symptoms, hepatotoxicity, Stevens-Johnson syndrome, anaphylaxis. Requires dose adjustment for renal impairment

Table 4.8. Recommended Doses of Parenteral and Oral Antifungal Drugs, continued

Drug	Route	Dose (per day)	Adverse Reactions[a,b]
		Cryptococcal meningitis (adults)[g]: Following induction therapy with amphotericin B plus flucytosine for at least 2 weeks, fluconazole 12 mg/kg/day (max 800 mg per day) in 2 divided doses for at least 8 weeks; 200 mg once daily is used for suppression of relapse of cryptococcal meningitis in patients with AIDS.	
		Coccidioidomycosis (adults): 400 mg once daily, can use up to 800 mg once daily in non-meningitis, and up to 1200 mg once daily in meningitis.	
Flucytosine	PO	100 mg/kg/day, divided dosing every 6 h (adjust dose for renal dysfunction and neonatal age); follow 2-h post peak levels closely (therapeutic range ≤100 μg/mL).	Bone marrow suppression, hepatotoxicity, renal dysfunction, gastrointestinal tract symptoms, rash, neuropathy, confusion, hallucinations. Cytosine arabinoside, a cytostatic agent, has been reported to inactivate the antifungal activity of flucytosine by competitive inhibition; drugs that impair glomerular filtration may prolong the biological half-life of flucytosine. The hematologic parameters and liver and kidney function should be monitored during therapy. Flucytosine should be used in combination with amphotericin B for the treatment of cryptococcosis because of the emergence of resistance to flucytosine.

Table 4.8. Recommended Doses of Parenteral and Oral Antifungal Drugs, continued

Drug	Route	Dose (per day)	Adverse Reactions[a,b]
Griseofulvin	PO	Ultramicrosize: 10–15 mg/kg, once daily; maximum dose per day, 750 mg. Microsize: 20–25 mg/kg per day divided in 2 doses; maximum dose per day, 1000 mg.	Rash, paresthesias, leukopenia, gastrointestinal tract symptoms, proteinuria, hepatotoxicity, mental confusion, headache.
Ibrexafungerp	PO	300 mg (2 tablets of 150 mg) twice a day for 1 day; for a total treatment dosage of 600 mg; not currently approved for use in children	The most frequent adverse reactions (≥2%) reported in clinical trials of vulvovaginal candidiasis treatment were diarrhea, nausea, abdominal pain, dizziness, and vomiting
Isavuconazole (prodrug is isavuconazonium sulfate)[h]	IV, PO	Adults: Approved in individuals ≥18 y of age. 200 mg, every 8 h for 6 doses, then 200 mg, once daily (corresponding to 372 mg of the sulfate compound every 8 h for 6 doses, then 372 mg daily), starting 12 to 24 h after the last loading dose. No target therapeutic concentration has been defined for isavuconazole. Pediatrics: Very limited pharmacokinetic and safety data available in children ≤17 y of age: Loading dose of 10 mg of isavuconazonium sulfate/kg/dose every 8 h for 6 doses (max 372 mg of isavuconazonium sulfate/dose), followed 12–24 h after last loading dose by maintenance dose of 10 mg of isavuconazonium sulfate/kg/dose IV every 24 h (max 372 mg of isavuconazonium sulfate/dose).	Most frequent adverse reactions are nausea, vomiting, diarrhea, headache, elevated aminotransferases, hypokalemia, constipation, dyspnea, cough, peripheral edema, and back pain. CYP3A4 inhibitors or inducers may alter the plasma concentrations of isavuconazole. Appropriate therapeutic drug monitoring and dose adjustment of immunosuppressants (ie, tacrolimus, sirolimus, and cyclosporine) may be necessary when coadministered with isavuconazole. Drugs with a narrow therapeutic window that are P-gp substrates, such as digoxin, may require dose adjustment coadministered concomitantly with isavuconazole.

Table 4.8. Recommended Doses of Parenteral and Oral Antifungal Drugs, continued

Drug	Route	Dose (per day)	Adverse Reactions[a,b]
Itraconazole[c]	PO	Children: 10 mg/kg per day divided into 2 doses; for endemic mycoses 2–5 mg/kg/dose three times a day for 3 days, then 2–5 mg/kg/dose twice daily (max of 200 mg/dose); acidic pH for better absorption; oral solution supplies more reliable bioavailability; serum trough concentrations of itraconazole should be 1 to 2 µg/mL. A trough level should be checked 10 days or later following initiation to ensure adequate drug exposure; when measured by high-pressure liquid chromatography, both itraconazole and its bioactive hydroxyitraconazole metabolite are reported, the sum of which should be considered in assessing the trough concentration; the itraconazole oral solution formulation is preferred over the capsule formulation because of improved absorption, and should be taken on an empty stomach; IFI prophylaxis[d]: 2.5 mg/kg twice a day, with minimum therapeutic level of 0.5 µg/mL. Adults: 200–400 mg/day once or twice a day for treatment of aspergillosis; 200 mg 3 times daily for 3 days and then 200 mg once or twice daily for treatment of endemic mycoses; 100–200 mg once daily for oropharyngeal and esophageal candidiasis. A super bioavailable (SUBA) itraconazole is now approved by the Food and Drug Administration for the treatment of pulmonary and extrapulmonary blastomycosis in individuals 18 years or older, with pharmacokinetic studies of this formulation demonstrating less variable absorption than conventional itraconazole capsules and a similar side effect profile; data in children are lacking.	Gastrointestinal tract symptoms, rash, edema, headache, hypokalemia, hepatotoxicity, tremor, thrombocytopenia, leukopenia; strong P450 CYP3A4 inhibitor; serious cardiovascular events, including QT prolongation, torsades de pointes, ventricular tachycardia, cardiac arrest, and/or sudden death have occurred in patients using cisapride, pimozide, levacetylmethadol (levomethadyl), methadone, or quinidine concomitantly with itraconazole and/or other CYP3A4 inhibitors, should not be used in patients with congestive heart failure.

Table 4.8. Recommended Doses of Parenteral and Oral Antifungal Drugs, continued

Drug	Route	Dose (per day)	Adverse Reactions[a,b]
Micafungin[i]	IV	Adults: 100 mg daily for treatment of candidemia, acute disseminated candidiasis, *Candida* peritonitis and abscesses; 150 mg daily for esophageal candidiasis; and 50 mg daily for prophylaxis of candida infections in hematopoietic cell transplant recipients. Pediatric: 2 mg/kg/day (max 100 mg daily) for candidemia and acute disseminated candidiasis, *Candida* peritonitis and abscesses; Doses up to 7 mg/kg/day have been used for disseminated candidiasis. 1 mg/kg/day (max 50 mg daily) for prophylaxis of *Candida* infections; for treatment of esophageal candidiasis, 3 mg/kg/day is used for children ≤30 kg and 2.5 mg/kg/day with a max 150 mg daily is used for children ≥30 kg; neonatal dosing is 10 mg/kg/day.	Fever, headache, nausea, vomiting, diarrhea, rash, thrombocytopenia, hepatic enzyme elevations, histamine-mediated symptoms including rash, pruritus, facial swelling, and vasodilatation can occur during infusion.
Nystatin	PO	Infants: 200 000 U, 4 times a day, after meals. Children and adults: 400 000–600 000 U, 3 times a day, after meals.	Gastrointestinal tract symptoms, rash.
Posaconazole[e]	PO, IV[j]	Adults and adolescents[k]: for prophylaxis of invasive *Aspergillus* and *Candida* infections[d]. IV formulation is approved only for use in patients 2 y or older, however there are no weight-based dosing recommendations. 300 mg, IV, twice a day on first day; followed by 300 mg, IV, once daily starting on second day.	Diarrhea, nausea, fever, vomiting, headache, coughing, hypokalemia, rash, edema, headache, anemia, neutropenia, thrombocytopenia, fatigue, thrombophlebitis, arthralgia, myalgia, fever; interactions with P450 CYP3A4 substrate drugs and can potentiate QT prolongation; posaconazole injection should be avoided in patients with moderate or severe renal impairment (creatinine clearance <50 mL/min).

Table 4.8. Recommended Doses of Parenteral and Oral Antifungal Drugs, continued

Drug	Route	Dose (per day)	Adverse Reactions[a,b]
		Delayed-release tablets can be used in children >2 y of age and weighing >40 kg; delayed- release oral suspension can be used in children ≥2 y and weighing ≤40 kg; Immediate release oral suspension can be used in children 13 y and older; 300 mg delayed-release tablets twice a day on the first day followed by 300 mg once daily, starting on the second day; or delayed-release oral suspension, dosing based on weight and loading dose on first day, then maintenance dosing starting on second day [10 to <12 kg: 90 mg twice daily on first day, then 90 mg once daily; ≥12 to <17 kg: 120 mg twice daily on first day, then 120 mg once daily; ≥17 kg to <21 kg: 150 mg twice daily on first day, then 150 mg once daily; ≥21 kg to <26 kg: 180 mg twice daily on first day, then 180 g once daily; ≥26 kg to <36 kg: 210 mg twice daily on first day, then 210 mg once daily; or ≥36 kg to 40 kg: 240 mg twice daily on first day, then 240 mg once daily]; 200 mg (5-mL) immediate release oral solution 3 times a day; duration of therapy for both IV and oral is based on recovery from neutropenia or immunosuppression; tablet and liquid forms are not interchangeable given bioavailability and dosing differences; give oral formulations with food. Delayed release tablet is better absorbed. For oropharyngeal candidiasis: oral suspension 100 mg (2.5 mL) twice a day on first day followed by 100 mg once daily for 13 days. For oropharyngeal candidiasis refractory to itraconazole and/or fluconazole: oral suspension 400 mg (10 mL) twice a day; duration of therapy is based on the severity of the patient's underlying disease and clinical response.	

Table 4.8. Recommended Doses of Parenteral and Oral Antifungal Drugs, continued

Drug	Route	Dose (per day)	Adverse Reactions[a,b]
		Serum trough concentrations of posaconazole should be 1 to 4 µg/mL, with a target of 1.25 µg/mL. For intravenous and oral tablet formulations, a trough level should be checked 3 days or later following initiation to ensure adequate drug exposure. For oral liquid formulation, a trough level should be checked 10 days or later following initiation to ensure adequate drug exposure.	
Terbinafine	PO	Children: once daily dosing Onychomycosis: 10–20 kg: 62.5 mg/day; 21–40 kg: 125 mg/day; >40 kg: 250 mg/day; treatment course of 12 wk for toenails, 6 wk for fingernails. Tinea capitis: <25 kg: 125 mg/day; 25–35 kg: 187.5 mg/day; >35 kg: 250 mg once daily; treatment course of 6 wk. Adults: 250 mg, once daily.	Common adverse events include headache, diarrhea, rash, dyspepsia, liver enzyme abnormalities, pruritus, taste disturbance, nausea, abdominal pain, and flatulence; liver failure, sometimes leading to liver transplant or death, has been reported with the use of oral terbinafine. Obtain pretreatment serum aminotransferases. Terbinafine is an inhibitor of CYP450 2D6 isozyme and has an effect on metabolism of desipramine. Drug interactions with cimetidine, fluconazole, cyclosporine, rifampin, and caffeine have also been reported.

Table 4.8. Recommended Doses of Parenteral and Oral Antifungal Drugs, continued

Drug	Route	Dose (per day)	Adverse Reactions[a,b]
Voriconazole[c]	IV, PO	Treatment or IFI prophylaxis[d]: • if 2–<12 y of age or 12–14 y of age and weight <50 kg: 9 mg/kg, IV, twice daily on day 1 of treatment; thereafter 8 mg/kg, IV, twice daily or 9 mg/kg, PO, twice daily; • if ≥15 y of age or 12–14 y of age and weight ≥50 kg: 6 mg/kg, IV, twice daily on day 1 of treatment; thereafter 4 mg/kg, IV, twice daily or 200 mg, PO, twice daily; • Trough levels should be obtained after 5 days of therapy; therapeutic trough levels are 2–6 μg/mL. Esophageal candidiasis: • If 2–<12 y of age or 12–14 y of age and weight <50 kg: 4 mg/kg IV every 12 h; PO 9 mg/kg every 12 h (max of 350 mg/dose PO every 12 h) • Not evaluated in ≥15 y of age or 12–14 y of age and weight ≥50 kg; adult dosing regimen is applied with max dosing of 200 mg, PO, every 12 h.	Concentration- or dose-related toxicities: hepatic toxicity, arrhythmias/QT prolongation, dermatologic reactions, visual disturbance, hallucinations, increased liver enzymes and bilirubin, encephalopathy; phototoxicity, rash; central nervous system-related toxicities are more associated with trough levels above 6 μg/mL. Close monitoring of voriconazole serum trough concentrations is critical for both efficacy and safety. Most experts agree that voriconazole trough concentrations should be measured on day 3 or later after initiating treatment and for children, therapeutic trough concentrations are 2–6 μg/mL. It is important to individualize dosing in patients following initiation of voriconazole therapy, because there is high interpatient variability in metabolism.

Table 4.8. Recommended Doses of Parenteral and Oral Antifungal Drugs, continued

Drug	Route	Dose (per day)	Adverse Reactions[a,b]
		A simpler proposed oral regimen for IFI prophylaxis[d]: 200 mg, PO, twice daily if weight is ≥40 kg and 100 mg, PO, twice daily if weight is <40 kg; if IV needed, then 4 mg/kg every 12 h is administered.	

CYP indicates cytochrome P; GVDH, graft versus host disease; IFI, Invasive fungal infection; IT, intrathecal; IV, intravenous; PO, oral.

[a] See package insert or listing in current edition of the *Physicians' Desk Reference* or **www.pdr.net** (for registered users only).

[b] Interactions with other drugs are common. Consult **www.fda.gov/drugs/development-resources/drug-interactions-labeling** and the Physicians' Desk Reference (a drug interaction reference or database) or a pharmacist before prescribing these medications.

[c] Limited efficacy and safety data in pediatric patients are available.

[d] Invasive fungal infection prophylaxis in at-risk pediatric patients with immunosuppression attributable to cancer or hematopoietic cell transplant.

[e] Safety and effectiveness of anidulafungin in patients ≤16 years of age has not been established.

[f] Experience with fluconazole in neonates is limited to pharmacokinetic studies in preterm newborn infants. Based on the prolonged half-life seen in preterm newborn infants (gestational age 26 to 29 weeks), these children, in the first 2 weeks of life, should receive the same dosage (mg/kg) as in older children, but administered every 72 hours. After the first 2 weeks, these children should be dosed once daily

[g] Perfect JR, Dismukes WE, Dromer F, et al. clinical practice guidelines for the management of cryptococcal disease: 2010 update by the Infectious Diseases Society of America. *Clin Infect Dis.* 2010;50(3):291–322.

[h] Safety and effectiveness of isavuconazole in patients younger than 18 years have not been established.

[i] Limited efficacy and safety data in pediatric patients younger than 4 months are available.

[j] IV formulation of posaconazole is recommended only for 18 years or older. For systemic *Candida* infections including candidemia, disseminated candidiasis, and pneumonia, optimal therapeutic dosage and duration of therapy have not been established. In open, noncomparative studies of small numbers of patients, doses of up to 400 mg daily have been used.

[k] Safety and effectiveness of posaconazole have been established in the age groups 13 years and older.

TOPICAL DRUGS FOR SUPERFICIAL FUNGAL INFECTIONS

Table 4.9. Topical Drugs for Superficial Fungal Infections

Drug	Strength	Formulation	Trade Name Examples	Application(s) per Day	Adverse Reactions/Notes
Basic fuchsin, phenol, resorcinol, and acetone (Rx and OTC)		S	Castellani Paint Modified	1	Excellent for intertriginous areas. Stains skin and clothing. Also available as a colorless solution with alcohol and without basic fuchsin. This is an alternative if the patient cannot tolerate other topical antifungals. Not FDA approved. Must be compounded.
Butenafine HCl (Rx and OTC)	1%	C	Mentax; Lotrimin Ultra	1–2, typically for 2 wk; Lotrimin Ultra may be used 2/day for 1 wk or 1/day for 4 wk	Safety and efficacy in patients younger than 12 y of age have not been established. Do not occlude.[a] Sensitivity to allylamines. Not to be used on scalp or nails.
Ciclopirox olamine (Rx)	0.77%; Nail lacquer 8%	C, L, S, Sh, P, G, NL	Loprox; Penlac nail lacquer; Ciclodan	2 for up to 4 wk; can be longer duration if applied to nails	Irritant dermatitis, hair discoloration; shake lotion vigorously before application; safety and efficacy in children younger than 10 y of age have not been established. Precautions: diabetes mellitus; immune compromise; seizures. Do not occlude.[a]
Clotrimazole (Rx and OTC)	1%	C, O, S, Com; check with pharmacist	Topical solution (more than 10 preparations); Lotrimin, Desenex, Microtrin/ Mycozyl AC, FungiCURE, Gyne-Lotrimin, Alevazol	1 (Rx) 2 (OTC) for 2–4 wk	Irritant dermatitis. Avoid topical steroid combinations.[b] Vaginal products contain excipients (eg, benzyl alcohol) not for use in other topical locations

Table 4.9. Topical Drugs for Superficial Fungal Infections, continued

Drug	Strength	Formulation	Trade Name Examples	Application(s) per Day	Adverse Reactions/Notes
Clotrimazole and betamethasone dipropionate (Rx)	1%/0.05%	C, L	Lotriderm, Lotrisone	2[b] for up to 2 wk for tinea corporis/cruris, 4 wk for pedis	Significant drug interactions exist, even with topical formulations; use caution Irritant dermatitis: Not FDA approved for patients younger than 17 y and not recommended for diaper dermatitis. In 2 studies in pediatric subjects, 39.5% of tinea pedis patients and 47.1% of tinea cruris patients demonstrated adrenal suppression as determined by cosyntropin testing. If used in the groin area, patients should use medication for 2 wk only and use sparingly. Do not occlude.[a] Safety and efficacy not established in children. Contraindication: avoid steroid in varicella.
Econazole nitrate (Rx)	1%	C, F	Zolpak, Ecoza	1 (dermatophyte) 2 (candidiasis) up to 4 wk	Irritant dermatitis; foam approved for tinea pedis in children 12 y and older. Concomitant administration of econazole and warfarin has resulted in enhancement of anticoagulation effect.
Efinaconazole (Rx)	10%	S	Jublia	1, for 48 wk applied to nails (*Trichophyton rubrum* and *Trichophyton mentagrophytes*)	Application site dermatitis; application site vesicles; application site pain. Safety and effectiveness in pediatric patients younger than 6 y have not been established.

Table 4.9. Topical Drugs for Superficial Fungal Infections, continued

Drug	Strength	Formulation	Trade Name Examples	Application(s) per Day	Adverse Reactions/Notes
Iodoquinol and 2% hydrocortisone acetate (Rx)	1%	G, C	Dermazene, Vytone	3–4	Burning/itching sensation. Local allergic reaction. Can stain skin and clothes. Can interfere with results of thyroid function tests. Not to be used under occlusion in the diaper area. Not intended for use on infants. Not FDA approved. Safety and efficacy in children have not been established. Most formulations contain benzyl alcohol derivatives
Ketoconazole (Rx and OTC)	1%, 2%	C, Sh, G, F	Nizoral, Nizoral AD, Sebizol, Xolegel, Extina, Ketodan, Ketoderm	1 (tinea dermatophyte) for 2–6 wk 2 (candidiasis) Once to treat (Rx S) Every 3–4 days (OTC S)	Potential sulfite reaction with anaphylactic or asthmatic reaction; shampoo can cause dry or oily hair and increase hair loss; irritant dermatitis. May interfere with permanent waving or changes in hair texture. Cream formulation only intended for patients 12 y and older; safety and efficacy not established for younger than 12 y. Foam must not be applied directly to hands, but onto a cool surface and applied using fingertips. OTC shampoo may be used for up to 8 wk to treat, and then used as needed to control dandruff.
Luliconazole (Rx)	1%	C	Luzu	1 (x 2 wk for tinea pedis; x 1 wk for tinea cruris and tinea corporis)	Application site reactions in <1% during Phase 3 clinical trials. Contact dermatitis and cellulitis have been reported during postmarketing surveillance. Safety and efficacy have been established in children 12 to <18 y with tinea pedis and tinea cruris and for children 2 to <18 y with tinea corporis.

Table 4.9. Topical Drugs for Superficial Fungal Infections, continued

Drug	Strength	Formulation	Trade Name Examples	Application(s) per Day	Adverse Reactions/Notes
Miconazole nitrate (Rx and OTC)	2%	O, C, P, S, Sp, SpP; check with pharmacist[c]	More than 10 preparations; Lotrimin, Cruex, Podactin, Desenex, Zeasorb AF, Micatrin	2 (seborrhea), apply 2–3 times/day for several months 2 (C, L) 2 (P, L) 1 (pityriasis versicolor)	Irritant and allergic contact dermatitis. Not recommended for children younger than 2 y. Also available as vaginal suppository intended only for patients 12 y and older.
Miconazole nitrate and 15% Zinc oxide (Rx)	0.25%	O	Vusion	Every diaper change for 1 wk	Skin irritation. Can be used in children 4 wk and older. Do not routinely use for more than 7 days. Do not use in infants or children who do not have a normal immune system.
Naftifine HCl (Rx)	1%, 2% gel	C, G	Naftin	1 (C) 1–2 (Gel) for 2 wk	Burning/stinging, irritant dermatitis. Safety and efficacy of gel formulation in children have not been established. Do not occlude.[a]
Nystatin (Rx and OTC	100 000 U/mL or 100 000 U/g	C, P, O, Com	Nystatin, Nystop powder, Nyamyc	2–4 (C) 2–3 (P)	Nontoxic except with topical steroid combinations.[d]

Table 4.9. Topical Drugs for Superficial Fungal Infections, continued

Drug	Strength	Formulation	Trade Name Examples	Application(s) per Day	Adverse Reactions/Notes
Nystatin and triamcinolone acetonide (Rx)	100 000 USP nystatin and 1 mg triamcinolone acetonide (0.1%)	C, O	Mycolog-II,	2[b]	Pediatric patients may demonstrate greater susceptibility to topical corticosteroid-induced hypothalamic-pituitary-adrenal (HPA) axis suppression and Cushing syndrome than mature patients because of a larger ratio of skin surface area to body weight. Contraindications: Hypersensitivity to component drug. Avoid steroid use in varicella or vaccinia. Do not occlude.[a] Use lowest effective dose. Do not routinely use for more than 2 wk.
Oxiconazole (Rx)	1%	C, L	Oxistat	1–2 (tinea dermatophyte), 2–4 wk depending on site; 1 (tinea (pityriasis) versicolor for 2 wk	Pruritus, burning, irritant dermatitis. Do not occlude. Intended for patients 12 y and older; safety and efficacy not established for younger than 12 y
Sertaconazole nitrate (Rx)	2%	C	Ertaczo	2 for 4 wk (pedis), 2 wk for corporis or candida	Dry skin, skin tenderness, contact dermatitis, local hypersensitivity. Safety and efficacy in children younger than 2 y have not been established.
Sulconazole (Rx)	1%	C, S	Exelderm	1–2 (pityriasis versicolor) for 3 wk 2 (tinea pedis) for 4 wk	Irritant dermatitis. Safety and efficacy in children have not been established.

Table 4.9. Topical Drugs for Superficial Fungal Infections, continued

Drug	Strength	Formulation	Trade Name Examples	Application(s) per Day	Adverse Reactions/Notes
Tavaborole (Rx)	5%	S	Kerydin	1, for 48 wk applied to nails (*Trichophyton rubrum* and *Trichophyton mentagrophytes*)	Application site exfoliation; application site erythema; application site dermatitis. Safety and efficacy have been established in children 6 y and older.
Terbinafine (Rx and OTC)	1%	C, Sp	Lamisil, Lamisil AT	1–2, tinea pedis can use up to 2 wk	Irritant dermatitis. Avoid use of occlusive clothing or dressings. Do not apply spray to face. Safety and efficacy in children younger than 12 y have not been established.
Tolnaftate (OTC)	1%	C, P, S, SpP, SpL; check with pharmacist[e]	>10 preparations; Tinactin, Podactin, Tinaspore	2	Irritant and allergic contact dermatitis. Not recommended if younger than 2 y.
Undecylenic acid and derivatives (OTC)	8%–25%	NL, O, S, SpP, P, (check with pharmacist for formulations and applications[e])	BioRx Sponix, Elon Dual Defense, Gordochom, Hongo Cura, Myco Nail A	2 for 4 wk applied to nails	Irritant dermatitis. Not recommended for children younger than 2 y.

Table 4.9. Topical Drugs for Superficial Fungal Infections, continued

Drug	Strength	Formulation	Trade Name Examples	Application(s) per Day	Adverse Reactions/Notes
Other Remedies					
Gentian violet (OTC)	1%	S	...	1–3 for 3 days	Staining. Oral mucosal ulceration reported in young children in as little as 4 days, only use as a last resort. Keep out of the reach of children. Safety and efficacy in children not established. OTC monograph not final.
Selenium sulfide (Rx and OTC)	1%, 2.3%, 2.5%	Sh, L	SelRx 2.3%	Use twice weekly for 2 wk (Sh) 1 for 7 days (L)	Irritant dermatitis and ulceration. For tinea capitis, to decrease spore formation and to decrease the potential spread of the dermatophyte. Hair loss, discoloration of hair, oiliness or dryness of scalp. Safety and efficacy in children not established. May damage jewelry. Not to be used when inflammation or exudation is present.
	1%	Sh, L	Head & Shoulders, Selsun Blue	Use twice weekly for at least 2 wk	For tinea capitis, to decrease spore formation and to decrease the potential spread of the dermatophyte.

C indicates cream; Com, combinations; F, foam; FDA, US Food and Drug Administration; G, gel; L, lotion; NL, nail lacquer; O, ointment; OTC, over the counter; P, powder; PKU, phenylketonuria; Rx, prescription; S, solution; Sh, shampoo; Sp, spray; SpL, spray lotion; SpP, spray powder.

[a] Indicates direct or indirect covering of skin with impermeable barrier (ie, petroleum, wound dressings).

[b] Topical steroids must be used with caution in young children and in areas of thin skin (eg, diaper area). In these circumstances, high systemic exposure may occur, resulting in endogenous synthesis suppression with the potential for serious adverse effects. Potential adverse effects include irritant dermatitis, folliculitis, hypertrichosis, acneiform eruptions, hypopigmentation, perioral dermatitis, allergic contact dermatitis, maceration, secondary infection, skin atrophy, striae, and miliaria. Topical steroids may worsen superficial fungal infections and cause tinea incognito and/or Majocchi granuloma.

[c] Pharmacists are an excellent resource to verify formulations that are available and new (they use *Facts and Comparisons* reference products).

[d] Any topical preparation has the potential to irritate the skin and cause itching, burning, stinging, erythema, edema, vesicles, and blister formation. For more information on individual drugs, see *Physician's Desk Reference* or **www.pdr.net** (for registered users only).

NON-HIV ANTIVIRAL DRUGS

Table 4.10. Non-HIV Antiviral Drugs[a]

Generic (Trade Name)	Indication	Route	Age	Usually Recommended Dosage
Acyclovir[b,c,d,e] (Zovirax)	Neonatal herpes simplex virus (HSV) infection	IV	Birth to ≤4 mo	Treatment dosing: 60 mg/kg per day, in 3 divided doses for 14 days (SEM disease) or 21 days (CNS or Disseminated disease) (durations >21 days are necessary if CSF PCR remains positive near end of treatment course)
		Oral	2 wk to 8 mo	Oral suppressive dosing following completion of IV treatment; dosing: 300 mg/m², 3 times per day for 6 mo
	HSV encephalitis	IV	>4 mo to 12 y	30–45 mg/kg per day, in 3 divided doses for 14–21 days; FDA-approved dose of 60 mg/kg per day for this age range and indication is not recommended, as risk of acute kidney injury may increase at incremental doses exceeding 500 mg/m² or 15 mg/kg; dosing per m² causes excessive weight-based dosing in younger children[f]; neurotoxicity (agitation, myoclonus, delirium, altered consciousness, etc) can occur with accumulated high acyclovir levels, often a result of renal dysfunction and unadjusted dosage
		IV	≥12 y	30 mg/kg per day, in 3 divided doses for 14–21 days[g]
	Varicella in immunocompetent host[h]	Oral	≥2 y	≤40 kg: 80 mg/kg per day, in 4 divided doses for 5 days; maximum daily dose of 3200 mg/day (800 mg/dose) >40 kg: 3200 mg, in 4 divided doses for 5 days (800 mg/dose) (Adult dose: 4000 g per day, in 5 divided doses for 5–7 days)
	Varicella in immunocompetent host requiring hospitalization	IV	≥2 y	30 mg/kg per day, in 3 divided doses for 7–10 days; or 1500 mg/m² per day, in 3 divided doses for 7–10 days[g]

Table 4.10. Non-HIV Antiviral Drugs,ᵃ continued

Generic (Trade Name)	Indication	Route	Age	Usually Recommended Dosage
	Varicella in immunocompromised host	IV	<2 y	30 mg/kg per day, in 3 divided doses for 7–10 days
		IV	≥2 y	1500 mg/m² per day, in 3 divided doses for 7–10 daysᵍ; some experts recommend the 30 mg/kg per day, in 3 divided doses for 7–10 days
	Zoster in immunocompetent host	IV (if requiring hospitalization)	All ages	Same as for varicella in immunocompetent host requiring hospitalization
		Oral	≥12 y	4000 mg/day (800 mg/dose), in 5 divided doses for 5–7 days
	Zoster in immunocompromised host	IV	All ages	30 mg/kg per day, in 3 divided doses, for 7–10 days; or 1500 mg/m² per day in 3 divided doses for 7–10 days
	HSV infection in immunocompromised host (localized, progressive, or disseminated)	IV	All ages	30 mg/kg per day, in 3 divided doses for 7–14 days
		Oral	≥2 y	1000 mg/day, in 3–5 divided doses for 7–14 days
	Prophylaxis of HSV, varicella, and zoster in immunocompromised hosts	Oral	≥2 y	80 mg/kg/day, in 2–3 divided doses (max dose: 800 mg) during period of risk; or 600–1000 mg/day, in 3–5 divided doses during period of risk. Some experts recommend 500 mg/m² per day, in 2–3 divided doses
		IV	All ages	15 mg/kg, in 3 divided doses during period of risk

Table 4.10. Non-HIV Antiviral Drugs,[a] continued

Generic (Trade Name)	Indication	Route	Age	Usually Recommended Dosage
	Genital HSV infection: first episode	Oral	≥12 y	1200 mg/day, in 3 divided doses for 7–10 days. Oral pediatric dose: 40–80 mg/kg per day, divided in 3–4 doses (max 1000 mg/day)
		IV	≥12 y	15 mg/kg per day, in 3 divided doses for 5–7 days
	Genital HSV infection: recurrence	Oral	≥12 y	1600 mg in 2 divided doses for 5 days, or 2400 mg in 3 divided doses for 2 days
	Chronic suppressive therapy for recurrent genital and cutaneous (ocular) HSV episodes	Oral	≥12 y	800 mg/day, in 2 divided doses for as long as 12 continuous mo; decisions to continue suppressive therapy should be revisited annually
	Recurrent herpes labialis	Oral	All ages	80 mg/kg per day, in 4 divided doses, for 5 to 7 days (max 3200 mg/day)
Adefovir[b,i] (Hepsera)	Chronic hepatitis B	Oral	≥12 y	10 mg, once daily, in patients with CrCL ≥50 mL/min (adult data suggest the following dosage adjustment: every 48 hours for CrCL = 30–49 mL/min; every 72 for CrCL = 10–29 mL/min)
				Test for HIV before treatment initiation
				Severe acute exacerbations of hepatitis have been reported in patients who have discontinued anti-hepatitis B therapy
				Nonpreferred regimen; Refer to AASLD 2018 hepatitis B guidance for preferred and nonpreferred treatment regimens and duration recommendations

Table 4.10. Non-HIV Antiviral Drugs,ª continued

Generic (Trade Name)	Indication	Route	Age	Usually Recommended Dosage
		Oral	2–12 y	≥7 y–12 y: 0.25 mg/kg, 2 y–<7 y: 0.3 mg/kg once daily (both to a max of 10 mg) gives similar systemic exposure as in adults Test for HIV before treatment initiation Severe acute exacerbations of hepatitis have been reported in patients who have discontinued anti-hepatitis B therapy Nonpreferred regimen; Refer to AASLD 2018 hepatitis B guidance for preferred and nonpreferred treatment regimens and duration recommendations
Baloxavir (Xofluza)	Influenza A and B treatment or prophylaxis	Oral	≥5 y	≥80 kg: 80 mg as single dose 20–79 kg: 40 mg as single dose <20 kg: 2 mg/kg as a single dose Longer treatment duration may be needed for severely ill patients Avoid concomitant antacids, dairy products, calcium-fortified beverages, polyvalent cation-containing laxatives, or oral supplements including iron, magnesium, selenium, or zinc
Brincidofovir (Tembexa)	Smallpox Mpox (through an emergency use investigational new drug request to FDA) (see Mpox, p 606)	Oral	Adult and children, including neonates	≥48 kg: 200 mg (two 100-mg tablets or 20-mL oral suspension for patients who cannot swallow tablets), once weekly for 2 doses 10–<48 kg: 4 mg/kg oral suspension, once weekly, for 2 doses <10 kg: 6 mg/kg oral suspension, once weekly, for 2 doses

Table 4.10. Non-HIV Antiviral Drugs,[a] continued

Generic (Trade Name)	Indication	Route	Age	Usually Recommended Dosage
Cidofovir (Vistide)	Cytomegalovirus (CMV) retinitis	IV	Adult dose[J] and adolescents	Induction: 5 mg/kg, once weekly, × 2 doses with probenecid 25–40 mg/kg (max 2 g) and appropriate hydration mandatory with each dose; seek alternative therapy if CrCL <55 mL/min or if ≥2+ proteinuria Maintenance: 3–5 mg/kg, once every 2 wk, with probenecid and hydration with each dose; duration dependent on CD4+ T-lymphocyte response to antiretroviral (ARV) therapy and regular ophthalmologic monitoring
Elbasvir and Grazoprevir (Zepatier)	Chronic hepatitis C (genotype 1 and 4)	Oral	≥12 y or weighing ≥30 kg	50 mg elbasvir and 100 mg grazoprevir, once daily, for 12–16 wk, with or without ribavirin Need for ribavirin is based on HCV genotype, baseline NS5A polymorphisms, and prior treatment status Test for HBV coinfection before treatment initiation Contraindicated in patients with moderate or severe hepatic impairment (Child-Pugh B or C) or those with any history of prior hepatic decompensation Hepatitis C therapy recommendations change rapidly; refer to most current AASLD/IDSA recommendations for appropriate treatment regimen

Table 4.10. Non-HIV Antiviral Drugs,ᵃ continued

Generic (Trade Name)	Indication	Route	Age	Usually Recommended Dosage
Entecavirᵇ (Baraclude)	Chronic hepatitis B	Oral	≥16 y	0.5 mg, once daily, in nucleoside-therapy-naïve patients; 1 mg once daily in patients who were previously treated with a nucleoside (not first choice in this setting); adult recommendations for renal dosage adjustment: For CrCL = 30–49 mL/min administer 50% of the usual dose or usual dose every 48 hours; For CrCL = 10–29 mL/min administer 30% of the usual dose or usual dose every 72 hours Test for HIV before treatment initiation Severe acute exacerbations of hepatitis B have been reported in patients who discontinue anti-hepatitis B therapy Refer to AASLD 2018 hepatitis B guidance for information on monitoring, toxicity, and duration of therapy
		Oral	2 to <16 y, naïve to treatment (normal renal function)	10–11 kg: 0.15-mg oral solution, once daily >11–14 kg: 0.2-mg oral solution, once daily >14–17 kg: 0.25-mg oral solution, once daily >17–20 kg: 0.3-mg oral solution, once daily >20–23 kg: 0.35-mg oral solution, once daily >23–26 kg: 0.4-mg oral solution, once daily >26–30 kg: 0.45-mg oral solution, once daily >30 kg: 0.5-mg oral solution or tablet, once daily

Table 4.10. Non-HIV Antiviral Drugs,ᵃ continued

Generic (Trade Name)	Indication	Route	Age	Usually Recommended Dosage
			Lamivudine-treated/-refractory OR with known lamivudine or telbivudine resistance mutations	Double the dosage in each above weight bracket, up to 1 mg daily for ≥16 y Test for HIV before treatment initiation Severe acute exacerbations of hepatitis B have been reported in patients who discontinue anti-hepatitis B therapy Refer to AASLD 2018 hepatitis B guidance for monitoring information, toxicity, and duration of therapy
Famciclovir,ᵇ	Genital HSV infection, recurrent episodes	Oral	Adult dose,ʲ adolescents	Immunocompetent: 2000 mg/day, in 2 divided doses for 1 day; CDC regimens featuring smaller incremental doses and greater number of treatment days are available. People with HIV: 1000 mg, in 2 divided doses for 7 days (CDC and NIH guidelines provide range of 5–14 days)
	Daily suppressive therapy	Oral	Adult dose,ʲ adolescents and children	Immunocompetent: 500 mg/day, in 2 divided doses for 1 y, then reassess for recurrence of HSV infection; HIV: 1000 mg/day, in 2 divided doses for minimum of 1 y; same dosage for children and adolescents old enough to receive adult doses
	Recurrent herpes labialis	Oral	Adult dose,ʲ adolescents	Immunocompetent: 1500 mg as a single dose People with HIV: 1000 mg/day, in 2 divided doses for 7 days (CDC and NIH guidelines provide range of 5–10 days); comparatively slower resolution seen in adolescent patients

Table 4.10. Non-HIV Antiviral Drugs,[a] continued

Generic (Trade Name)	Indication	Route	Age	Usually Recommended Dosage
	Herpes zoster	Oral	Adult dose,[h,j] adolescents	1500 mg/day, in 3 divided doses for 7 days (7–10 days in HIV patients with localized lesions, longer if lesions resolving slowly, or to complete 10–14 days total course with initial IV acyclovir if more severe skin or visceral infection)
Foscarnet[b] (Foscavir)	CMV retinitis in HIV infected patients (drug of choice in ganciclovir-resistant disease)	IV	Adult dose[j] and infants, children, and adolescents	180 mg/kg per day, in 2–3 divided doses for 14–21 days, then 90–120 mg/kg once a day for maintenance therapy and for secondary prophylaxis; may be added to ganciclovir as induction therapy, or as follow-up to failed ganciclovir monotherapy; if sight-threatening disease; IV infused no faster than 1 mg/kg/min
	HSV infection resistant to acyclovir in immunocompromised host	IV	Adult dose[j] and adolescents	80–120 mg/kg per day, in 2–3 divided doses for 3 wk or until infection resolves
	VZV infection resistant to acyclovir	IV	Adult dose[j] and adolescents	Patients with HIV: 120–180 mg/kg per day, in 2 divided doses
			Infants and children	120–180 mg/kg per day in 3 divided doses for 7–10 days or until no new lesions have appeared for 48 h

Table 4.10. Non-HIV Antiviral Drugs,[a] continued

Generic (Trade Name)	Route	Age	Usually Recommended Dosage
Ganciclovir[b] (Cytovene)	IV	Birth through 2 mo	12 mg/kg per day, divided every 12 h; duration of treatment is 6 mo, but most or all of the treatment should be accomplished with oral valganciclovir, as detailed below (there is no benefit to using ganciclovir instead of valganciclovir) for improved long-term developmental and hearing outcomes; dosage adjustment if neutropenia develops
	IV	Acquired CMV retinitis in immunocompromised host[k]	Adult dose[j]	Treatment: 10 mg/kg per day, in 2 divided doses for 14–21 days; long-term suppression 5 mg/kg per day for 7 days/wk or 6 mg/kg per day for 5 days/wk; HIV: duration of maintenance treatment is for at least 3–6 mo, with no active lesions, and with CD4+ T-lymphocyte count >100 cells/mm^3 for 3 to 6 mo in response to ART
	IV	Disseminated CMV and retinitis	Infants, children, and adolescents	10 mg/kg per day, in 2 divided doses for 14–21 days; increase to 15 mg/kg/day in 2 divided doses if needed, then 5 mg/kg body weight once daily for 5–7 days per wk for chronic suppression; discontinuation after 6 mo may be considered in children 1–5 y if CD4+ T-lymphocyte count >500/m^3 (or CD4+ T-lymphocyte percentage ≥15%); stated doses presume CrCL >50 mL/min/1.73 m^2; may add foscarnet (180 mg/kg per day divided into 2 or 3 doses) if vision at risk, or ganciclovir intravitreal injection or implant in children 9–12 y and adolescents

Table 4.10. Non-HIV Antiviral Drugs,ª continued

Generic (Trade Name)	Indication	Route	Age	Usually Recommended Dosage
	Prophylaxis of CMV in high-risk host (eg, post-transplant)	IV	All ages	10 mg/kg per day, in 2 divided doses for 5–7 days, then 5 mg/kg once daily for 100–120 days, or 6 mg/kg per day for 5 days/wk for 100 days
	Preemptive therapy of CMV in high-risk host (eg, <100 days post HCT)	IV	All ages	10 mg/kg per day, in 2 divided doses for 7–14 days, then 5 mg/kg once daily until CMV is not detectable (antigenemia, DNA PCR, or mRNA detection methods)
	>100 days post-HCT, OR receiving steroids for GVHD, OR if positive antigenemia or viremia/PCR x 2			10 mg/kg per day in 2 divided doses for 1–2 wk or until CMV undetectable
Glecaprevir/ Pibrentasvir (Mavyret)	Chronic hepatitis C (genotypes 1–6)	Oral	≥12 y, or weighing ≥45 kg	3 tablets (glecaprevir 100 mg/pibrentasvir 40 mg per tablet) (total daily dose: glecaprevir 300 mg/pibrentasvir 120 mg) once daily with food Duration: 8, 12, or 16 wk dependent on Rx-naïve vs Rx-experienced, genotype, prior vs concurrent therapy with NS3/4A protease inhibitor vs NS5A inhibitor, or other anti-hepatitis C drugs, and no cirrhosis vs compensated cirrhosis; refer to package insert for table of recommended lengths of treatment; numerous drug interactions complicates management

Table 4.10. Non-HIV Antiviral Drugs,[a] continued

Generic (Trade Name)	Indication	Route	Age	Usually Recommended Dosage
				Test for HBV coinfection before treatment initiation Contraindicated in patients with moderate or severe hepatic impairment (Child-Pugh B or C) or those with any history of prior hepatic decompensation Hepatitis C therapy recommendations change rapidly, refer to most current AASLD/IDSA recommendations for appropriate treatment regimen
		Oral	3–11 y	The oral pellet formulation is recommended for children weighing less than 45 kg. Each packet contains glecaprevir 50 mg and pibrentasvir 20 mg. <20 kg: 3 packets (total daily dose: glecaprevir 150 mg and pibrentasvir 60 mg) once daily 20–<30 kg: 4 packets (total daily dose: glecaprevir 200 mg and pibrentasvir 80 mg) once daily 30–<45kg: 5 packets (total daily dose: glecaprevir 250 mg and pibrentasvir 100 mg) once daily Test for HBV coinfection before treatment initiation Contraindicated in patients with moderate or severe hepatic impairment (Child-Pugh B or C) or those with any history of prior hepatic decompensation Hepatitis C therapy recommendations change rapidly, refer to most current AASLD/IDSA recommendations for appropriate treatment regimen

Table 4.10. Non-HIV Antiviral Drugs,[a] continued

Generic (Trade Name)	Indication	Route	Age	Usually Recommended Dosage
Lamivudine[b,i] (Epivir-HBV)	Chronic hepatitis B	Oral	Infants and children (HIV/HBV coinfected)	Children coinfected with HIV and hepatitis B should use the approved dose for HIV Dosing is weight based Refer to the package insert for details Tablets (150-mg scored tablets) are the preferred formulation 14 to <20 kg: 75 mg BID ≥20 to <25 kg: 75 mg AM dose + 150 mg PM dose ≥25 kg: 150 mg BID Oral solution dosing: 5 mg/kg/dose (max 150 mg/dose) twice daily; standard dosing for patients with CrCL >50 mL/min/1.73 m²; monitor for lamivudine-resistance Nonpreferred regimen. Refer to AASLD 2018 hepatitis B guidance for preferred and nonpreferred treatment regimens and duration of therapy
		Oral	Adolescents (HIV/HBV coinfected)	Children coinfected with HIV and hepatitis B should use the approved dose for HIV 300 mg, once daily, or 150 mg, twice daily; standard dosing for patients with CrCL >50 mL/min Nonpreferred regimen; Refer to AASLD 2018 hepatitis B guidance for preferred and nonpreferred treatment regimens and duration of therapy

Table 4.10. Non-HIV Antiviral Drugs,[a] continued

Generic (Trade Name)	Indication	Route	Age[c]	Usually Recommended Dosage
		Oral	Infants and children (HIV negative)	3 mg/kg/dose, once daily (max of 100 mg per day); use oral solution for doses <100 mg Nonpreferred regimen; Refer to AASLD 2018 hepatitis B guidance for preferred and nonpreferred treatment regimens and duration of therapy
		Oral	Adolescents (HIV negative)	100 mg, once daily Nonpreferred regimen. Refer to AASLD 2018 Hepatitis B Guidance for preferred and nonpreferred treatment regimens and duration of therapy
Ledipasvir (Harvoni as combination with sofosbuvir)	Chronic hepatitis C (genotypes 1, 4, 5, 6)	Oral	Children ≥3 y and adults	Harvoni dosing: <17 kg: 33.75 mg ledipasvir/150 mg sofosbuvir 17 kg to less than 35 kg: 45 mg ledipasvir/200 mg sofosbuvir ≥35 kg: 90 mg ledipasvir/400 mg sofosbuvir (adult dose: 90 mg ledipasvir/400 mg sofosbuvir) Ribavirin also may be added, based on genotype, cirrhosis, and liver transplant status; when used, ribavirin dosing is as follows (only available in 200-mg capsule in the US): Children: <47 kg: 15 mg/kg/day, in 2 divided doses 47–59 kg: 400 mg BID 60–73 kg: 400 mg in AM and 600 mg PM >73 kg: 600 mg BID

Table 4.10. Non-HIV Antiviral Drugs,[a] continued

Generic (Trade Name)	Indication	Route	Age	Usually Recommended Dosage
				Adults: <75 kg: 400 mg in AM and 600 mg in PM ≥75 kg: 600 mg in AM and PM Dosage modification of ribavirin based on treatment-emergent anemia (after interferon adjustment) and severe renal impairment; discontinue if severe blood dyscrasias or creatinine >2 g/dL Duration 12–24 wk dependent on genotype and prior treatment experience Test for HBV coinfection before treatment initiation Hepatitis C therapy recommendations change rapidly, refer to most current AASLD/IDSA recommendations for appropriate treatment regimen
Letermovir (Prevymis)	CMV prophylaxis in seropositive patients after HCT	IV, Oral	Adults	480 mg daily, IV or oral (240 mg per day in patients taking cyclosporine), starting 0–28 between days post-transplantation and continued through day 100 post-transplantation
Maribavir (Livtencity)	Treatment of refractory post-transplant CMV infection/disease	Oral	≥12 y and weighing ≥35 kg	400 mg twice daily
Nirmatrelvir plus ritonavir (Paxlovid)	Mild-to-moderate COVID-19 disease	Oral	≥12 y and weighing ≥40 kg	300 mg nirmatrelvir with 100 mg ritonavir; PO, twice daily for 5 days Available under emergency use authorization Has numerous drug-drug interactions; Consult listing on FDA or Pfizer websites prior to prescribing

Table 4.10. Non-HIV Antiviral Drugs,ᵃ continued

Generic (Trade Name)	Indication	Route	Age	Usually Recommended Dosage
Oseltamivirᵇ,ˡ (Tamiflu)	Influenza A and B: treatment (see Influenza, p 511)	Oral (suspension)	Birth to <9 moᵐ	3 mg/kg twice daily for 5 daysᵐ; longer treatment can be considered for patients still severely ill after 5 treatment days
		Oral (suspension)	9–11 mo	3.5 mg/kg twice daily for 5 days; longer treatment can be considered for patients still severely ill after 5 treatment days
		Oral (suspension and tablets)	1–12 y	≤15 kg: 30 mg, twice daily; 15.1–23 kg: 45 mg, twice daily; 23.1–40 kg: 60 mg, twice daily; >40 kg: 75 mg, twice daily. Treatment duration is for 5 days; longer treatment can be considered for patients still severely ill after 5 treatment days; half-dose given after dialysis session
		Oral (tablets)	≥13 y	75 mg, twice daily for 5 days; longer treatment can be considered for patients still severely ill after 5 treatment days; 30 mg given after dialysis session
	Influenza A and B: prophylaxis	Oral	3 mo–12 y	Same as the above treatment doses for patients 3 mo–12 y of age, except dose given once rather than twice daily; and given for 10 days rather than 5 (following known household exposure; 7 days for others) or for up to 6 wk (pre-exposure during community outbreak); not routinely recommended for infants <3 mo given lack of efficacy data
		Oral	≥13 y	75 mg, once daily for 10 days (following known household exposure; 7 days for others) or for up to 6 wk (pre-exposure during community outbreak); dosage adjustments for moderate to severe renal insufficiency in adults

Table 4.10. Non-HIV Antiviral Drugs,[a] continued

Generic (Trade Name)	Indication	Route	Age	Usually Recommended Dosage
Peramivir[b] (Rapivab)	Influenza A and B	IV	≥6 mo	6 mo to <13 y: 12 mg/kg, once (max dose: 600 mg) ≥13 y: 600 mg, once; full dose for CrCL of ≥50 mL/min/1.73 m²
				Renal dosing required for CrCl <50 mL/min
Remdesivir (Veklury)	SARS-CoV-2 infection requiring hospitalization, or not hospitalized but with mild-to-moderate COVID-19 and are at high risk for progression to severe COVID-19	IV	≥28 days and weighing ≥3 kg	Adults and pediatric patients weighing ≥40 kg: Single IV loading dose of 200 mg on day 1, followed by maintenance IV doses of 100 mg QD on and after day 2
				Pediatric patients ≥28 days weighing 3.0 kg through <40 kg: Single IV loading dose of 5.0 mg/kg on day 1, followed by maintenance IV doses of 2.5 mg/kg QD on and after day 2
				Treatment duration 10 days if requiring mechanical ventilation and/or ECMO, or 5 days if hospitalized but not requiring mechanical ventilation or ECMO, or 3 days if nonhospitalized with mild-to-moderate COVID-19 and at high risk for progression to severe COVID-19
Sofosbuvir (Sovaldi)	Chronic hepatitis C (genotype 1, 2, 3, 4, depending on adult (all four genotypes) or pediatric (genotypes 2 or 3)	Oral	Children ≥3 y and Adults	Sofosbuvir dosing: <17 kg: 150 mg 17 kg to less than 35 kg: 200 mg ≥35 kg: 400 mg (adult dose: 400 mg) Take once daily with or without food, as a component of combination therapy with other direct-acting antivirals (eg, daclatasvir), ribavirin, or with ribavirin plus pegylated interferon; length of treatment depending on HCV genotype and concomitant therapy used

Table 4.10. Non-HIV Antiviral Drugs,ᵃ continued

Generic (Trade Name)	Indication	Route	Age	Usually Recommended Dosage
				Ribavirin dosing (limited availability, 200-mg capsules only in US):
				Children:
				<47 kg: 15 mg/kg/day, in 2 divided doses
				47–59 kg: 400 mg BID
				60–73 kg: 400 mg in AM and 600 mg in PM
				>73 kg: 600 mg BID
				Adults:
				<75 kg: 400 mg in AM and 600 mg in PM
				≥75 kg: 600 mg in AM and PM
				Dosage modification of ribavirin based on treatment-emergent anemia (after interferon adjustment) and severe renal impairment; discontinue if severe blood dyscrasias or creatinine >2 g/dL
				Sofosbuvir available in a fixed-dose combination tablet with 90 mg ledipasvir (marketed as Harvoni) for use in children ≥3 y and adults
				Sofosvubir available in a fixed-dose combination tablet with 100 mg velpatasvir (marketed as Epclusa) for use in adults (includes ribavirin when decompensated cirrhosis present)
				Sofosbuvir has potential for reduced efficacy when combined with to P-glycoprotein inducers
				Test for HBV coinfection before treatment initiation
				Hepatitis C therapy recommendations change rapidly; refer to most current AASLD/IDSA recommendations for appropriate treatment regimen

Table 4.10. Non-HIV Antiviral Drugs,[a] continued

Generic (Trade Name)	Indication	Route	Age	Usually Recommended Dosage
Tecovirimat (TPOXX)	Smallpox Mpox (through expanded access Investigational New Drug protocol held by CDC) (see Mpox, p 606)	Oral, IV	Children ≥3 kg and adults	Intravenous: 3 kg to <35kg: 6 mg/kg IV, every 12 hours for 14 days 35 kg to <120 kg: 200 mg IV, every 12 hours for 14 days ≥120 kg: 300 mg IV, every 12 hours for 14 days Oral: 13 kg to <25 kg: 200 mg PO, 2 times daily for 14 days 25 kg to <40 kg: 400 mg PO, 2 times daily for 14 days 40 kg to <120 kg: 600 mg PO, 2 times daily for 14 days ≥120 kg: 600 mg PO, 3 times daily for 14 days Pediatric patients weighing 13 kg or more should be switched to oral dosing to complete the 14-day treatment course as soon as oral therapy can be tolerated
Tenofovir[b] disoproxil fumarate (Viread)	Chronic hepatitis B	Oral	Adolescents ≥12 y and weighing ≥35 kg, with or without HIV coinfection, adults	300 mg, once daily; adjustment of dosing interval recommended for CrCL <50 mL/min; monitor liver function and bone density
			≥2 y and at least 10 kg, with or without HIV coinfection	General dosing: 8 mg/kg/dose once daily; weight band dosing of reduced strength tablets and oral powder formulations. Test for HIV before treatment initiation Severe acute exacerbations of hepatitis B have been reported in patients who discontinue anti-hepatitis B therapy Refer to AASLD 2018 hepatitis B guidance for information on monitoring, toxicity, and duration of therapy

Table 4.10. Non-HIV Antiviral Drugs,ᵃ continued

Generic (Trade Name)	Indication	Route	Age	Usually Recommended Dosage
Tenofovir alafenamide fumarate (Vemlidy)	Chronic hepatitis B	Oral	Adult or ≥12 y	25 mg once daily with food; no need for renal dose adjustment but not recommended for CrCL<15 mL/min Test for HIV before treatment initiation Severe acute exacerbations of hepatitis B have been reported in patients who discontinue anti-hepatitis B therapy Refer to AASLD 2018 hepatitis B guidance for information on monitoring, toxicity, and duration of therapy
Valacyclovirᵇ (Valtrex)	Varicella	Oral	2 to <18 y	20 mg/kg, 3 times daily for 5 days, not to exceed 1 g per dose, longer if lesions unresolved; same dose for up to 6 wk after initial IV acyclovir treatment of acute retinal necrosis; HIV: same dose for 4–6 wk
	Genital HSV infection, first episode	Oral	Adult and adolescent dose	2 g/day, in 2 divided doses for 10 days (5–14 days in people with HIV); longer duration if lesions incompletely healed
		Oral	Children	<45 kg: 40 mg/kg/day in 2 divided doses ≥45 kg: 2 g/day, in 2 divided doses 7–10 days of treatment
	Episodic recurrent genital HSV infection	Oral	Adult	1 g/day, in 2 divided doses for 3 days, or 1 g/day, once daily, for 5 days; people with HIV should receive 2 g/day for 5–14 days
		Oral	Adolescent and children	>50 kg: 1000 mg once daily for 5 days <50 kg: 40 mg/kg/day in 2 divided doses

Table 4.10. Non-HIV Antiviral Drugs,ᵃ continued

Generic (Trade Name)	Indication	Route	Age	Usually Recommended Dosage
	Daily suppressive therapy for recurrent genital HSV infection	Oral	Adult doseʲ	Immunocompetent patients: 1000 mg, once daily for 1 y starting within 24 hours of symptom onset or assess history of recurrences (eg, 500 mg, once daily, in patients with ≤9 recurrences per y to reduce transmission) People with HIV (CD4+ T-lymphocyte count ≥100 cells/mm³): 500 mg, twice daily for at least 6 mo
			Adolescent and children	20 mg/kg/dose once daily (max daily dose: 500 mg or 1 g; the lower dose is less effective if frequent recurrences [eg, ≥10/y]) HIV: 500 mg, twice daily for indefinite duration; acyclovir for young children
	Recurrent herpes labialis	Oral	≥12 y	4 g/day, in 2 divided doses for 1 day HIV: 2 g/day in 2 divided doses for 5–10 days
	Herpes zoster	Oral	Adult and adolescent doseʲ	3 g/day, in 3 divided doses for 7 days
Valganciclovirᵇ (Valcyte)	Congenital CMV disease	Oral	Birth through 6 mo	32 mg/kg per day, in 2 divided doses, started within the first 13 wk following birth and continued for a total of 6 mo of treatment if moderate-severe symptomatic disease, or for a total of 6 wk of treatment if isolated sensorineural hearing loss; dosage adjustment if neutropenia or renal impairment develops; mildly symptomatic or asymptomatic patients should not receive antiviral therapy; see Table 3.4, p 349

Table 4.10. Non-HIV Antiviral Drugs,ᵃ continued

Generic (Trade Name)	Indication	Route	Age	Usually Recommended Dosage
	Acquired CMV retinitis in immunocompromised host	Oral	Adult and adolescent doseʲ	Induction treatment: 900 mg, twice daily for 2–3 wk Long-term suppression: 900 mg, once daily HIV: duration of maintenance treatment is for at least 3–6 mo, with lesions inactive, and with CD4+ T-lymphocyte count >100 cells/mm³ for 3 mo to 6 mo in response to ART
	Prevention of CMV disease in kidney, liver, or heart transplant patients	Oral	4 mo–16 y	Dose once a day within 10 days of transplantation according to dosage algorithm based on body surface area and creatinine clearance: Dose (mg) = 7 x body surface area x CrCL (calculated using the Schwartz equation with max value set at 150 mL/min/1.73 m²; see drug package insert; max 900 mg/day); round dose to the nearest 10-mg increment with solution; duration depends on type of transplant and risk status: 200 days after renal transplant, 100 days after heart or liver transplant Some experts recommend: 10 mg/kg/day, in 1 to 2 divided doses per day (max 900 mg/day), round dose to the nearest 10-mg increment with solution; duration depends on type of transplant and risk status: 200 days after renal transplant, 100 days after heart or liver transplant
		Oral	Adolescents ≥17 y	900 mg, once daily, for post-transplant patients; duration in children depends on type of transplant and risk status: 200 days after renal transplant, 100 days after heart or liver transplant

Table 4.10. Non-HIV Antiviral Drugs,ᵃ continued

Generic (Trade Name)	Indication	Route	Age	Usually Recommended Dosage
	Prevention of CMV disease in people with HIV (CMV-seropositive children ≥6 y with CD4+ T-lymphocyte counts <50 cells/mm³ or <6 y who are CMV-seropositive and have a CD4+ T-lymphocyte percentage <5%)	Oral	4 mo–16 y	Same calculated dose regimen as above; duration: stopping primary prophylaxis can be considered when the CD4+ T-lymphocyte count is >100 cells/mm³ for children ≥6 y; or CD4+ T-lymphocyte percentage is >10% in children <6 y
Velpatasvir (Epclusa as combination with sofosbuvir)	Chronic hepatitis C (genotypes 1–6)	Oral	Children ≥3 y and adults	<17 kg: 37.5 mg with 150 mg sofosbuvir once daily 17 kg to less than 30 kg: 50 mg with 200 mg sofosbuvir once daily ≥30 kg: 100 mg with 400 mg sofosbuvir once daily Duration 12–24 wk dependent on prior treatment experience, concurrent ribavirin use Test for HBV coinfection before treatment initiation Hepatitis C therapy recommendations change rapidly, refer to most current AASLD/IDSA recommendations for appropriate treatment regimen

Table 4.10. Non-HIV Antiviral Drugs,[a] continued

Generic (Trade Name)	Indication	Route	Age	Usually Recommended Dosage
Voxilaprevir (Vosevi as combination with sofosbuvir and velpatasvir)	Chronic hepatitis C (genotypes 1–6)	Oral	Adults	100 mg combined with 400 mg sofosbuvir and 100 mg velpatasvir once daily; taken with food; duration: 12 wk for all genotypes and treatment-experienced patient regimens Test for HBV coinfection before treatment initiation Hepatitis C therapy recommendations change rapidly, refer to most current AASLD/IDSA recommendations for appropriate treatment regimen
Zanamivir (Relenza)	Influenza A and B: treatment (see Influenza, p 511)	Inhalation	≥7 y (treatment)	10 mg (2 inhalations, one 5-mg powder blister per inhalation), twice daily for 5 days; first 2 doses can be separated by as little as 2 hours; only use Diskhaler device; longer treatment can be considered for patients still severely ill after 5 treatment days
	Influenza A and B: prophylaxis	Inhalation	≥5 y (prophylaxis)	10 mg (2 inhalations, one 5-mg powder blister per inhalation), once daily for 10 days; CDC recommends continuing chemoprophylaxis for 7 days after last known exposure

ART indicates combination antiretroviral therapy; BID, twice a day; CDC, Centers for Disease Control and Prevention; CrCL, creatinine clearance; CNS, central nervous system; CSF, cerebrospinal fluid; FDA, US Food and Drug Administration; GVHD, graft-versus-host disease; HBeAg, hepatitis B envelope antigen; HBV, hepatitis B virus; HCV, hepatitis C virus; HIV, human immunodeficiency virus; HCT, hematopoietic cell transplant; HSV, herpes simplex virus; IM, intramuscular; IV, intravenous; NIH, National Institutes of Health; PCR, polymerase chain reaction; QD, once a day; SC, subcutaneous; SEM, skin, eyes, and/or mouth; VZV, varicella-zoster virus.

[a] Drugs for human immunodeficiency virus infection are not included. See **https://hivinfo.nih.gov/home-page** for current information on HIV drugs and treatment recommendations.

[b] Dose should be decreased in patients with impaired renal function.

[c] Oral dosage of acyclovir in children should not exceed 80 mg/kg per day (3200 mg/day).

[d] Acyclovir doses listed in this table are based on clinical trials and clinical experience and may not be identical to doses approved by the FDA.

Table 4.10. Non-HIV Antiviral Drugs,[a] continued

Generic (Trade Name)	Indication	Route	Age	Usually Recommended Dosage

[e] In times of shortage of intravenous acyclovir, the American Academy of Pediatrics Committee on Infectious Diseases recommends that existing supplies of intravenous acyclovir be conserved to improve availability for neonatal HSV infections, herpes simplex encephalitis, or HSV and varicella-zoster virus infections in immunocompromised patients, including more ill pregnant women with visceral dissemination of either virus. If acyclovir is not available, intravenous ganciclovir should be substituted. Alternative regimens to the use of intravenous acyclovir and other options for priority and nonpriority conditions are outlined in an exclusive *Red Book Online* Intravenous Acyclovir Shortage Table (**https://publications.aap.org/redbook/resources/15648/Intravenous-Acyclovir-Shortage-Recommendations-for?searchresult=1**).

[f] Monitor for nephrotoxicity and neurologic irritation. Consider involving an infectious diseases or pharmacology specialist if weight-based dosing exceeds 800 mg per dose or if being administered with other nephrotoxic medications.

[g] Use estimate of ideal body weight in children and adolescents with severe obesity.

[h] Selective indications; see Varicella-Zoster Infections (p 938).

[i] "Nonpreferred" for treatment of chronic hepatitis B in the American Association for the Study of Liver Diseases 2018 hepatitis B guidance document (**https://journals.lww.com/hep/Fulltext/2018/04000/Update_on_prevention,_diagnosis,_and_treatment_of.34.aspx**).

[j] There are not sufficient clinical data to identify the appropriate dose for use in children.

[k] Some experts use ganciclovir in immunocompromised hosts with CMV gastrointestinal tract disease and CMV pneumonitis (with or without CMV immune globulin intravenous).

[l] See Influenza (p 511) and **www.cdc.gov/flu/professionals/antivirals/index.htm** for specific recommendations, which may vary on the basis of most recent influenza virus susceptibility patterns.

[m] Preterm, <38 weeks' postmenstrual age, oseltamivir, 1.0 mg/kg/dose, orally, twice daily; preterm, 38 through 40 weeks' postmenstrual age, 1.5 mg/kg/dose, orally, twice daily; preterm >40 weeks' postmenstrual age through 8 months' chronologic age, 3.0 mg/kg/dose, orally, twice daily.

For more information on individual drugs, refer to FDA package inserts (**www.accessdata.fda.gov/scripts/cder/daf/index.cfm**).

DRUGS FOR PARASITIC INFECTIONS

Table 4.11. Drugs for Parasitic Infections[1]

Disease	Drug	Adult Dosage	Pediatric Dosage	Links to CDC Website[2] and professional society guidelines
Ascariasis (*Ascaris lumbricoides*; intestinal roundworm)	Albendazole[3]	400 mg, orally, once (take with food)		www.cdc.gov/parasites/ascariasis/health_professionals/index.html
	OR			
	Mebendazole[4]	100 mg, orally, twice daily for 3 days OR 500 mg, orally, once		
	OR			
	Ivermectin[5]	150–200 µg/kg, orally, once (take on an empty stomach with water)		
	OR			
	Pyrantel pamoate[6]	11 mg/kg (up to a maximum of 1 g/dose), orally, daily for 3 days (may be given as a single dose for adults)		
	OR			
	Nitazoxanide[7]	500 mg, orally, twice daily for 3 days (take with food)	Age 1–3 y: 100 mg, orally, twice daily for 3 days Age 4–11 y: 200 mg, orally, twice daily for 3 days Age ≥12 y: 500 mg, orally, twice daily for 3 days (take with food)	

Table 4.11. Drugs for Parasitic Infections,[1] continued

Disease	Drug	Adult Dosage	Pediatric Dosage	Links to CDC Website[2] and professional society guidelines
Babesiosis[8]	Atovaquone[9] PLUS	750 mg, orally, twice daily (mild to moderate disease OR severe disease) for at least 7–10 days (take with food)	20 mg/kg/dose (up to 750 mg/dose), orally, twice daily (mild to moderate disease OR severe disease) for at least 7–10 days (take with food)	**www.cdc.gov/parasites/babesiosis/ health_professionals/index.html** **www.idsociety.org/practice-guideline/ babesiosis/**
	Azithromycin[10]	500 mg, orally, on day 1, then 250 mg, orally, once daily on subsequent days (mild to moderate disease) for 7–10 days; OR 500–1000 mg, IV, once daily (severe disease) until symptoms abate, then convert to all oral therapy; duration at least 7–10 days	10 mg/kg (up to 500 mg), orally, on day 1; then 5 mg/kg/day (max 250 mg/dose), orally, on subsequent days (mild to moderate disease) for 7–10 days OR 10 mg/kg (up to 500 mg), IV, daily (severe disease) until symptoms abate, then convert to all oral therapy; duration at least 7–10 days	
OR				

Table 4.11. Drugs for Parasitic Infections,[1] continued

Disease	Drug	Adult Dosage	Pediatric Dosage	Links to CDC Website[2] and professional society guidelines
	Clindamycin	600 mg, orally, 3 times daily (mild to moderate disease), **or** 600 mg, IV, 4 times daily (severe disease), for at least 7–10 days	7–10 mg/kg/dose (up to 600 mg), orally 3 times daily (mild to moderate disease) OR 7–10 mg/kg/dose (up to 600 mg), IV, 3 to 4 times daily (severe disease), for at least 7–10 days	
	PLUS			
	Quinine sulfate[11]	650 mg orally, 3 times daily, for at least 7–10 days	8 mg/kg/dose (max 650 mg), orally, 3 times daily, for at least 7–10 days	
Balantidiasis (*Balantidium coli*)	Tetracycline[12]	500 mg, orally, 4 times daily for 10 days	Age ≥8 y: 40 mg/kg/day (max 2 g per day or 500 mg/dose), orally, in 4 doses for 10 days	
	OR			
	Metronidazole	500–750 mg, orally, 3 times daily for 5 days	35–50 mg/kg/day, orally, in 3 doses for 5 days (max 750 mg/dose)	www.cdc.gov/parasites/balantidium/health_professionals/index.html
	OR			
	Nitazoxanide[7]	500 mg, orally, twice daily for 3 days	Age 1–3 y: 100 mg, orally, twice daily for 3 days Age 4–11 y: 200 mg, orally, twice daily for 3 days Age ≥12 y: 500 mg, orally, twice daily for 3 days	

Table 4.11. Drugs for Parasitic Infections,[1] continued

Disease	Drug	Adult Dosage	Pediatric Dosage	Links to CDC Website[2] and professional society guidelines
	OR			
	Iodoquinol[13]	650 mg, orally, 3 times daily for 20 days	30–40 mg/kg/day (max 650 mg per dose), orally, in 3 doses for 20 days	
Baylisascariasis (raccoon roundworm infection)	Albendazole[3]	25–50 mg/kg/day, orally, for 10–20 days[14] (take with food)		www.cdc.gov/parasites/baylisascaris/health_professionals/index.html
Blastocystis species infection[15]	Metronidazole	250 mg to 750 mg, orally, 3 times daily for 10 days OR 1500 mg, orally, once daily for 10 days	35–50 mg/kg/day, orally, in 3 doses for 10 days (max 500–750 mg/dose)	www.cdc.gov/parasites/blastocystis/health_professionals/index.html
	OR			
	Trimethoprim (TMP)-sulfamethoxazole (SMX)	160 mg TMP, 800 mg SMX, orally, twice daily for 7 days	Age ≥2 mo: 8 mg/kg TMP and 40 mg/kg SMX per day, orally, in 2 divided doses for 7 days	
	OR			

Table 4.11. Drugs for Parasitic Infections,[1] continued

Disease	Drug	Adult Dosage	Pediatric Dosage	Links to CDC Website[2] and professional society guidelines
	Nitazoxanide[7]	500 mg, orally, twice daily for 3 days	Age 1–3 y: 100 mg, orally, twice daily for 3 days Age 4–11 y: 200 mg, orally, twice daily for 3 days Age ≥12 y: 500 mg, orally, twice daily for 3 days	
	OR			
	Tinidazole	2 g, orally, once (take with food)	Age ≥3 y: 50 mg/kg (max 2 g) once (take with food)	
Capillariasis	Mebendazole[4]	200 mg, orally, twice daily for 20 days		www.cdc.gov/parasites/capillaria/health_professionals/index.html
	OR			
	Albendazole[3]	400 mg, orally, once daily for 10 days (take with food)		
Chagas disease; *Trypanosoma cruzi* infection	See Trypanosomiasis, American			
Chilomastix mesnili	No treatment is necessary; this protozoan is considered nonpathogenic but may be an indicator of ingestion of fecally contaminated food or water			www.cdc.gov/parasites/nonpathprotozoa/health_professionals/index.html
Clonorchiasis	Praziquantel[16]	75 mg/kg/day, orally, in 3 doses for 1–2 days (take with food)		www.cdc.gov/parasites/clonorchis/health_professionals/index.html
	OR			
	Albendazole[3]	10 mg/kg/day, orally, for 7 days (take with food)		

Table 4.11. Drugs for Parasitic Infections,[1] continued

Disease	Drug	Adult Dosage	Pediatric Dosage	Links to CDC Website[2] and professional society guidelines
Cryptosporidiosis	Nitazoxanide[17]	500 mg, orally, twice a day for 3 days	Age 1–3 y: 100 mg, orally, twice a day for 3 days Age 4 to 11 y: 200 mg, orally, twice a day for 3 days Age ≥12 y: 500 mg, orally, twice a day for 3 days Immunocompromised children with HIV may need a 14 day course, in addition to anti-retroviral therapy.	www.cdc.gov/parasites/crypto/treatment.html https://clinicalinfo.hiv.gov/en/guidelines/hiv-clinical-guidelines-adult-and-adolescent-opportunistic-infections/cryptosporidiosis?view=full
	If patient is immunocompromised or has diarrhea refractory to nitazoxanide, alternatives include using one or both of the drugs below, or adding one or both to prolonged (eg, 14 day) nitazoxanide treatment:			
	Paromomycin	500 mg, orally, 4 times/day, for 14–28 days	25–35 mg/kg/day, orally, in 2–4 divided doses per day, for 14 days	
	Azithromycin	500 mg orally, once daily, for 14 days	10 mg/kg orally on day 1, 5 mg/kg orally on days 2–10	
Cutaneous larva migrans (zoonotic hookworm)	Ivermectin[5]	200 µg/kg, orally, once daily for 1 day	Weight ≥15 kg: 200 µg/kg, orally, once daily for 1 day	www.cdc.gov/parasites/zoonotichookworm/health_professionals/index.html
	OR			
	Albendazole[3]	400 mg/day, orally, once daily for 3–7 days (take with food)	Age >2 y: 400 mg/day, orally, for 3 days (take with food)	

Table 4.11. Drugs for Parasitic Infections,[1] continued

Disease	Drug	Adult Dosage	Pediatric Dosage	Links to CDC Website[2] and professional society guidelines
Cyclosporiasis	Trimethoprim (TMP)-sulfamethoxazole (SMX)	160 mg TMP/800 mg SMX, orally, 2 times/day for 7–10 days[18]	Age >2 mo: 8–10 mg/kg TMP and 40–50 mg/kg SMX per day, orally, in 2 divided doses for 7–10 days[18]	www.cdc.gov/parasites/cyclosporiasis/health_professionals/index.html
Cysticercosis	See Neurocysticercosis			
Cystoisosporiasis (*Cystoisospora* infection; formerly isosporiasis)[19]	Trimethoprim (TMP)-sulfamethoxazole (SMX)	160 mg TMP/800 mg SMX, IV or orally, 2 times/day for 7–10 days	Age >2 mo: 8–10 mg/kg TMP and 40–50 mg/kg SMX per day, IV or orally, in 2 divided doses for 7–10 days	www.cdc.gov/parasites/cystoisospora/health_professionals/index.html

https://clinicalinfo.hiv.gov/en/guidelines/hiv-clinical-guidelines-pediatric-opportunistic-infections/isosporiasis |
| | OR | | | |
| | Pyrimethamine

PLUS

leucovorin (folinic acid) | 50–75 mg per day of pyrimethamine, either once daily or divided into 2 separate doses

10–25 mg per day of leucovorin (folinic acid) | -- | |
| | OR | | | |
| | Ciprofloxacin | 500 mg, orally, 2 times/day for 7 days | -- | |

Table 4.11. Drugs for Parasitic Infections,[1] continued

Disease	Drug	Adult Dosage	Pediatric Dosage	Links to CDC Website[2] and professional society guidelines
Dibothriocephalus infection (tapeworm)	Praziquantel[16]	5–10 mg/kg, orally, in a single dose (take with liquids during a meal)		www.cdc.gov/parasites/diphyllobothrium/health_professionals/index.html
	OR			
	Niclosamide (not available in the US)[20]	2 g, orally, once	50 mg/kg (max 2 g), orally, once	
Dientamoeba fragilis infection[21,22]	Metronidazole	500–750 mg, orally, 3 times/day for 10 days	35–50 mg/kg/day, orally, in 3 divided doses (max 500–750 mg/dose) for 10 days	www.cdc.gov/parasites/dientamoeba/health_professionals/index.html
	OR			
	Paromomycin	25–35 mg/kg/day, orally, in 3 divided doses, for 7 days		
	OR			
	Iodoquinol[13]	650 mg, orally, 3 times/day for 20 days	30–40 mg/kg/day (max 650 mg/dose), orally, divided 3 times/day for 20 days	
Dipylidium caninum infection (dog or cat flea tapeworm)	Praziquantel[16]	5–10 mg/kg, orally, in a single dose (take with liquids during a meal)		www.cdc.gov/parasites/dipylidium/health_professionals/index.html
	OR			
	Niclosamide (not available in the US)[20]	2 g, orally, once	50 mg/kg (max 2 g), orally, once	

Table 4.11. Drugs for Parasitic Infections,[1] continued

Disease	Drug	Adult Dosage	Pediatric Dosage	Links to CDC Website[2] and professional society guidelines
Echinococcosis[23]	Albendazole[3] (May not be appropriate for all forms of disease)	400 mg, orally, twice daily for 1–6 mo for cystic and 2 years for alveolar (take with food)	10–15 mg/kg/day (max 800 mg/day), orally, in 2 doses for 1–6 mo for cystic and 2 years for alveolar (take with food)	www.cdc.gov/parasites/ echinococcosis/health_professionals/ index.html
Endolimax nana	No treatment is necessary; this protozoan is harmless			www.cdc.gov/parasites/ nonpathprotozoa/
Entamoeba coli	No treatment is necessary; this protozoan is harmless			www.cdc.gov/parasites/ nonpathprotozoa/
Entamoeba dispar	No treatment is necessary; this protozoan is harmless			www.cdc.gov/parasites/ nonpathprotozoa/
Entamoeba hartmanni	No treatment is necessary; this protozoan is harmless			www.cdc.gov/parasites/ nonpathprotozoa/
Entamoeba histolytica (amebiasis) Asymptomatic intestinal colonization	Iodoquinol[13]	650 mg, orally, 3 times/day for 20 days	30–40 mg/kg/day (max 650 mg/dose), orally, divided 3 times/day for 20 days	www.cdc.gov/parasites/amebiasis/ index.html
	OR			
	Paromomycin	25–35 mg/kg/day, orally, divided 3 times/day for 7 days		
	OR			
	Diloxanide furoate[24]	500 mg, orally, 3 times/day for 10 days	20 mg/kg/day (max 500 mg/dose), orally, divided 3 times a day for 10 days	

Table 4.11. Drugs for Parasitic Infections,[1] continued

Disease	Drug	Adult Dosage	Pediatric Dosage	Links to CDC Website[2] and professional society guidelines
Entamoeba histolytica (amebiasis) Mild to moderate intestinal disease	Metronidazole	500 to 750 mg, orally, 3 times/day for 7–10 days	35–50 mg/kg/day, orally, divided 3 times/day for 7–10 days	**www.cdc.gov/parasites/amebiasis/index.html**
	OR			
	Tinidazole	2 g, orally, once daily for 3 days	Age >3 y: 50 mg/kg (max 2 g), orally, once daily for 3 days	
	OR			
	Nitazoxanide[7]	500 mg orally, twice daily for 3 days	Age 1–3 y: 100 mg, orally, 2 times/day for 3 days Age 4–11 y: 200 mg, orally, 2 times/day for 3 days Age ≥12 y: 500 mg, orally, 2 times/day for 3 days (take with food)	
	FOLLOWED BY EITHER:			
	Paromomycin	25–35 mg/kg/day, orally, divided 3 times/day for 7 days		
	OR BY			
	Iodoquinol[13]	650 mg, orally, 3 times/day for 20 days	30–40 mg/kg/day (max 650 mg/dose), orally, divided 3 times/day for 20 days	

Table 4.11. Drugs for Parasitic Infections,[1] continued

Disease	Drug	Adult Dosage	Pediatric Dosage	Links to CDC Website[2] and professional society guidelines
Entamoeba histolytica (amebiasis) Severe intestinal and extraintestinal disease	Metronidazole	500 to 750 mg, IV (switch to orally when tolerated), 3 times/day for 7–10 days	35–50 mg/kg/day, IV (switch to orally when tolerated), divided 3 times/day for 7–10 days (max 500–750 mg/dose)	www.cdc.gov/parasites/amebiasis/index.html
	OR			
	Tinidazole	2 g, orally, once daily for 5 days	Age >3 y: 50 mg/kg (max 2 g), orally, once daily for 5 days	
	OR			
	Nitazoxanide[7]	500 mg orally, twice daily for 3 days	Age 1–3 y: 100 mg, orally, 2 times/day for 3 days Age 4–11 y: 200 mg, orally, 2 times/day for 3 days Age ≥12 y: 500 mg, orally, 2 times/day for 3 days (take with food)	
	FOLLOWED BY EITHER:			
	Paromomycin	25–35 mg/kg/day, orally, divided 3 times/day for 7 days		
	OR BY			
	Iodoquinol[13]	650 mg, orally, 3 times/day for 20 days	30–40 mg/kg/day (max 650 mg/dose), orally, divided 3 times/day for 20 days	

Table 4.11. Drugs for Parasitic Infections,[1] continued

Disease	Drug	Adult Dosage	Pediatric Dosage	Links to CDC Website[2] and professional society guidelines
Entamoeba polecki	No treatment is necessary; this protozoan is harmless			www.cdc.gov/parasites/ nonpathprotozoa/health_ professionals/index.html
Enterobiasis (pinworm)	Mebendazole[4]	100 mg, orally, once; repeat in 2 wk		www.cdc.gov/parasites/pinworm/ health_professionals/index.html
	OR			
	Pyrantel pamoate[6]	11 mg/kg base, orally, once (max 1 g); repeat in 2 wk		
	OR			
	Albendazole[3]	400 mg orally once; repeat in 2 wk (take on an empty stomach)		
Fascioliasis (*Fasciola hepatica*; sheep liver fluke)	Triclabendazole[25]	10 mg/kg/dose, orally, every 12 hours for two doses in patients ≥6 y (take with food)		www.cdc.gov/parasites/fasciola/ health_professionals/index.html
	OR			
	Nitazoxanide[7]	500 mg, orally, 2 times/ day for 7 days (take with food)	Age 1–3 y: 100 mg, orally, 2 times/day for 7 days Age 4–11 y: 200 mg, orally, 2 times/day for 7 days Age ≥12 y: 500 mg, orally, 2 times/day for 7 days (take with food)	
Fasciolopsiasis (*Fasciolopsis buski*; intestinal fluke)	Praziquantel[16]	75 mg/kg/day; orally, in 3 divided doses for 1 day		www.cdc.gov/parasites/fasciolopsis/ health_professionals/index.html

Table 4.11. Drugs for Parasitic Infections,[1] continued

Disease	Drug	Adult Dosage	Pediatric Dosage	Links to CDC Website[2] and professional society guidelines
Giardiasis[26]	Tinidazole	2 g, orally, once	Age ≥3 y: 50 mg/kg (max 2 g), orally, once	www.cdc.gov/parasites/giardia/audience-health-professionals.html
	OR			
	Metronidazole	250 mg, orally, 3 times/day for 5–7 days	15 mg/kg/day (max 250 mg/dose), orally, divided 3 times/day for 5–7 days	
	OR			
	Nitazoxanide	500 mg, orally, 2 times/day for 3 days	Age 1–3 y: 100 mg, orally, 2 times/day for 3 days Age 4–11 y: 200 mg, orally, 2 times/day for 3 days Age ≥12 y: 500 mg, orally, 2 times/day for 3 days	
Gnathostomiasis (cutaneous)	Albendazole[3]	400 mg, orally, 1–2 times/day for 21 days (take with food)		www.cdc.gov/parasites/gnathostoma/health_professionals/index.html
	OR			
	Ivermectin[5]	100–200 µg/kg, orally, once daily for 1–2 days		
Heterophyiasis	Praziquantel[16]	75 mg/kg/day, orally, divided 3 times/day for 1 day		www.cdc.gov/dpdx/heterophyiasis/index.html

Table 4.11. Drugs for Parasitic Infections,[1] continued

Disease	Drug	Adult Dosage	Pediatric Dosage	Links to CDC Website[2] and professional society guidelines
Hookworm (Human; *Ancylostoma duodenale* and *ceylanicum*, *Necator americanus*)	Albendazole[3]	400 mg, orally once (take with food)	≥1 y: 400 mg, orally, once (take with food)	www.cdc.gov/parasites/hookworm/health_professionals/index.html
	OR			
	Mebendazole[4]	100 mg, orally, twice daily for 3 days; OR 500 mg, orally, once	100 mg, orally, twice daily for 3 days; OR 500 mg, orally, once	
	OR			
	Pyrantel pamoate[6]	11 mg/kg (max 1 g), orally, daily for 3 days		
Hymenolepiasis (*Hymenolepis nana*; dwarf tapeworm)	Praziquantel[16]	25 mg/kg in a single-dose therapy; orally; some experts recommend a second dose 10 days later		www.cdc.gov/parasites/hymenolepis/health_professionals/index.html
	OR			
	Niclosamide (not available in the US)[20]	2 g in a single dose for 7 days, orally	Weight 11–34 kg: 1 g in a single dose on day 1; then 500 mg per day, orally, for 6 days Weight >34 kg: 1.5 g in a single dose on day 1; then 1 g per day, orally, for 6 days	
	OR			

Table 4.11. Drugs for Parasitic Infections,[1] continued

Disease	Drug	Adult Dosage	Pediatric Dosage	Links to CDC Website[2] and professional society guidelines
	Nitazoxanide[7]	500 mg, orally, 2 times/day for 3 days	Age 1–3 y: 100 mg, orally, 2 times/day for 3 days Age 4–11 y: 200 mg, orally, 2 times/day for 3 days Age ≥12 y: 500 mg, orally, 2 times/day for 3 days	
Iodamoeba buetschlii	No treatment is necessary; this protozoan is harmless			www.cdc.gov/parasites/nonpathprotozoa/health_professionals/index.html
Leishmaniasis[27]				
Visceral (kala-azar)	Liposomal amphotericin B	3 mg/kg/day, IV, on days 1–5, 14, and 21 (total dose 21 mg/kg) If immunocompromised, 4 mg/kg/day, IV, on days 1–5, 10, 17, 24, 31, and 38 (total dose 40 mg/kg)		www.cdc.gov/parasites/leishmaniasis/health_professionals/index.html www.idsociety.org/practice-guideline/leishmaniasis/ www.cdc.gov/laboratory/drugservice/index.html https://clinicalinfo.hiv.gov/en/guidelines/hiv-clinical-guidelines-adult-and-adolescent-opportunistic-infections/leishmaniasis?view=full
	OR			
	Pentavalent antimonial drugs	See IDSA guidelines (web link in column on right)		
	OR			
	Miltefosine[27]	30 through 44 kg: 50 mg, orally, twice daily, for 28 consecutive days ≥45 kg: 50 mg, orally, 3 times daily, for 28 consecutive days (contraindicated in pregnant or breastfeeding people)		

Table 4.11. Drugs for Parasitic Infections,[1] continued

Disease	Drug	Adult Dosage	Pediatric Dosage	Links to CDC Website[2] and professional society guidelines
	Pentavalent antimonial drugs	See IDSA guidelines (web link in column on right)		www.cdc.gov/parasites/leishmaniasis/health_professionals/index.html www.idsociety.org/practice-guideline/leishmaniasis/ www.cdc.gov/laboratory/drugservice/index.html https://clinicalinfo.hiv.gov/en/guidelines/hiv-clinical-guidelines-adult-and-adolescent-opportunistic-infections/leishmaniasis?view=full
	OR			
	Miltefosine[27]	30 through 44 kg: 50 mg, orally, twice daily, for 28 consecutive days ≥45 kg: 50 mg, orally, 3 times daily, for 28 consecutive days (contraindicated in pregnant or breastfeeding people)		
	OR			
Complicated Cutaneous	Pentamidine Isethionate[28]	2–4 mg/kg/day base pentamidine IV or IM every other day for 4–7 doses (limitations include toxicity and variable effectiveness)		
	OR			
	Liposomal amphotericin B	3 mg/kg/day, IV, on days 1–5, and 10 or on days 1–7 (total dose 18–21 mg/kg)		
	OR			
	Azoles	Fluconazole, 200 mg, daily for 6 weeks (adult dose); or ketoconazole or itraconazole		
	OR			
	Intralesional or topical alternatives	See IDSA guidelines (web link in column on right)		

Table 4.11. Drugs for Parasitic Infections,[1] continued

Disease	Drug	Adult Dosage	Pediatric Dosage	Links to CDC Website[2] and professional society guidelines
Mucosal	Pentavalent antimonial drugs	See IDSA guidelines (web link in column on right)		www.cdc.gov/parasites/leishmaniasis/health_professionals/index.html
	OR			www.idsociety.org/practice-guideline/leishmaniasis/
	Liposomal amphotericin B	3 mg/kg/day IV for cumulative total of 20–60 mg/kg		www.cdc.gov/laboratory/drugservice/index.html
	OR			
	Miltefosine[27]	30–44 kg: 50 mg, PO, twice daily for 28 consecutive days ≥45 kg: 50 mg, PO, 3 times daily for 28 consecutive days (contraindicated in pregnant or breastfeeding people)		https://clinicalinfo.hiv.gov/en/guidelines/hiv-clinical-guidelines-adult-and-adolescent-opportunistic-infections/leishmaniasis?view=full
Lice infestation (Pediculus humanus, P capitis, P pubis)[29] See Fig 3.14, p 648	Pyrethrins with piperonyl butoxide[30]	Topically, twice, 9–10 days apart	Topically, twice, 9–10 days apart	www.cdc.gov/parasites/lice/pubic/health_professionals/index.html
	OR			
	0.5% Ivermectin lotion[31]	Topically, once	Topically, once	www.cdc.gov/std/treatment/default.htm
	OR			
	0.9% Spinosad suspension[32]	Topically, twice (if crawling lice present), 7 days apart	Topically, twice (if crawling lice present), 7 days apart	
	OR			

Table 4.11. Drugs for Parasitic Infections,[1] continued

Disease	Drug	Adult Dosage	Pediatric Dosage	Links to CDC Website[2] and professional society guidelines
	1% Permethrin[30] cream rinse	Topically, twice, 9–10 days apart	Topically, twice, 9–10 days apart	
	OR			
	5% Benzyl alcohol lotion[33]	Topically, twice, 7 days apart	Topically, twice, 7 days apart	www.cdc.gov/parasites/lice/pubic/health_professionals/index.html
	OR			
	0.5% Malathion[34] lotion	Topically, twice (if needed), 7–9 days apart	Topically, twice (if needed), 7–9 days apart	www.cdc.gov/std/treatment/default.htm
	OR			
	0.74% Abametapir[35] lotion	Topically, once	Topically, once	
	OR			
	Ivermectin[5,36]	200 µg/kg, orally, twice, 7–10 days apart	≥15 kg: 200 µg/kg, orally, twice, 7–10 days apart	
Loiasis (*Loa loa*)	Diethylcarbamazine (DEC)[37]	Symptomatic loiasis with microfilariae of *L loa* (MF)/mL <8000		www.cdc.gov/parasites/loiasis/health_professionals/index.html
		8–10 mg/kg/day, orally, in 3 divided doses for 21 days		www.cdc.gov/laboratory/drugservice/index.html

Table 4.11. Drugs for Parasitic Infections,[1] continued

Disease	Drug	Adult Dosage	Pediatric Dosage	Links to CDC Website[2] and professional society guidelines
	Albendazole[3]	Symptomatic loiasis, with MF/mL <8000 and failed 2 rounds of DEC OR Symptomatic loiasis, with MF/mL ≥8000 to reduce level to <8000 prior to treatment with DEC 200 mg, orally, twice daily for 21 days (take with food)		
	Apheresis followed by DEC[37,38]	Symptomatic loiasis, with MF/mL ≥8000		
Lymphatic filariasis (elephantiasis; *Wuchereria bancrofti, Brugia malayi, Brugia timori*)	Diethylcarbamazine (DEC)[37]	Treatment of lymphatic filariasis[39]: Adults and children >18 mo: 6 mg/kg/day, orally, in 3 divided doses for 12 consecutive days; OR 6 mg/kg as a single oral dose Treatment of tropical pulmonary eosinophilia (TPE): Adults and children ≥18 mo: 6 mg/kg/day, orally, in 3 divided doses for 14–21 days		**www.cdc.gov/parasites/ lymphaticfilariasis/health_ professionals/index.html** **www.cdc.gov/laboratory/drugservice/ index.html**

Table 4.11. Drugs for Parasitic Infections,[1] continued

Disease	Drug	Adult Dosage	Pediatric Dosage	Links to CDC Website[2] and professional society guidelines
Malaria (*Plasmodium* species)	Drug Susceptibility (Based on region infection acquired)			www.cdc.gov/malaria/resources/pdf/Malaria_Treatment_Table.pdf
Uncomplicated malaria *P falciparum* or species not identified If "species not identified" subsequently diagnosed as *P vivax* or *P ovale*, see below regarding radical cure with primaquine or tafenoquine	Chloroquine-resistant or unknown resistance[40,41] (All malarious regions except those specified as chloroquine-sensitive listed below.)			Updated guidance about treatment of severe malaria: www.cdc.gov/malaria/new_info/2021/artesunate_availability.html
	Preferred			
	Artemether-lumefantrine[42] 1 tablet = 20 mg artemether and 120 mg lumefantrine	A 3-day treatment schedule with a total of 6 oral doses is recommended for both adult and pediatric patients based on weight. The patient should receive the initial dose, followed by the second dose 8 hours later; then 1 dose, orally, 2 times/day, for the following 2 days. Weight 5 to <15 kg: 1 tablet per dose Weight 15 to <25 kg: 2 tablets per dose Weight 25 to <35 kg: 3 tablets per dose Weight ≥35 kg: 4 tablets per dose		CDC Malaria Hotline: (770) 488-7788 or (855) 856-4713 toll-free Monday–Friday 9 am to 5 pm EST; (770) 488-7100 after hours, weekends, and holidays
	Alternate options if above not available			

Table 4.11. Drugs for Parasitic Infections,[1] continued

Disease	Drug	Adult Dosage	Pediatric Dosage	Links to CDC Website[2] and professional society guidelines
	Atovaquone-proguanil[42] Adult tab: 250 mg atovaquone/100 mg proguanil Peds tab: 62.5 mg atovaquone/25 mg proguanil	1000 mg atovaquone/400 mg proguanil, orally, once daily for 3 days	Weight 5–<8 kg: 2 pediatric tablets, orally, once daily for 3 days Weight 8–<10 kg: 3 pediatric tablets, orally, once daily for 3 days Weight 10–<20 kg: 1 adult tab, orally, once daily for 3 days Weight 20–<30 kg: 2 adult tablets, orally, once daily for 3 days Weight 30–<40 kg: 3 adult tablets, orally, once daily for 3 days Weight ≥40 kg: 4 adult tablets, orally, once daily for 3 days	**www.cdc.gov/malaria/resources/pdf/Malaria_Treatment_Table.pdf** Updated guidance about treatment of severe malaria: **www.cdc.gov/malaria/new_info/2021/artesunate_availability.html** CDC Malaria Hotline: (770) 488-7788 or (855) 856-4713 toll-free Monday–Friday 9 am to 5 pm EST; (770) 488-7100 after hours, weekends, and holidays
	OR			

Table 4.11. Drugs for Parasitic Infections,[1] continued

Disease	Drug	Adult Dosage	Pediatric Dosage	Links to CDC Website[2] and professional society guidelines
	Quinine sulfate[43,44] plus one of the following: Doxycycline,[45] Tetracycline,[45] or, for pregnant people, Clindamycin	Quinine sulfate: 542 mg base (=650 mg salt), orally, 3 times/day for 3 or 7 days[44] Doxycycline: 100 mg, orally, 2 times/day for 7 days Tetracycline: 250 mg, orally, 4 times/day for 7 days Clindamycin: 20 mg base/kg/day, orally, divided 3 times/day for 7 days	Quinine sulfate: 8.3 mg base/kg (=10 mg salt/kg), orally, 3 times/day for 3 or 7 days Doxycycline: 2.2 mg/kg, orally, every 12 h for 7 days (max 200 mg/day) Tetracycline: 25 mg/kg/day, orally, divided 4 times/day for 7 days (max 250 mg/dose) Clindamycin: 20 mg base/kg/day, orally, divided 3 times/day for 7 days	www.cdc.gov/malaria/resources/pdf/Malaria_Treatment_Table.pdf Updated guidance about treatment of severe malaria: www.cdc.gov/malaria/new_info/2021/artesunate_availability.html CDC Malaria Hotline: (770) 488-7788 or (855) 856-4713 toll-free Monday–Friday 9 am to 5 pm EST; (770) 488-7100 after hours, weekends, and holidays
If above options not available				
	Mefloquine[46]	684 mg base (=750 mg salt), orally, as initial dose, followed by 456 mg base (=500 mg salt), orally, given 6–12 h after initial dose Total dose = 1250 mg salt	13.7 mg base/kg (=15 mg salt/kg; max 750 mg/dose), orally, as initial dose, followed by 9.1 mg base/kg (=10 mg salt/kg; max 500 mg/dose), orally, given 6–12 h after initial dose Total dose = 25 mg salt/kg	

Table 4.11. Drugs for Parasitic Infections,[1] continued

Disease	Drug	Adult Dosage	Pediatric Dosage	Links to CDC Website[2] and professional society guidelines
Uncomplicated malaria *P falciparum* or species not identified	Chloroquine-sensitive (Central America west of Panama Canal, Haiti, and the Dominican Republic)			
	Any of the antimalarials above, OR			
	Chloroquine phosphate[47]	600 mg base (=1000 mg salt), orally, immediately; followed by 300 mg base (=500 mg salt), orally, at 6, 24, and 48 h Total dose: 1500 mg base (=2500 mg salt)	10 mg base/kg (= 16.7 mg/kg salt; max 1000 mg salt/dose), orally, immediately; followed by 5 mg base/kg (=8.3 mg/kg salt; max 500 mg salt/dose), orally, at 6, 24, and 48 h Total dose: 25 mg base/kg (=41.6 mg/kg salt)	www.cdc.gov/malaria/resources/pdf/Malaria_Treatment_Table.pdf Updated guidance about treatment of severe malaria: www.cdc.gov/malaria/new_info/2021/artesunate_availability.html
	OR			
	Hydroxychloroquine	620 mg base (=800 mg salt), orally, immediately; followed by 310 mg base (=400 mg salt), orally, at 6, 24, and 48 h Total dose: 1550 mg base (=2000 mg salt)	10 mg base/kg (=12.9 mg/kg salt; max 800 mg salt/dose), orally, immediately; followed by 5 mg base/kg (=6.5 mg/kg salt; max 400 mg salt/dose), orally, at 6, 24, and 48 h Total dose: 25 mg base/kg (=32.4 mg/kg salt)	CDC Malaria Hotline: (770) 488-7788 or (855) 856-4713 toll-free Monday–Friday 9 am to 5 pm EST; (770) 488-7100 after hours, weekends, and holidays

Table 4.11. Drugs for Parasitic Infections,[1] continued

Disease	Drug	Adult Dosage	Pediatric Dosage	Links to CDC Website[2] and professional society guidelines
Uncomplicated malaria *P malariae* or *P knowlesi*	Chloroquine sensitive in all regions			**www.cdc.gov/malaria/resources/pdf/ Malaria_Treatment_Table.pdf** Updated guidance about treatment of severe malaria: **www.cdc.gov/malaria/new_info/2021/artesunate_availability. html** CDC Malaria Hotline: (770) 488-7788 or (855) 856-4713 toll-free Monday–Friday 9 am to 5 pm EST; (770) 488-7100 after hours, weekends, and holidays
	Any of the antimalarials above, OR			
	Chloroquine phosphate[47]	600 mg base (=1000 mg salt), orally, immediately; followed by 300 mg base (=500 mg salt), orally, at 6, 24, and 48 h Total dose: 1500 mg base (=2500 mg salt)	10 mg base/kg (= 16.7 mg/kg salt; max 1000 mg salt/dose), orally, immediately, followed by 5 mg base/kg (=8.3 mg/ kg salt; max 500 mg salt/ dose), orally, at 6, 24, and 48 h Total dose: 25 mg base/kg (=41.6 mg/kg salt)	
	OR			
	Hydroxychloroquine	620 mg base (=800 mg salt), orally, immediately; followed by 310 mg base (=400 mg salt), orally, at 6, 24, and 48 h Total dose: 1550 mg base (=2000 mg salt)	10 mg base/kg (=12.9 mg/kg salt; max 800 mg salt/dose), orally, immediately; followed by 5 mg base/kg (=6.5 mg/ kg salt; max 400 mg salt/ dose), orally, at 6, 24, and 48 h Total dose: 25 mg base/kg (=32.4 mg/kg salt)	

Table 4.11. Drugs for Parasitic Infections,[1] continued

Disease	Drug	Adult Dosage	Pediatric Dosage	Links to CDC Website[2] and professional society guidelines
	Chloroquine sensitive (All regions except Papua New Guinea and Indonesia. If chloroquine or hydroxychloroquine are not available, acceptable to use drugs listed under chloroquine resistant section below)			
Uncomplicated malaria *P vivax* or *P ovale*	Chloroquine phosphate[47]	600 mg base (=1000 mg salt), orally, immediately; followed by 300 mg base (=500 mg salt), orally, at 6, 24, and 48 h. Total dose: 1500 mg base (=2500 mg salt)	10 mg base/kg (=16.7 mg/kg salt; max 1000 mg salt/dose), orally, immediately; followed by 5 mg base/kg (=8.3 mg/kg salt; max 500 mg salt/dose), orally, at 6, 24, and 48 h. Total dose: 25 mg base/kg (=41.6 mg/kg salt)	www.cdc.gov/malaria/resources/pdf/Malaria_Treatment_Table.pdf Updated guidance about treatment of severe malaria: www.cdc.gov/malaria/new_info/2021/artesunate_availability.html CDC Malaria Hotline: (770) 488-7788 or (855) 856-4713 toll-free Monday–Friday 9 am to 5 pm EST; (770) 488-7100 after hours, weekends, and holidays
	PLUS EITHER			
	Primaquine phosphate[48] OR	Primaquine phosphate: 30 mg base, orally, once daily for 14 days	Primaquine phosphate: 0.5 mg base/kg, orally, once daily for 14 days (max 30 mg base/dose)	
	Tafenoquine[48]	Tafenoquine: 300 mg, orally, given once concurrently with chloroquine phosphate	Tafenoquine: Only for those ≥16 years; 300 mg, orally, given once concurrently with chloroquine phosphate	
	OR			

Table 4.11. Drugs for Parasitic Infections,[1] continued

Disease	Drug	Adult Dosage	Pediatric Dosage	Links to CDC Website[2] and professional society guidelines
	Hydroxychloroquine	620 mg base (=800 mg salt), orally, immediately, followed by 310 mg base (=400 mg salt), orally, at 6, 24, and 48 h Total dose: 1550 mg base (=2000 mg salt)	10 mg base/kg (=12.9 mg/kg salt; max 800 mg salt/dose), orally, immediately, followed by 5 mg base/kg (=6.5 mg/kg salt; max 400 mg salt/dose), orally, at 6, 24, and 48 h Total dose: 25 mg base/kg (=32.4 mg/kg salt)	**www.cdc.gov/malaria/resources/pdf/ Malaria_Treatment_Table.pdf** Updated guidance about treatment of severe malaria: **www.cdc.gov/malaria/new_ info/2021/artesunate_availability. html**
	PLUS EITHER			CDC Malaria Hotline: (770) 488-7788 or (855) 856-4713 toll-free Monday–Friday 9 am to 5 pm EST; (770) 488-7100 after hours, weekends, and holidays
	Primaquine phosphate[48] OR	Primaquine phosphate: 30 mg base, orally, once daily for 14 days	Primaquine phosphate: 0.5 mg base/kg, orally, once daily for 14 days (max 30 mg base/dose)	
	Tafenoquine[48]	Tafenoquine: 300 mg, orally, given once concurrently with hydroxychloroquine	Tafenoquine: Only for those ≥16 years; 300 mg, orally, given once concurrently with hydroxychloroquine	

Table 4.11. Drugs for Parasitic Infections,[1] continued

Disease	Drug	Adult Dosage	Pediatric Dosage	Links to CDC Website[2] and professional society guidelines
	Chloroquine-resistant[49] (Papua New Guinea and Indonesia)			www.cdc.gov/malaria/resources/pdf/ Malaria_Treatment_Table.pdf
Uncomplicated malaria *P vivax*	Artemether-lumefantrine[42] 1 tablet = 20 mg artemether and 120 mg lumefantrine PLUS	A 3-day treatment schedule with a total of 6 oral doses is recommended for both adult and pediatric patients based on weight. The patient should receive the initial dose, followed by the second dose 8 hours later, then 1 dose, orally, 2 times/day, for the following 2 days. Weight 5 to <15 kg: 1 tablet per dose Weight 15 to <25 kg: 2 tablets per dose Weight 25 to <35 kg: 3 tablets per dose Weight ≥35 kg: 4 tablets per dose		Updated guidance about treatment of severe malaria: www.cdc.gov/malaria/new_ info/2021/artesunate_availability. html
	Primaquine phosphate[48]	Primaquine phosphate: 30 mg base, orally, once daily for 14 days	Primaquine phosphate: 0.5 mg base/kg, orally, once daily for 14 days (max 30 mg base/ dose)	CDC Malaria Hotline: (770) 488-7788 or (855) 856-4713 toll-free Monday–Friday 9 am to 5 pm EST; (770) 488-7100 after hours, weekends, and holidays
	Quinine sulfate[43] PLUS EITHER	Quinine sulfate: 542 mg base (=650 mg salt),[44] orally, 3 times/day for 3 or 7 days[44]	Quinine sulfate: 8.3 mg base/ kg (=10 mg salt/kg), orally, 3 times/day for 3 or 7 days[44]	

Table 4.11. Drugs for Parasitic Infections,[1] continued

Disease	Drug	Adult Dosage	Pediatric Dosage	Links to CDC Website[2] and professional society guidelines
	Doxycycline[45]	Doxycycline: 100 mg, orally, 2 times/day for 7 days	Doxycycline: 2.2 mg/kg, orally, every 12 h for 7 days (max 200 mg/day)	**www.cdc.gov/malaria/resources/pdf/Malaria_Treatment_Table.pdf**
	OR Tetracycline[45]	Tetracycline: 250 mg, orally, 4 times/day for 7 days	Tetracycline: 25 mg/kg/day, orally, divided 4 times/day for 7 days (max 250 mg/dose)	Updated guidance about treatment of severe malaria: **www.cdc.gov/malaria/new_info/2021/artesunate_availability.html**
	OR in pregnant people			
	Clindamycin	Clindamycin: 20 mg base/kg/day, orally, divided 3 times/day for 7 days	Clindamycin: 20 mg base/kg/day, orally, divided 3 times/day for 7 days	CDC Malaria Hotline: (770) 488-7788 or (855) 856-4713 toll-free Monday–Friday 9 am to 5 pm EST; (770) 488-7100 after hours, weekends, and holidays
	PLUS Primaquine phosphate[48]	Primaquine phosphate: 30 mg base, orally, once daily for 14 days	Primaquine phosphate: 0.5 mg base/kg, orally, once daily for 14 days (max 30 mg base/dose)	

Table 4.11. Drugs for Parasitic Infections,[1] continued

Disease	Drug	Adult Dosage	Pediatric Dosage	Links to CDC Website[2] and professional society guidelines
	OR			
	Atovaquone-proguanil[42] Adult tab: 250 mg atovaquone/100 mg proguanil Peds tab: 62.5 mg atovaquone/25 mg proguanil	Atovaquone-proguanil: 1000 mg atovaquone/400 mg proguanil, orally, once daily for 3 days	Atovaquone-proguanil: 5–<8 kg: 2 pediatric tablets, orally, once daily for 3 days 8–<10 kg: 3 pediatric tablets, orally, once daily for 3 days 10–<20 kg: 1 adult tablet, orally, once daily for 3 days 20–<30 kg: 2 adult tablets, orally, once daily for 3 days 30–<40 kg: 3 adult tablets, orally, once daily for 3 days ≥40 kg: 4 adult tablets, orally, once daily for 3 days	**www.cdc.gov/malaria/resources/pdf/ Malaria_Treatment_Table.pdf** Updated guidance about treatment of severe malaria: **www.cdc.gov/malaria/new_info/2021/artesunate_availability. html** CDC Malaria Hotline: (770) 488-7788 or (855) 856-4713 toll-free Monday–Friday 9 am to 5 pm EST; (770) 488-7100 after hours, weekends, and holidays
	PLUS			
	Primaquine phosphate[48]	Primaquine phosphate: 30 mg base, orally, once daily for 14 days	Primaquine phosphate: 0.5 mg base/kg, orally, once daily for 14 days (max 30 mg base/dose)	

Table 4.11. Drugs for Parasitic Infections,[1] continued

Disease	Drug	Adult Dosage	Pediatric Dosage	Links to CDC Website[2] and professional society guidelines
	OR, if above antimalarials not available,			www.cdc.gov/malaria/resources/pdf/Malaria_Treatment_Table.pdf Updated guidance about treatment of severe malaria: www.cdc.gov/malaria/new_info/2021/artesunate_availability.html CDC Malaria Hotline: (770) 488-7788 or (855) 856-4713 toll-free Monday–Friday 9 am to 5 pm EST; (770) 488-7100 after hours, weekends, and holidays
	Mefloquine[46]		Mefloquine: 13.7 mg base/kg (=15 mg salt/kg; max 750 mg salt/dose), orally, as initial dose, followed by 9.1 mg base/kg (=10 mg salt/kg; max 500 mg salt/dose), orally, given 6–12 h after initial dose Total dose = 22.8 mg base/kg (=25 mg salt/kg)	
	PLUS			
	Primaquine phosphate[48]		Primaquine phosphate: 0.5 mg base/kg, orally, once daily for 14 days (max 30 mg base/dose)	

Table 4.11. Drugs for Parasitic Infections,[1] continued

Disease	Drug	Adult Dosage	Pediatric Dosage	Links to CDC Website[2] and professional society guidelines
	Chloroquine-sensitive (see uncomplicated malaria sections above for chloroquine-sensitive species by region)			
Uncomplicated malaria: alternatives for pregnant people[50,51,52]	Chloroquine phosphate[47]	600 mg base (=1000 mg salt), orally, immediately, followed by 300 mg base (=500 mg salt), orally, at 6, 24, and 48 h Total dose: 1500 mg base (=2500 mg salt)	Not applicable	www.cdc.gov/malaria/resources/pdf/Malaria_Treatment_Table.pdf Updated guidance about treatment of severe malaria: www.cdc.gov/malaria/new_info/2021/artesunate_availability.html CDC Malaria Hotline: (770) 488-7788 or (855) 856-4713 toll-free Monday–Friday 9 am to 5 pm EST; (770) 488-7100 after hours, weekends, and holidays
	OR			
	Hydroxychloroquine	620 mg base (=800 mg salt), orally, immediately, followed by 310 mg base (=400 mg salt), orally, at 6, 24, and 48 h Total dose: 1550 mg base (=2000 mg salt)	Not applicable	
	Chloroquine-resistant (see sections above for regions with chloroquine-resistant *P falciparum* and *P vivax*)			

Table 4.11. Drugs for Parasitic Infections,[1] continued

Disease	Drug	Adult Dosage	Pediatric Dosage	Links to CDC Website[2] and professional society guidelines
	Quinine sulfate[43]	Quinine sulfate: 542 mg base (=650 mg salt),[44] orally, 3 times/day for 3 or 7 days[44]	Not applicable	www.cdc.gov/malaria/resources/pdf/Malaria_Treatment_Table.pdf
	PLUS			
	Clindamycin	Clindamycin: 20 mg base/kg/day, orally, divided 3 times/day for 7 days		
	OR			
	Artemether-lumefantrine[42] (all trimesters)	1 tablet = 20 mg artemether and 120 mg lumefantrine. For 2nd or 3rd trimester of pregnancy and, if no other options or benefits outweigh risks, 1st trimester. A 3-day treatment schedule with a total of 6 oral doses (4 tablets per dose) is recommended; dose 1 followed by dose 2 8 hours later, then 1 dose twice daily for the following 2 days.	Not applicable	Updated guidance about treatment of severe malaria: www.cdc.gov/malaria/new_info/2021/artesunate_availability.html CDC Malaria Hotline: (770) 488-7788 or (855) 856-4713 toll-free Monday–Friday 9 am to 5 pm EST; (770) 488-7100 after hours, weekends, and holidays

Table 4.11. Drugs for Parasitic Infections,[1] continued

Disease	Drug	Adult Dosage	Pediatric Dosage	Links to CDC Website[2] and professional society guidelines
	OR			**www.cdc.gov/malaria/resources/pdf/ Malaria_Treatment_Table.pdf** Updated guidance about treatment of severe malaria: **www.cdc.gov/malaria/new_ info/2021/artesunate_availability. html**
	Mefloquine[46]	684 mg base (=750 mg salt), orally, as initial dose, followed by 456 mg base (=500 mg salt), orally, given 6–12 h after initial dose Total dose= 1250 mg salt	Not applicable	
Severe malaria[53,54,55]	All regions	Artesunate for Injection (manufactured by Amivas), IV, 2.4 mg/ kg/dose at hours 0, 12, and 24.[56] If additional doses needed, continue at 2.4 mg/kg/dose daily.	Artesunate for Injection, IV, 2.4 mg/kg/dose at hours 0, 12, and 24. If additional doses needed, continue at 2.4 mg/ kg/dose daily	CDC Malaria Hotline: (770) 488-7788 or (855) 856-4713 toll-free Monday–Friday 9 am to 5 pm EST; (770) 488-7100 after hours, weekends, and holidays

Table 4.11. Drugs for Parasitic Infections,[1] continued

Disease	Drug	Adult Dosage	Pediatric Dosage	Links to CDC Website[2] and professional society guidelines
		PLUS	PLUS	**www.cdc.gov/malaria/resources/pdf/Malaria_Treatment_Table.pdf**
		After at least 3 IV doses AND parasitemia ≤1% give oral regimen as listed above for uncomplicated, chloroquine-resistant *P falciparum*.	After at least 3 IV doses AND parasitemia ≤1% give oral regimen as listed above for uncomplicated, chloroquine-resistant *P falciparum*.	Updated guidance about treatment of severe malaria: **www.cdc.gov/malaria/new_info/2021/artesunate_availability.html**
		See CDC recommendations for further management.	See CDC recommendations for further management.	CDC Malaria Hotline: (770) 488-7788 or (855) 856-4713 toll-free Monday–Friday 9 am to 5 pm EST; (770) 488-7100 after hours, weekends, and holidays
Microsporidiosis				
Ocular				
Encephalitozoon hellem, E cuniculi, Vittaforma [Nosema] corneae	Fumagillin[57]	Fumagillin in saline equivalent to fumagillin 70 μg/mL eye drops 2 drops every 2 h for 4 days, then 2 drops 4 times per day		**https://clinicalinfo.hiv.gov/en/guidelines/hiv-clinical-guidelines-adult-and-adolescent-opportunistic-infections/microsporidiosis?view=full**

Table 4.11. Drugs for Parasitic Infections,[1] continued

Disease	Drug	Adult Dosage	Pediatric Dosage	Links to CDC Website[2] and professional society guidelines
	PLUS for management of systemic infection:			
	Albendazole[3]	400 mg, orally, twice a day (take with food)	15 mg/kg/day, orally, divided 2 times/day (max 400 mg/dose; take with food)	
Intestinal				
E bieneusi	Fumagillin[58]	20 mg, orally, 3 times/day for 14 days		
E intestinalis	Albendazole[3]	400 mg, orally, on empty stomach,[59] twice a day for 21 days	15 mg/kg/day orally, on empty stomach,[59] in 2 doses (max 400 mg/dose)	
Disseminated[60]				
E hellem, E cuniculi, E intestinalis, Pleistophora species,[60] Trachipleistophora species,[60] and Anncalia [Brachiola] vesicularum[60]	Albendazole[3]	Immunocompromised: 400 mg, orally, twice per day for 14 to 28 days (take with food). Continue treatment until CD4+ T-lymphocyte count >200 cells/μL for >6 mo after initiation of antiretroviral therapy	15 mg/kg/day (max 400 mg/dose), orally, divided 2 times/day (take with food)	

Table 4.11. Drugs for Parasitic Infections,[1] continued

Disease	Drug	Adult Dosage	Pediatric Dosage	Links to CDC Website[2] and professional society guidelines
Neurocysticercosis (*T solium*)[61]	Albendazole[3]	Immunocompetent: 400 mg, orally, twice a day for 7 to 14 days (take with food)		www.cdc.gov/parasites/cysticercosis/health_professionals/index.html www.idsociety.org/practice-guideline/neurocysticercosis/
		15 mg/kg/day (max 800 mg/day OR 1200 mg/day, depending on number and characteristics of lesions as detailed in IDSA guideline) for 10–14 days (take with food)	15 mg/kg/day (max 800 mg/day OR 1200 mg/day, depending on number and characteristics of lesions as detailed in IDSA guideline) for 10–14 days (take with food)	
	PLUS (when > 2 intraparenchymal lesions)			
	Praziquantel[16]	50 mg/kg/day, orally, for 10–14 days		
Onchocerciasis (*Onchocerca volvulus*; River Blindness)[62]	To kill microfilariae: Ivermectin[5]	150 µg/kg, orally, in 1 dose every 6mo until asymptomatic		www.cdc.gov/parasites/onchocerciasis/health_professionals/index.html
	To kill microfilariae: Moxidectin[63]	8 mg, orally, once (≥12 years)		
	To kill macrofilariae: doxycycline[45,64]	100–200 mg, orally, daily, for 6 wk	2.2 mg/kg/dose orally twice daily	

Table 4.11. Drugs for Parasitic Infections,[1] continued

Disease	Drug	Adult Dosage	Pediatric Dosage	Links to CDC Website[2] and professional society guidelines
Opisthorchis Infection (Southeast Asian liver fluke)	Praziquantel[16]	75 mg/kg/day, orally, divided 3 times/day for 1–2 days (take with liquids during meals)		www.cdc.gov/parasites/opisthorchis/health_professionals/index.html
	OR			
	Albendazole[3]	10 mg/kg/day, orally, for 7 days (take with food)		
Paragonimiasis (lung fluke)	Praziquantel[16]	75 mg/kg/day, orally, divided into 3 doses, for 2 days		www.cdc.gov/parasites/paragonimus/health_professionals/index.html
	OR			
	Triclabendazole[25]	10 mg/kg/dose, orally, every 12 hours for 2 doses in patients ≥6 y (take with food)		
Scabies (Mite Infestation)	Permethrin cream 5%	Topically, twice, at least 7 days apart (adults and children ≥2 months old)		www.cdc.gov/parasites/scabies/health_professionals/meds.html
	OR			
	Crotamiton lotion 10% or Crotamiton cream 10%	Topically, overnight, on days 1, 2, 3, and 8 (not FDA-approved for use in children)		
	OR			
	Sulfur (5%–10%) ointment	Apply overnight for 3 consecutive days		
	OR			
	Ivermectin[5]	200 µg/kg, orally, twice, at least 7 days apart (take with food)		

Table 4.11. Drugs for Parasitic Infections,[1] continued

Disease	Drug	Adult Dosage	Pediatric Dosage	Links to CDC Website[2] and professional society guidelines
Schistosomiasis (Bilharzia)		For *Schistosoma mansoni, S haematobium, S intercalatum:*		www.cdc.gov/parasites/ schistosomiasis/health_ professionals/index.html
	Praziquantel[16]	40 mg/kg/day, orally, in 2 divided doses for 1 day		
		For *S japonicum, S mekongi:*		
	Praziquantel[16]	60 mg/kg/day; orally, in 3 divided doses for 1 day		
Strongyloidiasis (*Strongyloides stercoralis*)	Ivermectin[5]	200 µg/kg, orally, daily for 1–2 days for uncomplicated infections; for hyperinfection/disseminated infection stop or reduce immunosuppressive therapy if possible and continue daily ivermectin until stool and/or sputum exams are negative for 2 weeks. The veterinary subcutaneous formulation of ivermectin has been used in patients who are severely ill with hyperinfection and are unable to take or reliably absorb oral medications. The subcutaneous formulation may be used under a single-patient IND protocol request to the FDA.		www.cdc.gov/parasites/strongyloides/ health_professionals/index.html
	OR			
	Albendazole[3]	400 mg, orally, 2 times/day for 7 days (take with food) for uncomplicated infections.		
Taeniasis [*Taenia saginata* (beef tapeworm), *Taenia solium* (pork tapeworm), and *Taenia asiatica* (Asian tapeworm)]	Praziquantel[16]	5–10 mg/kg, orally, once		www.cdc.gov/parasites/taeniasis/ health_professionals/index.html

Table 4.11. Drugs for Parasitic Infections,[1] continued

Disease	Drug	Adult Dosage	Pediatric Dosage	Links to CDC Website[2] and professional society guidelines
	OR			
	Niclosamide[20] (not available in the US)	2 g, orally, once	50 mg/kg (max 2 g), orally, once	
	OR			
	Albendazole[3]	400 mg daily for 3 days		
Toxocariasis[65] (Ocular Larva Migrans, Visceral Larva Migrans)	Albendazole[3]	400 mg, orally, 2 times/day for 5 days (take with food)		www.cdc.gov/parasites/toxocariasis/ health_professionals/index.html
	OR			
	Mebendazole[4]	100–200 mg, orally, 2 times/day for 5 days		
Toxoplasmosis (*Toxoplasma gondii*)[66]	See Tables in *Toxoplasma gondii* Infections (p 867)			www.cdc.gov/parasites/ toxoplasmosis/health_professionals/ index.html https://clinicalinfo.hiv.gov/ en/guidelines/hiv-clinical-guidelines-adult-and-adolescent-opportunistic-infections/toxoplasma-gondii?view=full
Trichinellosis (trichinosis; *Trichinella* species)[67]	Albendazole[3]	400 mg, orally, twice daily for 8 to 14 days (take with food)		www.cdc.gov/parasites/trichinellosis/ health_professionals/index.html
	OR			

Table 4.11. Drugs for Parasitic Infections,[1] continued

Disease	Drug	Adult Dosage	Pediatric Dosage	Links to CDC Website[2] and professional society guidelines
Trichuriasis (whipworm infection; *Trichuris trichiura*)	Mebendazole[4]	200–400 mg, orally, 3 times daily for 3 days; then 400–500 mg, orally, 3 times daily for 10 days		www.cdc.gov/parasites/whipworm/ health_professionals/index.html
	Albendazole[3]	400 mg, orally, for 3 days		
	OR			
	Mebendazole[4]	100 mg, orally, twice daily for 3 days		
	OR			
	Ivermectin[5]	200 μg/kg/day, orally, for 3 days		
Trypanosomiasis, American (Chagas disease; *Trypanosoma cruzi* infection)	Benznidazole[68]	5 mg/kg/day (or max 300 mg/day and prolong duration of therapy and complete a total dose equivalent to 5 mg/kg/day for 60 days), orally, in 2 divided doses for 60 days; doses for ages over 12 years are off-label	Age 2–12 y: 5–8 mg/kg/day, orally, in 2 divided doses for 60 days; doses for other ages are off-label; age >12 years: 5 mg/kg/day (or max 300 mg/day and prolong duration of therapy and complete a total dose equivalent to 5 mg/kg/day for 60 days), orally, in 2 divided doses for 60 days; doses for ages over 12 years are off-label	www.cdc.gov/parasites/chagas/ health_professionals/index.html
	OR			

Table 4.11. Drugs for Parasitic Infections,[1] continued

Disease	Drug	Adult Dosage	Pediatric Dosage	Links to CDC Website[2] and professional society guidelines
	Nifurtimox[68]	8–10 mg/kg/day, orally, in 3 divided doses for 60 days; doses for ages over 17 years are off-label	Age birth to <18 years of age and 2.5 kg to less than 41 kg: 10–20 mg/kg/day, orally, in 3 divided doses for 60 days. Age birth to <18 years of age and greater than or equal to 41 kg: 8–10 mg/kg/day, orally, in 3 divided doses for 60 days	
Trypanosomiasis, human African (HAT)(sleeping sickness; *Trypanosoma brucei rhodesiense* and *Trypanosoma brucei gambiense* infection)	Please see CDC guidance or WHO interim guidance for treatment of *gambiense* HAT; consultation with infectious disease or subject matter experts recommended when treating patients with HAT			www.cdc.gov/parasites/sleepingsickness/health_professionals/index.html CDC Drug Service: www.cdc.gov/laboratory/drugservice/formulary.html https://apps.who.int/iris/bitstream/handle/10665/326178/9789241550567-eng.pdf

CDC indicates Centers for Disease Control and Prevention; CNS, central nervous system; FDA, US Food and Drug Administration; IM, intramuscular; IV, intravenous.

[1] The contents of this table are provided to assist in decision making for patient management but are not a substitute for clinical judgment or expert consultation. The table may not address drug toxicities, drug-drug interactions, and issues pertinent to some special populations (eg, patients with HIV/AIDS). Recommendations in the table may not represent all potential treatment or dosage options. See CDC website for additional information on each disease and the treatment thereof. Not all recommended therapies and dosages included in this table match the recommendations on the pathogen-specific CDC web pages. Inclusion of the links to the CDC website does not suggest endorsement of the content of this table by the CDC.

[2] See CDC website for additional information on each disease and the treatment thereof.

Table 4.11. Drugs for Parasitic Infections,[1] continued

3 Safety of albendazole in children younger than 6 years is not certain. Studies of the use of albendazole in children as young as 1 year suggest that its use is safe. Albendazole should be taken with food when systemic absorption is desired. Some anthelmintics are very costly in the United States. The FDA website BeSafeRx (**www.fda.gov/drugs/buying-using-medicine-safely/quick-tips-buying-medicines-over-internet**) provides information for providers and patients who are considering online pharmacies that may provide drugs at lower cost.

4 Mebendazole is approved for some specific indications in children ages 2 and older. Safety has not been established in children; data are limited in children younger than 2 year. Some anthelmintics are very costly in the United States. The FDA website BeSafeRx (**www.fda.gov/drugs/buying-using-medicine-safely/quick-tips-buying-medicines-over-internet**) provides information for providers and patients who are considering online pharmacies that may provide drugs at lower cost.

5 Safety of ivermectin in treating pregnant people and children who weigh less than 15 kg has not been established. Ivermectin should be taken on an empty stomach with water.

6 Safety of pyrantel pamoate in children has not been established. According to WHO guidance on preventive chemotherapy, pyrantel may be used in children 1 year and older during mass treatment programs without diagnosis.

7 Not approved by the FDA for this indication.

8 The combination of clindamycin plus quinine, or the combination of IV azithromycin plus oral atovaquone, are options for treatment of babesiosis in patients who are severely ill.

9 Cases of cholestatic hepatitis, elevated liver enzymes, and fatal liver failure have been reported in patients treated with atovaquone.

10 Some immunocompromised adults with babesiosis have been treated with doses of azithromycin in the range of 600–1000 mg/day, in combination with atovaquone (750 mg twice per day).

11 Quinine treatment is associated with thrombocytopenia, QT prolongation, ventricular arrhythmias, hypoglycemia, and serious hypersensitivity reactions. Neuromuscular blocking agents should be avoided in patients receiving quinine sulfate. Use with caution in patients with atrial fibrillation or atrial flutter.

12 Tetracycline should be taken 1 hour before or 2 hours after meals containing dairy, and at least 1–2 hours before or 4 hours after an antacid. Tetracycline is not indicated for use in children younger than 8 years.

13 Iodoquinol tablets currently are not available in the United States.

14 In cases in which suspicion of exposure is high, immediate treatment with albendazole (25–50 mg/kg/day, orally, for 10–20 days) may be appropriate. Treatment is successful when administered soon after exposure to abort the migration of larvae and should be initiated as soon as possible after ingestion of infectious material, ideally within 3 days. When given in this setting, take albendazole on an empty stomach. For clinical baylisascariasis, treatment with albendazole (take with food) with concurrent corticosteroids to help reduce the inflammatory reaction is indicated to attempt to control the disease.

15 Clinical significance of *Blastocystis* species is controversial.

16 Praziquantel is not approved for treatment of children younger than 4 years. Take with water during meals.

17 There are no drug regimens with proven efficacy for the treatment of cryptosporidiosis in immunosuppressed patients.

18 HIV-infected patients may need longer courses of therapy for cyclosporiasis.

19 Expert consultation for treatment of cystoisosporiasis is recommended if the patient is immunosuppressed.

20 Niclosamide is not available for human use in the United States. Chew thoroughly or crush and mix with a small amount of water.

21 Asymptomatic infections generally do not require treatment; when *D fragilis* is the sole organism found in a patient with abdominal pain or diarrhea for a week or more treatment is appropriate.

22 Tetracycline or doxycycline also have been used for treatment.

23 See text in Other Tapeworm Infections (Including Hydatid Disease), p 845. Management depends on type and location of cysts, may involve surgery, and collaboration with specialists with experience treating this infection is advised. Albendazole is not appropriate for all forms of infection.

24 Diloxanide furoate is not commercially available in the United States.

25 Triclabendazole is approved by the FDA for treatment of fascioliasis in children 6 years and older. Safety and effectiveness of triclabendazole in children younger than 6 years have not been established.

26 Alternative treatments for giardiasis include albendazole, mebendazole, paromomycin, quinacrine, and furazolidone.

Table 4.11. Drugs for Parasitic Infections,[1] continued

27 Questions about treatment of leishmaniasis should be directed to Parasitic Diseases Inquiries (404-718-4745; e-mail **parasites@cdc.gov**). Only selected antileishmanial agents and regimens are listed in the table. Sodium stibogluconate is not currently being manufactured. Expert consultation about these and other potential treatment options for leishmaniasis is encouraged. For some cases of cutaneous leishmaniasis, no therapy may be needed or local (vs systemic) therapy may suffice or other systemic treatments may be considered. Miltefosine (IMPAVIDO) was approved in March 2014 by the FDA—for treatment of visceral leishmaniasis caused by *L donovani*; mucosal leishmaniasis caused by *L (Viannia) braziliensis*; and cutaneous leishmaniasis caused by *L (V) braziliensis, L (V) guyanensis,* and *L (V) panamensis* (ie, some New World cutaneous leishmaniasis species but no Old World cutaneous leishmaniasis species)—for patients who are at least 12 years of age; weigh at least 30 kg, and are not pregnant or breastfeeding during or for 5 months after the treatment course.

28 Pentam 300 contains 300 mg of pentamidine isethionate salt per vial.

29 Pediculicides should not be used for infestations of the eyelashes. Such infestations are treated with petrolatum ointment applied 2 to 4 times/day for 10 days. For pubic lice, treat with 1% permethrin, pyrethrins with piperonyl butoxide, or ivermectin.

30 Permethrin and pyrethrin are pediculicidal; retreatment in 9–10 days is needed to eradicate the infestation. Some lice are resistant to pyrethrins and permethrin. Pyrethrins with piperonyl butoxide are recommended for use in children ≥2 years of age; permethrin for children ≥2 months of age.

31 Ivermectin is not ovicidal, but lice that hatch from treated eggs die within 48 hours after hatching. Recommended for use in children ≥6 months of age.

32 Spinosad causes neuronal excitation in insects leading to paralysis and death. The formulation also includes benzyl alcohol, which is pediculicidal. Two applications 7 days apart are needed. Recommended for children ≥6 months of age.

33 Benzyl alcohol prevents lice from closing their respiratory spiracles, and the lotion vehicle then obstructs their airway, causing them to asphyxiate. It is not ovicidal. Two applications 9–10 days apart are needed. Recommended for use in children ≥6 months of age. Resistance, which is a problem with other drugs, is unlikely to develop.

34 Malathion is both ovicidal and pediculicidal; 2 applications 7–9 days apart are generally necessary to kill all lice and nits. Recommended for children ≥6 years of age and contraindicated in children <24 months of age. Malathion is flammable. Do not smoke or use electrical heat sources (ie, hair dryer, curling iron, flat iron) when applying and while the hair is wet.

35 Abametapir is ovicidal. Contains benzyl alcohol. Use is not recommended in pediatric patients younger than 6 months because of the potential for increased systemic absorption. Not available in the United States as of March 23, 2023.

36 Ivermectin is pediculicidal but not ovicidal; more than 1 dose is generally necessary to eradicate the infestation. The number of doses and the interval between doses have not been established; animal studies have shown adverse effects on the fetus. A single oral dose of 200 μg/kg, repeated in 7–10 days, has been shown to be effective against head lice. Most recently, a single oral dose of 400 μg/kg, repeated in 7 days, has been shown to be more effective than 0.5% malathion lotion.

37 Diethylcarbamazine (DEC) is not approved by the FDA but is available through the CDC Drug Service under an IND protocol; questions should be directed to Parasitic Diseases Inquiries (404-718-4745; e-mail **parasites@cdc.gov**). DEC is contraindicated in patients who may also have onchocerciasis. Before DEC therapy for lymphatic filariasis or loiasis, onchocerciasis should be excluded in all patients with a consistent exposure history because of the possibility of severe exacerbations of skin and eye involvement (Mazzotti reaction). People coinfected with *L loa* and *O volvulus* should not be treated with DEC until the onchocerciasis is treated; their onchocerciasis should not be treated with ivermectin if it is unsafe to treat their loiasis.

38 Apheresis should be performed at an institution with experience in using this therapeutic modality for loiasis.

39 Doxycycline is not standard treatment for lymphatic filariasis, but some studies have shown adult-worm killing with doxycycline therapy (200 mg/day for 4–6 weeks).

40 If a person develops malaria despite taking chemoprophylaxis, that particular medicine should not be used as a part of his or her treatment regimen. Use one of the other options instead.

41 There are 4 options available for treatment of uncomplicated malaria caused by chloroquine-resistant *P falciparum*. The first 3 options are equally recommended. Because of a higher rate of severe neuropsychiatric reactions seen at treatment doses, mefloquine is not recommended unless the other options cannot be used. Because there are more data on the efficacy of quinine in combination with doxycycline or tetracycline, these treatment combinations generally are preferred to quinine in combination with clindamycin.

42 Atovaquone-proguanil or artemether-lumefantrine should be taken with food or whole milk. If patient vomits within 30 minutes of taking a dose, the dose should be repeated. Atovaquone-proguanil not recommended during pregnancy or in people breastfeeding infants weighing <5 kg. May be considered if other treatment options are not available or not tolerated and benefits outweigh risks. Adult tablet = 250 mg atovaquone/100 mg proguanil. Pediatric tablet = 62.5 mg atovaquone/25 mg proguanil.

Table 4.11. Drugs for Parasitic Infections,[1] continued

43 US-manufactured quinine sulfate capsule is in a 324-mg dosage; therefore, 2 capsules should be sufficient for adult dosing. Pediatric dosing may be difficult because of unavailability of noncapsule forms of quinine.

44 For infections acquired in Southeast Asia, quinine treatment should continue for 7 days. For infections acquired elsewhere, quinine treatment should continue for 3 days.

45 Tetracycline is not indicated for use in children younger than 8 years. Doxycycline can be administered without regard to the patient's age or required duration of therapy (see Tetracyclines, p 975). For children younger than 8 years and weighing >5 kg with chloroquine-resistant *P falciparum*, atovaquone-proguanil and artemether-lumefantrine are recommended treatment options; mefloquine can be considered if no other options are available. For children younger than 8 years with chloroquine-resistant *P vivax*, mefloquine, or in those weighing >5 kg, atovaquone-proguanil or artemether-lumefantrine, are treatment options.

46 Treatment with mefloquine is not recommended in people who have acquired infections from Southeast Asia because of drug resistance.

47 When treating chloroquine-sensitive infections, chloroquine and hydroxychloroquine are recommended options. Regimens used to treat chloroquine-resistant infections may also be used if available, more convenient, or preferred.

48 Primaquine and tafenoquine are used to eradicate any hypnozoites that may remain dormant in the liver and, thus, prevent relapses in *P vivax* and *P ovale* infections. Because both drugs can cause hemolytic anemia in glucose-6-phosphate dehydrogenase (G6PD)-deficient people, G6PD screening must occur prior to starting treatment with primaquine or tafenoquine. For people with borderline G6PD deficiency or as an alternate to the above regimen, primaquine, 45 mg, orally, once per week for 8 weeks may be given; consultation with an expert in infectious disease and/or tropical medicine is advised if this alternative regimen is considered in G6PD-deficient people. Primaquine and tafenoquine must not be used during pregnancy. Tafenoquine can only be used in conjunction with chloroquine phosphate or hydroxychloroquine and is only approved for use in people 16 years and older. Dose of primaquine in patients ≥70 kg should be adjusted to a total dose of 6 mg/kg, divided into doses of 30 mg per day.

49 Four options are available for treatment of uncomplicated malaria caused by chloroquine-resistant *P vivax*. The first 3 options are equally recommended. Because of a higher rate of severe neuropsychiatric reactions seen at treatment doses, mefloquine is not recommended unless the other options cannot be used. High treatment failure rates attributable to chloroquine-resistant *P vivax* have been well documented in Papua New Guinea and Indonesia. Rare case reports of chloroquine-resistant *P vivax* also have been documented in Burma (Myanmar), India, and Central and South America. People acquiring *P vivax* infections outside of Papua New Guinea or Indonesia should be started on chloroquine. If the patient does not respond, treatment should be changed to a chloroquine-resistant *P vivax* regimen and the CDC should be notified (Malaria Hotline number listed previously).

50 For pregnant people diagnosed with uncomplicated malaria caused by chloroquine-resistant *P falciparum* or chloroquine-resistant *P vivax* infection, treatment with doxycycline or tetracycline generally is not indicated. Doxycycline or tetracycline may be used in combination with quinine (as recommended for nonpregnant adults) if other treatment options are not available or are not being tolerated and the benefit is judged to outweigh the risks.

51 Atovaquone-proguanil generally is not recommended during pregnancy; artemether-lumefantrine is recommended in the second and third trimester and may be used in the first trimester when benefits outweigh risks.

52 For *P vivax* and *P ovale* infections, primaquine phosphate or tafenoquine for radical treatment of hypnozoites should not be given during pregnancy. Pregnant patients with *P vivax* and *P ovale* infections should be maintained on chloroquine prophylaxis for the duration of their pregnancy. The chemoprophylactic dose of chloroquine phosphate is 300 mg base (=500 mg salt), orally, once per week. After delivery, patients with normal G6PD activity may be treated with primaquine or tafenoquine, depending on breastfeeding, or continue with chloroquine prophylaxis for a total of 1 year from acute infection. Primaquine can be used during breastfeeding if the infant is found to have normal G6PD activity; tafenoquine is not recommended during breastfeeding.

53 People with a positive blood smear OR history of recent possible exposure and no other recognized pathologic abnormality who have 1 or more of the following clinical criteria (impaired consciousness/coma, severe normocytic anemia, renal failure, pulmonary edema, acute respiratory distress syndrome, circulatory shock, disseminated intravascular coagulation, spontaneous bleeding, acidosis, hemoglobinuria, jaundice, repeated generalized convulsions, and/or parasitemia of >5%) are considered to have manifestations of more severe disease. Severe malaria is most often caused by *P falciparum*.

54 Patients with a diagnosis of severe malaria should be treated aggressively with parenteral antimalarial therapy. IV artesunate is now commercially available. If not in stock or available within 24 hours, contact CDC's Malaria Hotline.

Table 4.11. Drugs for Parasitic Infections,[1] continued

55 Pregnant people diagnosed with severe malaria should be treated aggressively with parenteral antimalarial therapy.

56 WHO guidelines recommend 3 mg/kg/dose IV artesunate for children <20 kg. See **https://app.magicapp.org/#/guideline/7661** and Haghiri A, Price DJ, Fitzpatrick P, et al. Evidence Based Optimal Dosing of Intravenous Artesunate in Children with Severe Falciparum Malaria. *Clin Pharmacol Ther.* 2023;114(6):1304-1312.

57 An investigational agent (non–FDA approved); not available in the United States at this time. For lesions attributable to *V corneae*, topical therapy generally is not effective and keratoplasty may be required (RM Davis, Font RL, Keisler MS, Shadduck JA. Corneal microsporidiosis. A case report including ultrastructural observations. *Ophthalmology.* 1990;97[7]:953-957). Data are insufficient to make recommendations on the use of fumagillin in children (see Guidelines for the Prevention and Treatment of Opportunistic Infections in Children with and Exposed to HIV. Department of Health and Human Services. Available at: **https://clinicalinfo.hiv.gov/en/guidelines/pediatric-opportunistic-infection)**

58 For gastrointestinal infections caused by *Enterocytozoon bieneusi*, fumagillin, 20 mg, orally 3 times daily, is the only drug with proven efficacy. Its use is associated with severe thrombocytopenia in 30% to 50% of patients, which is reversible on discontinuation of treatment. The drug is not currently available in the United States.

59 For intestinal infection without systemic involvement, albendazole should be taken on an empty stomach (for systemic infections, it should be taken with a fatty meal).

60 There is no established treatment for *Pleistophora*. For disseminated disease attributable to *Trachipleistophora* or *Anncaliia*, itraconazole, 400 mg, orally, once per day, plus albendazole 400 mg, orally, twice daily, may be tried.

61 Consultation with a specialist familiar with treatment of neurocysticercosis is advised. Although not all symptomatic patients with a single viable cyst of neurocysticercosis within brain parenchyma require antiparasitic medication, controlled studies demonstrate that clinical resolution and seizure recurrence rates are improved with albendazole. Two studies have demonstrated that in those with more than 2 viable intraparenchymal lesions, the response rate was better when albendazole was coadministered with praziquantel and corticosteroids. When a single agent is used, albendazole is preferred over praziquantel because it has fewer drug-drug interactions with anticonvulsants and steroids. The Centers for Disease Control and Prevention recommends 15 days of therapy, and suggests that more prolonged treatment courses (eg, 30 days of albendazole, which may be repeated) may be needed for extraparenchymal or extensive disease. Anti-inflammatory therapy is recommended when antiparasitic treatment is used though the optimal dose and duration have not been established. Commonly used regimens include dexamethasone 0.1 mg/kg/day (adult dose: 6 mg per day) or prednisone 1–2 mg/kg/day usually beginning at least 1 day before starting antiparasitic therapy, and continuing during treatment followed by a taper.

62 People coinfected with *O volvulus* and *L loa* should not be treated with diethylcarbamazine (DEC) until the onchocerciasis is treated; their onchocerciasis should not be treated with ivermectin if it is unsafe to treat their loiasis. Patients should only be treated with doxycycline if they no longer live in areas with endemic infection unless there is a contraindication for ivermectin.

63 Moxidectin approved in 2018 for children 12 years and older; not yet available commercially in the United States as of March 23, 2023. Screening for loiasis recommended before use. Safety and efficacy of repeat doses have not been studied. Safety and efficacy in children younger than 12 years have not been established.

64 Doxycycline is not standard therapy, but several studies support its use and safety. Treatment with a single oral dose of ivermectin (150 µg/kg) should be given 1 week before treatment with doxycycline to provide symptom relief to the patient. If the patient cannot tolerate the dosage of 200 mg, orally, daily of doxycycline, 100 mg, orally, daily is sufficient to sterilize female *Onchocerca organisms.* A dose of 2.2 mg/kg twice daily may be used for children. The safety of ivermectin in children weighing less than 15 kg and in pregnant people has not been established.

65 Albendazole preferred to mebendazole in ocular larva migrans (OLM) and CNS disease. Topical or systemic corticosteroids (prednisone 0.5–1 mg/kg/day) may be used to control inflammation in OLM and prednisone (0.5–1 mg/kg/day) may be used in severe visceral larva migrans. Length of therapy may be extended to 2 weeks in OLM; optimal dosing has not been established.

66 For treatment and chronic suppression of toxoplasmosis in human immunodeficiency virus (HIV) infected children, see Guidelines for the Prevention and Treatment of Opportunistic Infections in Children with and Exposed to HIV. Department of Health and Human Services. Available at: **https://clinicalinfo.hiv.gov/en/guidelines/pediatric-opportunistic-infection**.

67 In addition to antiparasitic medication, treatment with corticosteroids sometimes is required in more severe cases of trichinellosis.

68 The 2 drugs used to treat infection with *T cruzi* are benznidazole and nifurtimox. Benznidazole was approved in 2017 by the FDA for use in children 2–12 years of age for the treatment of Chagas disease. Use of benznidazole to treat a patient outside of the FDA-approved age range of 2–12 years is based on clinical diagnosis and decision making by a treating physician under practice of medicine. On August 6, 2020, the FDA announced approval of a nifurtimox product (LAMPIT [Bayer]) for treatment of Chagas disease in patients from birth to younger than 18 years weighing at least 2.5 kg. Use of nifurtimox to treat a patient outside of the FDA-approved age range of birth to younger than 18 years is based on clinical diagnosis and decision making by the treating physician under the practice of medicine. For both drugs, adverse effects are common and are more frequent and more severe with increasing age. Questions regarding treatment should be directed to Parasitic Diseases Public Inquiries (404-718-4745; email **parasites@cdc.gov**).

MEDWATCH–THE FDA SAFETY INFORMATION AND ADVERSE EVENT REPORTING PROGRAM

MedWatch, the Food and Drug Administration (FDA) Safety Information and Adverse Event Reporting Program, serves as a gateway for clinically important safety information and reporting of adverse events for human medical products, including FDA-regulated prescription and over-the-counter drugs, certain biologics (including gene therapies, human cells, tissues, and cellular and tissue-based products), medical devices (including in vitro diagnostics), special nutritional products, and cosmetics. MedWatch does not pertain to tobacco products, vaccines, or certain food products. MedWatch collects reports of drug adverse effects, product quality problems, product use errors, and therapeutic failures. Although reporting to MedWatch by health care professionals and consumers is voluntary, manufacturers of prescription medical products are required to submit adverse event reports to the FDA.

Because many prelicensure clinical trials are not large enough to reveal rare adverse events, postlicensure safety surveillance is used to identify and evaluate new safety concerns with drugs and devices after they are approved and widely used in clinical practice. MedWatch reports are used by the FDA as a pharmacovigilance data source. If a potential safety concern is identified through analysis of MedWatch reports, FDA's further evaluation might include conducting studies using other databases. On the basis of information from postmarketing safety surveillance, the FDA may take regulatory actions, such as revising and strengthening warnings, precautions, contraindications, and adverse reaction descriptions in medication package inserts or issuing "Dear Health Care Professional" letters. Safety alerts are published on the agency's website, and clinicians and the public can stay informed through email, X (formerly known as Twitter), and RSS feed updates. The FDA Adverse Event Reporting System (FAERS) Public Dashboard allows users to search publicly available information from adverse event reports submitted to the FDA.

Health care professionals and consumers are encouraged to report adverse events associated with medical products. Reports can be submitted online through the MedWatch Adverse Event Reporting system (**www.fda.gov/MedWatch/report.htm**) or the forms can be downloaded (**www.fda.gov/safety/medical-product-safety-information/medwatch-forms-fda-safety-reporting**) and sent by fax (800-FDA-0178) or mail. Phone reports can be made by calling 800-FDA-1088. A consumer-friendly reporting form (FDA3500B) is available to encourage increased reporting by patients. Vaccine-related adverse events should be reported to the Vaccine Adverse Event Reporting System (**http://vaers.hhs.gov/**).

ANTIMICROBIAL PROPHYLAXIS

Antimicrobial prophylaxis is defined as the use of antimicrobials in the absence of suspected or documented infection to prevent development of infection or disease. Antimicrobial prophylaxis is one of the most common indications for antimicrobial use in children, although its benefit has only been demonstrated for limited conditions or circumstances. Concerns about the emergence of resistant pathogens has led to a reexamination of the role of antimicrobial prophylaxis, especially for prevention of recurrent otitis media (OM) and urinary tract infection (UTI).

When using prophylactic antimicrobial therapy, the risks of development of antimicrobial resistance or having an adverse event from the antimicrobial must be weighed against potential benefits. Ideally, prophylactic agents should have a narrow spectrum of activity and be used for a brief period.

Infection-Prone Body Sites

Antimicrobial prophylaxis targeted at reducing infection at vulnerable body sites is most successful if the (1) period of risk is defined and brief; (2) expected pathogens have predictable antimicrobial susceptibility; and (3) antimicrobials achieve adequate concentrations in the targeted site.

ACUTE OTITIS MEDIA

Universal immunization of infants with pneumococcal conjugate vaccine has reduced the burden of acute otitis media (AOM) and recurrent OM and has altered the microbiology of AOM. The proportion of AOM attributable to *Streptococcus pneumoniae* has declined, while the proportion attributable to nontypeable *Haemophilus influenzae* and *Moraxella catarrhalis* has increased, potentially decreasing the effectiveness of antimicrobial prophylactic regimens relying on amoxicillin. Studies performed prior to the introduction of conjugate pneumococcal vaccines demonstrated that amoxicillin prophylaxis was modestly effective in reducing the frequency of recurrent episodes of OM in otitis-prone children, but once prophylaxis was discontinued, recurrent OM episodes occurred. In addition, greater understanding of the adverse impacts of antibiotic prophylaxis on the nasopharyngeal microbiome and colonization with resistant organisms has led to decreased use of antibiotic prophylaxis for the prevention of AOM.

No single strategy to prevent OM, including tympanostomy tube insertion, antimicrobial prophylaxis or episodic antimicrobial treatment, is superior and therefore an individualized approach for each child/family is appropriate. Guidelines for prevention of recurrent OM indicate that clinicians can offer tympanostomy tube insertion but should not prescribe antimicrobial prophylaxis, because it does not provide clear benefit and can cause development of antimicrobial resistance.[1]

---

[1] Lieberthal AS, Carroll AE, Chonmaitree T, et al. The diagnosis and management of acute otitis media. *Pediatrics.* 2013;131(3):e964-e999

Table 5.1. Circumstances in Which Antimicrobial Prophylaxis May or Should Be Considered[a]

Anatomic Site-Related Infections	Exposed Host; Time-Limited Exposure	Vulnerable Host (Pathogen); Ongoing Exposure
Urinary tract infection with vesicoureteral reflux (VUR) Endocarditis with certain underlying cardiac conditions Recurrent otitis media in select children	*Bordetella pertussis* exposure *Neisseria meningitidis* exposure Perinatal group B *Streptococcus* (perinatal) exposure Bite wound (human, animal, reptile) Infants whose birthing parent has HIV, to decrease the risk of HIV transmission Influenza virus, following close family exposure in those unimmunized Susceptible contacts of index cases of invasive *Haemophilus influenzae* type b disease or *Neisseria meningitidis* Exposure to aerosolized spores of *Bacillus anthracis* Exposure to tick bite in area with high prevalence of *Borrelia burgdorferi*[b] Ophthalmia neonatorum prophylaxis *(Neisseria gonorrhoeae)*	Immunosuppressed patients, eg, oncologic, rheumatologic, solid organ and hematopoietic cell transplant patients (*Pneumocystis jirovecii*, fungi, CMV, HSV, bacteremia from mucositis) HIV-infected children (*P jirovecii*, polysaccharide-encapsulated bacteria) Preterm neonates (*Candida* species) Anatomic or functional asplenia (polysaccharide-encapsulated bacteria)[c] Chronic granulomatous disease (*Staphylococcus aureus* and other catalase-positive bacteria and fungi) Congenital immune deficiencies (various pathogens) Rheumatic fever (group A *Streptococcus*) Treatment with eculizumab (*Neisseria meningitidis*) IgG and IgG subclass deficiency (respiratory pathogens)

CMV indicates cytomegalovirus; HIV, HSV, herpes simplex virus; IgG, immunoglobulin G.
[a]Antimicrobial prophylaxis regimens are described in each disease-specific chapter in Section 3.
[b]Prophylaxis of Lyme disease may be considered in specific circumstances (see Lyme Disease [p 549]).
[c]See Immunization and Other Considerations in Immunosuppressed Children (p 93).

URINARY TRACT INFECTION[1]

The role of chemoprophylaxis for UTI remains controversial because risk may outweigh benefit. The decision to provide prophylaxis requires weighing the benefit of modest reduction in recurrent UTI episodes and possible subsequent renal scarring versus the risk of colonization and infection with resistant organisms that may emerge during prophylaxis. Rather than ongoing prophylaxis, some experts prefer prompt diagnosis and effective treatment of each febrile UTI recurrence. The anatomic abnormalities of the urinary tract, the consequences of recurrent infection, the risks of

[1] American Academy of Pediatrics, Subcommittee on Urinary Tract Infections, Steering Committee on Quality Improvement and Management. Urinary tract infection: clinical practice guideline for the diagnosis and management of the initial UTI in febrile infants and children 2 to 24 months. *Pediatrics.* 2011;128(3):595-610

infection caused by a resistant pathogen, and the anticipated duration of prophylaxis need to be carefully assessed for each patient.

Children at highest risk for recurrence include those with first symptomatic UTI early in life, higher grades of vesicoureteral reflux (VUR), bilateral VUR, urinary stasis related to incomplete bladder emptying or anatomic conditions such as hydro-ureteronephrosis, and infection caused by pathogens other than *Escherichia coli*. Data do not support use of antimicrobial prophylaxis to prevent febrile recurrent UTIs in infants without VUR or conditions causing significant urinary stasis. The Randomized Intervention for Children with Vesicoureteral Reflux (RIVUR) study among children with grade I through grade IV VUR reported that chemoprophylaxis with trime-thoprim-sulfamethoxazole compared with placebo decreased recurrent UTI following a first or second febrile or symptomatic UTI by 50% but did not reduce renal scarring. Antibiotic prophylaxis to prevent recurrent UTI was most effective in children with bowel and bladder dysfunction and in those who were febrile at the time of presentation. However, among children who developed recurrent infection, those receiving prophylaxis had a higher rate of drug-resistant bacteria compared with children who did not receive prophylaxis. If prophylaxis is to be offered, children with high-grade reflux are most likely to benefit; low-grade reflux is believed to play little role in renal damage, and most studies show little benefit in prophylaxis with this group. Specific prophylaxis regimens should be based on antimicrobial susceptibility of prior infecting isolates. Trimethoprim-sulfamethoxazole or trimethoprim alone or nitrofurantoin can be used in infants and children over 2 months of age; beta-lactams are recommended for patients below 2 months of age.

Prophylaxis Following Exposure to Specific Pathogens

Prophylaxis may be indicated if an increased risk of serious infection with a specific pathogen exists and a specific antimicrobial agent has been demonstrated to decrease the risk of infection by that pathogen (eg, prophylaxis following exposure to *Neisseria meningitidis* [see Meningococcal Infections, p 585]). Pathogen-specific prophylaxis is addressed in Section 3. When prophylaxis is given, it is assumed that the benefit of prophylaxis is greater than the risk of adverse effects of the antimicrobial agent or the risk of subsequent infection by antimicrobial-resistant organisms. For some pathogens that colonize the upper respiratory tract, elimination of the carrier state can be difficult and may require use of a specific antimicrobial agent that achieves microbiologically effective concentrations in nasopharyngeal secretions (eg, rifampin).

Vulnerable Hosts

Attempts to prevent serious infections in immunocompromised patients with antimicrobial prophylaxis have been successful in some carefully defined at-risk populations. In some situations, such as prophylaxis of pneumococcal bacteremia/sepsis in children with asplenia or prophylaxis of sepsis caused by viridans group streptococci in children with leukemia, resistance to the prophylactic antibiotic may lead to decreased effectiveness of prophylaxis over time. In other situations, such as prophylaxis of *Pneumocystis* infection with trimethoprim-sulfamethoxazole in immunocompromised children, resistance has not developed despite years of continuous prophylaxis.

ANTIMICROBIAL PROPHYLAXIS IN PEDIATRIC SURGICAL PATIENTS

Surgical site infections (SSIs), which account for 20% of all hospital-acquired infections, prolong the length of hospitalization and increase the risk of death.[1] Prevention of SSIs are a priority for children's hospitals and surgical centers. Active surveillance targeting high-risk, high-volume procedures should be in place and requires education of surgeons and perioperative personnel, technological infrastructure, and use of a multidisciplinary team of trained personnel, including infection prevention specialists who are knowledgeable regarding SSI criteria. Institutions should monitor compliance with basic process measures and provide regular feedback to surgical personnel and hospital leadership.

Prevention of postoperative wound infections through perioperative prophylaxis is recommended for procedures with moderate or high infection rates or procedures in which a postoperative wound infection would have great consequences, such as implantation of prosthetic material into the heart. In contrast, for tissue sites already inoculated/infected, such as a ruptured appendix, antibiotics are used to treat rather than prevent infection. Consensus recommendations for prevention of SSIs in adults and children have been developed, although high-quality evidence for many of these recommendations is lacking. Although few data exist specifically for pediatric surgical prophylaxis, the principles of antimicrobial agent selection and exposure at surgical sites in adults should apply to children. Consequences of inappropriate use of prophylactic antimicrobial agents include increased costs, adverse events from toxicity, and emergence of resistant organisms. The emergence of drug-resistant organisms poses a risk not only to the recipient but also to other patients in whom a health care-associated infection could develop.

Guidelines for Appropriate Use

Guidelines for prevention of SSIs have been published.[2,3] General principles include the concepts that agents used for antimicrobial prophylaxis should prevent SSIs and related morbidity and mortality, reduce the duration and cost of care, minimize risk of adverse effects, minimize adverse consequences on the microbial flora, and not create SSIs from alternative pathogens. Published guidelines address indications, appropriate drug selection, dosing, preoperative timing and need for intraoperative redosing, and duration of prophylaxis. The Centers for Disease Control and Prevention (CDC) tracks and reports SSIs through the National Healthcare Safety Network (NHSN) and provides advice to prevent SSIs (**www.cdc.gov/hai/ssi/ssi.html**).

Indications for Prophylaxis

Major determinants of SSIs include the number of microorganisms in the wound during the procedure, the virulence of the microorganisms, the presence of foreign material in the wound, and host risk factors, including preoperative health status. The

---

[1] National Healthcare Safety Network. Surgical Site Infection Event (SSI). Centers for Disease Control and Prevention; January 2023. Available at: **www.cdc.gov/nhsn/pdfs/pscmanual/9pscssicurrent.pdf**

[2] Antimicrobial prophylaxis for surgery. *Med Lett Drugs Ther.* 2016;58(1495):63-68

[3] Berríos-Torres SI, Umscheid CA, Bratzler DW, et al. and the Healthcare Infection Control Practices Advisory Committee. Centers for Disease Control and Prevention Guideline for the Prevention of Surgical Site Infection, 2017. *JAMA Surg.* 2017;152(8):784-791

classification of surgical procedures is based on an estimation of bacterial contamination and, thus, risk of subsequent infection. The 4 classes are: (1) clean wounds; (2) clean-contaminated wounds; (3) contaminated wounds; and (4) dirty and infected wounds. Additional risk factors for SSIs include the operative site and the duration of the procedure. A patient risk index, which incorporates the preoperative physical status assessment score of the American Society of Anesthesiologists, the duration of the operation, and the aforementioned wound classification, has been demonstrated to be a good predictor of SSIs.[1] Others have summarized patients at "high risk" of surgical site infection.[2] Although a high-risk pediatric patient is not clearly defined, high-risk factors in adult patients include obesity, coexistent infections at a remote body site, altered immune response, colonization with pathogenic microorganisms, and diabetes mellitus.

CLEAN WOUNDS

Clean wounds are uninfected operative wounds in which no inflammation is encountered; the respiratory, alimentary, and genitourinary tracts or oropharyngeal cavity are not entered; and no break in aseptic technique occurred. The operative procedures usually are elective, and wounds are closed primarily and, if necessary, drained with closed drainage. Operative incisional wounds that follow nonpenetrating (blunt) trauma are included in this category, provided that the surgical procedure does not involve entry into the gastrointestinal or genitourinary tracts. The benefits of systemic antimicrobial prophylaxis do not justify the potential risks associated with antimicrobial use in most clean wound procedures, because the risk of infection is low (usually <1%). Some exceptions exist in which prophylaxis is administered because the risks or consequences of infection are high; examples include implantation of intravascular or deep tissue prosthetic material (eg, insertion of a prosthetic heart valve or a prosthetic joint), open-heart surgery for repair of structural defects, body cavity exploration in neonates, and most neurosurgical operations.

CLEAN-CONTAMINATED WOUNDS

In clean-contaminated wounds, the respiratory, alimentary, or genitourinary tracts are entered under controlled conditions without extensive contamination. Surgeries involving the gastrointestinal tract, biliary tract, appendix, vagina, or oropharynx, and urgent or emergency surgery in an otherwise clean procedure are included in this category, provided that no evidence of infection is encountered and no major break in aseptic technique occurs. Prophylaxis is limited to procedures in which a substantial amount of wound contamination is expected. The overall risk of infection for these surgical sites is 3% to 15%. On the basis of data from adults, procedures for which prophylaxis is indicated for pediatric patients include: (1) all gastrointestinal tract procedures in which there is obstruction, when the patient is receiving H_2 receptor

[1] Gaynes RP, Culver DH, Horan TC, Edwards JR, Richards C, Tolson JS. Surgical site infection (SSI) rates in the United States, 1992–1998: the National Nosocomial Surveillance System basic SSI risk index. *Clin Infect Dis.* 2001;33(Suppl 2):S69–S77

[2] Bratzler DW, Dellinger EP, Olsen KM, et al; American Society of Health-System Pharmacists; Infectious Disease Society of America; Surgical Infection Society; Society for Healthcare Epidemiology of America. Clinical practice guidelines for antimicrobial prophylaxis in surgery. *Am J Health Syst Pharm.* 2013;70(3):195-283

antagonists or proton pump blockers, or when the patient has a permanent foreign body; (2) selected biliary tract operations (eg, when there is obstruction from common bile duct stones); and (3) urinary tract surgery or instrumentation in the presence of bacteriuria or obstructive uropathy.

CONTAMINATED WOUNDS

Contaminated wounds are previously sterile tissue sites that are likely to be heavily contaminated with bacteria and include open, fresh wounds; operative wounds in the setting of major breaks in aseptic technique or gross spillage from the gastrointestinal tract; exposed viscera at birth from congenital anomalies; penetrating trauma of fewer than 4 hours duration; and incisions in which acute nonpurulent inflammation is encountered. The estimated rate of surgical site wound infection for these surgical sites is 15%, although it may be lower in healthy children. In wounds contaminated during procedures, antimicrobial prophylaxis is appropriate, but for those with acute nonpurulent inflammation isolated to, and contained within, an inflamed viscus (such as acute, nonperforated appendicitis or cholecystitis) with no wound contamination, prophylaxis is not necessary. For wounds in which contaminating bacteria have had an opportunity to establish inflammation and ongoing infection, antimicrobial use should be considered as treatment rather than prophylaxis.

DIRTY AND INFECTED WOUNDS

Dirty and infected wounds include penetrating trauma of more than 4 hours' duration from time of occurrence (the prolonged period assumes that the infection is already established), wounds with retained devitalized tissue, and wounds involving existing clinical infection or perforated viscera. This definition suggests that the organisms causing postoperative infection were present in the operative field before surgery, as noted above, and that antimicrobial use should be considered as treatment rather than prophylaxis. The estimated rate of infection for these surgical sites is 40%, although it may be lower in healthy children. In dirty and infected wound procedures, such as procedures for a perforated abdominal viscus (eg, ruptured appendix), a compound fracture, a laceration attributable to an animal or human bite >12 hours after injury, or when a major break in sterile technique occurs, antimicrobial agents are given as treatment rather than prophylaxis, although they may also prevent an infection of the surgical wound itself.

Surgical Site Infection Criteria

Specific classification criteria for SSIs have been developed by the National Healthcare Safety Network (NHSN) and are updated yearly (**www.cdc.gov/nhsn/index.html**). Reports from the NHSN are also posted periodically on the CDC website (**www.cdc.gov/nhsn/datastat/index.html**).

SUPERFICIAL INCISIONAL SSI

A superficial incisional SSI involves only the skin and subcutaneous layers of the incision and occurs within 30 days of the operation in a patient presenting with one of the following: (1) purulent drainage from the superficial incision; (2) an organism(s) that is (are) identified from an aseptically obtained specimen from the superficial incision or subcutaneous tissue by culture or molecular analysis; (3) surgical wound exploration (in the absence of laboratory results) when the patient presents with one of the following signs or symptoms: pain or tenderness, localized swelling, erythema, or pain; or (4) diagnosis of superficial incisional SSI by a physician, nurse practitioner, or physician assistant.

DEEP INCISIONAL SSI

A deep incisional SSI occurs within 30 or 90 days after the operative procedure, depending on the surgery; involves only the fascial or muscle layers; and results in at least 1 of the following: (1) purulent drainage from the deep incision but not from the organ/space component of the surgical site; (2) a deep incision that spontaneously dehisces or is deliberately opened by a physician, nurse practitioner, or physician assistant and at least 1 of the following signs or symptoms: fever (>38°C), localized pain, or localized tenderness; or (3) an abscess or other evidence of infection involving the deep incision that is found on direct examination, during reoperation, or by histopathologic or radiologic examination.

ORGAN/SPACE SSI

An organ or space SSI is defined by the specific site of infection that is opened and manipulated during the procedure (eg, endocarditis, mediastinitis, osteomyelitis). Organ/space SSI must occur within 30 or 90 days of the surgery (as defined by the specific procedure), and the patient must have 1 or more of the following: (1) purulent drainage from a drain that is placed through a stab wound into the organ/space; (2) organisms isolated from an aseptically obtained culture of fluid or tissue in the organ/space; or (3) an abscess or other evidence of infection involving the organ/space that is found on direct examination, during reoperation, or by histopathologic or radiologic examination.

Timing of Administration of Prophylactic Antimicrobial Agents

Effective chemoprophylaxis occurs only when the appropriate antimicrobial drug is present in tissues at sufficient local concentrations at the time of intraoperative bacterial contamination. Administration of an antimicrobial agent within 1 or 2 hours before surgery has been demonstrated to decrease the risk of wound infection. Accordingly, administration of the prophylactic agent is recommended within 60 minutes before surgical incision to ensure adequate tissue concentrations at the start of the procedure. When antimicrobial agents require longer administration times, such as glycopeptides (eg, vancomycin) or fluoroquinolones, administration should begin within 120 minutes prior to surgical incision.

Dosing and Duration of Administration of Antimicrobial Agents

Weight-based dosing for pediatric patients of all ages is routine. The preoperative doses should not exceed the usual dose for adults. Adequate antimicrobial concentrations should be maintained throughout the surgical procedure. In most instances, a single dose of an antimicrobial agent is sufficient, and the duration of prophylaxis after any procedure should not exceed 24 hours, with current data suggesting that no benefit can be documented for additional doses after surgery. Intraoperative dosing is required if the duration of the procedure is greater than 2 times the half-life of the antimicrobial agent or if there is excessive blood loss (eg, >1500 mL in adults). For example, cefazolin may be administered every 3 to 4 hours during a prolonged surgical procedure or one that involves large-volume blood loss. Postoperative doses after closure generally are not recommended in clean and clean-contaminated procedures, even in the presence of a drain.

Preoperative Screening and Decolonization

The use of preoperative surveillance to identify carriers of methicillin-susceptible *Staphylococcus aureus* (MSSA) or methicillin-resistant *S aureus* (MRSA) has been explored in the adult population. Recent changes in the epidemiology of MRSA suggest that risk of MRSA infections in children has decreased in the past decade, suggesting the targeted prophylaxis for MRSA may no longer be warranted. Use of preoperative nasal mupirocin and chlorhexidine baths for *S aureus* carriers may reduce the risk of deep SSI and is recommended as an adjunct to intravenous prophylaxis in adult cardiac and orthopedic surgery patients. Several small studies in children undergoing cardiac surgery have suggested similar benefit in using perioperative mupirocin.

Recommended Antimicrobial Agents

An antimicrobial agent is chosen based on bacterial pathogens most likely to cause infectious complications during and after the specific procedure, the antimicrobial susceptibility pattern of these pathogens, and the safety and efficacy of the drug. Antimicrobial agents administered prophylactically do not have to be active in vitro against every potential organism to be effective, because it is unlikely that all potential organisms are contaminating the wound. Doses are determined based on the need to achieve therapeutic blood and tissue concentrations throughout the procedure. Antimicrobial prophylaxis for most surgical procedures, including gastric, biliary, thoracic (noncardiac), vascular, neurosurgical, and orthopedic operations, can be achieved effectively using an agent such as a first-generation cephalosporin (eg, cefazolin) unless the risk for MRSA infection is high, in which case vancomycin may be indicated. For colorectal surgery or appendectomy, effective prophylaxis requires antimicrobial agents that are active against aerobic and anaerobic intestinal flora. Table 5.2 provides recommendations for drugs to be used in children undergoing surgical manipulation or invasive procedures. Physicians should be aware of potential interactions and adverse effects associated with prophylactic antimicrobial agents and other medications the patient may be receiving. Routine use of broad-spectrum agents (extended-spectrum cephalosporins, beta-lactam/beta-lactamase combinations, and carbapenems) for surgical prophylaxis generally is not necessary. Hospital antimicrobial stewardship programs should regularly update and evaluate compliance with antimicrobial prophylaxis protocols. There are no data to support the practice of continuing antibiotic prophylaxis until all invasive lines, drains, and indwelling catheters have been removed.

Routine use of vancomycin for prophylaxis is not recommended. However, vancomycin prophylaxis may be considered for patients with congenital heart disease who undergo cardiac surgery, patients who undergo certain orthopedic procedures (eg, spinal procedures, implantation of foreign materials), children known to be colonized

Table 5.2. Recommendations for Preoperative Antimicrobial Prophylaxis

Operation	Likely Pathogens	Recommended Drugs	Preoperative Dose
Neonatal (≤72 h of age)— all major procedures	Group B streptococci, enteric gram-negative bacilli,[a] enterococci	Ampicillin **PLUS** Gentamicin	50 mg/kg 4 mg/kg
Neonatal (>72 h of age)— all major procedures	Prophylaxis targeted to colonizing organisms, nosocomial organisms, and operative site		
Cardiac (cardiac surgical procedures, prosthetic valve or pacemaker, ventricular assist devices)	*Staphylococcus aureus*, *Corynebacterium* species, enteric gram-negative bacilli[a]	Cefazolin **OR** (if MRSA or MRSE is likely) Vancomycin	30 mg/kg (max 2 g; 3 g if ≥120 kg) 15 mg/kg
Gastrointestinal			
Esophageal and gastroduodenal	Enteric gram-negative bacilli,[a] gram-positive cocci	Cefazolin (high risk only[b])	30 mg/kg (max 2 g; 3 g if ≥120 kg)
Biliary tract	Enteric gram-negative bacilli,[a] enterococci	Cefazolin[c]	30 mg/kg (max 2 g; 3 g of ≥120 kg)
Colorectal or appendectomy (uncomplicated, nonperforated)	Enteric gram-negative bacilli,[a] enterococci, anaerobes (*Bacteroides* species)[d]	Cefoxitin or cefotetan **OR** Metronidazole **PLUS** Gentamicin **OR** Cefazolin **PLUS** Metronidazole	40 mg/kg (max 2 g) 15 mg/kg (max 500 mg) 2.5 mg/kg 30 mg/kg (max 2 g; 3 g if ≥120 kg) 15 mg/kg (max 500 mg)

Table 5.2. Recommendations for Preoperative Antimicrobial Prophylaxis, continued

Operation	Likely Pathogens	Recommended Drugs	Preoperative Dose
Ruptured viscus (regarded as treatment, not prophylaxis)	Enteric gram-negative bacilli,[a] enterococci, anaerobes (*Bacteroides* species)[d]	Cefoxitin **WITH OR WITHOUT** Gentamicin	40 mg/kg (max 2 g) 2.5 mg/kg
		OR	
		Gentamicin **PLUS** Metronidazole **PLUS** Ampicillin	2.5 mg/kg 15 mg/kg (max 500 mg) 50 mg/kg (max 2 g)
		OR	
		Piperacillin/tazobactam	80–100 mg/kg (max 3.375 g)
		OR	
		Other regimens for complicated appendicitis[e]	
Genitourinary	Enteric gram-negative bacilli,[a] enterococci, *S aureus*	Cefazolin	30 mg/kg (max 2 g; 3 if ≥120 kg)
		OR	
		Trimethoprim-sulfamethoxazole	4 mg/kg trimethoprim (max 160 mg), 20 mg/kg sulfamethoxazole (max 400 mg)

Table 5.2. Recommendations for Preoperative Antimicrobial Prophylaxis, continued

Operation	Likely Pathogens	Recommended Drugs	Preoperative Dose
Head and neck surgery (incision through oral or pharyngeal mucosa)	Anaerobes, enteric gram-negative bacilli,[a] S aureus	Cefazolin **PLUS** Metronidazole	30 mg/kg (max 2 g; 3 g if ≥120 kg) 15 mg/kg (max 500 mg)
		OR	
		Clindamycin **WITH OR WITHOUT** Gentamicin	10 mg/kg (max 900 mg) 2.5 mg/kg
		OR	
		Ampicillin-sulbactam	50 mg/kg (max 3g)
Neurosurgery (craniotomy, intrathecal baclofen shunt or ventricular shunt placement)	S aureus	Cefazolin	30 mg/kg (max 2 g; 3 g if ≥120 kg)
		OR	
		(if MRSA or MRSE is likely) Vancomycin	15 mg/kg

Table 5.2. Recommendations for Preoperative Antimicrobial Prophylaxis, continued

Operation	Likely Pathogens	Recommended Drugs	Preoperative Dose
Ophthalmic	*S aureus*, streptococci, enteric gram-negative bacilli;[a] *Pseudomonas* species	Gentamicin, ciprofloxacin, ofloxacin, moxifloxacin, tobramycin	Multiple drops topically for 2–24 h before procedure
		OR	
		Neomycin-gramicidin-polymyxin B	Multiple drops topically for 2–24 h before procedure
		OR	
		Cefazolin	100 mg, subconjunctivally at the end of the procedure
Orthopedic (internal fixation of fractures, implantation of materials including prosthetic joint and spinal procedures with and without instrumentation)	*S aureus*	Cefazolin	30 mg/kg (max 2 g; 3 g if ≥120 kg)
		OR	
		(if MRSA or MRSE is likely) Vancomycin	15 mg/kg
Thoracic (noncardiac)	*S aureus*, streptococci, gram-negative enteric bacilli[a]	Cefazolin	30 mg/kg (max 2 g; 3 g if ≥120 kg)
		OR	
		(if MRSA is likely) Vancomycin	15 mg/kg

Table 5.2. Recommendations for Preoperative Antimicrobial Prophylaxis, continued

Operation	Likely Pathogens	Recommended Drugs	Preoperative Dose
Traumatic wound (exceptionally varied pathogens, based on the anatomic site injured, and the instrument causing the trauma, particularly for penetrating injuries such as motor vehicle accidents or farm injuries)	Skin: *S aureus*, group A streptococci	Cefazolin	30 mg/kg (max 2 g; 3 g if ≥120 kg)
	Perforated viscus: gram-negative enteric bacilli, *Clostridium* species	Cefoxitin	40 mg/kg (max 2 g)
		WITH OR WITHOUT	
		Gentamicin	2.5 mg/kg
		OR	
		Gentamicin	2.5 mg/kg
		PLUS	
		Metronidazole	10 mg/kg (max 500 mg)
		PLUS	
		Ampicillin	50 mg/kg (max 2 g)
		OR	
		Piperacillin/tazobactam	80–100 mg/kg (max 3.375 g)
		OR	
		Other regimens for complicated appendicitis[e]	

MRSA indicates methicillin-resistant *Staphylococcus aureus*; MRSE, methicillin-resistant *Staphylococcus epidermidis*.

[a] Selection of antibiotics should take into consideration the susceptibility patterns of isolates found in the patient and at the institution.

[b] Esophageal obstruction, decreased gastric acidity, or gastrointestinal motility; see text for additional high risk factors.

[c] Acute cholecystitis, nonfunctioning gallbladder, obstructive jaundice, common duct stones.

[d] For *Bacteroides fragilis* group: high rates of resistance to clindamycin (only 25%–30% susceptible); lowest rates of resistance to metronidazole, carbapenems, ampicillin/sulbactam, and piperacillin/tazobactam. Resistance to cefoxitin reported at 30%.

[e] Solomkin JS, Mazuski JE, Bradley JS, et al. Diagnosis and management of complicated intra-abdominal infection in adults and children: guidelines by the Surgical Infection Society and the Infectious Diseases Society of America (erratum in *Clin Infect Dis*. 2010;50(12):1695; dosage error in article text). *Clin Infect Dis*. 2010;50(2):133-164.

or previously infected by MRSA, or children living in a community with a high rate of MRSA infections. Vancomycin is not as effective as cefazolin for the prevention of infection caused by many other organisms.

Misconceptions regarding penicillin allergies may result in patients receiving alternate and less-effective antibiotics for surgical prophylaxis. Efforts toward accurate labeling of patients with reported allergies include assessing the exact nature of the previous reaction, determining the likelihood that this reaction is a true immunoglobulin E (IgE)-mediated reaction, and determining the likelihood that the purported offending agent has cross-reactivity with the recommended perioperative antibiotic. Analysis of the chemical structure of the beta-lactams indicate little cross-reactivity between the penicillins and cefazolin, given differences in chemical side chains (see Fig 4.1, p 979). Institutions should develop programs (or at a minimum an algorithm) to assess, challenge (if appropriate) and delabel patients who do not have true penicillin allergy.

···

PREVENTION OF BACTERIAL ENDOCARDITIS

The Committee on Rheumatic Fever, Endocarditis, and Kawasaki Disease of the American Heart Association (AHA)'s Council on Cardiovascular Disease in the Young periodically issues detailed recommendations on the rationale, indications, and antimicrobial regimens for prevention of bacterial endocarditis for people at increased risk. The guidelines published in 2007[1] departed significantly from past recommendations in noting the lack of definitive evidence regarding the efficacy of antibiotic prophylaxis in preventing infective endocarditis (IE) after dental procedures. Bacteremia associated with most dental procedures represents only a very small fraction of bacteremia episodes that occur with events of daily living, such as brushing teeth, chewing, and other oral hygiene measures. The committee restricted recommendations for IE prophylaxis to a relatively narrow group of people who have certain cardiac abnormalities in which an episode of IE would likely carry a high risk of an adverse outcome. Additionally, IE prophylaxis was recommended for only a few procedures including only certain dental procedures and invasive airway procedures. Prophylaxis no longer is recommended for procedures involving the gastrointestinal and genitourinary tracts solely to prevent endocarditis.

In 2015, the AHA issued updated guidance on the epidemiology, clinical findings, pathogenesis, diagnosis, and treatment of pediatric bacterial endocarditis that included a short section on endocarditis prevention, which reiterated the 2007 published recommendations.[2] In 2017, a reconstituted expert AHA panel undertook a comprehensive review of the impact of 2007 endocarditis prophylaxis statement and whether, over the decade since original publication, the guidelines remained appropriate and valid.

---

[1] Wilson W, Taubert KA, Gewitz M, et al. Prevention of Infective Endocarditis. Guidelines from the American Heart Association. A Guideline From the American Heart Association Rheumatic Fever, Endocarditis, and Kawasaki Diseases Committee, Council on Cardiovascular Disease in the Young, and the Council on Clinical Cardiology, Council on Cardiovascular Surgery and Anesthesia, and the Quality of Care and Outcomes Research Interdisciplinary Working Group. *Circulation.* 2007;116(15):1736-1754

[2] Baltimore RS, Gewitz M, Baddour LM, et al; American Heart Association Rheumatic Fever, Endocarditis, and Kawasaki Disease Committee of the Council on Cardiovascular Disease in the Young and the Council on Cardiovascular and Stroke Nursing. Infective endocarditis in childhood: 2015 update: a scientific statement from the American Heart Association. *Circulation.* 2015;132(15):1487-1515

Table 5.3. Regimens for Antimicrobial Prophylaxis for selected Dental Procedures[a]

Clinical Circumstances	Antibiotic	Regimen: Single Dose 30 to 60 min Before Procedure	
		Children	Adults
Oral	Amoxicillin	50 mg/kg, PO	2 g, PO
Unable to take oral medication	Ampicillin	50 mg/kg, IM or IV	2 g, IM or IV
Allergic to penicillins or ampicillin	Cephalexin[b,c]	50 mg/kg, PO	2 g, PO
		OR	
	Clindamycin	20 mg/kg, PO	600 mg, PO
		OR	
	Azithromycin	15 mg/kg, PO	500 mg, PO
		OR	
	Clarithromycin	15 mg/kg, PO	500 mg, PO
		OR	
	Doxycycline	<45 kg, 2.2 mg/kg, PO ≥45 kg, 100 mg, PO	100 mg, PO
Allergic to penicillins or ampicillin and unable to take oral medication	Cefazolin or ceftriaxone[c]	50 mg/kg, IM (ceftriaxone) or IV (ceftriaxone or cefazolin)	1 g, IM or IV

IM, indicates intramuscular; IV, intravenous; PO, oral.

[a] Pediatric dosage should not exceed recommended adult dosage.

[b] Or other first- or second-generation oral cephalosporin in equivalent pediatric or adult dosage.

[c] Cephalosporins should not be used in a person with a history of anaphylaxis, angioedema, or urticaria with penicillins or ampicillin. In such cases, vancomycin 15 mg/kg IV (max 1 g) may be used in children.

Adapted from: Wilson WR, Gewitz M, Lockhart PB, et al; American Heart Association Young Hearts Rheumatic Fever, Endocarditis and Kawasaki Disease Committee of the Council on Lifelong Congenital Heart Disease and Heart Health in the Young; Council on Cardiovascular and Stroke Nursing; and Council on Quality of Care and Outcomes research. Prevention of viridans group streptococcal infective endocarditis: a scientific statement from the American Heart Association. *Circulation*. 2021;143(20):e963-e978.

This updated statement from the AHA was published in 2021[1] and focused specifically on viridans streptococcal IE, because those organisms are the principal pathogens in oral flora. The panel confirmed that the vast majority of data collected since 2017 indicated that reducing the indications for IE resulted in no increase in viridans group endocarditis and has been widely accepted by the dental and medical communities. Physicians should consult the published recommendations for further details **(https://doi.org/10.1161/CIR.0000000000000969)**.

Specific prophylactic regimens are presented in Table 5.3.

[1] Wilson WR, Gewitz M, Lockhart PB, et al; American Heart Association Young Hearts Rheumatic Fever, Endocarditis and Kawasaki Disease Committee of the Council on Lifelong Congenital Heart Disease and Heart Health in the Young; Council on Cardiovascular and Stroke Nursing; and Council on Quality of Care and Outcomes research. Prevention of viridans group streptococcal infective endocarditis: a scientific statement from the American Heart Association. *Circulation*. 2021;143(20):e963-e978

Cardiac conditions associated with the highest risk of an adverse outcome from endocarditis for which prophylaxis with dental procedures is reasonable include the following:

- Prosthetic cardiac valve or prosthetic material used for repair of valve.
- Durable mechanical circulatory support device (eg, ventricular assist device).
- Previous infective endocarditis.
- Congenital heart disease (CHD):
  - Unrepaired cyanotic CHD, including palliative shunts and conduits.
  - Completely repaired congenital heart defect with prosthetic material or device, whether placed by surgery or by catheter intervention, during the first 6 months after the procedure.
  - Repaired CHD with residual defect(s) at the site or adjacent to the site of a prosthetic patch or prosthetic device (which inhibits endothelialization).
  - Prosthetic pulmonary artery valve or conduit.
- Cardiac transplantation with subsequent cardiac valvulopathy.

Dental procedures for which endocarditis prophylaxis is reasonable for patients with a cardiac condition listed above include the following:

- All dental procedures that involve manipulation of gingival tissue or the periapical region of teeth or perforation of the oral mucosa. These procedures include cleaning, extractions, abscess drainage, biopsies, suture removal, and placement of orthodontic bands.
- The following procedures and events **do not** require prophylaxis: routine anesthetic injections through noninfected tissue, taking dental radiographs, placement of removable prosthodontic or orthodontic appliances, adjustment of orthodontic appliances, placement of orthodontic brackets, shedding of deciduous teeth, and bleeding from trauma to the lips or oral mucosa.

In addition, antibiotic prophylaxis is reasonable for the patients with cardiac conditions listed above who undergo an invasive procedure of the respiratory tract that involves incision or biopsy of the respiratory tract mucosa.

Neonatal Ophthalmia Prevention

Ophthalmia neonatorum is defined as conjunctivitis occurring within the first 4 weeks after birth. Infection usually is transmitted during passage through the birth canal. The causes and clinical characteristics of ophthalmia neonatorum are presented in Table 5.4. This chapter focuses on prevention of neonatal ophthalmia. Neonates with ophthalmia neonatorum disease require clinical evaluation with appropriate laboratory testing and prompt initiation of specific therapy if an infectious etiology is identified. See chapters on specific pathogens for appropriate laboratory testing, specific therapy, and other recommendations.

Primary Prevention

The current primary strategy for prevention of neonatal ophthalmia is based on antepartum identification and treatment of maternal infection, preventing exposure of the newborn infant. The Centers for Disease Control and Prevention (CDC) recommends routine first-trimester screening for chlamydia and gonorrhea in all

Table 5.4. Major and Minor Etiologies in Ophthalmia Neonatorum

Etiology of Ophthalmia Neonatorum	Proportion of Cases	Incubation Period (Days)	Severity of Conjunctivitis[a]	Associated Problems
Chlamydia trachomatis	2%–40%	5–12	+	Pneumonitis 3 wk–3 mo (see Chlamydial Infections, p 298)
Neisseria gonorrhoeae	Less than 1%	2–5	+++	Disseminated infection (see Gonococcal Infections, p 394)
Pseudomonas aeruginosa	Less than 1%	5–28	+++	Sepsis, meningitis
Other bacterial microbes[b]	30%–50%	5–14	+	Variable
Herpes simplex virus	Less than 1%	6–14	+[c]	Disseminated infection, meningoencephalitis (see Herpes Simplex, p 467); keratitis and ulceration also possible

[a] + indicates mild; +++, severe.

[b] Includes skin, respiratory, vaginal, and gastrointestinal tract pathogens such as *Staphylococcus aureus*, *Streptococcus pneumoniae*, nontypeable *Haemophilus influenzae*; group A and B streptococci, *Corynebacterium* species, *Moraxella catarrhalis*, *Escherichia coli*, and *Klebsiella pneumoniae*.

[c] Degree of purulence/local inflammatory response generally is not substantial, but consequences of untreated infection can be severe.

pregnant people 24 years or younger and older pregnant people at high-risk. Risk factors include having new or multiple sex partners, having a sex partner who has other concurrent partners or had a sexually transmitted infection, inconsistent condom use, previous or coexisting sexually transmitted infections, and exchanging sex for money or drugs. If there is uncertainty regarding risk during pregnancy, screening for *Chlamydia trachomatis* and *Neisseria gonorrhoeae* at the first prenatal visit can be considered, especially in areas of high prevalence of either pathogen. In addition, the CDC advises rescreening for chlamydia and gonorrhea during the third trimester for all pregnant people who remain at high risk as defined above, including all pregnant people 24 years and younger. When chlamydial infection is diagnosed during the first trimester, a test of cure to document chlamydial eradication should be performed approximately 4 weeks after treatment and repeated 3 months after treatment. When gonorrhea is diagnosed, it should be treated immediately, with repeat testing within 3 months.

Sex partners of infected individuals should also be tested and treated if positive. If a pregnant person has not been tested for *C trachomatis* and/or *N gonorrhoeae* before labor/delivery, testing should be performed during labor/delivery or immediately postpartum. If either pathogen is identified, the infant should receive therapy as outlined in the following sections.

Secondary Prevention

POSTEXPOSURE SYSTEMIC ANTIBIOTIC PROPHYLAXIS

To block transmission of infection, healthy infants whose birthing parent has untreated or inadequately treated gonococcal infection should receive 1 dose of ceftriaxone (25–50 mg/kg, intravenously [IV] or intramuscularly [IM], not to exceed 250 mg).[1] Ceftriaxone should be administered cautiously to hyperbilirubinemic infants, especially those born preterm. For infants in whom ceftriaxone is contraindicated (eg, receiving continuous intravenous calcium, as in parenteral nutrition), then 1 dose of cefotaxime (100 mg/kg, IV or IM), can be substituted for postexposure prophylaxis, if this agent is locally available. Other extended-spectrum cephalosporins, such as ceftazidime or cefepime, as a single dose, should be effective, although studies have not been performed. Note that gentamicin should not be used as treatment of neonates with gonococcal ocular disease because of inadequate penetration into the globe of the eye. Topical antimicrobial therapy alone is inadequate for *N gonorrhoeae*-exposed or -infected infants and is not necessary when systemic antimicrobial therapy is administered.

Infants whose birthing parent is known to have untreated chlamydial infection are at high risk of infection; however, prophylactic antimicrobial treatment is not indicated, because the efficacy of such treatment is unknown. Infants should be monitored clinically to ensure appropriate treatment if infection develops.

ROUTINE TOPICAL NEONATAL OPHTHALMIC PROPHYLAXIS

If gonorrhea is prevalent in the region and prenatal treatment cannot be ensured, or where required by law, a prophylactic agent of 0.5% erythromycin ointment should be instilled into the eyes of all newborn infants (including those born by cesarean delivery) to prevent sight-threatening gonococcal ophthalmia. Efficacy is unlikely to be influenced by delaying prophylaxis for as long as 1 hour to facilitate parent-infant bonding. Longer delays have not been studied for efficacy. Before administering local prophylaxis, each eyelid should be wiped gently with sterile cotton. A 1-cm ribbon of 0.5% erythromycin ointment should then be placed in each lower conjunctival sac. Ideally, ointment should be applied using single-use tubes or ampules rather than multiple-use tubes. The eyelids should then be massaged gently to spread the ointment. After 1 minute, excess ointment may be wiped away with sterile cotton. The ointment should not be flushed from the eyes after instillation, because flushing can decrease efficacy.

Periodic shortages of erythromycin ointment have occurred in recent years. If erythromycin ointment is not available, a birthing parent who is at risk for exposure to *N gonorrhoeae* or who had no prenatal care should be tested for *N gonorrhoeae* in the immediate peripartum setting using a nucleic acid amplification test (NAAT). If the birth parent's test is positive for gonorrheal infection or if the test result is pending at time of discharge with concerns for lack of follow-up, the neonate should receive ceftriaxone, 25 to 50 mg/kg of body weight, IV or IM, not to exceed 250 mg in a

---

[1] Centers for Disease Control and Prevention. Sexually transmitted infections treatment guidelines, 2021. *MMWR Recomm Rep*. 2021;70(RR-4):1-187. Available at: **www.cdc.gov/std/treatment-guidelines/gonorrhea-neonates.htm**

single dose[1-3]; if ceftriaxone is unavailable or contraindicated, a single dose of ceftazidime or cefepime may be substituted. Birthing parents at increased risk for gonococcal infection include those <25 years of age, and those 25 years or older who have a new partner, more than 1 sex partner, a sex partner with concurrent partners, or a sex partner who has an STI or lives in a community with high rates of gonorrhea; who practice inconsistent condom use when not in a mutually monogamous relationship; who have a previous or coexisting STI; who have a history of exchanging sex for money or drugs; or who have a history of incarceration. Information on current drug shortages in the United States can be found at **www.ashp.org/shortages**.[1,3]

Legal Mandates for Topical Prophylaxis for Neonatal Ophthalmia

The American Academy of Pediatrics supports ongoing reevaluation of the continued necessity of legislative mandates in the United States for universal neonatal eye prophylaxis[2] and advocates for the following preventive strategies:

- Diligent compliance with CDC recommendations for prenatal screening for and treatment of *N gonorrhoeae* and *C trachomatis* to prevent intrapartum exposures.
- Testing of unscreened individuals for *N gonorrhoeae* and *C trachomatis* infection at the time of labor or delivery, with treatment of infected birthing parents and their infants.
- Counseling of parents to bring conjunctival discharge and inflammation to immediate medical attention, resulting in optimal treatment of neonatal ophthalmia.
- Education of newborn care providers to ensure awareness that purulent conjunctivitis in a newborn infant requires thorough diagnostic evaluation and prompt specific treatment.
- Continuation of mandatory reporting of cases of gonococcal ophthalmia neonatorum to identify patterns of failure of primary prevention measures.

In regions where gonorrhea remains prevalent and prenatal screening and treatment is not routinely achievable, neonatal topical prophylaxis remains appropriate.

Pseudomonal Ophthalmia Neonatorum

Neonatal ophthalmia attributable to *Pseudomonas aeruginosa* is infrequent but may now be as common as gonococcal ophthalmia. This form of neonatal ophthalmia has a predilection for preterm infants and presents with eyelid edema and erythema, purulent discharge, and pannus formation. Because superficial infection can progress rapidly to corneal perforation, endophthalmitis, blindness, serious systemic infection (sepsis, meningitis), and death, this form of bacterial neonatal ophthalmia urgently requires a combination of systemic and topical therapy, because systemic antibiotics

---

[1] US Preventive Services Task Force. Screening for chlamydia and gonorrhea: US Preventive Services Task Force Recommendation Statement. *JAMA*. 2021;326(10):949-956

[2] Nolt D, O'Leary ST, Aucott SW; American Academy of Pediatrics, Committee on Infectious Diseases, Committee on Fetus and Newborn. Risks of infectious diseases in newborns exposed to alternative perinatal practices. *Pediatrics*. 2022;149(2):e2021055554

[3] Centers for Disease Control and Prevention. Sexually transmitted infections treatment guidelines, 2021. *MMWR Recomm Rep*. 2021;70(RR-4):1-187. Available at: **www.cdc.gov/std/treatment-guidelines/gonorrhea-neonates.htm**

alone have poor penetration into the anterior chamber of the eye. The diagnosis should be suspected when Gram-stained specimens of exudate contain gram-negative bacilli and should be confirmed by culture. Until *Pseudomonas* infection is excluded, evaluation for systemic infection and topical and systemic therapy are recommended. Ophthalmology consultation is also recommended.

Other Nongonococcal, Nonchlamydial Ophthalmia

Neonatal ophthalmia can be caused by many other bacterial pathogens (see Table 5.4). In general, uncomplicated resolution can be expected with topical treatment of these infections.

Herpes simplex keratoconjunctivitis should be considered in neonates with conjunctival inflammation and discharge, particularly when tests for bacterial and chlamydial infection are negative. The diagnosis should be suspected if there are also cutaneous vesicles or oral ulcers or vesicles and can be confirmed by demonstration of dendritic keratitis (requiring ophthalmology consultation for examination with fluorescein staining), or by virologic testing (eg, nucleic acid amplification test [NAAT] or culture). Specific treatment is indicated (see Herpes Simplex, p 467). Conjunctivitis caused by other viruses generally resolves without specific treatment.

APPENDIX I

Directory of Resources[a]

Organization	Telephone/Fax Number	Web Site
AIDSinfo	**1-800-HIV-0440 (1-800-448-0440** United States 1:00–4:00 pm Eastern time zone) 1-301-315-2816 (Outside US) TTY: 1-888-480-3739 Fax: 1-301-315-2818	**hivinfo.nih.gov**
American Academy of Pediatrics (AAP)	1-630-626-6000 1-800-433-9016 Fax: 1-847-434-8000 Publications/Customer Service: 1-866-THEAAP1 (1-866-843-2271)	**www.aap.org**
American Sexual Health Association	1-919-361-8400 Fax: 1-919-361-8425	**www.ashasexualhealth.org**
American Society of Health System Pharmacists current drug shortage listing		**www.ashp.org/shortages**
Canadian Paediatric Society (CPS)	1-613-526-9397 Fax: 1-613-526-3332	**www.cps.ca**
Centers for Disease Control and Prevention (CDC)	1-800-CDC-INFO (1-800-232-4636) TTY: 1-888-232-6348	**www.cdc.gov** **www.cdc.gov/cdc-info/index.html** **wwwn.cdc.gov/dcs/ContactUs/Form**
CDC Emergency Operations Center (24-Hour Service)	1-770-488-7100	
Advisory Committee on Immunization Practices		**www.cdc.gov/vaccines/acip**

Directory of Resources,[a] continued

Organization	Telephone/Fax Number	Web Site
Botulism case consultation and antitoxin	1-770-488-7100	www.cdc.gov/botulism/health-professional.html
Diphtheria case consultation and antitoxin	1-770-488-7100	www.cdc.gov/diphtheria/dat.html
Division of Foodborne, Waterborne, and Environmental Diseases		www.cdc.gov/ncezid/dfwed
Division of Healthcare Quality Promotion	1-404-639-4000	www.cdc.gov/ncezid/dhqp/index.html
Division of High-Consequence Pathogens and Pathology	1-404-639-3574	www.cdc.gov/ncezid/dhcpp
Division of Tuberculosis Elimination	1-404-639-8120	www.cdc.gov/tb
Division of Vector-Borne Diseases	1-970-221-6400	www.cdc.gov/ncezid/dvbd
Division of Viral Hepatitis		www.cdc.gov/hepatitis/index.htm
Drug Service	1-404-639-3670 (business hours) 1-770-488-7100 (after hours) Fax: 404-639-3717	www.cdc.gov/laboratory/drugservice
Influenza		www.cdc.gov/flu
Malaria Hotline	1-770-488-7788 1-855-856-4713 (toll free) 1-770-488-7100 (after hours)	www.cdc.gov/malaria
National Prevention Information Network	1-800-458-5231	https://npin.cdc.gov
Parasitic Diseases Branch	1-404-718-4745	www.cdc.gov/parasites
Travelers' Health	1-877-394-8747	wwwnc.cdc.gov/travel
Vaccines and Immunizations		www.cdc.gov/vaccines

Directory of Resources,[a] continued

Organization	Telephone/Fax Number	Web Site
Vaccine Information Statements		www.cdc.gov/vaccines/hcp/vis/index.html
Vaccines for Children Program		www.cdc.gov/vaccines/programs/vfc/index.html
Vaccine Safety		www.cdc.gov/vaccinesafety/index.html
Vaccine Shortages and Delays		www.cdc.gov/vaccines/hcp/clinical-resources/shortages.html
European Society for Paediatric Infectious Diseases		www.espid.org
Food and Drug Administration (FDA)	1-888-INFO-FDA (1-888-463-6332)	www.fda.gov
Drugs	1-855-543-3784 1-301-796-3400	www.fda.gov/drugs
Pediatrics		www.fda.gov/science-research/science-and-research-special-topics/pediatrics
Vaccines, Blood, and Biologics	1-800-835-4709 1-240-402-8010	www.fda.gov/BiologicsBloodVaccines/default.htm
MedWatch	1-800-FDA-1088 (1-800-332-1088)	www.fda.gov/safety/medwatch-fda-safety-information-and-adverse-event-reporting-program
Vaccine Adverse Event Reporting System (VAERS)	1-800-822-7967 Fax: 1-877-721-0366	https://vaers.hhs.gov/index.html

Directory of Resources,[a] continued

Organization	Telephone/Fax Number	Web Site
FDA-Approved Vaccine Package Inserts		www.fda.gov/vaccines-blood-biologics/vaccines/vaccines-licensed-use-united-states
Immunize.org [formerly the Immunization Action Coalition (IAC)]	1-651-647-9009 Fax: 1-651-647-9131	www.immunize.org
Infectious Diseases Society of America (IDSA)	1-703-299-0200 Fax: 1-703-299-0204	www.idsociety.org
Institute for Vaccine Safety		www.vaccinesafety.edu
National Academy of Medicine	1-202-334-2000	https://nam.edu
National Institutes of Health (NIH)	1-301-496-4000 TTY: 1-301-402-9612	www.nih.gov
Eunice Kennedy Shriver National Institute of Child Health and Human Development	1-800-370-2943 Fax: 1-866-760-5947	www.nichd.nih.gov
National Institute of Allergy and Infectious Diseases (NIAID)	1-301-496-5717 1-866-284-4107 TDD: 1-800-877-8339 Fax: 1-301-402-3573	www.niaid.nih.gov
National Library of Medicine	1-888-346-3656	www.nlm.nih.gov
National Network of STD Clinical Prevention Training Centers (NNPTC) STD Clinical Consultation Network		https://stdccn.org/render/Public
National Resource Center for Health and Safety in Child Care and Early Education	888-227-5125	nrckids.org

Directory of Resources,[a] continued

Organization	Telephone/Fax Number	Web Site
National Vaccine Injury Compensation Program	1-800-338-2382	www.hrsa.gov/vaccinecompensation/index.html
National Vaccine Program Office (NVPO)	1-202-690-5566	www.hhs.gov/nvpo
Pediatric Oncology Branch, Center for Cancer Research, National Cancer Institute	1-240-760-6560	https://ccr.cancer.gov/Pediatric-Oncology-Branch
Pediatric Infectious Diseases Society (PIDS)	1-703-299-6764 Fax: 1-703-299-0473	www.pids.org
Sociedad Latinoamericana de Infectología Pediátrica (SLIPE)		www.slipe.org
Vaccine Education Center of the Children's Hospital of Pennsylvania		www.chop.edu/centers-programs/vaccine-education-center
Voices for Vaccines	1-678-870-5877	www.voicesforvaccines.org
World Health Organization (WHO)	(+41 22) 791 21 11 Regional Office for the Americas: 1-202-974-3000 Fax: 1-202-974-3663	www.who.int

[a]Internet addresses and telephone/fax numbers are current at the time of publication.

....
APPENDIX II

Codes for Commonly Administered Pediatric Vaccines, Toxoids, and Immune Globulins

Vaccine, toxoid, and immune globulin codes use a specific vaccine *Current Procedural Terminology* (CPT) code to indicate which vaccine product was administered to the patient. A regularly updated listing of CPT product codes for commonly administered pediatric vaccines can be found at **https://downloads.aap.org/AAP/PDF/coding_vaccine_coding_table.pdf?_ga=2.32279294.1928077618.1652908186-1981473643.1640014472.**

CPT codes for vaccine administration ("Immunization Administration") are reported in addition to the CPT codes for specific vaccines and toxoid products. Codes 90460 and 90461 are only reported when the physician or other qualified health care professional provides face-to-face counseling during the encounter when a vaccine is administered to a patient through 18 years of age. Code 90460 should be reported for each vaccine administered, as it accounts for counseling on the first (or only) vaccine component. For vaccines with more than one component, code 90460 should be reported for the first component in conjunction with code 90461 for each additional component in a given vaccine (eg, DTaP counseling and administration will be reported with 90460 x 1 plus 90461 x 2). Multivalent antigens or multiple serotypes of antigens against a single organism are considered a single component of vaccines (eg, PCV-13 administration should use only one 90460). Without counseling by the physician or qualified health care professional, or if the patient is 18 years or older, report administration codes 90471–90474 instead based on the number of vaccines administered and the route of administration.

ICD-10-CM has only a single diagnosis code for reporting vaccines and vaccine administration, Z23. When reporting vaccines administered, ICD-10-CM requires use of code Z23 regardless of the reason for the encounter. For example, if vaccines are given as part of a childhood preventive care visit, code Z23 should be reported in addition to code Z00.121 or Z00.129 (encounter for routine child health examination, with or without abnormal findings). Codes Z00.110 (health examination for newborn under 8 days old) and Z00.111 (health examination for newborn 8 to 28 days old) can be used when parents defer the birth dose of hepatitis B vaccine. When a vaccine like tetanus is given during wound management, the code for the wound is primary and Z23 is secondary.

Immune globulin products are not considered vaccines, and the administration code 96372, therapeutic injection given intramuscularly or subcutaneously, should be used in all cases. For perinatal hepatitis B exposure, hepatitis B immune globulin (HBIG), use CPT code 90371 for the immunoglobulin product, and ICD-10-CM codes P00.2 (for perinatal exposure to maternal infection) and Z20.5 (for exposure to viral hepatitis). For rabies immune globulin (RIG) and rabies vaccine administration, ICD-10-CM code Z20.3 (contact with and [suspected] exposure to rabies) should be reported as well as the ICD-10-CM codes describing the nature of the injuries and circumstances surrounding the injury, including type of animal involved (ie, codes found in the V-Y categories). The ICD-10-CM code Z29.14, encounter for prophylactic RIG, can also be used.

For palivizumab (recombinant monoclonal RSV antibody), CPT code 90378 should be used for the product (with 1 unit per 50 mg administered), and the appropriate ICD-10-CM diagnoses of gestational age and/or other medical condition(s) that support the need to administer palivizumab should be reported. The ICD-10-CM code Z29.1, encounter for prophylactic immunotherapy, may be used in addition.

Although nirsevimab (the long-acting monoclonal RSV antibody) is categorized as a monoclonal antibody by CPT, ICD-10-CM's index suggests the appropriate diagnosis code is Z29.11, encounter for prophylactic immunotherapy for RSV. Report the administration of nirsevimab with code 96380 (administration of respiratory syncytial virus, monoclonal antibody, seasonal dose by intramuscular injection, with counseling by physician or other qualified health care professional) or with code 96381 (administration of respiratory syncytial virus, monoclonal antibody, seasonal dose by intramuscular injection). Do not report immunization administration codes 90461–90462 or 90471–90472 for the administration of nirsevimab, as these codes are limited to administering vaccine and toxoid products. To prevent cost share being passed on to the patient, append modifier 33 to the administration code to indicate to the payer that this was part of a preventive service.

・・・・・・・・・・・・・・・・・・・・・・
APPENDIX III

Nationally Notifiable Infectious Diseases in the United States

Nationally notifiable infectious diseases are those that public health officials from local, state, and territorial public health departments voluntarily report to the Centers for Disease Control and Prevention (CDC). Surveillance for nationally notifiable infectious diseases helps public health agencies monitor the occurrence and spread of disease across the nation and evaluate prevention and control measures, among other purposes. To ensure consistency in how the data are classified and enumerated, national surveillance case definitions are established and used for each disease. The Council of State and Territorial Epidemiologists (CSTE), with advice from the CDC, reviews the list of nationally notifiable infectious diseases on an annual basis and may recommend that a disease be added or deleted from the list or that a case definition be revised. Provisional nationally notifiable infectious disease data are published in weekly tables and finalized data are published in annual tables, available from the "Data and Statistics" section of the National Notifiable Diseases Surveillance System website (**www.cdc.gov/nndss/ data-statistics/index.html**). The CDC receives either daily or weekly case notifications for approximately 120 nationally notifiable diseases from all states, Washington, DC, New York City, and 5 US territories. For a subset of cases that meet the criteria for being a potential public health emergency of international concern, as per the 2005 revised International Health Regulations (**www.who.int/publications/i/ item/9789241580496**), the CDC Emergency Operations Center notifies the Department of Health and Human Services Secretary's Operations Center, which in turn notifies the World Health Organization. The World Health Organization makes the final determination about whether a public health emergency of international concern exists. The 2023 list of nationally notifiable infectious diseases, most of which are infectious, is included in Table 1. Should a more current list of such diseases be needed, visit **https://ndc.services.cdc.gov/**, select year of interest for the notifiable condition list year, check "Infectious" conditions, and click "Get Notifiable List by Year."

Case notifications submitted to the CDC are based on data collected at the local, state, and territorial levels as a result of legislation and regulations in those jurisdictions that require health care providers, clinical laboratories, hospitals, and other entities to submit health-related data on reportable diseases to public health departments. Case reporting to local, state, or territorial public health officials provides the information needed to investigate these diseases and to implement prevention and control strategies, among other purposes. Because the list of reportable infectious diseases is determined by local, state, and territorial law and varies by jurisdiction, health care providers, clinical laboratories, hospitals, and other required reporters are strongly encouraged to obtain specific reporting requirements from the appropriate public health department, including the timeliness required for case reporting.

If a reportable disease meets the criteria for a nationally notifiable infectious disease, the local, state, or territorial public health department will submit a case notification to the CDC. The timeliness of such case notifications to the CDC varies by disease, with some requiring notification within 4 hours of a case meeting the notification criteria. In addition, local or state reporting requirements for additional diseases may exist.

Table 1. Infectious Diseases and Conditions Designated as Notifiable at the National Level—United States, 2023[1,2]

- Anthrax
- Arboviral diseases, neuroinvasive and nonneuroinvasive
  - California serogroup virus diseases
  - Chikungunya virus disease
  - Eastern equine encephalitis virus disease
  - Powassan virus disease
  - St. Louis encephalitis virus disease
  - West Nile virus disease
  - Western equine encephalitis virus disease
- Babesiosis
- Botulism
  - Botulism, foodborne
  - Botulism, infant
  - Botulism, wound
  - Botulism, other
- Brucellosis
- Campylobacteriosis
- *Candida auris*, clinical
- *Candida auris*, screening
- Carbapenemase-producing organisms
- Carbapenemase-producing organisms, clinical
- Carbapenemase-producing organisms, screening
- Chancroid
- *Chlamydia trachomatis* infection
- Cholera
- Coccidioidomycosis
- Congenital syphilis
  - Syphilitic stillbirth
- Coronavirus disease 2019 (COVID-19)
- Cryptosporidiosis
- Cyclosporiasis

- Dengue virus infections
  - Dengue
  - Dengue-like illness
  - Severe dengue
- Diphtheria
- Ehrlichiosis and Anaplasmosis
  - *Anaplasma phagocytophilum* infection
  - *Ehrlichia chaffeensis* infection
  - *Ehrlichia ewingii* infection
  - Undetermined human ehrlichiosis/anaplasmosis
- Giardiasis
- Gonorrhea
- *Haemophilus influenzae*, invasive disease
- Hansen's disease
- Hantavirus infection, non-Hantavirus pulmonary syndrome
- Hantavirus pulmonary syndrome
- Hemolytic uremic syndrome, postdiarrheal
- Hepatitis A, acute
- Hepatitis B, acute
- Hepatitis B, chronic
- Hepatitis B, perinatal virus infection
- Hepatitis C, acute
- Hepatitis C, chronic
- Hepatitis C, perinatal infection
- HIV infection (AIDS has been reclassified as HIV Stage III)
- Influenza-associated pediatric mortality
- Invasive pneumococcal disease
- Legionellosis

- Leptospirosis
- Listeriosis
- Lyme disease
- Malaria
- Measles
- Melioidosis
- Meningococcal disease
- Monkeypox virus infection
- Mumps
- Novel influenza A virus infections
- Pertussis
- Plague
- Poliomyelitis, paralytic
- Poliovirus infection, nonparalytic
- Psittacosis
- Q fever
  - Q fever, acute
  - Q fever, chronic
- Rabies, animal
- Rabies, human
- Rubella
- Rubella, congenital syndrome
- *Salmonella* Paratyphi infection (*Salmonella enterica* serotypes Paratyphi A, B [tartrate negative], and C [*S* Paratyphi])
- *Salmonella* Typhi infection (*Salmonella enterica* serotype Typhi)
- Salmonellosis
- Severe acute respiratory syndrome-associated coronavirus disease
- Shiga toxin-producing *Escherichia coli*
- Shigellosis
- Smallpox
- Spotted fever rickettsiosis
- Streptococcal toxic shock syndrome

[1] **https://ndc.services.cdc.gov/**

[2] **www.cdc.gov/nndss/data-statistics/index.html**

Table 1. Infectious Diseases and Conditions Designated as Notifiable at the National Level—United States, 2023,[1,2] continued

- Syphilis
  - Syphilis, primary
  - Syphilis, secondary
  - Syphilis, early nonprimary nonsecondary
  - Syphilis, unknown duration or late
- Tetanus
- Toxic shock syndrome (other than streptococcal)
- Trichinellosis
- Tuberculosis
- Tularemia
- Vancomycin-intermediate *Staphylococcus aureus* and vancomycin-resistant *Staphylococcus aureus*

- Varicella
- Varicella deaths
- Vibriosis
- Viral hemorrhagic fever
  - Crimean-Congo hemorrhagic fever virus
  - Ebola virus
  - Lassa virus
  - Lujo virus
  - Marburg virus
  - New World arenavirus – Chapare virus
  - New World arenavirus – Guanarito virus
  - New World arenavirus – Junin virus

  - New World arenavirus – Machupo virus
  - New World arenavirus – Sabia virus
- Yellow fever
- Zika virus disease and Zika virus infection
  - Zika virus disease, congenital
  - Zika virus disease, noncongenital
  - Zika virus infection, congenital
  - Zika virus infection, noncongenital

[1] https://ndc.services.cdc.gov/

[2] www.cdc.gov/nndss/data-statistics/index.html

··············
Appendix IV

Guide to Contraindications and Precautions to Immunizations

A **contraindication** to vaccination is a condition in a patient that increases the risk of a serious adverse reaction and for whom this increased risk of an adverse reaction outweighs the benefit of the vaccine. A vaccine should not be administered when a contraindication is present. The only contraindication applicable to all vaccines is a history of anaphylaxis to a previous dose or to a vaccine component, unless the patient has undergone desensitization. Refer to the Description section of manufacturers' package inserts for components of each vaccine; package inserts for vaccines that are licensed for use in the United States are available at **www.fda.gov/ BiologicsBloodVaccines/Vaccines/ApprovedProducts/ucm093833.htm.**

The Centers for Disease Control and Prevention "Pink Book" (*Epidemiology and Prevention of Vaccine-Preventable Diseases* [**www.cdc.gov/vaccines/pubs/pinkbook/ genrec.html#contraindications**]) is also a helpful resource.

A **precaution** is a condition in a recipient that might increase the risk or seriousness of an adverse reaction, might interfere with vaccine effectiveness, or might complicate making another diagnosis because of a possible vaccine-related reaction. The only precaution applicable to all vaccines is moderate or severe acute illness, with or without fever.

People who administer vaccines should screen recipients for contraindications and precautions before administering vaccines, and this screening should be documented (eg, in the electronic health record).

A table that lists contraindications and precautions for commonly used vaccines can be found at **www.cdc.gov/vaccines/hcp/acip-recs/general-recs/ contraindications.html.** This information is based on recommendations of the Committee on Infectious Diseases of the American Academy of Pediatrics (AAP) and of the Advisory Committee on Immunization Practices (ACIP) of the Centers for Disease Control and Prevention (CDC). Sometimes, these recommendations differ from information in the manufacturers' package inserts. In addition, ACIP recommendations for influenza vaccine are updated on an annual basis and the most recent contraindications and precautions for influenza vaccines can be found at **www.cdc.gov/ vaccines/hcp/acip-recs/vacc-specific/flu.html.** Information on discussing vaccine recommendations with patients and families can be found in Understanding Vaccine Evaluation and Safety as an Approach to Addressing Parental Concerns, p 27.

....
APPENDIX V

Prevention of Infectious Disease From Contaminated Food Products

Foodborne diseases are associated with significant morbidity and mortality in people of all ages. The Foodborne Diseases Active Surveillance Network (FoodNet) of the CDC Emerging Infections Program conducts active, population-based surveillance at 10 sites in the United States, for all laboratory-diagnosed infections with select enteric pathogens transmitted commonly through food. The FoodNet program conducts surveillance for illnesses caused by *Campylobacter* species, *Cyclospora cayetanensis*, *Listeria monocytogenes*, *Salmonella* species, Shiga toxin-producing *Escherichia coli* (STEC) O157 and non-O157 STEC, *Shigella* species, *Vibrio* species, and enteric *Yersinia* species. FoodNet also conducts surveillance for hemolytic-uremic syndrome (HUS), which is a complication of STEC infection. In 2019, compared with the previous 3 years, the incidence of infections caused by pathogens transmitted commonly through food increased (for *Campylobacter*, *Cyclospora*, *Vibrio*, and *Yersinia* species, and STEC) or remained unchanged (for *Listeria*, *Salmonella*, and *Shigella* species).[1] Additional information about FoodNet can be found at **www.cdc.gov/foodnet/index.html.**

Outbreak surveillance provides insights into the causes of foodborne illness, types of implicated foods, and settings where transmission occurs. The CDC collects data on foodborne disease outbreaks submitted from all states and territories (**www.cdc. gov/foodsafety/fdoss/index.html**). In 2019, the Centers for Disease Control and Prevention (CDC) reported 873 foodborne disease outbreaks, resulting in roughly 12 000 illnesses, 1000 hospitalizations, and 2 deaths. Young children, pregnant people, elderly people, and immunocompromised people are especially susceptible to illnesses and complications caused by many of the organisms associated with foodborne illness.

Norovirus is the most common cause of outbreaks of foodborne illness in the United States. The system for surveillance and reporting for norovirus outbreak specimens is known as CaliciNet (**www.cdc.gov/norovirus/reporting/calicinet/ index.html**).

Public health, regulatory, and agricultural professionals can use this information when creating targeted control strategies and to support efforts to promote safe food preparation practices among food industry employees and the public. Data on foodborne disease outbreaks are available online through the National Outbreak Reporting System Dashboard (**wwwn.cdc.gov/norsdashboard**).

Four general rules should be followed for food safety:
1. **Clean:** Wash hands and surfaces thoroughly and often.
2. **Separate:** Do not cross-contaminate.
3. **Chill:** Refrigerate foods promptly.
4. **Cook:** Prepare and heat food to the proper temperature.

The following preventive measures can be implemented to decrease the risk of infection from specific foods.

---

[1] Tack DM, Ray L, Griffin PM, et al. Preliminary incidence and trends of infections with pathogens transmitted commonly through food—Foodborne Diseases Active Surveillance Network, 10 U.S. Sites, 2016–2019. *MMWR Morb Mortal Wkly Rep.* 2020;69(17):509-514

UNPASTEURIZED MILK AND MILK PRODUCTS

The American Academy of Pediatrics (AAP) endorses the use of pasteurized milk and recommends that parents be fully informed of the important risks associated with consumption of unpasteurized milk.[1] Interstate sale of unpasteurized (raw) milk and products made from unpasteurized milk (with the exception of certain hard cheeses) is banned by the US Food and Drug Administration (FDA). The most vulnerable populations, such as children, pregnant people, elderly people, and immunocompromised people, should not consume unpasteurized milk or products made from unpasteurized milk, including cheese, butter, yogurt, pudding, or ice cream, from any species, including cows, sheep, and goats. Serious infections attributable to *Salmonella* species, *Campylobacter* species, *Mycobacterium bovis*, *L monocytogenes*, *Brucella* species, STEC, *Y enterocolitica*, and *Cryptosporidium parvum* have been linked to consumption of unpasteurized milk. Although some states allow the sale of raw milk that meets state-designated arbitrary standards (certified milk), "certified" raw milk has also been linked to outbreaks. A number of outbreaks of *Campylobacter* infection among children have been associated with school field trips to farms during which children consumed raw milk. School officials should take precautions to prevent raw milk from being served to children during educational trips. Cheeses made from unpasteurized milk also have been associated with illnesses attributable to *Brucella* species, *L monocytogenes*, *Salmonella* species, *Campylobacter* species, *Shigella* species, *M bovis*, and STEC. Soft cheese made from pasteurized milk can be contaminated during production. Outbreaks of *Listeria* infections have more often been linked to soft cheese made from pasteurized milk rather than raw milk (**www.cdc.gov/ nationalsurveillance/pdfs/listeria-annual-summary-2014-508.pdf**).

RAW AND UNDERCOOKED EGGS

Children and other groups at high risk of severe foodborne disease should not eat raw or undercooked eggs, unpasteurized powdered eggs, or foods that may contain raw or undercooked eggs. Ingestion of raw or improperly cooked eggs can result in severe illness attributable to *Salmonella* species. Examples of foods that may contain raw or undercooked eggs include some homemade frostings and mayonnaise, homemade ice cream, tiramisu, eggs prepared "sunny-side up," Caesar salad dressing, Hollandaise sauce, cookie dough, and cake batter.

RAW DOUGH

Children should not eat raw dough, including unbaked goods such as cookies, tortillas, pizza, biscuits, or pancakes. Children should not play with raw dough, such as at home for crafts or at restaurants. Several regional outbreaks have been linked to STEC present in raw flour. Cookie dough in ice cream sold commercially is now treated to prevent transmission of pathogens.

RAW AND UNDERCOOKED MEAT

Children should not eat raw or undercooked meat or meat products. Various raw or undercooked meat products can commonly harbor harmful bacteria, including STEC, *Salmonella* species, and *Campylobacter* species. Specific meat products have

---

[1] American Academy of Pediatrics, Committee on Infectious Diseases and Committee on Nutrition. Consumption of raw or unpasteurized milk and milk products by pregnant women and children. *Pediatrics*. 2014;133(1):175-179. Reaffirmed November 2019

been linked with certain infections (pathogen-commodity pair): ground beef with
STEC and *Salmonella* species; hot dogs and deli meats with *L monocytogenes*; pork with
Trichinella species; and wild game with *Brucella* species, *Francisella tularensis*, STEC,
Trichinella species, and *Toxoplasma gondii*. Ground meats are especially risky, because
contamination on the outside of a cut of meat can end up in the center of a ham-
burger, the part least likely to be well cooked. Ground meats should be cooked to
an internal temperature of 160°F; roasts and steaks should be cooked to an internal
temperature of 145°F; and poultry should be cooked to an internal temperature of
165°F. Use of a food thermometer is the only accurate means of knowing that meat
has reached a high enough temperature to destroy pathogens. Color is not a reliable
indicator that ground beef patties have been cooked to a temperature high enough to
kill pathogens. Knives, cutting boards, plates, and other utensils used for raw meats
should not be used for preparation of fresh fruits or vegetables or for placement
of cooked meat until they have been cleaned properly (see websites at end of this
Appendix for details).

UNPASTEURIZED JUICES

Children should drink only fruit or vegetable juice that has been pasteurized or that
has been freshly squeezed from washed fruit or vegetables. Consumption of packaged
fruit juices that have not undergone pasteurization or a comparable treatment has
been associated with foodborne illness attributable to STEC, *Salmonella* species, and
Cryptosporidium parvum. To identify a packaged juice that has not undergone pasteurization or a comparable treatment, consumers should look for a warning statement that
the product has not been pasteurized.

RAW SEED SPROUTS

The CDC has reaffirmed health advisories that people who are at high risk of severe
foodborne disease, including children, people with compromised immune systems,
pregnant people, and elderly people, should avoid eating raw seed sprouts such as
alfalfa sprouts. Raw seed sprouts have been associated with outbreaks of illness attributable to *Salmonella* species, STEC, and *L monocytogenes*. The seeds themselves can harbor the pathogen, and many pathogens grow well in the warm, humid environments in
which seeds sprout.

FRESH FRUITS AND VEGETABLES AND RAW NUTS

Many fresh fruits and vegetables have been associated with illnesses caused by
Cryptosporidium species, *Cyclospora cayetanensis*, norovirus, hepatitis A virus, *Giardia duodenalis*, STEC, *Salmonella* species, *L monocytogenes*, and *Shigella* species. Raw nuts, commercially processed vegetable snacks, spinach, lettuce, tomatoes, cucumbers, melons,
basil, and cilantro have been associated with outbreaks of salmonellosis. Roasting
or otherwise treating nuts can minimize the risk of foodborne illness. Washing can
decrease bacterial contamination of fresh fruits and vegetables; however, washing even
in high concentrations of chlorine or other disinfectant is not guaranteed to remove
all pathogens, because pathogens can stick to surfaces and internalize into food items.
Knives, cutting boards, utensils, and plates used for raw meats should not be used for
preparation of fresh fruits or vegetables until the utensils have been cleaned properly
(see websites at end of this Appendix for details).

RAW SHELLFISH AND FISH

Children should not eat raw shellfish. Raw shellfish, including mussels, clams, oysters, scallops, and other mollusks, can carry many pathogens, including norovirus, *Vibrio* species, and hepatitis A virus as well as toxins (see Appendix VI, p 1150). *Vibrio* species contaminating raw shellfish may cause severe disease in people with liver disease or other conditions associated with decreased immune function. *Vibrio* species abundance appears to be increasing because of sea surface warming, thus posing increasing concern for these infections. Some experts caution against children ingesting raw fish, which has been associated with transmission of helminths (eg, *Anisakis simplex, Diphyllobothrium latum*).

HONEY

Children younger than 1 year should not consume honey. Honey is a raw agricultural product that can contain spores of *Clostridium botulinum*, the agent of botulism. The organism can grow and produce toxin in an infant's intestine; this type of pathogenesis is extremely rare in people beyond infancy.

POWDERED INFANT FORMULA

For many reasons, infants should be fed human milk rather than infant formula whenever possible. Powdered infant formula is not a sterile product and has been associated with severe illnesses attributable to *Cronobacter sakazakii* and *Salmonella* species. If infant formula is used, caregivers can reduce the risk of infection by choosing sterile, liquid formula products rather than powdered products, although this may not be practical for families with limited resources. This may be particularly important for those at greatest risk of severe infection, such as neonates and infants with immunocompromising conditions. Otherwise, water used for mixing infant formula must be from a safe water source, as defined by the state or local health department.[1,2] If there is concern or uncertainty about the safety of tap water, bottled water or cold tap water that has been brought to a rolling boil for 1 minute, then cooled to room temperature for no more than 30 minutes, may be used.

Prepared formula (including ready-to-feed products) must be discarded within 1 hour after serving to an infant. Prepared formula made from powder that has not been given to an infant may be stored in the refrigerator for 24 hours.

FOOD IRRADIATION[3]

Irradiation of food can be an effective tool to decrease transmission of pathogens. Irradiation involves exposing food briefly to ionizing radiation (eg, gamma rays, x-rays, or high-voltage electrons). More than 40 countries worldwide, including the United

---

[1] Woolf AD, Stierman BD, Barnett ED, et al; American Academy of Pediatrics, Council on Environmental Health and Climate Change, Committee on Infectious Diseases. Policy statement. Drinking water from private wells and risks to children. *Pediatrics.* 2023;151(2):e2022060644

[2] Woolf AD, Stierman BD, Barnett ED, et al; American Academy of Pediatrics, Council on Environmental Health and Climate Change, Committee on Infectious Diseases. Technical report. Drinking water from private wells and risks to children. *Pediatrics.* 2023;151(2):e2022060645

[3] **www.fsis.usda.gov/wps/portal/fsis/topics/food-safety-education/get-answers/
food-safety-fact-sheets/production-and-inspection/irradiation-resources/
irradiation-resources**

States, have approved the use of irradiation for various types of foods. Every governmental and professional organization that has reviewed the efficacy and safety of food irradiation has endorsed its use. Meat, spices, shell eggs, seeds for sprouting, and some produce items may be irradiated for sale in the United States. The risk of foodborne illness could be decreased significantly with the routine consumption of irradiated meat, poultry, and produce.

In addition to the websites previously cited in this section, detailed information on food safety issues and practices, including steps which consumers can take to protect themselves, is available on the following web sites:

- **www.foodsafety.gov**
- **www.cdc.gov/foodsafety**
- **www.fightbac.org**
- **www.fda.gov/food/resources-you-food**

··

Appendix VI

Clinical Syndromes Associated With Foodborne Diseases[1,2]

Foodborne disease results from consumption of contaminated foods or beverages and causes morbidity and mortality in children and adults. The epidemiology of foodborne disease is complex and dynamic because of numerous possible pathogens, the variety of disease manifestations, the increasing prevalence of immunocompromised children and adults, dietary habit changes, and trends toward centralized food production and widespread distribution. The cultural diversity of foods and food practices and international travel are also likely impacting the epidemiology of foodborne disease. Widespread availability of multiplex molecular diagnostic tests for gastrointestinal illness may lead to co-identification of multiple potential pathogens, complicating evaluation and treatment of diarrhea.

Consideration of a foodborne etiology is important in any patient with a gastrointestinal tract illness, as well as those with certain acute neurologic findings. Obtaining a detailed history is essential to assess time of onset and duration of symptoms, history of recent travel or antimicrobial use, food and water exposures, and presence of blood or mucus in stool. To aid in diagnosis, foodborne disease syndromes have been categorized by incubation period, predominant symptoms, causative agent, and foods commonly associated with specific etiologic agents (food vehicles) (see Table 1; also **www.cdc.gov/foodsafety/outbreaks/investigating-outbreaks/confirming_diagnosis.html**). Diagnosis can be confirmed by laboratory testing of stool, vomitus, or blood, depending on the causative agent. The Infectious Diseases Society of America Clinical Practice Guidelines for the Diagnosis and Management of Infectious Diarrhea can be found at **https://academic.oup.com/cid/article/65/12/e45/4557073.**

Sporadic (ie, non–outbreak-associated) cases account for the majority of foodborne illnesses. In localized outbreaks that affect individuals who shared a common meal, the incubation period can be estimated. In more widely dispersed outbreaks and in sporadic cases, the incubation period typically is unknown.

An outbreak should be considered when 2 or more people who have ingested the same food develop an acute illness characterized by nausea, vomiting, diarrhea, or neurologic signs or symptoms. If an outbreak is suspected, public health officials should be notified immediately to initiate an epidemiologic investigation, including diagnostic and management interventions, to curtail the outbreak.

---

[1] Dewey-Mattia D, Manikonda K, Hall AJ, Wise ME, Crowe SJ. Surveillance for foodborne disease outbreaks—United States, 2009–2015. *MMWR Surveill Summ.* 2018;67(10):1–11

[2] Centers for Disease Control and Prevention. Surveillance for foodborne disease outbreaks—United States, 1998–2008. *MMWR Surveill Summ.* 2013;62(SS-2):1-34

Table 1. Clinical Syndromes Associated With Foodborne Diseases

Clinical Syndrome	Incubation Period	Causative Agents	Commonly Associated Vehicles[a]
Nausea and vomiting	2–4 h	*Staphylococcus aureus* (preformed enterotoxins, A through V but excluding F)	Food contaminated by infected food handler that is not cooked or is improperly cooked and stored, including ham, poultry, beef, cream-filled pastries, potato and egg salads, mushrooms, unpasteurized cheese
	<1–6 h	Preformed *Bacillus cereus* (emetic toxin cereulide)	Contaminated food that is improperly stored after cooking, including rice
	<1 h	Heavy metals (copper, tin, cadmium, iron, zinc)	Acidic beverages, metallic container
	1 h	Vomitoxin (deoxynivalenol)	Foods made from grains such as wheat, corn, barley
	12–48 h	Astrovirus	Bivalve mollusks grown in polluted waters, fresh produce (greens, berries) irrigated with contaminated water, food contaminated by infected food handler that is not cooked or is improperly cooked and stored (ready-to-eat salads/sandwiches)
Flushing, dizziness, burning of mouth and throat, headache, gastrointestinal tract symptoms, urticaria and generalized pruritis	<1 h	Histamine (scombroid toxin)	Fish (bluefish, bonita, mackerel, mahi-mahi, marlin, tuna, skipjack, and many other fish types)
Usually gastrointestinal symptoms followed by neurologic symptoms (including facial and extremity paresthesias) and reversal of hot and cold temperature sensation (characteristic of ciguatera toxin)[c]	2–8 h[b] (can be up to 48 h)	Ciguatera toxin	Large reef-dwelling carnivorous fish (eg, amberjack, barracuda, grouper, snapper)
	Up to 18 h	Neurotoxic shellfish toxin (brevetoxin)	Shellfish (eg, mussels, oysters, clams)

Table 1. Clinical Syndromes Associated With Foodborne Diseases, continued

Clinical Syndrome	Incubation Period	Causative Agents	Commonly Associated Vehicles[a]
Symptoms similar to ciguatera and neurotoxic shellfish toxin, plus short-term memory loss[b]	1 day	Domoic acid (amnesic shellfish toxin)	Mussels, clams
Neurologic, including confusion, salivation, hallucinations; gastrointestinal tract manifestations	0–2 h	Mushroom toxins (short-acting)	Mushrooms
Neuromuscular weakness, symmetric descending paralysis, respiratory weakness, neurologic symptoms may be preceded by gastrointestinal tract manifestations[d]	18–36 h	Clostridium botulinum (preformed toxin)	Home-canned vegetables, fruits and fish, salted fish, meats, bottled garlic, potatoes baked in aluminum foil, cheese sauce
Neurologic, constipation in infant younger than 1 y[d]	3–30 days	Clostridium botulinum (ingestion of spores with production of toxin in the intestine)	Honey
Neurologic, gastrointestinal tract[b]	10–45 min	Tetrodotoxin (ascending paralysis)	Puffer fish
	0.5–3 h	Paralytic shellfish toxins (saxitoxins, etc)	Shellfish (clams, mussels, oysters, scallops, other mollusks)
Abdominal cramps and watery diarrhea, vomiting	6–24 h	Bacillus cereus (diarrheal enterotoxin)	Meats, stews, gravies, vanilla sauce
	6–24 h	Clostridium perfringens	Meat, poultry, gravy, dried or precooked foods
	12–48 h	Norovirus	Feces-contaminated shellfish, salads, ice, cookies, water, sandwiches, fruit, leafy vegetables, ready-to-eat foods handled by infected food worker
	1–3 days	Rotavirus	Feces-contaminated salads, fruits, ready-to-eat foods handled by infected food worker

Table 1. Clinical Syndromes Associated With Foodborne Diseases, continued

Clinical Syndrome	Incubation Period	Causative Agents	Commonly Associated Vehicles[a]
Abdominal cramps, watery diarrhea	1–3 days[e]	Enterotoxigenic *Escherichia coli*	Feces-contaminated seafood, herbs, fruits, vegetables, water, often acquired abroad—"travelers' diarrhea"
	Unknown	*Listeria monocytogenes*	Soft cheeses, raw milk, hot dogs, cole slaw, ready-to eat delicatessen meats, produce (eg, sprouts, cantaloupe)
	4–30 h	*Vibrio parahaemolyticus*	Shellfish, especially oysters
	12–72 h	*Vibrio vulnificus*	Shellfish, especially oysters
	1–5 days	*Vibrio cholerae* O1 and O139	Shellfish (including crabs and shrimp), fish, water
	1–5 days	*V cholerae* non-O1 and non-O139	Shellfish, especially oysters
	1–14 days	*Cyclospora* species	Raspberries, vegetables, fresh herbs, water
	2–28 days	*Cryptosporidium* species	Vegetables, fruits, milk, water, in particular recreational water exposures
	1–3 weeks	*Giardia duodenalis*	Water, ready-to-eat foods handled by infected food worker
Diarrhea, fever, abdominal cramps, blood and mucus in stools, bacteremia	6–48 h	*Salmonella* species (nontyphoidal)	Poultry; pork; beef; eggs; dairy products, including ice cream; raw vegetables, alfalfa sprouts; fruit, including unpasteurized juices; peanut butter
	2–4 days	*Shigella* species	Feces-contaminated lettuce-based salads, potato and egg salads, salsas, dips, and oysters, ready-to-eat foods handled by infected food worker
	7–14 days	*Salmonella* Typhi	Food contaminated by infected food handler (acutely ill or chronic carrier)
	2–4 wk	Amebiasis (*Entamoeba histolytica*)	Feces-contaminated food or water

Table 1. Clinical Syndromes Associated With Foodborne Diseases, continued

Clinical Syndrome	Incubation Period	Causative Agents	Commonly Associated Vehicles[a]
Bloody diarrhea, abdominal cramps, hemolytic-uremic syndrome (HUS)	3–4 days	Shiga toxin-producing *E coli* (STEC)	Undercooked beef (hamburger); raw milk; roast beef; salami; salad dressings; lettuce and other leafy greens; game meats, unpasteurized juices, including apple cider; sprouts; water
Febrile diarrhea or, especially in older children, abdominal pain resembling that of appendicitis	4–6 days	*Yersinia enterocolitica*	Pork chitterlings, other pork products, tofu, milk
Hepatorenal failure, watery diarrhea	6–24 h	Mushroom toxins (long-acting)	Mushrooms (especially *Amanita* species)
Other extraintestinal manifestations (fever, myalgias, arthralgias, fatigue)	Varied, up to months (usually >30 days)	*Brucella* species	Goat cheese, queso fresco, raw milk, meats
Fever, chills, headache, pharyngitis, arthralgia	1–4 days	Group A *Streptococcus*	Egg and potato salad, pasta
Fever, malaise, anorexia, jaundice	15–50 days	Hepatitis A virus	Shellfish, raw produce (eg, strawberries, lettuce, green onions)
Meningoencephalitis, sepsis, fetal loss	2–6 wk	*Listeria monocytogenes*	Soft cheeses, raw milk, hot dogs, coleslaw, ready-to eat delicatessen meats, produce (eg, sprouts, cantaloupe)
Muscle soreness and pain	Varied, up to 4 wk	*Trichinella spiralis*	Wild game, pork, meat

Table 1. Clinical Syndromes Associated With Foodborne Diseases, continued

Clinical Syndrome	Incubation Period	Causative Agents	Commonly Associated Vehicles[a]
Fever, lymphadenopathy, encephalitis, retinitis (may be reactivation disease for the latter two)	5–23 days	*Toxoplasma gondii*	Undercooked meat (especially pork, lamb, and game meat), fruits, vegetables, raw shellfish
Sepsis, meningitis among infants	Unknown	*Cronobacter sakazakii*	Powdered infant formula
	Unknown	*Salmonella* species	Powdered infant formula
Seizures, behavioral disturbances, and other neurologic signs and symptoms	Months	*Taenia solium* (neurocysticercosis)	Food contaminated with feces from a human carrier of adult pork tapeworm
Epigastric discomfort, abdominal pain, cholangitis, obstructive jaundice, pancreatitis	Varied (several days to months)	*Clonorchis sinensis* (liver fluke); *Opisthorchis* species (liver fluke)	Eating raw or undercooked infected freshwater fish, crabs, crayfish
Guillain-Barré syndrome (ascending paralysis)	2–10 days	*Campylobacter* species *Shigella* Enteroinvasive *E coli* *Yersinia enterocolitica* *Vibrio parahaemolyticus*	Poultry, raw milk, water Feces-contaminated food or water Vegetables, hamburger, raw milk Pork chitterlings, tofu, raw milk Fish, shellfish

Table 1. Clinical Syndromes Associated With Foodborne Diseases, continued

Clinical Syndrome	Incubation Period	Causative Agents	Commonly Associated Vehicles[a]
Postdiarrheal HUS (acute renal failure, hemolytic anemia, thrombocytopenia)	7 days–2 wk after onset of diarrhea	Shiga toxin-producing *E coli* (especially serotype O157:H7), or shiga-toxin 2-producing strains of non-O157 *E coli*	Beef (hamburger); raw milk; roast beef; salami; salad dressings; lettuce and other leafy greens; unpasteurized juices, including apple cider; alfalfa and radish sprouts; water
	1–5 days after onset of diarrhea	*Shigella dysenteriae* type 1	Water; milk, other contaminated food, rare in the United States
Reactive arthritis	Varies	*Campylobacter* species	Poultry, raw milk, water
	Varies	*Salmonella* species	Poultry, pork, beef, eggs, dairy products, including ice cream; vegetables (alfalfa sprouts and fresh produce); fruit, including unpasteurized juices; peanut butter
	Varies	*Shigella* species	Feces-contaminated food or water
	Varies	*Yersinia enterocolitica*	Pork chitterlings, tofu, raw milk

[a] List of vehicles in several categories is not exhaustive, because any number of foods can be contaminated; current online literature may be helpful to sort through commonly associated vehicles.
[b] See **www.cdc.gov/habs/illness-symptoms-marine.html.**
[c] See **https://emergency.cdc.gov/agent/brevetoxin/casedef.asp.**
[d] See **www.cdc.gov/botulism/symptoms.html.**
[e] See **www.cdc.gov/ecoli/etec.html.**

....
APPENDIX VII

Diseases Transmitted by Animals (Zoonoses)

Morbidity resulting from selected zoonotic diseases in the United States is reported annually by the Centers for Disease Control and Prevention (CDC; see "Summary of Notifiable Diseases" at **www.cdc.gov/mmwr/mmwr_nd/**). Information also can be obtained via the website of the National Center for Emerging and Zoonotic Infectious Diseases (**www.cdc.gov/ncezid/about-ncezid.html**) or through the main CDC website (**www.cdc.gov**). There are many opportunities to acquire zoonotic diseases, including companion animal exposure and occupational, recreational, or other exposures to animals or their products. Zoonotic diseases also include vector-borne, foodborne, and waterborne diseases. Anthropogenic factors that contribute to the increasing spillover of zoonotic infections from animal reservoirs into humans include habitat destruction, which upsets the balance controlling animal vectors in healthy ecosystems; the increasing penetration of humans into once remote areas of the planet where they encounter previously sequestered species; the consumption of "bush meat;" and the clandestine global trade in endangered species.

Table 1. Diseases Transmitted by Animals

Disease and/or Organism	Animal Sources/Reservoirs	Vector or Modes of Transmission
Bacterial Diseases		
Aeromonas species	Aquatic animals, especially shellfish, fish, medical leeches; has also been isolated from feces of horses, pigs, sheep, and cows	Wound infection; ingestion of contaminated water or food, including seafood, meat and dairy products; direct contact with infected animals or their environment
Anthrax *(Bacillus anthracis)*	Domestic and wild herbivores (cattle, goats, horses, sheep, antelope, deer) Outbreaks associated with heavy rainfall, flooding, or drought; spores remain viable in soil or animal products, such as wool or hides, for decades	Direct contact with infected animals or their carcasses, or contact with products from infected animals (eg, meat, hides, hair, or wool) contaminated with *B anthracis* spores; ingestion of contaminated meat, inhalation of aerosolized spores from contaminated materials; injection of *B anthracis* contaminated materials (via injection drug use)
Bartonellosis		
Cat-scratch disease *(Bartonella henselae)*	Cats (especially kittens) and other felids, infrequently other animals	Scratches, bites, licks; fleas play a role in cat-to-cat transmission (evidence for transmission from cat fleas to humans is lacking)
Bartonella quintana	Cats, dogs, rodents, and nonhuman primates	Bite from human body louse, infestation in clothing or bedding in high density populations with poor access to hygienic services, sanitation
Bartonella bacilliformis	Unknown	Bite of sand flies
Brucellosis *(Brucella* species)	Cattle, coyotes, hares, chickens, goats, sheep, pigs, dogs, elk, bison, deer, camels, desert woodrats and other rodents, marine mammals	Direct or indirect contact with aborted fetuses, tissues, or fluids of infected animals; inoculation through mucous membranes or cuts or abrasions of the skin; inhalation of contaminated aerosols; ingestion of raw (unpasteurized) dairy products

Table 1. Diseases Transmitted by Animals, continued

Disease and/or Organism	Animal Sources/Reservoirs	Vector or Modes of Transmission
Campylobacteriosis (*Campylobacter jejuni*)	Poultry, dogs (especially puppies), kittens, ferrets, pigs, nonhuman primates, pet rodents, cattle, sheep, birds	Ingestion of contaminated food or water; improperly cooked poultry, raw dairy products, direct contact with animals or environment, person-to-person (fecal-oral), fomites
Capnocytophaga canimorsus	Dogs and cats	Wound infections, bites, scratches; prolonged contact with dogs and cats
Erysipeloid (*Erysipelothrix rhusiopathiae*)	Pigs, horses, dogs, cats, rats, sheep, cattle, wild and domestic birds (including poultry), fresh and saltwater fish, shellfish	Direct contact with animals or contaminated animal products or contaminated water
Hemolytic-uremic syndrome (eg, Shiga toxin-producing *Escherichia coli*) (STEC)	Cattle, sheep, goats, deer, pigs, and poultry	Ingestion of undercooked contaminated ground beef, raw milk or dairy products, unpasteurized ale cider, leafy vegetables, alfalfa sprouts; other contaminated foods or water; contact with infected animals or their environments (eg, farms and ranches); contact with animals in public settings including petting zoos and agricultural fairs; person-to-person (fecal-oral)
Leptospirosis (*Leptospira* species)	Cattle, sheep, goats, pigs, horses, dogs, rodents, and all other mammals (including aquatic species)	Contact with or ingestion of water, food, or soil contaminated with urine or body fluids from infected animals, or direct contact with infected animals or their organs; increased risk with seasonal flooding
Lyme disease (*Borrelia burgdorferi*, *Borrelia mayonii* in United States, *Borrelia afzelii* and *Borrelia garinii* in Eurasia)	White-footed mice, squirrels, shrews, and other small rodents; opossums, raccoons, birds; although deer are important in the life cycle of *Ixodes* ticks, deer do not get infected	Tick bite (blacklegged/deer tick [*Ixodes scapularis* or *Ixodes pacificus*] in United States, castor bean tick [*Ixodes ricinus*] in Europe, taiga tick [*Ixodes persulcatus*] in Asia)
Mycobacterium marinum	Fresh water, brackish water, and saltwater; fish	Contaminated water sources; skin injury or contamination of existing wound, cleaning aquariums

Table 1. Diseases Transmitted by Animals, continued

Disease and/or Organism	Animal Sources/Reservoirs	Vector or Modes of Transmission
Mycobacterium bovis	Cattle, sheep, goats, elephants, giraffes, rhinoceroses, bison, deer, elk, feral pigs, possums, nonhuman primates	Eating or drinking contaminated raw dairy products; direct contact with infected animals, wound infection; inhalation
Mycobacterium tuberculosis	Nonhuman primates, elephants, guinea pigs, swine, sporadic cases in other species, including cattle	*M tuberculosis* is uncommon in nonhuman species, although when it is identified it is typically found in nonhuman primates and elephants. Transmission is by the airborne route; other routes may be involved in zoonotic transmission (although these have not been documented)
Pasteurellosis (*Pasteurella multocida*)	Cats, dogs, rabbits, pigs, birds, many other wild and domestic animals	Bites, scratches, licks, saliva, respiratory droplets from animals (primarily cats and dogs), and contaminated meat
Plague (*Yersinia pestis*)	Rodents, (eg, prairie dogs, chipmunks, squirrels, mice, voles, rats) cats, dogs, rabbits, wild carnivores (eg, bobcats, coyotes)	Most commonly via bite of infected rodent fleas; direct contact with infected animals, including their tissues; inhalation of respiratory droplets from other human or animal (eg, cat) with pneumonic plague
Q fever (*Coxiella burnetii*)	Sheep, goats, cows, buffalo, and camels are primary reservoirs; cats, dogs, rabbits, rodents, horses, pigs, pigeons, geese, other wild fowl, ticks	Contact with birth products, urine, feces, milk of infected animals, inhalation of contaminated dust, ingestion of raw dairy products; and contact with contaminated materials (wool, straw, bedding); possible role of ticks not well defined; rarely by blood transfusions, sexual contact in humans, intrauterine transmission
Rat-bite fever (*Streptobacillus moniliformis, Spirillum minus*)	Rodents (especially rats, occasionally squirrels), gerbils, weasels, and rodent-eating animals	Bites, scratches, contact with urine and secretions, aerosols, direct contact with rodent, or its environment; contaminated food or water; raw milk

Table 1. Diseases Transmitted by Animals, continued

Disease and/or Organism	Animal Sources/Reservoirs	Vector or Modes of Transmission
Relapsing fever (Borrelioses) Soft tick-borne relapsing fever (*Borrelia hermsii; Borrelia turicatae*) Hard tick-borne relapsing fever (*Borrelia miyamotoi*)	Wild rodents White-footed mice, squirrels, shrews, and other small rodents; opossums, raccoons, birds	Bites from soft-bodied tick (*Ornithodoros* species) in rodent infested environments Bites from blacklegged hard ticks (*Ixodes* species)
Salmonellosis (*Salmonella* species)	Cattle, poultry, turtles, frogs, lizards, snakes, salamanders, geckos, iguanas, fish, invertebrates, dogs, cats, pigs, sheep, horses, hedgehogs, hamsters, guinea pigs, mice, rats and other rodents, ferrets, other wild and domestic animals	Fecal-oral transmission most common; ingestion of contaminated food (eg, meat, poultry, dairy, eggs, produce, processed foods including nut butters); raw dairy products, or contaminated water; contact with infected animals or their environments (including healthy reptiles); contaminated animal products including dry dog and cat food and pet treats
Streptococcus iniae	Fish from many regions of the world	Skin wound during handling and preparation of infected fish
Streptococcus suis	Pigs	Direct contact; consumption of undercooked meat
Tetanus (*Clostridium tetani*)	Any animal indirectly via soil containing animal feces	Wounds, especially deep tissue, puncture or crush injuries or compound fractures with inoculation of bacterial spores (from contaminated soil, dust or other material)
Tularemia (*Francisella tularensis*)	Wild rabbits, hares, sheep, dogs, cats, pigs, horses, voles, squirrels, prairie dogs, beaver, lemmings, muskrats, moles, hamsters, birds, reptiles, and fish	Tick bites (wood tick [*Dermacentor andersoni*], dog tick [*D variabilis*], Lone-star tick [*Amblyomma americanum*]), deerfly bites; direct contact with infected animals or their tissues, ingestion of contaminated water or meat; mechanical transmission from claws or teeth (cats/dogs), inhalation

Table 1. Diseases Transmitted by Animals, continued

Disease and/or Organism	Animal Sources/Reservoirs	Vector or Modes of Transmission
Vibrio species	Shellfish	Ingestion of raw or undercooked seafood; skin injury or exposure of existing wound to contaminated seawater
Yersiniosis (*Yersinia enterocolitica, Yersinia pseudotuberculosis*)	Pigs, deer, elk, horses, goats, sheep, cattle, rodents, birds, rabbits, dogs	Ingestion of contaminated food (particularly raw or undercooked pork products such as chitterlings), raw dairy products, contaminated water; rarely direct contact
Fungal Diseases		
Cryptococcosis (*Cryptococcus neoformans*)	Excreta of birds, including pigeons, canaries, parakeets, and chickens	Inhalation of aerosols from accumulations of bird feces; can also be isolated from fruit and vegetables, house dust, air conditioners, air, and sawdust; can also enter body through skin
Histoplasmosis (*Histoplasma capsulatum*)	Excreta of bats or birds such as chickens, pigeons, and starlings	Inhalation of aerosolized spores from accumulations of bat or bird feces, including those released during construction involving old buildings; spores can also be ingested
Ringworm/tinea corporis (*Microsporum* and *Trichophyton* species)	Cats, dogs, chickens, pigs, mice, moles, guinea pigs, horses, rodents, cattle, monkeys, goats	Direct contact with animal or contaminated soil or fomite; pathogenic fungi found worldwide; hot and humid climates generally increase incidence
Parasitic Diseases		
Angiostrongylus cantonensis (rat lungworm)	Rodents and mollusks (eg, slugs and snails)	Ingestion of larvae in raw or undercooked snails or slugs, freshwater shrimp, land crabs or frogs or contaminated raw produce
Anisakiasis (*Anisakis* species) (herring worm disease)	Crustaceans eat infective larvae from marine mammal feces; fish or squid eat the infected crustaceans.	Ingestion of larvae in raw or undercooked fish or squid (eg, sushi)
Babesiosis (several *Babesia* species)	Mice, other rodents, and small mammals; wildlife	Tick bite (in the United States, *Babesia microti* is transmitted mainly by *Ixodes scapularis*; in Europe, *Babesia divergens* is mainly transmitted by *Ixodes* tick bites)

Table 1. Diseases Transmitted by Animals, continued

Disease and/or Organism	Animal Sources/Reservoirs	Vector or Modes of Transmission
Balantidiasis (*Balantidium coli*)	Pigs	Ingestion of contaminated food or water
Baylisascariasis (*Baylisascaris procyonis*)	Raccoons	Ingestion of eggs shed in raccoon feces found in dirt or animal waste
Clonorchiasis/Opisthorchiasis (*Clonorchis*/*Opisthorchis* species)	Fish, crabs, crayfish, snails, cats, dogs	Ingestion of metacercariae in raw or undercooked fish, crabs, or crayfish
Cryptosporidiosis (*Cryptosporidium* species)	*Cryptosporidium parvum* can infect all mammals; common in calves and other young ruminants; pigs, rarely in cats, dogs, and horses; other *Cryptosporidium* species can infect birds and reptiles	Fecal-oral; ingestion of contaminated water (especially groundwater) or foods, contaminated soil or surfaces; infection by inhaling aerosols can also occur
Cutaneous larva migrans (primarily *Ancylostoma* species hookworms)	Dogs, cats	Penetration of skin by larvae, which develop in soil or sand contaminated with animal feces
Dog tapeworm (*Dipylidium caninum*)	Dogs and cats, other animals (eg, foxes) can also be hosts	Ingestion of fleas infected with cysticercoid stage
Dwarf tapeworm (*Hymenolepis nana*) and rat tapeworm (*Hymenolepis diminuta*)	Rodents (humans are more important reservoirs than rodents for *H nana*; for *H diminuta*, rodents are primary and human infection is infrequent); arthropods including beetles and fleas can serve as intermediate hosts	Ingestion of eggs in contaminated food or water; animal-to-person (fecal-oral); person-to-person (fecal-oral); ingestion of cysticercoid-infected arthropods Autoinfection may also occur in humans if eggs remain in intestine (*H nana*)

Table 1. Diseases Transmitted by Animals, continued

Disease and/or Organism	Animal Sources/Reservoirs	Vector or Modes of Transmission
Echinococcosis, hydatid disease (*Echinococcus* species)	Definitive hosts are canids including dogs, coyotes, foxes, dingoes, jackals, hyenas, and wolves. Intermediate hosts encompass many domestic and wild animals, including herbivores such as sheep, goats, cattle, and deer; rodents	Ingestion of eggs shed in animal feces contaminating soil, water, or food
Fascioliasis (*Fasciola* species)	Sheep, cattle	Ingestion of larvae in contaminated water, on raw watercress and other contaminated water plants, vegetables, or eating raw or undercooked sheep or goat liver
Fish tapeworm (*Diphyllobothrium latum*)	Saltwater and freshwater fish	Ingestion of larvae in raw or undercooked fish (eg, sushi)
Giardiasis (*Giardia duodenalis*)	Wild and domestic animals, including dogs, cats, cattle, sheep, goats, pigs, beavers, muskrats, racoons, rats, pet rodents, rabbits, nonhuman primates	Ingestion of contaminated water or food, contact with contaminated surfaces, and animal-to-person and person to person (fecal-oral)
Leishmaniasis (*Leishmania* species)	Rodents, dogs, foxes, wolves, sloths, opossum, and other mammals (including humans) are reservoir hosts	Inoculation by bite of infected female phlebotomine sand fly
Myiasis (*Dermatobia, Cochliomyia, Chrysomya, Cordylobia, Cuterebra,* Oestrus, and *Wohlfahrtia* species)	Flies	Eggs laid near or on open wound or sore; accidental ingestion of larvae or transmission of larvae by mosquito or tick which harbors larvae; with *Chrysomya* screwworm flies, exposure of flies to unbroken soft skin

Table 1. Diseases Transmitted by Animals, continued

Disease and/or Organism	Animal Sources/Reservoirs	Vector or Modes of Transmission
Taeniasis/beef tapeworm (*Taenia saginata*)	Cattle (intermediate host)	Ingestion of larvae in raw or undercooked beef; cysticercosis in cattle is caused by ingestion of embryonated eggs excreted by humans with *Taenia* infection
Taeniasis and cysticercosis/pork tapeworm (*Taenia solium*; *Taenia asiatica* less common)	Pigs (intermediate host)	Ingestion of larvae in raw or undercooked pork resulting in intestinal infection in humans with adult tapeworms (taeniasis); porcine cysticercosis (infection in pigs) is caused by ingestion of embryonated eggs excreted by humans with *Taenia* infection, human cysticercosis is caused by ingestion of eggs through fecal contamination of food or water, or by autoinfection
Toxocariasis ocular or visceral larva migrans (*Toxocara canis* and *Toxocara cati*)	Dogs, cats; puppies are a major source of environmental contamination	Ingestion of infected, larvated eggs, usually from soil, dirty hands, or food contaminated by animal feces
Toxoplasmosis (*Toxoplasma gondii*)	Members of the *Felidae* family (including domestic cats) are definitive hosts; many mammals (eg, sheep, goats, and swine) and birds can serve as intermediate hosts	Transmission can be foodborne, zoonotic, congenital, or in rare instances through organ transplantation Zoonotic transmission can occur through ingestion of infective oocysts from hands after cleaning litter boxes or gardening (soil), or ingestion of anything that has become contaminated with cat feces, such as ingestion of vegetables or low growing fruits; consumption of cysts in raw or undercooked meat (such as lamb, pork, venison) or shellfish (clams, mussels, oysters) Consumption of contaminated water, consumption of raw dairy products (particularly goat's milk)
Trichinellosis (*Trichinella spiralis* and other *Trichinella* species)	Pigs, bears, moose, wild boars, seals, walruses, rodents, horses, foxes, wolves	Ingestion of larvae in raw or undercooked meat, particularly pork or wild game meat

Table 1. Diseases Transmitted by Animals, continued

Disease and/or Organism	Animal Sources/Reservoirs	Vector or Modes of Transmission
Chlamydial and Rickettsial Diseases		
Human ehrlichiosis (*Ehrlichia chaffeensis, Ehrlichia ewingii,* and *Ehrlichia muris eauclairensis*)	Dogs, red foxes, deer, wolves, coyotes, sheep, goats, raccoons, opossums, and lemurs (*E chaffeensis*); dogs may be reservoir hosts along with wolves and jackals (*Ehrlichia canis* and *E ewingii*); unknown (*E muris eauclairensis*)	Tick bites [Lone star tick [*A americanum*] for *E chaffeensis, E ewingii*; blacklegged tick [*I scapularis*] for *E muris eauclairensis*); in rare cases *Ehrlichia* species have been spread through blood transfusion and organ transplantation
Human anaplasmosis (*Anaplasma phagocytophilum*)	Small mammals including woodrats and deer mice; larger mammals such as deer, elk, moose, and bison	Tick bites (*I scapularis* and *I pacificus*)
Psittacosis (*Chlamydia psittaci*)	Domestic and wild birds (especially psittacine birds such as parakeets, parrots, macaws, and cockatoos); including poultry	Inhalation of aerosols from feces or dried respiratory secretions of infected birds as well as fecal-oral transmission.
Rickettsialpox (*Rickettsia akari*)	Common house mouse	Mite bites (house mouse mite, *Liponyssoides sanguineus*)
Rocky Mountain spotted fever (*Rickettsia rickettsii*)	Dogs, wild rodents, rabbits	Tick bites (American dog tick, *Dermacentor variabilis*; Rocky Mountain wood tick, *D andersoni*; and brown dog tick, *Rhipicephalus sanguineus*)
Rickettsia parkeri infection (maculatum disease, American boutonneuse fever)	Unknown; perhaps cattle, dogs, small wild rodents	Tick bites (Gulf coast tick [*Amblyomma maculatum*])
Typhus, fleaborne endemic typhus, Murine typhus (*Rickettsia typhi*)	Rats, opossums, cats, dogs	Infected flea feces scratched into abrasions; oriental rat fleas (*Xenopsylla cheopis*) and cat fleas (*Ctenocephalides felis*) are vectors
Typhus, louseborne epidemic typhus (*Rickettsia prowazekii*)	Flying squirrels (sylvatic typhus)	Person-to-person via infected body louse, contact with flying squirrels, their nests, or ectoparasites (role and species of ectoparasites undefined)

Table 1. Diseases Transmitted by Animals, continued

Disease and/or Organism	Animal Sources/Reservoirs	Vector or Modes of Transmission
Viral Diseases		
B virus (formerly herpes B, monkey B virus, herpesvirus simiae, or herpesvirus B)	Macaque monkeys (excluding Cynomolgus macaques of Mauritian origin)	Bite or exposure to secretions or tissues
Cache Valley virus	Deer, cattle, horses, elk, and sheep	Mosquito bites (many species); rarely through blood transfusion
Colorado tick fever virus	Rodents (eg, squirrels, chipmunks, mice)	Tick bites (Rocky Mountain wood tick [*Dermacentor andersoni*]); rarely through blood transfusion
Crimean Congo hemorrhagic fever (orthonairovirus)	Many wild and domestic animals including cattle, hares, goats, sheep	Ixodid (hard) ticks, genus *Hyalomma*, are reservoir and vector; infection from tick bite or contact with infectious blood and body fluids from animal slaughter; person-to-person is possible via direct contact or contact with blood or bodily fluids of an infected person; improperly sterilized medical equipment
Eastern equine encephalitis virus	Birds; possibly rodents; horses and other domesticated mammals can become infected and develop disease but are not believed to amplify virus	Mosquito bites (*Coquillettidia* species, *Aedes* species, *Culex* species, *Ochlerotatus* species), rarely through organ transplantation
Ebola virus disease (Zaire ebolavirus, Sudan ebolavirus, Taï Forest ebolavirus, Bundibugyo ebolavirus)	Fruit bats; nonhuman primates and other animals may become infected	Direct contact with infected fruit bats or nonhuman primates; person-to-person transmission via direct contact or contact with blood or bodily fluids of an infected person or dead body; prolonged presence in semen of infected individuals (sexual transmission possible); intrauterine transmission; intrapartum transmission, transmission through human milk

Table 1. Diseases Transmitted by Animals, continued

Disease and/or Organism	Animal Sources/Reservoirs	Vector or Modes of Transmission
Hantaviruses	Wild and peridomestic rodents (cotton rat, deer mouse, rice rat, white-footed mouse)	Inhalation of aerosols of infected rodent secreta and excreta; contact with infected rodents or infected droppings and urine, contaminated food; person-to-person transmission of Andes virus (South America) is possible via close contact or inhalation of respiratory secretions from an infected person
Heartland virus	Unknown	Tick bites (Lone-star tick [*A americanum*])
Hendra virus	Fruit bats (*Pteropus* genus) are the natural reservoir; horses can become infected	Contact with body fluids of infected horses, close contact with fruit bats
Novel influenza A viruses (eg, H5N1, H7N9, H9N2, H3N2 variant)	Chickens, birds, pigs	Contact with secretions of infected animals, contaminated surfaces or aerosols (markets, slaughterhouse)
Jamestown Canyon virus	Deer	Mosquito bites (many species)
Japanese encephalitis virus	Water birds; pigs and other mammals can become infected and develop disease but are not believed to amplify virus	Mosquito bites (*Culex tritaeniorhynchus*); rarely through blood transfusion
Kyasanur forest disease/Alkhurma hemorrhagic fever (Flavivirus)	Monkeys, rodents, and shrews are common hosts after being bitten by infected ticks	Primarily tick bites (*Haemaphysalis spinigera*), contact with infected animal
La Crosse virus	Rodents (eg, chipmunks, squirrels)	Mosquito bites (*Aedes triseriatus*)
Langya henipavirus	Shrews	Unknown

Table 1. Diseases Transmitted by Animals, continued

Disease and/or Organism	Animal Sources/Reservoirs	Vector or Modes of Transmission
Lassa fever (Lassa virus)	Multimammate rat (*Mastomys natalensis*)	Inhalation of aerosols or direct contact with infected rodent secreta or excreta; consumption of food contaminated by rodents; person-to-person transmission is possible via direct contact or contact with blood or bodily fluids of an infected person
Lujo hemorrhagic fever (Lujo virus)	Rodents	Inhalation of aerosols or direct contact with infected rodent secreta or excreta; consumption of food contaminated by rodents; person-to-person transmission is possible via direct contact or contact with blood or bodily fluids of an infected person
Lymphocytic choriomeningitis virus	Rodents, particularly house mice and pet hamsters (includes feeder rodents used as reptile food), guinea pigs	Inhalation of aerosols; direct contact with infected rodent secreta or excreta; consumption of food contaminated by rodents; vertical transmission if infected during pregnancy
Marburg hemorrhagic fever (Marburg virus)	African fruit bat (*Rousettus aegyptiacus*), infected nonhuman primates	Contact with fruit bats, their excreta, saliva, or infectious aerosols (eg, entering caves or mines inhabited by bats); contact with infectious blood or tissue of infected monkeys; person-to-person transmission is possible via direct contact or contact with blood or bodily fluids of an infected person
Middle East respiratory syndrome (MERS coronavirus)	Camels are host species in several countries	Respiratory secretions, possible airborne transmission in some cases, direct contact
Monkeypox virus	Natural reservoir unknown; African rodent species and nonhuman primates play a role in transmission	Direct contact with an infected animal or person, including bites or scratches; contact with infected body fluids or lesions (including during sex), or contact with contaminated bedding; inhalation of respiratory droplets and aerosolized particles

Table 1. Diseases Transmitted by Animals, continued

Disease and/or Organism	Animal Sources/Reservoirs	Vector or Modes of Transmission
Nipah virus	Fruit bats; pigs can become infected	Direct contact with infected bats or pigs, or their body fluids; consumption of bat contaminated fruit/sap; person-to-person transmission is possible via direct contact or contact with blood or body fluids of an infected person
Omsk hemorrhagic fever virus	Infected rodents including muskrats and voles	Handling infected muskrats (eg, hunting, trapping, skinning), bites from infected ticks (*Dermacentor reticulatus, Ixodes persulcatus, Dermacentor marginatus*); raw dairy products from infected goats or sheep
Orf virus	Sheep, goats, and occasionally other ruminants	Direct contact with infected animals; contact with contaminated saliva or fomites, especially through damaged skin
Powassan virus	Small to medium-sized rodents (eg, groundhogs, squirrels, mice)	Tick bites *(Ixodes cookei, Ixodes marxi, I scapularis)*; rarely through blood transfusion
Rabies (Lyssavirus)	In the United States, primarily mammalian wildlife (bats, raccoons, skunks, foxes, coyotes, mongooses) or, less frequently, domestic animals (dogs, cats, cattle, horses, sheep, goats, ferrets)	Bites from infected animals; rarely contact of open wounds, abrasions (including scratches), or mucous membranes with saliva or other infectious materials (eg, neural tissue), corneal and organ transplantation
Rift Valley fever virus	Domesticated livestock (eg, cattle, sheep, goats, buffalo, and camels)	Contact with blood, body fluids, or tissues of infected animals; bites from infected mosquitoes; rarely bites from other insects with virus on their mouthparts; possibly consumption of raw dairy products

Table 1. Diseases Transmitted by Animals, continued

Disease and/or Organism	Animal Sources/Reservoirs	Vector or Modes of Transmission
Severe acute respiratory virus-1 (SARS-CoV-1)	Bats, civet cats, potentially other animal species	Respiratory droplets (airborne transmission believed to occur in some cases), direct contact
Severe acute respiratory virus-2 (SARS-CoV-2)	Unknown	Respiratory secretions (droplets and aerosol particles, including airborne transmission); direct contact with exposed mucous membranes; risk of animal- to-human transmission is low
South American arenaviruses (Junin, Machupo, Guanarito, Sabia, Chapare)	Rodents	Inhalation of aerosols or direct contact with infected rodent secreta or excreta; consumption of food contaminated by rodents; person-to-person transmission is possible
St. Louis encephalitis virus	Birds	Mosquito bites (*Culex* species); rarely through blood transfusion
Tick-borne encephalitis virus	Primarily small rodents; large animals such as cows, goats and sheep become infected but do not play a role in virus maintenance	Tick bites (*Ixodes* species); consumption of infected raw dairy products; rarely intrauterine, blood transfusion, or organ transplantation transmission
Venezuelan equine encephalitis virus	Sylvatic rodents, possibly birds; horses are dead-end hosts	Mosquito bites (*Aedes* species, *Anopheles* species, *Culex* species, *Deinocerites* species, *Mansonia* species, and *Psorophora* species)
West Nile virus	Birds; horses and other mammals can become infected and develop disease but are not believed to amplify virus	Mosquito bites (*Culex* species); rarely through blood transfusion; organ transplantation; intrauterine; risk of transmission through human milk is unknown
Western equine encephalitis virus	Birds; possibly reptiles; horses and other mammals can become infected and develop disease but are not believed to amplify virus	Mosquito bites (*Culex tarsalis*)
Yellow fever virus	Nonhuman primates	Mosquito bites (*Haemagogus* species, *Sabethes* species, *Aedes [Stegomyia]* species); rarely intrapartum

Index

Page numbers followed by "t" indicate a table. Page numbers followed by "f" indicate a figure.

C

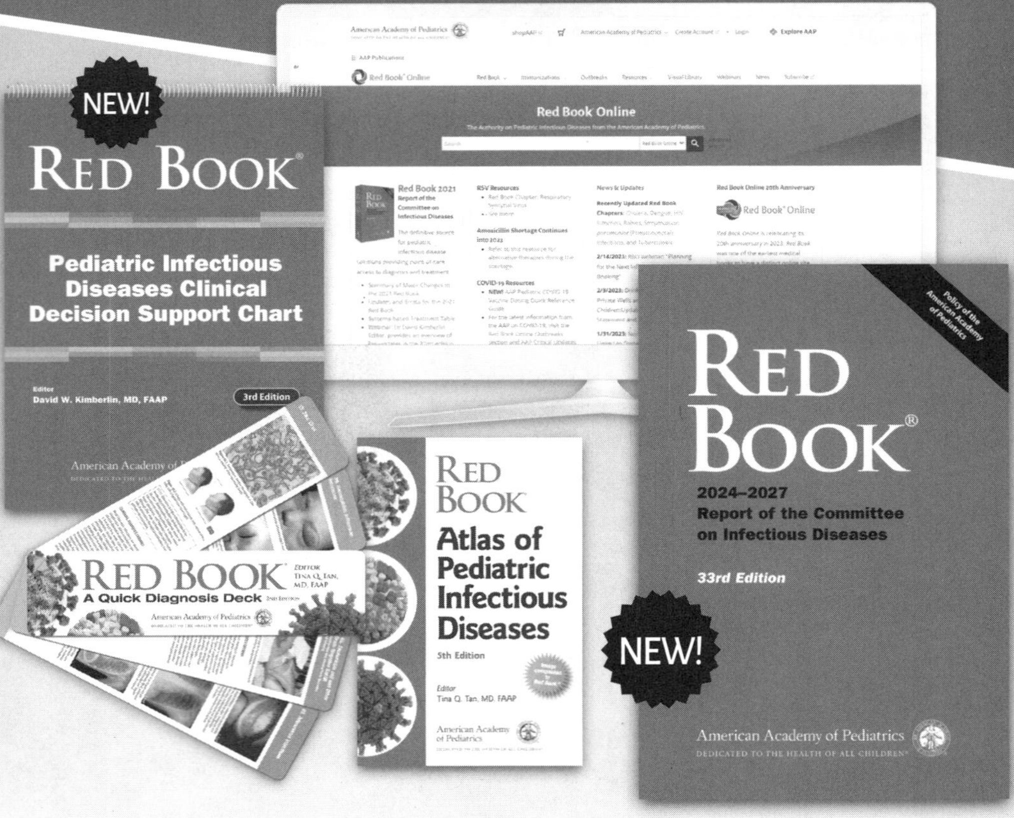

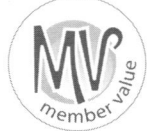
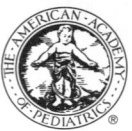